Musculoskeletal Imaging

The Core Requisites

FIFTH EDITION

David A. May MD, FACR
Radiology Associates of Richmond
Richmond, Virginia

William B. Morrison MD, FACR
Professor of Radiology
Chief of Musculoskeletal Radiology
Thomas Jefferson University
Philadelphia, Pennsylvania

Jeffrey A. Belair MD
Assistant Professor of Radiology
Musculoskeletal Radiology Fellowship Director
Thomas Jefferson University
Philadelphia, Pennsylvania

Contributors

B.J. Manaster MD, PhD
David G. Disler MD

ELSEVIER

Elsevier
1600 John F. Kennedy Blvd.
Ste 1800
Philadelphia, PA 19103-2899

MUSCULOSKELETAL IMAGING: THE CORE REQUISITES, FIFTH EDITION

ISBN: 978-0-323-68059-2

Previous editions copyrighted 1996, 2002, 2007, and 2013.

Library of Congress Control Number: 2021942180

Senior Content Strategist: Kayla Wolfe/Melanie Tucker
Content Development Manager: Meghan Andress
Publishing Services Manager: Shereen Jameel
Project Manager: Aparna Venkatachalam
Design Direction: Amy L. Buxton

Printed in India

Last digit is the print number: 9 8 7 6 5 4 3 2 1

Working together
to grow libraries in
developing countries

www.elsevier.com • www.bookaid.org

With love to Julie, with gratitude to mentors John Tampas, Col. Tom Johnson, and BJ Manaster, and with encouragement to trainees. I hope our work helps you learn.

-DM

I would like to acknowledge my family for tolerating me as I spent way too much time in the office. Thank you Jeanne, Michael, Bobby, and Louis (as well as my mother Dorothy—thanks mom!). Also my feline coauthors Binx and Boots, who enjoyed stepping on the keyboard; they apologize for any typographical errors you might find.

-WM

To my wife, DeAnna, for her unconditional love and endless patience.
To my parents, Al and Kathy, for the opportunities they've afforded me in life.
And to my countless mentors, colleagues, and friends who have provided immeasurable guidance, support, and encouragement.

-JB

Preface

We are pleased to present *Musculoskeletal Imaging: Core Requisites*. Bill Morrison, Chief of Musculoskeletal Radiology at Thomas Jefferson University, and his colleague Jeff Belair join David May as coauthors. Content has been extensively updated from the fourth edition of *Musculoskeletal Imaging: The Requisites*. Under the direction of series editor James Thrall, the text format has been substantially revised as well. Most of the text is now presented in bullet list format, and when appropriate, chapters are organized using a specific template. Content is more focused on the American Board of Radiology (ABR) Core Exam. Consequently, most esoteric topics are absent or barely mentioned unless listed in the ABR study guide. We hope that this new edition is a welcome study aid to Radiology residents preparing for the ABR Core Exam, as well as a useful reference for Orthopedic and Rheumatology trainees and practicing radiologists and clinicians.

Foreword

Musculoskeletal Imaging: Core Requisites

Congratulations to Drs May, Morrison, and Belair for producing *Musculoskeletal Imaging: Core Requisites*, the second book in the newly reimagined *Core Requisites* series. The authors have successfully pivoted from a traditional narrative or prose-based approach for knowledge sharing to an outline format that immediately brings forward and highlights the most important facts and concepts for each topic. The outline format makes the material covered readily accessible to readers, a key attribute for textbooks and a major objective for the redesign of the *Requisites* series.

Musculoskeletal Imaging: Core Requisites builds on the outstanding tradition of the previous editions on this topic in the Requisites series, most recently the fourth edition contributed by Drs McMaster, May, and Disler. The chapter layout of the new fifth edition logically begins with presentations of the imaging anatomy in the respective musculoskeletal regions, followed by chapters addressing major disease categories, and finishes with a discussion of musculoskeletal interventions. This layout also facilitates the goal of being able to rapidly find desired information.

In looking at different subspecialty areas of radiology, none have seen more continuous change in the last several decades than musculoskeletal radiology, creating an obvious challenge in crafting up-to-date texts. From an almost entirely plane film and diagnosis only orientation of 50 years ago, the field has not only adopted multiple new imaging technologies including computed tomography, magnetic resonance imaging, ultrasound and positron emission tomography, but has also become one of the most vibrant in terms of both diagnostic and therapeutic interventions. In *Musculoskeletal Imaging: Core Requisites*, Drs May, Morrison, and Belair have brought these rapidly evolving methods and their applications up to date and placed them into the perspective of current practice.

While the format of the *Core Requisites* series differs substantially from the traditional *Radiology Requisites* series, the philosophy remains the same—the production of a series of books covering the core material required across the spectrum of what radiologists need to know; from their first encounters as residents with subject material in different subspecialty areas, to studying for board exams and later for reference during clinical practice. We hope that radiologists, whether in training or practice, will find the books useful as well as trainees and practitioners in the related fields of orthopedics and rheumatology. The books in the *Core Requisites* series continue to be richly illustrated. The books are intended to be practical, not encyclopedic.

Congratulations again to Drs May, Morrison, and Belair for adding their excellent text to the new *Core Requisites* series. I hope that this and the following books in the series will become regarded with the same fondness and familiarity as earlier books in the *Radiology Requisites* family that have been used by radiologists at all career stages now for over 30 years.

James H. Thrall, MD
Chairman Emeritus
Department of Radiology
Massachusetts General Hospital;
Distinguished Taveras Professor of Radiology
Harvard Medical School
Boston, Massachusetts

Acknowledgments

Former coauthors B.J. Manaster and Dave Disler did not directly participate in writing this edition, but some of their work and cases are included, and we acknowledge that here. This edition contains new artwork by radiologist James Snyder, MD and the art staff at Elsevier. As always, we thank our colleagues who contributed cases and the technologists who skillfully obtained these studies. Special thanks to Meghan Andress, Erika Ninsin, Kayla Wolfe, Melanie Tucker, and Aparna Venkatachalam and her production team at Elsevier, and Jeannine Carrado at Spring Hollow Press, who patiently and skillfully guided this new edition through the editing and layout process.

Contents

1 Introduction to Musculoskeletal Imaging

Part 1: Bones

Bone Anatomy

Bone is composed of mineral (*calcium hydroxyapatite*) deposited on a matrix (*osteoid*) made mainly of collagen. Bones have a thick outer *cortex* that surrounds an inner network of *trabeculae*.

- Synonyms:
  - Cortical bone = compact bone. Dense and strong, accounts for most of the weight of a bone.
  - Cancellous bone = trabecular bone = spongy bone.
- Both cortex and trabeculae are composed of *lamellar bone*, and both contribute to bone strength.

- Precursor to lamellar bone is *woven bone.*
  - Less well ordered, with disordered osteoid and less mineral.
  - Formed initially during intrauterine growth and some fracture healing, later remodels into mature lamellar bone.
  - Woven bone is also seen in high bone turnover conditions and *Paget disease* and hyperparathyroidism (Chapter 13).

LONG BONES (FIG. 1.1):

- *Epiphyses* at the ends.
- *Diaphysis* (shaft) in the middle.
- *Metaphyses* in between, transition between the relatively narrower shaft and wider epiphysis, normally with concave contour.

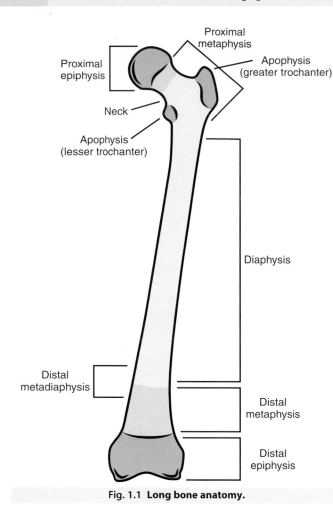

Fig. 1.1 **Long bone anatomy.**

(Labels in figure: Proximal metaphysis; Apophysis (greater trochanter); Proximal epiphysis; Neck; Apophysis (lesser trochanter); Diaphysis; Distal metadiaphysis; Distal metaphysis; Distal epiphysis)

- *Diametaphysis = Metadiaphysis =* the transition between metaphysis and diaphysis.
- Long bones of growing children also have at least one *physis* (*growth plate, epiphyseal growth plate*), composed primarily of cartilage, located transversely between a metaphysis and epiphysis.
  - The physis allows for bone elongation during growth.
  - Weaker than surrounding bone, so a frequent site of fracture in children.

MARROW CAVITY

- Contains trabecular bone and varying amounts of cellular and fatty marrow.
- Normal site of hematopoiesis.

PERIOSTEUM

- Covers the bone surface, except at the joints.
- Composed of tough fibrous outer layer and lined with an inner layer (*osteogenic layer,* or *cambium*) that produces bone as needed, allowing bone diameter to increase with growth (and throughout life to some degree), and rapidly in case of fracture.
- Periosteum is tightly bound to underlying bone in adults, but less so in children (except at the physes, where it is tightly bound).

- Cortical bone contains a network of microscopic channels, including *Haversian canals*, that extend through the cortex. Haversian canals provide a route out of the medullary space for tumors or infection, which can elevate the periosteum.

Around joints the *articular cartilage* covers most of the bone surface along with the joint capsule and ligaments.

Embryology and Bone Growth After Birth

- Development of the skeleton begins during the first trimester of gestation.
- *Mesoderm* differentiates into *sclerotome* (eventually forms the bones), *myotome* (muscles), and *dermatome* (skin).
- Aggregation of *mesenchymal cells* during the first trimester forms the limb buds that subsequently become the bones, joints, muscles, and tendons.

BONE FORMATION

Bones are formed by either *intramembranous ossification* or *enchondral ossification*, both of which involve replacement of connective tissues by bone.

Intramembranous Ossification

- Bone is formed by direct transformation of primitive mesenchyme into bone.
- Forms most of the skull, mandible, most of the facial bones, portions of the clavicles, and pubis.
- Contributes to most fracture healing.
- Periosteum can make new bone by intramembranous and enchondral ossification.

Enchondral Ossification

- Bone is formed in a two-step process:
  1. Chondrocytes form a cartilage model
  2. Osteocytes replace the chondrocytes and convert the cartilage model into bone.
- Forms the bones of the extremities, skull base, spine, and most of the pelvis.
- The *physis* (growth plate) in the long bones of children creates bone by enchondral ossification, which allows for long bone growth before and after birth. The physis is reviewed in detail in Part 3 of this chapter.
- Most fracture healing occurs by enchondral ossification.

The bone formed by either process initially is immature *woven bone*. The immature woven bone is subsequently remodeled in a coordinated process of bone resorption by *osteoclasts* and bone formation by *osteoblasts* into stronger, mature *lamellar bone*.

Similar coordinated osteoclast bone resorption and osteoblast bone formation is essential throughout life:

- During growth: *remodels* (reshapes) bones as they grow into the adult configuration.
- Throughout life: maintains bone strength in adults by continuously replacing older bone weakened by microfractures with new bone. This process is called *bone turnover*.

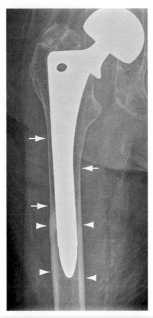

Fig. 1.2 Wolff's law: bone loss as a result of disuse. The hip arthroplasty femoral stem is stiffer than the surrounding proximal femur, effectively shielding the proximal femur from routine stress. The resulting bone loss is seen as cortical thinning *(arrows)*. In contrast, bone loading around the stem tip is increased because stress is concentrated at this point, resulting in new bone formation with cortical thickening *(arrowheads)*. There are many potential causes of bone loss; the stress shielding illustrated here is just one.

Bone growth and bone turnover are governed by multiple factors:

- Hormones, including growth hormone and the sex hormones.
- Genetics.
- Metabolic conditions.
- Mechanical stress.
  - **Wolff's law**: An increase in bone stress shifts the bone resorption/bone production balance toward greater bone production. Cortex thickens. Trabeculae thicken and become more numerous. In contrast, decreased bone loading causes bone resorption to exceed bone production ('use it or lose it'). If unchecked, this leads to decreased bone mass, cortical thinning, and loss of trabeculae (Fig. 1.2).

Pathophysiology: Bone Trauma

Bone is a dynamic tissue performing essential roles in biomechanics, calcium homeostasis, and normal hematopoiesis. The following discussion concentrates on bone trauma.

BASIC BONE BIOMECHANICS

- Normal mature bone is strong and rigid. If enough force is applied, a normal adult bone will break rather than permanently deform.
- Children's bones and, to a lesser degree, adult bones weakened by certain disease states such as *osteomalacia* or *osteoporosis* are 'softer' and can permanently deform

without breaking into two separate fragments. Such deformities are the result of numerous microscopic fractures.

There are three primary forces in bone trauma: *compression*, *tension*, and *shear*.

- *Compression* is force that pushes two portions of a bone together.
- *Tension* is the opposite: it is force that pulls two portions of a bone apart.
- *Shear* is force that slides two portions of a bone past one another.

These forces act on both gross and microscopic levels. Any material—be it metal, wood, or bone—has a unique threshold at which it will fail (fracture, in the case of bone) with each of these forces.

- Bones and joints are *anisotropic* (i.e., not the same in each direction). Specifically, bones are stronger in compression and weaker in tension and shear.
- A fracture can be caused by just one of the three basic mechanical forces or by a combination.
- An example of a fracture resulting from *isolated tension*: transverse fracture of the patella, in which violent contraction of the quadriceps muscles places the patella under extreme tension. If the patella fails, the resulting fracture will be transverse (Fig. 1.3).
  - This example illustrates the general rule that fractures resulting from tension tend to occur perpendicular to the direction of the applied force.
- The common cortical avulsion fracture is another example of a tension fracture, due to tension by an inserting ligament.

Pure *compression force* in a long bone usually produces an oblique fracture (Fig. 1.4).

- In the spine, pure compression produces a vertebral body compression or burst fracture (Fig. 1.5).

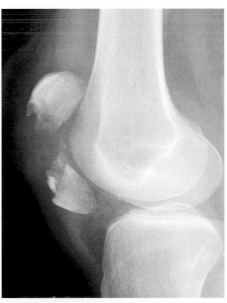

Fig. 1.3 Transverse fracture of the patella caused by tension failure during extreme quadriceps contraction.

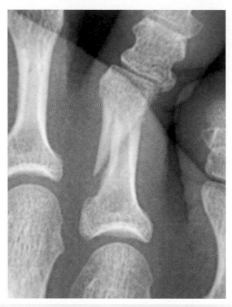

Fig. 1.4 Oblique fracture of the fourth toe proximal phalanx.

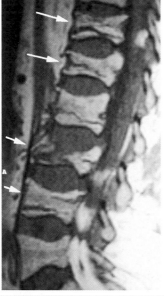

Fig. 1.5 Multiple compressions of the lumbar vertebral bodies *(arrows)* in a patient with osteoporosis (sagittal T1-weighted MR image). The irregular transverse low-signal lines within the vertebral bodies are fracture lines.

Shear forces tend to create fracture lines oblique to the line of force. Shear forces are present on a microscopic level in most fractures, because some of the multidirectional bone trabeculae are placed under shear stress regardless of whether the primary force is compression or tension.

Many fractures are caused by some combination of the three basic mechanical forces.

- *Example 1*: Bone bending. If a curved long bone is compressed, the force tries to bend the bone. Tension forces develop along the convex portion of the cortex and compressive forces develop along the concave portion of the cortex. Bone is better able to withstand compression forces than tension forces, so the convex margin tends to fail first. Examples are childhood *pure plastic bowing* fracture and childhood *greenstick fracture* (Fig. 1.6) and the butterfly-shaped comminuted fracture in adults (Fig. 1.7).
- *Example 2*: A twisting or rotational injury in which torsion force is applied around the circumference of a bone. This mechanism combines compression, tension, and shear, resulting in a *spiral fracture* (Fig. 1.8).

An additional important biomechanical property of bone is that the fracture threshold is inversely related to the rate at which a load is applied.

- In other words, bone is more resistant to force that builds slowly than to a rapidly applied force.
- A rapidly delivered, sharp impact such as from a bullet or a direct blow to a bone is more likely to cause a fracture than a greater force that builds slowly.
- On the other hand, because a bone can tolerate a greater load if applied slowly, more energy is stored. If the bone does eventually fracture, the damage may be more severe.
- In the soft tissues a rapidly applied force also is more likely to cause tissue failure. This is why the shock wave from a high-velocity gunshot wound can cause so much damage to the soft tissues.

IMAGING TECHNIQUES IN BONE TRAUMA

Radiographs

- First-line, and often the best and only imaging exam that is needed.
  - Main exception: spine (computed tomography [CT] is better).
- Orthogonal views are needed to detect fracture and characterize deformity.
- A single radiograph as a screening exam decreases sensitivity and is not encouraged.
- Ionizing radiation.
- Radiographs may not provide sufficient fracture characterization to guide therapy.

CT

- Current generation CT with multiplanar reformats has excellent sensitivity.
- More sensitive than radiographs. Useful when radiographs are negative but clinical suspicion is high, especially for body parts where radiography has lower sensitivity such as the midfoot and spine.
- Excellent depiction of fracture fragments.
- Helpful in characterizing complex fractures such as comminuted intraarticular fractures and planning surgery. 3D reconstructions can be useful.
- Fast; often readily available.
- Dual energy CT scanners can identify marrow edema, increasing sensitivity for nondisplaced fractures in osteoporotic patients.
- Ionizing radiation.
- Less sensitive for nondisplaced fractures in osteoporotic patients.
- Can be limited by artifact from orthopedic hardware.

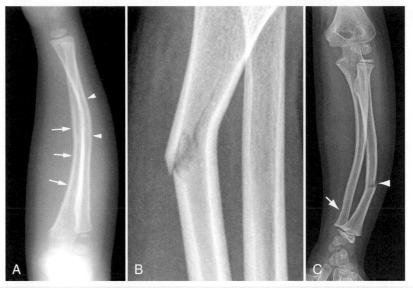

Fig. 1.6 Bowing fractures in children. (A) Pure plastic bowing fracture of the forearm in a 5-year-old. The ulna is laterally bowed *(arrows)* and the radius is dorsally bowed *(arrowheads)*. These bones are normally mildly bowed in these directions, but the degree of bowing, combined with a history of fall and forearm pain, establishes the diagnosis. **(B)** Greenstick fracture of the distal radius. **(C)** Plastic bowing deformities of the ulna and radius. Also note essentially complete radius fracture *(arrowhead)* and the minimal buckle fracture of the distal medial ulna *(arrow)*.

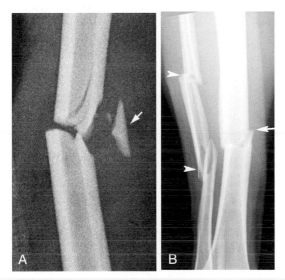

Fig. 1.7 Comminuted fractures. (A) Adult equivalent of bowing fracture: butterfly comminution fracture. *Arrow* points to the butterfly fragment in a humerus midshaft fracture. **(B)** Segmental fracture. Lateral view of the leg shows two fracture sites in the fibula *(arrowheads)* separated by a segment of normal bone. The tibia fracture *(arrows)* is nearly transverse, in this case reflecting a high-force injury.

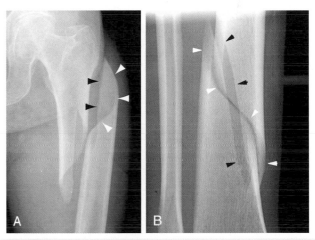

Fig. 1.8 Spiral fractures. Laterally displaced **(A)** and mildly displaced **(B)** fractures. Note the typical combination of a spiral component *(white arrowheads)* and a straight, longitudinal component *(black arrowheads)*.

Magnetic Resonance Imaging

- Excellent problem solver in acute trauma when other studies are negative due to very high sensitivity and high specificity.
  - Magnetic resonance imaging (MRI) findings in an otherwise occult fracture: Marrow edema on *fluid-sensitive sequences* such as inversion recovery or fat-suppressed T2-weighted images. The low-signal fracture line is often best seen on T1-weighted images (Fig. 1.9)
- Good depiction of larger fracture fragments.
- Can show pediatric fractures through unossified cartilage.
- Also demonstrates soft tissue injuries.

- No ionizing radiation.
- Image quality degraded by motion and metal artifacts.
- Need sedation in younger children.
- Many electronic implants (pacemakers, cochlear implants) are not MRI compatible.

Radionuclide Bone Scan

- Insensitive to acute fractures, but becomes positive after about 3 days (healing response).
- Allows whole body imaging.
- Useful if joint replacement or other metal implant creates artifact on CT or MRI.
- Often used for suspected stress fractures (if negative excludes a stress fracture)
- Can be helpful in suspected child abuse.
- Less sensitive than MRI.

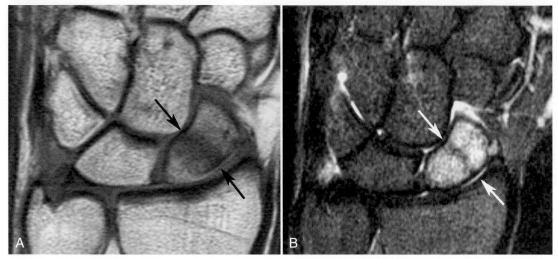

Fig. 1.9 MR imaging of a radiographically occult fracture. Young adult with snuff box tenderness and normal radiographs. Coronal T1-weighted **(A)** and inversion recovery **(B)** images show a scaphoid waist fracture *(arrows)*. Note the diffuse high-signal marrow edema in **B**.

- Ionizing radiation.
- Need sedation in younger children.

FRACTURE DESCRIPTION TERMINOLOGY

Accurate description is extremely important and requires conventional terminology to facilitate communication of the findings.

Fracture Location

- Which bone?
- Which part of the bone (diaphysis, metaphysis, etc.)?
  - Long bone shaft fractures: divide the length of the shaft into thirds. Localize the fracture to the proximal third, the junction of the proximal and middle thirds, the middle third, the junction of the middle and distal thirds, or the distal third.
  - In bones with specific anatomy (neck, trochanter, etc.), use that term.
- Does the fracture extend to a joint surface (*intraarticular*)?
- In children: does the fracture involve a physis? Physeal fractures and their classification system are discussed in Part 3.

Open Versus Closed Fracture

- *Closed fracture*: osseous fragments do not breach the skin surface.
- *Open fracture* is associated with skin disruption and exposure of a bone fragment (Fig. 1.10).
  - Due to infection risk, open fracture is an emergent situation needing lavage and surgical reduction.

Complete Versus Incomplete Fractures

Complete Fractures

- Two or more separate bone fragments.
- *Transverse*: fracture perpendicular or up to 30 degrees oblique to the bone long axis.
- *Oblique*: fracture is at an angle > 30 degrees to the long bone axis.
- *Spiral*: combination of curved oblique and longitudinal.

- *Comminuted*: more than two fragments (only mention when present).
  - *Segmental* fracture: the same bone is fractured in two separate sites, with an intact segment of bone between the fracture sites (see Fig. 1.7B).
  - *Butterfly-comminuted (wedge)* fracture: a wedge-shaped 'butterfly' fragment of intervening bone is present (see Fig. 1.7A). This fragment is at risk for osteonecrosis, and these fractures often require hardware fixation.

Incomplete Fractures

- Cortex is incompletely interrupted.
- Occur most often in children because of the different mechanical properties of bone in children compared with those of adults, as noted earlier.
  - *Buckle fracture*: focal compression of cortex caused by an axial load (Fig. 1.11; see also Figs. 1.1 to 1.5).

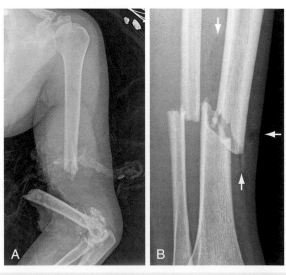

Fig. 1.10 Open fractures. (A) Some open fractures are obvious. **(B)** Most are more subtle. Notice the tell-tale subtle low-density soft tissue gas near the tibia fracture *(arrows).*

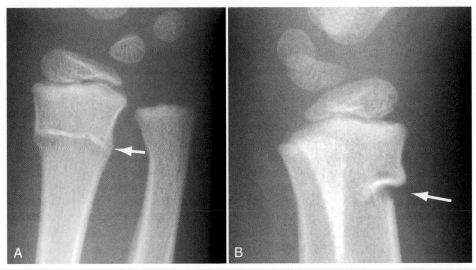

Fig. 1.11 **Childhood buckle fracture.** PA **(A)** and lateral **(B)** views show a dorsal-distal-radial metaphyseal buckle fracture *(arrows)*.

- *Torus fracture*: circumferential type of buckle fracture.
- *Greenstick fracture*: results from bending force with distraction of cortex fragments on the convex side of the bone (see Fig. 1.6B).
- *Pure plastic bowing deformity (plastic deformation)*: a bending of bone without a visible fracture line (see Fig. 1.6A). This injury represents innumerable micro-fractures of a long segment of bone.
- *Toddler's fracture*: Usually nondisplaced lower extremity fracture in a newly ambulating toddler. May be difficult to detect on radiographs (Fig. 1.12).
- Incomplete fractures in adults are less common and are usually nondisplaced. Such fractures may have unusual mechanisms or may occur in bone weakened by disease such as osteoporosis or osteomalacia (Fig. 1.13).

Fracture Displacement

By convention, *displacement* is described by the position of the more distal fragment relative to the more proximal fragment.

Translation (Position)
- Anterior/posterior, medial/lateral, proximal/distal.
- Anterior/posterior and medial/lateral displacement can be described in terms of percentage of shaft diameter.
- If displacement is greater than 100% of the shaft diameter, muscle pull can cause the fracture fragments to slide past one another (*overriding, overlap,* or *bayonet apposition*).
- *Distraction* is longitudinal separation of the fracture fragments. This may result from muscle pull or interposed soft tissue.
- The length of any fragment overlap or distraction should be included in the report.

Angular Deformity (Alignment). Directional change of the long axis of the distal fragment relative to the long axis of the proximal fragment. This is described in one of two ways:

1. Orientation of the apex of the angle formed by the fracture fragments

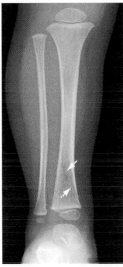

Fig. 1.12 **Toddler's fracture.** AP radiograph shows an oblique fracture of the distal tibia *(arrows)*. These nondisplaced fractures of the lower extremities of toddlers are always subtle and are often only detected on follow-up radiographs by the development of tell-tale periosteal reaction. Most toddler's fractures occur in the tibia.

2. Orientation of the distal fracture fragment relative to the proximal fragment

Orthopedic surgeons often use the latter system.

- *Medial angulation (varus)*: The distal fracture fragment is pointing relatively more toward the midline of the body when compared with the proximal fragment. This is the same as 'apex lateral angular deformity'.
- *Lateral angulation (valgus)* is the opposite; the distal fracture fragment is pointing relatively more away from the midline of the body than is the proximal fragment. This is the same as 'apex medial angular deformity'.
  - Anterior and posterior angulation are similar.
  - Other common descriptors: volar/dorsal, radial/ulnar.
- Report the angular deformity in degrees.

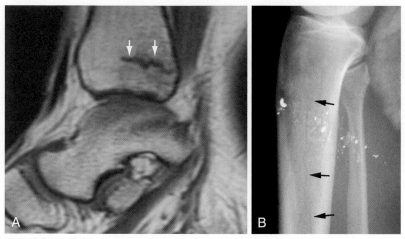

Fig. 1.13 Incomplete fractures in adults. (A) Sagittal T1-weighted MR image shows irregular linear low signal in the distal posterior tibia *(arrows)* representing a nondisplaced, incomplete trabecular fracture, in this case caused by impaction. **(B)** Incomplete tibial fracture in an adult *(arrows)* because of a gunshot wound. Note the metal fragments that mark the bullet tract.

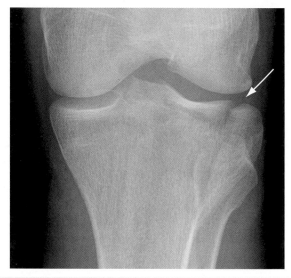

Fig. 1.14 Intraarticular fracture. Shallow oblique AP knee radiograph shows a lateral tibial plateau fracture *(arrow)* with mild diastasis and depression of the lateral fragment.

Rotation or Torsion. Twisting of the distal fracture fragment relative to the proximal around the bone long axis.
- Can be difficult to determine with radiographs.
- Often evaluated clinically.
- MRI or low-dose CT can be helpful in difficult cases (see Fig. 5.33).

Additional Fracture Descriptors

Impaction
- Often with local comminution.

Intraarticular Fracture
- Any fracture that extends to an articular surface.
- Intraarticular fractures are more likely to need surgical intervention and less likely to have a normal outcome (Fig. 1.14).
- Can be very subtle on routine radiographs, requiring special views or CT or MRI for diagnosis or exclusion.

- Hemarthrosis is suggestive but not specific.
  - Fluid-fluid level on horizontal beam radiograph or CT.
  - Cells layer dependently, with lower density serum on top.
- *Fat-fluid level* is specific.
  - Caused by escape of marrow fat into the joint space through an articular fracture.
  - Three levels may be seen: fat on top, serum, and the cellular layer on the bottom (Fig. 1.15).
- *Articular split fracture* cleaves a joint surface into two or more separate fragments.
- *Die-punch fragment.*
  - An articular surface fragment that is driven into the epiphysis or metaphysis.
  - The fragment may be rotated or tilted.
  - Die-punch fragments occur most commonly in distal radius and tibial plateau fractures (Fig. 1.16).

Osteochondral Fracture
- Compression or shear fracture of the subchondral bone and that is confined to the peripheral portion of an epiphysis.
- The equivalent term *osteochondral lesion* is now used.
- Shear injuries may result in a displaced osteochondral fragment. The fragment may remain in or close to its original position or may be displaced into the joint (Fig. 1.17).

One of the most important complications of an intraarticular fracture is posttraumatic osteoarthritis. An articular surface step-off or a gap of more than 2 mm is associated with a significantly increased rate of development of posttraumatic osteoarthritis. Therefore a complete report measures and reports all joint surface gaps and step-offs.

Avulsion Fracture
- Caused by tension (traction) by a tendon or ligament (Fig. 1.18).
- *Chip fracture* is sometimes used to describe any small cortical fragment, but it is more precisely limited to fractures caused by focal impaction or shearing rather than avulsion.

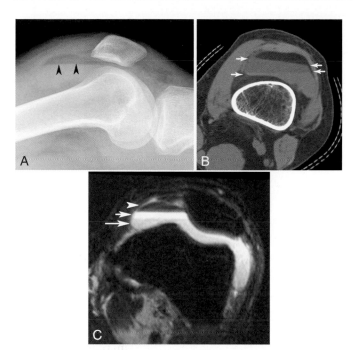

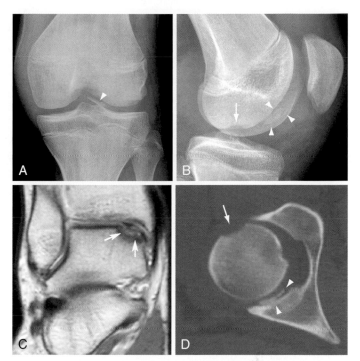

Fig. 1.15 Traumatic joint effusions with fluid levels. (A) Cross-table lateral knee radiograph in a patient with a tibial plateau fracture. Note the fat-fluid level *(arrowheads)* with low-attenuation fat layer on top and the dependent blood below. **(B)** Axial CT image in a different patient with an intraarticular distal femur fracture (not visible on this image) shows three layers *(arrows)*, with low-attenuation fat on top, a dense serum layer in the middle, and a slightly denser layer containing serum and blood cells at the bottom. The layers are not exactly parallel in this image, a temporary phenomenon seen with modern high-speed CT scanners related to patient motion just before the scan and differing fluid viscosities. **(C)** Lipohemarthrosis on MRI. Axial fat-suppressed T2-weighted MR image in the knee of a patient with a tibial plateau fracture shows layering identical to that seen in **B**. The fat layer has low signal intensity because of fat suppression. If this image had been obtained without fat suppression, the fat would be bright. The cellular (most dependent) layer is slightly darker than the serum (middle) layer because of susceptibility artifact due to intracellular hemoglobin. See also Fig. 6.6.

Fig. 1.17 Osteochondral fractures. (A and B) Displaced osteochondral fragment *(arrowheads)* in the knee joint. This is a typical osteochondral fragment in that it is narrow and the subcortical bone is clearly visible. (The cartilage is not visible on radiographs.) Lateral view **(B)** shows the donor site on the lateral femoral condyle *(arrow)*. **(C)** Coronal T2-weighted MR image shows a minimally displaced medial talar dome osteochondral fracture *(arrows)*. Note high T2 signal between the fragment and the talus. **(D)** Displaced osteochondral fragment the hip joint *(arrowhead)* after hip dislocation. Note the donor site *(arrow)*.

- Avulsion fractures are more significant, because they may be associated with joint instability.
- Knowledge of the normal sites of ligament attachment can be helpful in distinguishing avulsion fractures from the less significant chip fractures.

Fragility Fracture
- Fracture resulting from a ground level fall or similar minor trauma in bones weakened by osteoporosis, osteomalacia, osteogenesis imperfecta, and other widespread conditions.
- Common sites include the proximal femur, proximal humerus, and distal radius.

Pathologic Fracture
- Fracture caused by normal stresses on an abnormal bone.
- Fragility fractures and insufficiency fractures discussed later technically are pathologic fractures, but in general usage the term *pathologic fracture* is reserved to describe a fracture through bone weakened by a tumor (Fig. 1.19), osteomyelitis, or other focal lesion.
- Pathologic fractures tend to be transverse. Diaphyseal transverse fractures warrant extra scrutiny for a possible underlying lytic lesion.

Trabecular Fracture
- Fracture confined to trabecular bone.

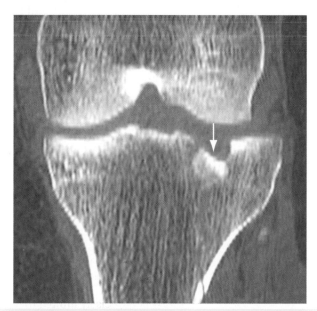

Fig. 1.16 Die-punch fragment. Coronal CT reconstruction of a tibial plateau fracture shows depressed lateral plateau fragment *(arrow)*.

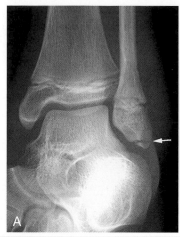
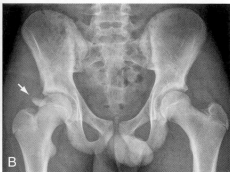

Fig. 1.18 Avulsion fracture. (A) Avulsion fracture of the tip of lateral malleolus *(arrow)* following a supination ankle injury. **(B)** Right anterior inferior iliac spine (AIIS) avulsion. The fragment *(arrow)* is displaced distally by the rectus femoris.

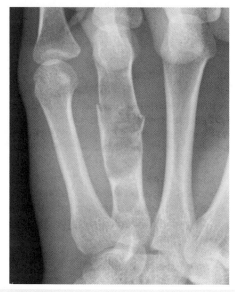

Fig. 1.19 Pathologic fracture through a fourth metacarpal shaft enchondroma.

- May be incomplete and nondisplaced or minimally displaced.
- Typically occur in bone weakened by osteoporosis.
- Subchondral and metaphyseal locations are typical.
- May be visible on radiographs as a sclerotic band.
- MRI: fracture has low signal on T1-weighted images. Surrounding marrow edema may be extensive.

Bone Bruise (Bone Contusion)
- Edema, hemorrhage, and trabecular microfractures caused by a direct blow.
- MRI: marrow edema on fluid-sensitive sequences.

Sample Reports
- Spiral fracture proximal humeral shaft. Distal fragment is displaced medially by greater than one shaft width and the fragments override 3 cm. 15 degrees varus alignment.

- Oblique fracture tibial midshaft. Distal fragment is displaced medially by one-half shaft width with 20 degrees apex anteromedial angular deformity. Adjacent soft tissue gas consistent with an open fracture.
- Buckle fracture dorsal distal radial metadiaphysis with 30 degrees dorsal angulation.
- Transverse fracture proximal femoral shaft through a lytic lesion highly concerning for malignancy.

FRACTURE REDUCTION

- Ideal goal is restoration of anatomic (normal) alignment.
- However, compromises must often be made to achieve the best possible outcome.
- A host of factors determine the desired fragment positions after reduction.
  - Maximize the likelihood of healing.
  - Minimize the risk of complications.
  - Maintaining the function of nearby joints is one of the most important goals.
- Angulation of a long bone shaft fracture is generally undesirable but may be tolerated if it is in the same plane as the motion of an adjacent joint. For example, little if any varus or valgus malalignment or rotation is acceptable in a tibial fracture, because both the ankle and knee are sagittal-plane hinge joints and unable to compensate. The highly mobile shoulder joint is better able to compensate for adjacent deformity.
  - An intraarticular fracture with a step-off or diastasis of greater than 2 mm has a significantly increased risk of developing posttraumatic osteoarthritis.

When reducing a fracture, the orthopedic surgeon reverses the forces that caused the fracture. For example, a *Colles fracture* is caused by compression of the dorsal aspect of the distal radius. When reducing a Colles fracture, the surgeon must distract the dorsal radius, which is accomplished by distraction and palmar flexion of the wrist.

Closed Reduction
- Manipulation to improve alignment.
- The improved alignment is maintained with a cast or splint.

Open Reduction

- Operative access to the injured bone.
  - To assist reduction, especially of intraarticular fragments.
  - To apply fixating hardware.
- The improved alignment may be maintained with hardware fixed to the bone.
- ORIF = open reduction with internal fixation.

Internal Fixation

- Screws that cross an oblique fracture, cortical plate on the bone surface fixed with transverse screws, encircling cerclage wires, or intramedullary fixation with a nail or rod (Figs. 1.20 to 1.22).

External Fixation

- Achieved by pins or wires placed through the skin into the bone remote from the fracture site.
- The pins or wires are fixed to one another externally (Fig. 1.23).

- Used when the fracture site may be infected and, rarely, for fractures near the end of a bone.

Compression across the fracture improves contact between the fragments which speeds healing and reduces the risk of nonunion. A variety of techniques may be used to achieve such compression (Figs. 1.23 and 1.21).

- On the other hand, compression must sometimes be limited.
  - Example: comminuted long bone fracture would telescope and shorten if compressed. The bone length can be controlled by fixation with a cortical plate or an intramedullary nail (rod) with proximal and distal interlocking screws (Fig. 1.22).

Dynamic fixation means that fragment motion is allowed in one direction but constrained in all others. Examples:

- Dynamic hip screw (discussed further in Chapter 5).
- 'Dynamizing' an interlocked intramedullary nail. After a tibial or femoral shaft fracture has partially healed enough to resist compression, bone apposition may be improved by removal of the interlocking

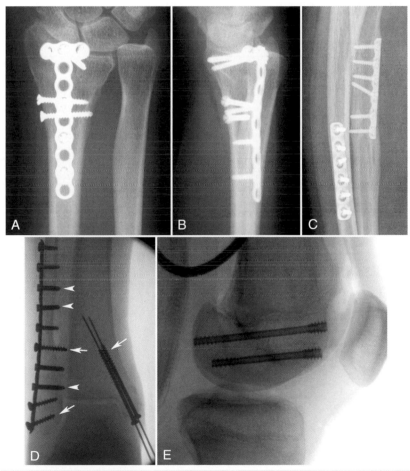

Fig. 1.20 Internal fixation with plates and screws. AP **(A)** and lateral **(B)** radiographs show dorsal T-plate fixation of distal radius fracture. Also note the two lateromedial transverse screws. **(C)** Forearm fractures in adult bones fixed with cortical compression plates. The slots for the screw heads are designed to force the fragments toward the center of the plate. Such compression increases apposition of bone fragments and thus speeds healing. **(D)** Screw types. Screws designed to gain purchase in cortex have fine threads *(arrowheads)*. Screws designed to gain purchase in softer trabecular bone have wider threads *(arrows)*. The medial malleolus screws are lag screws. The gap (lag) between the threads and the head allows compression as the screw is tightened. **(E)** Differential thread screws. This child had a coronal plane fracture across the femoral condyles. The screws were placed from an anterior approach. Note the difference in the threads: the leading edge (more posterior) threads have higher pitch (i.e., are spaced farther apart). As both threads bite, the anterior and posterior bone fragments are compressed together. A similar but smaller screw called a Herbert screw is frequently used to fix scaphoid waist fractures.

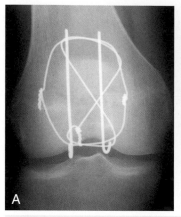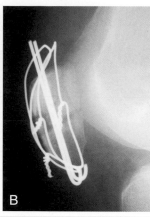

Fig. 1.21 Internal fixation with cerclage wires and pins. (A) AP radiograph and **(B)** lateral radiograph of compression wiring fixation of patellar fracture. Same patient as in Fig. 1.2.

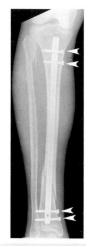

Fig. 1.22 Internal fixation with intramedullary nail. Frontal radiograph of the tibia demonstrates intramedullary rod with interlocking screws *(arrowheads)*, which prevent rotation and shortening after reduction.

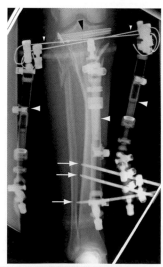

Fig. 1.23 External fixation. Note the fixation of the main proximal tibial fragment with crossing wires *(small white arrowheads)*, the main distal fragment with pins *(white arrows)*, and the adjustable external frame *(large white arrowheads)*. This patient also has a tibial plateau fracture that is fixed with two transverse screws *(black arrowhead)*.

screws at one end of the nail. This allows the fragments to slide along the nail and impact against one another (Fig. 1.24), thereby improving bone apposition and healing.

Sample Reports

- Comminuted femoral shaft fracture fixed by an interlocked intramedullary nail. Alignment is anatomic.
- Comminuted intraarticular distal radius fracture has been surgically reduced and fixed with a volar plate and multiple screws.

FRACTURE HEALING

The process described here, known as *secondary fracture healing*, occurs in the large majority of fractures (Fig. 1.25). In contrast, tightly apposed fracture fragments can heal without callus formation (*primary healing*).

The Process

Inflammatory

- Initially a hematoma forms at the fracture site, which provides a source of growth factors and stimulates neovascularization.
- Granulation tissue forms around the fracture site.
  - Contains fibroblasts and stem cells that are supplied in part from the periosteum and endosteum.
- Radiographic findings: Initially none (except for the fracture). Later, blurring or softening of the fracture margins, local demineralization.

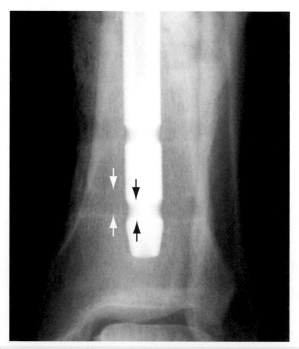

Fig. 1.24 Dynamized intramedullary nail. This distal tibial fracture is in the late stages of healing. The fracture was initially fixed with an intramedullary nail with proximal and distal interlocking screws. After the healing process had begun and partial fracture stability was achieved, the distal interlocking screws were removed. This allowed the distal fragment to slide proximally along the nail until fully impacted against the proximal fragment, causing the old screw tracts *(white arrowheads)* to shift proximally relative to the screw holes in the nail *(black arrowheads)*.

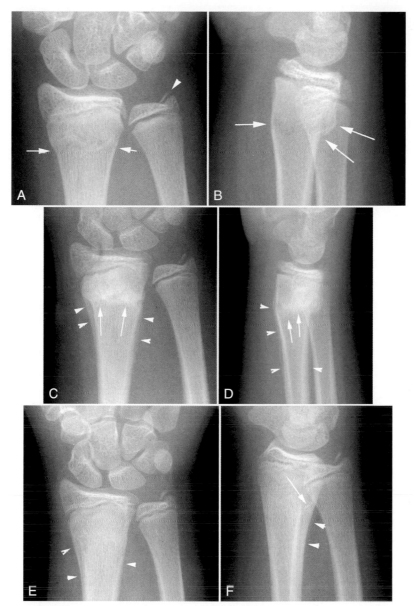

Fig. 1.25 Fracture healing in a child. PA **(A)** and lateral **(B)** views show an acute distal radius buckle fracture *(arrows)*. Also note the ulnar styloid avulsion *(arrowhead* in **A)**. **(C and D)** Follow-up views obtained 3 weeks later show trabecular healing seen as increased density along the fracture line *(arrows)*. Also note the periosteal new bone formation *(arrowheads)*. The periosteum is loosely adherent to the underlying bone in children, except at the physis, where it is tightly attached. Childhood fractures often result in periosteal elevation because of hematoma associated with the fracture. The elevated periosteum begins to form new bone soon after the fracture. **(E and F)** Follow-up views obtained 5 weeks later show further maturation and remodeling of the periosteal new bone and remodeling of the old fractured cortex *(arrow* in F). On subsequent radiographs (not shown), the bone remodeled to anatomic alignment with no evidence that the fracture had ever occurred.

Repair

- *Primary (immature, soft) callus* forms around the fracture.
  - Contains fibroblasts and chondroblasts that produce cartilage.
- Next, the primary callus is converted to *hard (mature) callus* by enchondral ossification.
  - Woven (immature) bone.
- Note that motion at the fracture site increases callus formation.
- Radiographic findings:
  - *Gap healing*: spaces between fragments fill in with callus.

- Callus progressively calcifies.
- The periosteum elevated by hematoma may produce bone that is initially a thin shell and is seen on radiographs as a slender line. (Periosteal new bone formation is also termed *periosteal reaction* or *periostitis*.) The hematoma is eventually converted to bone (Fig. 1.25).

Remodeling

- The callus is remodeled into mature lamellar bone (Fig. 1.25).
- Remodeling goes on for months to years, long after the biomechanical stability is restored, usually toward the prefracture configuration.

- Radiographic findings: amorphous callus replaced by mature bone with cortex and trabeculae.

The *rate of fracture healing* is affected by several factors, including:

- Blood supply.
  - Degree of local bone and soft tissue devitalization.
  - Fracture site.
- Patient age.
  - Children fastest, elderly slowest.
- Fracture location.
  - Metaphysis has the best blood supply.
  - Tibial shaft fractures are notoriously slow to heal (months vs. 6–8 weeks for most fractures).
  - Segmental fractures heal less well.
- Degree of immobilization and apposition of bone fragments after reduction.
  - A small amount of mobility at the fracture site speeds healing.
  - Too much or too little mobility (very rigid internal fixation) slows healing.
  - Too much mobility is also associated with abundant callus formation.
- Smoking slows healing.
- Inadequate nutrition.
  - Vitamin D.
  - Gastric bypass limits calcium absorption.
  - Generalized malnourishment delays healing.
- Drugs.
  - Corticosteroids slow healing and can produce abundant callus (Box 1.1).
  - Nonsteroidal antiinflammatory drugs (NSAIDs) interfere with the early healing process.
- Presence of local complicating factors such as infection or tumor at the fracture site, and bone necrosis.
- Soft tissues interposed between the fracture fragments can delay or block healing.

Interventions that promote fracture healing:

- Electrical stimulation ('bone stimulator').
- Ultrasound (US).
- Various biomaterials, some radiodense, may be placed at the fracture during open reduction. These materials improve fracture healing.

Follow-up Imaging in Routine Uncomplicated Fractures

- Radiographs usually adequate.
  - CT can be used as a problem solver (Fig. 1.26).

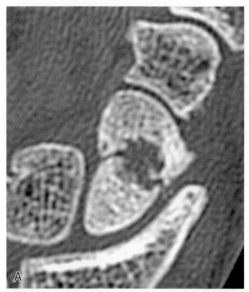

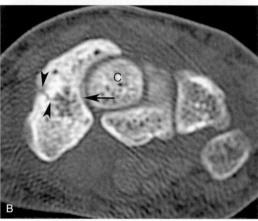

Fig. 1.26 **CT for assessing fracture union. (A)** Ununited scaphoid waist fracture. Oblique coronal CT reconstruction in a patient who sustained a scaphoid waist fracture 10 weeks previously. No bridging bone was present on this image, nor on any other. **(B)** Partial union of a scaphoid waist fracture. Axial CT image in a different patient obtained several weeks after a scaphoid waist fracture shows partial union, with bridging bone along the medial cortex *(arrow)*, but most of the fracture line is still visible *(arrowheads)*. C, Capitate.

- Fragment alignment: report change or no change. If changed, describe.
- Hardware (if present): report change or no change. Look for lucency around screws and other hardware, which is evidence of loosening or infection. This is discussed further below.
- Assess maturity of fracture healing.
  - Earliest: softened fracture lines.
  - Callus first seen at 2+ weeks.
  - Maturing callus.
  - Callus converting to bone (cortex and trabeculae) as early as 3 weeks in children.
  - Late: remodeling (may last for years).

Sample report

- Distal fifth metacarpal fracture is unchanged in position and alignment. Fracture lines have softened and faint callus surrounds the fracture.

Box 1.1   **Excessive Callus Formation**

Corticosteroids (exogenous, Cushing)
Neuropathic joint
Congenital insensitivity to pain
Paralysis
Osteogenesis imperfecta
Renal osteodystrophy
Burn patients
Subperiosteal bleed in scurvy

FRACTURE HEALING COMPLICATIONS AND IMAGING

Key Concepts

Fracture Healing Complications

Delayed union
Nonunion
Malunion
Osteonecrosis (avascular necrosis)
Soft tissue injury
Infection (open fracture, open reduction, orthopedic hardware)
Hardware failure
Complex regional pain syndrome (reflex sympathetic dystrophy)
Myositis ossificans, heterotopic ossification

DELAYED UNION

- Fracture ununited at 6 months (more or less).
- Delayed union is a clinical diagnosis, with time to union affected by a number of issues that are not evident on the radiograph. These may include:
  - Nutritional status.
  - Alcohol use.
  - Steroids.
  - Smoking.
  - Patient age.
  - Metabolic state.
  - Soft tissue damage.
  - Devascularization.
  - Particular bone involved.

- This term should be used with caution by a radiologist because it may be incorrectly applied to a fracture that is healing slowly but satisfactorily.

NONUNION

- Healing process terminates before osseous union is achieved.
- Radiographic diagnosis.
- No *bridging bone* joining the fracture fragments (Fig. 1.27).
- Can be hypertrophic or atrophic.
  - *Hypertrophic*: sclerotic with excessive new bone formation
  - *Atrophic*: associated with demineralization.
- Rounding and cortication of the fracture edges ('neocortication').
- *Pseudarthrosis* may result.
- *Incomplete union* can be expressed as a percentage, for example '30% osseous union' (Fig. 1.26).

Imaging of suspected nonunion or incomplete union can be difficult in some fractures, even with CT with reformats.

- Comminuted fractures are multiple fractures. Many of the fractures may be well healed, but careful evaluation may show no or only limited continuous bridging bone uniting the most proximal and distal fragments.
- Fixation hardware may obscure fracture lines on radiographs and creates artifact on CT.
  - May need to use much higher CT dose in order to obtain diagnostic images.
  - Dual energy CT and other strategies can reduce this need.

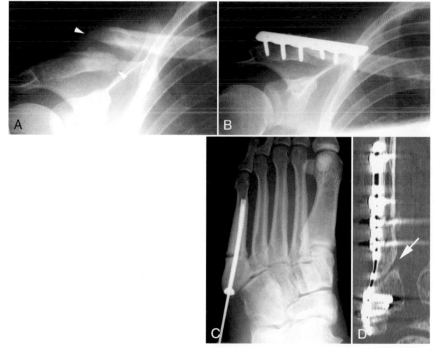

Fig. 1.27 Fracture nonunion. (A and B) Atrophic nonunion of a clavicle fracture. Note the smooth, tapering margins of the fragments (*arrowheads* in A). Surgical fixation was elected **(B). (C)** Nonunion of fracture of the fifth metatarsal proximal shaft. Note the smooth, sclerotic fracture margins. This radiograph also illustrates the technique of placement of a cannulated lag screw. The guide pin is placed under fluoroscopic observation, then the screw is placed over the pin. Because only the tip of the screw is threaded ('lag' screw), tightening the screw compresses the fragments together. **(D)** Nonunion in an internally fixed distal fibular fracture *(arrow)*.

MALUNION
- Fracture healing with angular or positional deformity.
- Can result in a limb-length discrepancy or limb deformity that may limit function or cause pain.
- As noted in the discussion of fracture reduction, angular deformity in the plane of motion of adjacent joints is better tolerated than angular deformity outside this plane.
- Anterior or posterior angular deformities in children may be corrected over time by the normal remodeling of ongoing bone growth.
- However, varus or valgus angular deformity in children tends to remodel less well and rotational deformity very little.
- Imaging is usually straightforward. CT or MRI can better demonstrate articular surface deformity.

OSTEONECROSIS (AVASCULAR NECROSIS, AVN)
- Potential fracture complication.
- Most common in bones or portions of bones with a tenuous blood supply.
  - Examples include the scaphoid proximal pole (Fig. 1.28), talar dome, and femoral head. These bones have in common extensive covering by articular cartilage, which limits the available sites for blood vessels to enter the bone.
- Diminished bone blood supply can sometimes be detected on radiographs obtained during the initial days and weeks following the fracture.

- The devascularized bone appears denser than surrounding, vascularized bone.
- It is not actually denser than that before the fracture. Rather, the vascularized surrounding bone becomes osteopenic due to local hyperemia.
- Although increased fragment density is a sign of AVN, it is not pathognomonic.
  - For example, mild sclerosis of the proximal pole of the scaphoid can be a benign finding in a healing scaphoid fracture.
- Fractures complicated by AVN may require grafting or surgical removal for treatment.
- AVN is discussed further in Chapter 13.

OSTEOMYELITIS
- Open fractures are at especially high risk.
- Risk associated with orthopedic hardware placement is small (Fig. 1.29).
- Look for the development of soft tissue gas, swelling, and bone resorption or other radiographic signs of osteomyelitis.
- Osteomyelitis related to screw placement is usually manifested radiographically as an area of osteolysis surrounding the screw or tract enlargement on follow-up imaging after hardware removal.
- Osteomyelitis is discussed in more detail in Chapter 14.

ORTHOPEDIC HARDWARE LOOSENING AND FAILURE
The potential causes are many. This is a partial list

- Inadequate fracture reduction, which results in undue strain on applied hardware.
- Inadequate hardware.
- Noncompliant patients who place excessive loads on their reduced fractures and hardware before the bone can heal.
- Even the strongest hardware may eventually fail if the fracture fails to heal.
- Imaging findings:
  - Loosening: Look for bone resorption around screws and adjacent to hardware (Fig. 1.30).
  - Hardware fracture (Fig. 1.31).
  - Screw backing out.

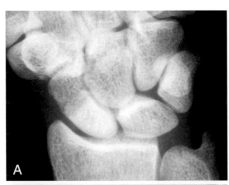
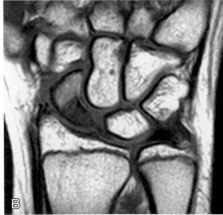

Fig. 1.28 Posttraumatic avascular necrosis. (A) AP wrist radiograph obtained after a nondisplaced scaphoid fracture shows dense proximal pole due to lack of hyperemic healing response. **(B)** Coronal T1-weighted MR image in a different patient shows lack of normal fat signal in the proximal pole because of avascular necrosis.

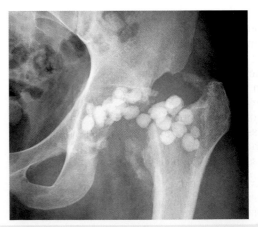

Fig. 1.29 Antibiotic-impregnated methyl methacrylate beads. After the patient underwent a total hip arthroplasty, the hardware became infected and was removed. The hip is allowed to 'float' during long-term antibiotic therapy before a new arthroplasty is performed. The beads theoretically create high local antibiotic concentration.

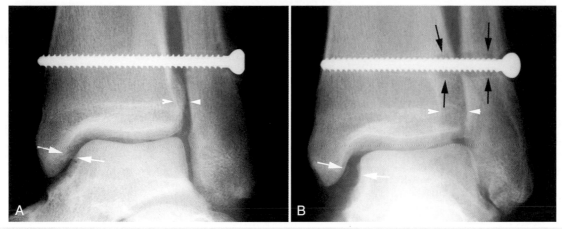

Fig. 1.30 Hardware loosening. (A) Initial AP radiograph of the ankle shows an intact syndesmotic screw fixing a distal tibiofibular diastasis injury. Note the normal alignment of the distal tibiofibular joint *(arrowheads)* and the medial ankle mortise *(arrows)*. **(B)** Radiography repeated several weeks later shows bone resorption seen as lucency around the lateral aspect of the screw, especially in the fibula and lateral tibia *(black arrows)*. Note the widening of the distal tibiofibular joint *(arrowheads)* and the medial mortise *(white arrows)*. Infection or mechanical loosening could cause this appearance.

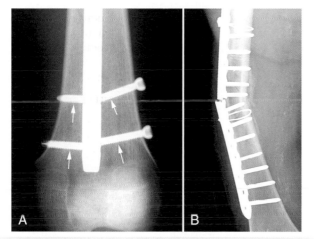

Fig. 1.31 Hardware failure. (A) AP radiograph in a patient with a femoral shaft fracture that was fixed with an interlocking intramedullary nail. He resumed weight-bearing earlier than advised, which placed shearing force across the interlocking screws. The distal screws failed *(arrows)*. **(B)** Hardware fracture. Failed fixation of proximal femur fracture with compression plate and screws.

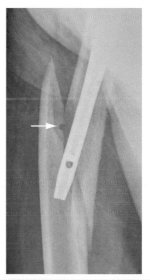

Fig. 1.32 Stress riser fracture. Oblique proximal femoral shaft fracture near the distal end of intramedullary fixation for a hip fracture. Note that the fracture line crosses—and may have originated at—the hole for the distal interlocking screw *(arrow)*.

STRESS RISER (STRESS CONCENTRATION)

- A small defect in a bone such as an orthopedic screw tract or a foramen where a blood vessel penetrates the cortex can allow force to be magnified at that single point.
- A stress riser can significantly lower the fracture threshold of a long bone shaft, and some fractures begin at a stress riser (Fig. 1.32).
- Orthopedic hardware fractures also often occur at a stress riser in the hardware.

COMPLEX REGIONAL PAIN SYNDROME (CRPS, REFLEX SYMPATHETIC DYSTROPHY [RSD], SUDECK ATROPHY)

- Poorly understood alteration in the nervous system that causes regional hyperemia, pain, osteoporosis, soft tissue trophic changes, and alteration in temperature control.
- Frequently is initiated by a fracture or other trauma.
- This condition is discussed further in Chapter 13.

Soft tissue Injury Associated With Fracture

- Frequently occurs with a fracture, particularly if there is significant fragment displacement or associated dislocation.
- Suspected arterial injury is an indication for emergent angiography, usually CT angiography.
- Nerve or ligament injury can result in poor limb function despite satisfactory fracture healing.
- Additional forms of posttraumatic soft tissue injury are discussed in Part 2.

Stress Injury

- *Fatigue fractures* result from abnormal stresses placed on normal bone.
- *Insufficiency fractures* result from normal stresses placed on bone that is weakened by a generalized process such as osteoporosis.

- The term *stress fracture* is usually reserved for fatigue fractures, although this is not universally agreed upon. Many authors regard both fatigue and insufficiency fractures as stress fractures.
- In some cases, the distinction between fatigue fracture and insufficiency fracture is blurred. An example is lower extremity stress fracture in a young female runner with the *female athletic triad* of eating disorder, diminished or absent menses, and deceased bone mineral density. These stress fractures have features of both fatigue and insufficiency fractures.
- *Stress injury* is an umbrella term that covers the wide clinical and imaging spectrum from minimal injury to complete fracture.

Fatigue Fractures

Occur when abnormal stresses are placed on normal bone, typically multiple and frequent repetition of an otherwise normal force.
- Contributing factors:
  - Muscles, tendons, and ligaments normally help to redistribute forces applied to the bones and joints. Muscle fatigue during prolonged exercise diminishes this protection.
  - Increased bone loading stimulates a normal adaptive process that leads to new bone formation (Wolff's law). The shift toward greater bone formation requires the activity of both osteoblasts and osteoclasts. Unfortunately, the osteoclasts begin first, so an increase in bone stress such as increased physical activity initially results in the bones becoming weaker for a few weeks before ultimately becoming stronger. This creates a window of vulnerability during which microfractures already present can coalesce into a discrete fracture.

Stress Fractures Evolve Over Time

- Begin as microcracks on the bone surface. Undetectable on clinical imaging studies at this stage.
- Initial healing response removes some cortical bone and may incite a periosteal reaction. This stage is sometimes termed a *stress reaction* or, in the tibia, a *shin splint*, but the terminology is not standardized.
  - Radiographs at this stage are usually normal, but faint cortical resorption may be seen.
  - MRI: periosteal edema that may be subtle. Normal marrow signal
  - Bone scan: longitudinal cortical tracer uptake.
- With injury progression, microfractures in a focal segment within the stress reaction may weaken more rapidly. This weaker segment becomes a focal point for bone deformation during repeated loading, because it is less able to resist deformation than adjacent bone. This concentration of microscopic bone deformation at the focally weakened segment has two important consequences.
  - First, the stresses applied to the remainder of the bone are partially relieved, potentially allowing these portions of the bone to heal.
  - Second, the microfractures in the weakened segment are subject to greater deformation, so they are more likely to progress.
  - Radiographs at this stage show periosteal reaction (new bone formation) and cortical demineralization.
  - MRI: periosteal and endosteal edema.
  - Bone scan: trace uptake becomes focal.
- If the injury progresses, there is further fracture progression through the cortex into the medullary space.
  - Radiographs at this stage show cortical bone loss.
  - MRI: more extensive marrow edema. Cortical edema may also be seen.
  - Bone scan: focally hot.
- Further fracture progression results in the fracture line visible on radiographs (the *dreaded black line*). The fracture line may be very faint, but in any terminology this is a true stress fracture (Figs. 1.33 to 1.39).

If untreated, a stress fracture can progress to a complete fracture.

- *Tensile stress fracture* is a stress fracture at a site of distracting force, for example, on the convex side of a curved weight-bearing long bone. Examples include

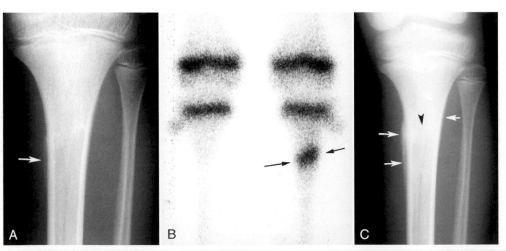

Fig. 1.33 Proximal tibia stress fracture. (A) Radiograph shows ill-defined lamellar periosteal bone formation in proximal medial tibial diaphysis *(arrow).* **(B)** Bone scan shows oblique transverse stress fracture in the proximal tibia *(arrows).* **(C)** Frontal tibial radiograph obtained 3 weeks later demonstrates progressive formation of periosteal new bone formation *(arrows)* and appearance of subtle linear sclerosis at the stress fracture site *(arrowhead).*

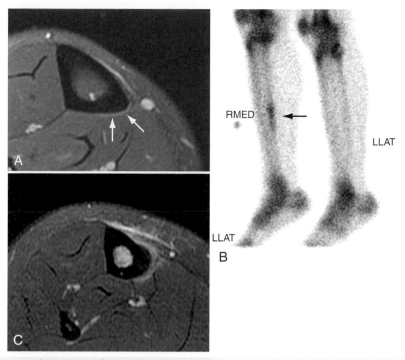

Fig. 1.34 Tibia shin splint progressing to stress fracture in a long-distance runner. (A) Initial axial fat-suppressed T2-weighted MR image shows subtle periosteal edema on the posterior tibial shaft *(arrows)*. **(B)** Bone scan obtained the next day confirms classic stress reaction pattern with localized longitudinal tracer uptake in the posterior proximal tibial cortex *(arrow)*. Despite these findings, the patient chose to continue running. **(C)** Repeat MRI using the same sequence 3 weeks later shows intense bone marrow and periosteal edema of a stress fracture.

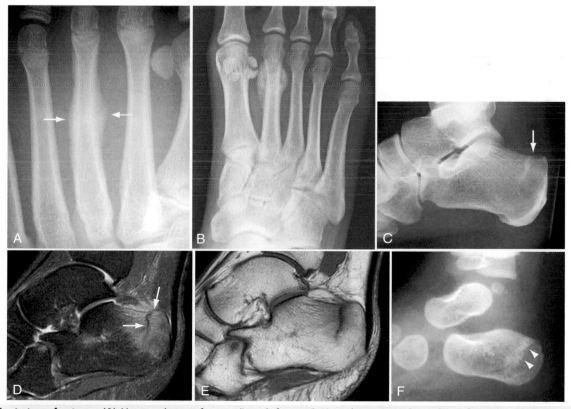

Fig. 1.35 Foot stress fractures. (A) Metatarsal stress fracture ('march fracture'). Note the periosteal new bone formation in the metatarsal shaft *(arrows)* and the subtle sclerosis caused by healing response to the metatarsal fracture. **(B)** Healing metatarsal stress fracture. Radiographs 3 weeks earlier were completely normal, but the diagnosis was made with MRI and the foot was casted. (C–E) Calcaneus stress fracture. **(C)** Note the sclerotic incomplete fracture line *(arrow)*. **(D)** A sagittal fat-suppressed T2-weighted MR image shows low-signal fracture and intense surrounding bone marrow edema. **(E)** Sagittal T1-weighted MR image also shows low-signal fracture. **(F)** Calcaneus stress fracture in a young child. Note the sclerotic zone in the posterior calcaneus *(arrowheads)*. This can be considered a type of toddler's fracture.

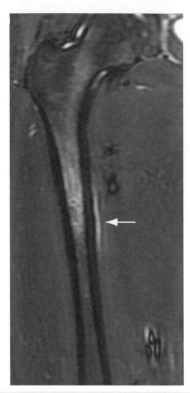

Fig. 1.36 Femoral shaft stress fracture. Coronal inversion recovery image shows medial periosteal edema *(arrow)* and bone marrow edema.

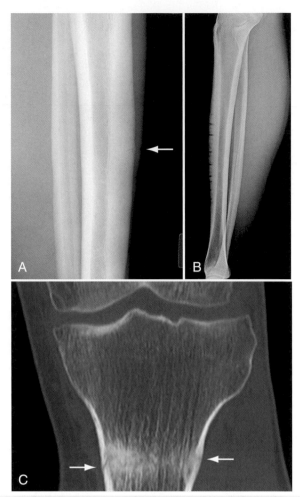

Fig. 1.38 Severe tibial stress fractures. (A) Lateral radiograph shows a visible transverse cleft in the thickened anterior tibial cortex *(arrow)*. **(B)** Unusual example with multiple visible anterior cortical stress fractures. **(C)** Coronal CT reconstruction shows nondisplaced complete stress fracture across the proximal metadiaphysis *(arrows)*.

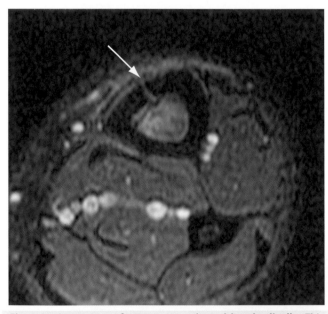

Fig. 1.37 Some stress fractures are oriented longitudinally. This axial fat-suppressed T2-weighted MR image shows interruption of the anterior tibial cortex *(arrow)*. This finding was present on multiple consecutive images. Radiographs were normal.

the anterior tibia, superior femoral neck, and proximal femoral shaft. These fractures are at high risk for completion.
■ *Compressive stress fracture* is a stress fracture at a site of compressive force, for example, the inferior femoral neck. These fractures are at low risk for completion.

Stress Injury Imaging

■ Radiographs are insensitive and do not accurately evaluate injury severity. However, they are obtained as a first-line test, in part to search for alternative diagnoses such as a lytic lesion.
■ CT is more sensitive than radiographs in demonstrating the fracture, periosteal elevation, and surface or endosteal callus.
■ Radionuclide bone scanning with TC99m tagged bisphosphonates has high sensitivity and a negative scan has very high negative predictive value. Specificity is lower.
■ MRI is highly sensitive for stress injury and fracture because of the associated marrow, periosteal, and/or cortical edema, and it is highly specific when a fracture line is shown. MRI also may demonstrate an injury in an adjacent tissue, such as a muscle strain that clinically simulates a bone stress injury. MRI has the additional advantage of no ionizing radiation. MRI is now generally obtained rather than bone scan when the region of concern is a single site or adjacent sites such as bilateral tibias.

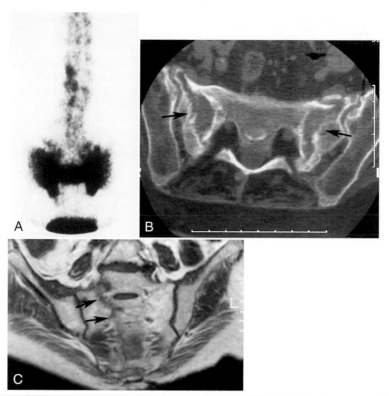

Fig. 1.39 Insufficiency fracture of the sacrum. (A) Radionuclide bone scan demonstrates intense uptake in sacrum in an H configuration. This pattern is typical of sacral insufficiency fracture. **(B)** Axial CT image of the same patient demonstrates chronic fractures in both sacral alae *(arrows)*. Sclerotic opposing margins indicate chronic nature of these insufficiency fractures. **(C)** Oblique coronal T1-weighted spin-echo image in a different patient demonstrates low-signal insufficiency fracture line in the right sacral wing *(arrows)*.

Stress fractures can occur in almost any stressed bone. Some classic locations include:

- Femoral neck.
- Tibial shaft.
- Metatarsals (*march fracture*; see Fig. 1.35A and B).
- Femoral shaft.
- Fibular shaft.
- Calcaneus.
- Tarsal navicular.
- Lumbar spondylolysis in activities with forceful spine hyperextension.
- Some bifid first metatarsophalangeal sesamoid bones are stress fractures.
- Some less common sites have particular associations:
  - Hamate hook in golf, baseball, and tennis players.
  - Medial pubic bone in soccer players and gymnasts.
  - Obturator ring and pediatric wrist in gymnasts.
  - Proximal humerus and around the elbow in pediatric baseball pitchers.
  - Ribs in rowers.

Stress Fracture Mimics

- Osteoid osteoma is painful and produces periosteal new bone with marrow edema.
- Other bone tumors.
- Osteomyelitis, especially in children.

Stress Fracture Management

- Rest and, in more advanced cases, immobilization.

- Internal fixation for the most severe cases.
- Successful conservative treatment requires the cooperation of the patient.
  - Many stress fractures are self-inflicted overuse injuries in which patients ignore the warning signs because of their passion for the injurious activity (see Fig. 1.34). Knowledge that earlier intervention results in more rapid healing may help to persuade the injured patient to allow the fracture to heal.

Insufficiency Fracture

- Caused by normal stresses placed on bone that is weakened by a generalized process such as osteoporosis.
- Also seen in osteomalacia, hyperparathyroidism, corticosteroids, Paget disease, and numerous other conditions that weaken bones.
- Like a fatigue-type stress fracture, an insufficiency fracture can often be diagnosed by clinical history, but imaging is helpful for confirmation and assessment of severity.
- As with fatigue-type stress fracture, tensile fractures are at greater risk for completion than compressive fractures.
- Most common at sites with high trabecular bone content because trabecular bone is disproportionately lost in osteoporosis.
- Common locations:
  - Vertebral osteoporotic compression fracture (Fig. 1.5)
  - Ends of weight-bearing long bones.
  - Pelvic ring.
  - Sacrum.
    - Sagittal plane alar fractures.

- Transverse fracture across the mid-upper sacrum.
  - These may coalesce into an H-shaped pattern (Fig. 1.39).
- Proximal lateral femoral shaft, associated with long-term bisphosphonate therapy for osteoporosis. A characteristic laterally oriented spike of bone resembling a beak is usually seen at the fracture line. These fractures can be bilateral.

Insufficiency Fracture Imaging

- Radiographs are insensitive. Detection of a nondisplaced insufficiency fracture on radiographs can be quite difficult because of osteopenia. Initial films are negative approximately 80% of the time.
- CT is much more sensitive than radiographs, but less sensitive than bone scan or MRI. Findings may include lucent fracture line, cortical interruption, deformity, increased trabecular bone density (healing response in trabecular fractures), and subtle callus adjacent to the cortex. Dual energy scanners can detect marrow edema in osteoporotic bones, increasing sensitivity.
- Radionuclide bone scanning is sensitive but less specific unless a specific pattern of tracer uptake can be identified, such as the H-shaped pattern of activity seen with a sacral insufficiency fracture (Fig. 1.39).
- MRI is highly sensitive to the presence of a fracture and more specific than radionuclide imaging because a fracture line usually can be shown.

Insufficiency Fracture Management

- Rest.
- Internal fixation for some.
- Methyl methacylate injection for acute vertebral and sacral fractures (vertebroplasty, kyphoplasty, sacroplasty).
- Management of the underlying condition (usually osteoporosis).

Part 2: Joints and Soft Tissues

Joint Basics
Ligament Basics
Tendon Basics
Muscle Basics
Articular Cartilage Basics
Nerve Basics
Foreign Body Imaging

This section provides an overview of imaging findings in normal and injured musculoskeletal soft tissues. Many of the generalizations and specific injuries introduced in this section are discussed in greater detail in later chapters.

Joint Basics

- Structures that connect adjacent bones.
- Function: allow motion.

There are three types of joints:
Synovial joint (diarthrosis)

- Most of the joints of the extremities, facet joints of the spine, inferior portion of the sacroiliac joints.

- Freely mobile with a wide range of motion.
- Three basic components:
  - Articular cartilage covering the ends of the bones.
    - Cushions the bones and allows for nearly frictionless joint motion.
  - Flexible, synovium-lined fibrous joint capsule.
    - Synovium produces synovial fluid, which lubricates and nourishes the articular cartilage.
  - Stabilizing ligaments.

Cartilaginous joint

- Intervertebral discs of the spine, symphysis pubis.
- Limited range of motion.
- Articulating bones are covered with fibrocartilage.
- No synovial lining.
- Usually invested with a central disc.

Fibrous joint

- Cranial sutures, superior portions of the sacroiliac joints.
- Strongest type of joint.
- Allows almost no motion and has only fibrous tissue between the bones.

JOINT PATHOLOGY TERMINOLOGY (PARTIAL LIST)

Valgus

- Abnormal angulation of the distal bone away from the midline, for example, genu valgum (knock knees).
- The term is used in context, as some valgus is present normally in the adult knee and elbow.

Varus

- Distal bone is oriented more toward the midline than normal, for example, genu varum (bow legs).
- The term is used in context, as some varus is present normally in the pediatric knee.

Dislocation

- Complete loss of contact between the articular surfaces.

Subluxation

- Partial loss of contact between the articular surfaces.
- Causes:
  - Acute or chronic ligamentous injury (Fig. 1.40).
  - Laxity due to a generalized process such as Ehlers–Danlos syndrome (discussed in Chapter 15).
  - Articular cartilage thinning in the setting of arthritis.

Diastasis

- Separation or widening of a slightly mobile joint such as the acromioclavicular joint or the symphysis pubis.
- The term diastasis is also used to describe gaps between articular surface fragments of an intraarticular fracture.

Internal Derangement

- Disruption of normal joint anatomy.
- In common usage also associated with pain and/or limited joint function.
- Examples: rotator cuff tear in the shoulder, meniscal tear in the knee.

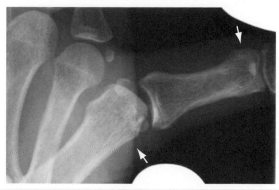

Fig. 1.40 **Instability of the thumb metacarpophalangeal (MCP) joint related to chronic ulnar collateral ligament tear.** Radiograph without stress was normal (not shown). Valgus stress *(arrows)* applied across the thumb MCP joint by the examiner's gloved hands results in valgus alignment across the joint.

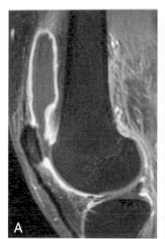 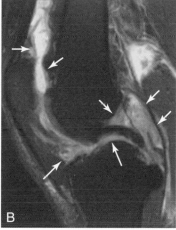

Fig. 1.41 **Synovitis. (A)** Sagittal fat-suppressed gadolinium-enhanced T1-weighted MR image of the knee in a patient with a septic knee shows intense enhancement of uniformly thickened synovium. **(B)** Sagittal fat-suppressed T2-weighted MR image of the knee in a different patient with new onset of inflammatory arthritis shows bulky synovial hypertrophy. The thickened synovium is seen as intermediate signal intensity *(arrows)*, compared with the higher signal intensity of joint fluid.

Synovitis

- Synovial inflammation.
- Many potential causes, including infection, autoimmune, intraarticular hemorrhage, and trauma.
- Synovium can thicken and become hyperemic (Fig. 1.41).

JOINT IMAGING TECHNIQUES

- Radiographs: evaluate alignment, detect intraarticular fractures, joint effusion, degenerative changes.
- CT: same as radiographs, but much more sensitive than radiographs for joint effusion and intraarticular fracture.
- US: effusion, synovial hypertrophy, can detect some ligament injuries.
- MRI: same as CT combined with US, plus better detection of many soft tissue injuries (Fig. 1.42).
- CT and MR arthrography: enhanced detection of some internal derangements such as labral or meniscal tears

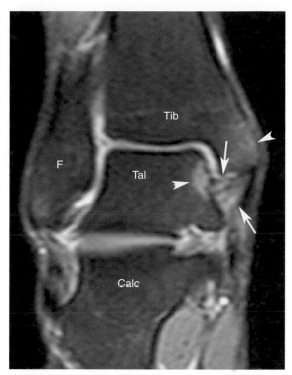

Fig. 1.42 **Ankle ligament sprain.** Coronal fat-suppressed T2-weighted MR image of the right ankle in a 30-year-old woman who sustained an ankle inversion injury shows edema in the deltoid ligament (between *arrows*). Also note bone marrow edema in the medial malleolus and talus at the ligament insertions *(arrowheads)*. *calc*, Calcaneus; *f*, fibula; *tal*, talus; *tib*, tibia.

and articular cartilage defects. Can also be helpful in postoperative imaging.

INTRAARTICULAR BODIES (LOOSE BODIES)

- Can cause joint pain and locking (Fig. 1.43; see also Fig. 1.17).
- A common source is displaced articular cartilage fragments or, in the knee, a displaced meniscal fragment.
- Not all intraarticular bodies are truly loose, because many are fixed to the synovium.
- May grow, change shape, calcify, or ossify over time.

Imaging of Intraarticular Bodies

- Radiography and CT:
  - Visible if calcified or ossified.
  - Bone portion of an acute, displaced osteochondral fragment also visible.
  - CT arthrogram can show low-density bodies.
- US can show intraarticular bodies but is not a first-line test.
- MRI: often low signal on all sequences. Ossified bodies may contain marrow fat.

Ligament Basics

- Strong, flexible bands or cords of fibrous tissue composed of highly ordered collagen fibers.
- Anisotropic (not the same in every direction).

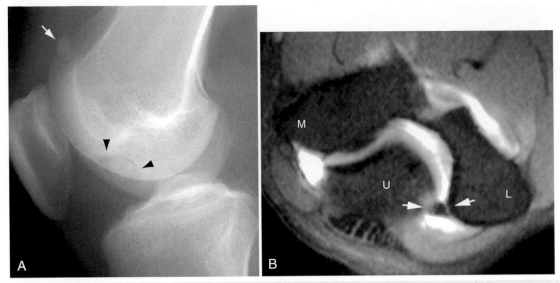

Fig. 1.43 Intraarticular bodies. (A) Lateral knee radiograph shows a small bone fragment in the superior joint recess *(arrow)*. Also note the donor site of this osteochondritis dissecans fragment on the medial femoral condyle defect *(arrowheads)*. **(B)** Elbow intraarticular body diagnosed by use of MR arthrography. Axial fat-suppressed T1-weighted MR arthrogram shows a small filling defect (between *arrows*) between the ulna and humerus in the lateral aspect of the olecranon fossa. This body caused pain on the elbow extension and therefore was removed. *L*, Lateral epicondyle; *M*, medial epicondyle; *U*, ulna.

- Connects a bone to another bone.
- Function: provides joint stability by resisting tension.
- Most ligaments are contiguous with the joint capsule.
  - Notable exceptions are the *anterior* and *posterior cruciate ligaments* of the knee, which are located inside the joint capsule (although they are technically extraarticular because they are separated from the joint compartment by the synovium)

Enthesis

- The site of attachment of a ligament or a tendon to a bone.
- Two types:
  - *Fibrous* (most common).
    - Calcified collagen fibers (*Sharpey fibers*) form the intraosseous root.
  - *Fibrocartilagenous.*
    - Complex anatomy allows stresses to be spread over a larger volume.
    - Example: rotator cuff.

LIGAMENT INJURY (SPRAIN)

- Occurs with tension.
- Simplified grading system:
  - Grade 1: injury without macroscopic tear.
  - Grade 2: partial tear.
  - Grade 3: complete ligament interruption.
- *Avulsion fracture:*
  - Ligament and its bony attachment are detached, with intact or partially intact ligament (Fig. 1.18A).
  - The associated bone fragment is usually small and can be difficult to identify on radiographs and invisible on MRI.

- Knowledge of the sites of ligament attachments to bone is helpful.
- A complete ligament tear or avulsion often occurs with transient joint subluxation or dislocation.
- Traumatic dislocation with residual joint subluxation or distraction generally implies the presence of significant ligament injury and the potential for chronic joint instability.

IMAGING OF LIGAMENT INJURIES

Radiographs and CT

- Limited direct visualization.
- Secondary findings:
  - Malalignment (Fig. 1.40).
  - Subtle avulsion fracture fragment.
  - Adjacent soft tissue edema and swelling, joint effusion.

US

- Excellent for superficial ligaments.
- Can distinguish partial from complete tears.
- Real-time stress imaging increases sensitivity.
- May detect a small avulsion fragment that is invisible on MRI.

MRI

Most normal ligaments and tendons are dark on all MRI sequences because of their highly ordered, *anisotropic ultrastructure*. This is discussed further in the section on 'normal tendon imaging'.

- Fluid-sensitive sequences demonstrate sprain severity.
  - Mild sprains (grade 1): edema with intact fibers (Fig. 1.42).

- Partial tears (grade 2): edema and some of the ligament fibers may appear to be lax, wavy, or obviously interrupted. Surrounding edema and hemorrhage frequently present.
- Complete ligament tears (grade 3): may show either obvious interruption or edema with laxity of all fibers. Surrounding edema and hemorrhage are variable and may be extensive.
- Avulsion fracture of a ligament insertion may mimic a complete ligament tear on MR images, with a ligament clearly discontinuous from bone. Marrow edema at the avulsion donor site is usually minimal, in contrast to the intense and extensive edema associated with bone bruises due to impaction. When visible, the small cortical avulsion fragment is low-signal, thin, and linear or curvilinear.

Note that while imaging plays a major role in evaluation of ligament injuries, clinical examination for pain and stability is the gold standard.

Tendon Basics

- Tendons connect a muscle to a bone.
- Function: allows muscle contraction to act on a bone.
- Structurally and biomechanically similar to ligaments.
    - Surgeons routinely exploit this similarity by harvesting a tendon to replace a damaged ligament.
- Some tendons are surrounded by a synovial lined *tendon sheath.*
    - Examples: most tendons of the hand, wrist, feet, and ankles.
    - Allows the tendon to glide without friction around corners and in narrow spaces such as the carpal tunnel and around bony prominences such as the malleoli of the ankles.
    - Prone to wear-and-tear injuries (poor blood supply) and laceration (superficial and peripheral location).
- Other tendons have no sheath.
    - Examples: quadriceps, patellar, Achilles.
    - Loose fatty tissue (*paratenon*) surrounds the tendon.
        - Better blood supply, heal well.
    - Prone to injuries at the insertion and myotendinous junction.

Tendon attachment to bone:

- Is an enthesis, just like ligament attachments.
- Sometimes termed the *tendon footprint.*
- Generalization: tendons that attach to an epiphysis or an apophysis have a wide range of angular motion at the insertion through the range of motion.
    - This makes them more vulnerable to overuse and wear-and-tear injury.
    - Examples: rotator cuff, distal biceps tendon, Achilles.
- In contrast, tendons that attach to a long bone metaphysis or diaphysis generally have a narrow range of insertion angle.
    - Less prone to injury at the insertion.
    - Example: deltoid insertion on the humerus.

IMAGING OF NORMAL TENDONS (AND LIGAMENTS)

Key Concepts

Normal Tendon

US: echogenic, uniform pattern of parallel fibers
MRI: normally dark on all sequences
Exceptions:
1. Specific areas of normal variation, often where tendons fan out or merge
2. Magic angle. Solution: evaluate tendons with T2-weighted images

US

- Excellent for superficial tendons.
- Readily displays the parallel fibers of a normal tendon.
- Tendon echogenicity depends on the angle of the transducer.
    - If the transducer is held exactly perpendicular to a normal tendon, the tendon appears hyperechoic because of specular reflections from the parallel tendon fibers (Fig. 1.44).
    - Inability to induce these specular echoes can indicate tendon pathology.

MRI

- Normal tendons and ligaments are dark on all MRI sequences because of their highly ordered, anisotropic ultrastructure (Fig. 1.45). Explanation: The extremely highly ordered, anisotropic ultrastructure of tendons and ligaments results in very rapid T2 signal decay, markedly diminishing signal intensity on T2-weighted images. In other words, the normal low signal of ligaments and tendons on MRI can be considered an artifact, albeit a very useful artifact.
- Intermediate or high signal intensity in a tendon or ligament usually indicates loss of the normal highly ordered anisotropic ultrastructure and thus tendon injury.
- Important exceptions:
    - Some tendons normally have intermediate signal at or near the insertion or origin or at sites where the tendon normally fans out or merges with other tendons. The

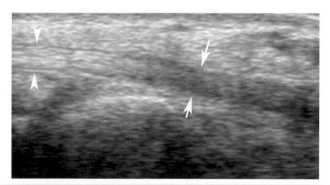

Fig. 1.44 Normal tendon on US. Normal flexor hallucis longus tendon in the foot. Note the normal high echogenicity of normal tendon that is perpendicular to the transducer (between *arrowheads*) and lower echogenicity of tendon that is not perpendicular to the transducer (between *arrows*).

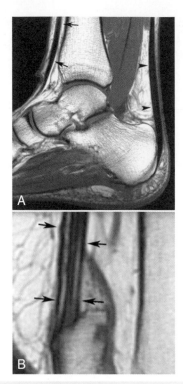

Fig. 1.45 Normal tendons on MRI. (A) Normal tendons have low signal intensity on all MRI sequences, with a few specific exceptions. Sagittal T1-weighted MR image of the ankle and hindfoot shows normal Achilles *(arrowheads)* and tibialis anterior *(arrows)* tendons. **(B)** As shown in this sagittal T1-weighted MR image, one exception is the distal quadriceps tendon, which is formed from four muscles in three layers *(arrows)*.

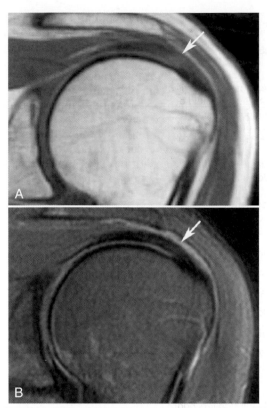

Fig. 1.46 Magic angle effect. (A and B) Oblique coronal T1-weighted **(A)** and fat-suppressed fast spin-echo T2-weighted **(B)** (echo time effective, 60 msec) MR images show the normal curved course of the supraspinatus tendon over the humeral head. Images were obtained in a high-field magnet with β_0-oriented head-to-toe. Note increased tendon signal in A but normal low signal in B, where the tendon is oriented about 55 degrees away from β_0 *(arrow)*.

tendon fibers at these sites are less anisotropic and thus do not normally have low signal. Example: the distal semimembranosis tendon at the proximal tibia.
- The distal quadriceps tendon often has a striated appearance on sagittal images as a normal finding. This reflects the quadriceps anatomy, because this tendon is formed from the tendons of four muscles.
- *Magic angle*: Due to a quirk in MRI physics, a normal ligament or tendon will have an intermediate or bright signal when oriented 55 degrees relative to the bore of the magnet (β_0) on short-echo time (TE) sequences such as gradient echo, T1, or proton density. This is known as the *magic angle effect* or *phenomenon* (Fig. 1.46). The magic angle effect occurs in the ankle tendons as they curve around the malleoli and in the supraspinatus tendon as it curves over the humeral head. Increasing TE reduces magic angle effect, so T2-weighted images are essential when imaging the rotator cuff and ankle.

Radiography and CT
- Tendons have higher attenuation than joint fluid and muscle

TENDON INJURY AND ASSOCIATED IMAGING FINDINGS (BOX 1.2)

Tendons can be injured by acute or chronic overloading, extrinsic compression such as impingement, laceration, tenosynovitis, infection, crystal deposition, and tumors. Tendons have a poor blood supply, so an injured tendon tends to heal poorly, especially sheathed tendons in the extremities. Microscopic injuries may accumulate over many years, with associated gradual tendon weakening. Thus, clinically apparent tendon injuries in patients in their 20s and 30s tend to be associated with a high-force acute injury, whereas tendon injuries in older patients often present after minimal trauma or overuse.

Tendon Tears
- May be complete or partial.
- An *intrasubstance tear* is a partial tear that does not extend to a tendon surface.
  - Some intrasubstance tear subtypes (terminology varies):
    - *Interstitial tear*: longitudinally oriented along the course of the tendon.
    - *Laminar* or *cleavage tear*: a sheetlike interstitial tear in a flat tendon such as the rotator cuff.

Imaging Findings
RADIOGRAPHS
- Direct tendon evaluation is limited.
- Some injuries visible on radiographs can imply a tendon tear.
- Examples: extreme patella alta (high position of the patella) in patellar tendon tear or patella baja (low position of the patella) with quadriceps tendon tear.

Box 1.2   Tendon Injury Patterns

Complete tear

MRI

Tendon interruption visible
Bright T2 signal (fluid or granulation) fills the gap between torn tendon fragments
Retraction may or may not be present
Chronic tear: Muscle fatty atrophy

US

Tendon interruption visible
Anechoic or hypoechoic fluid may fill gap between tendon fragments
Fragments move separately
Retraction may or may not be present

Partial tear

Similar to complete tear, but tendon partially intact

Chronic partial tear

Tendon may be too thick or thin, with normal signal

Tendinosis

Spectrum of abnormal findings due to degeneration, tendinitis, partial tears, repair
Too thick
Too thin
Abnormal signal/echogenicity

Tenosynovitis

Increased fluid and/or synovial hypertrophy in the tendon sheath

Stenosing tenosynovitis

MRI and US

Focal tendon thickening or fibrosis adjacent to the tendon sheath
US can show tendon tethering in real time
Tendon sheath fluid may be in pockets or absent
Fibrosis may be visible around sheath

Calcific tendinitis

Radiography: Amorphous calcification
MRI: Low signal on all sequences
US: Hyperechoic with shadowing

MRI, magnetic resonance imaging; *US,* ultrasound.

US AND MRI
- A completely interrupted tendon usually has fluid or granulation tissue between the torn fragments that has very bright T2 signal, or on US has low echogenicity (see Fig. 1.47).
- Partial tendon tears may be seen as a focal defect or tendon thinning, but not all partial tears are readily demonstrated.
- Some chronic partial tears manifest only as tendon thickening, thinning, and/or elongation.

Tendinosis

- Umbrella term for chronic tendon tearing and repair.
- Histologically, there is replacement of normal collagen fibers with mucoid tissue, granulation, or fibrosis.
- The tendon may become thicker or thinner, or have variable thickness.

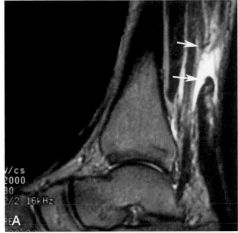
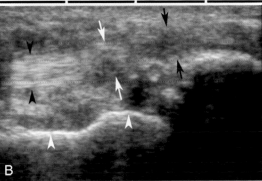

Fig. 1.47 Complete tendon tears. (A) MR image of Achilles tendon rupture. Sagittal T2-weighted spin-echo image shows a complete tear at the musculotendinous junction of the Achilles. Note wide, fluid-filled gap due to retraction of the distal muscle fibers *(arrows).* **(B)** Ultrasonogram of complete tear of the posterior tibial tendon in the foot. Note normal tendon proximally *(black arrowheads,* at the left side of the image), but low echogenicity at the torn tendon margin *(white arrows)* and empty tendon sheath more distally *(black arrows).* Also note the medial cortex of talus *(white arrowheads).*

- Loss of normally highly ordered ultrastructure and tendon edema.
  - US: loss of normal specular echoes, decreased echogenicity.
  - MRI: variably increased signal on fluid-sensitive sequences, but usually less bright than fluid (Fig. 1.48)
- *Tendinitis* is a clinical term for a tender, painful tendon. Tendinitis is usually associated with imaging findings in the tendinosis spectrum.

Impingement

- Abnormal tissue compression.
- In sports medicine, the term is most often applied to transient pathologic compression of soft tissues in or near a joint that occurs with a specific motion or activity, and that has the potential to cause pain and lead to more serious injury.
- Example: the supraspinatus tendon of the shoulder is vulnerable to impingement between the humeral head and the acromion, especially during overhead activities such as throwing a ball.
- Impingement is a clinical diagnosis.
- It is a common condition.

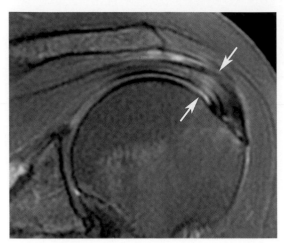

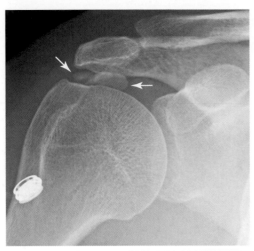

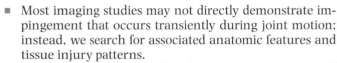

Fig. 1.48 **Tendinosis.** Compare with Fig. 1.46B. Coronal fat-suppressed T2-weighted fast spin-echo MR image shows increased signal intensity in the rotator cuff (between *arrows*). This is an example of mild tendinosis. More severe cases might show tendon thickening or thinning.

Fig. 1.49 **Calcific tendinitis.** Left shoulder AP radiograph shows the typical uniform calcification *(arrows)* of calcific tendinitis of the rotator cuff.

- Most imaging studies may not directly demonstrate impingement that occurs transiently during joint motion; instead, we search for associated anatomic features and tissue injury patterns.
- US has the potential to directly visualize some types of impingement.
- Imaging findings depend on the specific site and are reviewed later in this book.

Tendon Subluxation and Dislocation

Many tendons, as they curve around osseous structures at a joint, are held in position by a groove in the adjacent bone and an overlying retinaculum. If the bony groove is malformed or the retinaculum is lax or deficient, the tendon may sublux or dislocate from its normal position, either transiently or continuously.

Examples:

- Extensor carpi ulnaris (ECU) at the ulnar styloid.
- Peroneus longus and brevis at the lateral malleolus.
- Tibialis posterior at the medial malleolus.
- Biceps long head tendon from its groove between the humeral tuberosities in the setting of a subscapularis tendon tear.
- Recurrent subluxation may cause tendon degeneration, dysfunction, and pain.

Imaging: tendon is displaced, and may also have abnormal appearance due to related injury.

Calcific Tendinitis

- Calcium hydroxyapatite deposits within a degenerated tendon.
- Can be very painful.

Imaging

- The calcium deposit usually has uniform high density on radiographs (see Fig. 1.49), is hyperechoic with posterior acoustic shadowing on US, and has low signal intensity on all MRI sequences (which can be subtle or confusing until the radiographs are reviewed).

- The involved tendon often is highly edematous on MRI. The calcium deposit has low signal on all sequences.
- Calcific tendinitis is discussed further in Chapter 2, because the rotator cuff is the prototypic site for this condition. The numerous causes of soft tissue calcification are listed in Box 1.3 and are discussed throughout this book.

Tenosynovitis

- Inflammation of a tendon sheath.
- Tenosynovitis may result from more generalized synovitis (e.g., rheumatoid arthritis) or may be localized because of tendon degeneration, inflammation, tear, overuse, or tendon sheath trauma or infection.
- An effusion and/or thickening and hyperemia of the synovium may be present.
- Imaging: US and MRI show tendon sheath effusion and/or synovial hypertrophy (Fig. 1.50).

Stenosing Tenosynovitis

- Abnormal friction between a tendon and surrounding the tendon sheath.
- May be due to focal tendon thickening or tendon sheath narrowing.
- Examples:
  - *Trigger finger*, which classically occurs in the ring finger long flexor tendon
  - *De Quervain's tenosynovitis* in the abductor pollicis longus and extensor pollicis brevis tendons (wrist first extensor compartment)
- Also termed *tendon entrapment.*

Tendon Entrapment Between Fracture Fragments
- Different from stenosing tenosynovitis.
- A tendon may be trapped between bone fragments following a fracture or fracture reduction, notably at the ankle.
- The entrapped tendon may be visible on CT due to its relatively high density.
- Detection requires diligent review of all tendons—are they all where they should be?

Box 1.3   Soft Tissue Calcification

1. Trauma
   a. Heterotopic ossification: Most often after trauma or surgery. Also seen with brain or spinal cord injury, especially about the hips
   b. Myositis ossificans: Distinctive subtype of heterotopic ossification. Characteristic timing and maturation with peripheral calcification
   c. Burns: Often associated with contractures and acroosteolysis
   d. Frostbite: Thumb is often spared; acroosteolysis
2. Tumor
   a. Synovial cell sarcoma
   b. Liposarcoma
   c. Fibrosarcoma and malignant fibrous histiocytoma
   d. Soft tissue osteosarcoma
   e. Phleboliths in vascular tumors
   f. A soft tissue tumor may have dystrophic calcification.
3. Collagen vascular diseases
   a. Scleroderma: Usually subcutaneous, with other changes including acroosteolysis
   b. Dermatomyositis: Sheetlike in muscle or fascial planes, but other calcification patterns are also seen
   c. Systemic lupus erythematosus: Calcification is uncommon, but may occur, especially in lower extremities; consider when avascular necrosis is also seen
   d. CREST syndrome: Calcinosis cutis, Raynaud phenomenon, esophageal dysmotility, scleroderma, telangiectasias
   e. Calcinosis cutis
4. Arthritis
   a. Calcium pyrophosphate deposition arthropathy: triangular fibrocartilage complex, menisci, pubic symphysis, hyaline cartilage
   b. Hydroxyapatite deposition disease: Especially calcific tendinitis, bursitis, juxtaarticular
   c. Gout: Tophus is usually juxtaarticular
   d. Synovial chondromatosis: Intraarticular
5. Congenital
   a. Tumoral calcinosis: Periarticular
   b. Myositis ossificans progressiva: Usually axial, bridging between bones of the thorax
   c. Pseudohypoparathyroidism, pseudo-pseudohypoparathyroidism
   d. Progeria
   e. Ehlers–Danlos disease
6. Metabolic disorders
   a. Hyperparathyroidism (primary or secondary)
   b. Hypoparathyroidism
   c. Renal dialysis sequelae: Periarticular
7. Infectious disorders
   a. Granulomatous: Tuberculosis, brucellosis, coccidioidomycosis
   b. Dystrophic calcification in abscesses
   c. Leprosy: Linear calcification in digital nerves
   d. Cysticercosis: Small calcified oval bodies in muscle
   e. *Echinococcus* infection: Usually liver or bone, but occasionally in soft tissue
8. Drugs
   a. Hypervitaminosis D
   b. Milk-alkali syndrome

Bursa

- Synovium-lined potential space that allows reduced friction so that adjacent tissues such as ligaments or tendons can slide easily past one another or an adjacent bone.
- Also common between skin and bony prominences.

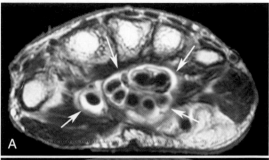
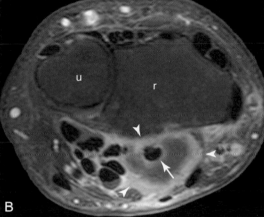

Fig. 1.50 **Tenosynovitis. (A)** Carpal tunnel tenosynovitis due to overuse. Axial T2-weighted fast spin-echo MR image shows fluid distention of the carpal tunnel tendon sheaths *(arrows)*. **(B)** Infectious tenosynovitis. Axial fat-suppressed contrast-enhanced T1-weighted MR image through the distal forearm at the distal radioulnar joint shows distended, enhancing tendon sheath *(arrowheads)* and low–signal-intensity fluid surrounding the flexor pollicis longus tendon *(arrow)*. The nonenhancing fluid in the tendon sheath in this case was pus related to *Staphylococcus aureus* infection. *r*, Radius; *u*, ulna.

- In addition to the numerous normally occurring bursae, bursae may be created de novo in areas of unusual shear stress (*adventitial bursa*), for example, around the ankles in figure skaters.

Bursitis

- Inflammation of a bursa.
- Causes: trauma, calcium salt deposition (*calcific bursitis*), infection, or causes of generalized synovial inflammation such as rheumatoid arthritis.
- Normal bursae are nearly invisible on imaging studies, but an inflamed bursa is readily apparent because of the presence of fluid, synovial thickening, and/or calcification (Fig. 1.51).

Skeletal Muscle Basics

- Function: allows motion through contraction.
- Composed of ordered bundles of muscle fibers and an investing fascial sheath.
- Supplied by blood vessels, lymphatics, and nerves.
- Attaches to bone by a tendon. The tendon usually extends far into the muscle belly.
  - *Myotendinous junction* is the junction of tendon and muscle.

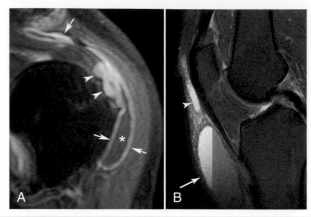

Fig. 1.51 Bursitis. (A) Sagittal fat-suppressed T1-weighted MR image with intravenous gadolinium of the left shoulder shows synovial enhancement of subacromial subdeltoid bursa *(arrows)* in this patient with bursitis. The bursal fluid *(asterisk)* does not enhance. Also note enhancement of granulation tissue *(arrowheads)* in a supraspinatus tendon tear. **(B)** Sagittal fat-suppressed T2-weighted MR image shows a hemorrhagic effusion with a fluid-fluid level in the infrapatellar bursa *(arrow)* and a smaller effusion in the prepatellar bursa *(arrowhead)*.

IMAGING OF NORMAL SKELETAL MUSCLE

- Radiography: soft tissue density.
- CT: muscle attenuation is lower than tendons. Fat may be found between the muscle fibers, especially in obese patients or in chronically injured muscle. Intravenous contrast is very useful for evaluating certain conditions such as intramuscular abscess.
- US: excellent demonstration of the normal multibundle anatomy.
- MRI: intermediate signal on T1w and low to intermediate signal intensity on T2w images (Fig. 1.52). As with CT, intramuscular fat may be present.
- Nerves and blood vessels are visible and may be assessed with US, CT, and MRI.

MUSCLE PATHOLOGY AND ASSOCIATED IMAGING FINDINGS

- MRI is the most sensitive modality for evaluating most types of muscle injuries.
- US can show many of the same injuries as MRI, in superficial muscles, but with much lower contrast.
- Radiography and CT can display intramuscular calcification, which can be a subacute or late finding after many types of muscle injury. These modalities also allow assessment of the pattern of calcification, as in the peripheral calcification of myositis ossificans or the streaky, sheetlike pattern of polymyositis.

Muscle Strain

- An *intrinsic* muscle injury that is produced by an intrinsic force generated by the muscle itself (in contrast with an *extrinsic injury* such as a contusion or stab wound).
- Strains are most common in muscles that elongate while they contract (*eccentric contraction*), such as the hamstrings and the biceps.
- A strain begins as a microscopic muscle fiber tearing, usually at the musculotendinous junction, caused by forceful contraction while under load. More severe strains include tearing of the myotendinous junction and can, when still more severe, extend into the muscle belly.

Imaging

- MRI is most sensitive due to high contrast (Box 1.4). US can detect many of the same findings, especially in more severe strains, but the findings are more subtle.
- Mild (grade 1) strain: feathery edema between the muscle fibers, usually centered along the musculotendinous junction (see Fig. 1.53).
- Moderate (grade 2) strains: have more extensive edema and fluid collections (see Fig. 1.54).
- Severe (grade 3) strains involve disruption of the musculotendinous junction with loss of muscle function. Both

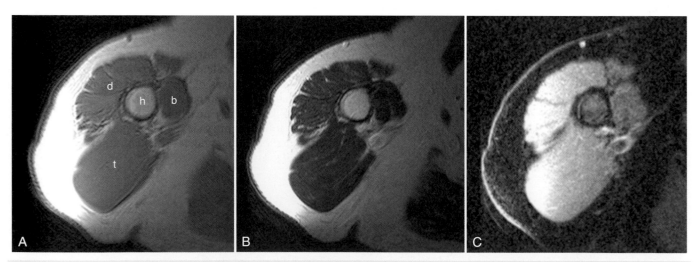

Fig. 1.52 Normal muscle and fat. (A–C) Axial MR images obtained through the proximal right arm. T1-weighted (A), T2-weighted **(B)**, and inversion recovery **(C)** images. Note intermediate signal intensity of muscle on all sequences. Fat is much brighter than muscle, except on the inversion recovery sequence **(C)**, which uses an inversion time of 140 msec at 1.5 T to null fat signal. A selective presaturation pulse can accomplish the same effect. Inversion recovery using a shorter inversion time of 110–130 msec suppresses but does not eliminate fat signal, resulting in images that many radiologists find easier to interpret. Most of the inversion recovery images in this text use a shorter inversion time. The fat signal intensity in **A** and **B** and muscle signal in **C** artifactually much higher laterally because of proximity to the receiver coil. *b*, Biceps; *d*, deltoid; *h*, humerus; *t*, triceps.

Box 1.4   Muscle Injury Patterns

Localized fluid collection at musculotendinous junction

Strain

Anywhere

Hematoma
Abscess
Myonecrosis
- Myonecrosis causes
  - Severe trauma
  - Compartment syndrome
  - Infection
  - Autoimmune disorders
  - Diabetes mellitus

Edema without fluid collection

Diffuse

Overuse (delayed-onset muscle soreness [DOMS])
Subacute denervation (after 2–4 weeks)
Radiation therapy

Focal

At musculotendinous junction:
- Strain
Anywhere:
- Trauma
- Early myonecrosis
- Infection without abscess
- Tumor

Atrophy with fatty infiltration

Paralysis, chronic denervation
Chronic tendon tear
End-stage autoimmune disease
Muscular dystrophy
Chronic corticosteroid use

Muscle calcification

Mass with peripheral calcification: Myositis ossificans
Sheetlike: Autoimmune disorder
Small nodules: Parasites
Tumors: Various patterns

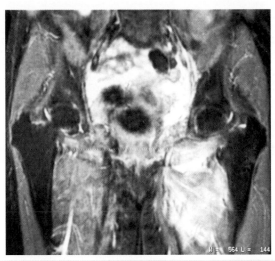

Fig. 1.54 Muscle strain in an elderly patient who fell. Coronal inversion recovery MR image shows high signal intensity in the left hip adductors. (Reprinted with permission from May DA, Disler DG, Jones EA, et al. Abnormal signal within skeletal muscle in magnetic resonance imaging: patterns, pearls, and pitfalls. *Radiographics.* 2000;20:S295–S315.)

MRI and US images reveal the musculotendinous disruption, as well as fluid collections and extensive regional edema (Box 1.4).

Extrinsic muscle injuries caused by trauma include contusion or penetrating injuries such as a knife wound. Intramuscular hematoma may result.

- A **muscle contusion** produces intramuscular edema and small fluid collections, usually centered at the site of injury.
- An **intramuscular hematoma** may contain a fluid-fluid level and/or have high signal on T1-weighted images because of the presence of methemoglobin (Fig. 1.55). An older hematoma may have a low signal intensity rim resulting from the presence of hemosiderin which results in marked signal loss on all MRI sequences, especially gradient-echo images.

Heterotopic Ossification

- Bone formation in soft tissue (Fig. 1.56).
- Common sites include around the hip or knee joint after arthroplasty, or around the hip after placement of an intramedullary nail in the femur. Soft tissues around the elbow are especially vulnerable to heterotopic ossification (HO).
- Can also occur when joint motion is profoundly reduced as, for example, in patients paralyzed by a spinal cord or brain injury.
- Rare progressive genetic forms also exist.
- Initial presentation is pain with an appropriate history. Late presentation is painless reduced range of motion.
- Heterotopic bone can limit the range of motion of an adjacent joint and, in extreme cases, effectively fuse the joint.
- Early management is with indomethacin or other NSAIDs.
- Preoperative or postoperative radiation is sometimes used as prophylaxis before hip arthroplasty. The effectiveness of this therapy is debated.

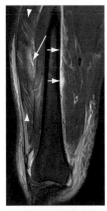

Fig. 1.53 Muscle strain. Coronal inversion recovery (short-tau inversion recovery [STIR]) MR image of the right thigh shows quadriceps strains. Note edema within the vastus lateralis oriented with the muscle fibers (between *arrowheads*), small fluid collection in a musculotendinous junction tear *(long arrow)*, and intense edema along the vastus intermedius femoral origin *(short arrows)*. The femur bone marrow signal is normal.

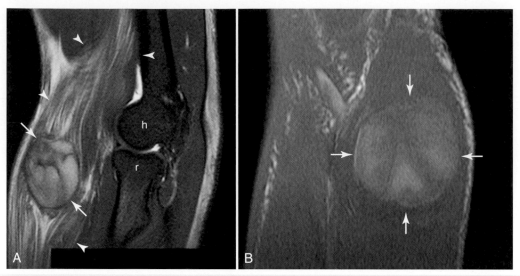

Fig. 1.55 Muscle laceration and hematoma. MR images in a patient with brachialis muscle injury. Sagittal fat-suppressed T2-weighted MR image **(A)** shows bright edema signal interposed between brachialis muscle fibers *(arrowheads)*. A masslike hematoma *(arrows)* with complex signal is located between interrupted muscle fibers. Coronal T1-weighted image **(B)** shows elevated signal of methemoglobin in the hematoma *(arrows). h,* Distal humerus; *r,* proximal radius.

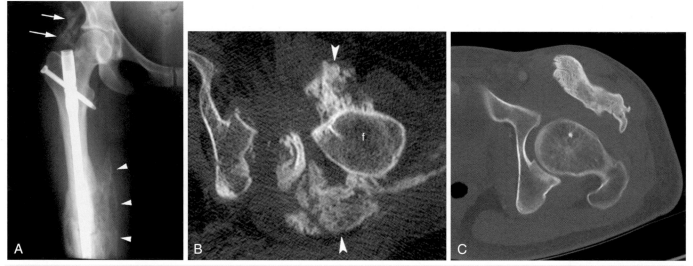

Fig. 1.56 Posttraumatic heterotopic ossification. (A) AP radiograph of the right thigh and hip shows mature bone above the femoral neck *(arrows)* and medial thigh *(arrowheads).* **(B)** Heterotopic ossification *(arrowheads)* surrounding chronically dislocated left hip. **(C)** Heterotopic ossification anterior to the proximal left femur. *f,* Proximal femur.

- Imaging in early HO:
  - Radiography: soft tissue calcification develops 3–4 weeks after onset of symptoms.
  - Bone scan allows earlier diagnosis.
  - US also can detect calcification before radiographs: echogenic interface and limited posterior acoustic shadowing.
- Imaging in late HO: mature bone with cortex, trabeculae, and marrow.

Myositis Ossificans

- A distinctive and poorly understood form of HO that occurs in muscle after blunt trauma or intramuscular hematoma (Fig. 1.57).
- Trauma initiates conversion of local cells into osteocytes and chondrocytes.

- Bone formation may be detected by bone scan or US as early as 2 weeks. US initially shows a hypoechoic mass with subtle peripheral hyperechogenicity with limited posterior acoustic shadowing. Bone scan is initially hot on blood flow and blood pool, but becomes progressively hotter on delayed images as the lesion matures.
- At 3–4 weeks, sometimes later, soft tissue calcification becomes visible on radiographs.
  - Initially it is amorphous.
- After about 8 weeks, soft tissue calcification evolves into characteristic maturing *peripheral* calcification that reveals the true, benign nature of this process.
- There also may be periosteal reaction new bone formation in an adjacent long bone, but no bone destruction is seen.
- Over the course of weeks to months, the soft tissue bone may resolve or diminish, migrate toward and

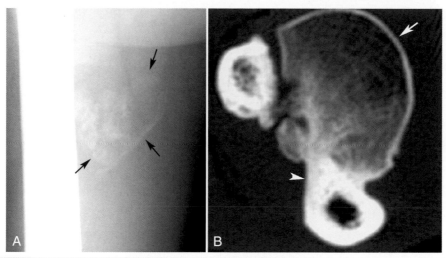

Fig. 1.57 Myositis ossificans. (A) AP radiograph of the right midthigh shows calcification that is densest at the periphery *(arrows)*. **(B)** Axial CT image in a different patient with myositis ossificans in the forearm shows mature ossification with cortex and trabeculae *(arrow)* that is fusing with the ulna *(arrowhead)*. (**A** reprinted with permission from May DA, Disler DG, Jones EA, et al. Abnormal signal within skeletal muscle in magnetic resonance imaging: patterns, pearls, and pitfalls. *Radiographics*. 2000;20:S295-S315. **B** courtesy of William Pommersheim, MD.)

ultimately merge with the adjacent bone, or remain unchanged.

- MRI can be misleading, showing a masslike intramuscular lesion that can be confused at imaging and at biopsy with an aggressive sarcoma. Careful evaluation that includes patient history may mitigate potentially confusing biopsy findings.
- Myositis ossificans is discussed in greater detail in Chapter 12.

Key Concepts

MRI to evaluate an unknown myopathy

Axial T1 is used to assess for fatty infiltration (usually indicates nonspecific end stage).

Axial fluid-sensitive sequence such as T2 with fat suppression or inversion recovery is used to assess for edema.

Including both sides for comparison can be helpful.

Use gadolinium enhancement if necrosis or abscess is suspected.

Edema without fatty infiltration indicates a good site for biopsy.

Denervation

- Muscle deprived of normal innervation undergoes degeneration and atrophy.
- MRI is highly sensitive in detection of muscle denervation and can provide prognostic information (Fig. 1.58).
- During the first 2–4 weeks after denervation, muscle signal is normal.
- After about 2–4 weeks, the denervated muscle becomes diffusely and uniformly edematous, with elevated signal on fluid-sensitive images.
- If normal innervation is restored within a few weeks, the muscle returns to normal both clinically and on MR images.

- However, denervation that persists for several weeks to months results in irreversible muscle wasting that manifests as fatty atrophy.
  - CT and MRI show decreased muscle bulk with fatty infiltration (*muscle fatty atrophy*). A chronic complete tendon tear results in a similar appearance but may also show muscle and tendon retraction

Other causes of muscle fatty atrophy:

- Long-term high-dose corticosteroid use, especially in trunk and proximal extremity muscles.
- Degenerative neuromuscular conditions (e.g., muscular dystrophy).
- Autoimmune inflammatory conditions (e.g., *dermatomyositis* or *polymyositis*) may also progress from edema during the active phase of the disease to end-stage irreversible fatty atrophy. These processes may be patchy or irregular in distribution.
- MRI is useful in guiding a biopsy when these conditions are suspected, because an optimal biopsy site should not show nonspecific end-stage fatty atrophy but rather edema related to active inflammatory cell infiltration.
- Late-stage dermatomyositis or polymyositis may show streaky or sheetlike calcifications.
- These conditions are illustrated and discussed further in Chapter 9.

Muscle infection may cause diffuse or focal edema.

- Infectious myositis due to pyogenic organisms can result in formation of an intramuscular abscess (Fig. 1.59). This condition is well known in the tropics but also occurs in temperate climates. Patients with immune dysfunction are the most vulnerable.
- An intramuscular abscess is similar in appearance to an abscess elsewhere in the body, with central fluid surrounded by an enhancing margin.
- Intramuscular gas bubbles suggest infection with a highly aggressive organism such as a *Clostridium* species; this condition is a surgical emergency requiring prompt debridement.
- Muscle infection is discussed further in Chapter 14.

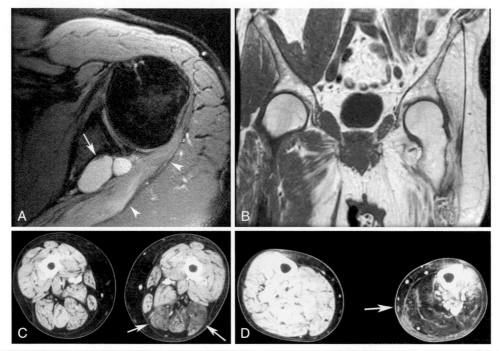

Fig. 1.58 Muscle denervation. (A) Acute muscle denervation. Acute infraspinatus denervation caused by nerve compression. Axial fat-suppressed T2-weighted MR image shows diffusely increased signal intensity in the infraspinatus muscle *(arrowheads)* caused by compression of the suprascapular nerve in the scapular spinoglenoid notch by a large paralabral cyst *(arrow)*. T1-weighted images (not shown) showed no fatty infiltration, indicating that the muscle injury is reversible. **(B)** Chronic muscle denervation, coronal T1-weighted MR image in an adult who had polio as a child shows profound fatty atrophy of left pelvic and thigh musculature. **(C and D)** Sciatic nerve injury. Axial CT images in the thighs **(C)** and calves **(D)** show fatty atrophy *(arrows)* of the hamstrings in **C** and ankle flexors in **D**. Fatty atrophy indicates irreversible muscle injury.

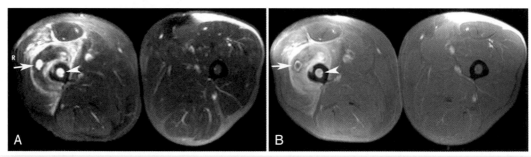

Fig. 1.59 Infectious myositis, intramuscular abscess, and osteomyelitis. Axial fat-suppressed T2-weighted (A) and contrast-enhanced fat-suppressed T1-weighted (B) MR images show small abscess in the right vastus intermedius *(arrow)* with surrounding muscle edema and enhancement, and femur midshaft marrow edema and enhancement *(arrowheads)* due to *Staphylococcus aureus* infection. (Reprinted with permission from May DA, Disler DG, Jones EA, et al. Abnormal signal within skeletal muscle in magnetic resonance imaging: patterns, pearls, and pitfalls. *Radiographics*. 2000;20:S295–S315.)

Necrotizing Fasciitis

- Infection along fascial planes that can be explosively progressive and highly lethal.
- When suspected, there is no time for imaging. The patient is taken directly to the OR for extensive debridement.
- Should imaging be obtained, fluid accumulation along fascial planes with or without enhancement may be seen. Gas bubbles may be present.

Myonecrosis

- Imaging findings vary: can resemble a mass on noncontrast CT and MRI.
- With intravenous contrast, a nonacute muscle infarct may resemble an abscess, with an enhancing rim surrounding a central region of edema or fluid.

- Outcomes also vary, can range from permanent muscle loss to complete recovery.
- Potential causes include:
  - Sickle cell disease.
  - Rhabdomyolysis.
  - Severe blunt trauma.
  - Venomous snake bite.
  - *Compartment syndrome* (discussed later in this chapter).
  - *Diabetic myonecrosis.*
    - An incompletely understood condition that resembles severe infectious myositis in imaging studies (Fig. 1.60).
    - Not due to infection and does not require aspiration, antibiotics, or surgical drainage. Extremely

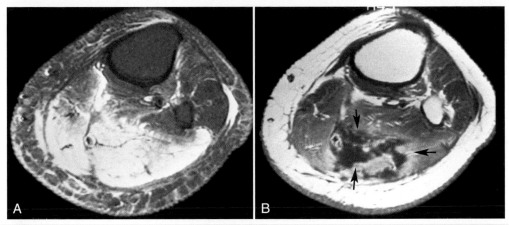

Fig. 1.60 Diabetic myonecrosis. Axial fat-suppressed T2-weighted **(A)** and contrast-enhanced T1-weighted **(B)** MR images show intense edema in the left soleus in **A** and heterogeneous enhancement and an irregularly shaped muscle infarct (*arrows* in **B**). (Reprinted with permission from May DA, Disler DG, Jones EA, et al. Abnormal signal within skeletal muscle in magnetic resonance imaging: patterns, pearls, and pitfalls. *Radiographics.* 2000;20:S295-S315.)

painful. Additional clues to the diagnosis are a history of poorly controlled diabetes mellitus and a normal or near-normal leukocyte count.

Acute Compartment Syndrome

- Muscles of the leg and volar forearm, as well as several other sites in the extremities are invested in indistensible fascia.
- Fracture, blunt or sharp trauma, a surgical procedure, or other insult can cause muscle swelling or hemorrhage that in extreme cases lead to a vicious cycle of increasing intracompartmental pressure, ischemia, more edema and swelling, further increased pressure, and, ultimately, tissue necrosis due to ischemia.
- If undetected, the compartment contents including muscles and nerves atrophy and scar, with contracture and irreversible complete loss of function. Early detection is imperative to avoid this devastating outcome.
- Acute compartment syndrome is treated by decompression with fasciotomy.
- When acute compartment syndrome is suspected, direct measurement of intracompartmental pressure is the appropriate test. This should not be delayed to obtain MRI or other imaging studies. If obtained, MRI shows muscle edema.

Exertional Compartment Syndrome

- Reversible muscle ischemia that manifests as reproducible pain during exercise.
- Running athletes.
- Anterior compartment of the leg is a common site.
- Sometimes can be detected with MRI. The symptomatic extremity can be scanned during or immediately after the offending activity. Muscle edema, often subtle, develops transiently in the affected muscle.
- The main role of MRI is to exclude other pathology.

Subacute compartment syndrome and *chronic compartment syndrome* are less precise terms that are sometimes used for milder cases of compartment syndrome (Fig. 1.61) or for exertional compartment syndrome. Some may still require fasciotomy.

A tight cast can produce compartment syndrome–like symptoms, due to swelling after cast placement. Treatment is simple: The cast is revised or simply divided longitudinally into two pieces ('bivalve' the cast, like a clam's shell) and wrapped with elastic wrap. This allows the soft tissues to swell without necessitating replacement of the cast.

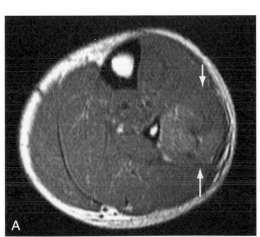

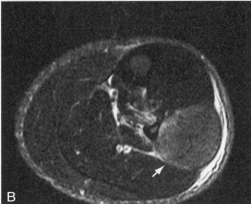

Fig. 1.61 Chronic compartment syndrome. Axial T1-weighted **(A)** and axial inversion recovery **(B)** MR images show enlargement of the peroneus longus muscle in the proximal lateral calf (*arrows*). Note edema signal in **B** and mildly elevated T1 signal in **A** suggesting hemorrhage.

Radiation Therapy

- Produces long-lasting soft tissue edema throughout the radiation field.
- MR images often show a sharp, straight margin between the edematous radiated tissue and the normal adjacent tissue (Fig. 1.62). This finding helps to distinguish incidental radiation therapy–induced edema from other causes of muscle and adjacent soft tissue edema.

Myofascial Defect

- Presents as a bump or protrusion along the surface of a muscle, often in the calf.
- Caused by muscle bulging through a defect in the muscle fascia (Fig. 1.63).
- Often incidental but may cause concern for a neoplasm and occasionally are symptomatic during exercise.
- Because some lesions can be reproduced with muscle contraction, US or rapid MRI with the muscle relaxed and contracted may show the muscle bulging through the defect.
- Symptomatic defects occasionally show muscle edema on MRI.

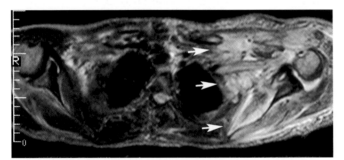

Fig. 1.62 Radiation therapy. Axial T2-weighted MR image of the upper chest in a patient previously treated with radiation therapy to the left shoulder and axilla region shows diffuse edema in the radiated soft tissues. Note sharp, straight margin between the radiated and normal tissues *(arrows)*. (Reprinted with permission from May DA, Disler DG, Jones EA, et al. Abnormal signal within skeletal muscle in magnetic resonance imaging: patterns, pearls, and pitfalls. *Radiographics.* 2000; 20:S295-S315.)

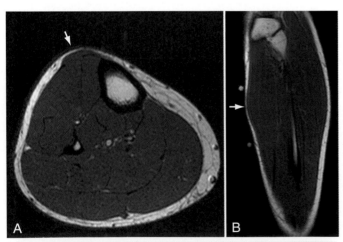

Fig. 1.63 Myofascial defect. Axial **(A)** and coronal **(B)** T1-weighted MR images in a 25-year-old patient with a palpable lump in the anterior proximal right calf show subtle anterior muscle protrusion *(arrows)*.

- More often, MRI shows nothing at all. The absence of a mass and edema are key findings in an incidental myofascial defect.

Morel-Lavallée Lesion

- Separation of skin and subcutaneous fat from underlying muscle fascia caused by a closed shear ('degloving') injury.
- This interrupts the blood vessels and lymphatics supplying the overlying fat and skin.
- Lymph, blood products, and sometimes necrotic/liquified fat from the overlying more superficial tissues distend the potential space and block healing. This fluid may often be complex and may contain fat globules (Fig. 1.64).
- Size varies from a few millimeters to several centimeters in thickness.
- May develop a thick or thin pseudocapsule.
- The fluid may become infected.
- Overlying skin is vulnerable to necrosis.
- May exert mass effect on adjacent muscle, but adjacent muscle otherwise is unaffected.
- Most common sites: proximal lateral thigh and hip followed by other sites around the pelvis and the knee.
- CT, US, or MRI shows the fluid collection between superficial muscle fascia in a characteristic location in the lateral thigh, around the hip or pelvis, or by the knee.

Articular Cartilage Basics

- Articular cartilage covers the ends of bones in synovial joints.
- Function: cushions the bone ends and allows essentially frictionless motion in a joint.
- Composed of a complex matrix of collagen and large proteoglycan molecules, chondrocytes, and water that is bound by hydrogen bonds.
- A simplified model of articular cartilage anatomy consists of four layers, distinguished by the orientation of the collagen fibers (Fig. 1.65).
  - Most superficial layer (*superficial zone*): mainly collagen fibers oriented parallel to the cartilage surface. This layer is very thin.
  - Intermediate layer (*transitional zone*): collagen fiber orientation is overall relatively random as the fibers transition from perpendicular to parallel to the cartilage surface. Moderate proteoglycan concentration.
  - Deep layer (*radial zone*): collagen fibers are oriented radially—that is, mostly perpendicular to the subchondral bone. High proteoglycan concentration.
  - The *calcified zone* anchors the radial zone which is anchored to underlying subchondral bone by calcified collagen.
- Articular cartilage has no blood, lymphatic, or nerve supply and must rely on the diffusion of nutrients from the synovial fluid and, to a lesser extent, the extracellular space of subchondral bone.
  - Joint motion with normal loading assists in cartilage nourishment by driving in nutrients from the synovial fluid.

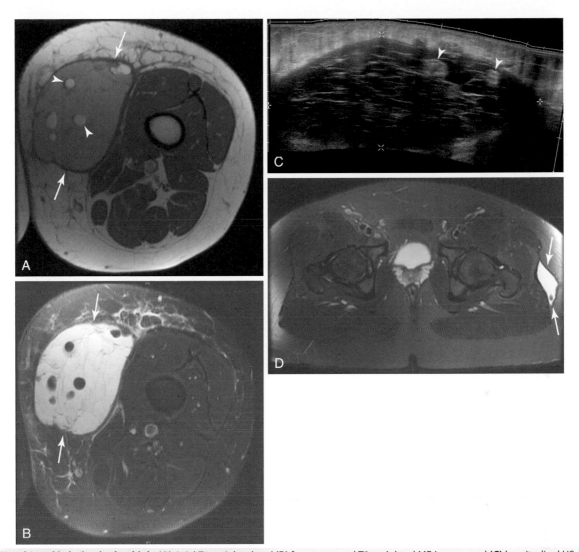

Fig. 1.64 Morel-Lavalée lesion in the thigh. (A) Axial T1-weighted and **(B)** fat-suppressed T2-weighted MR images and **(C)** longitudinal US. This lesion has many of the features that are variably present in Morel-Lavalée lesions, including a surrounding low-signal pseudocapsule *(arrows)*, innumerable internal thin septations, fat lobules within the lesion *(arrowheads)*, and mass effect on adjacent musculature. Note the characteristic location between subcutaneous fat and superficial muscle fascia. The medial location of this lesion is somewhat atypical, as most lesions occur laterally. **(D)** Smaller lesion in a different patient, lateral to the left hip.

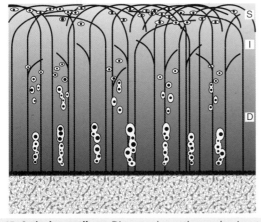

Fig. 1.65 Articular cartilage. Diagram shows the predominant orientation of collagen and proteoglycan fibers in the superficial, intermediate, and deep layers. This diagram exaggerates the thickness of the superficial layer, which is actually very thin. Calcified cartilage anchors the deep layer to underlying bone. *D*, Deep; *I*, intermediate; *S*, superficial.

IMAGING OF ARTICULAR CARTILAGE

MRI

- The gold standard imaging tool for articular cartilage.
- Lightly T2-weighted (intermediate) fast spin-echo.
  - The most widely used sequence.
  - An optimal TE is about 45 msec.
  - Often obtained with fat suppression.
    - Fat suppression increases dynamic range and reduces chemical shift artifact.
  - Normal articular cartilage has low to intermediate signal intensity on this sequence (Fig. 1.66A).
  - The deep cartilage layer may display slightly lower signal intensity because of its anisotropic ultrastructure.
- Fat-suppressed three-dimensional spoiled gradient-echo sequence (3D SPGR, FLASH).
  - Provides higher spatial resolution than a fast spin-echo sequence.

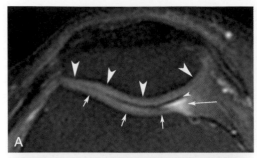

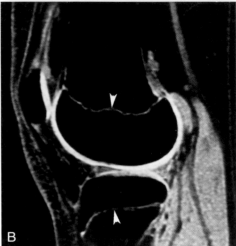

Fig. 1.66 Normal articular cartilage. (A) Axial fat-suppressed T2-weighted fast spin-echo (echo time, 45 msec) MR image obtained through the patella shows patellar *(large arrowheads)* and femoral trochlea *(short arrows)* cartilage. Careful observation shows slightly higher signal intensity in the intermediate layer (due to lack of anisotropy in this layer). The dark line between the patellar and trochlear cartilage *(small arrowhead)* is due to susceptibility artifact. Contrast the overall intermediate signal intensity of the normal articular cartilage with the high signal intensity of joint fluid *(long arrow)*. Cartilage defects are seen as high-signal regions. **(B)** Sagittal fat-suppressed three-dimensional spoiled gradient-echo MR image (repetition time, 60 msec; echo time, 5 msec; flip angle, 40 degrees) shows normal articular cartilage of the knee. Also note similar, normal signal of distal femoral and proximal tibial growth plates *(arrowheads)*. Hyaline cartilage is bright on this imaging sequence. Cartilage defects are seen as low-signal regions.

- Normal cartilage is bright on this sequence (see Fig. 1.66B).
- Downsides: long acquisition time, does not help in assessing other tissues, and displays only cartilage morphology. It is thus less widely used than fast spin-echo

Numerous other pulse sequences have been developed and validated for articular cartilage imaging. Example of more advanced techniques:

- T2 mapping.
  - Articular cartilage damage allows influx of free water, which prolongs T2.
  - Provides quantitative or semiquantitative assessment of cartilage T2 with high resolution.
  - Can detect cartilage degeneration earlier than fast spin-echo sequences.
  - Works best on 3T scanners.
  - Is becoming more available outside of research settings.

Other imaging options: both CT and MR arthrography can depict articular cartilage surface defects with excellent resolution.

Radiographs

- Poor sensitivity.
- The radiolucent cartilage space or joint space narrows with gross cartilage loss.
  - By the time such changes are visible on radiographs, cartilage loss is often extensive.

ARTICULAR CARTILAGE DEFECTS: DIAGNOSIS AT ARTHROSCOPY

- The current gold standard for articular cartilage assessment is arthroscopy.
- At arthroscopy, normal articular cartilage is smooth, firm, and glistening.
- The surgeon searches for visible articular cartilage defects and probes for abnormal cartilage softening.

Chondromalacia (Soft Cartilage)

- The earliest surgically detectable form of cartilage derangement is softness to a metal probe at arthroscopy. The cartilage may be swollen.
- More severe cartilage defects are classified by the defect *size* and *depth*.
- The most severe defects are full thickness with exposed subchondral bone.

Some cartilage defects have specific features that require additional terminology.

- *Fissure*: a crack in the cartilage surface of variable depth.
- *Fibrillation*: partial thickness cartilage loss with an irregular surface likened to crab meat.
- *Delamination*: separation of the cartilage from the subchondral bone.
  - These can be subtle or occult at arthroscopy if overlying superficial cartilage is intact.
  - Has high potential to progress to a full thickness defect.
  - MRI shows fluid signal intensity in deep articular cartilage (Fig. 1.67).
- *Flap tear*: delamination defect that extends to the cartilage surface at one or more sides.
  - The torn cartilage can be partially lifted off the bone.
- *Osteochondral fracture (lesion, defect)*: includes both cartilage and subchondral bone (Fig. 1.68).

Key Concepts

Describing Articular Cartilage Defects

Defect size, grade, location
Other features when applicable: fissure, flap tear, delamination, osteochondral lesion
Underlying subchondral bone: edema, sclerosis, cysts
Associated lesions such as synovitis, meniscal tears

IMAGING OF ARTICULAR CARTILAGE DEFECTS

- Easiest and most successful in the knee.
  - The knee has the thickest cartilage, up to 5 mm thick in the patella.

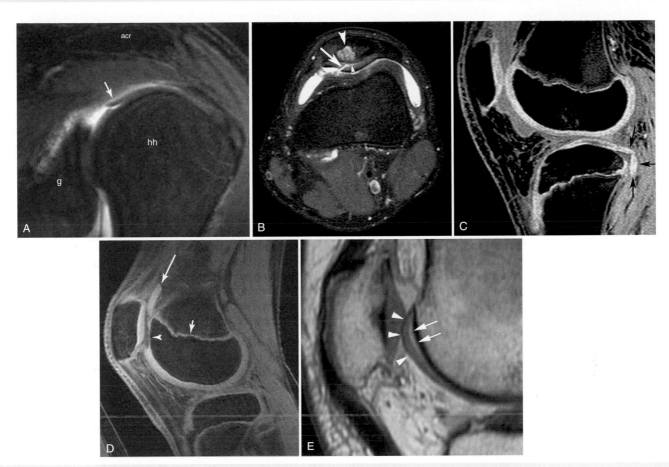

Fig. 1.67 Articular cartilage defects: flap tears and delamination. (A) Small humeral head flap tear. Oblique sagittal fat-suppressed T2-weighted fast spin-echo MR image shows flap tear *(arrow)* outlined by high-signal joint fluid. **(B)** Fissure with flap tear and partial delamination. Axial fat-suppressed fast spin-echo T2-weighted MR image (echo time, 60 msec) of a painful left knee shows an oblique fissure in the medial patellar facet *(arrow)* that extends laterally *(small arrowhead)*. Also note the adjacent patellar subchondral cyst *(large arrowhead)*. **(C)** Delamination of posterior lateral tibial plateau *(arrows)*. Sagittal fat-suppressed spoiled gradient-echo (SPGR) MR image in an adolescent who also sustained an anterior cruciate ligament tear with this injury. **(D)** Displaced full-thickness cartilage fragment. Fat-suppressed three-dimensional SPGR sequence. Recall that cartilage is bright on this sequence. Note the femoral trochlea chondral defect *(arrowhead)* and superiorly displaced fragment *(long arrow)*. Also note that the physis (growth plate) has similar bright signal, a normal finding *(short arrow)*. **(E)** Subtle delamination. Femoral trochlea cartilage *(arrowheads)* is separated from subchondral bone *(dark stripe)* by a thin layer of bright fluid signal *(arrows)*. *acr*, Acromion process; *g*, glenoid; *hh*, humeral head.

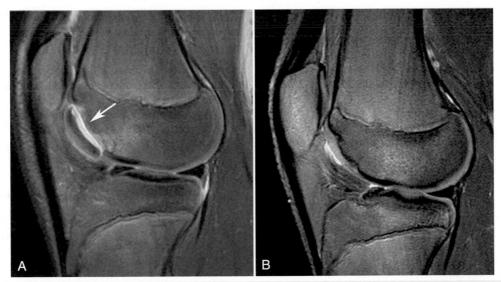

Fig. 1.68. Osteochondral fracture with successful repair. (A) Sagittal fat-suppressed lightly T2-weighted fast spin-echo MR image (echo time, approximately 45 msec) shows a detached lateral femoral trochlea osteochondral lesion *(arrow)*. **(B)** Follow-up MR study performed several months after surgical fragment reattachment shows successful repair, with healing of the bone fragments and smooth articular cartilage contour.

- In contrast, cartilage at the ankle joint, for example, is only about 1.5 mm on each surface and is harder to resolve.

MRI evaluation of focal cartilage defects:

- A cartilage defect may be seen as a region of increased T2 signal intensity or decreased cartilage thickness.
- Experience has shown that a reproducible and reliable MRI classification system of articular cartilage defects benefits from slight modification of the arthroscopic schemes.
- Defect evaluation includes defect signal intensity, depth and size, and signal change in the underlying bone.
- Most commonly used are adaptions of the arthroscopic grading system described by Outerbridge. Of these, the system adopted by the International Cartilage Regeneration and Joint Preservation Society (formerly known as the International Cartilage Repair Society and still goes by ICRS) is probably the most commonly used (Box 1.5 and Fig. 1.69; see also Fig. 1.67).
  - Grade 1 defect:
    - Mild irregularity and/or increased T2 signal of the cartilage surface on MRI images.
    - Most often due to cartilage surface degradation or microscopic disruption of the cartilage matrix deep to the cartilage surface. The damaged cartilage may *imbibe* (literally, 'drink') free water from the joint fluid.
  - Grade 2 defect:
    - Deeper than grade 1 but extends through less than 50% of the cartilage thickness or are localized areas of cartilage edema and swelling.
  - Grade 3 defect:
    - Greater than 50% thickness but not full thickness.
  - Grade 4 defect:
    - Full-thickness defects.
- Variations on the ICRS grading system are common. Examples:
  - Some authors consider any defect associated with a subchondral cyst or edema to be a grade 4 defect, regardless of the apparent depth of the defect on MR images.
  - Some authors simplify the ICRS system by lumping together grades 1 and 2 or grades 2 and 3 into a single grade, with a grade 3 being a full-thickness defect in these systems and grades 1 and 2 being something less.
- Simply describing a defect is another alternative.
  - Sample report: '12 by 7 mm 50% thickness articular cartilage defect posterior weight-bearing lateral femoral condyle. Underlying marrow signal is normal'.

Box 1.5　Magnetic Resonance Imaging Grading of Articular Cartilage Defects

Grade 0: Normal
Grade 1: Superficial edema and/or surface irregularity
Grade 2: Partial-thickness defect less than 50% thickness
Grade 3: Partial-thickness defect greater than 50% thickness
Grade 4: Full-thickness defect

Global joint evaluation systems such as WORMS (*Whole-Organ Magnetic Resonance Imaging Score*) and MOAKS (*MRI Osteoarthritis Knee Score*) combine assessment of articular cartilage loss with other knee pathology such as osteophytes, intraarticular bodies, effusion, and ligament and meniscal tears. These grading systems were developed as research tools to monitor potential effects of nonsurgical osteoarthritis therapies specifically in the knee, but in theory they could be modified to evaluate any joint.

MANAGEMENT OF ARTICULAR CARTILAGE DEFECTS

Articular cartilage is one of the few tissues of the musculoskeletal system that is incapable of regeneration.

The eventual response to articular cartilage injury is osteoarthritis. Osteoarthritis is the most common disability in the Western world and is associated with enormous direct and indirect costs to society, not only from treatment costs but also from economic loss of productivity. Ideal management arrests or reverses articular cartilage loss.

- *Delamination fragments* are sometimes successfully reattached to the subchondral bone. However, they may eventually break away or are resected when diagnosed, resulting in a full-thickness defect.
- An *osteochondral fracture fragment* has a higher likelihood of successful reattachment (see Fig. 1.68), because bone heals to bone much better than cartilage heals to anything.

Microfracture, Drilling, and Related Procedures

- Breaching subchondral bone in a full-thickness articular cartilage defect allows pluripotential cells to enter the exposed subchondral bone surface from underlying marrow.
- This allows for a cytokine-generated repair response that produces fibrocartilage in the defect. Fibrocartilage is inferior to articular (hyaline) cartilage but is better than no cartilage.
- Patients can increase their activity level with less pain.

Osteochondral Autologous Transplantation (OATS, Mosaicplasty, or Autologous Osteochondral Transplantation [AOTS], Fig. 1.70A)

- Cylindrical osteochondral plugs harvested from non–weight-bearing parts of the joint are transplanted to the site of a chondral or osteochondral lesion.
- Allografts made from biomaterials are also available.
- At present, this technique is limited to lesions that are about 2 cm² or less in size, although some surgeons use this approach for larger lesions.

Osteochondral Allograft Transplantation

- Used for large articular cartilage and osteochondral lesions.
- Requires careful matching of donor to recipient contours.
- Cadaver implants have not performed well.
- Grafts with living cells perform better, but availability is limited and these carry some risk of disease transmission.

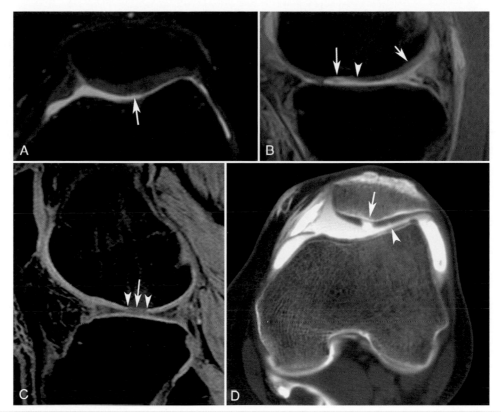

Fig. 1.69. **Articular cartilage defects. (A)** Axial fat-suppressed fast spin-echo T2-weighted MR image (echo time, 42 msec) shows grade 1 or shallow grade 2 defect of the median ridge of the patella *(arrow)*. **(B)** Sagittal fat-suppressed fast spin-echo T2-weighted MR image (echo time, 60 msec) of the knee shows grade 4 *(long arrow)* and grade 2 *(arrowhead)* defects of the lateral femoral condyle. Contrast this with the normal cartilage more posteriorly *(short arrow)*. **(C)** Sagittal fat-suppressed spoiled gradient-echo MR image shows grade 4 defect of the lateral femoral condyle *(arrow)*. The *arrowheads* mark the margins of this sharply marginated cartilage defect. **(D)** Axial computed tomographic arthrogram of the left knee shows grade 4 defect of the medial patellar facet *(arrow)*. Also note small, grade 1 defect of the lateral patellar facet *(arrowhead)*.

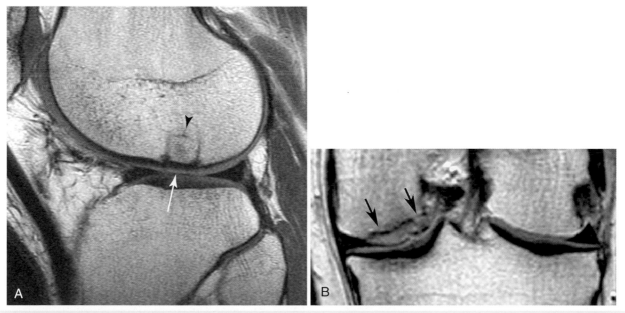

Fig. 1.70. **Cartilage repair techniques. (A)** Autologous osteochondral transplant (OATS). Sagittal proton-density MR image. *Arrowhead* marks the deep margin of the cylindrical bone and cartilage plug that was harvested from the high medial femoral trochlea and placed 6 months previously to repair a high-grade lateral condyle articular cartilage defect. The plug margin is visible as parallel low-signal lines perpendicular to the articular surface. The normal graft cartilage *(arrow)* blends smoothly with adjacent intact cartilage. **(B)** Autologous chondrocyte implantation (ACI). Coronal proton-density fast spin-echo MR image shows successful repair of a medial femoral condyle osteochondral lesion. Note the intermediate–signal-intensity new cartilage *(arrows)* filling the defect. The mildly irregular and raised articular surface is considered to be an acceptable finding.

Autologous Chondrocyte Implantation (ACI)

- Chondrocytes are harvested from the patient and cultivated ex vivo.
- The cultured chondrocytes are implanted into an articular cartilage defect under a protective periosteal flap (see Fig. 1.70B).
- The new cartilage requires months to mature, which requires long protected weight-bearing.
- Two operations required.

Matrix-associated ACI

- As with ACI, chondrocytes are harvested and cultured ex vivo.
- Cultured cells are embedded in a collagen scaffold that is glued into the cartilage defect.
- Two operations required.

ADDITIONAL ARTICULAR CARTILAGE PATHOLOGY

Acute Chondrolysis

- Sudden diffuse uniform loss of articular cartilage.
- Rare.
- May occur after trauma (including slipped capital femoral epiphysis) or arthroscopy.
- Also seen in immobilized patients.
- Most frequently in the hip joint, also the shoulder and elbow.
- Etiology is uncertain. Potential causes:
  - Increased intraarticular pressure and/or high intraarticular concentration of analgesics during arthroscopy.
    - Marcaine and related analgesics are toxic to chondrocytes in vitro.
  - Thermal capsule-tightening procedures used to manage shoulder laxity.
  - Lack of cyclic loading that nourishes cartilage in ambulatory patients might contribute in immobilized patients.
- Main differential diagnosis: infection, which can be identical in uniform, rapid, articular cartilage thinning and joint space narrowing. Large joint effusion suggests infection. Laboratory and clinical evaluation can distinguish.

Chondrocalcinosis

- Calcification of cartilage.
- Can be seen in association with:
  - Hypercalcemia in hyperparathyroidism.
  - Crystal deposition arthropathies, especially *calcium pyrophosphate deposition disease* (CPPD).
  - Hemochromatosis.
  - Various rare inborn errors of metabolism.
  - Older age as a degenerative but otherwise incidental finding.

Nerve Basics

- The peripheral nerves are composed of bundles of nerve fibers termed *fascicles*.

- Some of the major nerves of the extremities are part of a *neurovascular bundle* consisting of a nerve, artery, and vein or veins.

NORMAL NERVE IMAGING

- The myelin within the nerve sheaths has imaging features similar to fat.
  - CT: nerves have lower attenuation than muscle or water.
  - MRI: high signal intensity on T1- and T2-weighted MR images without fat suppression. Nerve signal intensity drops considerably on fat-suppressed or inversion recovery MR images.
  - High-resolution CT, MRI, and US demonstrate the individual fascicles within a peripheral nerve.

PERIPHERAL NERVE INJURY

Peripheral nerves are vulnerable to injury by direct trauma, compression, tension, tumor, autoimmune conditions, infection, radiation, and a variety of neuropathies.

- *Direct trauma* can be caused by an external source such as a knife wound or by a bone fragment following a fracture.
  - Example: the radial nerve of the arm is vulnerable to laceration or displacement by a humeral shaft fracture because it courses along the posterior margin of this bone. Surgeons may choose not to attempt to reduce a humeral midshaft fracture to avoid the risk of injuring this nerve while manipulating the fracture fragments.
- *Peripheral nerve entrapment* refers to a variety of clinical nerve dysfunction syndromes caused by nerve compression in relatively narrow anatomic spaces (Box 1.6; see Fig. 1.71).
  - The most common example is carpal tunnel syndrome, in which the median nerve is compressed within the carpal tunnel by a mass or mass effect—for example, by tendon sheaths enlarged by rheumatoid arthritis (see Chapter 4).
- *Tumors* may affect a nerve by compression or encasement. Some tumors such as a neurofibroma or schwannoma arise within a nerve. Careful attention to the status of nerves near a tumor is an essential part of evaluating surgical options for tumor treatment. Nerve and nerve sheath tumors are discussed in Chapter 12.
- *Neuritis* may be caused by peripheral nerve infection, notably by viral agents, or by immune-mediated inflammation, often following a systemic viral infection.
  - An injured or inflamed nerve may be associated with edema, enhancement, or swelling.
  - '*MR neurography*', using hybrid inversion recovery sequences in 3T scanners, can show nerve edema and swelling better than more conventional techniques on lower field strength magnets.
  - Muscle innervated by an injured motor nerve may show MRI findings of denervation (see Fig. 1.58).
  - Electromyelography is generally superior to imaging studies for assessing nerve injury or dysfunction, but can only be used in superficial nerves.

Box 1.6 Peripheral Nerve Entrapment Syndromes

Median nerve

Wrist: Carpal tunnel syndrome
  Causes: Congenitally narrow tunnel, overuse, synovitis (e.g., rheumatoid arthritis), mass, hypothyroidism, fracture, idiopathic
Proximal forearm: Pronator syndrome
  Cause: Compression within pronator teres
Distal arm: Ligament of Struthers
  Cause: Anatomic variant, avian spur

Radial nerve

Proximal forearm: Posterior interosseous nerve syndrome
  Cause: Compression of deep branch within the supinator muscle
Midarm: Compression or injury by humerus shaft fracture
Axilla: Sleep palsy
  Cause: Compression while sleeping on side

Ulnar nerve

Elbow: Cubital tunnel syndrome
  Cause: Nerve subluxation, mass, trauma, inflammation
Wrist: Guyon canal syndrome
  Cause: Mass, trauma, inflammation

Axillary nerve

Quadrilateral space syndrome
  Cause: Fibrotic bands, mass

Suprascapular nerve

Suprascapular notch syndrome
  Cause: Mass or inflammation in spinoglenoid or suprascapular notch

Posterior tibial nerve

Tarsal tunnel syndrome
  Cause: Nerve subluxation, mass, trauma, inflammation

Sciatic nerve

Piriformis syndrome

Lateral femoral cutaneous nerve

"Meralgia paresthetica"
  Cause: Compression as nerve courses over inguinal ligament adjacent to anterior superior iliac spine

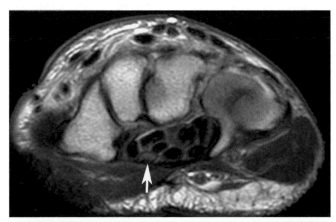

Fig. 1.71 Normal nerve. Axial T2-weighted fast spin-echo MR image obtained through the wrist shows the intermediate–signal-intensity median nerve *(arrow)* in the carpal tunnel. Contrast with the low signal of the carpal tunnel tendons.

Foreign Body Imaging

- The term *foreign body* includes both surgical implants and unwanted objects, such as metal or wood splinters that are usually introduced by direct penetration.
- Sufficiently radiodense foreign bodies including most glass fragments may be detected with radiographs (Fig. 1.72).
  - A skin marker at the penetration site is useful for localization.
- US is helpful for localization of superficial foreign bodies (Fig. 1.73).
- The MRI appearance of foreign bodies varies widely depending on their composition.
  - Microscopic metallic fragments are common after arthroscopy and can be numerous if a drill or burr

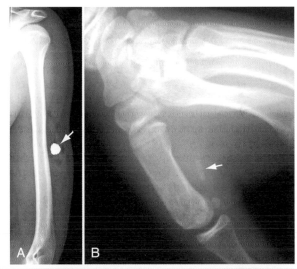

Fig. 1.72 Foreign bodies seen at radiography. (A) Bullet in soft tissues of the arm. **(B)** Smaller and less-dense foreign bodies can be subtle on radiographs. Oblique hand radiograph shows a linear foreign body in the soft tissues medial to the thumb *(arrow)*. This was the graphite core of a pencil. Foreign bodies with density similar to surrounding tissues such as most wood fragments can be invisible on radiographs.

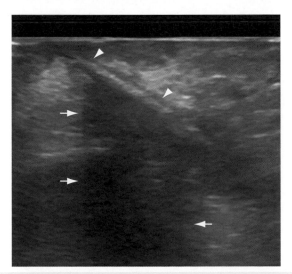

Fig. 1.73 Foreign body seen at US. Image of the calf shows an echogenic wood splinter *(arrowheads)*. Note the posterior acoustic shadowing *(arrows)*.

Box 1.7   Magnetic Resonance Imaging Techniques to Minimize Metal Artifact

Do

Increase receiver bandwidth.
Use fast spin-echo rather than conventional spin-echo.
Increase matrix.
Orient frequency encoding direction parallel to long axis of the metal object.
Use low field strength magnet.

Do not

Use gradient echo.
Use chemical fat suppression.

Note: The amount of metal artifact is greatly influenced by the type of metal alloy. Cobalt chromium steel alloys tend to cause much greater metal artifact than titanium and zirconium oxide alloys.

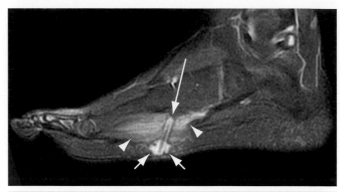

Fig. 1.75 Radiographically occult foreign body seen at MRI. Sagittal T2-weighted spin-echo MR image of the foot demonstrates a long, thin low-signal foreign body *(long arrow)* with adjacent soft tissue edema *(arrowheads)* and a small fluid collection around the plantar end of the foreign body *(short arrows)*. The foreign body proved to be a wood fragment.

was used. These fragments are too small to be seen with radiography or CT. However, they cause susceptibility artifact and local field inhomogeneities that can be conspicuous on MR images, especially on gradient-echo images where they are seen as small areas of low signal intensity. This artifact can be minimized by using fast spin-echo sequences and other techniques (Box 1.7).

- Wood splinters are often simply invisible on MR images. When visible, they usually have low signal intensity on all sequences.
- Foreign bodies may develop a surrounding rim of granulation, sterile fluid, or pus with high T2 signal intensity that greatly increases lesion conspicuity on MRI (Figs. 1.74 and 1.75; see also Fig. 1.75).

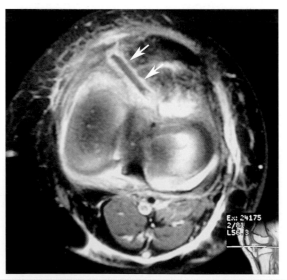

Fig. 1.74 Radiographically occult foreign body seen at MRI. Axial T2-weighted MR image of the knee in a child who sustained an anterior left knee puncture wound by a tree branch 2 weeks previously shows a linear low–signal-intensity splinter with surrounding high–signal-intensity granulation tissue *(arrows)* at the level of the knee joint (note the localizer image at the *lower right corner* of the image). MRI is insensitive to small nonmetallic foreign bodies. However, reaction to the foreign body may include edema and granulation that can be detected with MRI.

Part 3: Special Considerations in Imaging of Musculoskeletal Injury in Children

Children's bones are biomechanically different than adult bones

1. Children's bones are 'softer' (have greater plasticity), especially in younger children, and can permanently deform without fracturing into separate fragments. This plasticity decreases with age. Analogy: bones are like a bagel. Newborn bones are like a fresh bagel, soft and easily bent with only minimal disruption of the outer 'cortex'. As a child grows, the bones become progressively stronger and stiffer—like a bagel that has been left out on the kitchen counter for a few days. The analogous bagel is stiffer yet can still be bent, but with multiple cracks and circumferential disruption of the outer cortex. Adult bones are like a bagel that has been left out on the kitchen counter for weeks. The bagel is strong enough to support a stack of cookbooks, but it cannot bend, at least not perceptibly. If enough bending force is applied, the bagel, like an adult bone, will break into separate fragments rather than permanently bend. (Appreciation to the late pediatric radiologist Robert Wilkinson for this analogy.)
2. The *physis* (growth plate) is weaker than adjacent bone when exposed to shear or tension, so fractures often involve the physis.
3. Fractures in the immature skeleton have much greater potential for remodeling during later growth (see Fig. 1.32). Remodeling potential toward anatomic after a fracture depends upon:
   - The age of the child (younger is better, with more time to remodel toward normal during further growth).
   - Location (metaphyseal is best, best blood supply).
   - When present, the orientation of any angular deformity.
     - Angular deformity in the plane of motion of adjacent joints remodels better than angular deformity perpendicular to the plane of motion of adjacent joints.

■ Example: a tibial shaft fracture with angular deformity in the coronal plane (valgus or varus) tends to remodel less than a fracture with angular deformity in the sagittal plane (apex anterior or posterior). This is unfortunate, because the knee and ankle can partially compensate for angular deformity in the sagittal plane but not in the coronal plane.

4. The periosteum of children's bones is loosely attached to the underlying bone except at the physis, where it is very tightly attached. This allows blood, pus, or tumor to accumulate between the periosteum and metaphyseal and/or diaphyseal cortex without extension into adjacent soft tissues.

   ■ *Periosteal reaction (periostitis, periosteal new bone formation)*: New bone formed by periosteum displaced away from the cortex by tumor, hematoma, or pus. If the process elevates the periosteum then stops, early new bone that is created by the displaced periosteum may be seen on radiographs initially as a thin line or arc of calcification roughly parallel to the shaft (Fig. 1.76, see also Fig. 1.32). In contrast, sustained periosteal displacement, for example due to an enlarging tumor, results in different patterns that provide important clues to the nature of the underlying process. This is discussed further in Chapter 11.

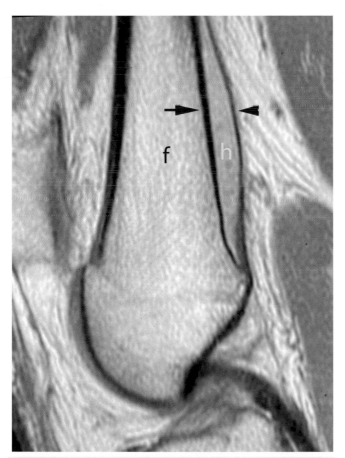

Fig. 1.76 Periosteal elevation by a traumatic hematoma. Sagittal PD-weighted MR image of the distal femur *(f)* in an adolescent shows a hematoma *(h)* between the posterior femoral cortex *(arrow)* and the elevated periosteum *(arrowhead)*.

Long Bone Growth and Remodeling

Longitudinal bone growth occurs at the physis.

THE PHYSIS IN GREATER DETAIL

■ Also termed *growth plate, primary physis, epiphyseal growth plate*.
■ Specialized site of enchondral ossification that allows long bone longitudinal growth (Fig. 1.77).
■ The physis functions as a rolling assembly line that pushes the epiphysis away from the ossified metaphysis and diaphysis as it manufactures new bone in a multistep process.

A Summary of the Process

1. Chondrocytes are located along the epiphyseal margin of the physis (the *resting zone*).
2. These chondrocytes proliferate and produce a cartilage template.
3. This template becomes calcified (*zone of provisional calcification*, visible on radiographs and is a marker for some disease processes).
4. The chondrocytes die and the calcified cartilage is subsequently invaded by osteocytes. An intact metaphyseal blood supply is essential for this step.
5. The osteocytes convert the calcified cartilage to bone at the metaphyseal side of the physis.
   ■ The new bone deposited along the metaphyseal side of the physis is immature (woven) bone, and undergoes extensive remodeling to become cortex and trabeculae of mature lamellar bone
   ■ New cartilage is produced along the epiphyseal side of the physis at the same rate that it is converted to bone along the metaphyseal side. This equilibrium results in uniform width of the healthy physis throughout growth.

SECONDARY PHYSIS

Allows growth in the *secondary growth centers* (epiphyses and *epiphyseal equivalents*, i.e., apophyses and the small bones of the wrist and foot).
■ Histologically similar to the primary physis.
■ Not a linear plate like the primary physis, rather a thin circumferential shell around the ossified center of an epiphysis or epiphyseal equivalent.
■ Creates radial rather than linear growth.
■ Most do not appear until after birth.
■ Not visible on radiographs but can be seen on high resolution T2-weighted MRI as a thin band of brighter signal around the ossified portion of the epiphysis.

LONGITUDINAL GROWTH RATE

■ Depends on circulating hormones, notably growth hormone, and poorly understood local factors that maintain proportional skeletal growth.
■ Fastest longitudinal growth in the appendicular skeleton occurs at the distal femur, where new bone is formed at up to 1–1.5 cm per year.

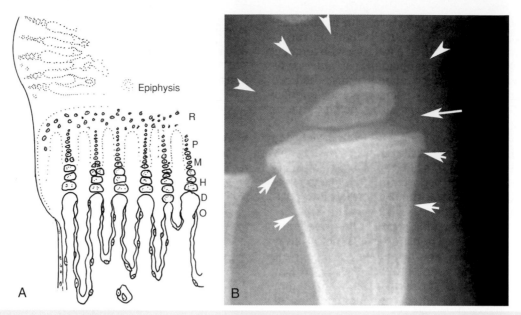

Fig. 1.77 The physis. (A) Diagram shows the histologic organization of the physis. The resting zone *(R)* adjacent to the epiphysis contains small clusters of cartilage cells. The proliferation zone *(P)* contains dividing and enlarging cartilage cells organized into longitudinal columns. Cell division ceases in the maturation zone *(M)*, but the cartilage cells continue to enlarge. The cells greatly enlarge in the hypertrophic zone *(H)*, and the surrounding cartilage becomes calcified (termed *provisional calcification* because it is not yet bone). The cartilage cells degenerate and die in the cartilage degeneration zone *(D)* and are replaced by osteoblasts. In the osteogenic zone *(O)* the osteoblasts begin the process of conversion of the calcified cartilage into bone. This zone marks the transition from the physis to the metaphysis. The term *bone bark* is sometimes used to describe the lateral margin of the physis, which occasionally calcifies and is seen on radiographs as a small spicule of bone extending distally from the metaphysis. **(B)** Radiograph of a child's distal radius shows the corresponding radiographic anatomy. The *long arrow* marks the physis. The convex contour of the metaphysis *(short arrows)* is the result of bone remodeling by osteoclasts and osteoblasts. If osteoclast activity is diminished, then this concave contour is not produced (undertubulation; see text and Fig. 1-79). The *arrowheads* mark the true margins of the epiphysis, which is composed mostly of cartilage in this young child.

CESSATION OF LONG BONE LENGTHENING

The chondrocytes in the resting zone of the physis stop dividing. Consequently, no new cartilage is formed and longitudinal growth ceases. The remaining cartilage is converted to bone as the physis closes.

- A dense transverse line on radiographs, sometimes termed a *physeal scar*, marks the final position of the physis.
  - This line may persist into adulthood but is eventually removed by normal adult bone remodeling.

The timing of physeal closure varies at different sites.

- Most bones stop lengthening by about age 14 in girls and 16 in boys.
- The medial clavicle physes are among the last to close, typically in the third decade, years after adult stature has been achieved.

Growth Arrest Lines

- Also termed *growth recovery lines, Park lines, Harris lines, or stress lines*
- Thin transverse sclerotic line across the metaphysis parallel to the physis.
  - Uniform, sharply defined, straight.
  - Does not abut the physis.
- Associated with periods of childhood stress such as illness, injury, or immobilization. Formed during the recovery phase after such episodes.
- Like the rings of a tree, the physis grows away from the line over time.

- Typically are single, but in the setting of repeated insults can be multiple (Fig. 1.78).
- Often persist into adulthood but are eventually removed by routine bone remodeling.

In contrast, *transverse metaphyseal bands* are broader, less well-defined, and abut the physis.

- *Sclerotic* transverse metaphyseal bands can be seen as a normal finding when found only in weight-bearing bones, or as an abnormal finding when found in all bones as a consequence of heavy-metal poisoning (see Fig. 13.53).
- *Lucent* transverse metaphyseal bands can occur in rickets, leukemia, and metastatic neuroblastoma.

LONG BONE LATERAL GROWTH AND REMODELING

- The periosteum produces bone that allows a bone to increase in diameter.
- *Tubulation*: As the bone lengthens, metaphyses are converted into a tube-like diaphyses.
  - Tubulation is mediated by coordinated function of osteoclasts and osteoblasts.
  - Disorders of tubulation may result in a wide metaphysis (*undertubulation, Erlenmeyer flask deformity*; Fig. 1.79 and Box 1.8; see Fig. 15.80), or a narrow, tubular metaphysis (*overtubulation*; Fig. 1.80 and Box 1.9).
  - For example, the diminished osteoclastic activity associated with osteopetrosis and marrow packing in storage diseases result in undertubulation.

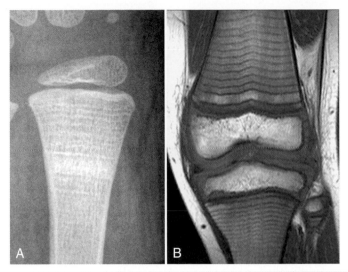

Fig. 1.78 Growth arrest lines (Park lines, Harris lines). (A) AP radiograph of the distal radius in a 5-year-old shows multiple thin, sharp lines parallel to the physis. **(B)** Coronal T1-weighted MR image of the knee in a different patient shows similar findings, although extraordinarily prominent. This child has osteogenesis imperfecta that has been treated with periodic bisphosphonate injections. The growth recovery lines are formed by impaired osteoclast function during therapy. The growth recovery lines are more widely spaced in the femurs than in the tibias because the femurs grow more rapidly.

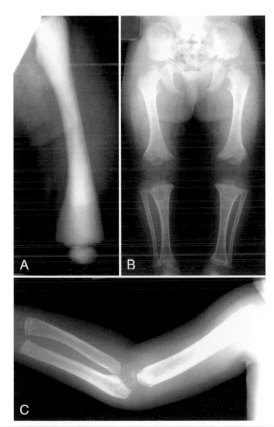

Fig. 1.79 Undertubulation. (A) Osteopetrosis. Failure of osteoclast function results in wide metaphyses. **(B)** Achondroplasia. Note the short, squat bones with wide metaphyses. **(C)** Hurler syndrome (mucopolysaccharidosis 1H). The marrow is packed with abnormal metabolites, causing expansion of the diaphyses and metaphyses. See also Fig. 15.80. (**B** courtesy of Stephanie Spottswood, MD.)

Box 1.8 Common Causes of Undertubulation

Bones of normal length
  Rickets
  Osteopetrosis
  Fibrous dysplasia
  Multiple osteochondromas
Short, often squat bones
  Dwarfism (numerous types, achondroplasia most common)
  Storage diseases
  Multiple osteochondromas

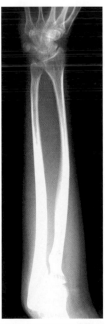

Fig. 1.80 Overtubulation. Note the short transition from epiphysis to diaphysis in the forearm of this child with osteogenesis imperfecta. Also note the long, narrow diaphyses. This overall appearance is often described as 'gracile bones' and is most commonly seen in neuromuscular conditions with chronic absence of weight-bearing, such as cerebral palsy.

■ Overtubulation is seen most commonly in neuromuscular conditions with absent or diminished weight-bearing, such as cerebral palsy.

Neuromuscular conditions (e.g., cerebral palsy, myelomeningocele)
Osteogenesis imperfecta
Juvenile idiopathic arthritis
Marfan syndrome
Homocystinuria
Arthrogryposis

Key Concepts

Tubulation

Process of remodeling the shaft of a long bone into a normal configuration.
Overtubulation: cylindrical portion of the shaft is too long, with short and narrowed metaphysis (e.g., absent weight-bearing, neuromuscular conditions).
Undertubulation: cylindrical portion of the shaft is too short, with wide and long metaphysis (e.g., osteopetrosis, Gaucher disease).

Physeal Fractures

The physis is weaker than adjacent bone in resistance to shearing and torsional forces, but it is not weaker in resistance to compression. Fractures that cross or extend along a physis account for 15% of all pediatric fractures. The percentage is not higher because most pediatric fractures are caused by compression resulting from a fall.

SALTER–HARRIS SYSTEM OF FRACTURES INVOLVING THE PHYSIS (FIG. 1.81)

Salter–Harris I

- Involve only the physis, with displacement of the epiphysis relative to the metaphysis.
- Displacement may be minimal or imperceptible on radiographs. Comparison with the contralateral side and/or follow-up radiographs may make the diagnosis.
- MRI usually is definitive when needed.

Salter–Harris II

- Extend through a portion of the physis and a portion of the metaphysis.
- This is the most frequent pattern, 85% of physeal fractures.

Salter–Harris III

- Involve the physis and epiphysis. Thus, these are intraarticular fractures.

Salter–Harris IV

- Extend through the epiphysis, physis, and metaphysis.

Salter–Harris V

- Compression injury of the physis, which may be missed or resemble a Salter–Harris I fracture at initial diagnosis.
- Rare.

Some authors extend the Salter–Harris system with a variety of pure metaphyseal and epiphyseal fractures that do not extend into the physis. These additional Salter–Harris categories are not widely used.

IMAGING DIAGNOSIS OF FRACTURES INVOLVING THE PHYSIS

Radiography
- First-line test.

CT
- Mainly used for preoperative planning in some fractures in adolescents.

MRI
- Highly sensitive.
- Can show fractures in unossified epiphyseal cartilage.
- Requires sedation in younger children.

US
- Can show fractures in unossified epiphyseal cartilage.
- Can show cortical disruption and periosteal elevation by hematoma.

Bone Scan
- Hampered by normal intense tracer uptake at the physes. Pinhole imaging and careful comparison with the

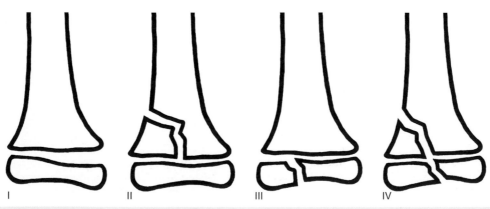

Fig. 1.81 Salter–Harris classification system of pediatric fractures that involve the physis. Salter–Harris V is a crush injury of the physis.

contralateral side improve the accuracy of bone scintigraphy, but this modality is inferior to MRI and US, and uses ionizing radiation.

PHYSEAL INJURY COMPLICATIONS

Direct trauma to the physis can result in osseous healing across the physis (*bone bridge* or *bone bar*) or injury to the chondrocytes that are needed to produce the cartilage model. Either complication can cause growth arrest or growth deformity (Figs. 1.82 to 1.85).

Bone Bridge Across the Physis (Bone Bar)

- Bone that crosses the physis and connects the epiphysis to the metaphysis.
- Can be large or small.
  - Large: growth arrest.
  - Small: the bridge tethers only a portion of the physis, resulting in a cup like or angular deformity.

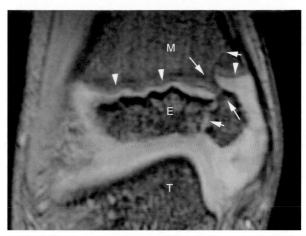

Fig. 1.83 Physeal bar and deformity after distal tibial physeal injury. Coronal fat-suppressed spoiled gradient-echo MR image shows the bony bridge *(long arrows)*, old Salter–Harris IV fracture line *(short arrows)*, and the physis *(arrowheads)*. Note the angular deformity between the talar dome (T) and distal tibial epiphysis (E). M, metaphysis.

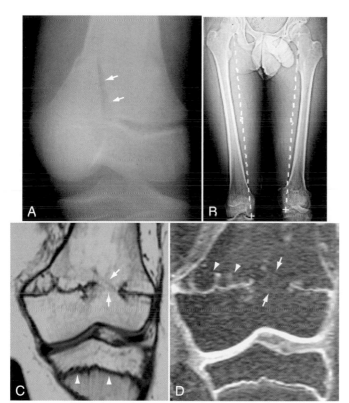

Fig. 1.82 Growth plate arrest after distal femur physeal fracture. (A) Frontal radiograph obtained at the time of injury shows Salter–Harris II fracture of the distal left femur *(arrows)*. **(B)** CT scanogram obtained 3 years later demonstrates shortening of left femur, the site of previous fracture. *Dashed lines* of each femur indicate the degree of left-sided shortening. **(C)** Coronal T1-weighted MR image shows substantial irregularity of distal femoral physis and focal absence of growth plate *(arrows)*. Note smooth contour of proximal tibial physis *(arrowheads)*. **(D)** Coronal fat-suppressed three-dimensional spoiled gradient-echo MR image (repetition time, 60 msec; echo time, 5 msec; flip angle, 40 degrees) shows cartilaginous irregularities of medial aspect of distal femoral physis *(arrowheads)* and focal absence of growth plate cartilage *(arrows)*. Note smooth contour of proximal tibial physis. (**D** adapted and reproduced, with permission, from Disler DG. Fat-suppressed three-dimensional spoiled gradient-recalled MR imaging: assessment of articular and physeal hyaline cartilage. *AJR.* 1997;169:1117-1123.)

Main risk factors for development of a bone bridge:

- Vertical fracture.
  - Longitudinally oriented Salter–Harris IV fracture.
  - Just a few millimeter displacement along the fracture can allow a metaphyseal fragment to abut and heal directly to an epiphyseal fragment.
- Physis with a normally undulating contour.
  - The distal tibia and femur are the most common sites of growth arrest.
  - The physes at these sites have an undulating contour, which allows slight fracture displacement to appose metaphyseal and epiphyseal bone.

Imaging a Suspected Bone Bridge

Radiographs

- Obvious bone bridge across the physis and growth arrest or deformity are later findings.
- Earlier detection: observe any *growth recovery lines* (defined earlier).
  - The growth recovery line initiated by the fracture should uniformly separate from the physis on subsequent radiographs.
  - If focal physeal tethering is present, the growth recovery line may merge with the bone bridge (Fig. 1.85).
- A bone bridge in the center of the physis will cause growth arrest without an angular deformity but may cause a ball-in-cup appearance.
- A more peripheral bone bridge results in angular deformity as the uninjured portion of the physis continues to grow (see Fig. 1.85).

MRI

- Can confirm or exclude a bone bridge earlier and better than radiographs.
- Mature bone bridge:
  - Continuous marrow fat signal across the physis on T1w.
  - Pathognomonic but not always present.

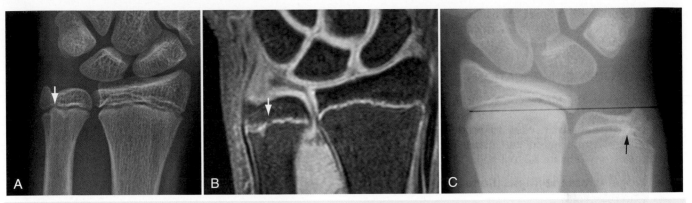

Fig. 1.84 Ulnar physeal bar. (A) Radiograph shows subtle narrowing of the ulnar growth plate, suspicious for a bony bar. **(B)** Coronal fat-suppressed spoiled gradient-echo MR image 4 weeks later confirms interruption of the bright growth plate by a small bar. This lesion was treated promptly with no resulting growth disturbance. **(C)** Similar lesion identified later, in a different patient. Note ulnar shortening without other deformity, due to a bony bridge *(arrow)*.

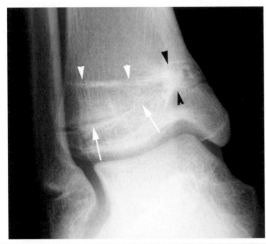

Fig. 1.85 Growth deformity after a distal tibial physeal injury. This AP view was obtained several months after a distal tibia fracture that healed with casting. Note the osseous healing across the medial physis, forming a continuous bony bridge between the metaphysis and epiphysis *(black arrowheads)*. Also note the growth recovery line in the distal tibial metaphysis, which was formed as a result of the fracture *(white arrowheads)*. Since the fracture, there has been normal growth laterally but absent growth medially due to physeal tethering by the bony bridge. As a result, the growth recovery line is seen to merge with the physis *(white arrows)* at the bony bridge.

- Earlier detection:
  - Fat-suppressed 3D SPGR (FLASH), the same sequence used for articular cartilage imaging.
    - Both articular and physeal cartilage are bright on this sequence.
    - A bone bridge is seen as an interruption of the bright signal of the normal physis (Figs. 1.82 and 1.83).
    - Allows precise localization of the bridge (Figs. 1.82 and 1.83). (For an excellent discussion of MRI for preoperative planning of growth plate injuries, see Ecklund and Jaramillo, 2002.).

Management of a Bone Bridge

- Goal is to prevent the development of deformity.
- If the bone bridge involves less than 50% of the physis, physeal growth may be salvaged by resection of the bridge with a drill, using an oblique approach through the metaphysis.
  - Preoperative MRI with fat-suppressed 3D SPGR allows precise localization of the bridge (Figs. 1.82 and 1.83).
  - This procedure is reserved for younger children with more growth potential.
- *Epiphysiodesis*
  - Fusion of the physis to arrest all growth, to prevent the development of angulation.
  - Can result in a leg length discrepancy.
  - Contralateral epiphysiodesis can keep the extremities of equal or at least length.
  - Alternatively, a bone lengthening procedure can be performed on the injured bone.
  - This is discussed further in Chapter 15.

OTHER CAUSES OF GROWTH ARREST

Injury to the chondrocytes that produce the cartilage model:

- Direct trauma (Salter V fracture), thermal injury (osteoid osteoma or osteoblastoma thermal ablation).
- Injury to the epiphyseal blood supply to the chondrocytes.
  - Trauma.
  - Focal infection.
  - Disseminated intravascular coagulation (DIC), as may result from *meningococcemia* (Fig. 1.86).
    - Limb amputation is a common sequela of meningococcemia but if a child survives with the limbs intact, growth deformities may become apparent over subsequent months.
    - The growth arrest in DIC often begins at the central portion of each physis, probably because of greater vulnerability of the blood supply, resulting in a cupped shape of the physes.
- Intact metaphyseal blood supply to the physis is essential to converting the cartilage model into bone.
  - Damage to metaphyseal blood supply by trauma, infection, or other insult can result in focal or generalized widening of the physis, because the newly

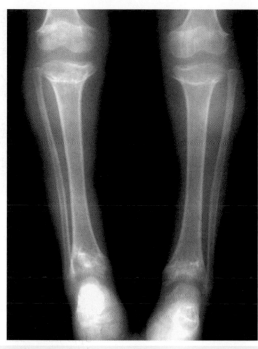

Fig. 1.86 Growth arrest after meningococcemia. Radiograph shows irregular, premature fusion of all physes.

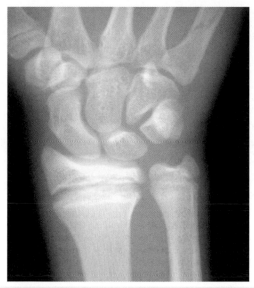

Fig. 1.87 Chronic Salter–Harris I injury of the distal radius in a young female gymnast. Note the sclerosis and irregularity around the physis.

produced cartilage cannot be transformed into bone. Growth disturbance and deformity may result.

PHYSEAL STRESS INJURY

- Can be considered a chronic Salter–Harris I injury.
- Radiographs: widening and irregularity of the growth plate.
- MRI: widening and irregularity of the growth plate and adjacent marrow edema, especially in the metaphysis.
- Overuse injuries in high-performance child and adolescent athletes.
  - Gymnasts: distal radius and ulna (Fig. 1.87).
  - Baseball pitchers: proximal humerus, humeral medial epicondyle.
  - Runners: lower extremities.
- These injuries usually resolve with conservative therapy.

GROWTH CARTILAGE

- Unossified epiphyseal (and apophyseal) cartilage in younger children located between the superficial articular cartilage and the ossified central portion of the epiphysis (the *ossific nucleus*).
- Mainly fibrocartilage.
- MRI of growth cartilage.
  - Lower signal intensity on T2-weighted MR images than articular cartilage.
  - Highly vascular and enhances following gadolinium administration.
  - Absent enhancement is a sign of injury or infection.
- Fractures that involve unossified growth cartilage can be invisible on radiographs.
- Detection of a fracture through unossified cartilage requires MRI, US, or intraoperative arthrography (for intraarticular fractures).

Key Concepts

Osteochondritis dissecans (OCD)

Distinctive form of osteochondral injury of older children and adolescents
Subchondral stress injury
May heal with or without deformity or result in a fragment that is loose in situ or displaced into the joint

Osteochondritis Dissecans

- OCD overlaps with but is not exactly the same as *osteochondral* lesion or OCL.
- Distinctive type of osteochondral injury that occurs in older children and teenagers.
- Likely cause is chronic/repetitive shear stress injury, and specifically injury to the secondary physis, with subsequent disturbed enchondral ossification. Advanced cases result in fragmentation and involve the overlying articular cartilage.
- Becoming more prevalent in younger children due to increased participation in high-level sports at a younger age.
- Present with joint pain of months or longer duration.
- More advanced cases present with joint pain, swelling, clicking, and locking.
- The knee is by far the most common site for OCD, especially at the lateral aspect of the medial femoral condyle.
  - Mnemonic: LAME, for **l**ateral **a**spect of the **m**edial femoral (**e**pi)condyle (Fig. 1.88)
  - Other sites are listed in Box 1.10

The disease process and imaging findings in OCD are mostly similar at all sites, but most literature is focused on the knee.
OCD is a process:

- Begins as a subchondral injury with intact overlying articular cartilage.
  - MRI may initially show only edema in unossified subchondral cartilage, which is nonspecific because

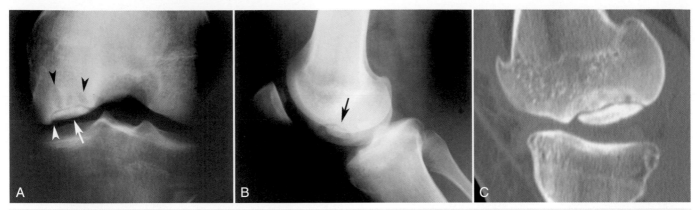

Fig. 1.88 Osteochondritis dissecans (OCD), knee. (A and B) Classic radiographic appearance. AP **(A)** and lateral **(B)** radiographs demonstrate typical location of osteochondritis dissecans along lateral aspect of the medial femoral condyle. Note osteochondral fragment *(arrows)* and linear lucency separating fragment from underlying bone. Note also adjacent cystlike bone lucencies *(black arrowheads* in **A)**, which suggest instability of bone fragments. Incongruence of osteochondral fragment and underlying bone *(white arrowhead* in **A)** also suggests instability of fragment. **(C)** Sagittal CT reformat in a different patient shows similar findings: sclerotic OCD fragment separated from the host femur by soft tissue attenuation that could be fluid, granulation tissue, or fibrous or cartilaginous connective tissue.

Box 1.10   Osteochondritis Dissecans: Sites

Knee (most common site):
    Lateral aspect of medial femoral condyle (mnemonic: LAME)
    Less common: patella, any surface of the femoral condyles
Elbow: Distal capitellum
Shoulder: Humeral head
Ankle: Talar dome, most often medial

---

edema can be seen as a benign transient finding (see Fig. 1.89).

- If the normal thin high T2-signal signature of the secondary physis is no longer visible at the adjacent chondro-osseous junction, secondary physeal injury may be present. This is associated with risk for progression.
- If the process continues in younger children:
  - Fragmentation of unossified growth cartilage and/or epiphyseal bone.

- Eventual extension into overlying articular cartilage, creating fragments.
- Fragment displacement.
- If the process continues in older children, classic OCD findings develop:
  - Thickening of unossified cartilage due to the secondary physis injury.
  - Epiphyseal trabecular microfractures develop and may coalesce into a subchondral fracture line that is roughly parallel to the subchondral cortex (see Figs. 1.90 to 1.92).
  - The fracture can focally extend to the joint surface (see Figs. 1.91 and 1.92).
  - This may progress to a complete separation of the osteochondral fragment. The fragment may remain in place ('loose in situ' *or 'in situ loose'*) (Figs. 1.92 to 1.95), or may displace into the joint (Fig. 1.96).

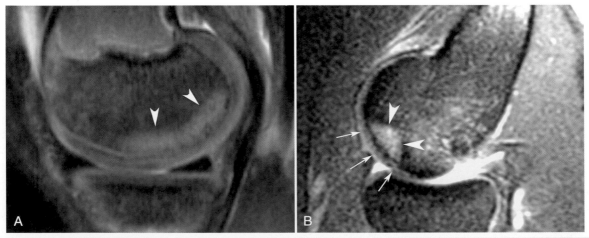

Fig. 1.89 Early osteochondritis dissecans (OCD). (A) Very early OCD. Sagittal fat-suppressed T2-weighted MR image shows subchondral marrow edema in the medial femoral condyle *(arrowheads)*. This edema is not specific and may resolve. In this child, painful subchondral fragmentation typical of OCD subsequently developed. **(B)** Early OCD of the humeral capitellum (Panner disease). Sagittal fat-suppressed T1-weighted MR image obtained after administration of intravenous contrast medium and elbow exercise shows enhancement of the OCD lesion *(arrowheads)*, which indicates an intact blood supply and thus a good potential for resolution without further progression. Note the intact overlying cartilage *(small arrows)*. This image also illustrates the technique of indirect arthrography, which delivers gadolinium to the joint via diffusion through the synovium.

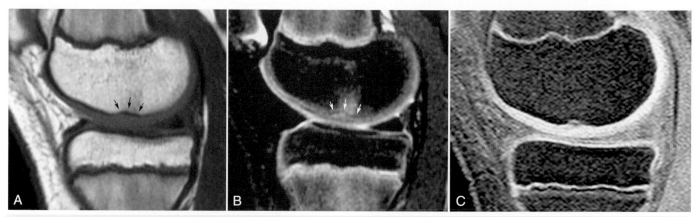

Fig. 1.90 **Early osteochondritis dissecans with intact overlying articular cartilage.** Sagittal T1-weighted **(A)**, fat-suppressed T2-weighted **(B)**, and sagittal fat-suppressed spoiled gradient-echo MR images **(C)** show subchondral irregular low-signal line *(small arrows)* with adjacent marrow edema. Note intact overlying articular cartilage, best seen in **C**, with normal signal intensity. This could be a subchondral impaction fracture along with early osteochondritis dissecans.

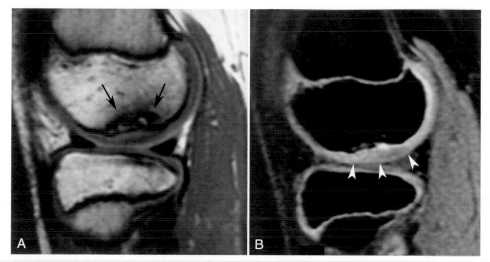

Fig. 1.91 **Osteochondritis dissecans with intact overlying articular cartilage. (A and B)** Sagittal T1-weighted **(A)** and fat-suppressed spoiled gradient-echo **(B)** MR images show the osteochondral fracture lines *(arrows* in **A)**. The overlying articular cartilage is intact *(arrowheads* in **B)**.

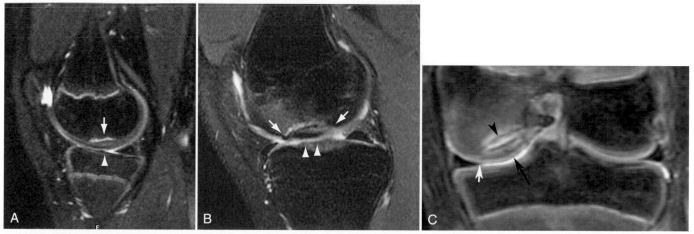

Fig. 1.92 **Osteochondritis dissecans (OCD) progression over time to loose in situ fragment. (A)** Sagittal fat-suppressed T2-weighted MR image shows incomplete transverse fracture in subchondral trabecular bone *(arrow)* with completely intact overlying articular cartilage *(arrowhead)*. **(B)** Same patient 7 years later, now a young adult. The OCD lesion has progressed to a loose in situ fragment. Edema completely separates the host bone from the OCD fragment, including through articular cartilage at the lesion margins *(arrows)*. Also note edema in degenerating fragment cartilage *(arrowheads)*. **(C)** Coronal fat-suppressed proton-density MR image of the left knee in a different child shows medial femoral condyle OCD fragment *(long arrow)* and high T2 signal between the fragment and the host femur *(arrowhead)*, indicating that the fragment is loose, despite intact medial articular cartilage *(short white arrow)*.

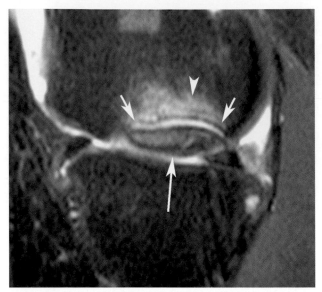

Fig. 1.93 Osteochondritis dissecans (OCD) with loose in situ fragment. Sagittal fat-suppressed T2-weighted MR image shows medial femoral condyle OCD fragment *(long arrow)* with uniform high signal intensity consistent with fluid *(short arrows)* surrounding the fragment. Also note the intense marrow edema in the adjacent femur *(arrowhead)*. Same patient as shown in Fig. 1.88C.

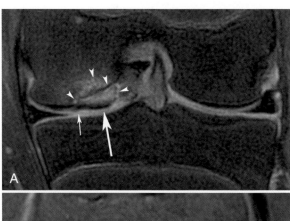

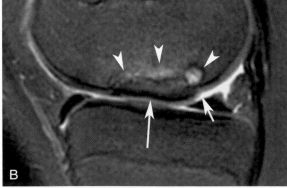

Fig. 1.94 Osteochondritis dissecans (OCD) with loose in situ fragment. MRI findings in a loose fragment are not always as unambiguous as seen in Fig. 1.93. Coronal fat-suppressed proton-density **(A)** and sagittal fat-suppressed T2-weighted **(B)** MR images of the left knee show medial femoral condyle OCD fragment *(large arrow)*, with surrounding high signal, small cystlike lesions, and marrow edema at the margin of the fragment and the host bone *(arrowheads)*. Also note the small articular step-off posteriorly *(short arrows)*. These findings are highly suggestive of a loose fragment, but a fragment that is healing in place could have a similar appearance. Arthroscopy was needed to confirm that this fragment was loose in situ.

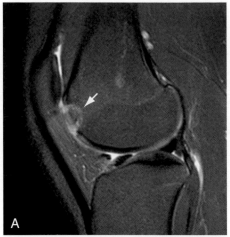

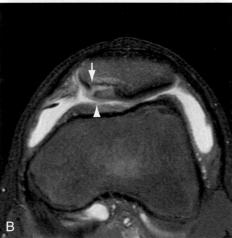

Fig. 1.95 Patellofemoral osteochondritis dissecans (OCD). (A) Sagittal fat-suppressed T2-weighted MR image shows lateral femoral trochlea OCD lesion *(arrow)*. **(B)** Axial T2-weighted spin-echo MR image obtained after intraarticular saline injection in a different patient shows partially displaced patellar OCD fragment *(arrowhead)*. Note that the intermediate signal material between the fragment and the host patella *(arrow)* has lower signal than the joint fluid. This tissue may be granulation, fibrous tissue, cartilage, or a combination. Joint fluid does not flow between the fragment and the host bone. At arthroscopy, the fragment was fixed in position.

Imaging of Osteochondritis Dissecans

Radiographs

- Subchondral fracture in a characteristic location (Box 1.10).
- Notch (tunnel, intercondylar) view, i.e. an anteroposterior view with the knee flexed at 40 degrees is the best view for detection.
- Fragment and/or adjacent epiphysis may be sclerotic (associated with a worse outcome).
- Note that some apparent fragmentation of epiphyseal bone can be a normal variant in the posterior femoral condyles in younger children (further discussed later).
- MRI findings range from subchondral bone marrow edema and thickened unossified cartilage to subchondral fractures and fragmentation to displacement of an osteochondral fragment.
- A main indication of MRI in OCD is to evaluate the stability of the osteochondral fragment. Fragments that are prone to displacement are managed surgically.

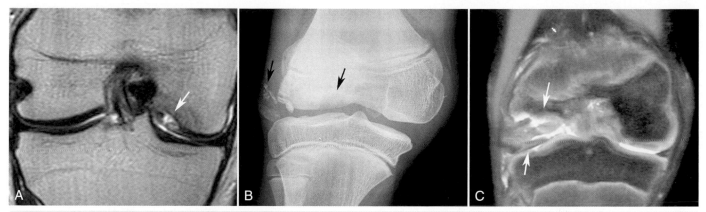

Fig. 1.96 Osteochondritis dissecans (OCD) with displaced fragments. (A) Coronal T2-weighted MR image of the right knee shows fluid filling medial femoral condyle OCD defect *(arrow)*. The fragment was displaced into the joint. (Same patient as shown in Fig. 1.88A.) Anteroposterior radiograph **(B)** and coronal fat-suppressed proton-density MR image **(C)** in a different patient show severe fragmentation of the medial femoral condyle *(arrows)*.

- Findings indicating an unstable ('loose in situ') fragment are less well defined in OCD than for an adult osteochondral lesion:
  - Bright T2 signal that surrounds the fragment (may be joint fluid, granulation, or edematous fibrous tissue, but the distinction is not important). This finding is highly specific for a loose fragment in an adult but less so in OCD.
  - Cystlike change in adjacent epiphyseal bone.
- MRI arthrography or high-resolution CT arthrography is occasionally requested. Joint contrast that surrounds part or the entire fragment is evidence of an unstable fragment.
- Additional findings in advanced OCD:
  - Fragment signal varies, but frequently has decreased T1 signal and sclerosis on CT.
  - Fragment may be mildly displaced, resulting in articular surface contour step-off.
  - Overlying articular cartilage may be intact, fractured at the fragment margin, and/or degenerated with decreased thickness and increased T2 signal.
  - Enhancement with intravenous contrast early in the process suggests better potential for healing.

OCD Management

- Based on the stability of the OCD lesion.
- Stable lesions are treated with non–weight-bearing and have a good prognosis.
- Unstable lesions require surgery.
  - Fragment stabilization with a pin or screw.
  - Fragment debriding or resection.
  - Osteochondral graft (see previous section).
  - Less severe lesions may be managed with drilling through the fragment into underlying host bone. This stimulates fibrocartilage growth and potentially bone that may adequately stabilize the fragment.
  - Prognosis of unstable lesions is better in OCD than in adult osteochondral lesion.

IMPORTANT OCD MIMIC

- Normal variation in epiphyseal ossification can overlap the imaging appearance of OCD (Fig. 1.97).

- Radiographs frequently show irregularity of the margin of the condylar ossification centers in 3- to 6-year-olds. Magnetic resonance images often show elevated T2 signal in the unossified growth cartilage in the posterior femoral condyles of younger children.
- In 10- to 13-year-olds, mild apparent fragmentation of the posterior portion of the femoral condyles may be seen as a normal variant.
  - Incidental cases usually are bilaterally symmetric and asymptomatic, with intact overlying cartilage and no edema on MRI.
  - However, this normal variant occasionally progresses to OCD, especially if the fragmentation is extensive, the joint is painful, and the child maintains a high level of activity. MRI shows edema in the fragments and unossified cartilage.

Child Abuse

- Inflicted or nonaccidental trauma, battered child syndrome, shaken baby syndrome, trauma X.
- Imaging findings in child abuse is essential knowledge for any radiologist who interprets pediatric images.
- This discussion briefly reviews the skeletal findings that are most specific for child abuse. Other organ systems, notably the central nervous system, may also sustain injuries that are fairly specific for child abuse.

IMAGING ASSESSMENT OF CHILD ABUSE

Techniques

- Radiographic skeletal survey.
  - First-line exam in children younger than 2 years.
  - Complete set of high-quality radiographs of the entire body, as recommended by the American College of Radiology (Box 1.11).
  - Adding lateral views of the extremities increases fracture detection but adds radiation.
  - High-detail equipment is required.
  - Obtaining these radiographs is time-consuming and requires a highly skilled and diplomatic technologist.

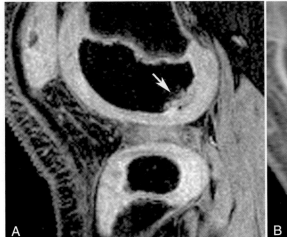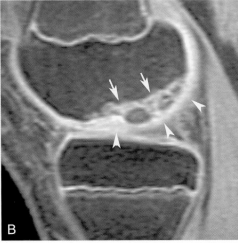

Fig. 1.97 Disorders that mimic osteochondritis dissecans (OCD). Subchondral bone irregularity or fragmentation is a frequent finding in the posterior femoral condyles of children. **(A)** Sagittal fat-suppressed spoiled gradient-echo MR image shows corresponding finding of subchondral irregularity, with cartilage filling the defect. Note the normal contour of overlying articular cartilage. Also, fluid-sensitive sequences showed no marrow edema, which is another clue to a benign process. **(B)** More extensive fragmentation *(arrows)* in a different child, in this case with potential to progress to OCD. Note the intact overlying cartilage *(arrowheads)*. Other sequences showed normal marrow signal, and the child had only minimal symptoms. These rather extreme findings resolved with restriction of the child's activities.

Box 1.11   Radiographic Series for Suspected Child Abuse

AP skull and lateral skull, additional skull views if needed
AP and lateral cervical spine
AP and lateral thorax
Oblique rib views optional but recommended
Lateral lumbosacral spine
AP pelvis
AP humeri
AP forearms
PA hands
AP femurs
AP tibias
PA or AP feet

AP, anteroposterior; PA, posteroanterior.

- In children younger than 2 years of age, a repeat examination after 2 weeks can be helpful to detect healing fractures that were originally occult.
- In older children, the examination can be tailored to 'where it hurts', but some sort of whole-body screening may still be appropriate.
- Bone scintigraphy.
  - Used as a complement to the skeletal survey.
  - Improves sensitivity for detecting periosteal reaction and rib, spine, pelvic, and acromion fractures.
  - Used when skeletal survey is negative but clinical suspicion remains high, either at presentation or more optimally 2 weeks later.
  - Normal physeal tracer uptake limits detection of adjacent fractures. Pinhole collimator imaging improves sensitivity.
- CT improves the detection of rib and spine fractures, but requires additional radiation and may require sedation.
- MRI can be helpful in detecting marrow and subperiosteal edema.

- Both MRI and US can detect fractures of unossified epiphyseal cartilage that are not visible on radiographs.

Findings

- The most specific fractures associated with child abuse are summarized in Box 1.12. Other fractures are less specific but still may be nonaccidental.
- The *classic metaphyseal lesion* (CML) is also known as the metaphyseal corner fracture and the bucket handle fracture. These are actually the same injury as seen from different perspectives (Fig. 1.98A and B).
  - The CML is radiographically similar to a Salter–Harris II fracture, but the transverse component extends through the immature bone of the distal metaphysis rather than through the cartilaginous physis as in a true Salter–Harris II fracture.
  - The mechanism is a combination of twisting and tension, as can occur when a child is violently shaken or when an extremity is violently pulled and twisted.
- Fractures around the infant thorax, especially the posterior ribs, result from forceful squeezing of the thorax by adult hands (Fig. 1.98C).
  - Highly specific for child abuse.

Box 1.12   Fractures Highly Suggestive of Physical Abuse

Classic metaphyseal lesions
Rib fractures, especially posterior
Scapular fractures
Spinous process fractures
Sternal fractures
Skull fractures that are complex or involve bones other than the parietal bone
Multiple fractures involving more than one skeletal area
Fractures of different age

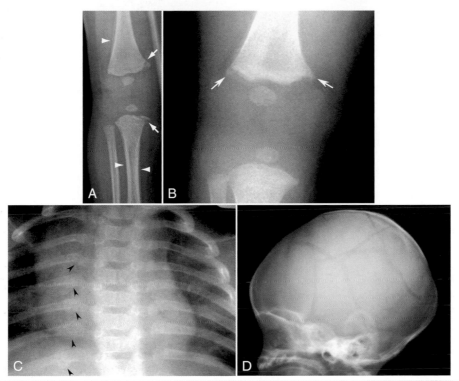

Fig. 1.98 Child abuse, skeletal findings. (A and B) Classic metaphyseal lesions *(arrows)*. Also note the periosteal new bone formation in **A** *(arrowheads)*. **(C)** Posterior rib fractures. The fracture lines are not visible, but the callus formation indicates their presence *(arrowheads)*. These can be undetectable at the time of injury, illustrating the usefulness of follow-up radiographs. Even on delayed radiographs, subtle fractures of child abuse may remain nearly occult and must be carefully sought. **(D)** Multiple skull fractures. This finding is less specific for child abuse than the classic metaphyseal lesion and posterior rib fractures.

- Cardiopulmonary resuscitation of infants does not cause posterior rib fractures.

FRACTURE DATING

Fractures of different of ages is highly suspicious for child abuse. Also, precise fracture dating would provide important forensic evidence.

- As a result, radiologists are often asked to date healing fractures.
- Radiographs: callus usually first appears within 7–14 days but can be seen as early as 4 days.
- Most other generalizations are not reliably applied to an individual fracture, especially a fracture that has not been treated with immobilization. Therefore the following should be considered only as vague generalizations.
- Immature endosteal callus develops along the fracture, resulting in increased density within 10–14 days, and is maximal at 2–3 weeks.
- The endosteal callus matures and is subsequently removed by remodeling by 7–13 weeks after the fracture.
- Remodeling of a deformity begins by 3 months and can take up to 2 years.
- Repeated injury can prolong all of these time periods.

POTENTIAL MIMICKERS OF CHILD ABUSE

- Birth injury.
  - Often associated with shoulder dystocia or breech vaginal delivery.
    - Can cause clavicle and rib fractures and the CML in the extremities.
    - Review of the birth history and clinical follow-up are usually adequate to exclude abuse.
- Vigorous physical therapy in disabled children can cause fractures, including the CML.
- Other types of fractures are frequently seen in child abuse but are less specific (see Fig. 1.98D).
- Rickets.
  - Has characteristic radiographic and features such as rachitic rosary and metaphyseal flaring, reviewed in Chapter 13.
  - Rib fractures are rare in rickets.
- Metabolic bone disease of prematurity.
  - Basically rickets.
  - Very low birth weight infants are born without adequate stores of calcium, phosphate, and vitamin D. Oral delivery after birth is inadequate at first.
  - Most evident between 6 and 12 weeks postnatal.
- Osteogenesis imperfecta (OI), which is discussed in Chapter 15.
  - 95% of children with OI have blue sclerae.
  - Genetic evaluation for the associated mutation.

Other exceedingly rare syndromes also may produce findings suggestive of child abuse in the absence of true abuse, including Schmid-type metaphyseal chondrodysplasia, Langer-type spondyloepiphyseal dysplasia, Caffey disease (discussed in Chapter 15), Menkes syndrome (abnormal copper metabolism leading to weak bones), and congenital indifference to pain.

Box 1.13   Periosteal New Bone Formation in Children

Infection/inflammation
Healing fracture
Healing subperiosteal hematoma
Metabolic (scurvy, hypervitaminosis A and D, Gaucher disease, others)
Juvenile rheumatoid arthritis
Physiologic (during rapid growth, symmetric)
Solid tumors (often aggressive periosteal reaction)
Leukemia
Premature birth (prostaglandin E, physiologic, metabolic disease of prematurity)
Caffey disease (Chapter 15)
Melorheostosis (Chapter 15) can mimic periosteal new bone formation

Periosteal elevation in children can be associated with trauma, but there are numerous other potential causes (Box 1.13).

Congenital infection (e.g., due to syphilis) and scurvy, like rickets, also may produce features suggestive of child abuse. Clinical and laboratory workup and/or follow-up skeletal surveys are usually adequate to diagnose or exclude these conditions. Other entities such as 'brittle bone disease' and radiographically occult rickets due to vitamin D deficiency have been hypothesized but are not generally accepted.

Measuring Skeletal Maturity

- Essential information for diagnosis and management of many pediatric conditions.
  - Important examples:
    - Growth or sex hormone deficiency or excess.
    - Timing of surgery for childhood growth disturbances or scoliosis.
- The process of skeletal maturation tends to follow an orderly progression, even when accelerated or delayed by endocrine conditions, nutritional deficiencies, or other disease states.
- Thus, evaluation of just one part of the skeleton can serve as a reasonable surrogate for the entire skeleton.

GREULICH AND PYLE'S RADIOGRAPHIC ATLAS OF SKELETAL DEVELOPMENT OF THE HAND AND WRIST

- Widely adopted in the US as a standard reference for determining the skeletal age of children older than 1 year.
- Atlas of reference images of the maturing left hand.
- Derived from a longitudinal study of healthy children of northern European decent living in the Cleveland area during the 1930s.
  - This may not represent an optimal data set, but current appreciation of the potential harm of ionizing radiation makes it unlikely that a similar study will ever be performed in other racial or ethnic groups.
- Contemporary evaluations of this atlas have verified its accuracy, at least in children of European descent.

- Provides bone age and standard deviations. Chronologic age within two standard deviations of bone ages is considered to be normal.
- Automated versions are available.
- As a general rule, children of African descent tend to skeletally mature faster than white children. Girls mature faster than boys, and the difference becomes greater as they grow.

TANNER–WHITEHOUSE METHODS 2 AND 3

- Evaluates the hand and wrist.
- Based on a data set of British children from the 1950s and 1960s.
- This method is used more commonly in Europe.
- Arguably more precise than Greulich and Pyle, but time-consuming when done manually.
- Artificial intelligence apps reduce the analysis time to a few seconds with either technique.

METHOD OF SONTAG, SNELL, AND ANDERSON

- For infants and very young children not covered by Greulich and Pyle.
- Radiographs of one upper and one lower extremity are evaluated for the number of secondary growth centers (epiphyses, apophyses, and small round bones) that have started to ossify.
- Relies on a yes-or-no determination of the presence of visible ossification in each secondary growth center (Table 1.1).
  - The *Elgenmark method* is similar, but it uses only unilateral carpal and tarsal bones.

RISSER TECHNIQUE

Is used to estimate skeletal maturity of the spine in adolescents with scoliosis.

- Based on the radiographic appearance of the iliac crest apophyses.
- The iliac crest apophyses ossify in an orderly sequence from lateral to medial before fusing to the crest when or shortly after spinal growth is complete.
- Discussed further in the Scoliosis Management section in Chapter 15.

Table 1.1   Skeletal Age in Infants: the Method of Sontag, Snell, and Anderson

MEAN TOTAL NUMBER OF CENTERS ON THE LEFT SIDE OF BODY OSSIFIED AT GIVEN AGE LEVELS

Age (months	Boys		Girls	
	Mean No.	SD	Mean No.	SD
1	4.11	1.41	4.58	1.76
3	6.63	1.86	7.78	2.16
6	9.61	1.95	11.44	2.53
9	11.88	2.66	15.3	4.92
12	13.96	3.96	22.40	6.93
18	19.27	6.61	34.10	8.44

SD, standard deviation.

Sample Report

History: short stature.

Comparison: 6 months previously.

The child's chronologic age is 9 years, 4 months.

Using the standards of Greulich and Pyle, the child's skeletal age is 8 years, 5 months. The standard deviation is 8 months.

Skeletal age on the prior exam was 8 years.

Impression: Normal skeletal maturation.

Sources and Suggested Readings

Adamsbaum C, Méjean N, Merzoug V, Rey-Salmon C. How to explore and report children with suspected non-accidental trauma. *Pediatr Radiol.* 2010;40(6):932–938.

American College of Radiology ACR Appropriateness Criteria® Suspected Physical Abuse–Child. https://acsearch.acr.org/docs/69443/Narrative/.

Beaman FD, Bancroft LW, Peterson JF, et al. Imaging characteristics of bone graft materials. *RadioGraphics.* 2006;26:373–388.

Beaty JH, Kasser JR, Shaggs DL, et al., eds. *Rockwood and Green's Fractures in Children.* Philadelphia: Lippincott-Raven; 2009.

Beck BR, Bergman AG, Miner M, et al. Tibial stress injury: relationship of radiographic, nuclear medicine bone scanning, MR imaging, and CT severity grades to clinical severity and time to healing. *Radiology.* 2012; 263(3):811–818.

Brittberg M, Winalski CS. Evaluation of cartilage injuries and repair. *J Bone Joint Surg Am.* 2003;85-A(Suppl 2):58–69.

Bucholz RW, Court-Brown CM, Heckman JD, Tornetta P, eds. *Rockwood and Green's Fractures in Adults.* Philadelphia: Lippincott-Raven; 2009.

Christian CW, States LJ. Medical mimics of child abuse. *Am J Roentgenol.* 2017;208(5):982–990.

Crema MD, Roemer FW, Marra MD, et al. Articular cartilage in the knee: current MR imaging techniques and applications in clinical practice and research. *Radiographics.* 2011;31(1):37–61.

Deshmukh S, Carrino JA, Feinberg JH, et al. Pins and needles from fingers to toes: high-resolution MRI of peripheral sensory mononeuropathies. *AJR Am J Roentgenol.* 2017;208(1):W1–W10.

Disler DG. Articular cartilage in the knee: current MR imaging techniques and applications in clinical practice and research. Invited commentary. *Radiographics.* 2011;31(1):61–62.

Ecklund K, Jaramillo D. Patterns of premature physeal arrest: MR imaging of 111 children. *AJR Am J Roentgenol.* 2002;178:967–972.

Gold GE, Chen CA, Koo S, et al. Recent advances in MRI of articular cartilage. *AJR Am J Roentgenol.* 2009;193(3):628–638.

Gorbachova T, Melenevsky Y, Cohen M, Cerniglia BW. Osteochondral lesions of the knee: differentiating the most common entities at MRI. *Radiographics.* 2018;38:1478–1495.

Guermazi A, Roemer FW, Alizai H, et al. State of the art: MR imaging after knee cartilage repair surgery. *Radiology.* 2015;277(1):23–43.

Hu H, Zhang C, Chen J, et al. Clinical value of MRI in assessing the stability of osteochondritis dissecans lesions: a systematic review and meta-analysis. *AJR Am J Roentgenol.* 2019;213:147–154.

Jaimes C, Jimenez M, Shabshin N, et al. Taking the stress out of evaluating stress injuries in children. *Radiographics.* 2012;32:537–555.

Jarraya M, Hayashi D, de Villiers RV, et al. Multimodality imaging of foreign bodies of the musculoskeletal system. *Am J Roentgenol.* 2014;203(1):W92–W102.

Jo S, Sammet S, Thomas S, et al. Musculoskeletal MRI pulse sequences: a review for residents and fellows. *Radiographics.* 2019;39:2038–2039.

Joint ACR/Society for Pediatric Radiology/Society of Skeletal Radiology guidelines. https://www.acr.org/-/media/ACR/Files/Practice-Parameters/Scoliosis.pdf.

Kleinmann P, ed. *Diagnostic Imaging of Child Abuse.* 3rd ed. Cambridge: Cambridge University Press; 2015.

Laor T, Zbojniewicz AM, Eismann EA, Wll EJ. Juvenile osteochondritis dissecans: is it a growth disturbance of the secondary physis of the epiphysis? *AJR Am J Roentgenol.* 2012;199(5):1121–1128.

Lonergan GJ, Baker AM, Morey MK, Boos SC. From the archives of the AFIP. Child abuse: radiologic-pathologic correlation. *Radiographics.* 2003;23:811–845.

Marshall RA, Mandell JC, Weaver MJ, et al. Imaging features and management of stress, atypical, and pathologic fractures. *Radiographics.* 2018; 38:2173–2192.

May DA, Disler DG, Jones EA, et al. Abnormal signal within skeletal muscle in magnetic resonance imaging: patterns, pearls, and pitfalls. *Radiographics.* 2000;20:S295–S315.

McCarthy EF, Sundaram M. Heterotopic ossification: a review. *Skeletal Radiol.* 2005;34:609–619.

Miller TT, Reinus WR. Nerve entrapment syndromes of the elbow, forearm, and wrist. *AJR Am J Roentgenol.* 2010;195(3):585–594.

Narayanasamy S, Krishna S, Sathiadoss P, et al. Radiographic review of avulsion fractures. *Radiographics.* 2018;38:1496–1497.

Nguyen JC, Markhardt BK, Merrow AC, et al. Imaging of pediatric growth plate disturbances. *Radiographics.* 2017;37:1791–1812.

Offiah A, van Rijn R, Perez-Rossello JM, Kleinman P. Skeletal imaging of child abuse (non accidental injury). *Pediatr Radiol.* 2009;39(5):461–470.

Outerbridge RE. The etiology of chondromalacia patellae. *J Bone Joint Surg Br.* 1961;43-B:752–757.

Pathria MN, Chung CB, Resnick DL. Acute and stress-related injuries of bone and cartilage: pertinent anatomy, basic biomechanics, and imaging perspective. *Radiology.* 2016;280:21–38.

Peterfy CG, Guermazi A, Zaim S, et al. Whole-organ magnetic resonance imaging score (WORMS) of the knee in osteoarthritis. *Osteoarthritis Cartilage.* 2004;12(3):177–190.

Sargar KM, Singh AK, Kao SC. Imaging of skeletal disorders caused by fibroblast growth factor receptor gene mutations. *Radiographics.* 2017;37:1813–1830.

Schulze M, Kötter I, Ernemann U, et al. MRI findings in inflammatory muscle diseases and their noninflammatory mimics. *AJR Am J Roentgenol.* 2009;192(6):1708–1716.

Smitaman E, Flores DV, Mejía Gómez C, Pathria MN. MR imaging of atraumatic muscle disorders. *Radiographics.* 2018;38:500–522.

van Vucht N, Santiago R, Lottmann B, et al. The Dixon technique for MRI of the bone marrow. *Skeletal Radiol.* 2019;48:1861.

Vassalou E, Zibis AH, Raoulis VA, et al. Morel-Lavallée lesions of the knee: MRI findings compared with cadaveric study findings. *AJR Am J Roentgenol.* 2018;210(5):W234–W239.

White CL, Chauvin NA, Waryasz GR, et al. MRI of native knee cartilage delamination injuries. *Am J Roentgenol.* 2017;209(5):W317–W321.

Winalski CS, Rajiah P. The evolution of articular cartilage imaging and its impact on clinical practice. *Skeletal Radiol.* 2011;40(9):1197–1222.

Wooten-Gorges SL, Soares BP, Alazraki AL, et al. ACR appropriateness criteria: suspected physical child abuse. Expert Panel on Pediatric Imaging. *J Am Coll Radiol.* 2017;14:S338–S349.

2 *Shoulder*

Anatomy

OSSEOUS

The major osseous structures of the shoulder include the *scapula*, *proximal humerus*, and *clavicle*, which are supported by surrounding muscles and connective tissues. The two joints of the shoulder include the *glenohumeral joint* and the *acromioclavicular (AC) joint*. Normal shoulder anatomy on radiography is outlined in Figs. 2.1 and 2.2. Anatomy of the chest wall is also briefly discussed in this chapter, which includes the *sternoclavicular (SC) joint*. Reference to an anatomy atlas may be helpful while reading this section.

The *scapula* is anatomically comprised of the body, spine, acromion process, scapular neck, glenoid, and coracoid process. Two important landmarks adjacent to the scapular neck are the spinoglenoid notch posterosuperiorly and the suprascapular notch superiorly.

- *Suprascapular nerve* passes through these notches, providing neurovascular supply to the supraspinatus and infraspinatus muscles.

- Mass lesion, ganglion cyst, or displaced fracture fragment in this region can compress this neurovascular bundle, causing muscle weakness that can simulate rotator cuff pathology.

The *scapula* develops from multiple ossification centers, which can simulate a fracture in children, adolescents, and young adults.

- Separate ossification centers form the tip of the coracoid process, the acromion process, the glenoid rim, the inferior angle of the scapular body, and the vertebral border of the scapular body.
- Failure of fusion of an acromial ossification center results in an *os acromiale*.

The *proximal humerus* is composed of the articular surface or humeral head (which is bordered by the anatomic neck), the greater and lesser tuberosities, the vertically oriented intertubercular (bicipital) groove between the tuberosities, and the proximal humeral shaft.

- *Anatomic neck* is designated by the proximal humeral physeal scar, separating the epiphysis and articular surface from the metaphysis and humeral tuberosities.

60

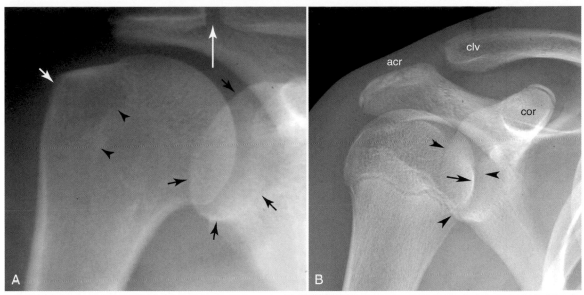

Fig. 2.1. Normal shoulder anatomy on radiography. (A) AP view in external rotation in an adult shows the greater tuberosity *(short white arrow)*, glenoid rim *(short black arrows)*, bicipital groove *(black arrowheads)*, and acromioclavicular joint *(long white arrow)*. **(B)** AP view in internal rotation in a child shows glenoid rim *(arrowheads)*, lesser tuberosity *(arrow)* and acromion *(acr)*, distal clavicle *(clv)*, and coracoid process *(cor)*.

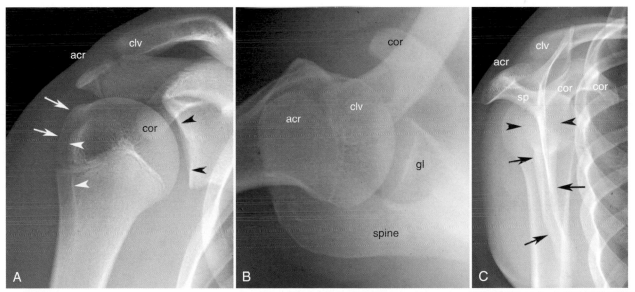

Fig. 2.2 Shoulder anatomy on radiography. (A) Grashey (true AP) view is obtained 40 degrees oblique in the horizontal plane to align the x-ray beam with the glenoid *(black arrowheads)*. Note that the radiolucent glenohumeral joint space is visible. The humerus is in external rotation in this example. Note the acromion, clavicle, tip of coracoid process, and the greater *(arrows)* and lesser *(white arrowheads)* tuberosities. The bicipital groove is between these tuberosities. **(B)** Axillary view is obtained with the arm abducted and the beam passing vertically through the shoulder. Note the normal alignment of the humeral head with the glenoid. Also note the distal clavicle, coracoid process tip, scapular spine, and acromion. **(C)** Scapular Y-view is obtained with the patient turned approximately 45 degrees oblique to the x-ray beam with patient's hand resting on the opposite shoulder to align the beam with the scapula. The "Y" is formed by the spine of the scapula posteriorly, the coracoid process anteriorly, and the body or blade of the scapula *(arrows)*. Note that the humeral head is centered normally over the glenoid *(black arrowheads)* at the center of the Y. Also note the acromion process and distal clavicle. *acr*, Acromion; *clv*, clavicle; *cor*, coracoid; *gl*, glenoid; *sp*, scapular spine.

- *Surgical neck* is a much more common site of fracture and is the ill-defined transverse junction of the humeral head and proximal shaft, located just below the greater and lesser tuberosities; fractures at this site may result in injury to the:
  - *axillary nerve* (innervates the deltoid and teres minor muscles).
  - *posterior circumflex artery* (supplies the teres minor, teres major, deltoid, and long head of the triceps muscles).
- *Greater tuberosity* is located lateral to the humeral head articular surface, serving as an attachment site for the supraspinatus, infraspinatus, and teres minor tendons.

- *Lesser tuberosity* is located anteroinferior to the humeral head articular surface, serving as an attachment site for the subscapularis tendon.
- *Intertubercular (bicipital) groove* is located between the tuberosities, in which the long head biceps tendon (LHBT) is normally located.
- *Proximal humeral shaft* includes the broad deltoid tuberosity on its proximal lateral surface (Fig. 2.3).

The *clavicle* is an S-shaped long bone, with an anterior convex margin along its medial half.

- Clavicle articulates with the manubrium medially and with the acromion process of the scapula laterally.
- *Rhomboid fossa* is a variable and frequently irregular concavity in the undersurface of the medial clavicle above the costal cartilage of the first rib and is more common in males (Fig. 2.4).
  - Normal variant; should not be mistaken for a lytic or erosive process.

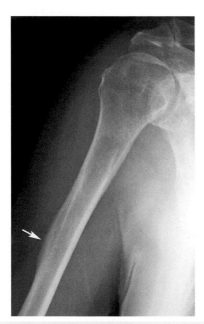

Fig. 2.3 Normal deltoid tuberosity (*arrow*).

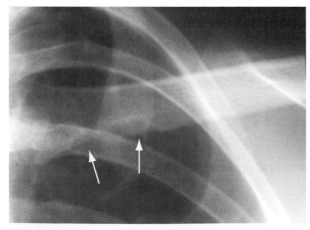

Fig. 2.4 Rhomboid fossa. Note the irregular defect in the inferior medial clavicle adjacent to the first rib (arrows).

GLENOHUMERAL JOINT

The *glenohumeral joint* is formed by the articulation of the humeral head and glenoid fossa, a ball-and-socket synovial joint. The glenohumeral joint is the most mobile, least stable major joint in the body, and consequently is a frequent site of pain and dysfunction. The glenohumeral joint anatomy is outlined in Figs. 2.5 through 2.7 (see footnoted key* for an explanation of the abbreviations used in these figures).

- *Glenoid* articular surface is roughly perpendicular to the scapular body, slightly concave, and pear-shaped when viewed *en face* (wider inferiorly), forming the 'socket' of the glenohumeral joint.
  - Subchondral bone of the glenoid is nearly flat, with a shallow central depression.
  - Overlying glenoid articular cartilage is thinnest at its central portion, which slightly enhances the concavity of the glenoid fossa.
  - Anatomy results in a shallow socket with extraordinary mobility but poor intrinsic stability.
  - When viewed *en face*, the glenoid fossa may be compared to the face of a clock, always with 12:00 superiorly, 3:00 anteriorly, 6:00 inferiorly, and 9:00 posteriorly (Fig. 2.8).
    - Clock face orientation is used commonly by orthopedic surgeons and is recommended for reporting imaging findings, such as location of a labral tear.
- *Humeral head* articular surface is rounded, forming the 'ball' of the glenohumeral joint.
  - Articular surface is hemispherical and directed superomedially and slightly posterior to the humeral axis.

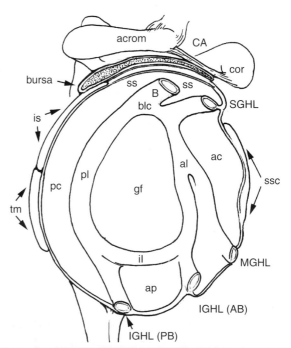

Fig. 2.5 Glenohumeral joint anatomy. This diagram views the glenoid fossa *en face* with the humeral head removed. Anterior is to the viewer's right, by a convention used by orthopedic surgeons. The MR images in this chapter display anterior to the viewer's left, by a convention often used by radiologists.*

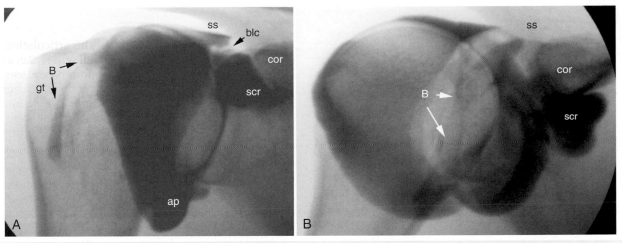

Fig. 2.6 Glenohumeral joint: normal arthrographic anatomy. (A) AP external rotation. **(B)** AP internal rotation.*

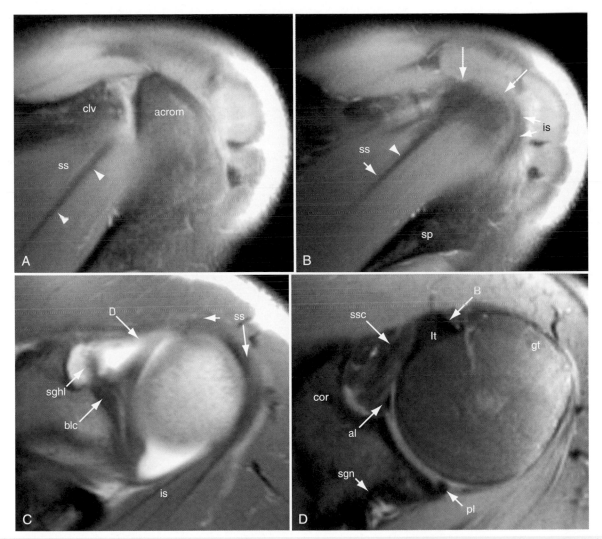

Fig. 2.7 Glenohumeral joint: normal anatomy shown on MRI and CT. Axial images **(A–I)**. **(A)** Fat-suppressed proton density image obtained through the acromioclavicular joint. The most superior image should include this joint to assess for os acromiale and anterior spurs. Note the central slip of the supraspinatus tendon *(arrowheads)*. The oblique coronal scans should be aligned with this portion of the tendon. **(B)** Image obtained just below image A, same study. Note how the supraspinatus tendon becomes broad distally, like a cuff *(long arrows)*. **(C)** MR arthrogram obtained through the top of the humeral head is perpendicular to the supraspinatus tendon as it curves over the head toward its insertion onto the greater tuberosity. For this reason, distal supraspinatus tears may be best seen on axial images. **(D)** Fat-suppressed proton density image at the level of the base of the coracoid.

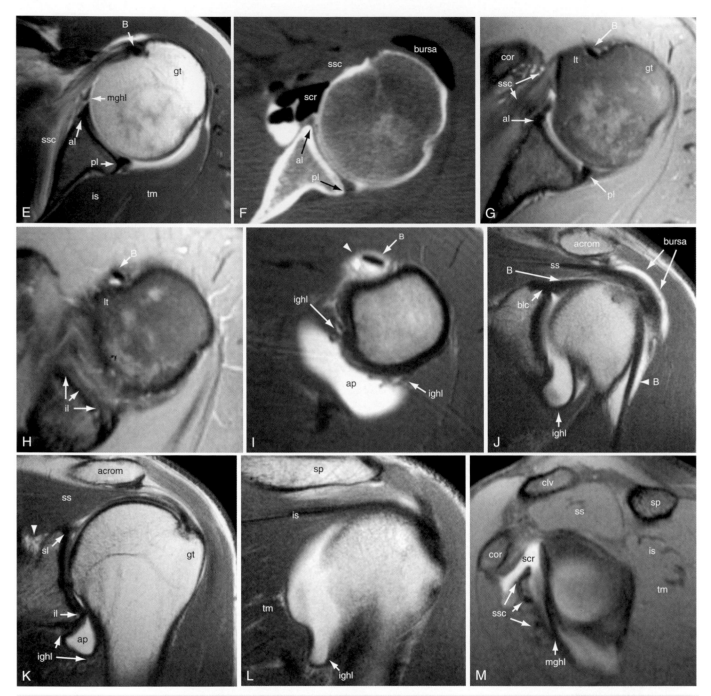

Fig. 2.7, cont'd (E) T1-weighted MR arthrogram obtained at approximately the 9:00 and 3:00 levels. The increased signal intensity in the subscapularis tendon and muscle was due to a combination of harmless contrast extravasation from the joint and direct injection during needle placement. **(F)** CT air-contrast arthrogram in a different patient performed at approximately the same level as the image in E. The gas in the subdeltoid bursa was due to a rotator cuff tear (not shown). **(G)** Fat-suppressed proton density image at approximately the 4:00 to 8:00 levels. **(H)** Fat-suppressed proton density image obtained through the inferior glenoid. **(I)** T1-weighted MR arthrogram obtained through the axillary pouch. Note that contrast fills the biceps tendon sheath *(arrowhead)*, a normal finding. **(J–L)** Oblique coronal images. All images are T2-weighted arthrograms obtained from the same study. **(J)** Anterior image. **(K)** Central image. Note the suprascapular notch *(arrowhead)* that contains the suprascapular nerve, which innervates the supraspinatus and infraspinatus muscles. **(L)** Posterior image. Oblique sagittal images **(M–P)**. All images are T1-weighted MR arthrograms but were not obtained from the same study. **(M)** Slightly medial to the glenoid fossa.

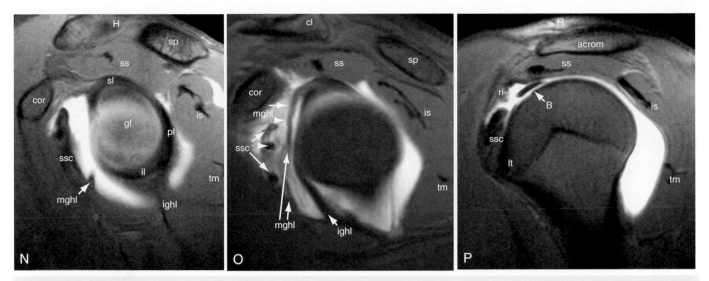

Fig. 2.7, cont'd **(N)** At the glenoid fossa. **(O)** Lateral to the glenoid fossa. **(P)** Through the center of the humeral head.* *Key to Figs. 2.5 to 2.7: Bones: *acrom*, acromial arch; *clv*, clavicle; *cor*, coracoid process; *gt*, greater tuberosity; *lt*, lesser tuberosity; *sgn*, spinoglenoid notch (posterior scapular neck); *sp*, spine of scapula; *ssn*, suprascapular notch (superior scapular neck). Muscles and tendons: *B*, biceps long head; *is*, infraspinatus; *ri*, rotator interval; *ss*, supraspinatus; *ssc*, subscapularis; *tm*, teres minor. Ligaments: *CA*, coracoacromial ligament; *IGHL*, inferior glenohumeral ligament; *IGHL (AB)*, inferior glenohumeral ligament anterior band; *IGHL (PB)*, inferior glenohumeral ligament posterior band; *MGHL*, middle glenohumeral ligament; *SGHL*, superior glenohumeral ligament. Capsule: *ac*, anterior capsule; *ap*, axillary pouch; *pc*, posterior capsule; *scr*, subscapular recess or bursa (subcoracoid recess). Labrum: *al*, anterior labrum; *blc*, biceps labral complex; *bursa*: subacromial subdeltoid bursa; *gf*, glenoid fossa; *il*, inferior labrum; *pl*, posterior labrum.

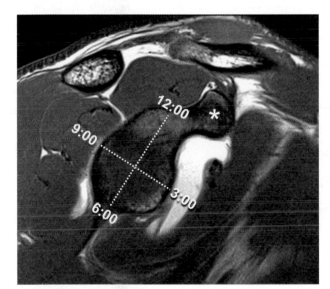

Fig. 2.8 Clock face orientation of the glenoid. Clock positions of the glenoid are as follows: 12:00 superiorly, 3:00 anteriorly, 6:00 inferiorly, and 9:00 posteriorly. The coracoid process can be used as an anatomic landmark, as it always points anterior (*asterisk*). Note that the glenoid fossa may be tilted off-axis on the sagittal sequence, as in this case.

LABRUM, CAPSULE, AND LIGAMENTS

The *glenoid labrum* is a fibrocartilaginous 'suction cup' that forms a rim around the glenoid, deepening the glenoid fossa and increasing the joint contact area. The labrum varies in terms of normal shape and fixation to the glenoid.

- Most frequently triangular in cross section, though the posterior labrum often has a rounded lateral contour.
- Generally fixed to the glenoid periosteum and underlying glenoid articular cartilage.

- Several patterns of normal labral variants occur fairly commonly:
  - *Sublabral foramen* is an absent fixation of the labrum between the 1:00 and 3:00 positions (Fig. 2.9A).
  - *Sublabral recess* or *sulcus* is a cleft between the superior labrum and the glenoid (Fig. 2.9B).
  - *Buford complex* is an absent anterosuperior labrum and a thickened, cordlike middle glenohumeral ligament (MGHL) that may simulate a labral detachment (Fig. 2.10).
- Variants may imitate a superior labral tear, i.e., a SLAP (superior labrum anterior posterior) tear.
  - Note: absence or detachment of the labrum outside of the anterosuperior quadrant (12:00 to 3:00 positions) generally indicates labral pathology.
- Hypertrophy of the posterior labrum may be seen in overhead throwing athletes as an adaptive response.
  - *Bennett lesion* (Fig. 2.11) is a rim of calcification along the posterior glenoid that is associated with chronic posterior capsule avulsive injury in such athletes.

The glenohumeral *joint capsule* is difficult to assess on imaging studies unless the capsule is distended by a joint effusion or intraarticular contrast solution (direct arthrography).

- Posterior capsular anatomy is fairly simple and constant.
  - Medial posterior joint capsule is attached to the glenoid labrum and adjacent glenoid periosteum and is bounded by the rotator cuff.
  - Occasionally, the medial posterior capsule inserts medial to the glenoid rim (Fig. 2.12).
- Anterior capsule is more complex and variable.
  - Medial anterior capsule may attach to the glenoid rim or may insert onto the scapula medial to the labrum.
  - Such medial attachment may occur as a normal variant or as a consequence of a previous anterior shoulder dislocation due to stripping of the capsule and periosteum from the glenoid.

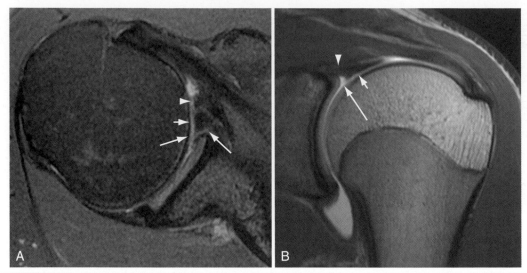

Fig. 2.9 Common anterior and superior labrum normal variants. (A) Sublabral foramen. Axial T2-weighted MR image shows narrow high-signal band *(long arrows)* between the anterior labrum *(short arrow)* and the glenoid. This finding is a normal variant only between the 1:00 and 3:00 positions. Also note the middle glenohumeral ligament *(arrowhead)*. This could be a labral tear, but in this location this finding is more likely to be a normal variant. **(B)** Sublabral sulcus. Coronal T1-weighted arthrogram image. Note smooth gap *(long arrow)* between the meniscus-like superior labrum laterally *(short arrow)* fixed to the proximal biceps long head tendon *(arrowhead)*. This normal sulcus is oriented superiorly and slightly medially, toward the AC joint, in contrast with many superior labral tears that are oriented superiorly and laterally, toward the deltoid.

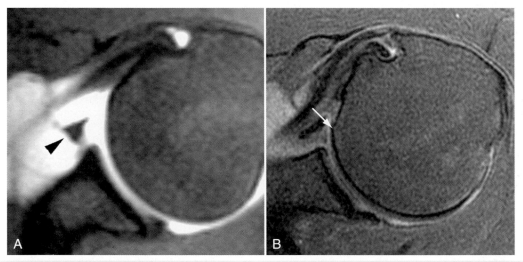

Fig. 2.10 Buford complex. (A) MR arthrogram image. Note the absence of the anterosuperior labrum and thick middle glenohumeral ligament *(arrowhead)*. **(B)** Axial fat-suppressed T2-weighted image. Note the thick middle glenohumeral ligament *(arrow)* and absent labrum.

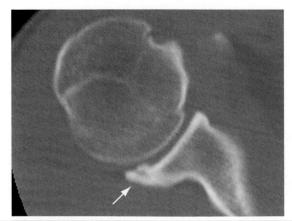

Fig. 2.11 Bennett lesion in a baseball pitcher. Note the rim of calcification along the posterior inferior glenoid *(arrow)*.

- Glenohumeral joint capsule varies in redundancy.
    - Some capsular redundancy is required to allow for a normal range of motion.
    - Excessive redundancy may predispose the shoulder to instability, dislocation, rotator cuff degeneration and tears, and labral tears.
    - An overly tight joint capsule, as can occur after inflammatory processes (*adhesive capsulitis*; Fig. 2.13) or surgical 'tightening' procedures performed to correct shoulder instability, can cause pain and limited range of motion.
    - Estimation of capsular laxity on imaging studies is subjective and arguably should be avoided unless the findings are extreme.
- Normal synovial recesses, or pouches, extending from the glenohumeral synovial compartment include the saddle-shaped *subscapularis recess* anterosuperiorly and the *axillary recess* inferiorly (see Figs. 2.6 and 2.7).

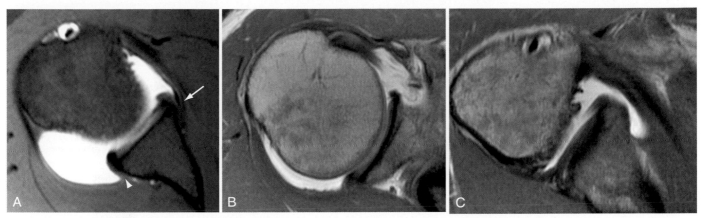

Fig. 2.12 Capsule insertion variation. Axial MR arthrogram images in different patients. **(A)** External rotation. Relatively lateral anterior capsule insertion *(arrow)* with unusually far medial posterior capsule insertion *(arrowhead)*. **(B)** This is the normal posterior capsule insertion, adjacent to the labrum, seen in the vast majority of patients. The anterior capsule insertion in this patient is not seen on this image. **(C)** Internal rotation. Relatively medial anterior capsule insertion with the normal posterior capsule insertion. Contrast these examples with Fig. 2.7F, a CT arthrogram image of a patient who suffered a prior anterior shoulder dislocation with stripping of the anterior capsule and periosteum off of the glenoid. In that image, note how the anterior capsule joins the anterior glenoid at an abrupt, sharp angle rather than the smooth, curved transition in **C** here.

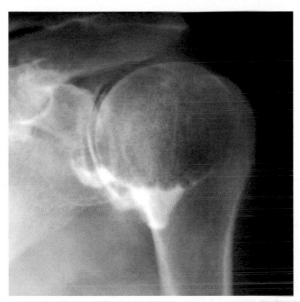

Fig. 2.13 Adhesive capsulitis ('frozen shoulder'). Radiograph following arthrogram injection shows a very-low-capacity joint capsule.

- The *subcoracoid bursa* is a separate, distinct potential space from the subscapularis recess that normally does not communicate with the glenohumeral joint.
- Fluid in the *subcoracoid bursa* may reflect subcoracoid bursitis or abnormal communication with the glenohumeral joint, typically in the setting of anterior rotator cuff tears or traumatic rotator interval lesions.

The glenohumeral ligaments are thick fibrous bands within the anterior and inferior portion of the joint and are important contributors to anterior shoulder stability.

- *Inferior glenohumeral ligament (IGHL).*
  - Thickest and most important glenohumeral ligament.
  - Extends from the inferior glenoid labrum to the proximal humeral shaft in a sling-like arrangement of thick *anterior* and *posterior bands*, connected by a thin capsular membrane termed the *axillary pouch*.
  - Lax and redundant when the arm is adducted, which contributes to the normal axillary recess (see Figs. 2.6 and 2.7).
  - Tightens when the arm is abducted and becomes the primary static stabilizer of the glenohumeral joint.
- *Middle glenohumeral ligament (MGHL).*
  - Originates at the anterosuperior labrum or adjacent glenoid neck and attaches to the base of the lesser tuberosity of the humerus, often blending with the deep fibers of the subscapularis.
  - May be of variable thickness and is occasionally duplicated; absent in about 25–30% of people.
  - Normal-variant *Buford complex* consists of an absent anterosuperior labrum and a thickened, cordlike MGHL (see Fig. 2.10).
- *Superior glenohumeral ligament (SGHL).*
  - Located superior to the MGHL and arises from the anterosuperior labrum, glenoid, and coracoid process.
  - Attaches distally to the superior aspect of the lesser tuberosity, at the medial edge of the bicipital groove.
  - Helps stabilize the LHBT.
- MGHL and SGHL contribute to anterior glenohumeral stability but are not as critical as the IGHL.
- Glenohumeral ligaments are best visualized on imaging studies with distention of the joint capsule using computed tomography (CT) or magnetic resonance (MR) arthrography.

ROTATOR CUFF

The muscles of the *rotator cuff* originate from the medial scapula and their tendons insert on the humeral head, where they are broad and sheetlike. The rotator cuff contributes to the motion of the upper extremity and also serves as a dynamic stabilizer of the humeral head within the glenoid fossa. The rotator cuff muscles contribute to shoulder motion. Primarily, the subscapularis internally rotates the shoulder, the teres minor and infraspinatus externally rotate the shoulder, and the supraspinatus abducts the shoulder. The supraspinatus, infraspinatus, and teres minor tendons insert onto the greater tuberosity, whereas the subscapularis tendon inserts onto the lesser tuberosity.

- *Supraspinatus*
  - Muscle originates from the supraspinatus fossa along the dorsal aspect of the scapula, located above the scapular spine.
  - Innervation: *suprascapular nerve.*
  - Tendon inserts onto the highest facet of the greater tuberosity, anterior to the infraspinatus tendon.
- *Infraspinatus*
  - Muscle originates from the infraspinatus fossa along the dorsal aspect of the scapula, located below the scapular spine.
  - Innervation: *suprascapular nerve.*
  - Tendon inserts onto the middle facet of the greater tuberosity, posterior to the supraspinatus tendon.
- *Teres minor*
  - Muscle originates along the dorsal aspect of the lateral margin of the scapula, making up the most inferior portion of the rotator cuff posteriorly.
  - Innervation: posterior branch of the *axillary nerve.*
  - Tendon inserts onto the inferior facet of the greater tuberosity, posteroinferior to the infraspinatus tendon.
- *Subscapularis*
  - Broad triangular multipennate muscle, originates from the subscapular fossa at the anterior scapula.
  - Largest rotator cuff muscle; approximately as large as the infraspinatus and teres minor muscles combined.
  - Innervation: *upper* and *lower subscapular nerves.*
  - Tendon has a complex insertion on the lesser tuberosity.
    - Also intimately associated with the glenohumeral ligaments and coracohumeral ligament.
    - *Transverse humeral ligament*, a continuation of the subscapularis tendon fibers, crosses the bicipital groove to the greater tuberosity and helps to contain the LHBT within the groove.
    - Dislocation of the LHBT generally indicates a subscapularis tear or detachment from the lesser tuberosity.
    - Main action is to adduct and internally rotate the arm.

The primary function of the rotator cuff is to act as a *dynamic stabilizer* of the glenohumeral joint; that is, to resist glenohumeral subluxation during shoulder motion.

- Powerful contraction of the deltoid muscle during shoulder abduction applies a superior force to the humeral head, which, if not counterbalanced, would result in impingement of the supraspinatus and infraspinatus tendons between the humeral head and the coracoacromial arch.
- Muscles of the rotator cuff apply compressive force across the glenohumeral joint, helping maintain normal joint alignment.

The *central cuff* refers to central region of the rotator cuff consisting of the posterior supraspinatus and anterior infraspinatus tendon fibers, which form a *conjoined tendon* as they insert on the greater tuberosity.

- This is a common site for degenerative rotator cuff tears.

The *rotator cable* is a frequently present thickening of the supraspinatus and infraspinatus tendon critical zones consisting of undersurface transverse fibers.

- Disperses forces applied to the rotator cuff and likely accounts for an interesting variant of large tears: a near-complete tear of the supraspinatus and infraspinatus tendons that spares the anterior supraspinatus and posterior infraspinatus tendons.
- Torn portions of these tendons may retract substantially, forming a crescent-shaped tear when viewed from above, but good function may be maintained, and surgery may not be necessary.

ROTATOR INTERVAL

The rotator interval is a small, triangular shaped gap between the anterior margin of the supraspinatus tendon and the superior margin of the subscapularis tendon, lateral to where they are separated by the coracoid process.

- Roof of the rotator interval is composed of the sheetlike coracohumeral ligament (CHL) and SGHL.
- Intraarticular portion of the LHBT sits within the rotator interval, with the CHL and SGHL serving as primary stabilizers.
- Traumatic rotator interval lesions in which there is disruption of these ligaments may destabilize the biceps tendon or glenohumeral joint.
- Edema and infiltration of the normal rotator interval fat, thickening of the CHL, and thickening of the axillary pouch (inferior joint capsule) are findings associated with *adhesive capsulitis* (discussed later in this chapter).

BICEPS TENDON

As its name implies, the biceps muscle has two heads. The *short head* of the biceps originates at the coracoid process along with the tendon of the coracobrachialis. The *LHBT* originates at the supraglenoid tubercle and the superior glenoid labrum at the 12:00–1:00 position (termed the *biceps anchor* or *biceps labral complex*), arches obliquely over the humeral head within the joint capsule through the *rotator interval*, and then courses inferiorly into the intertubercular groove where it becomes extraarticular.

- *Biceps pulley* is a 'sling' that stabilizes the LHBT at the level of the proximal bicipital groove, comprising the SGHL, CHL, and the distal superficial fibers of the subscapularis tendon.
- As the LHBT courses more distally it encounters secondary stabilizers, including the transverse humeral ligament proximally and the pectoralis major tendon distally.
- LHBT resists anterior and superior humeral head subluxation and thus contributes to glenohumeral joint stability.
- Synovial sheath of the LHBT communicates with the glenohumeral joint.
- Pathology of the LHBT is much more frequently encountered than the short head.

ACROMIOCLAVICULAR JOINT

The *AC joint* is a plane-type synovial joint at the articulation between the distal clavicle and acromion.

- Tightly invested with connective tissue, which results in a strong joint with limited mobility.

- Strong coracoclavicular ligaments nearby add to the stability of the AC joint.
- The AC joint is a synovial joint and is vulnerable to osteoarthritis; osteophytes projecting inferiorly from the AC joint can narrow the subacromial space and cause rotator cuff impingement.
- Traumatic injury to the AC joint (*acromioclavicular joint separation*) is graded by clinical and radiographic findings.

STERNOCLAVICULAR JOINT

- The *SC joint* is a saddle-type synovial joint at the articulation between the medial clavicle with the superolateral manubrium.
- Lined with fibrocartilage and contains a small fibrocartilage disc.
- Difficult to evaluate with radiographs because of overlapping structures.
- Best imaged by CT with breath-hold or magnetic resonance imaging (MRI)-obtained prone, which immobilizes the sternum and reduces breathing artifact.

Imaging Techniques

RADIOGRAPHY

Radiographs are the initial imaging study of choice for shoulder pain, particularly in the posttraumatic setting. Radiographs may demonstrate dislocation, fracture, glenohumeral joint osteoarthritis, osseous findings associated with rotator cuff impingement and sequelae of rotator cuff arthropathy, abnormalities of the AC joint, calcific tendinosis, calcified or ossified intraarticular bodies, osseous lesions, and other acute and nonacute findings. Routine radiographic projections include:

- *Anteroposterior (AP) internal rotation view*—projects the greater tuberosity over the head, resulting in a rounded contour (see Fig. 2.1).
- *AP external rotation view*—profiles the greater tuberosity laterally and the articular surface medially, with the lesser tuberosity projecting over the center of the humeral head.
- *Grashey (true AP) view*—obtained at a 40-degree mediolateral angle, imaging the glenohumeral joint in profile (see Fig. 2.2A).
- *Axillary view*—obtained with the x-ray beam passing caudocranially with the arm abducted (see Fig. 2.2B), useful for localizing the humeral head and glenoid to detect glenohumeral dislocation; may also identify an os acromiale.
- *Scapular Y-view*—obtained by angling the x-ray beam parallel to the scapula (see Fig. 2.2C), also useful for detecting glenohumeral dislocation and does not require manipulation of the shoulder; may also identify scapular fractures.

MAGNETIC RESONANCE IMAGING

MRI has become the mainstay of imaging the shoulder for soft tissue and occult osseous injuries. While protocols may vary between institutions, routine MRI of the shoulder includes imaging in the coronal and sagittal planes (prescribed parallel to the rotator cuff and glenoid fossa, respectively) and axial plane (prescribed perpendicular to the long axis of the humeral shaft). Imaging is acquired using T1-weighted, short tau inversion recovery (STIR), and proton density (PD) or T2-weighted fat-suppressed pulse sequences. Sequence selection is largely a matter of personal preference and the capabilities of the available MRI scanner.

- Every examination should include fast spin-echo (FSE) sequences with long echo time (TE), either PD or T2-weighted, in the coronal and sagittal planes to assess for abnormal signal within the rotator cuff tendons.
- Moderate TE values of 50–60 msec is long enough to avoid the magic angle effect and also allows for assessment of articular cartilage defects.
- Fat suppression improves detection of abnormal fluid-equivalent signal within rotator cuff tears, as well as soft tissue and marrow edema.
- Sample shoulder MRI protocol routinely used in our practices includes: axial PD fat-suppressed, coronal oblique STIR or fat suppressed T2, coronal oblique T1, sagittal oblique T2 sequences, and sagittal oblique PD fat-suppressed or T1-w sequences.

MRI performed after intraarticular injection of gadolinium-based contrast solution (*direct MR arthrography*) is the gold standard for radiologic evaluation of the labrum.

- For technique, see Chapter 16—Musculoskeletal Procedures and Techniques.
- Contrast solution distends out the joint capsule and outlines the intraarticular structures, providing improved detection of labral tears, capsuloligamentous injuries, and undersurface rotator cuff tears.
- Gadolinium in the appropriate concentration is a T1-hyperintense agent, thus shoulder MR arthrography includes the addition of T1-weighted fat-suppressed sequences, typically both in the coronal and axial planes.
- Axial oblique imaging may also be performed perpendicular to the axis of the glenoid for better visualization of the labrum.
- Sample shoulder MR arthrography protocol routinely used in our practices includes: axial T1 fat-suppressed, coronal oblique T1 fat-suppressed, coronal oblique PD fat-suppressed, and sagittal oblique T1 sequences.
  - Optional sequences to better assess the labrum include an ABER (abduction and external rotation) T1 fat-suppressed sequence or axial oblique T1 fat-suppressed sequence prescribed along the axis of the glenoid.

Indirect MR arthrography may be performed when a radiologist is unavailable to provide intraarticular injection.

- Accomplished by intravenous (IV) injection of contrast followed by exercise of the joint.
- Imaging is typically delayed 15–20 minutes following IV injection to allow the gadolinium to diffuse across the synovium into the joint.
- Less invasive than direct arthrography but less reliable in delivering contrast into the joint and does not distend the joint capsule.

MRI tailored to the chest wall may be appropriate when assessing for muscle strains, occult rib injuries, pectoralis major tears, or SC joint pathology.

- Chest wall MRI protocol typically includes imaging in all three anatomic planes using both T1-weighted and fluid-sensitive sequences.
- Large field-of-view (FOV) imaging of the chest is acquired for side-to-side comparison, and small FOV imaging is targeted to the affected side.
- Pectoralis major protocol MRI is even more specialized, with coronal and sagittal imaging planes prescribed parallel and perpendicular to the orientation of the pectoralis major muscle, respectively.
  - Sample pectoralis MRI protocol routinely used in our practices includes: axial T1, axial STIR, axial T2, coronal oblique STIR, and sagittal oblique T2 fat-suppressed sequences.

ULTRASOUND

The shoulder is one of the most frequently imaged joints using musculoskeletal ultrasound (US) due to exceptional visualization of the rotator cuff. US can reliably diagnose most rotator cuff tears, pathology of the LHBT, and joint effusions. While US of the shoulder requires a high degree of operator experience and requires more physician time than does MRI, many patients prefer US to MRI. In some regions, musculoskeletal US has become ubiquitous for diagnostic evaluation of the shoulder, surpassing MRI in popularity. Shoulder interventional procedures are often performed under US guidance, such as joint injections, subacromial/subdeltoid bursa injections, calcific tendinosis barbotage, and paralabral cyst aspirations.

COMPUTED TOMOGRAPHY

CT is useful for characterizing fractures, dislocations, glenoid and humeral head morphology, and soft tissue calcifications such as calcific tendinitis. CT is also useful for detecting osseous bridging if there is clinical concern for delayed fracture healing.

CT following the intraarticular injection of iodinated contrast solution (CT arthrography) may be utilized in patients where MRI is contraindicated or prohibited due to susceptibility artifact from metallic hardware.

- CT arthrography using the latest generation multislice scanners allows for multiplanar reformations in the traditional coronal, sagittal, and axial planes, and is therefore is a viable alternative to MRI.
- CT arthrography may also be used for assessment of hardware component loosening in patients who have undergone shoulder arthroplasty.

Pathophysiology

GLENOHUMERAL JOINT INSTABILITY

Glenohumeral joint stability depends on a combination of static and dynamic mechanisms.

- *Static stabilizers* include the labrum, the joint capsule and glenohumeral ligaments, and negative pressure at the area of contact of the articular surfaces.

- *Dynamic stabilizers* include the rotator cuff and long head biceps tendons and muscles.

Shoulder instability, or more precisely glenohumeral instability, is the tendency of the humeral head to subluxate or dislocate. Glenohumeral instability can occur in any direction, but the most common pattern is *anterior instability*.

- Anterior instability is usually the consequence of prior anterior shoulder dislocation with disruption of the anterior shoulder stabilizers (discussed earlier in this chapter).
- Recurrent anterior dislocation is the classic feature of anterior instability, although a history of dislocation is not present in all individuals with anterior instability.
- Treatment of anterior instability is usually surgical; the goal is to restore normal anatomy by repairing or augmenting the damaged structures.

Posterior instability, like the posterior dislocation or subluxation that may precede it, is relatively rare by comparison.

- MR findings include disruption of the posterior labrum, a lax posterior joint capsule, and interruption of the posterior band of the IGHL.
- Treatment is also surgical.

Multidirectional instability is glenohumeral joint laxity due to a lax joint capsule; it is often exacerbated by poorly coordinated action of the rotator cuff muscles.

- Frequently bilateral and occurring in younger individuals; generalized joint laxity throughout the body may be present.
- Humeral head subluxation can result in pain, labral injuries, and rotator cuff impingement.
- Imaging findings often absent, although the labrum may be small and the capsule lax/redundant; may observe capacious joint capsule on direct arthrography.
- Treatment consists of rotator cuff strengthening exercises; surgical tightening of the joint capsule is sometimes needed.

Glenoid dysplasia, or *glenoid hypoplasia*, is a spectrum of developmental deformity of the scapular neck and glenoid (Fig. 2.14).

- Ranges in degree, from mild to severe with gross shoulder instability.
- Best depicted on axial CT or MRI, with typical findings including hypoplasia of the posterior glenoid and glenoid retroversion.
- Associated with posterior shoulder instability, posterior labral tears, and posterior labral hypertrophy.
- May be accompanying deformity of the acromion or humeral head in severe cases.

Many labral tears are associated with shoulder dislocation or instability, but labral tears can occur in the absence of shoulder instability.

For example, only about 20% of superior labral tears are associated with shoulder instability.

ROTATOR CUFF IMPINGEMENT

The *subacromial space* is the space between the humeral head and the coracoacromial arch.

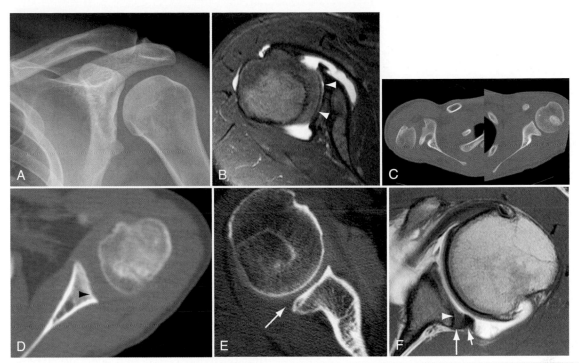

Fig. 2.14 Glenoid dysplasia. (A) Idiopathic. AP radiograph shows a deficient glenoid neck and a mildly flat humeral head. The right shoulder had the same appearance. **(B)** Axial fat-suppressed T2-weighted saline arthrogram in a different patient shows similar findings. Note the broad glenoid articular surface that is aligned in the sagittal plane *(arrowheads)*. **(C)** Composite CT image of a young adult with right Erb palsy shows small, dysplastic humeral head and glenoid related to disuse since birth. **(D)** CT image of less severe dysplasia in a child with Erb palsy shows deficient posterior glenoid *(arrowhead)*. **(E and F)** Mild dysplasia. CT image **(E)** shows medial slope of the posterior glenoid *(arrow)*, considered by many authors to be glenoid dysplasia. This mild dysplasia may be associated with posterior instability and posterior labral tear. MR arthrogram image in a different patient **(F)** shows similar bone morphology *(arrowhead)*. Note the compensatory hypertrophy of posterior articular cartilage *(long arrow)* and labrum *(short arrow)*.

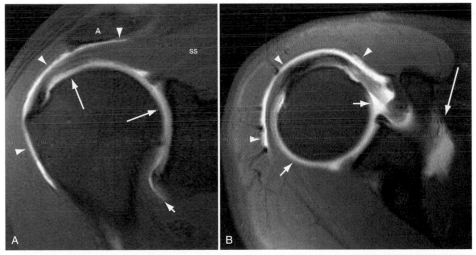

Fig. 2.15 Subdeltoid subacromial bursa, normal anatomy. Oblique coronal **(A)** and axial **(B)** T1-weighted MR arthrogram images after combined contrast injection of the bursa *(arrowheads)* and the glenohumeral joint *(arrows)*. **(A)** Note the supraspinatus muscle (ss) and tendon further laterally separating the bursa and joint. Also note the axillary pouch or recess *(short arrow)*, which is not distended in this image. **(B)** Note the subscapularis recess *(long arrow)*, which is part of the shoulder joint.

- Contents of the subacromial space, from superficial to deep: subacromial bursa → supraspinatus and infraspinatus tendons → glenohumeral joint capsule.
- Subacromial bursa communicates with the more lateral subdeltoid bursa and are therefore considered a single bursa (*subacromial/subdeltoid bursa*; Fig. 2.15).
- This bursa allows the rotator cuff to glide beneath the coracoacromial arch and the deltoid muscle.

The acromion process and the coracoacromial ligament form the *coracoacromial arch* (Fig. 2.16), which overlies the subacromial space. The *coracoacromial ligament* is variable in thickness, about 2–5 mm, best seen on MR images as a low-signal-intensity structure that can be traced between the anterior acromion process and the coracoid on sequential coronal or sagittal images. The coracoacromial arch contributes to shoulder stability by limiting superior

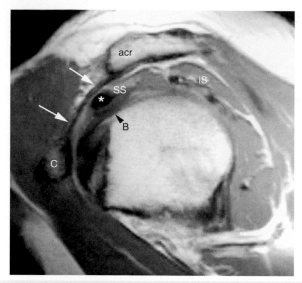

Fig. 2.16 Coracoacromial arch. Oblique sagittal MR image happens to include the entire coracoacromial ligament on one image *(arrows)*. Note that the supraspinatus tendon is deep to the coracoacromial ligament, which is often a factor in supraspinatus impingement. In this case the supraspinatus tendon is focally thickened with low signal intensity *(asterisk)* because of a calcium deposit. Also note the infraspinatus tendon and biceps long head tendon. *acr*, Acromion; *c*, coracoid; *is*, infraspinatus tendon; *SS*, supraspinatus tendon.

Box 2.1	**Modified Bigliani Classification System**	
Type	**Morphology**	**Comments**
1	Flat	
2	Curved (concave)	Most common type
3	Anteriorly hooked	Associated with rotator cuff impingement
4	Reverse curved (convex)	Rarest type

subluxation of the humeral head, but this is also a major factor in rotator cuff impingement.

- Any process that narrows the subacromial space has the potential to compress the rotator cuff and other soft tissues in the subacromial space.
- Acromial features associated with impingement include *subacromial spurs*, os acromiale, hooked anterior undersurface of the acromion process (*type 3 acromion*, see Box 2.1), inferior AC joint osteophytes (Fig. 2.17) or capsular hypertrophy, and lateral downsloping of the acromion.
  - A *subacromial spur* is a traction spur (enthesophyte) at or adjacent to the acromial attachment of the coracoacromial ligament.
    - Visible on radiographs or MRI (sagittal oblique or coronal oblique) sequences.
    - Extends anteriorly and inferiorly from the anterior acromion process (Fig. 2.18A).
    - Distinguished from the coracoacromial ligament on MRI, which is a dark structure on all sequences, whereas a subacromial spur contains marrow fat (Fig. 2.18B).

- *Os acromiale* (see Fig. 2.58) is associated with rotator cuff impingement and rotator cuff tears.
  - Unstable os acromiale may narrow the subacromial space due to downward pull from the deltoid.
  - Degenerative osteophytes at the os acromiale synchondrosis may likewise narrow the subacromial space.
- Contour of the acromial undersurface can contribute to rotator cuff impingement.
  - Acromial undersurface contour best determined by an outlet radiograph or may be seen on sagittal oblique MR images (Fig. 2.19).
  - Somewhat dependent on the orientation of the images, as well as on which image is selected.
  - Use only the two most lateral images from the sagittal oblique sequence.
  - *Modified Bigliani classification* used to characterize the acromial undersurface morphology (Box 2.1).
- Acromial slope is a separate morphologic consideration, depicted best on coronal oblique images.
  - *Lateral downsloping* thought to contribute to rotator cuff impingement, although this has not been convincingly proven.

Impingement-related pain is due to compression of the rotator cuff tendons and the subacromial/subdeltoid bursa between the humeral head and the coracoacromial arch.

- Rotator cuff impingement syndrome occurs more frequently in older patients but may also be seen in younger individuals.
- Cardinal feature is reproducible pain with overhead maneuvers (when the shoulder is abducted).
- Occurs more frequently in individuals who perform repetitive overhead activities, such as throwing athletes or certain workers.
- Impingement syndrome is a clinical diagnosis, although anatomic factors that contribute to rotator cuff impingement and sequelae of impingement may be seen on imaging studies.
  - Imaging findings on MRI and US include subacromial/subdeltoid bursitis, rotator cuff tendinopathy, and rotator cuff tears.
  - Supraspinatus tendon is the most vulnerable rotator cuff tendon because of its anatomic location at the most frequent site of impingement between the anterior acromion and humeral head.

Coracohumeral impingement is an uncommon cause of rotator cuff impingement that results from the compression of the subscapularis tendon due to narrowing of the coracohumeral space.

- Measured on axial images when imaged with MRI or CT.
- Normal distance between the anterior aspect of the humeral head and the posterior margin of the coracoid process is approximately 8–11 mm, which may be slightly lower in women.
- Coracohumeral distance of less than 7 mm may result in entrapment of the subscapularis tendon between the anterior humeral head and the coracoid process.
- US is useful for demonstrating narrowing of the coracohumeral distance and dynamic impingement of the

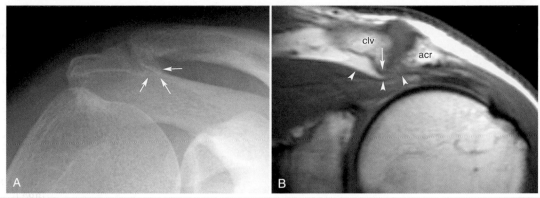

Fig. 2.17 **Acromioclavicular osteophytes. (A and B)** AP radiograph **(A)** and oblique coronal T1-weighted MR image in a different patient **(B)** show osteophytes protruding inferiorly from the acromioclavicular joint *(arrows)*, with deformation of the supraspinatus tendon in B *(arrowheads)*. *acr*, Acromion; *clv*, clavicle.

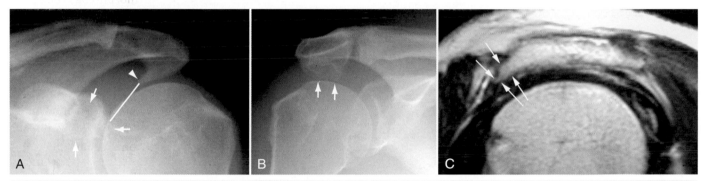

Fig. 2.18 **Anterior acromial spur. (A)** AP radiograph shows an unusually long anterior enthesophyte *(arrowhead)* originating from the anterior acromion. The *line* marks the location of the coracoacromial ligament. *Arrows* mark the coracoid, which is superimposed on the glenoid. **(B)** AP radiograph oriented mildly caudad in another individual with an anterior subacromial spur *(arrows)*. The lordotic x-ray beam angulation better displays an anterior acromial spur. **(C)** Oblique sagittal T2-weighted MR image shows a spur *(arrows)* at the attachment of the coracoacromial ligament. Note that the spur contains marrow, which allows it to be distinguished on MR images from the coracoacromial ligament, which has low signal intensity on all sequences.

subscapularis tendon during shoulder adduction and internal rotation.

Internal impingement is another form of rotator cuff impingement, seen in overhead throwing athletes, especially baseball pitchers.

- Painful posterosuperior glenoid impingement of the rotator cuff during late cocking/early acceleration phase of throwing.
- Associated with undersurface (articular-sided) tears of the posterior supraspinatus and/or anterior infraspinatus tendons, cystic change and/or marrow edema at the posterosuperior humeral head, and tears of the posterosuperior glenoid labrum.

OSTEOARTHRITIS

In general, osteoarthritis develops over time as a chronic degenerative process due to 'wear and tear', with damage to the articular surfaces. Osteoarthritis in the shoulder is a common cause of symptoms in middle-aged and older individuals, though seen less frequently than in weight-bearing joints, such as the knee. Common pathoetiologies of glenohumeral joint osteoarthritis include the following:

- *Chronic instability*—chronic tears of the glenoid labrum and/or capsuloligamentous structures may result in

instability of the glenohumeral articulation, leading to accelerated cartilage wear and damage.
- *Rotator cuff arthropathy*—rotator cuff tears, particularly when large and chronic, destabilize the glenohumeral joint (due to unopposed upward forces of the deltoid muscle), manifest by cephalad migration of the humeral head and accelerated glenohumeral joint osteoarthritis.
- *Posttraumatic osteoarthritis*—trauma may result in direct damage to the articular cartilage, such as in the setting of intraarticular fractures or osteochondral lesions (OCLs). Fractures may also result in incongruity of the articular surface or result in osseous deformity, altering normal biomechanics and leading to accelerated osteoarthritis.

Disease Processes

FRACTURE

Fractures are commonly encountered in the shoulder and may involve the proximal humerus, clavicle, or scapula. A widely used classification of proximal humeral fractures in adults, the *Neer system*, provides prognostic information and aids in treatment planning based on

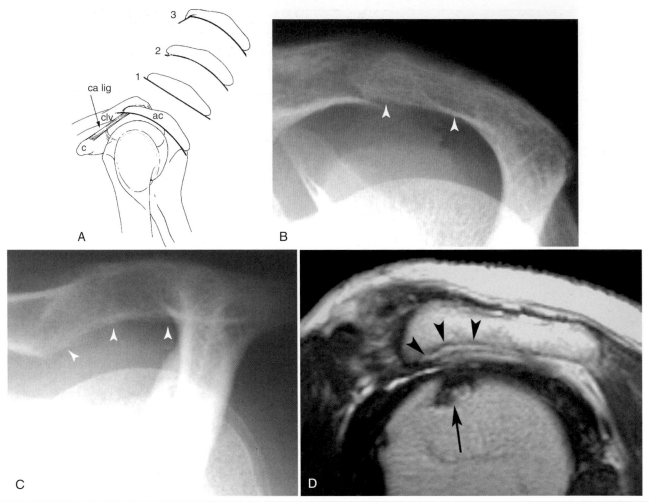

Fig. 2.19 Bigliani classification of the shape of the undersurface of the acromion. (A) Diagram with anterior to the viewer's left shows the contour of type 1 (flat), type 2 (concave), and type 3 (anterior hook). **(B)** Type 1. Outlet view shows a flat acromial undersurface *(arrowheads)*. **(C)** Type 2. Outlet view shows a concave acromial undersurface *(arrowheads)*. **(D)** Type 3. Oblique sagittal T2-weighted MR image shows anterior hook *(arrowheads)*. Also note the signal changes in the humeral head marrow *(arrow)* caused by chronic impingement. The subacromial space is narrow because there is a complete rotator cuff tear with retraction (not shown). *ac,* Acromion; *c,* coracoid process; *ca lig,* coracoacromial ligament; *clv,* clavicle.

anatomic site, number of fracture 'parts', and fracture fragment displacement. Humeral neck fractures are the most common proximal humeral fracture in adults and are especially frequent in older patients with osteoporosis (Fig. 2.20A).

- Most *Surgical neck fractures* have a good prognosis because the blood supply to the humeral head usually is preserved.
- *Anatomic neck fractures* less common and have a poor prognosis because the blood supply to the humeral head is compromised, resulting in poor healing, humeral head avascular necrosis, and secondary osteoarthritis.

Proximal humeral fractures are much less common in children than in adults.

- *Buckle (torus) fractures* of the surgical neck and proximal shaft region are most common (Fig. 2.21).
- Humeral head and greater tuberosity are formed from separate ossification centers that unite during childhood, resulting in an inverted V shape of the combined physis that may simulate a fracture on radiographs (see Fig. 2.21).

- True Salter–Harris fractures are most frequently type I fractures in children up to approximately 5 years of age (Fig. 2.22) or type II fractures in preteens.
- Salter I injury of the proximal humeral physis (epiphysiolysis) can occur as an overuse injury in older children (typically baseball pitchers), essentially a stress fracture known as *Little Leaguer's shoulder* (see Fig. 2.22D).

Fractures of the humeral shaft are predictably displaced by traction from the muscles that insert at different locations on the humerus (Fig. 2.23).

- Surgical neck fractures can result in abduction of the proximal fragment by the rotator cuff.
- Fractures between the pectoralis major and deltoid insertions result in adduction of the proximal fragment by the pectoralis.
- Fractures distal to the deltoid insertion result in abduction of the proximal fragment by the deltoid (Fig. 2.24).

Humeral fractures (or attempts at closed reduction of a humeral fracture) may injure adjacent nerves.

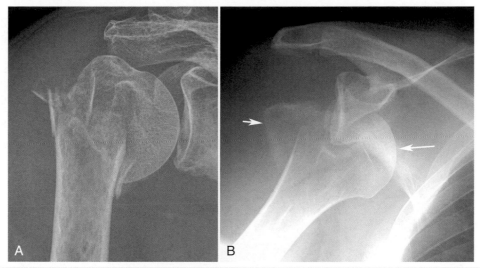

Fig. 2.20 Proximal humerus fractures in adults. (A) Surgical neck fracture. **(B)** Fracture dislocation. The humeral head *(long arrow)* is anteriorly dislocated. The greater tuberosity *(short arrow)* was sheared off and is laterally displaced from the remainder of the proximal humerus.

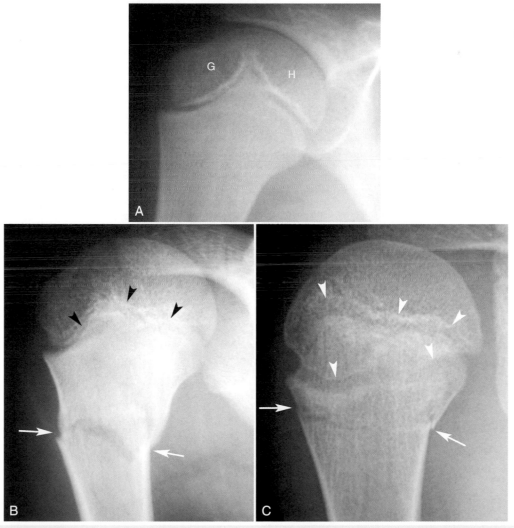

Fig. 2.21 Proximal humerus fractures in children. (A) External rotation, normal appearance. Note that the separate ossification centers for the humeral head and the greater tuberosity result in an inverted V shape of the physis. **(B)** External rotation view in a child with a metaphyseal fracture. Note the normal physis *(arrowheads)* and the more distal fracture *(arrows)*. **(C)** Internal rotation view in a different child with a metaphyseal fracture. Internal rotation causes the physis to have a complex appearance *(arrowheads)* that should not be confused with a fracture. Note the metaphyseal fracture *(arrows)*. *G*, Greater tuberosity; *H*, humeral head.

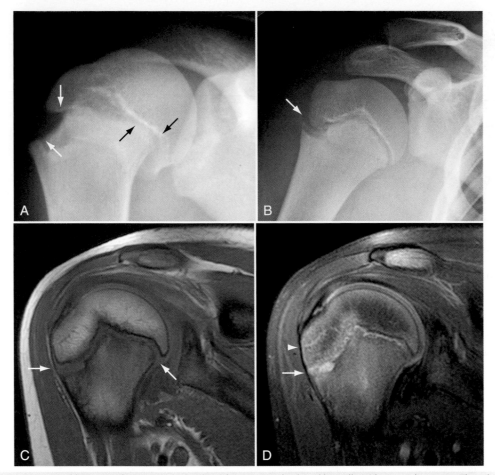

Fig. 2.22 Salter–Harris I proximal humerus fracture. (A) The distal fragment is displaced laterally with varus alignment. The *white* and *black* pairs of *arrows* show the displacement. **(B and C)** These fractures can be extremely subtle. Radiograph in a different child **(B)** shows a minimal step off with lateral displacement of the proximal shaft at the physis *(arrow)*. This radiograph was subtly asymmetric with the contralateral shoulder. **(C)** Oblique coronal T1-weighted MR image shows widened physis *(arrows)*. T2-weighted image (not shown) showed adjacent edema. **(D)** Stress fracture of the proximal humeral physis, also known as Little Leaguer's shoulder, in a 13-year-old baseball pitcher. Oblique coronal fat-suppressed T2-weighted image shows high-signal edema *(arrow)* along the lateral physis and edema within the lateral epiphysis *(arrowhead)*. Radiographs in this case were normal but can sometimes show widening of the physis and adjacent sclerosis.

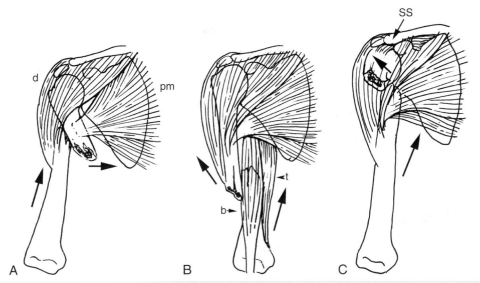

Fig. 2.23 Displacement of humeral fractures. (A) Fractures between the pectoralis major and deltoid insertions result in adduction of the proximal fragment by the pectoralis. **(B)** Fractures distal to the deltoid insertion result in abduction of the proximal fragment by the deltoid (see also Fig. 2.24). The fragments may override, as shown in the diagram. The distal fragment is pulled proximally by the biceps and triceps muscles and medially by the pectoralis major muscle. **(C)** Displaced surgical neck fractures can result in abduction of the proximal fragment by the supraspinatus muscle, as well as proximal displacement of the distal fragment, similar to B. *b*, Biceps; *d*, deltoid; *pm*, pectoralis major; *ss*, supraspinatus muscle; *t*, triceps.

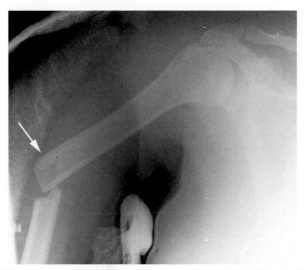

Fig. 2.24 Humeral fracture. Fracture distal to the deltoid tuberosity (*arrow*) results in abduction of the proximal fragment.

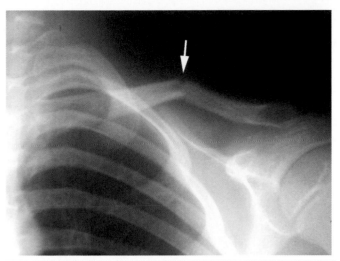

Fig. 2.25 Clavicle fracture in a child (*arrow*). As in an adult, the sternocleidomastoid muscle pulls the proximal fragment superiorly.

- *Axillary nerve* courses around the surgical neck.
- *Radial nerve* courses along the posterior humeral shaft.

Depending on the location and severity, humeral fractures may be treated with an arm sling, cast immobilization, or surgery.

- Most patients tolerate less than anatomic alignment quite well because the highly mobile shoulder joint can compensate for some rotational and angular deformity.
- Internal fixation is usually reserved for severe or complex fractures, such as segmental or intraarticular fractures, or for cases with associated neurovascular injury.
- Severe humeral head fractures may also be treated with arthroplasty, particularly in elderly patients or when fractures are markedly comminuted and involve the articular surface; humeral hemiarthroplasty or total shoulder arthroplasty may be used.

In both children and adults, most clavicle fractures are caused by a fall on an outstretched hand, and most fractures occur at the middle third.

- Fracture fragments are frequently displaced because the sternocleidomastoid muscle pulls the medial fragment superiorly and the weight of the arm pulls the distal fragment inferiorly (Fig. 2.25).
- Muscles that attach the shoulder to the chest wall, such as the pectoralis major and latissimus dorsi, often medially displace the distal fragment, causing the fragments to override.
- Despite such displacement, most clavicle fractures heal rapidly without complication and with minimal immobilization required.
- Childhood clavicle fractures may be incomplete (see Fig. 2.25).
- Surgical fixation of clavicle fractures is usually reserved for open fractures, fractures in high-level athletes, cases of delayed union or nonunion (see Fig. 1.27A), and distal fractures associated with AC or coracoclavicular ligament disruption.

Scapula fractures are usually the result of direct high-impact trauma. Scapula fractures can be a challenge to identify on radiographs in the acute traumatic setting due to overlapping anatomy and support devices, and presence of other fractures (Fig. 2.26).

- Knowledge of the mechanism of injury and careful scrutiny of the scapula is needed.
- Scapular body fractures are usually treated with immobilization.
- Fractures of the glenoid, scapular neck, and coracoid process are often treated with surgical reduction and fixation.
- CT is particularly helpful in detecting and characterizing scapula fractures and for identifying involvement of the glenoid articular surface (see Fig. 2.26B).

GLENOHUMERAL DISLOCATION

The shoulder is the most frequently dislocated major joint. Glenohumeral dislocation may occur in almost any direction, but most dislocations (95%) are anterior (Fig. 2.27). Posterior glenohumeral dislocation is much less common than anterior dislocation. Radiographs are diagnostic when a properly positioned scapular Y-view, axillary, or transthoracic view is performed. Shoulder dislocation in directions other than anterior and posterior are unusual. A distinctive form of inferior dislocation, termed *luxatio erecta*, occurs after forceful abduction of the humerus and results in fixed abduction of the arm (Fig. 2.28).

Anterior dislocation

- Mechanism: forced extension, abduction, and external rotation of the arm; also, anterior distraction or a direct blow to the posterior shoulder.
- On radiographs, humeral head is positioned anterior, medial, and slightly inferior to the glenoid fossa.
- Posterosuperior humeral head contacts the anteroinferior glenoid rim, which may result in a wedge-shaped

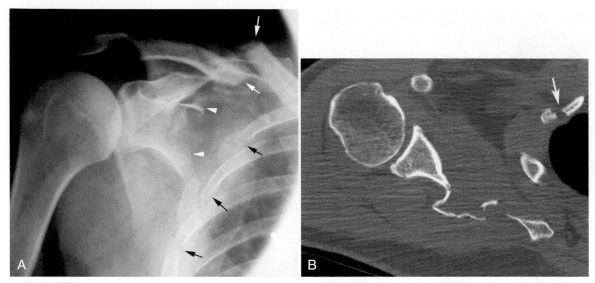

Fig. 2.26 Scapula fracture. (A) Radiograph shows scapula fracture *(white arrowheads)*. Also note the rib fractures *(black arrows)* and the clavicle fracture *(white arrows)*. **(B)** Axial CT in a different patient shows typical comminution of the scapular blade. Also note superior rib fracture *(arrow)*. Scapula fractures often occur in high-force injuries such as motor vehicle accident ejections, with frequent associated fractures.

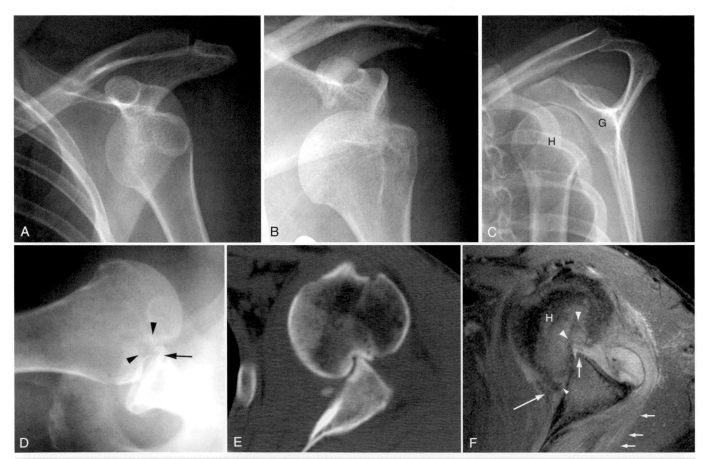

Fig. 2.27 Anterior shoulder dislocation in different patients. (A) AP view shows the humeral head inferior and medial to the coracoid. **(B)** Grashey (true AP) view in a different patient also shows the subcoracoid and medial position of the humeral head. **(C)** Y-view shows the humeral head *(H)* anterior to the glenoid *(G)*. **(D)** Axillary view shows a Hill–Sachs lesion *(arrowheads)* caused by impaction against the anterior glenoid *(arrow)*. **(E)** Axial CT scan shows similar findings. **(F)** Axial fat-suppressed proton density MR image also shows the anteriorly dislocated humeral head *(H)* impacted against the anterior glenoid *(short arrow)* and a Hill–Sachs lesion *(large arrowheads)*. The anterior labrum is displaced medially *(small arrowhead)*. Also note stripped anterior capsule *(long arrow)* and edema in the infraspinatus and teres minor muscle bellies *(small arrows)* due to muscle strains.

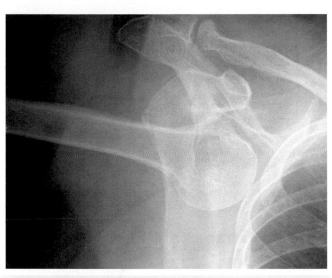

Fig. 2.28 Luxatio erecta. Frontal radiograph shows humeral head dislocated inferiorly with the humerus locked in abduction.

humeral head impaction fracture, termed a *Hill–Sachs lesion* (Fig. 2.29).

- Hill–Sachs lesion may be quite subtle and apparent only on radiographs obtained after the dislocation is reduced.
- Radiographs obtained in internal rotation are more sensitive for detection, because the fracture is located posterolaterally.
- Both CT and MRI are highly sensitive in depicting Hill–Sachs lesions.
- Associated marrow edema on MRI typically seen when imaged in the acute-to-subacute period (< 6–8 weeks following injury).
- Size of a Hill–Sachs lesion should be noted (width and depth); larger lesions are more strongly associated with subsequent anterior glenohumeral instability and may engage with the glenoid (off-track lesions).
- Potential pitfall: posterolateral humeral head has a normal indentation above the surgical neck, potentially simulating a Hill–Sachs lesion.

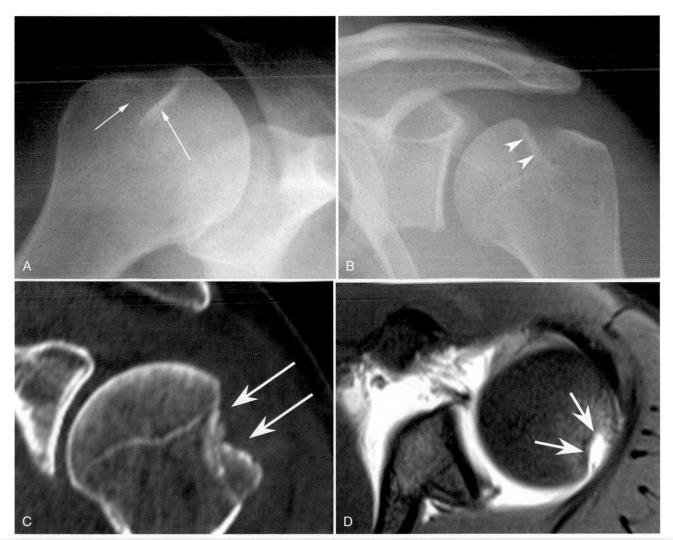

Fig. 2.29 Hill–Sachs lesions in different patients. (A) AP radiograph in internal rotation shows a notchlike defect in the posterosuperior humeral head *(arrows)*. **(B)** Grashey view shows a Hill–Sachs lesion *(arrowheads)*. **(C)** Coronally reformatted CT image shows similar defect *(arrows)*. **(D)** Axial T1-weighted MR arthrogram shows notchlike defect. Note that the Hill–Sachs lesion is seen at the level of the base of the coracoid process. More inferior notched contours are developmental in nature and should not be confused with a Hill–Sachs lesion. *C*, Coracoid process.

- Indentation occurs below the level of the coracoid process as seen on axial images, whereas Hill–Sachs lesions are seen at or above the level of the coracoid process.
- Anterior dislocation also injures the anterior structures of the shoulder.
  - *Bankart lesion* (Figs. 2.30 to 2.32) is a tear or separation of the anteroinferior glenoid labrum, sometimes found with a fracture of the adjacent glenoid rim (*osseous Bankart lesion* or *Bankart fracture*).
  - A variety of patterns of anterior labral tear may be seen (see Fig. 2.31).
    - *Perthes lesion*—nondisplaced anteroinferior labral tear with periosteal stripping from the glenoid rim (see Fig. 2.31).
    - *ALPSA lesion* (anterior labroligamentous periosteal sleeve avulsion)—detachment of the anteroinferior labrum from the glenoid with more extensive periosteal stripping and medial displacement of the torn labrum (see Fig. 2.31).
    - *GLAD lesion* (glenolabral articular disruption)—anteroinferior labral tear with adjacent cartilage lesion (see Fig. 2.31).
- Associated soft tissue injuries include glenohumeral ligament tears, CHL tear or avulsion, subscapularis tears (with/without subluxation of the LHBT), avulsion fracture of the lesser tuberosity (Fig. 2.33), and stripping of the anterior joint capsule.
- A *Bankart fracture*, or "bony Bankart", may be a subtle finding on radiographs but is more easily identified with CT or MRI (Fig. 2.30B).
  - Bankart fractures may result in a displaced fragment or impaction of the anteroinferior glenoid rim.
  - Presence of glenoid marrow edema indicates that an osseous Bankart lesion is likely to be acute or subacute.
- Bankart lesions and related soft tissue injuries are the most important sequelae of an anterior shoulder dislocation because they damage the anterior glenohumeral stabilizers.
  - Results in instability and potential for recurrent dislocations, particularly in teenagers and young adults.
  - Associated soft tissue injuries can be difficult to detect on routine MR images unless the joint capsule is distended by an effusion or by arthrographic contrast.

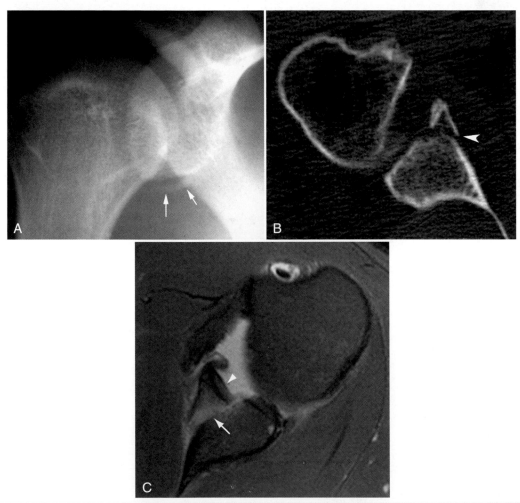

Fig. 2.30 Bankart fractures in different patients. (A) Radiograph shows a subtle fracture fragment inferior to the glenoid *(arrows)*. **(B)** CT shows anterior inferior glenoid fracture *(arrowhead)*. **(C)** Axial fat-suppressed T1-weighted MR arthrogram image shows Bankart fracture *(arrow)* with large medially displaced fragment *(arrowhead)*.

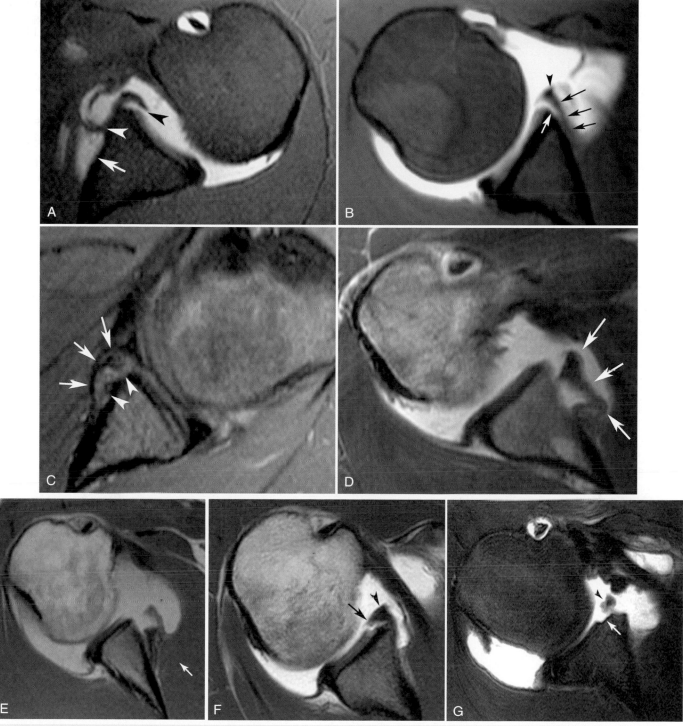

Fig. 2.31 Bankart lesions in different patients. (A) Anteroinferior labral tear *(black arrowhead)* shown on fat-suppressed T1-weighted MR arthrogram. This patient has a normal attachment of the anterior capsule *(white arrowhead)* without periosteal stripping. *Arrow* denotes extravasated contrast beyond the joint capsule. **(B)** Labral tear with periosteal stripping (Perthes lesion). Axial T1-weighted MR arthrogram shows that the anteroinferior labrum *(arrowhead)* is stripped away from the glenoid with glenoid periosteum *(arrows)*. In this variant the labrum remains attached to the periosteum, which is stripped off the anterior glenoid. Note high signal intensity of contrast medium between the glenoid and the stripped periosteum and labrum *(white arrow)*. **(C)** Another Perthes lesion, shown on unenhanced fat-suppressed T2-weighted MR image. The stripped capsule and labrum *(arrows)* appear separated from the scapula by intermediate-signal material *(arrowheads)* that was granulation tissue and hemorrhage at arthroscopy. **(D)** Anterior labroligamentous periosteal sleeve avulsion (ALPSA lesion). This lesion *(arrows)* may be considered a medially displaced Perthes lesion. The labrum, anterior band of the inferior glenohumeral ligament, and associated stripped periosteum have displaced medially. This Bankart variant has a high association with anterior instability and recurrent shoulder dislocation. **(E)** Another ALPSA lesion *(arrow)*. **(F)** Glenolabral articular disruption (GLAD lesion). The anteroinferior labrum *(arrowhead)* and a fragment of underlying articular cartilage *(arrow)* have detached as a unit from the glenoid. **(G)** Another GLAD lesion. The anteroinferior labrum and a fragment of underlying articular cartilage have completely detached as a unit *(arrowhead)* from the glenoid. Note chondral defect *(arrow)*.

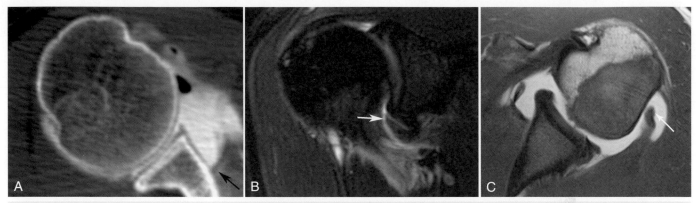

Fig. 2.32 Additional anterior soft tissue injuries following anterior shoulder dislocation. (A) Anterior capsular stripping. CT arthrogram shows medial displacement of the anterior capsule margin; an acute angle is formed by the anterior capsule and the scapula *(arrow)*. Contrast this finding with the obtuse angle in Fig. 2.31A. **(B)** Humeral avulsion of the inferior glenohumeral ligament (HAGL) lesion. Coronal fat-suppressed T2-weighted MR image shows interrupted lateral attachment of the inferior glenohumeral ligament (GHL) *(arrow)*, which is curved into a J shape. **(C)** Axial MR arthrogram image in a different patient shows abnormal position of the posterior band inferior GHL *(arrow)*. Tears of the GHLs are common after dislocation, and tears of the inferior GHL are the most clinically significant.

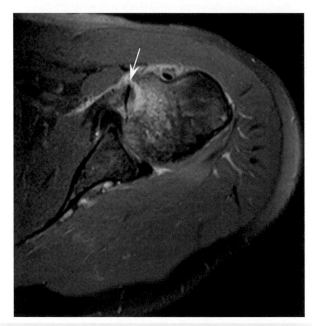

Fig. 2.33 Lesser tuberosity avulsion fracture. Axial proton density fat-suppressed MR image demonstrates an acute avulsion of the lesser tuberosity *(arrow)* at the subscapularis attachment site, with intense marrow edema in the anteromedial humeral head.

- MR arthrography is often performed prior to surgery to fully assess soft tissue injury.
- Several potential pitfalls may falsely suggest anterior capsular injury on MR arthrography.
  - Can be difficult to differentiate traumatic capsular stripping from an atraumatic, normal-variant medial capsular attachment.
  - Appearance of the joint capsule on imaging studies depends on the amount of fluid in the joint and the position of the humerus.
  - Previously stripped joint capsule may join the scapula at a shallow angle, whereas an atraumatic normal-variant medial capsular attachment often forms an obtuse angle (see Figs. 2.31 and 2.32; see also Fig. 2.12).

- Injected contrast medium may 'extravasate' along the anteromedial scapula, simulating capsular stripping (Fig. 2.31A); such extravasated contrast often dissects into the subscapularis muscle, resulting in a distinctive pattern (see Fig. 2.7E).
- Normal subscapularis and axillary recesses should not be mistaken for a pathologically redundant capsule.
- Normal labral variants are seen in the anterosuperior quadrant (12:00 to 3:00), as discussed in the **Anatomy** section.
- Normal synovial folds or inadvertently injected air bubbles may simulate an intraarticular loose body on MR arthrography.

Posterior dislocation

- Mechanism: forceful muscle contraction (seizure or electrocution), fall onto a flexed and adducted arm, or a forceful direct blow to the anterior shoulder.
  - Seizures and electrocution can result in bilateral dislocations.
- Humeral head usually dislocates directly posteriorly and is locked in internal rotation.
- AP radiographs may be misleading because the posteriorly dislocated humeral head can project over its normal position on this view.
- Scapular Y-view or axillary view is diagnostic (Fig. 2.34).
- Anterior humeral head impacts against the posterior glenoid rim, which may result in an anterior humeral head impaction fracture *(reverse Hill–Sachs lesion)*.
  - Reverse Hill–Sachs lesion may be appreciated on an AP radiograph as a vertically oriented linear impression *(trough sign, Fig. 2.35; see also Fig. 2.34A and C)*.
- Associated osseous and soft tissue injuries mirror those of anterior dislocation.
  - Posterior joint capsule is stripped off of the glenoid and the posterior labrum is often torn.
    - Results in posterior glenohumeral instability, leaving the patient vulnerable to recurrent posterior dislocations.

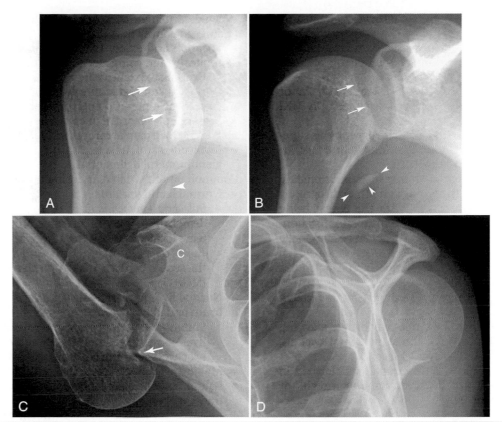

Fig. 2.34 Posterior shoulder dislocations. (A) Grashey view shows overlap of the humeral head and glenoid, indicating that a dislocation is present. Note the subtle humeral head impaction fracture *(arrows)*, termed the *trough sign*, and the small reverse Bankart fracture *(arrowhead)*. **(B)** Postreduction AP view shows the trough sign (reverse Hill–Sachs fracture) *(arrows)*. Also note the reverse Bankart fracture fragment *(arrowheads)*. **(C)** Axillary view in a different patient shows reverse Hill–Sachs fracture *(arrow)*. Note that the dislocation is opposite from the coracoid process *(C)*. **(D)** Y-view in another patient with posterior dislocation. Compare with Fig. 2.27C.

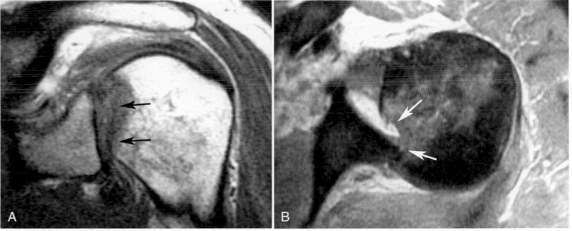

Fig. 2.35 Posterior shoulder dislocation on MRI. (A and B) Coronal T1-weighted **(A)** and axial fat-suppressed T2-weighted **(B)** MR images show posterior dislocation with impaction fracture *(arrows)* and adjacent marrow edema.

■ May also see posterior glenoid rim fracture (*reverse Bankart fracture*; see Fig. 2.34C).

LABRAL TEAR

Imaging diagnosis of labral tears is complicated by the normal variation of labral shape and fixation to the glenoid, particularly the anterosuperior labrum, discussed earlier in the **Anatomy** section. Labral tears may result in shoulder pain, weakness, mechanical symptoms (locking, grinding, or catching), particularly in younger patients and athletes. Degeneration of the superior labrum characterized by tearing or fraying may occur with aging; abnormalities of the superior labrum in middle-aged and older individuals are generally not treated surgically. The labrum is best evaluated by MRI.

- Normal labrum has low signal intensity on all MRI sequences.
- Magic angle effect results in increased signal intensity on short TE sequences in portions of the labrum oriented 55 degrees to the bore of the magnet.
- Linear or amorphous high signal intensity on PD or T2-weighted imaging suggests a labral tear on MRI (Fig. 2.36).
- Direct MR arthrography (and CT arthrography) is superior to conventional MRI for diagnosing a labral tear, increasing conspicuity and sensitivity.
  - Abnormal T1-hyperintense contrast signal extending into the substance of the labrum on MR arthrography is diagnostic of a labral tear, with the caveat being normal labral variants in the anterosuperior location.
- Detection of an anteroinferior labral tear can be marginally improved by placing the arm in the *ABER position*, which places tension on the anteroinferior labroligamentous complex (see Fig. 2.36C and D).
- *Paralabral cysts* may form in the setting of an underlying labral tear.
  - Labral tear functions as a one-way valve, allowing joint fluid to pass through the tear but not back in, resulting in a fluid-filled cystic mass.
  - Can result in compression neuropathy if located in the spinoglenoid notch, suprascapular notch, or quadrilateral space (see Fig. 2.64).

- When describing a labral tear, there are several pertinent findings to convey in the report.
  - Location and extent (should be described both anatomically and using clock faces, to avoid confusion).
    - Example: 'Extensive tear of the superior and anterior labrum extending from 11:00 posterosuperiorly through 4:00 anteroinferiorly'.
  - Presence of a labral flap or displaced fragment.
  - Presence of a paralabral cyst, including size and location.
  - Involvement of adjacent structures (biceps anchor, glenohumeral ligaments).
- Common pitfalls when diagnosing a labral tear include:
  - Normal labral variants
    - *Sublabral foramen*, *sulcus*, or *recess*—such variants demonstrate smooth margins and are almost always located between the 12:00 and 3:00 positions.
    - *Buford complex* — absent anterosuperior labrum and thickened, cordlike middle glenohumeral ligament (MGHL).
  - Normal finding of articular cartilage between the labrum and glenoid at the chondrolabral junction.
    - Smooth, tapering, intermediate-signal-intensity hyaline cartilage immediately subjacent to dark fibrocartilage of the labrum.
  - Magic angle effect.
  - Labral tears in older individuals are often incidental and not clinically significant.

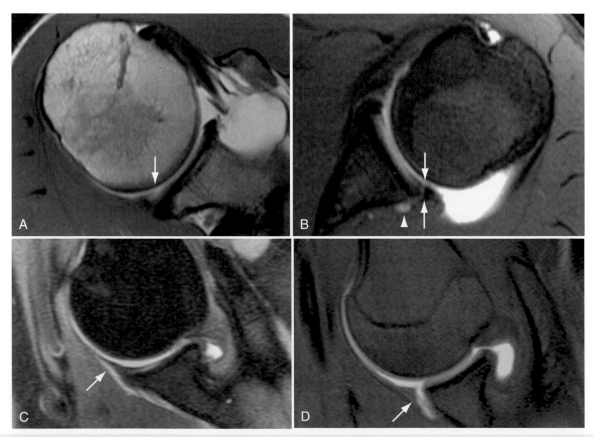

Fig. 2.36 Labral tears. (A) Axial fat-suppressed T1-weighted arthrogram in a baseball pitcher with internal impingement shows a posterior labral tear *(arrow)*. **(B)** MR arthrogram image in a different patient shows a subtle posterior labral tear (between *arrows*), confirmed by finding of intraarticular contrast medium beginning to fill an adjacent paralabral cyst *(arrowhead)*. **(C and D)** Abduction and external rotation (ABER) position to enhance detection of anterior labral tear. **(C)** Normal ABER view. Fat-suppressed T1-weighted MR arthrogram in ABER position shows intact inferior labrum and inferior glenohumeral ligament *(arrow)*. **(D)** MR arthrogram ABER view shows a tear of the anterior inferior labrum *(arrow)*. See also Fig. 2.31A.

SLAP *tears* represent a subset of commonly encountered labral tears that invariably involve the superior labrum, a frequent indication for MR arthrography (Fig. 2.37).

- Proximal biceps tendon, and biceps attachment to the labrum (*biceps anchor*) are variably involved.
- Many SLAP tears occur after a forced extension injury or during rapid arm abduction during a fall.
- SLAP tears also occur during the deceleration phase of overhead throwing and are thus an occupational hazard of athletes who throw, such as baseball pitchers.
- The following classification system is used for SLAP tears:
  - Type 1: degenerative superior labral fraying, with a normal LHBT.
    - Type 1 tears have amorphously increased signal in the superior labrum on coronal oblique MR images.
    - This can be a "normal" finding in older patients, especially patients with a chronically high-riding shoulder, such as those with chronic rotator cuff tear.
  - Type 2: superior labral tear with involvement of the biceps anchor.
  - Type 3: superior labral bucket handle tear with intact biceps anchor.
  - Type 4: superior labral bucket handle tear that extends into the LHBT (see Fig. 2.37).

SLAP tears can extend beyond the superior labrum and adjacent biceps into the anterior labrum, posterior labrum, or the glenohumeral ligaments. There are evolving arthroscopic classification systems of these more extensive tears.

- SLAP tears (other than Type 1) show a discrete defect in the superior labrum that extends from anterior to posterior, which must be distinguished from the previously discussed normal-variant sublabral sulcus (see Fig. 2.9B).
  - On coronal oblique MR images, the normal-variant sublabral sulcus is typically oriented in an inferolateral to superomedial direction (toward the patient's head).
  - In contrast, many (but not all) SLAP tears are oriented in a superolateral to inferomedial direction (toward the acromion).
  - Sublabral sulcus should not extend posterior to the biceps anchor, and usually not posterior to the 11:00 position.
  - Width of the space between the superior labrum and the glenoid greater than 2–3 mm usually indicates a SLAP tear rather than a sulcus.

Symptomatic labral tears in younger individuals are usually repaired arthroscopically. The torn labrum is

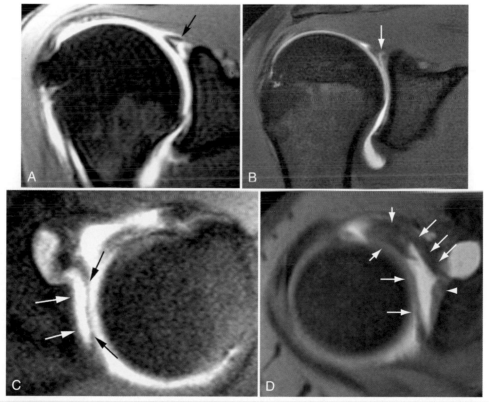

Fig. 2.37 Superior labral anterior to posterior (SLAP) tears in different patients. (A) Oblique coronal fat-suppressed T1-weighted MR arthrogram shows high signal intensity within the superior labrum, oriented toward the acromion *(arrow)*. **(B)** More subtle SLAP tear in a different patient. **(C)** Axial T2-weighted saline arthrogram image obtained at the level of the superior labrum in a different patient shows fluid tracking between the labrum *(black arrows)* and the glenoid *(white arrows)*. The separation of the labrum and the glenoid is greater than 2–3 mm and extends posteriorly to the 10:00 position; it is therefore likely to represent a SLAP tear rather than a sublabral sulcus. **(D)** Type 4 (bucket handle) SLAP tear. Axial fat-suppressed T1-weighted MR arthrogram image. Note the retracted biceps labral complex (between *short arrows*) and only contrast where the biceps long head normally attaches to the glenoid *(arrowhead)*. The partially detached labrum *(long arrows)* connects the avulsed biceps labral complex to the glenoid in a bucket handle configuration.

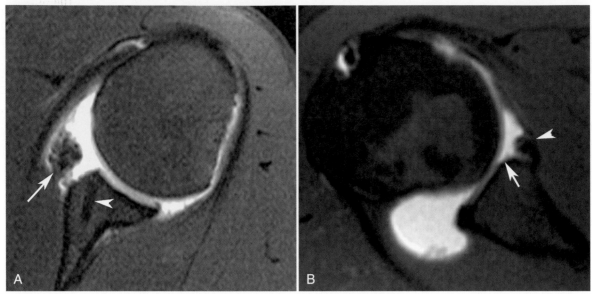

Fig. 2.38 Failed Bankart repairs in different patients. Axial MR arthrograms. **(A)** Detached Bankart fragment *(arrow)*. Note suture anchor seen as a subtle linear low signal in the glenoid *(arrowhead)*. **(B)** Recurrent GLAD (glenolabral articular defect, *arrowhead*), with defect of anterior glenoid cartilage *(arrow)*. Note anterior subluxation of the humeral head.

reattached by suturing the labrum to suture anchors that are set into the glenoid. Debridement of irregular or loose labral margins may also be performed during arthroscopy. Special considerations for imaging of the postoperative labrum must be taken into account.

- Direct MR arthrography can be of considerable value in evaluating the postoperative labrum (Fig. 2.38).
- Normal postoperative appearance may include fraying and blunting of the repaired labrum, as the labrum is often debrided.
- Abnormal signal within the substance of the labrum may represent postoperative granulation tissue or fibrosis.
- Labral retear is diagnosed when contrast extends completely beneath the repaired labrum, there is uncovering of a suture anchor, or there is displacement of the labrum.

OSTEOCHONDRAL INJURY

- Osteochondral injuries of the shoulder include osseous Bankart and reverse Bankart fractures, already discussed, as well as GLAD lesions (see Fig. 2.31F).
- Although the shoulder is not a weight-bearing joint, considerable loads are placed across the shoulder joint during abduction, and osteochondral lesions (*OCLs*) or articular cartilage injuries may result.
- Most articular cartilage defects of the glenohumeral joint occur in the setting of osteoarthritis, though discrete OCLs may be seen in younger individuals, particularly high-level athletes (Fig. 2.39).

CAPSULOLIGAMENTOUS INJURIES

- Injuries to the glenohumeral joint capsule and glenohumeral ligaments may occur in the setting of glenohumeral dislocation, in combination with labral tears, or in isolation.

- Injuries to the IGHL may occur at the medial (glenoid) or lateral (humeral) attachment sites.
  - IGHL tear from its humeral attachment is termed a *HAGL lesion* (humeral avulsion of the glenohumeral ligament) (Fig. 2.32B and C).
  - IGHL tear from its glenoid attachment is termed a *GAGL lesion* (glenoid avulsion of the glenohumeral ligament).

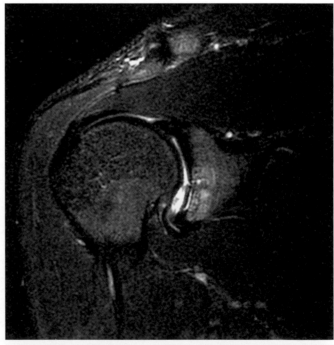

Fig. 2.39 Osteochondral lesion (OCL) of the glenoid. Coronal STIR MR image shows an OCL at the inferior glenoid with fluid undermining the osteochondral fragment, consistent with instability. Small glenohumeral joint effusion is noted.

- MR arthrogram imaging demonstrates irregularity and/or disruption of the IGHL with contrast extravasation inferiorly from the joint capsule into the axillary soft tissues.
- Traumatic rotator interval lesions include injuries to the rotator interval capsule, biceps pulley, CHL, or SGHL.
  - MRI may demonstrate edema and infiltration of the rotator interval fat, similar to adhesive capsulitis.
  - MR arthrography provides better visualization of structures of the rotator interval by distending the joint capsule.

GLENOHUMERAL OSTEOARTHRITIS

Glenohumeral joint osteoarthritis is typically diagnosed on radiographs but is also frequently encountered in older individuals on MRI.

- Glenohumeral joint osteoarthritis may result from chronic instability, rotator cuff insufficiency, or in the posttraumatic setting.
- Similar to osteoarthritis in other joints, MRI findings include articular cartilage loss, subchondral changes (cystic change, marrow edema, sclerosis), and marginal osteophytes (see **Chapter 9 - Arthritis**).
- In severe osteoarthritis, there is often remodeling of the humeral head and glenoid and there may be accompanying intraarticular bodies within the joint recesses or LHBT sheath.

Total shoulder arthroplasty is performed for painful arthritis when conservative management has failed. There are two main types of shoulder arthroplasties: anatomic and reverse.

- If the rotator cuff is functional, *anatomic total shoulder arthroplasty* is typically performed.
- If there is a large rotator cuff tear or the rotator cuff is otherwise insufficient, a *reverse total shoulder arthroplasty* is generally performed.

- Glenoid component is converted into a 'ball' and the humeral head component is converted into a 'socket', moving the center of rotation of the shoulder inferomedially.
- Improves joint stability and mobility by enhancing action of the deltoid muscle.
- MRI is typically requested in the setting of end-stage osteoarthritis prior to surgery to evaluate integrity of the rotator cuff.

ROTATOR CUFF TENDINOSIS

Recurrent impingement causes tendon edema and hemorrhage, and can lead to tendinitis, fibrosis, and degeneration. *Tendinitis* is a clinical term for an acutely painful tendon, but is a bit of a misnomer as inflammatory cellular infiltrates in the symptomatic tendon are usually not a prominent feature. Thus, the alternative umbrella terms *tendinopathy* or *tendinosis* are generally preferable.

- Changes result in an increase in free water within the tendon, seen on MRI as increased signal intensity on both T1- and T2-weighted sequences (Fig. 2.40).
- Tendinopathy is also often characterized by abnormal tendon thickening (*hypertrophic tendinosis*), although eventually tendon attenuation may occur (*attritional tendinosis*).
- Healing is possible but is limited by poor tendon blood supply; the *critical zone* of the rotator cuff (approximately 1 cm medial to the greater tuberosity insertion) is a watershed zone between arterial supplies.
- Severity or degree of tendinosis may be estimated but lacks standardization and is susceptible to interobserver variability.
- Ongoing tendon impingement may ultimately progress to partial and full-thickness rotator cuff tear.

Surgical treatment of rotator cuff impingement usually is accomplished by surgical decompression of the subacromial space (Fig. 2.41).

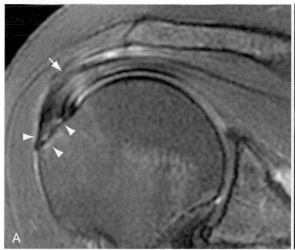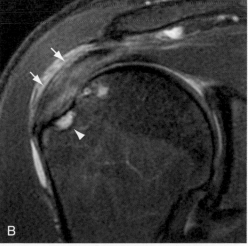

Fig. 2.40 Rotator cuff tendinosis (tendinopathy). (A) Mild. Oblique coronal fat-suppressed T2-weighted MR image shows increased signal in the rotator cuff tendons *(arrow)*, but no areas of very high signal intensity to indicate tear. Also note areas of insertional tendon high signal intensity and mild marrow edema *(arrowheads)*. Arthroscopy showed no tear, and the signal changes were due to tendon degeneration. **(B)** More severe tendinosis in a different patient. Note the thickened and edematous supraspinatus tendon *(arrows)*. Also note subcortical cystlike changes in the adjacent greater tuberosity *(arrowhead)* and lateral humeral head.

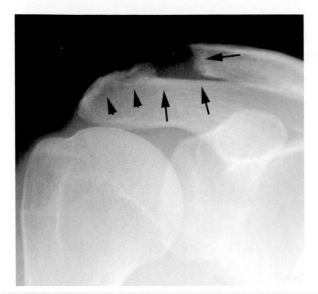

Fig. 2.41 Acromioplasty and resection of the distal clavicle. The acromial undersurface *(arrowheads)* and the distal clavicle and acromioclavicular joint *(arrows)* and accompanying spurs were resected to relieve rotator cuff impingement. Compare with Fig. 2.18A and B.

- *Acromioplasty* may be performed in cases of chronic rotator cuff impingement, or during rotator cuff repair surgery to correct a contributing factor of the rotator cuff tear.
- Inferior surface of the anterolateral acromion is resected along with any associated subacromial spur, anterior hook, or AC joint osteophytes.
- Hypertrophic changes at the AC joint may also be addressed by resection of the distal clavicle (*Mumford procedure*) or entire AC joint (see Fig. 2.41).
- Coracoacromial ligament may be debrided, resected, or released at its attachment to the acromion.
- Current surgical technique favors performing this procedure through an arthroscope placed in the subacromial bursa, a procedure termed *arthroscopic subacromial decompression*.

ROTATOR CUFF TEAR

Ongoing tendon impingement in the presence of one or more of the anatomic factors discussed earlier can result in a partial thickness tendon tear.

- Partial thickness tear may have an MRI appearance similar to that of tendinosis or may be seen as a discrete defect, usually with higher signal intensity than is seen with tendon degeneration (Figs. 2.42 and 2.43).
- Focal signal abnormality that is near fluid bright on fluid-sensitive MRI sequences likely represents a tear rather than tendinosis.
- Careful attention to window and level settings and cross-referencing with other imaging planes is helpful in confirming a subtle tear.
- Ultrasonography can also reliably depict rotator cuff tears (Fig. 2.44) and is becoming increasingly popular for initial assessment.

Partial thickness tears should be described using the following criteria:

- Type
    - Partial-thickness tear may occur along the bursal surface, along the articular surface, within the substance of the tendon (intrasubstance tear), or in some combination.
    - Some partial thickness tears are intrasubstance and extend along the length of the tendon (*delaminating tear*), with or without extension to the tendon surface (see Fig. 2.43).
        - Fluid-filled *intramuscular cysts* within the muscle belly are associated with such tears, typically at the distal myotendinous junction.
- Location
    - Location of a tear within a given tendon should be described, such as at the insertion (*footprint*) or medial to the footprint (for example, at the *critical zone*).
    - Tears may involve more than one tendon and/or propagate into adjacent tendons.
    - *Anterosuperior rotator cuff tear* refers to a commonly encountered scenario in which an anterior

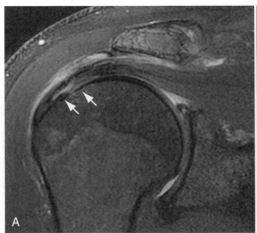 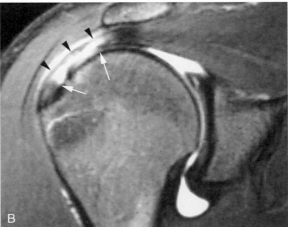

Fig. 2.42 Rotator cuff partial thickness tears. (A) Oblique coronal fat-suppressed T2-weighted image shows small partial-thickness undersurface tear *(arrows).* **(B)** Extensive partial-thickness supraspinatus undersurface tear *(arrows).* Coronal T2-weighted MR arthrogram shows extensive partial-thickness undersurface tear with only a thin layer of intact tendon *(arrowheads).* Note that there is no muscle retraction. The subacromial bursal fluid was due to a minute perforation of the infraspinatus (not shown).

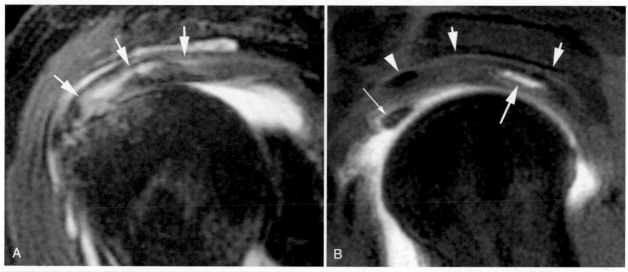

Fig. 2.43 Laminar interstitial rotator cuff tears. (A) Oblique coronal fat-suppressed T2-weighted MR image shows longitudinal intrasubstance high signal within the supraspinatus tendon *(arrows)*. Another term for this type of tear is *interstitial delamination*. **(B)** Oblique sagittal fat-suppressed T1-weighted MR arthrogram in a different patient shows contrast medium within the infraspinatus tendon *(long arrow)* that entered the tendon from a distal undersurface tear. For orientation note the acromial undersurface *(short arrows)*, supraspinatus tendon *(arrowhead)*, and biceps long head tendon *(thin arrow)*.

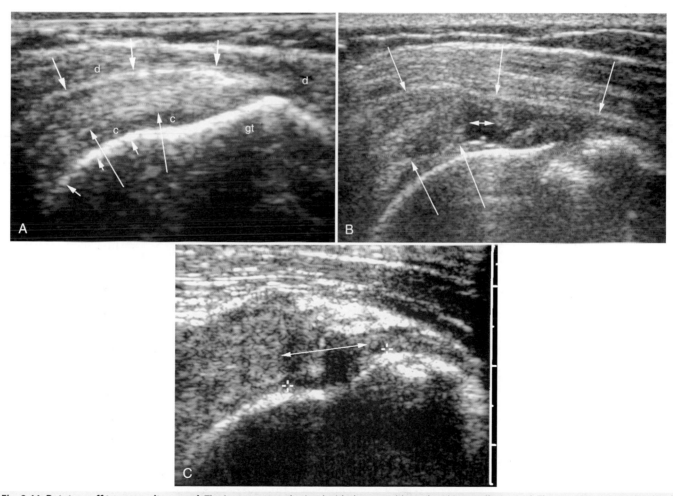

Fig. 2.44 Rotator cuff tears on ultrasound. The images were obtained with the arm adducted and internally rotated. This position moves the distal supraspinatus tendon out from under the acromion, allowing it to be imaged with ultrasound. **(A)** Longitudinal image of normal supraspinatus tendon *(long arrows)*. A normal tendon shows mildly hyperechoic uniform echotexture. Note the greater tuberosity *(gt)*, deltoid muscle *(d)*, subchondral cortex of the humeral head *(short arrows)*, and articular cartilage *(c)*. **(B)** Partial thickness undersurface tear *(double arrow)* seen as hypoechoic defect within the supraspinatus tendon *(arrows)*. **(C)** Complete tear *(double arrow)*.

supraspinatus tear extends through the rotator interval to involve the superior subscapularis tendon.

- Degenerative rotator cuff tears often occur at the *central cuff* or *conjoined tendon* formed by the posterior supraspinatus and anterior infraspinatus tendons.
- Tears of the supraspinatus *anterior leading edge* are also commonly encountered, best seen on coronal images through the anterior margin of the tendon and on sagittal images.

- Grade
  - As a general rule of thumb, *high-grade partial-thickness* tears involve greater than 50% of tendon thickness.
  - Tears involving less than 50% of tendon thickness may be considered *low-grade partial-thickness* tears, or further subcategorized into *low-grade* (<25%) and *intermediate-grade* (25–50%) partial-thickness tears.

Full-thickness tears refer to rotator cuff tears that extend from the articular surface to the bursal surface, though they may vary in size (width of involvement).

- *Complete tendon tears* (full-thickness, full-width tears) are characterized by complete disruption of a particular tendon.

- *Full-thickness tears* that do not involve the entire tendon are measured in width, that is, AP dimension for supraspinatus and infraspinatus tears, and craniocaudal (CC) dimension for subscapularis tears.
- Anatomic description also provides valuable information, for example 'full-thickness tear of the supraspinatus anterior leading edge' or 'full-thickness tear of the superior third subscapularis tendon'.
- Full-thickness tears are reliably detected on routine MRI and MR arthrography.
  - Noncontrast MRI demonstrates a full-thickness tendon defect that is fluid bright, as the tear fills with joint fluid or granulation tissue, both of which have high signal intensity on T2-weighted images (Fig. 2.45).
    - Increased fluid in the subacromial bursa is frequently an associated finding but is not specific and may simply reflect bursitis.
  - MR arthrography demonstrates contrast medium passing through the full-thickness defect into the overlying subacromial/subdeltoid bursa.
- Large full-thickness tear and a complete tear allow for varying degrees of tendon retraction; this finding should be noted in the report because retraction in

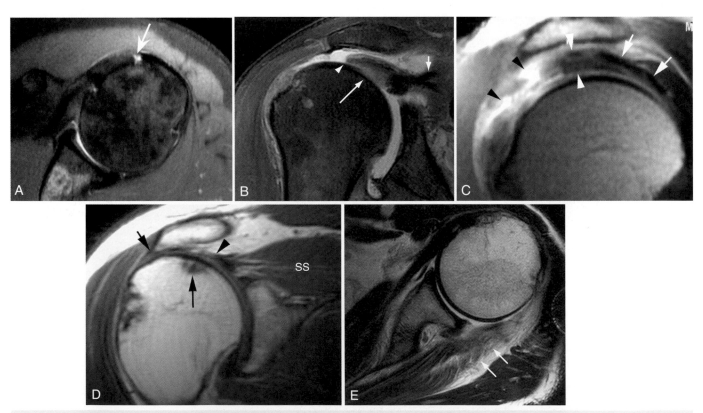

Fig. 2.45 Supraspinatus full-thickness and complete tears. (A) Small perforation. Axial fat-suppressed T2-weighted MR image shows a small tear at the anterior supraspinatus insertion *(arrow)*. **(B)** Complete tear with retraction. Note the retracted tendon free edge *(arrowhead)* and musculotendinous junction *(short arrow)*. The retracted tendon is edematous and irregular *(long arrow)*. When describing this tear, it is helpful to the surgeon to measure retraction of the free edge and the longer distance to normal-appearing tendon. **(C)** Large tear, but not complete. Oblique sagittal fat-suppressed T1-weighted MR arthrogram in a different patient shows an anterior supraspinatus tear *(black arrowheads)* with intact posterior tendon *(white arrowheads)* and intact infraspinatus *(white arrows)*. **(D)** Complete tear. Oblique coronal T1-weighted MR image in a different patient shows a supraspinatus complete tear with retraction, but no supraspinatus muscle atrophy *(SS)*. Note the retracted tendon margin *(arrowhead)*, signal changes in the superior humeral head due to impaction against the acromion *(long arrow)*, and lateral acromial spur *(short arrow)*. This patient's tear was successfully repaired. **(E)** Axial T2-weighted MR image shows complete infraspinatus tear with retraction *(arrows)* in a 32-year-old man who suffered a severe seizure. The contralateral shoulder (not shown) had an identical tear.

excess of 3–4 cm has a reduced potential for successful surgical repair.

- Chronic tears may have associated fatty atrophy of the muscle belly, which is unlikely to benefit from surgical repair, especially when fat signal has replaced 50% or more of normal muscle signal (Goutallier grade 3 or 4).
  - *Goutallier grading system* is commonly used to grade rotator cuff muscle atrophy.
    - Grade 0—normal muscle.
    - Grade 1—fatty streaking without loss of muscle bulk.
    - Grade 2—fatty atrophy with <50% loss of muscle bulk.
    - Grade 3—fatty atrophy with approximately 50% loss of muscle bulk.
    - Grade 4—fatty atrophy with <50% loss of muscle bulk.

Most frequently, rotator cuff tears occur in the supraspinatus tendon, usually at its anterior insertion onto the greater tuberosity, synonymous with *rim rent* or *footprint* tears. Tears also often occur in the *critical zone* of the tendon, which is approximately 1 cm medial to the distal insertion.

- Critical zone is the watershed area between blood supplies.
- Area most vulnerable to chronic tendinopathy and tearing because of poor blood supply.

Subscapularis tears can be challenging to understand and describe because of the complex insertion anatomy (Fig. 2.46).

- Subscapularis tendon inserts primarily onto the lesser tuberosity but also has superficial fibers which continue across the intertubercular groove onto the greater tuberosity, which contribute to the *transverse humeral ligament*.
- Fibers from the CHL and the SGHL also contribute to the superior portion of the transverse humeral ligament, including the important superomedial portion that forms part of the *biceps pulley*, where the biceps long head tendon changes orientation from vertical to horizontal.
- Subscapularis tears can be associated with biceps long head subluxation and dislocation (see Fig. 2.46B and C).

Massive full-thickness rotator cuff tears (involving more than one tendon) most frequently begin in the anterior supraspinatus tendon and extend posteriorly into the infraspinatus tendon and anteroinferiorly into the superior subscapularis tendon.

- Chronic massive rotator cuff tear with retracted supraspinatus and/or infraspinatus tendons results in a chronically high-riding humeral head (Fig. 2.47).
  - Radiographs typically reveal the subacromial space to be obviously narrowed (6 mm or less).

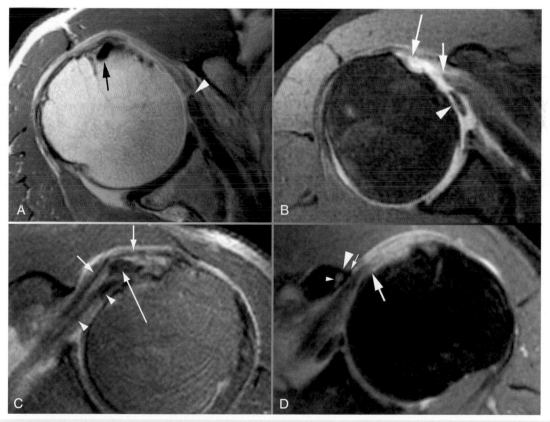

Fig. 2.46 Subscapularis tears. Axial T1-weighted MR arthrograms in four different patients. **(A)** Tear with retraction. Note torn tendon *(arrowhead)*. The biceps long head tendon is normally positioned *(arrow)*. **(B)** Complete tear with retraction *(short arrow)*. Also note medial biceps dislocation *(arrowhead)* and empty bicipital groove *(long arrow)*. **(C)** Partial tear with dislocation of the biceps long head tendon into the subscapularis *(long arrow)*. The anterior subscapularis *(medium arrows)* is detached from the lesser tuberosity but is continuous with the greater tuberosity. The posterior subscapularis *(arrowheads)* is attached to the lesser tuberosity. **(D)** Coracohumeral impingement with subscapularis tear with retraction *(long arrow)*. Note the narrow space between the coracoid process tip *(large arrowhead)* and the humerus. Also note the small spur *(small arrow)* and adjacent cyst *(small arrowhead)* in the coracoid tip caused by mechanical impingement against the humerus.

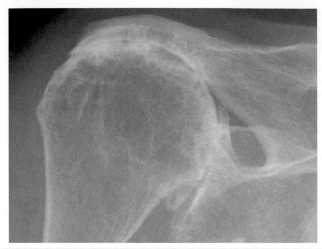

Fig. 2.47 Chronic massive rotator cuff tear. AP radiograph shows superior subluxation of the humeral head and matching concave contour of the acromial undersurface due to chronic impaction by the humeral head. No additional imaging study is needed to diagnose the tear.

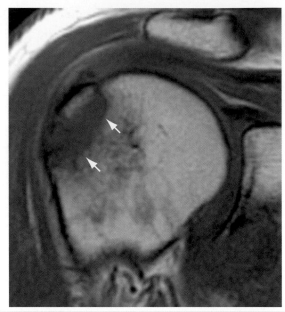

Fig. 2.48 Greater tuberosity fracture. Radiographs (not shown) did not reveal a fracture. Oblique coronal T1-weighted MR image shows a nondisplaced fracture, seen as a low-signal line *(arrows)*. The rotator cuff was intact.

■ May reveal remodeling of the acromial undersurface into a concave contour that matches the contour of the humeral head due to chronic impaction and mechanical erosion.

Important considerations when evaluating an MRI for rotator cuff tear (i.e., what the clinician wants to know) include:

■ Tear: present or absent.
■ If tear is present: site (e.g., insertion, critical zone), partial or full-thickness, tendon(s) involved.
■ If partial thickness: extent, including greater or less than 50% tendon thickness.
■ Retraction.
■ Muscle belly atrophy.
■ Status of biceps long head tendon.
■ Presence of cystic change in the greater tuberosity (may affect suture anchor placement).
■ Acromiohumeral outlet findings.
  ■ Modified Bigliani classification (see Box 2.1).
  ■ Subacromial spur or AC osteophytes.
  ■ Os acromiale.
  ■ Bursal effusion.

Common pitfalls of rotator cuff tears that may simulate a tear include:

■ Magic angle phenomenon.
■ Overlap of adjacent tendon fibers.
■ Normal composition of tendon layers.
■ Rotator interval gap.

Patients with other clinical conditions may present similarly to those with rotator cuff impingement and tears. Imaging studies in these patients can exclude rotator cuff disease and frequently can help identify the true cause of symptoms.

■ Suprascapular nerve injury or neuritis (MRI shows muscle signal changes of denervation; may show underlying cause).
■ Nondisplaced greater tuberosity avulsion fracture (may be occult on radiographs; MRI shows the fracture; Fig. 2.48).
■ Bursitis (MRI or US shows bursal fluid or thickening).

Rotator cuff repairs were originally performed using open and mini-open surgical techniques, but are now almost universally performed arthroscopically. Sutures are used to reattach the torn tendon to bone, with suture anchors placed in the humeral head. In the setting of massive rotator cuff tears that are irreparable by traditional tendon-to-bone repair, tendon transfer or graft reconstruction may be employed. Grafts may be used to bridge large tears with significant medial tendon retraction, using xenograft, allograft, and synthetic patches.

■ Rotator cuff repair is typically reserved for high-grade partial thickness and full-thickness rotator cuff tears.
■ Lower-grade tears may be treated with rotator cuff debridement and by surgically addressing underlying causes of impingement, such as performing subacromial decompression.

Postoperative appearance of the rotator cuff following repair on MRI may be characterized by tendon distortion, signal alteration, and shortening of the repaired tendon.

■ Intermediate signal abnormality within the repaired tendon may represent granulation tissue or fibrosis.
■ Repaired tendon may demonstrate tendon thickening or fibrosis, or tendon attenuation and irregularity, depending on quality of the repaired tendon.
■ Postoperative imaging is usually ordered to evaluate for rotator cuff re-tear, which is characterized by a tendon defect, uncovering of the suture anchor(s), or tendon retraction in the setting of a full-thickness retear (Fig. 2.49).
■ Occasionally, a repaired tendon may tear in a new location, for example medial to the repair site at the critical zone.
■ Intraarticular contrast (MR arthrography) may aid in diagnosis of rotator cuff retear, although contrast

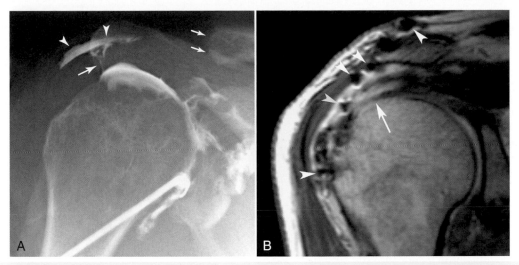

Fig. 2.49 Rotator cuff retears after repair. (A) Spot image obtained during shoulder arthrography shows contrast medium passing through a small rotator cuff tear *(large arrow)* to the subacromial/subdeltoid bursa *(arrowheads)*. Also note the distal clavicle resection *(small arrows)* and acromioplasty. **(B)** Coronal T1-weighted MR arthrogram shows delaminating tear with retraction *(arrow)*. Note the multiple low-signal postoperative artifacts *(arrowheads)*.

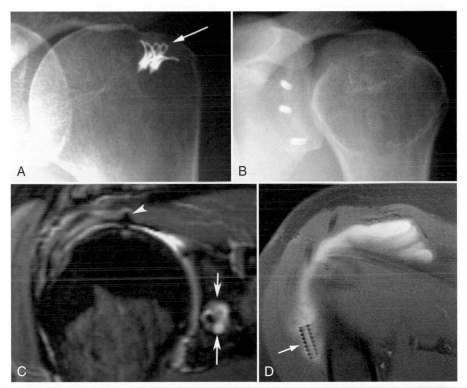

Fig. 2.50 Suture anchors and tacks. (A) Rotator cuff repair with metallic suture anchors in the greater tuberosity *(arrow)*. The suture anchors provide a site to reattach the torn supraspinatus tendon. **(B)** Anterior capsular repair. The suture anchors were placed in the anterior glenoid to allow reattachment of a stripped anterior capsule and labrum. **(C)** Suture anchor complications after anterior capsule repair. Sagittal fat-suppressed T2-weighted MR image shows fluid signal surrounding low signal of a suture anchor *(arrows)*, representing granulomatous reaction. Metallic anchors have been supplanted by various radiolucent bioabsorbable polymers, some of which are prone to granulomatous reaction. Also note a displaced suture anchor above the humeral head, partially within the rotator cuff *(arrowhead)*. **(D)** Oblique coronal fat-suppressed T1-weighted MR arthrogram image in a different patient shows a bioabsorbable suture anchor *(arrow)* in the posterior inferior subacromial/subdeltoid bursa.

extension into the subacromial/subdeltoid bursa is not always indicative of a full-thickness retear as repairs are not always watertight.

■ Other postoperative complications of rotator cuff (and labral) repairs include granulomatous reaction to the bioabsorbable suture anchors and displacement of suture anchors (Fig. 2.50).

HYDROXYAPATITE DEPOSITION (CALCIFIC TENDINITIS)

Hydroxyapatite deposition disease (HADD) is a condition characterized by abnormal deposition of calcium hydroxyapatite crystals in periarticular soft tissues, most commonly within tendons, referred to clinically as *calcific tendinitis*.

The tendons of the rotator cuff are the most common site of HADD. The pathophysiology of HADD remains unclear but seems to involve a cell-mediated process due to local tendon trauma or ischemia.

- Initially, small asymptomatic calcium deposits may develop ('silent phase').
- If calcium deposits enlarge, there is impingement on the subacromial space, and impingement symptoms of variable severity develop ('mechanical phase').
- Calcium crystals may subsequently erupt from the tendon and extrude into the subacromial/subdeltoid bursa, joint space, periarticular soft tissues, or even into the subcortical bone.
  - Intrabursal rupture causes a clinical syndrome of acute bursitis, with an inflammatory response and severe pain.
  - Eruptions of calcific deposits may occur repeatedly until the tendon is cleared of such deposits.
- Bursal fibrosis can occur as a late-stage complication.

Special mention of *calcific bursitis* and *calcific tendinitis* must be made in the imaging report. Although the two conditions may be seen in combination, bursitis often follows tendinitis as part of the typical progression (Fig. 2.51).

- Calcific tendinitis and bursitis is usually diagnosed with radiographs (see Fig. 2.51A).
- MRI typically demonstrates globular foci of hypointense signal on all imaging sequences (see Fig. 2.51B).

Calcium deposits in HADD typically resolve naturally over time, which can take several months or longer.

- Calcium deposits can be treated with US-guided percutaneous aspiration and lavage (*barbotage*), typically performed using an 18- or 20-gauge needle (Fig. 2.52).
  - Procedure is performed by repeatedly pulsating a saline solution into the calcium deposit, which is often in suspension.
  - Some operators follow this lavage with a corticosteroid injection into the overlying subacromial/subdeltoid bursa.
- Surgical enucleation is an option if conservative treatment or barbotage fails.

SUBACROMIAL/SUBDELTOID BURSITIS

Subacromial bursitis is often associated with rotator cuff impingement.

- Repeated mechanical compression of the bursa causes bursal thickening and increased fluid within the bursa.

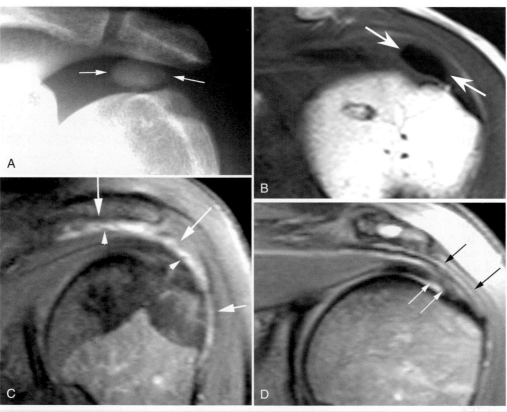

Fig. 2.51 Calcific tendinitis. (A and B) Mechanical phase. AP radiograph **(A)** shows typical uniform calcification in expected position of the supraspinatus tendon *(arrows)*. Oblique coronal proton density–weighted MR image **(B)** shows supraspinatus tendon thickening and very low signal intensity in the region of mineralization *(arrows)*. Tendon calcium deposits have similar low signal on all MR sequences. The patient subsequently underwent surgical debridement with significant symptomatic improvement. **(C)** Follow-up oblique coronal fat-suppressed T2-weighted MR image obtained 4 months later shows a more normal appearance of the tendon *(arrowheads)*. Radiographs (not shown) also showed resolution of the calcium deposit. However, now note the bursal fluid *(arrows)* with tiny, low-signal-intensity filling defects, thought to represent residual hydroxyapatite crystals and other debris. The patient was only mildly symptomatic. **(D)** Oblique coronal fat-suppressed T2-weighted MR image obtained 2 months later shows only a trace amount of fluid in the subacromial bursa *(black arrows)* and only mild supraspinatus tendinosis *(white arrows)*. Bursal fibrosis is a potential late-stage complication of calcific tendinitis, but this patient clinically did not have such fibrosis.

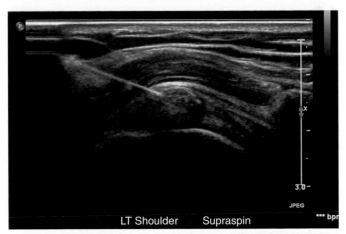

Fig. 2.52 **Calcific tendinosis percutaneous aspiration and lavage (barbotage).** Intraprocedural US image demonstrates a needle positioned within a large calcium deposit in the supraspinatus tendon.

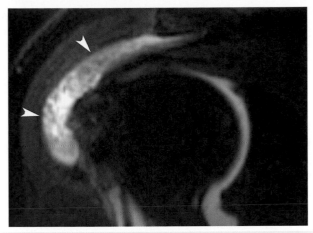

Fig. 2.53 **Subacromial/subdeltoid bursitis.** Oblique coronal fat-suppressed T2-weighted MR arthrogram shows distention of the subacromial/subdeltoid bursa *(arrowheads)* with fluid and lower signal synovial hypertrophy. T1-weighted images showed no gadolinium in the bursa. Thus there is no communication between the joint and the bursa, indicating that the cause of the bursal fluid is bursitis rather than rotator cuff tear.

- MRI reveals increased fluid in the bursa (Fig. 2.53).
- US may also demonstrate bursal thickening and/or hyperemia.
- Bursal thickening may also contribute to rotator cuff impingement as a cause, for example, bursal enlargement due to rheumatoid arthritis that reduces the subacromial space.
- Note: fluid within the subacromial/subdeltoid bursa is a nonspecific finding in the presence of a full-thickness rotator cuff tear given communication with the glenohumeral joint.

BICEPS TENDON SUBLUXATION

Medial subluxation or frank dislocation of the *LHBT* occurs with tearing of the CHL, transverse ligament, and/or subscapularis tendon.

- *Intraarticular dislocation*: in the setting of a full-thickness or undersurface subscapularis tendon tear, the LHBT may dislocate into the joint (see Fig. 2.46B).
- *Intrasubstance dislocation*: The LHBT may dislocate into the substance of the subscapularis tendon in the setting of an interstitial tear (see Fig. 2.46C).
- In the setting of a transverse ligament tear and/or tearing of the superficial (bursal-sided) subscapularis tendon fibers, the LHBT may dislocate anterior to the subscapularis tendon.
- LHBT subluxation or dislocation out of the bicipital groove can be distinguished from biceps tendon rupture by tracing the tendon from its origin distally into the upper arm.

BICEPS TENDON TEAR

As previously mentioned, the *LHBT* originates at the supraglenoid tubercle and the superior glenoid labrum at the 12:00–1:00 position (termed the *biceps anchor* or *biceps labral complex*).

- Superior labral tears may involve the biceps anchor, and even propagate into the proximal intraarticular LHBT.

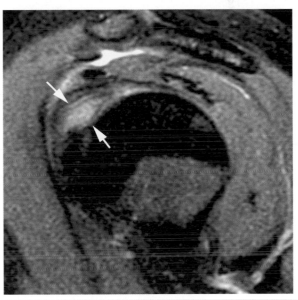

Fig. 2.54 **Long head biceps tendinosis.** Oblique sagittal fat-suppressed T2-weighted MR image shows a thick, edematous long head biceps tendon (between *arrows*).

The intraarticular portion of the LHBT is vulnerable to impingement, degeneration, and tearing by the same mechanisms as rotator cuff impingement (Fig. 2.54).

- Severe biceps tendinosis or partial tearing may be treated surgically with biceps tenodesis, which is often performed at the time of rotator cuff repair if indicated.
  - Tenodesis involves resecting the diseased portion of the tendon and reattaching the tendon to the proximal humerus using a suture anchor.

The extraarticular portion of the LHBT may also demonstrate tendinopathy, tearing, or associated biceps tenosynovitis.

- Extraarticular portion of the LHBT is best evaluated on axial MRI.

- LHBT should be evaluated for thickening, intrinsic signal abnormality, partial or full-thickness tear, adjacent fluid out of proportion to the joint fluid, loose bodies, and medial subluxation.
  - Note: fluid within the tendon sheath with an intact tendon may represent normal extension of glenohumeral joint fluid or tenosynovitis.
- An occasional normal variant is duplicated LHBT, in which there is a flat accessory tendon slip anterior to the main tendon in the bicipital groove.
  - This can be difficult to distinguish from a longitudinal split tendon tear but may be suggested if there is an otherwise normal appearance of the LHBT.
  - Accessory long head biceps may arise from the rotator cuff or anterior glenohumeral joint capsule.

An empty intertubercular groove that contains only fluid indicates either a LHBT dislocation (discussed previously) or complete tendon rupture with distal retraction.

- Complete tendon rupture usually occurs at the LHBT origin, with nonvisualization of the intraarticular segment.
- An extremely rare variant, congenital absence of the LHBT, is typically seen in combination with other congenital anomalies.

ADHESIVE CAPSULITIS

Adhesive capsulitis, colloquially called 'frozen shoulder', is a pathologic entity of unclear etiology characterized by progressive worsening of shoulder pain and restricted motion.

- Onset of symptoms may be idiopathic, related to a prior trauma, repetitive minor trauma, previous surgery, or seen in patients with underlying diabetes or rheumatologic conditions.
- Typically occurs in middle-aged and older individuals, more common in women.
- Pathophysiology involves synovitis of the glenohumeral joint capsule, with typical imaging features on MRI (Fig. 2.55).
  - Edema and infiltration of the rotator interval fat +/− thickening of the CHL.
  - Thickening of the inferior glenohumeral joint capsule/axillary pouch (normally <4 mm).
  - Low-capacity joint capsule on arthrography (see Fig. 2.13).
- Treatment options include physical therapy, glenohumeral joint steroid injection or hydrodilatation, closed shoulder manipulation under anesthesia, or arthroscopic capsular release.

OS ACROMIALE

The acromion normally develops from multiple ossification centers, which are usually fused by age 22–26 (Fig. 2.56). Failure of fusion of the acromial ossification centers can result in an *os acromiale*, which is almost always at the junction of the meso-acromion and meta-acromion. Repetitive microtrauma across the acromial physis during development may contribute to development, a process termed *acromial apophysiolysis* (Fig. 2.57). Os acromiale is present in 2–3% of the population and is bilateral in 60% of cases.

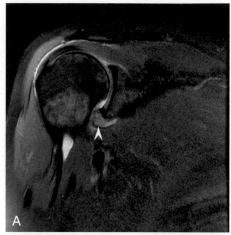

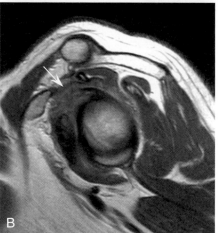

Fig. 2.55 Adhesive capsulitis. (A) Coronal STIR MR image demonstrates a markedly thickened, edematous inferior joint capsule (*arrowhead*). **(B)** Sagittal T2-weighted MR image demonstrates extensive infiltration of the rotator interval fat (*arrow*).

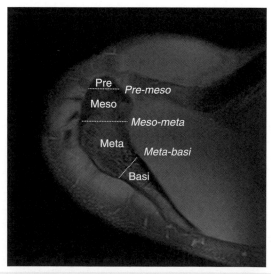

Fig. 2.56 Acromial ossification centers. The three main acromial ossification centers include the pre-acromion, meso-acromion, and meta-acromion. The adjacent basi-acromion is located at the lateral scapula. *Acromial apophysiolysis* and *os acromiale* almost always occur at the meso-meta location. *basi*, Basi-acromion; *meso*, meso-acromion; *meta*, meta-acromion; *pre*, pre-acromion.

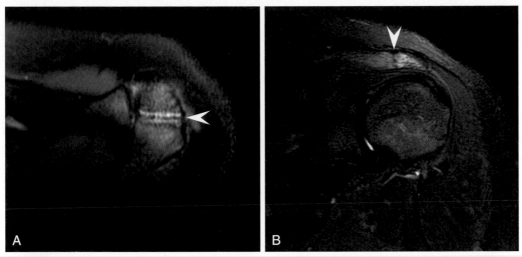

Fig. 2.57 Acromial apophysiolysis in a 14-year-old girl. Axial proton density fat-suppressed **(A)** and coronal STIR **(B)** MR images demonstrate marrow edema spanning the meso-meta growth plate.

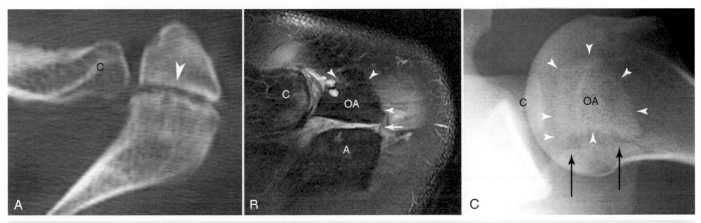

Fig. 2.58 Os acromiale. (A) Axial CT shows typical straight cleft with mildly sclerotic margins *(arrowhead)* across the acromion process. *C* marks the clavicle. **(B)** Fat-suppressed T2-weighted MR image and axillary radiograph **(C)** in different patients also show os acromiale (*OA* [*white arrowheads*]). Note the variable but generally straight shape of the cleft between the os acromiale and the remainder of the scapula *(arrows)*. A, Acromion, C, distal clavicle.

Os acromiale is readily identified on axillary shoulder radiographs and shoulder CT or MRI.

- Best depicted on axial images, although may be inadvertently excluded if the imaging volume is set too low.
- On sagittal or coronal imaging, the os acromiale has been described as simulating a 'double' AC joint due to the presence of the accessory synchondrosis, which is located posterior to the true AC joint.
- Os acromiale may be distinguished from an acromial fracture by its smooth, sclerotic margins and orientation perpendicular to the axis of the acromion (Fig. 2.58).

Os acromiale is important to identify and report given its association with rotator cuff impingement and tears.

- An unstable os acromiale can act as a fulcrum and may displace downwards during contraction of the deltoid muscle, narrowing the subacromial space.
- Degenerative changes may develop across the os acromiale synchondrosis, characterized by marginal osteophytes, cystic change, and marrow edema on MRI.

- Degenerative osteophytes at the synchondrosis may narrow the subacromial space.
- An unrecognized os acromiale is a known cause of failed rotator cuff repair.

ACROMIOCLAVICULAR JOINT SEPARATION

AC separation injuries can occur with direct trauma or fall onto the shoulder, most commonly seen in contact sports. Traumatic injury disrupts the relatively weaker AC ligaments before the stronger coracoclavicular ligaments, resulting in a predictable pattern of injury that is described by a standard grading system.

- Radiographs are the initial imaging study of choice.
- Normal findings include a continuous line or arc across the inferior margins of the acromion and clavicle at the AC joint, and symmetry of the right and left AC joints.
  - AC joint separation injuries are characterized by asymmetric widening of the AC joint +/- displacement of the distal clavicle with widening of the coracoclavicular distance (Fig. 2.59).

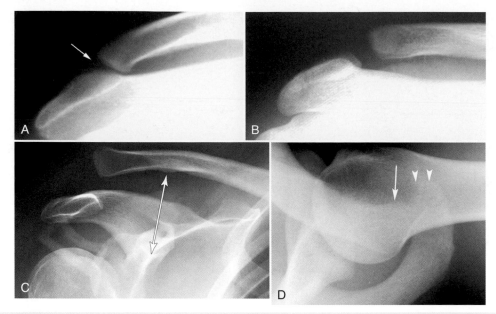

Fig. 2.59 Acromioclavicular joint injury. (A and B) Grade 2 acromioclavicular (AC) sprain. AP radiograph without **(A)** and with **(B)** distraction of the AC joint (*arrow* in A) shows widening in B. **(C)** Grade 3 AC sprain. Dislocated AC joint and widened coracoclavicular distance *(arrow)*. **(D)** Grade 4 AC separation. AP view (not shown) showed no definite abnormalities. Axillary view shows that the distal clavicle *(arrow)* is displaced posteriorly relative to the acromion *(arrowheads)*.

- AC joint space is usually 5 mm wide or less, with right and left differing by no more than 2–4 mm.
    - Coracoclavicular distance normally 11–13 mm.
  - Passive inferior traction on the arm, usually accomplished by attaching a weight to the wrist, may reveal or upgrade an AC injury that is not apparent without traction.
- MRI can be obtained to fully assess extent of injury (Box 2.2).
- AC injuries are treated based on severity of injury.
    - Grade 1 and 2 AC injuries are treated conservatively.
    - Grade 3 may be treated conservatively or with surgery.
    - Grade 4 and higher injuries are treated surgically, which may include internal fixation with a hook plate, distal clavicular resection, and/or CC ligament reconstruction.
- Old AC injuries may heal with persistently abnormal alignment, and injured ligaments may calcify or ossify.
- Differential for AC joint widening on x-ray includes AC joint separation, distal clavicular osteolysis (DCO), or erosion due to rheumatoid arthritis, hyperparathyroidism, or infection.

ACROMIOCLAVICULAR OSTEOARTHRITIS

- AC joint osteoarthritis may be a source of pain or extrinsic impingement of the rotator cuff.
- Findings on MRI include capsular hypertrophy, joint effusion, subchondral marrow edema, or cystic change, in addition to osseous productive change.
- Changes in AC joint osteoarthritis are typically demonstrated on both sides of the joint, which may help differentiate from *DCO* (see below).

Box 2.2   Acromioclavicular Joint Separation Grading on MRI

- Grade 1 injury
    - Sprain or partial tearing of joint capsule, AC ligaments
    - AC joint *not* widened
- Grade 2 injury
    - Complete disruption of AC ligaments
    - Coracoclavicular (CC) ligaments sprained or partially torn, comprised of the conoid and trapezoid components
    - Widening of AC joint may be evident
- Grade 3 injury
    - Complete disruption of AC and CC ligaments
    - Widening of AC joint with superior displacement of the distal clavicle, increased CC distance
    - Strain/low-grade tearing of proximal deltoid, distal trapezius (clavicular attachment) may be evident
- Grade 4 injury
    - Grade 3 injury + posterior displacement of the distal clavicle with 'buttonholing' into the trapezius muscle (see Fig. 4.15C)
- Grade 5 injury
    - Grade 3 injury + extensive tearing of deltoid and trapezius muscles
    - Unopposed upward pull by the sternocleidomastoid muscle resulting in more significant superior displacement of the clavicle and increased coracoclavicular distance
- Grade 6 injury
    - Inferior displacement of clavicle due to superior blow with complete tear of AC ligaments
    - Associated clavicle and rib fractures, brachial plexus injuries

DISTAL CLAVICULAR OSTEOLYSIS

- DCO is a painful condition characterized by resorption of the distal clavicle.
- Can be seen in the posttraumatic setting or with repetitive microtrauma (classically seen in weightlifters).

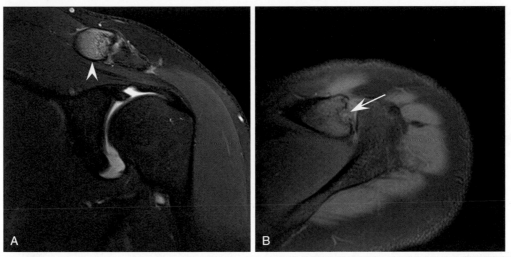

Fig. 2.60 Distal clavicular osteolysis. (A) Coronal proton density fat-suppressed image obtained as part of an MR arthrogram study demonstrates intense marrow edema in the distal clavicle (*arrowhead*) with adjacent capsular edema. **(B)** Axial T1-weighted fat-suppressed sequence demonstrates osseous irregularity and resorption of the distal clavicle (*arrow*).

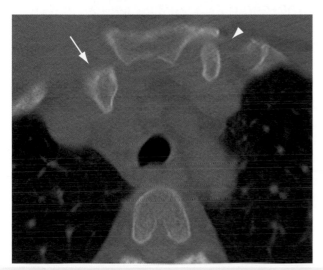

Fig. 2.61 Sternoclavicular joint posterior dislocation. Axial CT shows posterior dislocation of the right sternoclavicular joint (*arrow*). The left medial clavicular head (*arrowhead*) remains normal in position.

- Radiographs may demonstrate soft tissue swelling about the AC joint, demineralization of the distal clavicle, loss of cortical margins, and widening of the AC joint.
- MRI findings include intense marrow edema isolated to the distal clavicle with osseous resorption and surrounding soft tissue edema (Fig. 2.60).
- Treatment is usually conservative, including nonsteroidal antiinflammatory medications (NSAIDs) and immobilization; distal clavicle resection may be considered in refractory cases.
- Distal clavicle may reconstitute following treatment, or the AC joint may remain widened.

STERNOCLAVICULAR JOINT DISLOCATION

- SC joint supported by strong capsular ligaments.
- SC joint can be dislocated in a high-speed motor vehicle crash or similarly violent injury (Fig. 2.61).

- Medial clavicle can dislocate in various directions.
    - Superior dislocation may be detected with radiographs.
    - Posterior dislocation (which can result in compression/injury of the great vessels or trachea) may be difficult to diagnose on radiographs and is best evaluated with CT.
    - Dislocation results in damage to the intraarticular disc and posttraumatic SC joint osteoarthritis.
- Potential pitfall: medial clavicle fracture in a young adult.
    - Medial clavicular epiphysis does not begin to ossify until 18–20 years, does not fuse with the remainder of the clavicle until approximately age 25.
    - Salter–Harris I or II fractures may be misinterpreted as SC dislocations or vice versa.
    - Careful attention on CT images for a smoothly marginated, calcified epiphysis versus irregularly marginated fracture fragment can avoid this pitfall.

STERNOCLAVICULAR OSTEOARTHRITIS

- Most frequent pathologic condition of the SC joint is degenerative osteoarthritis.
- SC osteoarthritis is fairly common in older individuals and usually incidental but can be painful.
- Prominent osteophytes may simulate a chest wall mass on physical exam.

JOINT INFECTION

- Septic arthritis can involve any joint in the shoulder, including the glenohumeral, AC, and SC joints.
- Infection may be introduced via *direct inoculation*, typically in the setting of recent joint injection or surgery, or *hematogenous spread*, particularly IV drug users, immunocompromised patients, and bacteremic patients.
- Findings on radiographs may be subtle, including periarticular osteopenia (due to increased blood flow), joint space loss, and osseous erosions.

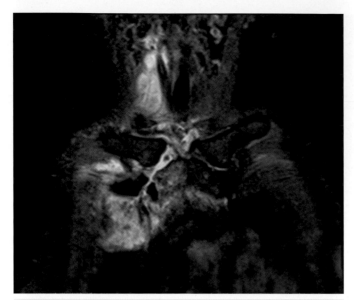

Fig. 2.62 Sternoclavicular joint septic arthritis. Coronal STIR image of the anterior chest demonstrates florid septic arthritis of the right sternoclavicular joint with joint effusion, marrow edema in the right superior sternum, and extensive surrounding phlegmon/abscess extending contiguously into the right upper mediastinum and cephalad along the right neck.

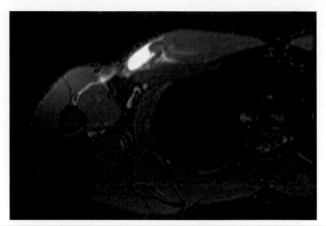

Fig. 2.63 Complete rupture of the pectoralis major tendon. Axial STIR image of the right chest wall demonstrates complete rupture of the pectoralis major tendon with medial retraction of the distal myotendinous junction and fluid/hematoma surrounding the retracted tendon stump.

- MRI reveals several characteristic findings:
  - Joint effusion, synovial thickening and enhancement (if contrast administered), and osseous erosions.
  - Reactive subchondral marrow edema and/or adjacent osteomyelitis.
  - Extensive periarticular soft tissue edema, including intramuscular edema, sometimes with adjacent abscess (Fig. 2.62).
- Joint aspiration is the gold standard for confirming the diagnosis and should be performed expeditiously.
- Septic arthritis in a native joint is a medical emergency, treated with IV antibiotics and urgent surgical intervention (arthroscopic washout/drainage, debridement).

PECTORALIS MAJOR TEAR

- Pectoralis major musculotendinous injuries are most frequently encountered in weightlifters and high-level athletes.
- Pectoralis major is a fan-shaped muscle composed of three muscular heads (clavicular, sternal, and abdominal), which converge to form a short tendon that inserts on the proximal humerus at the lateral ridge of the bicipital groove.
  - Partial tears more common at the myotendinous junction (most commonly involving the sternal head).
  - Complete ruptures are more common at the distal tendon insertion.
- MRI using a pectoralis major protocol reliably demonstrates site of injury, degree of tearing (partial versus complete), retraction, and accompanying hematoma (Fig. 2.63).

SPINOGLENOID AND SUPRASCAPULAR NOTCH IMPINGEMENT

- The suprascapular nerve is vulnerable to entrapment in the *spinoglenoid notch* and the adjacent *suprascapular notch*.
  - The suprascapular notch is contiguous with and just anterior to the spinoglenoid notch.
  - Compression may occur due to paralabral cyst, soft tissue mass, or displaced fracture.
- Impingement at the level of the *spinoglenoid notch* results in denervation of the *infraspinatus muscle* (Fig. 2.64).
- Impingement at the level of the *suprascapular notch* results in denervation of both the *supraspinatus* and *infraspinatus muscles*.
- Suprascapular nerve dysfunction can cause a syndrome of supraspinatus and/or infraspinatus denervation that clinically mimics a rotator cuff tear.
  - Denervation results in diffuse intramuscular edema beginning about 2–4 weeks after initial insult.
  - Chronic denervation causes irreversible fatty infiltration and muscle atrophy.

QUADRILATERAL SPACE IMPINGEMENT

- *Quadrilateral space* is formed by the teres minor muscle superiorly, teres major muscle inferiorly, humerus laterally, and triceps muscle medially.
- The *axillary nerve* passes through the quadrilateral space, where it is vulnerable to entrapment due to fibrous bands, mass lesions, fracture, or abduction of the arm.
- Such entrapment may cause denervation of the posterior deltoid and teres minor muscles.
  - MRI may show evidence of deltoid and teres minor denervation (intramuscular edema, fatty infiltration, muscle atrophy) and can reveal a mass if present.
- Isolated atrophy of the teres minor muscle may be seen without findings of quadrilateral space impingement, thought to result from entrapment of the *nerve to the teres minor* (a branch of the axillary nerve) due to fibrous bands or adhesions (Fig. 2.65).

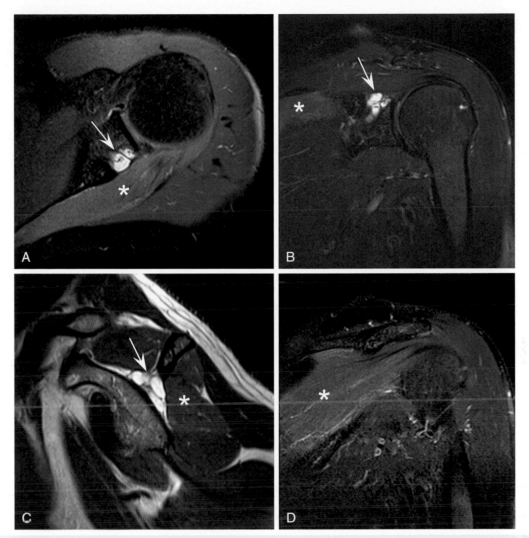

Fig. 2.64 Suprascapular nerve impingement at the spinoglenoid notch. Axial proton density fat-suppressed **(A)**, coronal STIR **(B)**, sagittal T2 **(C)**, and coronal STIR **(D)** MR images demonstrate a multilocular ganglion cyst in the spinoglenoid notch (*arrow*), with subtle denervation edema throughout the infraspinatus muscle (*asterisks*).

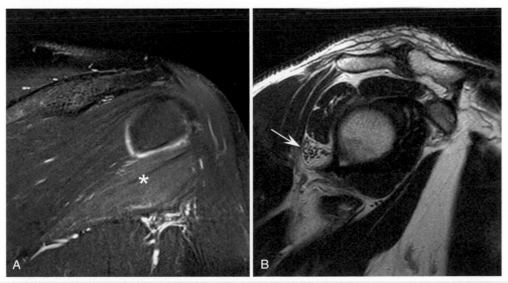

Fig. 2.65 Isolated teres minor denervation and atrophy. (A) Coronal STIR MR image demonstrating early denervation edema within the teres minor muscle (*asterisk*) in a patient with history of prior traction injury. **(B)** Sagittal T2-weighted MR image in a different patient showing severe isolated fatty atrophy of the teres minor muscle (*arrow*). No mass lesion was identified in the quadrilateral space in either patient.

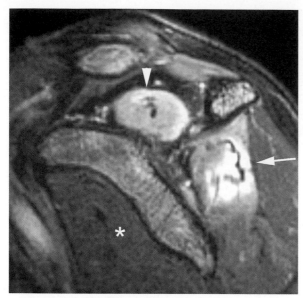

Fig. 2.66 Parsonage–Turner syndrome. Oblique sagittal fat-suppressed T2-weighted MR image shows edema in the supraspinatus *(arrowhead)* and infraspinatus *(arrow)* muscles. Contrast this finding with the normal signal intensity of the adjacent muscles, such as the subscapularis *(asterisk)*. The patient had recently experienced a viral illness; no mass was present and there was no history of trauma.

BRACHIAL NEURITIS

- *Brachial neuritis*, also known as *Parsonage–Turner syndrome*, can cause selective nerve dysfunction and accompanying muscular denervation patterns (Fig. 2.66).
  - Idiopathic, possibly postviral or immunologic-mediated condition that occurs more frequently in males.
  - Most cases spontaneously resolve after several months.
  - Suprascapular nerve involved in almost all cases; additional nerves may be involved in combination.
- Traction injury of the suprascapular nerve may result in an identical MRI appearance and should be considered in the posttraumatic setting.

Structured Report

REPORTING TIPS AND RECOMMENDATIONS

- Related findings may be separated in the body of the report due to template structure, but impression should tie findings together.
  - For example, in the setting of a recent anterior shoulder dislocation, findings may include both osseous abnormalities (Hill–Sachs lesion, osseous Bankart lesion) and soft tissue injuries (labral tear, capsuloligamentous injury).
- Impression should summarize findings that may be elaborated on further in the body of the report; avoid direct copying and pasting into the impression.
- Mention findings clinically relevant to the clinician, such as tendon retraction or rotator cuff muscle atrophy in the setting of rotator cuff tear.
- Organize impression points by order of importance.
- Directly answer any specific clinical questions in the impression.

Example Normal Shoulder Report Template

Exam Type: MRI SHOULDER WITHOUT CONTRAST
Exam Date and Time: Date and Time
Indication: Clinical History
Comparison: Prior Studies

IMPRESSION: Impression

TECHNIQUE: MRI of the side shoulder was performed on a scanner type system in three planes (axial, sagittal, and coronal) using a standard noncontrast protocol.

FINDINGS:

ROTATOR CUFF: The supraspinatus, infraspinatus, subscapularis, and teres minor tendons are intact without tendinosis or tear. No partial or full-thickness rotator cuff tear is identified.

OSSEOUS STRUCTURES: Alignment is anatomic. No acute fracture or osseous contusion. No Hill–Sachs deformity or osseous Bankart defect.

LABRUM and GLENOHUMERAL JOINT: Labrum: No labral tear by nonarthrogram MRI.
Glenohumeral joint: No joint effusion. No focal cartilage defects or osteoarthritis. No intraarticular bodies.

LONG HEAD BICEPS TENDON: Normally positioned in the bicipital groove without subluxation. No tendinosis or tendon tear. No tenosynovitis.

MUSCLES: Rotator cuff musculature normal in bulk and signal without edema or atrophy.

ACROMION and ACROMIOCLAVICULAR JOINT: No acromioclavicular joint osteoarthritis. No subacromial spur. No os acromiale.

SUBACROMIAL/SUBDELTOID BURSA: No subacromial/subdeltoid bursitis.

OTHER: Fat in the rotator interval is preserved. No mass effect in the spinoglenoid, suprascapular notch, or quadrilateral space. No soft tissue edema.

Sources and Suggested Readings

Aina R, Cardinal E, Bureau N, et al. Calcific shoulder tendinitis: treatment with modified US-guided fine-needle technique. *Radiology.* 2001;221:455–461.

Beaty JH, Kasser JR, Shaggs DL, et al. eds. *Rockwood and Green's Fractures in Children.* Philadelphia: Lippincott-Raven; 2009.

Bergin D, Parker L, Zoga A, et al. Abnormalities on MRI of the subscapularis tendon in the presence of a full-thickness supraspinatus tendon tear. *AJR Am J Roentgenol.* 2006;186:454–459.

Bucholz RW, Court-Brown CM, Heckman JD, et al. *Rockwood and Green's Fractures in Adults.* Philadelphia: Lippincott-Raven; 2009.

Cook TS, Stein JM, Simonson S, Kim W. Normal and variant anatomy of the shoulder on MRI. *Magn Reson Imaging Clin N Am.* 2011;19(3):581–594.

Drakos MC, Rudzki JR, Allen AA, et al. Internal impingement of the shoulder in the overhead athlete. *J Bone Joint Surg Am.* 2009;91(11):2719–2728.

Fritz J, Fishman EK, Small KM, et al. MDCT arthrography of the shoulder with datasets of isotropic resolution: indications, technique, and applications. *AJR Am J Roentgenol.* 2012;198(3):635–646.

Gondim Texeira PA, Balaj C, Chanson A, et al. Adhesive capsulitis of the shoulder: value of inferior glenohumeral ligament signal changes on

T2-weighted fat-saturated images. *AJR Am J Roentgenol.* 2012;198(6): W589–W596.

Ha AS, Petscavage-Thomas JM, Tagoylo GH. Acromioclavicular joint: the other joint in the shoulder. *AJR Am J Roentgenol.* 2014;202(2):375–385.

Harper K, Helms C, Haystead C, Higgins L. Glenoid dysplasia: incidence and association with posterior labral tears as evaluated by MRI. *AJR Am J Roentgenol.* 2005;184:984–988.

Helms CA, Major NA, Anderson MW, Kaplan PA. *Musculoskeletal MRI.* 2nd ed. Philadelphia: Saunders; 2008.

Jacobson JA, Miller B, Bedi A, Morag Y. Imaging of the postoperative shoulder. *Semin Musculoskelet Radiol.* 2011;15(4):320–339.

Jacobson JA. Shoulder US: anatomy, technique, and scanning pitfalls. *Radiology.* 2011;260:6–16.

Jamadar DA, Robertson BL, Jacobson JA, et al. Musculoskeletal sonography: important imaging pitfalls. *AJR Am J Roentgenol.* 2010;194(1):216–225.

Kassarjain A, Torriani M, Ouellette H, Palmer W. Intramuscular rotator cuff cysts: association with tendon tears on MRI and arthroscopy. *AJR Am J Roentgenol.* 2005;185:160–165.

Kim YJ, Choi JA, Oh JH, et al. Superior labral anteroposterior tears: accuracy and interobserver reliability of multidetector CT arthrography for diagnosis. *Radiology.* 2011;260:207–215.

Kon DS, Darakjian AB, Pearl ML, Kosco AE. Glenohumeral deformity in children with internal rotation contractures secondary to brachial plexus birth palsy: intraoperative arthrographic classification. Radiology. 2004;231:791–795.

Krief OP. MRI of the rotator interval capsule. *AJR Am J Roentgenol.* 2005; 184:1490–1494.

Kwong S, Kothary S, Poncinelli LL. Skeletal development of the proximal humerus in the pediatric population: MRI features. *AJR Am J Roentgenol.* 2014;202(2):418–425.

Massengill AD, Seeger LL, Yao L, et al. Labrocapsular ligamentous complex of the shoulder: normal anatomy, anatomic variations, and pitfalls of MR imaging and MR arthrography. *Radiographics.* 1994;14:1211–1223.

Mohana-Borges AVR, Chung C, Resnick D. MR imaging and MR of the postoperative shoulder: spectrum of normal and abnormal findings. *Radiographics.* 2004;24:69–85.

Mohana-Borges AVR, Chung C, Resnick D. Superior labral anteroposterior tear: classification and diagnosis on MRI and MR arthrography. *AJR Am J Roentgenol.* 2003;181:1449–1462.

Morag Y, Jacobson JA, Miller B, et al. MR imaging of rotator cuff injury: what the clinician needs to know. *Radiographics.* 2006;26(4):1045–1065.

Morag Y, Jacobson JA, Shields G, et al. MR arthrography of rotator interval, long head of the biceps brachii, and the biceps pulley of the shoulder. *Radiology.* 2005;235:21–30.

Morag Y, Jamadar DA, Boon TA, et al. Ultrasound of the rotator cable: prevalence and morphology in asymptomatic shoulders. *AJR Am J Roentgenol.* 2012;198:W27–W30.

Morag Y, Jamadar DA, Miller B, et al. The subscapularis: anatomy, injury, and imaging. *Skeletal Radiol.* 2011;40(3):255–269.

Park S, Lee DH, Yoon SH, et al. Evaluation of adhesive capsulitis of the shoulder with fat-suppressed T2-weighted MRI: association between clinical features and MRI findings. *AJR Am J Roentgenol.* 2016;207(1): 135–141.

Polster JM, Schickendantz MS. Shoulder MRI: what do we miss? *AJR Am J Roentgenol.* 2010;195(3):577–584.

Rhee RB, Chan KK, Lieu JG, et al. MR and CT arthrography of the shoulder. *Semin Musculoskelet Radiol.* 2012;16(1):3–14.

Robinson R. Sonography of common tendon injuries. *AJR Am J Roentgenol.* 2009;193(3):607–618.

Roedl JB, Morrison WB, Ciccotti MG, et al. Acromial apophysiolysis: superior shoulder pain and acromial nonfusion in the young throwing athlete. *Radiology.* 2015;274(1):201–209.

Ropp AM, Davis DL. Scapular fractures: what radiologists need to know. *AJR Am J Roentgenol.* 2015;205(3):491–501.

Shah N. Imaging signs of posterior glenohumeral instability. *AJR Am J Roentgenol.* 2009;192(3):730–735.

Sheah K, Bredella MA, Palmer WE. Transverse thickening along the articular surface of the rotator cuff consistent with the rotator cable: identification with MR arthrography and relevance in rotator cuff evaluation. *AJR Am J Roentgenol.* 2009;193(3):679–686.

Tuite MJ, Cirillo RL, De Smet AA, et al. Superior labrum anterior-posterior (SLAP) tears: evaluation of three MR signs on T2-weighted images. *Radiology.* 2000;21:841–845.

Vinson EN, Wittstein J, Garrigues GE, et al. MRI of selected abnormalities at the anterior superior aspect of the shoulder: potential pitfalls and subtle diagnoses. *AJR Am J Roentgenol.* 2012;199(3):534–545.

Yanny S, Toms AP. MR patterns of denervation around the shoulder. *AJR Am J Roentgenol.* 2010;195(2):W157–W163.

3 Elbow

Anatomy

OSSEOUS

The three bones that comprise the elbow are the distal humerus, proximal radius, and proximal ulna. The normal radiographic anatomy of the elbow is illustrated in Fig. 3.1.

The distal humerus widens medially and laterally to form the *epicondyles*.

- *Lateral epicondyle* is the common origin of the wrist extensor muscles.
- *Medial epicondyle* is the common origin of the wrist flexor muscles and the pronator teres (PT) muscle.

Humeral *condyles* form the rounded capitellum laterally and the V-shaped trochlea medially, which articulate with the radius and ulna, respectively.

- Condyles are anteriorly positioned relative to the epicondyles.
- On the lateral radiograph, a line drawn along the anterior humeral shaft cortex, the *anterior humeral line*, normally passes through the middle third of the capitellum (Fig. 3.2).

  - Deviation from this suggests a supracondylar fracture.
- Distal humerus has concavities on both its anterior and posterior surfaces.
  - Shallow *coronoid fossa* anteriorly accommodates the ulnar coronoid process during elbow flexion.

- Deeper *olecranon fossa* posteriorly accommodates the ulnar olecranon process during elbow extension.
- A normal variant foramen may connect the coronoid and olecranon fossae.

The *radial tuberosity* on the proximal-medial radial shaft is the insertion site of the distal biceps tendon.

- Medial insertion allows the biceps to function as a wrist supinator (turns palm anteriorly) in addition to an elbow flexor.
- When viewed *en face*, the radial tuberosity may simulate a lytic lesion (Fig. 3.3).
  - Normal nature of this finding is confirmed by characteristic location and convex contour on an orthogonal view.

The *olecranon process* is a large bony eminence at the proximal ulna, which sits in the olecranon fossa during elbow extension.

- Serves as the primary attachment site of the distal triceps musculotendinous insertion.

The 'carrying angle' of the elbow is formed by the humerus and ulna in the coronal plane when the elbow is extended.

- Normal fully extended elbow is in about 165 degrees of valgus alignment—slightly greater in women and less in men.

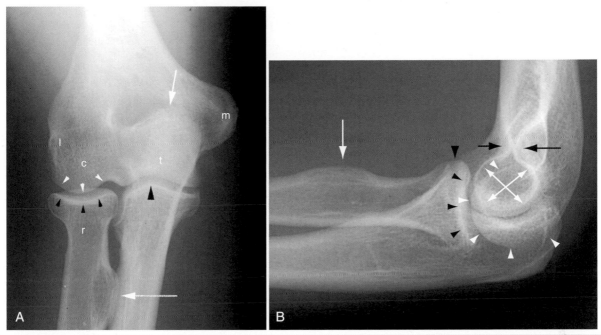

Fig. 3.1 Normal radiographic anatomy of the elbow. **(A)** AP view. **(B)** Lateral view. *Small black arrowheads*, radial head articular surface; *small white arrowheads*, capitellum articular surface; *large black arrowhead*, coronoid process of the ulna; *short white arrow*, olecranon process of the ulna; *long white arrow*, radial tuberosity (insertion site of biceps); *short black arrow* (in B only), coronoid fossa; *long black arrow* (in B only), olecranon fossa; *white double arrows* (in B only), trochlea. *c*, Capitellum; *l*, lateral epicondyle; *r*, radial neck; *m*, medial epicondyle; *t*, trochlea (superimposed over the olecranon).

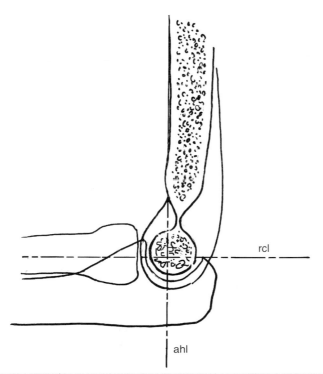

Fig. 3.2 Radiocapitellar and anterior humeral lines. The anterior humeral line is drawn along the anterior cortex of the humeral shaft cortex. If this line does not pass through the middle of the capitellum, then a fracture is likely. The radiocapitellar line is drawn along the center of the radial shaft. If this line does not bisect the capitellum, then a radial head dislocation or subluxation is present. This diagram also illustrates the normal relationship of the trochlea (seen in cross-section) and the ulna. Note that the capitellum articular surface projects slightly anterior to the trochlea. *ahl*, Anterior humeral line; *rcl*, radiocapitellar line.

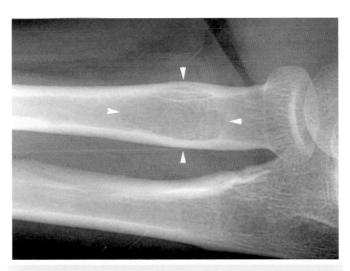

Fig. 3.3 Pseudolesion of the proximal radius *(arrowheads)* caused by the normal appearance of the radial tuberosity when seen *en face*.

A *supracondylar process*, or 'avian spur', is an uncommon developmental variant (1% incidence) characterized by a bony excrescence on the anteromedial distal humeral shaft (Fig. 3.4).

- Supracondylar process points toward the elbow, in contrast with an osteochondroma, which usually points away from the nearest joint.
- May serve as an attachment site for a vestigial structure, the *ligament of Struthers*, thereby forming a *supracondylar canal*.
  - Can cause symptoms due to compression of the median nerve or brachial artery, which pass through the supracondylar canal.

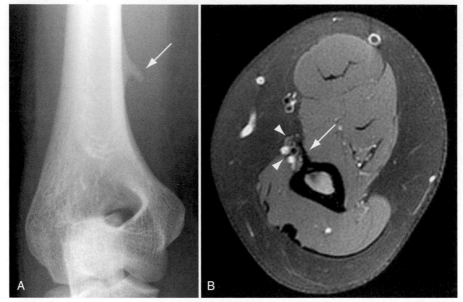

Fig. 3.4 Supracondylar process (avian spur). **(A)** Radiograph. This normal variant bony excrescence *(arrow)* projects anteriorly and slightly medially from the distal humeral shaft. **(B)** Axial fat-suppressed T2-weighted MR image shows the low-signal spur *(arrow)*. Note the brachial neurovascular bundle *(arrowheads)* adjacent to the spur, which includes the median nerve.

Understanding normal maturation of ossification centers in the elbow is critical to identifying apophyseal avulsion injuries in a pediatric patient.

- The order of appearance on radiographs of the six ossification centers of the elbow may be recalled with the mnemonic CRITOE (Fig. 3.5).
- The <u>c</u>apitellum begins to ossify at about age 1 year, followed by the <u>r</u>adial head after age 3 years, the medial ('<u>i</u>nternal') epicondyle around age 4–5 years, the <u>t</u>rochlea around age 7–8 years, the <u>o</u>lecranon around age 8–10 years, and finally the lateral ('<u>e</u>xternal') epicondyle around age 9–13 years.
- Ossification of each center tends to begin a year or two earlier in girls than in boys.
- Exact ages are fairly variable and are not absolutely essential to memorize; rather it is the order of appearance of the ossification centers that is important to know.

ELBOW JOINT

The elbow joint is enclosed by a single synovial compartment that includes the articulations of the radial head with the humeral capitellum (*radiocapitellar* or *radiohumeral joint*), the proximal ulna with the humeral trochlea (*ulnotrochlear* or *ulnohumeral joint*), and the *proximal radioulnar joint*.

- *Radiocapitellar (radiohumeral) joint.*
  - Cylindrical radial head articulates with the rounded capitellum.
  - A line drawn through the center of the radial shaft, the *radiocapitellar line*, should bisect the capitellum on any view (see Fig. 3.2).
    - Failure of the radiocapitellar line to bisect the capitellum indicates a radial head dislocation or subluxation.
- *Ulnotrochlear (ulnohumeral) joint.*
  - Proximal ulna, including the olecranon process posteriorly and the coronoid process anteriorly, forms the

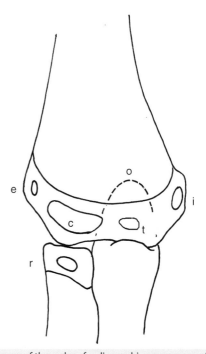

Fig. 3.5 Diagram of the order of radiographic appearance of ossification centers around the elbow ('CRITOE'). *c*, Capitellum; *r*, radial head; *i*, medial ('internal') epicondyle; *t*, trochlea; *o*, olecranon; *e*, lateral ('external') epicondyle.

trochlear (or *semilunar*) *notch*, which articulates broadly with the humeral *trochlea*.
- *Proximal radioulnar joint.*
  - Pivot joint between the radial head and the concave radial notch of the ulna, allowing for pronation and supination.

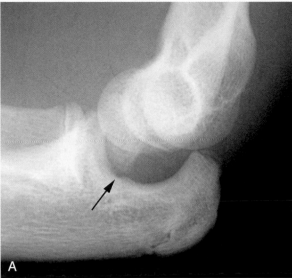

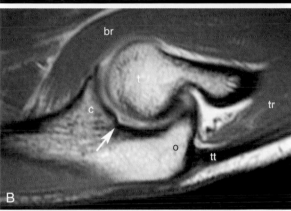

Fig. 3.6 Normal 'pseudodefect' of the ulnar trochlear groove at the base of the coronoid process. **(A)** Lateral radiograph in a patient with an elbow dislocation shows a small notchlike defect in the subchondral bone at the base of the coronoid process *(arrow)*. **(B)** Sagittal T1-weighted MR arthrogram also demonstrates the normal variant pseudodefect *(arrow)*. This image also illustrates normal anatomy. *br*, Brachialis muscle; *c*, coronoid process; *o*, olecranon; *t*, trochlea; *tr*, triceps muscle; *tt*, triceps tendon.

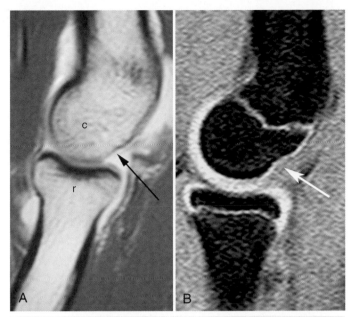

Fig. 3.7 Normal 'pseudodefect' of the dorsal capitellum. **(A)** Sagittal T1-weighted MR arthrogram from the same study as shown in Fig. 3.6A shows a shallow concave 'defect' in the dorsal capitellum *(arrow)*. **(B)** Sagittal fat-suppressed spoiled gradient-echo sequence in a child shows the same finding *(arrow)*. This normal variant should not be confused with an osteochondral lesion. *c*, Capitellum; *r*, radial head.

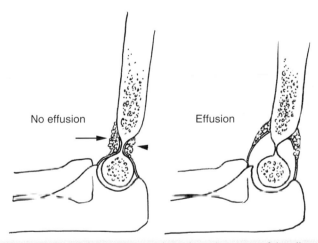

Fig. 3.8 The fat pad sign. Diagram shows how distention of the elbow joint capsule displaces the posterior fat pad *(arrowhead)* out of the olecranon fossa, making it visible on a lateral view, and distorts the anterior fat pad *(arrow)*, potentially causing it to have a convex margin anteriorly that is known as the 'sail sign'.

Small notchlike *pseudodefects* in the elbow articular cartilage are seen normally and should not be mistaken for cartilage defects or osteochondral defects.

- Trochlear notch at the base of the coronoid process (Fig. 3.6).
- Dorsal capitellum (Fig. 3.7).

Normal extrasynovial anterior and posterior fat pads exist within the elbow joint.

- *Posterior fat pad* resides within the olecranon fossa, which is normally <u>not</u> visible on lateral radiographs obtained with the elbow flexed 90 degrees because it is superimposed over the distal humerus.
  - Joint effusion, hemarthrosis, or another process that distends the joint capsule, such as synovitis or pigmented villonodular synovitis, can displace this fat pad posteriorly out of the olecranon fossa.
  - Produces the *posterior fat pad sign* on a lateral radiograph (Figs. 3.8 and 3.9).
- *Anterior fat pad* resides at the anterior margin of the distal humerus and can be a normal finding on lateral radiographs.
  - Normal anterior fat pad should have a straight anterior contour.
  - Joint effusion or other synovial-based process may cause the anterior fat pad to bulge anteriorly, creating the *sail sign* (see Figs. 3.8 and 3.9).
- If a posterior fat pad sign or sail sign is seen in the posttraumatic setting without definite fracture, a radiographically occult fracture may be present (think radial head fracture in adults and supracondylar fracture in children).

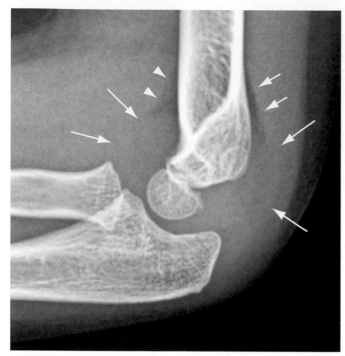

Fig. 3.9 Fat pad sign in child with a nondisplaced supracondylar fracture. Lateral radiograph shows posterior *(short arrows)* and anterior *(arrowheads)* fat pad signs due to hemarthrosis. *Long arrows* outline the distended joint capsule.

LIGAMENTS

The major ligaments of the elbow are the *ulnar, or medial, collateral ligament (UCL) complex,* and the *radial, or lateral, collateral ligament (RCL) complex.* The medial and lateral ligament structures are shown in Figs. 3.10 through 3.12. The RCL complex blends with the *annular ligament* that surrounds the radial head.

Medial Ligaments

The UCL complex (see Fig. 3.10) is composed of three separate components, the easiest to see and functionally most important being the *anterior bundle.* The *posterior* and *transverse bundles* are thin and closely apposed to the trochlea and ulna, making them difficult to distinguish as distinct structures even with high-resolution ultrasound (US) or magnetic resonance imaging (MRI).

- *Anterior bundle.*
  - Cordlike bundle that attaches to the medial epicondyle proximally and sublime tubercle distally.
  - Functionally composed of anterior and posterior components, which are not resolved by MRI.
  - Primary restraint to valgus forces, therefore vulnerable to injury with acute or chronic valgus stress.
  - Best seen on coronal MR images obtained with the elbow in extension (see Fig. 3.12B and C).
  - Normal anterior bundle has sharp margins and low signal intensity on all sequences.
- *Posterior bundle.*
  - Fan-shaped bundle that attaches to the medial epicondyle proximally and the medial margin of the trochlear notch of the ulna distally.
  - Secondary stabilizer of the elbow during flexion.

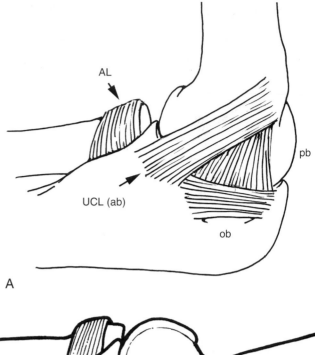

A

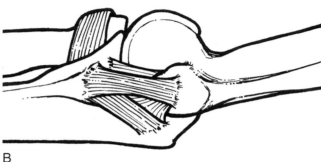

B

Fig. 3.10 Diagram of medial ligaments of the elbow. **(A)** Elbow flexed. **(B)** Elbow extended. *AL,* Annular ligament; *UCL (ab),* ulnar collateral ligament anterior bundle or band (the strongest and most important component of the UCL); *ob,* oblique (transverse) band of the UCL; *pb,* posterior bundle of the UCL.

- *Transverse bundle.*
  - Attaches to the olecranon proximally and the coronoid process distally, just posterior to the anterior bundle attachment site.
  - Plays least important role in medial elbow stability.

Lateral Ligaments

The RCL complex (see Fig. 3.11) includes both the RCL proper and the *lateral ulnar collateral ligament* (LUCL), both of which blend with the *annular ligament.*

- *Radial collateral ligament.*
  - Extends in a fan-like configuration from the lateral epicondyle proximally to the annular ligament distally (see Fig. 3.12A and B).
  - Primary lateral stabilizer and restraint to varus forces.
  - Best seen on coronal MR images obtained with the elbow in extension.
  - Lies just deep to the common extensor tendon origin; thus, abnormalities of the RCL are commonly seen in combination with chronic common extensor origin pathology (i.e. lateral epicondylitis).

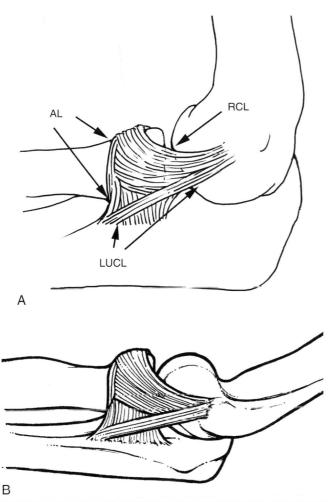

Fig. 3.11 Diagram of lateral ligaments of the elbow. **(A)** Elbow flexed. **(B)** Elbow extended. *AL*, Annular ligament; *LUCL*, lateral ulnar collateral ligament; *RCL*, radial collateral ligament (note that the RCL blends into the annular ligament).

- *Lateral ulnar collateral ligament.*
  - Extends from the posterior aspect of the RCL origin on the lateral epicondyle, coursing medially and distally along the posterior aspect of the radial head and neck, attaching distally onto the posterolateral ulna (see Fig. 3.12C).
  - Blends imperceptibly with the RCL at its proximal attachment site, which cannot be distinguished by MRI.
  - Forms a sling along the posterior margin of the radial head and serves as an important posterolateral elbow stabilizer.
  - Best seen on coronal MR images obtained with the elbow in extension.
  - May be injured during posterior elbow dislocation or subluxation and result in posterolateral rotatory instability (PLRI).
- *Annular (or orbicular) ligament.*
  - Attaches to the radial notch of the proximal ulna and wraps around the radial head in the transverse plane (see Fig. 3.12A and B; see also Fig. 3.13B).
  - Forms a collar around the radial head, stabilizing the radial head and preventing dislocation during supination and pronation.

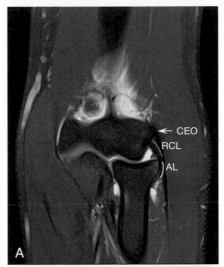
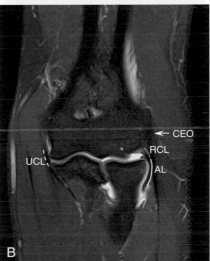
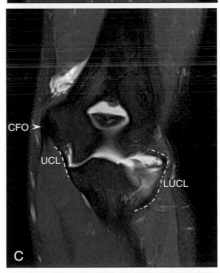

Fig. 3.12 Medial and lateral structures of the elbow. Three sequential coronal proton density fat-suppressed MR arthrogram images **(A–C,** anterior to posterior) demonstrate the main medial and lateral ligament and tendon structures. *AL*, Annular ligament (*solid line*); *CEO*, common extensor tendon origin (*arrow*); *CFO*, common flexor-pronator tendon origin (*arrowhead*); *LUCL*, lateral ulnar collateral ligament (*dot-dashed line*); *RCL*, radial collateral ligament (*dotted line*); *UCL*, ulnar collateral ligament (*dashed line*). Image modified with permission from Sulcus, Inc.

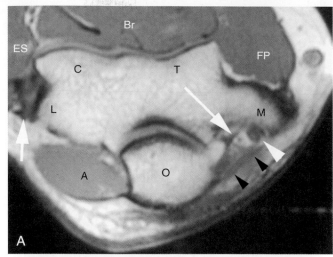

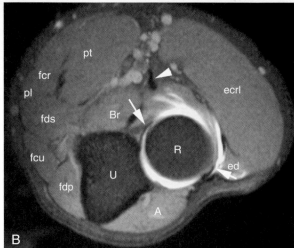

Fig. 3.13 Normal MR anatomy of the elbow: axial images. **(A)** Axial T1-weighted MR image obtained through the distal aspect of the humeral epicondyles. *White arrowhead,* ulnar nerve; *black arrowheads,* cubital tunnel retinaculum; *short white arrow,* common extensor tendon; *long arrow,* floor of the cubital tunnel formed by the transverse and posterior bands of the ulnar collateral ligament. **(B)** Fat-suppressed T1-weighted MR arthrogram more distal than in A, through the radial head. *Arrowhead,* biceps tendon; *short arrows,* annular ligament. Muscles: *A,* Anconeus; *Br,* brachialis; *ecrl,* extensor carpi radialis longus; *ed,* extensor digitorum; *ES,* extensor-supinator group; *fcr,* flexor carpi radialis; *fcu,* flexor carpi ulnaris; *fdp,* flexor digitorum profundus; *fds,* flexor digitorum superficialis; *FP,* flexor pronator group; *pl,* palmaris longus; *pt,* pronator teres. Bones: *C,* Capitellum; *L,* lateral epicondyle; *M,* medial epicondyle; *O,* olecranon; *R,* radial head; *T,* trochlea; *U,* ulna.

- Serves as the distal attachment site for the RCL and as the origin for the superficial head of the supinator muscle.
- Most commonly disrupted by radial head dislocation in adults.

COMMON EXTENSOR ORIGIN

The lateral epicondyle serves as the common tendon origin for the wrist extensor muscles (see Fig. 3.12A and B).

- Tendons of the common extensor origin include:
  - Extensor carpi radialis brevis (ECRB).
  - Extensor digitorum communis (EDC).

- Extensor carpi ulnaris (ECU).
- Extensor digitorum minimi (EDM).
- ECRB and EDC share an origin along the most superior and anterior aspect of the lateral epicondyle and are the primary sites of common extensor tendon pathology (clinically termed *lateral epicondylitis*).
  - Note that it is difficult to separate out the origins of the common extensor tendons on MRI.
- The brachioradialis and extensor carpi radialis longus (ECRL) muscles arise from the supracondylar ridge and lie anterior and superficial to the common extensor tendon origin.
- The anconeus muscle originates at the posterior margin of the lateral epicondyle.
- The supinator muscle originates at the anterior margin of the lateral epicondyle.

COMMON FLEXOR-PRONATOR ORIGIN

The medial epicondyle is larger than the lateral epicondyle and serves as the common tendon origin for the wrist flexor-pronator muscle group (commonly referred to in the orthopedic literature as the *flexor-pronator mass*) (see Fig. 3.12C).

- Structures of the flexor-pronator muscle group (from radial to ulnar) include:
  - PT.
  - Flexor carpi radialis (FCR).
  - Palmaris longus (PL).
  - Flexor digitorum superficialis (FDS).
  - Flexor carpi ulnaris (FCU).
- PT and FCR share an origin along the anterior margin of the medial epicondyle and are the primary sites of common flexor-pronator tendon pathology (clinically termed *medial epicondylitis*).

BICEPS TENDON

- The main function of the *biceps* muscle is to flex the elbow joint and supinate the forearm.
- The biceps muscle is composed of two separate heads:
  - *Long head* originates at the supraglenoid tubercle and superior labrum.
  - *Short head* originates from the coracoid process.
- The two heads of the biceps converge to form a common tendon approximately 7 cm from the distal attachment site, which crosses the elbow joint and inserts on the radial tuberosity.
  - Each tendon head component has a distinct footprint on the radial tuberosity.
  - Long head component is positioned posterior to the short head component, inserting more proximal and ulnar on the radial tuberosity than the short head.
- The *bicipitoradial bursa* lies between the biceps tendon and radial tuberosity, and is usually collapsed.
  - Distal biceps tendon does NOT have a tendon sheath; fluid identified about an intact distal biceps tendon is typically within the bicipitoradial bursa.
- The *lacertus fibrosus,* or *bicipital aponeurosis,* is a broad medial expansion of the distal biceps myotendinous junction.

- Descends medially, covering the brachial artery and median nerve, and blending with the deep fascia of the forearm flexor muscle group.
- In the setting of a complete biceps tendon rupture, an intact lacertus fibrosis may limit tendon retraction and falsely simulate an intact tendon on clinical exam.

TRICEPS TENDON

- The *triceps* muscle is the primary extensor of the elbow joint (the *anconeus* also plays a minor role in elbow extension).
- The triceps muscle is composed of three separate heads:
  - *Long head* originates from the infraglenoid tubercle of the scapula.
  - *Lateral head* originates from the posterior humeral shaft, above the radial groove.
  - *Medial head* originates from the posterior humeral shaft, below the radial groove.
- The distal triceps has a broad insertion on the olecranon process, with two distinct olecranon attachments:
  - Thick posterior tendon insertion formed by the combined lateral and long head contributions.
  - Anterior, predominantly muscular insertion formed by the medial head contribution.
- The *olecranon bursa* is located superficial to the distal triceps insertion and the olecranon process.

CUBITAL TUNNEL

- The ulnar nerve is located posterior to the medial epicondyle of the humerus in a small groove medial to the olecranon, the *cubital tunnel* (Fig. 3.13A).
  - Superficial location exposes the ulnar nerve to direct trauma.
  - Subluxation of the ulnar nerve out of the cubital tunnel during flexion/extension may result in ulnar neuropathy.
  - Injury to the nearby UCL and flexor-pronator muscle group can result in concomitant ulnar nerve pathology.
- The posterior and transverse bundles of the UCL form the floor of the cubital tunnel and thus are adjacent to the ulnar nerve.
- The cubital tunnel retinaculum (also termed the *ligament of Osborne*) forms the roof of the cubital tunnel, extending from the medial epicondyle to the olecranon.
- Proximal to the cubital tunnel, the ulnar nerve descends between the medial head of triceps muscle and the medial intermuscular septum.
- Distal to the cubital tunnel, the ulnar nerve extends into the forearm between the superficial and deep heads of the FCU muscle.

Imaging Techniques

RADIOGRAPHY

Radiographs are the initial imaging study of choice for elbow pain, particularly in the posttraumatic setting. Radiographs may demonstrate fracture, dislocation, osteoarthritis, calcific tendonitis, calcified or ossified intraarticular bodies, osseous lesions, and other acute and nonacute findings.

- All elbow series should include at least anteroposterior (AP) and lateral views, the latter obtained with the elbow flexed 90 degrees to assess for a joint effusion.
- AP oblique views can increase detection of subtle fractures.
- Oblique radial head view may be useful if a radial head fracture is suspected (see Fig. 3.14C).

MAGNETIC RESONANCE IMAGING

MRI of the elbow is extremely useful for evaluating soft tissue structures in the elbow, including ligaments, muscles, tendons, and nerves. MRI is also exquisitely sensitive for the detection of marrow edema and may demonstrate radiographically occult fractures.

- MRI of the elbow is performed with the elbow fully extended.
- Use of a surface coil that allows the elbow to be scanned at the patient's side may enhance patient comfort but places the elbow away from the magnet isocenter.
- Positioning the elbow in the center of the magnet with the arm fully abducted (elbow above the patient's head) is an alternative if off-axis imaging is unsuccessful.

While protocols may vary between institutions, routine MRI of the elbow includes imaging in the coronal, sagittal, and axial planes, using the medial and lateral epicondyles as anatomic landmarks. Imaging is acquired using T1-weighted, short tau inversion recovery (STIR), and proton density (PD) or T2-weighted fat-suppressed pulse sequences.

- Anterior and posterior compartment structures best evaluated using the sagittal and axial images.
- Medial and lateral elbow structures best evaluated on coronal and axial images.
- Sample elbow MRI protocol routinely used at our practices includes: axial T1, axial STIR, coronal T1, coronal PD fat-suppressed, and sagittal PD fat-suppressed sequences.

A special *FABS* (flexion abduction supination) view may be performed to better evaluate the distal biceps tendon. This is performed with the arm positioned above the head, flexed at 90 degrees. Imaging plane is prescribed coronal to the distal humerus, perpendicular to the proximal radius, using either PD or T2 weighting, with and without fat suppression.

MRI performed after intraarticular injection of gadolinium-based contrast solution (direct MR arthrography) is the preferred technique for assessment of collateral ligament injury in athletes and can also be useful for evaluation of articular cartilage and osteochondral defects.

- Imaging principles similar to those discussed in Chapter 2—Shoulder.
- Protocols rely on T1-weighted fat-suppressed and PD or T2-weighted fat-suppressed sequences to best assess the articular cartilage and ligaments.
- Sample elbow MR arthrogram protocol routinely used at our practices includes: axial T1, axial PD fat-suppressed,

coronal T1 fat-suppressed, coronal PD fat-suppressed, and sagittal T1 fat-suppressed sequences.

ULTRASOUND

Musculoskeletal US of the elbow is best utilized as a targeted examination to answer a specific question about a particular anatomic structure. US is useful to evaluate for:

- Distal biceps and triceps tendon insertion tendinopathy and tears.
- Common flexor-pronator and common extensor tendon origin pathology (medial and lateral epicondylitis).
- Radial and UCL integrity.
- Cubital tunnel and ulnar nerve abnormalities.
- Joint effusion, synovitis, and olecranon bursitis.

A major advantage of US over MRI is the ability to evaluate the dynamic status of structures in real time, such as ulnar nerve subluxation or abnormal gapping of the medial joint space with valgus loading (in the setting of UCL insufficiency).

US is often utilized for image-guided elbow interventional procedures, such as joint aspiration, corticosteroid injections, and percutaneous needle tenotomy.

COMPUTED TOMOGRAPHY

Computed tomography (CT) is useful for characterizing complex intraarticular fractures and posttraumatic complications, such as intraarticular bodies, fracture fragment malalignment, and osteophytes. CT may also detect soft tissue calcifications or ossification within tendons or ligaments. Direct CT arthrography may aid in detection of intraarticular bodies and chondral defects if MRI is contraindicated.

Pathophysiology

EPICONDYLITIS

Epicondylitis is a chronic injury involving the common extensor or common flexor-pronator tendon origins at the lateral or medial epicondyles, respectively. The term *epicondylitis* is a misnomer, as the disease process is manifest by tendinopathy and/or tendon tearing, rather than an inflammatory condition. Nonetheless, the terms *medial epicondylitis* (or '*golfer's elbow*') and *lateral epicondylitis* (or '*tennis elbow*') remain pervasive throughout the literature and in clinical practice.

- Repetitive microtrauma results in microtears and breakdown of the tendon collagen fibers with subsequent ingrowth of fibroblasts and granulation tissue, referred to as *angiofibroblastic tendinosis*.
- *Angiofibroblastic hyperplasia* is the term used to describe the histologic changes that occur within the tendon caused by chronic repetitive trauma:
  - Normal collagen architecture is damaged by fibroblast infiltration, immature vascular response, and an incomplete reparative process, with few acute or chronic inflammatory cells.

- Ultimately progresses to structural failure with tendon degeneration, microtearing, fibrosis, and/or calcification.
- Findings on MRI include tendon thickening, increased intrasubstance signal, and/or tendon tearing.

Disease Processes

TRAUMA

Elbow radiographs are the initial imaging study of choice in the posttraumatic setting. A normal elbow radiograph checklist is included in Box 3.1. Elbow fractures often occur in the setting of fall on an outstretched hand or due to direct high-impact trauma. Common sites include supracondylar fractures in children and radial head fractures in adults.

Fractures in Adults

- Radial head and neck fractures.
  - Fall on an outstretched hand is the most common cause in adults (Fig. 3.14).
  - Normal elbow valgus angulation concentrates axial loads laterally; the radial head and neck are the weakest links in adults.
  - Radial head fractures may be nondisplaced and subtle on radiographs, but typically show an accompanying joint effusion.
    - Additional radial head or oblique views may reveal the fracture.
    - MRI or CT is diagnostic in equivocal cases, and may be recommended if occult fracture is suspected (Fig. 3.15).
  - Impaction of the radial head articular surface is common.
    - Fracture displacement resulting in an articular surface step-off of 2 mm or greater is associated with development of secondary osteoarthritis.
    - Open reduction with internal fixation may be used to improve congruency of the articular surfaces.
  - Highly comminuted or displaced radial head and neck fractures are typically caused by high-impact trauma.
    - In such cases, additional fractures, elbow dislocation, and concomitant soft tissue injuries may be present.

Box 3.1   Normal Elbow Radiographic Anatomy Checklist

Anteroposterior (AP) view checklist	Lateral view checklist
Radial head aligned with capitellum	Fat pad sign (effusion)
Ulna aligned with trochlea	Radial head aligned with capitellum
Radial head articulates with ulna	Anterior humeral line intersects middle third of capitellum
Normal valgus ('carrying angle') approximately 165 degrees	Ulna congruent with trochlea
In children: Ossification centers normally positioned	

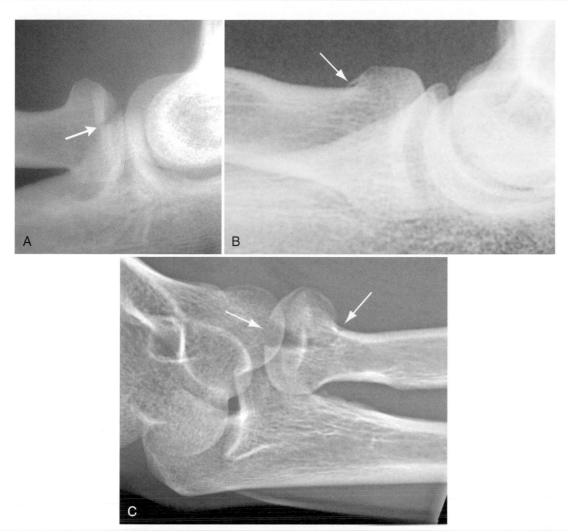

Fig. 3.14 Adult radial head fractures. **(A)** Linear fracture across the radial head *(arrow)*. **(B)** Subtly impacted radial head fracture *(arrow)* with intact articular surface. These fractures are treated conservatively. **(C)** Displaced head fracture *(arrows)*. This fracture may be treated with internal fixation or resection of the displaced anterior head fragment.

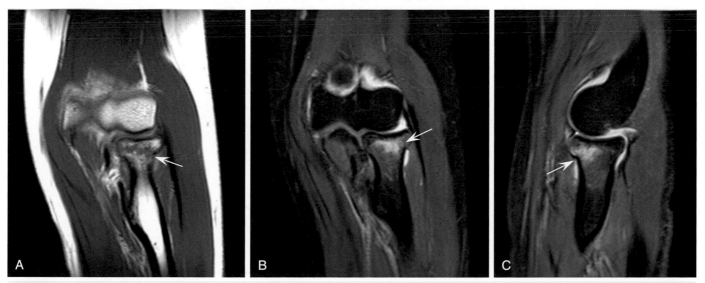

Fig. 3.15 Radiographically occult radial head fracture: diagnosis with MRI. Coronal T1-weighted MR image **(A)** shows an acute nondisplaced radial head fracture *(arrow)*, which was not evident on radiographs. Coronal **(B)** and sagittal **(C)** T2-weighted fat-suppressed MR images demonstrate associated intense marrow edema *(arrows)*. Note the associated joint effusion.

- *Essex-Lopresti fracture* is a comminuted fracture of the radial head and neck, acute tear of the interosseous ligament of the forearm, and dislocation of the distal radioulnar joint (Fig. 3.16).
- Olecranon process fractures.
  - Intraarticular fractures of the olecranon can occur as a result of direct trauma or due to avulsion of the distal triceps tendon (Fig. 3.17A).
    - Traction by the triceps displaces the proximal fragment proximally, potentially resulting in wide diastasis.
    - This fracture is treated with internal fixation (Fig. 3.17B).
- Distal humerus fractures.
  - Typically seen in older, osteoporotic patients and often simple transverse fractures.

- Fractures in younger adults typically also include a longitudinal intraarticular component in a Y or T configuration.
  - In such situations, an intraarticular fracture line usually extends through the trochlea, requiring surgical internal fixation usually with transcondylar screws and medial and lateral plates.
  - Complex intraarticular fractures may require an olecranon osteotomy for adequate visualization and access to the articular fragments during surgery.
- Forearm fractures.
  - *Nightstick fracture.*
    - Isolated fracture of the ulnar shaft caused by a direct blow to the forearm, such as when protecting oneself from the blow of a police officer's nightstick.

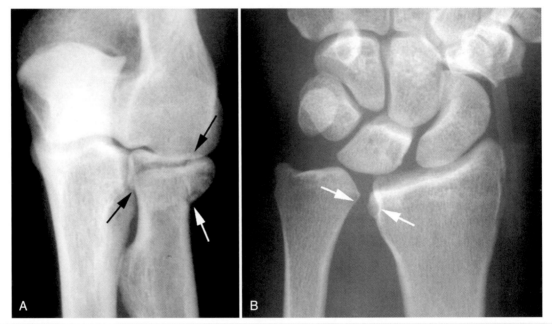

Fig. 3.16 Essex-Lopresti fracture-dislocation. The elbow **(A)** shows a comminuted radial head fracture *(arrows)*. The wrist **(B)** shows distal radioulnar joint dislocation seen as joint widening and distal displacement of the ulna *(arrows)*. The primary injury is an acute tear of the interosseous ligament of the forearm. This is an unstable fracture that requires specialized orthopedic management.

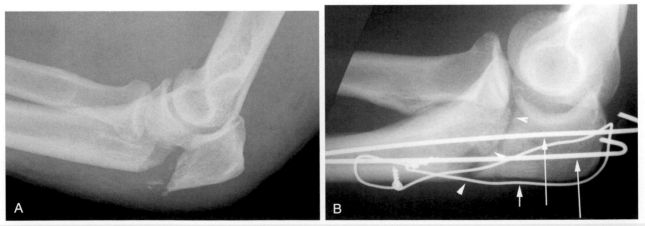

Fig. 3.17 Olecranon avulsion fracture. **(A)** Transverse fracture due to avulsion by the triceps muscle. **(B)** Postoperative appearance in a different patient. Fixation can be accomplished with a longitudinal screw or, as in this case, wires *(long arrows)* with a figure-of-eight tensioning band *(short arrows)*. Note the fracture *(arrowheads)*.

- *Galeazzi fracture.*
  - Fracture of the radial shaft and dislocation of the distal ulna (Fig. 3.18).
  - Distal radioulnar joint is injured and may result in chronic instability.
- *Monteggia fracture.*
  - Dislocation of the radial head and fracture of the proximal ulnar shaft (Fig. 3.19).
- Most commonly, forearm shaft fractures involve both bones (radius and ulna).
  - Both-bone fractures in children are often treated with casting, given their inherent ability to heal rapidly and continue to remodel after healing is complete.

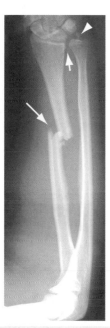

Fig. 3.18 Galeazzi fracture. Note the radial shaft fracture *(long arrow)* and distal ulnar dislocation *(short arrow)*. This patient also has an ulnar styloid fracture *(arrowhead)*.

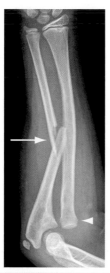

Fig. 3.19 Monteggia fracture dislocation. Lateral radiographic view of the forearm shows anterior dislocation of the radial head *(arrowhead)* and a fracture of the proximal ulna *(arrow)*.

- Both-bone fractures in adults are usually treated by internal fixation of each bone.
- In the setting of forearm fractures, the anterior (volar) forearm musculature is vulnerable to compartment syndrome.
  - Early detection is imperative, accomplished best by direct measurement of intracompartmental pressure rather than by imaging.
  - Treatment of acute compartment syndrome is by decompressive fasciotomy.
  - *Volkmann contracture* is a devastating result of volar forearm compartment syndrome, whereby the fingers and wrist develop progressive fixed flexion deformity due to fibrosis of the necrosed forearm muscles.

Fractures in Children

- *Supracondylar fractures.*
  - Most elbow fractures in children are the result of a fall on an outstretched hand, with the axial load resulting in forced hyperextension of the elbow.
  - Hyperextension forces the ulna to lever against the posterior distal humerus, resulting in a transverse fracture above the humeral condyles, a *supracondylar fracture* (Fig. 3.20).
  - Most common elbow fracture encountered in children.
  - May be obvious or subtle on radiographs, with two cardinal signs often present:
    - Posterior fat pad sign.
    - Posterior displacement of the capitellum relative to the anterior humeral line.
  - Alignment on the AP radiograph should also be assessed for evidence of abnormal cubitus valgus or varus because either of these findings may alter treatment.
    - May be quantitatively measured using *Baumann's angle*, formed by the humeral shaft and the capitellar physis.
    - Comparison with the contralateral elbow may be required; a difference of 5 degrees or more between injured and uninjured sides is considered significant.
- *Lateral condyle fractures.*
  - Fractures of the lateral humeral condyle are the second most common type of elbow fracture in children.
  - Lateral condyle fractures are caused by varus stress, which may be due to lateral blow to the forearm or when a child falls laterally with the arm at the side.
  - Varus stress causes distraction force across the lateral side of the elbow that can result in an avulsion-like fracture that may be complete or incomplete.
  - Typically, these fractures extend along or across the lateral distal humeral physis, usually with a small metaphyseal fragment (Fig. 3.21).
  - The distal extent of the fracture may be incomplete or complete, though distinguishing between the two can be difficult because there is often a large component involving unossified cartilage, which is not visible on radiographs (Fig. 3.22).
    - Additional imaging with MRI or intraoperative arthrography may be useful for distinguishing between the two.
  - If *incomplete*, the fracture may not extend beyond the physis, or may extend distally into the lateral condyle,

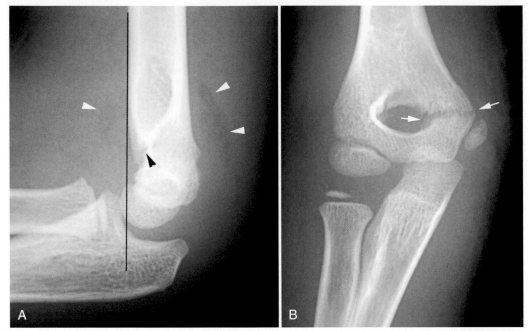

Fig. 3.20 Displaced supracondylar fracture. **(A)** Lateral radiographic view shows displaced anterior and posterior fat pads *(white arrowheads)* and posterior displacement of the capitellar growth center relative to the anterior humeral line. A portion of the fracture line is faintly seen *(black arrowhead)*. **(B)** AP view shows the lateral aspect of the fracture line. The AP view of a supracondylar fracture often does not show the fracture. Careful attention to the appearance of the fat pads and alignment on the lateral view is necessary to make the diagnosis.

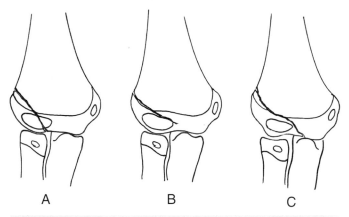

Fig. 3.21 Diagram of childhood lateral humeral condylar fractures. **(A)** True Salter–Harris IV fracture with osseous fracture of the capitellar growth center. **(B)** Incomplete fracture with extension into the condylar cartilage. The fracture line might also terminate within the physis without extension into the condylar cartilage. **(C)** Complete fracture through the condylar cartilage. This fracture can be difficult to diagnose with radiographs. This pattern is more common than that seen in A and is also potentially unstable.

either through the ossified portion of the capitellum or, far more frequently, medial to the capitellum through unossified cartilage.

- Incomplete lateral condyle fractures generally are stable and are treated with casting.
- If *complete*, the fracture line continues distally to the articular surface.
  - Complete lateral condyle fractures generally are unstable and require operative fixation.
- Distal humeral physeal separation injury.
  - Fracture-separation of the distal humeral physis (also termed a transphyseal distal humerus fracture)

represents a displaced Salter–Harris I (or rarely Salter–Harris II) fracture of the distal humerus.

- Displacement of the epiphysis is usually medial or posteromedial, in contrast with the posterolateral displacement usually seen in adult elbow dislocation.
- Significant force is required, often with a twisting component.
- Can occur during a difficult delivery and is associated with child abuse in infants and toddlers.
- Clinical and radiographic diagnosis can be difficult, especially in infants because the displaced bones are unossified, and therefore difficult to distinguish from elbow dislocation.
  - US or MRI can confirm the diagnosis in infants and toddlers.
- Medial epicondyle ossification center avulsion injury.
  - Valgus stress can result in avulsion of the medial epicondyle ossification center (Figs. 3.23 to 3.25).
  - Can occur as an acute avulsion with obvious displacement or as a chronic stress injury due to repetitive traction (see Little Leaguer's elbow).
  - Valgus stress causes traction on the medial epicondyle by the strong UCL and the wrist flexor-pronator muscle group.
  - The apophysis physis is the weakest link, thus it yields before the other structures are injured.
  - The avulsed medial epicondyle is typically displaced distally by the pull of the UCL and flexor-pronator muscles.
    - Radiographs reveal displacement of the medial epicondyle ossification center, which may be subtle and require comparison with the uninjured side.
    - Either MRI or US can be helpful in diagnosing avulsion of an unossified medial epicondyle in a younger child.

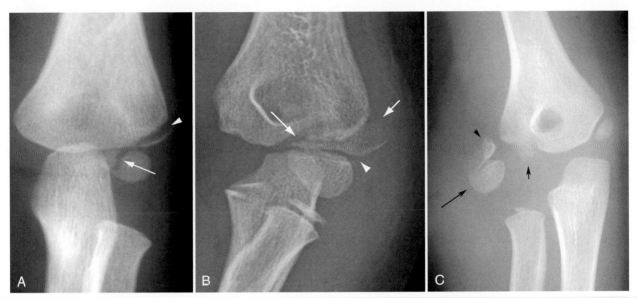

Fig. 3.22 Lateral condylar fractures. **(A)** Salter–Harris IV fracture. AP radiograph shows the fracture extending through the distal lateral metaphysis *(arrowhead)* and the capitellar growth center *(arrow)*, similar to Fig. 3.21A. **(B)** Displaced complete fracture. Note the fracture *(arrows)* proximal to the capitellar physis *(arrowhead)*. The fragment is displaced laterally. The fracture extended distally and medially through unossified trochlear cartilage similar to Fig. 3.21C. **(C)** Complete fracture. The fragment is displaced laterally and rotated. Note the small metaphyseal fragment *(arrowhead)* and the capitellar growth center *(long arrow)*. Although the capitellar growth center appears to be intact on this view, there is a small nondisplaced capitellar fragment *(short arrow)*. Also note the extensive lateral soft tissue swelling. (Image **C** courtesy of L. Das Narla, MD)

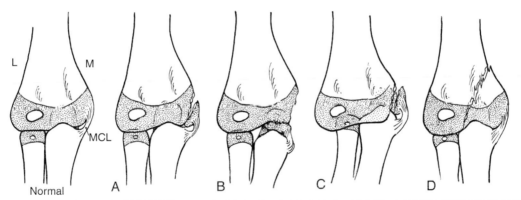

Fig. 3.23 Diagram shows types of fractures involving medial epicondyle in children. Right elbow is illustrated. **(A)** Simple avulsion of medial epicondyle. **(B)** Avulsion with entrapment of medial epicondyle between ulna and trochlea. **(C)** Avulsion in association with elbow dislocation. **(D)** Salter–Harris IV fracture of medial humeral condyle. *L,* Lateral; *M,* medial; *MCL,* medial (ulnar) collateral ligament. (Reprinted with permission from May DA, Disler DG, Jones EA, Pearce DA. Using sonography to diagnose an unossified medial epicondyle avulsion in a child. *AJR.* 2000;174:1115-1117. Modified with permission from Rogers LF. *Radiology of Skeletal Trauma.* New York: Churchill Livingstone; 1992, pp 772-779.)

- Prompt healing with normal function is achieved simply by placing the arm in a sling, although radiographs often reveal persistent widening and irregularity of the injured physis.
- Surgical repair is generally reserved for high-level athletes, patients with elbow instability, or if there is displacement of the medial epicondyle by greater than 5 mm.
- An important variant of medial epicondyle ossification center avulsion is intraarticular *medial epicondyle entrapment* (see Fig. 3.24).
  - The elbow may transiently dislocate posterolaterally during a medial epicondylar avulsion, opening the medial joint space and allowing the avulsed medial epicondyle fragment to slip between the trochlea and ulna, where it becomes entrapped.
- Rapid identification of this condition is essential because an entrapped medial epicondyle will fuse to the ulna within a few weeks, resulting in permanent disability.
- Radiographs of medial epicondylar entrapment may be deceptive; a joint effusion may not be present and the entrapped medial epicondylar ossification center may simulate a normal trochlear ossification center if the trochlea is unossified.
- Knowledge of the normal maturation of the elbow ossification centers is necessary to avoid this pitfall (recall the mnemonic CRITOE; see Fig. 3.5).

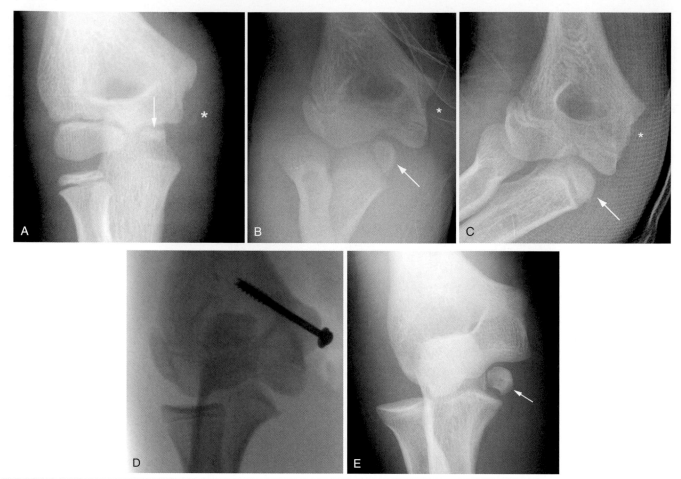

Fig. 3.24 Medial epicondyle avulsion injuries in children. **(A)** Medial epicondyle entrapment after transient elbow dislocation. The entrapped medial epicondyle simulates a normal trochlear ossification center *(arrow)*. The medial soft tissue swelling is a clue to the diagnosis, but the important finding is that a normal medial epicondyle growth center is not seen *(asterisk)*. **(B–D)** Medial epicondyle entrapment in an older child after elbow dislocation. **(B)** Initial frontal radiograph shows elbow dislocation. The medial epicondyle is absent from its normal location *(asterisk)* and is displaced distally and medially *(arrow)*. **(C)** Repeat radiograph after dislocation reduction shows medial epicondyle entrapment *(arrow)*. Again note the absence of the medial epicondyle from its normal location *(asterisk)*. Diagnosis in this case is easier than in the younger child shown in A. **(D)** Postoperative radiograph. The medial epicondyle was reduced and, in this older child, fixed with a lag screw. **(E)** Entrapped medial epicondyle in an older child after spontaneous partial reduction of an elbow dislocation *(arrow)*. Note that all the other ossification centers have fused. The medial epicondyle is the last elbow ossification center to fuse.

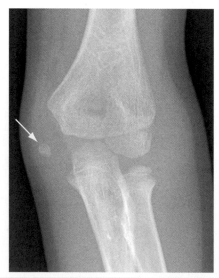

Fig. 3.25 Medial epicondyle avulsion. AP radiograph shows medial and distal displacement of the medial epicondyle ossification center *(arrow)*.

- If what appears to be a normal trochlear ossification center is seen without a normally positioned, partially ossified medial epicondylar center, the diagnosis of medial epicondylar entrapment is likely.
- If this diagnosis is suspected in a younger child, in whom neither the medial epicondyle nor the trochlea has begun to ossify, then US or MRI can be used to locate the medial epicondyle.

Elbow Dislocation in Children

- The elbow is the most frequently traumatically dislocated joint in children younger than 10 years.
- Complete dislocation of both the ulna and radius can occur during a fall with the elbow slightly flexed.
  - The radius and ulna usually dislocate posteriorly, although displacement in other directions may occur.
- If only the radial head is dislocated, then a proximal ulnar fracture (*Monteggia fracture*) must be excluded (see Fig. 3.19).

- Childhood elbow dislocation can also occur on a congenital basis, either as a sporadic finding or in association with onycho-osteodysplasia (discussed in Chapter 15—Congenital and Developmental Conditions).
- *Nursemaids' elbow*, also termed 'jerked elbow' or 'pulled elbow', is anterior subluxation or dislocation of the radial head in a young child with no disruption or only partial disruption of the annular ligament.
    - A distracting force applied to the forearm or hand with the arm extended can allow the radial head to slip out of the collar formed by the annular ligament.
    - The typical child with this condition is between 2 and 3 years old, although it may occur in older children up to age 6 or 7 years.
    - Careful scrutiny of radiographs may reveal subtle subluxation of the radial head, but radiographs are frequently normal, and an elbow joint effusion is usually absent.
    - The child often holds the injured elbow in flexion and pronation and refuses to allow extension or supination.
    - This condition is usually self-limited and may spontaneously reduce (including when positioning the child for x-rays) but may require closed reduction, which is accomplished by supination with the elbow flexed.

Elbow Dislocation in Adults

- Elbow dislocation is less frequent in adults than in children.
- As in children, the radius and ulna usually dislocate posteriorly, although dislocation in almost any direction may occur.
- Associated fractures are frequent, and there often is significant associated ligamentous, neurovascular, and muscular injury (Fig. 3.26).

- Myositis ossificans in the muscles that surround the elbow, notably in the brachialis muscle, is a frequent sequela of elbow dislocation.
- Prompt reduction of the elbow dislocation reduces the risk of posttraumatic heterotopic ossification and associated limited range of motion.

OSTEOCHONDRAL INJURY

- Varying osteochondral pathologies occur in the elbow.
- *Panner disease* is a usually benign and self limited condition affecting the articular cartilage, unossified cartilage, and subchondral bone of the capitellum, with fragmentation and often edema.
    - Seen in children aged 5–10 years (commonly in the dominant arm of throwing athletes) during active endochondral ossification of the capitellar growth center.
    - Characterized by flattening, fragmentation, fissuring, and sclerosis of the capitellar growth center, usually affecting the entire capitellar epiphysis (Fig. 3.27).
    - Healing may require cessation of the offending activity.
    - Usually does *not* result in an unstable osteochondral fragment or intraarticular body.
- *Osteochondritis dissecans* (OCD) of the capitellum is a separate clinical entity characterized by osteonecrosis or osteochondral separation.
    - Seen in individuals older than 10 years, and most often adolescents, after the capitellar growth center has ossified.
    - Thought to result from acute trauma or repetitive microtrauma compounded by relatively poor epiphyseal blood supply.
        - Most commonly seen in the dominant arm throwing athletes, particularly baseball pitchers, and those participating in sports requiring substantial upper extremity use.

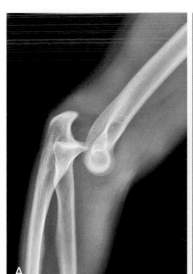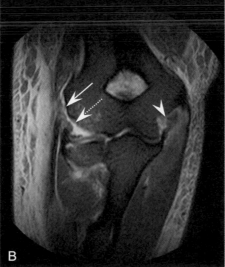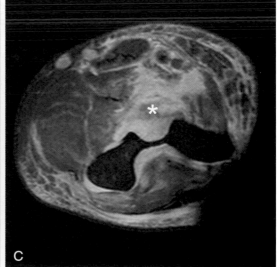

Fig. 3.26 Posterior elbow dislocation. (A) Lateral radiograph demonstrating an acute posterior elbow dislocation. (B) Coronal proton density fat-suppressed MR image demonstrates avulsion of the common extensor tendon *(arrow)* and radial collateral ligament (RCL, *dotted arrow*), as well as tearing of the ulnar collateral ligament (UCL, *arrowhead*). (C) Axial STIR MR image shows extensive tearing of the brachialis muscle with interposed fluid/hematoma *(asterisk)*.

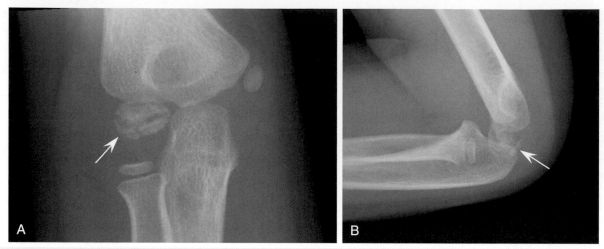

Fig. 3.27 Panner disease (osteochondrosis of the capitellum). AP **(A)** and lateral **(B)** radiographs of the elbow in a 5-year-old demonstrate irregularity and fragmentation of the capitellar growth center *(arrows)*.

- ▪ Identical to osteochondritis dissicans occurring elsewhere in the body, although less common than in the knee and ankle.
  - ▪ Characterized by fragmentation of capitellar articular cartilage and bone, and subchondral marrow edema and cystic change, usually affecting the anterolateral capitellum (Fig. 3.28).
  - ▪ May be stable or develop an unstable osteochondral fragment or fragments, characterized by an in situ fragment with undermining fluid signal (or contrast if arthrography is performed).
  - ▪ Displacement of an unstable osteochondral fragment into the joint results in an intraarticular body (Fig. 3.29).
- ▪ Osteochondral injuries must be distinguished from the normal variant *pseudodefect of the capitellum*, which is seen at the posterolateral capitellum (see Fig. 3.7).

INTRAARTICULAR BODY

- ▪ Intraarticular bodies in the elbow joint are most commonly seen in the setting of articular cartilage injury,

displaced osteochondral fragment, or underlying osteoarthritis.
- ▪ May cause pain and mechanical symptoms (locking, catching, etc.) and can be removed arthroscopically in symptomatic individuals.
- ▪ Multiple intraarticular bodies resulting from articular cartilage damage or osteoarthritis (secondary synovial chondromatosis) must be differentiated from primary synovial chondromatosis.
- ▪ *Primary synovial chondromatosis* is a benign idiopathic condition characterized by synovial metaplasia resulting in multiple intraarticular cartilage bodies, which may ossify over time (Fig. 3.30).
  - ▪ Typically seen in younger patients (aged 30–50) compared to secondary chondromatosis, with lesser degrees of osteoarthritis (though can lead to secondary osteoarthritis related to mechanical erosion of articular cartilage).
  - ▪ Numerous small, uniformly sized intraarticular bodies.
- ▪ *Os supratrochleare dorsale* is a small ossicle that resides in the olecranon fossa, generally considered to be a normal variant.

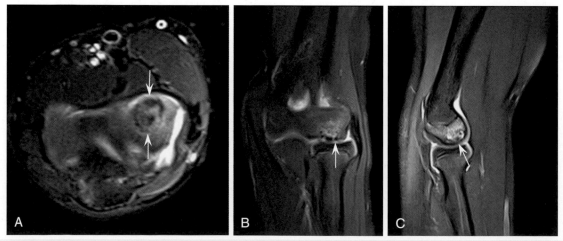

Fig. 3.28 Osteochondritis dissecans of the capitellum. Axial STIR **(A)** and coronal **(B)** and sagittal **(C)** proton density fat-suppressed MR images show osteochondritis dissecans of the anterior capitellum *(arrows)*, characterized by intense subchondral marrow edema, cystic change, and irregularity of the subchondral bone plate.

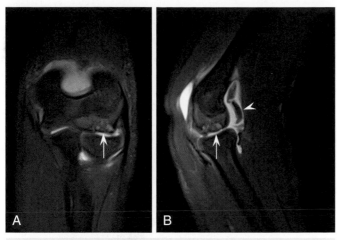

Fig. 3.29 Osteochondral lesion of the capitellum with displaced fragment. Coronal **(A)** and sagittal **(B)** proton density fat-suppressed MR images show a large osteochondral defect of the capitellum *(arrows)* with the corresponding displaced osteochondral fragment in the anterior joint recess *(arrowhead)*. Note the large joint effusion.

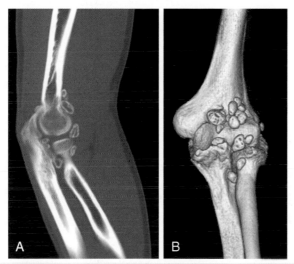

Fig. 3.30 Primary synovial chondromatosis of the elbow. Sagittal reconstruction CT image **(A)** and 3D volume-rendered image **(B)** of the elbow demonstrate numerous ossified intraarticular bodies throughout the elbow joint, consistent with primary synovial (osteo) chondromatosis.

- Can be asymptomatic or cause impingement and pain during elbow extension.
- May have an identical appearance to an ossified intraarticular body, though the distinction is not important, as a symptomatic ossicle will be removed whereas an asymptomatic ossicle generally will not.

LATERAL EPICONDYLITIS

- *Lateral epicondylitis* (colloquially referred to as *'tennis elbow'*) is a tendinopathy of the common extensor tendon origin, where the wrist extensor muscles attach at the lateral epicondyle (Figs. 3.31 and 3.32).
- Common affliction of many active individuals in addition to tennis players, typically presenting in the 4th and 5th decades of life.

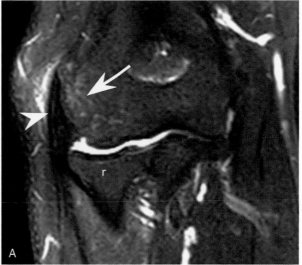

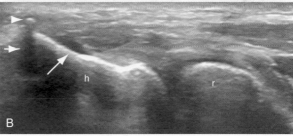

Fig. 3.31 Lateral epicondylitis. **(A)** Coronal inversion recovery MR image shows marrow edema in the lateral epicondyle *(arrow)* and subtle edema adjacent to the mildly thickened common extensor tendon *(arrowhead)*. This is a mild case. **(B)** Coronal US image in a different patient shows acute and chronic findings. Note the hyperechoic calcification *(arrowhead)* in thickened proximal tendon with posterior acoustic shadowing *(short arrow)*, compatible with chronic injury. Further distally, note a small hypoechoic acute partial tear *(long arrow)* h, Lateral humerus; r, radial head.

- Overuse injury caused by repetitive extension and/or supination of the wrist and forearm.
- Onset of symptoms usually insidious, presenting with lateral elbow pain exacerbated by gripping, lifting, and extension of the wrist.
- Most cases recover with conservative therapy; percutaneous tenotomy or surgical debridement may be used in refractory cases.
- Imaging is reserved for patients who do not respond adequately to initial conservative treatment.
  - Radiographs may be normal or show dystrophic tendon calcification with chronic disease (see Fig. 3.32A).
  - US may show tendon hypoechogenicity and thickening with loss of the normal fiber pattern, intratendinous or peritendinous hyperemia, tendon calcification, and tendon tearing.
  - MRI can be useful in assessing the extent of injury and exclude other causes of lateral elbow pain.
    - Common extensor tendon is best evaluated on PD or T2-weighted fat-suppressed imaging in the coronal plane; sagittal and axial imaging planes are complimentary.
    - Common extensor origin tendinosis is characterized by increased signal intensity on PD or T2-weighted

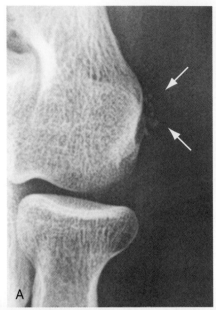

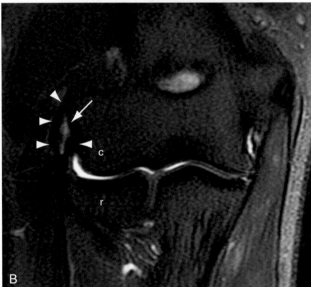

Fig. 3.32 Chronic lateral epicondylitis. **(A)** Radiograph shows numerous small calcifications in degenerated tendon *(arrows)*. **(B)** Coronal fat-suppressed T2-weighted MR image in a different patient shows interstitial tearing *(arrow)* in the substance of thickened tendon *(arrowheads)* c, Capitellum; r, radial head.

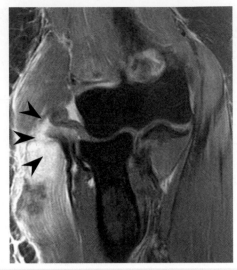

Fig. 3.33 Tear of the common extensor tendon. Coronal STIR MR image shows high signal intensity in and adjacent to the tendon *(arrowheads)* c, Capitellum; r, radial head. See also Fig. 3.38.

imaging, tendon thickening, peritendinous edema, and sometimes subentheseal marrow edema in the lateral epicondyle.
- More severe cases will show near-fluid bright intrasubstance T2 signal, which may represent fluid or granulation tissue within a tendon tear.
- Complete tears or avulsion of the common tendon may be seen in extreme cases or as an acute injury (Fig. 3.33, see also Fig. 3.38C).
- Potential pitfalls of lateral epicondylitis on MRI include the following:
  - Recent corticosteroid or platelet-rich plasma (PRP) injection can result in edema-like signal or fluid within the peritendinous soft tissues, which can persist for several days.

- Severity of MRI findings does not always correlate with severity of pain.
- Degeneration or tearing of the RCL complex often accompanies findings of lateral epicondylitis but are rarely of clinical significance and should not be overstated.

MEDIAL EPICONDYLITIS

- *Medial epicondylitis* (colloquially referred to as '*golfer's elbow*') is a tendinopathy of the common flexor-pronator tendon origin, where the wrist flexor and pronator muscles attach at the lateral epicondyle (Fig. 3.34).
- Occurs less commonly than lateral epicondylitis, but in a similar demographic.
- Overuse injury caused by repetitive valgus stress at the elbow, flexion, and/or pronation of the wrist and forearm.
- Imaging findings and treatment algorithm are identical to lateral epicondylitis.
- May be seen in combination with UCL and valgus extension overload injuries, particularly in throwing athletes.
- Must differentiate from ulnar nerve pathology, which is an alternative cause of medial pain.

DISTAL BICEPS TENDON RUPTURE

- Distal biceps tendon pathology ranges from tendinosis to partial- or full-thickness tear, summarized in Box 3.2.
- Chronic repetitive stress and injury results in tendinosis and weakening the tendon increasing the risk of later partial or complete tear (Fig. 3.35).
- Most frequently encountered tear is a *complete rupture* (full-thickness tear) at the insertion on the radial tuberosity, with proximal tendon retraction (Fig. 3.36).
  - Demographics and presentation:
    - Tears are most commonly seen in middle-aged males, particularly weightlifters.

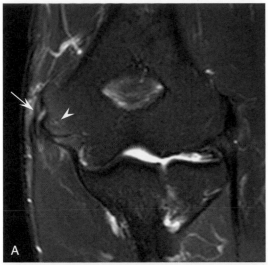

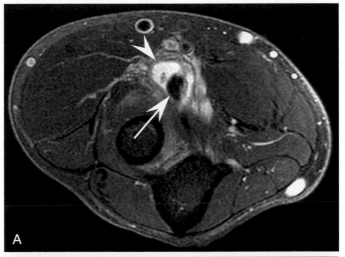

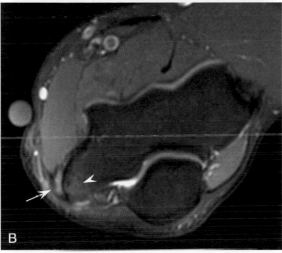

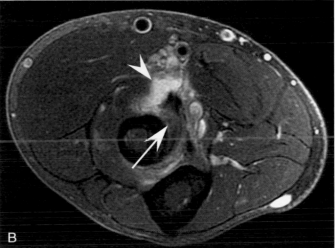

Fig. 3.34 Medial epicondylitis. Coronal **(A)** and axial **(B)** T2-weighted fat-suppressed MR images demonstrate thickening and interstitial tearing of the common flexor-pronator tendon origin *(arrows)* and mild subentheseal marrow edema *(arrowheads)*.

Fig. 3.35 Distal biceps tendinosis. Two sequential axial STIR MR images of the elbow **(A** and **B**, proximal to distal) demonstrate severe distal biceps tendinosis *(arrows)* with associated bicipitoradial bursitis *(arrowheads)*.

Box 3.2   Distal Biceps Tendon Injuries

Demographics	▪ Dominant arm
	▪ 40–70 years old
	▪ Male > female
Mechanism of injury	Axial loading with elbow flexed 90 degrees
Tendon's distal attachment site	Radial tuberosity
Injury pattern	Complete tear most common
MR evaluation	
▪ T2 axial images	▪ Complete versus incomplete tear
▪ T2 sagittal images	▪ Measure extent of tendon retraction
Pitfalls	
▪ Lacertus fibrosus	→ May prevent retraction of torn tendon mimicking an incomplete tear
▪ Bicipitoradial bursitis	→ Mimic of tendon pathology

▪ Local corticosteroid injection, use of anabolic steroids, and underlying inflammatory conditions such as rheumatoid arthritis increase the risk of biceps tendon tear.

▪ Patient often describes a 'pop' followed by acute onset of pain, swelling, and ecchymosis in the antecubital fossa.

▪ Physical exam may reveal a palpable tendon defect and bulging of the contracted muscle belly (*Popeye sign*).

▪ Best imaged with MRI of the elbow, which may require an increased field of view (FOV) to include the distal biceps myotendinous junction.

  ▪ MRI of the humerus is typically not adequate for evaluating the distal insertion on the radial tuberosity; imaging 5 cm distal to the elbow joint reliably includes the entire distal biceps tendon.

▪ Axial fluid-sensitive MR images demonstrate complete interruption of the distal biceps tendon, which is absent at the insertion.

▪ Sagittal fluid-sensitive MR images demonstrate the torn, retracted tendon.

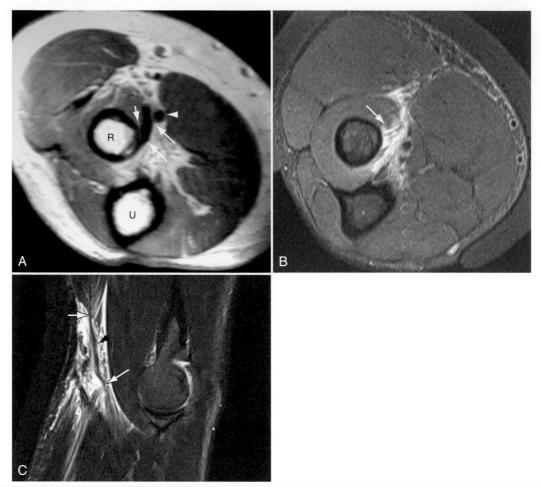

Fig. 3.36 Biceps tendon insertion and tear. **(A)** Normal distal biceps tendon. Axial T2-weighted MR image shows the distal tendon *(long arrows)* inserting onto the radius. Most biceps tendon tears occur at the insertion. The *short arrow* marks the location of the cubital bursa, which is normal in this case and therefore is not seen. Inflammation of this bursa causes local fluid accumulation and can clinically simulate a distal biceps tear or tendinitis. The *arrowhead* marks the ulnar artery. *R*, Radius; *U*, ulna. **(B)** Biceps tendon insertion tear. Axial fat-suppressed T2-weighted MR image shows intense edema in the expected location of the distal tendon *(arrow)* with surrounding edema. Most tears are distal and require surgical reattachment. **(C)** Partial tear. Sagittal fat-suppressed T2-weighted MR image shows edematous, elongated distal biceps tendon *(arrows)* with surrounding edema. Note some intact fibers *(arrowhead)*.

- Specialized coronal *FABS* sequence provides a longitudinal view of the tendon from the distal musculotendinous junction to the insertion; can be helpful in assessment and for measuring retraction, though often unnecessary to make the diagnosis.
  - Fluid and/or blood products are typically seen within the tear defect and surrounding the retracted tendon stump.
  - Degree of proximal retraction may be limited if the *lacertus fibrosus* remains intact.
- MRI of a degenerated or partially torn tendon reveals increased signal intensity on all sequences, tendon thickening, bicipitoradial bursitis, and/or peritendinous edema (see Fig. 3.35).
  - Distal biceps tendon has contributions from both the short and long heads, each with distinct footprints; tears may involve one tendon contribution more than the other.
- Biceps tendon tears are generally repaired surgically if complete (full-thickness) or high-grade partial-thickness (>50% of tendon involved).

- Note that distal biceps tendon tears are much less common than proximal long head biceps tendon tears (in the shoulder).

DISTAL TRICEPS TEAR

- The distal triceps has two olecranon insertions: a posterior tendon insertion (formed by the combined lateral and long heads), which is more vulnerable to tear/avulsion, and an anteromedial muscular insertion (arising from the medial head) that is torn much less commonly.
  - Distal triceps tendon tears, while rare, are usually characterized by complete avulsion (full-thickness tear) of the posterior tendon component at the insertion on the olecranon process.
  - Complete avulsions may have an accompanying displaced avulsion fracture fragment from the olecranon process.
  - The anterior muscular component (medial head component) may remain completely or partially

intact, which can limit the degree of proximal tendon retraction.

- Olecranon bursitis or hemorrhage may accompany a distal triceps tear.
- Predisposing factors for triceps tendon degeneration and tears include repetitive resisted extension (weightlifters and certain athletes, such as football linemen), as well as exogenous steroid use.
- Full-thickness triceps tears are often clinically apparent, but MRI and US can assist in determining the extent of injury (Fig. 3.37).
- Partial tendon tears or tendinosis are likewise best evaluated by MRI or US.
  - On MRI, the distal triceps tendon is best evaluated on the sagittal and axial fluid-sensitive sequences.
  - Findings of distal triceps tendinosis include increased signal intensity on all sequences, tendon thickening, reactive marrow edema within the olecranon process, and/or overlying olecranon bursitis.
  - Normal tendon contains thin longitudinal streaks of fibro-fatty tissue, giving the distal tendon a typical striated appearance, which should not be mistaken for interstitial tearing.

ULNAR COLLATERAL LIGAMENT TEAR

- Recall that the anterior bundle of the UCL is the primary restraint to valgus stress in the elbow.
  - UCL injuries are commonly seen in overhead throwing athletes, particularly baseball pitchers.
  - UCL is more susceptible to injury during high pitch counts when the dynamic medial stabilizers

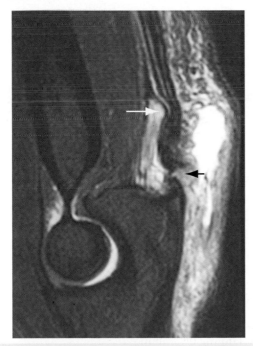

Fig. 3.37 Triceps tendon tear. Sagittal T2-weighted fat-suppressed MR image shows distal tear (black arrow), with wavy fibers further proximally (white arrow) and surrounding edema and fluid. Note that the tendon is not retracted, because the muscular medial insertion (not shown) was intact (as it often is), and intact lateral tendon fibers blend into lateral fascia, also tethering the tendon.

(common flexor muscles) are fatigued, which results in increased valgus stress transmitted to the UCL.

- Normally, the anterior bundle of the UCL has sharp margins and low signal intensity on all MRI sequences, best seen on coronal T2 or PD fat-suppressed sequences, or coronal T1-weighted fat-suppressed sequences on MR arthrography (see Fig. 3.12B and C).
- Low-grade sprains of the anterior bundle are characterized by increased signal intensity within the ligament, ligament thickening, periligamentous edema, and sometimes with edema in the overlying common flexor-pronator muscle group.
- Partial-thickness tears are characterized by partial disruption of ligament fibers, which may occur at the proximal, middle, or distal portions (Fig. 3.38).
  - Intraarticular contrast on MR arthrography may enter but not pass completely through a partial-thickness tear.
  - T sign on MR arthrography is characterized by contrast fluid undermining the distal UCL anterior bundle at the sublime tubercle attachment site due to partial-thickness undersurface tearing (although this finding can occasionally represent a normal variant distal insertion).
  - Approximately 50% of partial-thickness UCL tears in high-level athletes will heal with conservative treatment, the other 50% require UCL reconstruction.
- Complete tears reveal interruption and possibly laxity of ligament fibers, with escape of joint fluid or injected contrast into the overlying extraarticular soft tissues (see Fig. 3.38A).
  - Most will require UCL reconstruction, colloquially known as 'Tommy John surgery' (Fig. 3.39).
- Additional findings associated with UCL injuries at the medial elbow include marrow edema in the sublime tubercle, common flexor-pronator origin tendinosis, strains of the proximal flexor-pronator muscle group, and ulnar neuritis.
- Prior chronic UCL injuries may demonstrate calcification or ossification within the ligament, best visualized on radiographs, CT, or US.
- These transverse and posterior bundles of the UCL are thin and closely apposed to the trochlea and ulna, poorly seen even with high-resolution US or MRI.
  - Tears of these bundles can be inferred if intraarticular contrast medium escapes from the medial aspect of the elbow in the presence of a normal-appearing anterior bundle.
- Note that compensatory thickening of the UCL can be a normal finding in overhead throwing athletes, which may be seen in combination with hypertrophy/prominence of the medial epicondyle.

VALGUS EXTENSION OVERLOAD

- Valgus extension overload (or pitcher's elbow) refers to a clinical syndrome seen in the overhead throwing athlete and may include a variety of injuries:
- Injury of the medial elbow stabilizers due to tensile forces, including degeneration and tears of the UCL and common flexor-pronator tendon origin.

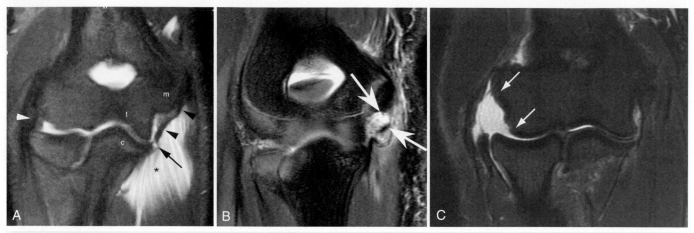

Fig. 3.38 Elbow collateral ligament tears. **(A)** Ulnar collateral ligament tear (UCL). Coronal fat-suppressed T2-weighted MR arthrogram obtained in a professional baseball pitcher who developed medial elbow pain while pitching. Note the focal tear *(black arrow)* in the distal UCL with extension of contrast medium into the medial musculature *(asterisk)*. Also note the normal low signal intensity of the remainder of the UCL *(black arrowheads)* and the normal radial collateral ligament *(white arrowhead)*. **(B)** Complete UCL tear in a different patient. Coronal inversion recovery MR image shows proximal tear *(arrows)*. **(C)** Lateral ligament complex complete tear. Coronal fat-suppressed T2-weighted MR image in a different patient shows 'bare' lateral epicondyle *(arrows)*, because the lateral collateral and lateral ulnar collateral ligaments and the common extensor tendon origin have avulsed. *c*, Coronoid process; *m*, medial epicondyle; *t*, trochlea.

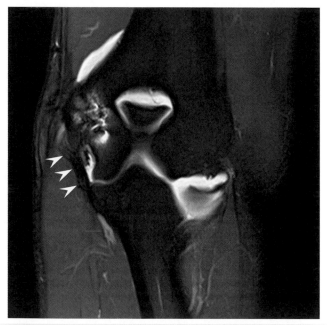

Fig. 3.39 Ulnar collateral ligament (UCL) reconstruction. Coronal T1-weighted fat-suppressed MR arthrogram image of the elbow demonstrates an intact UCL ligament reconstruction graft *(arrowheads)*. The graft is robust and there is no contrast extravasation into the medial soft tissues.

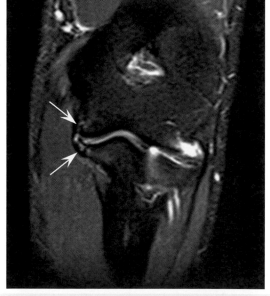

Fig. 3.40 Posteromedial impingement. Coronal proton density fat-suppressed MR image in a baseball pitcher demonstrates reciprocal osteophytic spurring and subchondral marrow edema *(arrows)* at the posteromedial aspect of the ulnotrochlear articulation.

- Injury at the posteromedial elbow joint due to shear forces, termed *posteromedial impingement*.
  - Characterized by osteophytes at the posteromedial olecranon and olecranon fossa, often with adjacent synovitis (Fig. 3.40).
  - May result in degenerative changes at the posteromedial ulnotrochlear articulation and intraarticular bodies.
- Injury at the lateral elbow joint due to compressive forces at the radiocapitellar articulation.
  - May result in chondrosis or osteochondral injury at the radial head or capitellum.
  - May ultimately progress to osteoarthritis at the radiocapitellar joint, including subchondral degenerative changes, marginal osteophytes, or intraarticular bodies.
- Traction, compression, and subluxation injuries of the ulnar nerve resulting in ulnar neuritis.
- Avulsive apophysitis at the medial epicondyle in skeletally immature athletes.

POSTEROLATERAL ROTATORY INSTABILITY

- *PLRI* is the most common form of elbow instability, seen most frequently after elbow trauma or elbow dislocation in which there was injury to the RCL complex, specifically the LUCL.
- May also be seen in patients with chronic lateral epicondylitis due to degeneration of the ligament or in the postsurgical setting.
- Insufficiency of the LUCL, the primary static lateral stabilizer, allows distraction of the ulnotrochlear joint and posterior subluxation of the radial head relative to the capitellum during extension-supination.
- Patients typically report elbow pain, clicking, and instability when pushing off with the affected arm.
- Diagnosis is typically made based on clinical and MRI findings (Fig. 3.41).

LITTLE LEAGUER'S ELBOW

- *Little Leaguer's elbow* is a chronic repetitive traction injury at the medial epicondyle seen in young baseball pitchers, other throwing athletes, and hockey players.
- Due to extreme tensile forces during valgus loading.
- Radiographs typically reveal displacement, fragmentation, or sclerosis of the medial epicondyle (Fig. 3.42).
- MRI demonstrates marrow edema at the medial epicondyle apophysis and variable physeal widening.
- Because the medial epicondyle is the last elbow secondary ossification center to fuse, Little Leaguer's elbow can occur late into adolescence (Fig. 3.43).

CUBITAL TUNNEL SYNDROME

- *Cubital tunnel syndrome* is ulnar neuropathy caused by nerve trauma in the cubital tunnel, located posterior to the medial epicondyle.

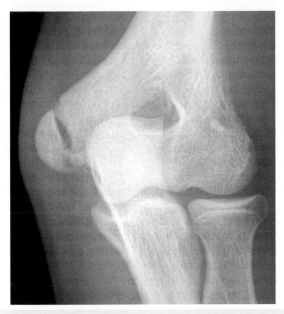

Fig. 3.42 Little Leaguer's elbow. AP radiograph shows wide physis of the medial epicondyle. This was a chronic, painful finding in a 17-year-old baseball pitcher.

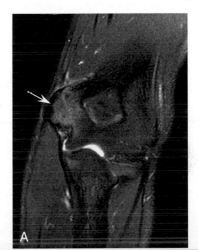

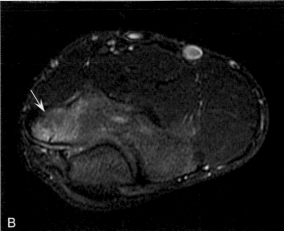

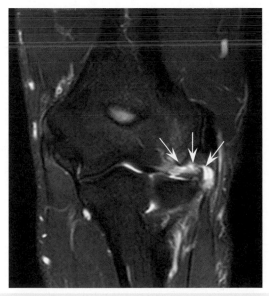

Fig. 3.41 Posterolateral rotatory instability (PLRI). Coronal proton density fat-suppressed MR image shows high-grade tearing of the lateral ligamentous structures *(arrows)* in a patient presenting with clinical findings of PLRI.

Fig. 3.43 Little Leaguer's elbow on MRI. Coronal proton density fat-suppressed **(A)** and axial STIR **(B)** MR images in a 14-year-old little league baseball pitcher demonstrate intense marrow edema in the medial epicondyle apophysis, reflecting a chronic traction overuse injury.

■ Causes of cubital tunnel syndrome include ulnar nerve subluxation, traction injuries, ulnar bone spurs, ganglion cyst or other mass lesion, perineural fibrosis, fracture, inflammatory process, or other anatomic derangements.

■ Clinical features include weakness of the FCU muscle and the intrinsic muscles of the hand, and pain/numbness/tingling along the ulnar aspect of the forearm and hand.

■ MRI may reveal a compressive mass lesion or infiltration of the fat that normally surrounds the ulnar nerve within the tunnel.

■ Fluid-sensitive MRI features of ulnar neuritis include nerve enlargement and intraneural or perineural edema (Fig. 3.44).

  ■ Note that T2-hyperintense signal in the ulnar nerve in or near the cubital tunnel as an isolated finding is not specific for ulnar neuropathy, as this finding also occurs in normal nerves.

■ US may reveal abnormal nerve enlargement, prominence of fascicles, and hypoechogenicity.

■ Dynamic US may reveal abnormal subluxation of the ulnar nerve out of the cubital tunnel during elbow flexion-extension maneuvers.

■ Treatment depends on the cause and may be conservative or surgical.

  ■ Surgical options include cubital tunnel decompression with release of the overlying retinaculum (Fig. 3.45), medial epicondylectomy, and anterior ulnar nerve transposition, which may be subcutaneous or submuscular.

MEDIAN NERVE ENTRAPMENT

■ The median nerve is vulnerable to entrapment neuropathy as it courses between the two heads of the PT muscle, termed *pronator syndrome*.

■ Other sites of compression include the lacertus fibrosus (bicipital aponeurosis), ligament of Struthers (vestigial structure usually arising from an anomalous supracondylar process, discussed previously), and the proximal arch of the FDS.

■ Clinical features of median nerve entrapment include numbness and weakness of the first three fingers, weakness of the thenar muscles, and pain in the volar forearm, particularly with activities using the PT muscle.

■ MR images are usually unrevealing unless a mass lesion is present, but may show denervation edema or atrophy within the muscles innervated by the median nerve.

■ *Anterior interosseous nerve syndrome.*

  ■ Anterior interosseous nerve (AIN) is a branch of the median nerve that supplies the deep muscles of the anterior forearm.

  ■ Compression of the AIN can occur by tendinous bands, a deep head of the PT, accessory muscles, aberrant radial artery branches, and fractures.

  ■ Symptoms include pain in the proximal forearm and weakness of the flexor pollicis longus (FPL), pronator quadratus, and the radial half of the flexor digitorum profundus (FDP) muscles.

  ■ MRI may reveal denervation edema or atrophy within the muscles innervated by the AIN.

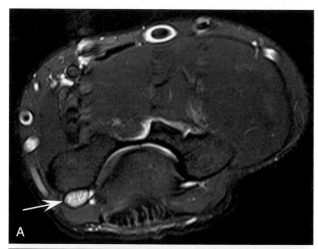

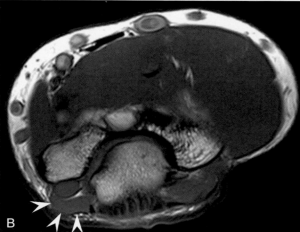

Fig. 3.44 Ulnar neuritis. **(A)** Axial STIR MR image shows a markedly enlarged, edematous ulnar nerve in the cubital tunnel *(arrow)*. **(B)** Axial T1-weighted MR image shows an accessory anconeus epitrochlearis muscle in the cubital tunnel *(arrowheads)*, causing mechanical compression of the ulnar nerve in this case.

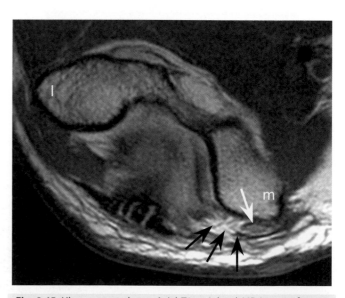

Fig. 3.45 Ulnar nerve release. Axial T2-weighted MR image after release of the cubital tunnel retinaculum. Note surgically divided retinaculum *(black arrows)* and ulnar nerve, which is displaced medially *(white arrow)*. *l*, Lateral epicondyle; *m*, medial epicondyle.

RADIAL NERVE ENTRAPMENT

- The radial nerve is vulnerable to compression neuropathy throughout its course, most commonly at the level of the elbow or proximal forearm.
- The radial nerve bifurcates just proximal to the elbow joint into the superficial radial nerve and the deep radial nerve, also called the posterior interosseous nerve (PIN).
- Potential causes of compression include previous elbow dislocation or fracture, extrinsic compression by a mass lesion, or entrapment by various anatomic structures.
- Symptoms are dependent on the location of nerve compression.
- *Superficial radial nerve syndrome (Wartenberg syndrome).*
  - Superficial radial nerve is the sensory branch of the radial nerve, which innervates the first three digits (thumb, index, and middle fingers).
  - Usually compressed between the brachioradialis and extensor carpi radialis longus (ECRL) muscles at the distal forearm during pronation.
  - Results in pain, numbness, and paresthesias affecting the first three digits.
- *Posterior interosseous nerve (PIN) syndrome.*
  - Deep radial nerve, or PIN, is the motor branch of the radial nerve, which innervates the supinator muscle and extensor muscles of the wrist and hand.
  - Results in weakness of the extensor muscles and lateral forearm pain but no sensory deficit.
  - MRI revels denervation edema or atrophy of the affected muscles (Fig. 3.46).
  - Most common site of compression is at the *arcade of Frohse*, or supinator arch, which represents the proximal fibrous edge of the supinator muscle.
  - Other less common sites of compression include the fibrous capsule of the radiocapitellar joint, radial recurrent artery and the *venae comitantes (leash of Henry)*, fibrous edge of the ECRB muscle, and the distal fibrous edge of the supinator muscle.
  - *Radial tunnel syndrome* is thought to represent an early manifestation of PIN syndrome, in which there is lateral forearm pain but no motor deficit, which may simulate lateral epicondylitis.
- Entrapment of the radial nerve proximal to its bifurcation will result in both motor and sensory deficits.

OLECRANON BURSITIS

- The subcutaneous olecranon bursa overlies the olecranon process and is the most common site of bursitis in the body.
- Causes of olecranon bursitis include direct trauma, hemorrhage, inflammatory processes (e.g., rheumatoid arthritis or gout), and infection, presenting with pain and swelling over the olecranon process (Fig. 3.47).
- Infectious (septic) bursitis comprises up to 20% of cases, most commonly from direct inoculation of *Staphylococcus aureus*.
  - Aspiration is usually required to differentiate between septic and nonseptic bursitis.
  - Bone marrow edema in olecranon process can be reactive in nature, but osteomyelitis must be excluded in the setting of septic bursitis.

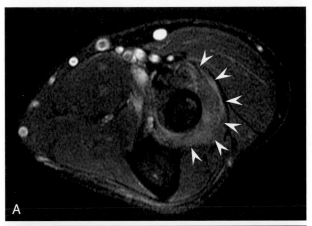

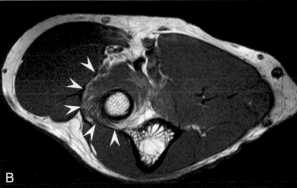

Fig. 3.46 Posterior interosseous nerve (PIN) syndrome. **(A)** Axial STIR MR image demonstrates diffuse edema throughout the supinator muscle *(arrowheads)*, a finding suggestive of PIN syndrome. **(B)** Axial T1-weighted MR image in a different patient presenting with forearm weakness demonstrates fatty infiltration of the supinator muscle *(arrowheads)*, suggestive of chronic denervation atrophy secondary to PIN entrapment.

Structured Report

REPORTING TIPS AND RECOMMENDATIONS

- Impression points should succinctly summarize findings, which may be further described in detail in the body of the report.
  - For example, findings of 'severe lateral epicondylitis' may be further described in the body of the report as 'severe common extensor origin tendinosis with high-grade tearing involving approximately 70% of tendon cross-sectional area'.
- Related structures, such as the medial (or lateral) tendons and ligaments, may be separated in the body of a templated report but should be scrutinized in tandem.
  - For example, degeneration or tearing of the medial or lateral collateral ligament complexes often accompany findings of epicondylitis but are rarely of clinical significance and should not be overstated.
- Elbow dislocations often represent the most complex injuries encountered on elbow MRI and are best approached in a systematic and organized fashion.
- Organize impression points by order of importance.
- Directly answer any specific clinical questions in the impression.

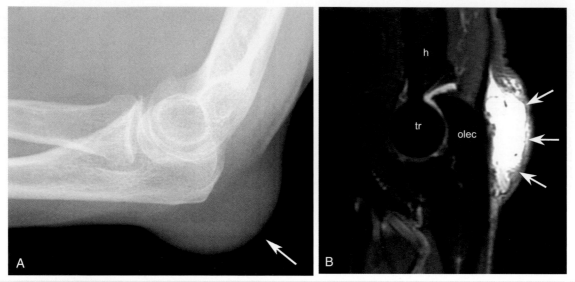

Fig. 3.47 Olecranon bursitis. **(A)** Lateral radiograph shows soft tissue swelling centered over the olecranon process *(arrow)*. This case was due to hemorrhage into the bursa caused by direct trauma. **(B)** Sagittal fat-suppressed T2-weighted MR image in a different patient shows fluid-filled bursa *(arrows)* due to infection. *h*, Distal humeral shaft; *olec*, olecranon; *tr*, trochlea.

Example Normal Elbow Report Template

Exam Type: MRI ELBOW WITHOUT CONTRAST
Exam Date and Time: Date and Time
Indication: Clinical History
Comparison: Prior Studies

IMPRESSION: Impression

TECHNIQUE: MRI of the side elbow was performed on a scanner type system in three planes (axial, sagittal, and coronal) using a standard noncontrast protocol.

FINDINGS:

JOINT/BONES: No acute fracture or bone bruise. No elbow joint effusion. No focal cartilage defects. No osteochondral lesion. Alignment is anatomic.

LIGAMENTS:
UCL: Intact.
RCL: Intact.
LUCL: Intact.

Annular ligament: Intact.

TENDONS: Common extensor tendon origin: No tendinosis or tear.
Common flexor-pronator tendon origin: No tendinosis or tear.
Biceps tendon: No tendinosis or tear.
Brachialis tendon: No tendinosis or tear.
Triceps tendon: No tendinosis or tear.

CUBITAL TUNNEL: Ulnar nerve is normal in location, morphology, and signal intensity. No mass or mass effect in the cubital tunnel. No accessory muscles.

MUSCLES: No atrophy or edema.

SOFT TISSUES: No soft tissue edema. No fluid collection or soft tissue mass.

Sources and Suggested Readings

Beaty JH, Kasser JR, Shaggs DL, et al. eds. *Rockwood and Green's Fractures in Children.* Philadelphia: Lippincott-Raven; 2009.

Beltran LS, Bencardino JT, Beltran J. Imaging of sports ligamentous injuries of the elbow. *Semin Musculoskelet Radiol.* 2013;17(5):455–465.

Bredella MA, Tirman PF, Fritz RC, et al. MR imaging findings of lateral ulnar collateral ligament abnormalities in patients with lateral epicondylitis. *AJR Am J Roentgenol.* 1999;173(5):1379–1382.

Bucholz RW, Court-Brown CM, Heckman JD, Tornetta P, eds. *Rockwood and Green's Fractures in Adults.* Philadelphia: Lippincott-Raven; 2009.

Bucknor MD, Stevens KJ, Steinbach LS. Elbow imaging in sport: sports imaging series. *Radiology.* 2016;279(1):12–28.

Demertzis JL, Rubin DA. Upper extremity neuromuscular injuries in athletes. *Semin Musculoskelet Radiol.* 2012;16(4):316–330.

Dunning CE, Zarzour ZD, Patterson SD, et al. Ligamentous stabilizers against posterolateral rotatory instability of the elbow. *J Bone Joint Surg Am.* 2001;83(12):1823–1828.

Hayter CL, Adler RS. Injuries of the elbow and the current treatment of tendon disease. *AJR Am J Roentgenol.* 2012;199(3):546–557.

Helms CA, Major NA, Anderson MW, Kaplan PA. *Musculoskeletal MRI.* 2nd ed. Philadelphia: Saunders; 2008.

Jacobson JA, Fessell DP, Lobo Lda G, et al. Entrapment neuropathies I: upper limb (carpal tunnel excluded). *Semin Musculoskelet Radiol.* 2010;14(5):473–486.

Jacobson JA. *Fundamentals of Musculoskeletal Ultrasound.* Philadelphia: Saunders; 2008.

Jamadar DA, Robertson BL, Jacobson JA, et al. Musculoskeletal sonography: important imaging pitfalls. *AJR Am J Roentgenol.* 2010;194(1):216–225.

Kijowski R, DeSmet AA. MRI findings of osteochondritis dissecans of the capitellum with surgical correlation. *AJR Am J Roentgenol.* 2005;185:1453–1459.

Kim SJ, Hong SH, Jun WS, et al. MR imaging mapping of skeletal muscle denervation in entrapment and compressive neuropathies. *Radiographics.* 2011;31(2):319–332.

Konin GP, Nazarian LN, Walz DM. US of the elbow: indications, technique, normal anatomy, and pathologic conditions. *Radiographics.* 2013;33(4):E125–E147.

Levin D, Nazarian L, Miller T, et al. Lateral epicondylitis of the elbow: US findings. *Radiology.* 2005;237:230–234.

Madsen M, Marx RG, Millett PJ, et al. Surgical anatomy of the triceps brachii tendon: anatomical study and clinical correlation. *Am J Sports Med.* 2006;34(11):1839–1843.

Mulligan SA, Schwartz ML, Broussard MF, Andrews JR. Heterotopic calcification and tears of the ulnar collateral ligament: radiographic and MR findings. *AJR Am J Roentgenol.* 2000;175:1099–1102.

Munshli M, Pretterklleber ML, Chung CB, et al. Anterior bundle of the ulnar collateral ligament: evaluation of anatomic relationships by using MR imaging, MR arthrography, and gross anatomic and histologic analysis. *Radiology.* 2004:231:797–803.

Nirschl RP, Pettrone FA. Tennis elbow. The surgical treatment of lateral epicondylitis. *J Bone Joint Surg Am.* 1979;61(6):832–839.

Robinson R. Sonography of common tendon injuries. *AJR Am J Roentgenol.* 2009;193(3):607–618.

Sheehan SE, Dyer GS, Sodickson AD, et al. Traumatic elbow injuries: what the orthopedic surgeon wants to know. *Radiographics.* 2013;33(3):869–888.

Sonin AH, Tutton SM, Fitzgerald SW, Peduto AJ. MR imaging of the adult elbow. *Radiographics.* 1996;16:1323–1336.

Anatomy

WRIST

The wrist consists of the structures between the distal radius and ulna and the metacarpal bases, including the: eight carpal bones; distal radioulnar joint (DRUJ); radiocarpal, midcarpal, and carpometacarpal (CMC) joints; intrinsic (or intercarpal) and extrinsic ligaments of the wrists; triangular fibrocartilage complex (TFCC); flexor and extensor tendon compartments; and neurovascular structures, including the median and ulnar nerves.

The wrist is an extraordinarily complex joint, made all the more challenging for the radiologist by the comparatively small size of many important structures that test the limits of both our scanners and diagnostic skills. Normal wrist anatomy is reviewed in Figs. 4.1 and 4.2. Normal wrist alignment is summarized in Box 4.1.

Osseous and Articular

- *Distal radius.*
  - The articular surface of the distal radius is normally tilted toward the ulna (termed *radial inclination*) by approximately 20–25 degrees and toward the palm (*volar tilt*) by approximately 11 degrees (see Fig. 4.1).
  - Deviation from this pattern is most frequently the result of an old fracture that healed with deformity,

although developmental conditions such as *Madelung deformity* should also be considered.
  - *Madelung deformity* is usually caused by premature arrest of the ulnar aspect of the distal radial physis, resulting in shortening of the radius with positive ulnar variance, increased radial inclination, and increased volar tilt of the radiocarpal articulation (see Fig. 15.74).
- The articular surface of the radius frequently contains two shallow depressions that correspond to the scaphoid and lunate bones and are known as the *scaphoid fossa* (or facet) and the *lunate fossa* (or facet).
  - These are useful landmarks for localizing an intraarticular fracture of the distal radius.
- The *ulnar* (or *sigmoid*) *notch* is a concave depression in the distal radius, which articulates with the head of the ulna, forming the DRUJ.
- *Distal ulna.*
  - The distal ulna has a cylindrical cross-sectional contour that forms the *ulnar head*, which articulates with *ulnar* (or *sigmoid*) *notch* of the distal radius.
    - This is exactly the reverse of the arrangement at the elbow between the smaller, cylindrical radial head and the concave articular surface of the proximal ulna.
  - The distal surface of the ulnar head articulates with the undersurface of the central TFCC, which is interposed

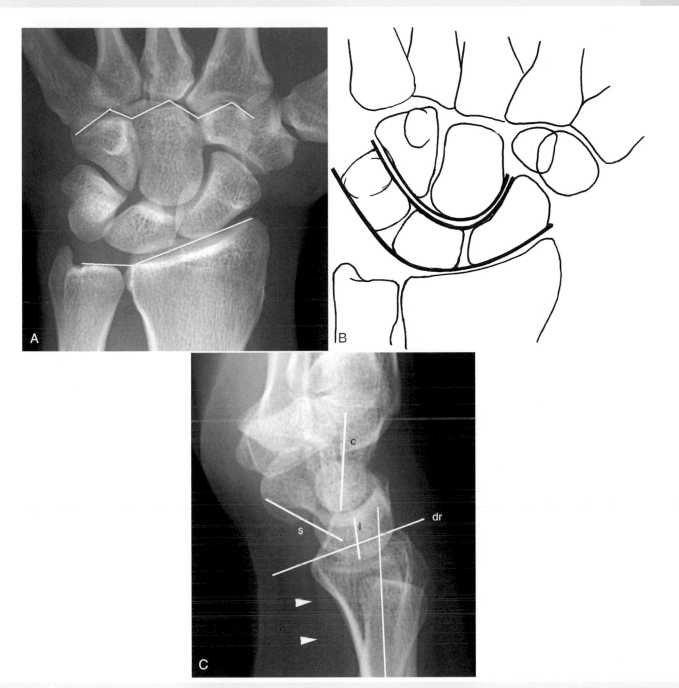

Fig. 4.1 Normal radiographic anatomy of the wrist. (A) PA view. Note the normal ulnar inclination of the distal radius *(long white line)*. Also note the approximately equal length of the distal ulna and radius *(short transverse line)* and the *zigzag* contour formed by the carpometacarpal (CMC) joints. **(B)** Diagram of the normal smooth carpal arcs. Interruption of one of these arcs is evidence of a ligamentous injury or carpal dislocation. **(C)** Lateral view. The long axes of the radius, capitate, scaphoid, and lunate are marked with *lines*. Note how the long axis of the scaphoid is estimated by connecting the two most volar projections, which are relatively easy to identify. The radius, capitate, and lunate are approximately colinear. The scaphoid is angled approximately 45 degrees volar compared with the lunate. Note the volar tilt of the distal radial articular surface. Also note the normal fat pad volar to the pronator quadratus muscle *(arrowheads)*. *c*, capitate; *dr*, distal radial articular surface; *l*, lunate; *s*, scaphoid.

between the ulnar head and the lunate and triquetrum, separating the DRUJ from the radiocarpal joint.
- The *ulnar styloid process* is a small nonarticular osseous protuberance at the ulnar aspect of the distal ulna, serving as one of the attachment sites of the peripheral TFCC.
- The *ulnar fovea* is situated just radial to the base of the ulnar styloid process, serving as another attachment site of the peripheral TFCC.

- The *ulnar groove* is a shallow depression at the dorsal-ulnar aspect of the distal ulna formed by the ulnar styloid process and ulnar head, within which the extensor carpi ulnaris (ECU) tendon lies.
- *Ulnar variance* refers to the length of the distal ulna with respect to the distal radius, designated as *neutral*, *positive* (ulna longer than radius), or *negative* (ulna shorter than radius).
  - The distal ulna is normally equal to or a few millimeters shorter than the adjacent radius; pathology

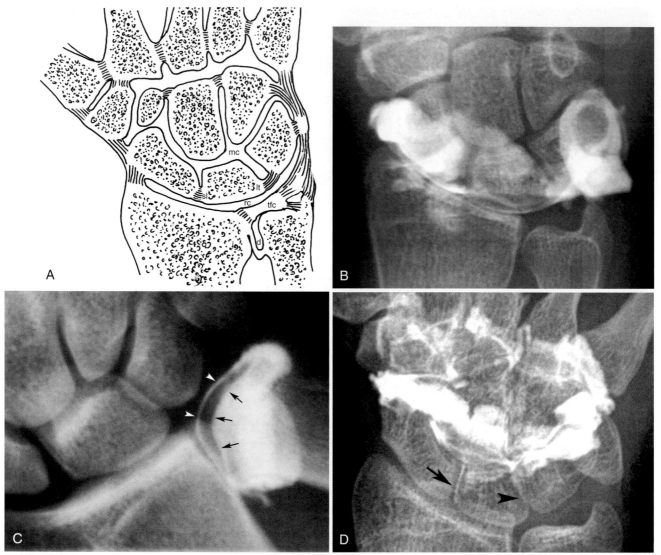

Fig. 4.2 Wrist compartmental anatomy. (A) Diagram shows the synovial compartments of the wrist. Note the soft tissues that separate the compartments: the scapholunate *(sl)* and lunotriquetral *(lt)* interosseous ligaments separate the radiocarpal *(rc)* and midcarpal *(mc)* compartments. The triangular fibrocartilage complex (TFCC) separates the radiocarpal joint from the distal radioulnar joint *(d)*. Note the ligamentous fixation of the TFCC articular disc *(tfc)* to the radius, ulna, and medial joint capsule. **(B)** Normal radiocarpal arthrogram. Note that contrast medium does not flow through the interosseous ligaments of the proximal carpal row into the midcarpal joint or through the TFCC into the distal radioulnar joint. **(C)** Normal distal radioulnar joint arthrogram. Note the radiolucent articular cartilage of the distal ulna *(arrows)*. *Arrowheads* mark the proximal margin of the triangular fibrocartilage. **(D)** Midcarpal joint arthrogram. Contrast medium extends between the scaphoid and lunate *(arrow)* and lunate and triquetrum *(arrowhead)*, but is contained by the scapholunate and lunotriquetral interosseous ligaments.

Box 4.1   Normal Wrist Alignment

- Distal radius articular surface: Volar tilt, ulnar inclination
- Distal ulna: May be a few millimeters shorter than distal radius, not longer
- Carpal bone alignment (wrist in neutral position)
- PA view:
  - Proximal and distal rows form smooth arcs
- Lateral view:
  - Scaphoid tilted volar, scapholunate angle 30 to 60 degrees
  - Lunate aligned within 10 degrees of capitate
- Carpometacarpal joints: Normal zigzag pattern on PA radiograph

PA, Posteroanterior.

associated with abnormal (positive or negative) ulnar variance is discussed later in this chapter.

- *DRUJ.*
  - The DRUJ is anatomically and functionally distinct from the more distal synovial compartments around the carpal bones.
  - The DRUJ, paired with the proximal radioulnar joint at the elbow, allows wrist pronation and supination.
  - The DRUJ has a relatively small volume (1–2 mL when maximally distended), bounded distally and separated from the radiocarpal joint by the TFCC (see Fig. 4.2).
  - The primary stabilizers of the DRUJ are the dorsal and volar radioulnar ligaments (part of the TFCC); injury

to these structures may result in DRUJ instability, discussed later in this chapter.

- Communication between the DRUJ and the radiocarpal compartment at arthrography indicates a full-thickness defect in the TFCC.

- *Carpus.*
  - Understanding the carpus (i.e., the carpal bones as a unit) begins with the concept of carpal rows.
  - The carpal bones are arranged in two rows: from radial to ulnar, the *proximal carpal row* consists of the scaphoid, lunate, triquetrum, and pisiform, and the *distal carpal row* consists of the trapezium, trapezoid, capitate, and hamate.
  - A posteroanterior (PA) radiograph of a normal wrist shows the margins of the carpal rows to form smooth arcs, termed *carpal arcs* or *Gilula arcs* in honor of the late radiologist Louis Gilula, who described them (see Fig. 4.1B).
  - The lateral view of the wrist superimposes most of the carpal bones; however, a well-positioned lateral wrist radiograph *in neutral alignment* (essential!) will allow identification of the radius, scaphoid, lunate, capitate, and third metacarpal.
    - The radius, lunate, and capitate should be roughly colinear when the wrist is in neutral alignment (see Fig. 4.1C).
    - The long axis of the scaphoid is normally angled volar by approximately 30–60 degrees relative to the mid-axis of the lunate at neutral wrist positioning (termed the *scapholunate [SL] angle*).
    - The long axis of the capitate is normally angled within 30 degrees of the mid-axis of the lunate at neutral wrist positioning (termed the *capitolunate angle*).
  - Carpal motion is complex but may be simplified by considering the concept of carpal rows; a useful simplification is that each carpal row functions as a unit, with carpal motion occurring at the radiocarpal joint and at the midcarpal joint between the carpal rows.
  - Approximately 50% of wrist flexion and extension occurs at the radiocarpal joint and 50% at the midcarpal joint.
    - Thus, a lateral radiograph of the wrist in volar flexion should show the lunate volar flexed relative to the radius and the capitate volar flexed relative to the lunate.
  - Motion in the coronal plane—that is, ulnar and radial deviation—is more complex (Fig. 4.3), because the carpus pivots around a center of rotation in the proximal capitate.
    - When the wrist is in neutral position, the lunate straddles the junction of the radius and the TFCC.
  - Ulnar deviation slides the proximal carpal row *radially* (laterally) as the fingers angle medially; in addition, the scaphoid and lunate tilt dorsally during ulnar deviation.
    - The lunate articulates exclusively with the radius when the wrist is in ulnar deviation.
  - Radial deviation slides the proximal carpal row *medially* as the hand angles laterally; in addition, the scaphoid and lunate tilt volarly during radial deviation.
    - Only about 30–50% of the lunate articulates with the radius when the wrist is in radial deviation.

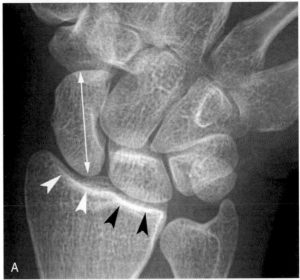

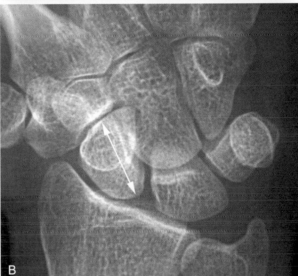

Fig. 4.3 Effects of carpal motion on radiographic appearance. Normal carpal motion in ulnar **(A)** and radial **(B)** deviation. Note that the proximal carpal row slides along the radius. Also note that the scaphoid appears to shorten with radial deviation as it tilts more volarly and appears to elongate with ulnar deviation as it tilts toward the coronal plane. The spaces between the scaphoid, lunate, and triquetrum change only slightly between the two images. Also note the concavities in the articular surface of the distal radius; these are the normal scaphoid and lunate fossae and are marked with *white* and *black arrowheads*, respectively, in A. These fossae may be well developed, as in this patient, or nearly absent. Slight angulation of the x-ray beam also can make these fossae more or less apparent.

- Variation from these normal patterns of carpal alignment and motion may be the only telltale sign of a significant ligamentous injury or carpal instability (discussed later in this chapter).
- *Carpal coalition* is a congenital fusion involving two or more carpal bones, most commonly occurring between the lunate and triquetrum (lunotriquetral [LT] coalition; see Fig. 15.55A).
  - 60% of LT coalitions are bilateral.
  - Carpal coalition occurs more frequently in females (2:1 female-to-male ratio) and in patients of African or Caribbean descent.

- *Radiocarpal joint.*
  - The *radiocarpal joint* is formed by the articulation of the distal radius with the scaphoid and lunate.
  - The radiocarpal joint synovial compartment is bounded by the proximal carpal row distally and the radius and the TFCC proximally (see Fig. 4.2).
  - The capacity of the radiocarpal joint at maximal distention is approximately 3–5 mL.
  - Communication between the radiocarpal and midcarpal joints at arthrography generally indicates a tear of the SL or LT interosseous ligaments.
    - Such tears are usually significant in younger individuals but also can occur in the form of asymptomatic perforations in older individuals.
  - Communication between the radiocarpal joint and the DRUJ indicates a full-thickness tear or perforation of the TFCC articular disc, which can also be seen as an incidental, age-related finding.
- *Carpometacarpal (CMC) joints.*
  - The first metacarpal base articulates with the trapezium, constituting the first carpometacarpal (CMC) joint of the thumb (the first CMC joint).
    - The first CMC joint is a saddle-shaped joint that allows movement in multiple planes.
    - The ligamentous anatomy of the first CMC joint is complex and includes the anterior oblique ligament (*AOL*, or *beak ligament*), posterior oblique ligament (*POL*), intermetacarpal ligament (*IML*), and dorsoradial ligament (*DRL*); injuries to these structures are beyond the scope of this chapter.
  - The second metacarpal base articulates with the trapezoid, the third metacarpal base articulates with the capitate, and the fourth and fifth metacarpal bases articulate with the hamate.
  - The proximal second through fifth metacarpal bases also articulate with adjacent metacarpal bases.
  - The articulation of the second through fifth metacarpals and the distal carpal row form a single synovial compartment, the second through fifth CMC joints.
    - This compartment frequently communicates with the midcarpal joint as a normal variant.
    - The articulations of the second through fifth CMC joints normally have a zigzag pattern on a true posteroanterior (PA) radiograph obtained with the palm and fingers flat against the x-ray detector plate (see Fig. 4.1A).
    - Disruption of this pattern suggests a dislocation (Fig. 4.4).
    - Second through fifth CMC joint dislocations are usually dorsal, may be multiple, and are often associated with small fractures.
    - Conversely, the presence of a small fracture fragment at or adjacent to a CMC joint suggests that a dislocation is or was present.

Ligaments

The ligamentous anatomy of the wrist is extremely complex. The ligaments best known to radiologists and functionally most important are the SL and LT interosseous ligaments (see Fig. 4.2A). Other interosseous ligaments unite the bones of the distal carpal row and are rarely interrupted. The SL and LT ligaments are best evaluated

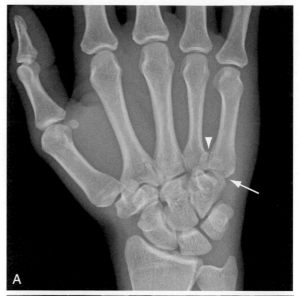
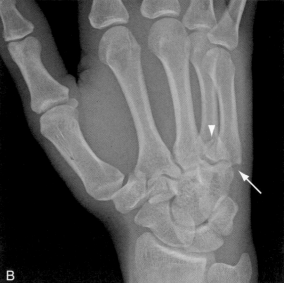

Fig. 4.4 Fracture-dislocation of the base of the fifth metacarpal. (A) PA radiograph shows subtle medial displacement of the base of the fifth metacarpal with disruption of the normal zigzag pattern of the carpometacarpal joints. Also note the fracture fragment projecting over the fourth metacarpal base *(arrowhead).* **(B)** Oblique view shows similar findings. The base of the fifth metacarpal is also displaced posteriorly *(arrow).*

with high-quality MRI, MR arthrography, or computed tomography (CT).

- *SL ligament.*
  - The SL ligament is a U-shaped structure centered at the proximal SL articulation, anatomically composed of volar and dorsal bandlike components and a central membranous component proximally.
  - The *dorsal component* is the thickest component of the SL ligament and functionally is most important for SL (and overall wrist) stability.
- *LT ligament.*
  - The LT ligament is similar in structure to the SL ligament, centered at the proximal LT articulation and also composed of volar, dorsal, and membranous components.

- The *volar component* of the LT ligament is thickest and functionally most important for LT stability, though the dorsal component also plays an important role as a rotational constraint.
- Perforation of the thin membranous central portions of the SL or LT ligaments can occur as an incidental finding, especially in older patients; such perforations do not indicate ligament failure and therefore are a potential pitfall in interpreting arthrograms in older patients.
- Thin-section MRI often shows the membranous portions of these ligaments to be triangular in cross section.
- Ligaments may appear on MR images to attach directly onto the articular hyaline cartilage or through the cartilage into bone.
- Both the LT and SL ligaments can stretch by approximately 50% to 100% of their length before tearing.

The extrinsic wrist ligaments are a complex set of organized thickenings of the volar and dorsal joint capsule (Fig. 4.5); these ligaments are very important functionally but are difficult to assess on imaging.

- The volar capsular ligaments are thought to be stronger and more important in maintaining wrist stability than the dorsal ligaments.
- Many of the capsular ligaments are named by the bones they connect.
  - The main volar ligaments include the radioscaphocapitate, radiolunotriquetral, ulnotriquetral, and ulnar collateral ligaments.
  - The main dorsal ligaments include the dorsal radioscaphoid and dorsal radiolunotriquetral ligaments and a variable dorsal intercarpal (transverse) ligament or ligaments that extend from the triquetrum laterally across the capitate to the scaphoid and trapezoid.
  - Capsular ligament anatomy can vary between patients; adding to potential confusion for radiologists, there are alternate names for many of these ligaments.
- Limited demonstration of these ligaments is possible with thin-section MRI. Some acute injuries may be visible on MRI (Fig. 4.5B) or may manifest on radiographs as easily overlooked small dorsal cortical avulsion fractures.

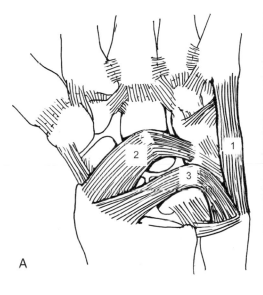

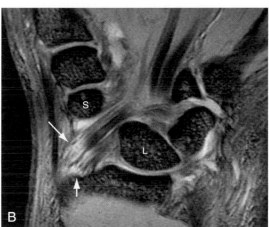

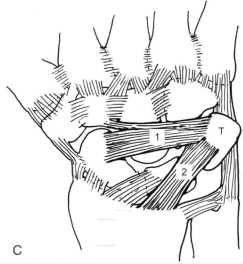

Fig. 4.5 **Capsular carpal ligament anatomy. (A)** Diagram of the volar carpal ligaments. The most important are labeled: *1,* ulnar carpal complex (includes the ulnar collateral ligament); *2,* distal arc (radioscaphocapitate and capitotriquetral, blends into 1); *3,* proximal arc (radiolunotriquetral, also termed *long radiolunate,* and ulnotriquetral). **(B)** Coronal gradient-echo magnetic resonance image shows edema related to sprains of the volar radioscaphocapitate *(long arrow)* and radiolunate *(short arrow)* ligaments. **(C)** Diagram of the dorsal carpal ligaments. The most important are labeled: *1,* dorsal intercarpal (transverse) ligament; *2,* dorsal radiocarpal (radiolunotriquetral) ligament. Note that both insert onto the triquetrum. *L,* Lunate; *S,* scaphoid distal pole; *T,* triquetrum.

- Much can be inferred about the functional status of wrist ligaments by assessment of carpal alignment and motion on radiographs (see Figs. 4.11 to 4.13).

Triangular Fibrocartilage Complex

- The TFCC is located between the distal ulna and the proximal carpal row (Fig. 4.6; see also Fig. 4.2).
- The TFCC is the primary stabilizer of the DRUJ and also allows wider distribution of forces across the radiocarpal joint.
- The TFCC consists of several components that are not discrete structures but rather blend continuously.
- The TFCC includes a central disc-shaped fibrocartilaginous portion, termed the *triangular fibrocartilage (TFC) articular disc*, the TFC proper, or simply the *articular disc*.
- The articular disc blends into the thick, strong *dorsal* and *volar radioulnar ligaments* that fix the articular disc to the radius laterally and to the *ulnar fovea* and *styloid process* medially (the *peripheral* attachments).
- The *ECU tendon sheath* and the volar-ulnar portions of the wrist capsular ligaments, the *ulnotriquetral* and *ulnolunate ligaments*, also are considered components of the TFCC.
- The *meniscus homologue* is a wedge-shaped fibrofatty thickening of the medial joint capsule distal to the articular disc that is occasionally identified at wrist arthrography, considered by some authors to be a component of the TFCC.

Tendons

- Nine of the flexor tendons of the hand/wrist are located within the carpal tunnel (see the section on *Carpal tunnel*).
- Three flexor tendons of the wrist are outside of the carpal tunnel:
  - *Flexor carpi radialis (FCR) tendon*, which inserts on the second and third metacarpal bases.

- *Flexor carpi ulnaris (FCU) tendon*, which inserts on the pisiform, hook of the hamate, and the fifth metacarpal base.
- *Palmaris longus tendon*, which inserts on the palmar aponeurosis and flexor retinaculum of the hand.
  - May be absent as an anatomic variant in approximately 14% of individuals.
- The extensor tendons of the hand/wrist are separated into six compartments, each invested with their own synovial tendon sheaths (Fig. 4.7); from radial to ulnar these include:
  - *Compartment 1*: abductor pollicis longus (APL) tendon and extensor pollicis brevis (EPB) tendon.
  - *Compartment 2*: extensor carpi radialis longus (ECRL) tendon and extensor carpi radialis brevis (ECRB) tendon.
  - *Compartment 3*: extensor pollicis longus (EPL) tendon.
  - *Compartment 4*: extensor indicis proprius (EIP) tendon and extensor digitorum communis (EDC) tendons.
  - *Compartment 5*: extensor digiti minimi (EDM) tendon.
  - *Compartment 6*: ECU tendon.
- *Lister's tubercle* is a bony prominence at the dorsal radius, separating the second and third extensor compartments.
- Extensor tendon pathology is most frequently encountered at the first extensor compartment (*De Quervain's syndrome* or *tenosynovitis*) and sixth extensor compartment (*ECU* tendon abnormalities), which are discussed later in this chapter.

Carpal Tunnel

- The *carpal tunnel* is a fibro-osseous tunnel at the volar aspect of the wrist containing the flexor pollicis longus tendon, four flexor digitorum profundus and four flexor digitorum superficialis tendons, and the median nerve (Fig. 4.8A).

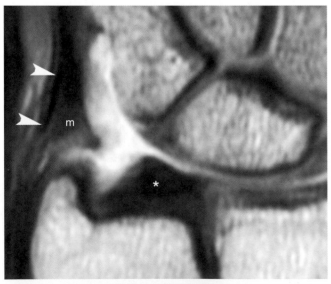

Fig. 4.6 **The triangular fibrocartilage complex (TFCC).** Coronal T1-weighted MR arthrogram shows normal appearance of the TFCC articular disc *(asterisk)*, with low signal intensity and smooth margins. This patient has a normal variant 'meniscal homologue' attached to the ulnar collateral ligament *(arrowheads)*. The meniscal homologue is partially composed of fibrocartilage and is triangular in shape, hence its name. *m*, Meniscal homologue. (Image courtesy of Charles Pappas, MD)

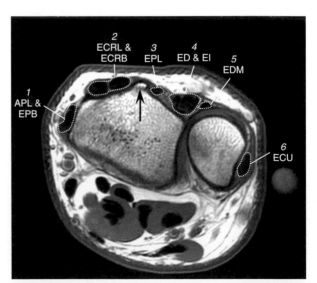

Fig. 4.7 **Wrist extensor tendon compartments.** Axial T1-weighted MR image shows the six extensor tendon compartments. Clockwise, from the left (radial) side of the image: *APL*, abductor pollicis longus; *EPB*, extensor pollicis brevis; *ECRL*, extensor carpi radialis longus; *ECRB*, extensor carpi radialis brevis; *EPL*, extensor pollicis longus; *ED*, extensor digitorum; *EI*, extensor indicis; *EDM*, extensor digiti minimi; *ECU*, extensor carpi ulnaris. Prior to their decussation, the second and third extensor tendon compartments are separated by Lister's tubercle *(arrow)*.

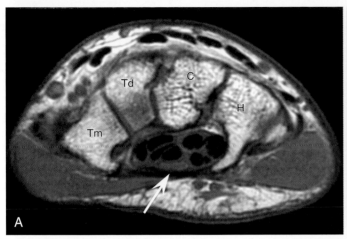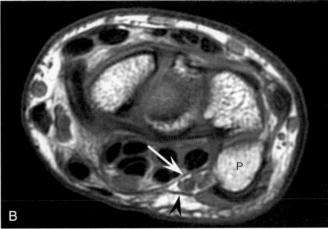

Fig. 4.8 Carpal tunnel and Guyon's canal. (A) Axial T1-weighted MR image of the wrist at the level of the distal carpal row demonstrates the carpal tunnel, bounded by the carpal bones and transverse carpal ligament, or flexor retinaculum *(white arrow)*. The carpal tunnel contains the flexor pollicis longus tendon, four flexor digitorum profundus and four flexor digitorum superficialis tendons, and the median nerve. **(B)** Axial T1-weighted MR image of the wrist at the level of the proximal carpal row shows Guyon's canal, a triangular space located volar-ulnar to the hook of the hamate containing the ulnar nerve, artery, and vein. Guyon's canal is bounded dorsally by the transverse carpal ligament, or flexor retinaculum *(white arrow)*, volarly by the palmar carpal ligament *(black arrowhead)*, and ulnarly by the pisiform. *C*, capitate; *H*, hamate; *P*, pisiform; *Td*, trapezoid; *Tm*, trapezium.

- Boundaries of the carpal tunnel are as follows:
  - *Radial*: scaphoid and trapezium.
  - *Ulnar*: pisiform and hamate.
  - *Dorsal*: carpal bones.
  - *Volar*: transverse carpal ligament (flexor retinaculum).

Guyon's Canal

- *Guyon's canal* is a fibro-osseous tunnel at the volar-ulnar aspect of the wrist containing the ulnar nerve, artery, and vein (Fig. 4.8B).
- Boundaries of Guyon's canal are as follows:
  - *Radial*: hook of the hamate and transverse carpal ligament (flexor retinaculum).
  - *Ulnar*: pisiform, FCU tendon, and abductor digiti minimi muscle.
  - *Dorsal*: transverse carpal ligament (flexor retinaculum), pisohamate, and pisotriquetral ligaments.
  - *Volar*: palmar (volar) carpal ligament and palmaris brevis muscle.

HAND

The hand consists of the structures distal to the CMC joints, including the: five metacarpals and phalanges of the first through fifth digits; metacarpophalangeal (MCP) and interphalangeal joints of the first through fifth digits; joint capsules and ligaments; flexor and extensor tendons (including the flexor pulley system); and the intrinsic muscles and surrounding soft tissues. Like the wrist, the hand is extraordinarily complex in both anatomy and function.

Osseous

- There are normally five digits, including the thumb (first digit), index finger (second digit), middle or long finger (third digit), ring finger (fourth digit), and pinky or little finger (fifth digit).
- The thumb (first digit) is composed of the first metacarpal and proximal and distal phalanges; the articulations between these bones form the first MCP and first interphalangeal (IP) joints.

- The second through fifth digits are composed of metacarpals and proximal, middle, and distal phalanges; the articulations between these bones form the MCP, proximal interphalangeal (PIP), and distal interphalangeal (DIP) joints.
- Several anatomic variants can occur.
  - Having more than five digits is termed *polydactyly* and associated with numerous syndromic conditions.
  - Having fewer than five digits is termed *oligodactyly* and is extremely rare.
  - *Syndactyly* refers to fusion of the digits, which may be osseous or soft tissue; when occurring in combination with polydactyly, this is termed *polysyndactyly*.
  - Congenital osseous fusion of the interphalangeal joints (or less commonly the MCP joints) is termed *symphalangism* (see Fig. 15.56).

Joint Capsules and Ligaments

- Each MCP joint has a strong fibrous capsule with cord-like radial and ulnar collateral ligaments (*RCL* and *UCL*, respectively), which are further subdivided into the proper and accessory collateral ligaments.
  - The UCL and RCL resist valgus (abduction) and varus (adduction) forces, respectively.
- The *volar plate* is a capsular thickening that stabilizes the volar MCP and interphalangeal joints and prevents hyperextension.
  - The *deep transverse metacarpal ligaments* extend between the metacarpal heads in the coronal plane, connecting the adjoining volar plates of the second through fifth MCP joints.
- The *extensor hood* is located at the dorsal aspect of each MCP joint and is formed by an aponeurotic expansion of the extensor tendon, the dorsal joint capsule, and the radial and ulnar *sagittal bands*.
  - The *sagittal bands* extend from each side of the extensor tendon and attach to the volar plate and the deep transverse metacarpal ligaments, stabilizing the extensor tendon and preventing medial or lateral tendon subluxation.

- The capsular anatomy of the interphalangeal joints is similar to the MCP joints, composed of thickened RCL and UCL and volar plates.
  - The *dorsal extensor apparatus* of the first IP and second through fifth PIP and DIP joints differs from the MCP joints, formed by the various extensor tendon insertions.

Tendons

Second through fifth digits

- The *EDC*, or simply *extensor digitorum*, tendons supply the second through fifth digits, though can be variable in their anatomy.
  - Most commonly, the EDC tendons supply the second (index), third (middle), and fourth (ring) fingers; a separate fifth (pinky) finger EDC tendon is usually absent.
- The *EDM*, also called the *extensor digiti quinti proprius*, is usually a double tendon slip that supplies the fifth (pinky) finger, joined by an EDC tendon slip from the fourth (ring) finger.
- The *EIP*, or simply *extensor indicis*, tendon supplies the index finger and inserts on the ulnar side of the index finger EDC tendon.
- *Juncturae tendinum* (or *connexus intertendinei*) are bands of connective tissue that connect the EDC tendons to each other and sometimes to the EDM tendon, found between the second through fifth metacarpals, proximal to the MCP joints.
- The distal attachment sites of the EDC tendons are variable, but typically include insertions along the dorsal digit at the level of the MCP, DIP, and PIP joints via slips that attach to the adjacent joint capsule and collateral ligaments.
  - The central (or middle) tendon slip inserts on the middle phalanx base at the PIP joint (Fig. 4.9); tear or avulsion results in a *boutonnière deformity*, characterized by flexion at the PIP joint and extension at the DIP joint (see Figs. 4.31 and 4.32).
  - The lateral tendon slips converge and insert on the distal phalanx base at the DIP joint (see Fig. 4.9); tear or avulsion results in a *mallet finger*, characterized by flexion at the DIP joint with inability to actively extend (see Fig. 4.30).
- Flexion of the second through fifth digits is facilitated by the combined action of two separate tendons, the *flexor digitorum profundus* (FDP) and the *flexor digitorum superficialis* (FDS).

- After exiting the carpal tunnel, the FDP and FDS tendons travel together, entering a common tendon sheath at the level of the MCP joint, with the FDP located just deep to the FDS.
- Proximal to the PIP joint, the FDS tendon splits into two slips to allow passage of the FDP tendon, which becomes superficial at this level; this normal split in the FDS tendon through which the FDP passes is referred to as *Camper's chiasm*.
- Distally, the separate tendon slips of the FDS then reunite deep to the FDP and insert as radial and ulnar slips onto the middle phalanx base at the volar aspect.
- The FDP tendon continues on and inserts on the distal phalanx base at the volar aspect.
- With this anatomic configuration, the FDS tendon controls flexion of the PIP joint, while the FDP tendon controls flexion of the DIP joint.
- Avulsion of the FDP tendon from its insertion results in *jersey finger*, seen clinically as a slight extension of the DIP joint with inability to actively flex.
- The *flexor pulleys* are a complex system of fibrous bands or retinacular sheaths, responsible for maintaining the proper position of the flexor tendons firmly against the volar aspect of the phalanges, preventing 'bowstringing' of the tendons during flexion of the digits (Fig. 4.10).

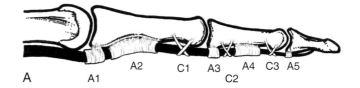

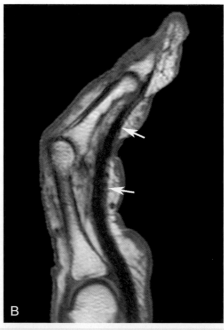

Fig. 4.10 Flexor pulley system. (A) Diagram of the flexor pulleys of the finger, which hold the flexor tendons close to the palmar surface of the phalanges. The annular pulleys (A1–A5) are of greater interest to surgeons than the cruciate pulleys (C1–C3). **(B)** Pulley failure. Sagittal T1-weighted MR image shows abnormal volar displacement of the long flexor tendon *(arrows)* due to failure of the distal A2, A3, and A4 pulleys.

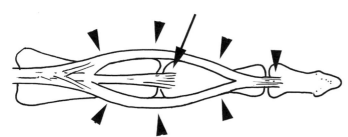

Fig. 4.9 Diagram of the extensor tendon anatomy of the fingers. This dorsal view shows the middle slip *(arrow)* inserting onto the middle phalanx and the lateral slips *(arrowheads)* that unite distally before inserting onto the distal phalanx. (Modified with permission from Manaster BJ. *Handbook of Skeletal Radiology.* 2nd ed. St. Louis: Mosby; 1997.)

- The pulley system of each finger (second through fifth digits) is composed of five *annular* and three *cruciate* pulleys.
  - The A1, A3, and A5 pulleys are located at the level of the MCP, PIP, and DIP joints, respectively.
  - The A2 and A4 pulleys are located at the level of the proximal phalanx and middle phalanx shafts, respectively.
  - The C1, C2, and C3 pulleys are located between A2 and A3, A3 and A4, and A4 and A5, respectively.
- The A2 and A4 pulleys are most critical for providing normal digit flexion and preventing tendon bowstringing.
- The cruciate pulleys are functionally less important, facilitating approximation of annular pulleys and structurally supporting the tendon sheath during flexion of the digit.
- The *vincula tendina* are thin fibrous bands that connect the FDS and FDP tendons to each other and to the phalanges and joint capsules, as well as carry blood supply to the flexor tendons.

Thumb (first digit).

- The *EPL* tendon inserts on the first distal phalanx base at the dorsal aspect.
- The *EPB* tendon lies radial to the EPL tendon and inserts on the first proximal phalanx base at the dorsal aspect.
- The *flexor pollicis longus (FPL)* tendon passes between the opponens pollicis and oblique head of the adductor pollicis and inserts distally on the first distal phalanx at the volar aspect.
- The flexor tendon pulley system of the thumb differs from the second through fifth digits, consisting of two main *annular pulleys* (A1 and A2), a *variable annular pulley* (Av), and an *oblique pulley*.
  - The A1 pulley is located at the level of the first metacarpal head and first MCP joint.
  - The Av pulley (if present) is just distal to the A1 pulley, at the level of the first proximal phalanx base.
  - The oblique pulley runs obliquely at the level of the first proximal phalanx shaft.
  - The A2 pulley is located at the level of the first proximal phalanx head and first IP joint.
- The aponeurosis of the ad̲ductor pollicis brevis tendon inserts on the ulnar aspect of the first MCP joint, which may become interposed between the torn edges of the UCL (*Stener lesion*), discussed later in this chapter.
- The aponeurosis of the ab̲ductor pollicis brevis tendon inserts on the radial aspect of the first MCP joint.

Imaging Techniques

RADIOGRAPHY

Conventional radiography is the first-line imaging modality for evaluation of hand and wrist pain. In a setting of trauma, radiographs are useful for detection of acute fractures, dislocations, and foreign bodies. Radiographs are likewise invaluable for evaluation of the atraumatic hand and wrist. Osteoarthritis and other various arthritides can be characterized based on pattern of joint involvement and specific findings of joint space narrowing, marginal osteophytes, osseous erosions, periostitis, subluxations, and soft tissue calcifications, which may all help narrow the differential diagnosis. Standard radiographic projections of both the hand and wrist include: *posteroanterior (PA)*, *oblique*, and *lateral* projections. Neutral alignment is optimal for all views, but is essential for the lateral view of the wrist. For hand radiographs, care must be taken to avoid overlap of the digits on the lateral view. Special modified views of the hand and wrist include:

- Wrist.
  - *Scaphoid series*—used to better evaluate for scaphoid fracture; includes PA and angled PA views with ulnar deviation, an external oblique view, and a lateral view.
  - *Clenched-fist view*—used to evaluate for SL dissociation; includes PA views of both wrists while both hands are clenched.
  - *Carpal tunnel view*—axial view of the wrist along the axis of the carpal tunnel, used to evaluate for hook of the hamate, pisiform, and trapezial ridge fractures.
  - *Carpal bridge view*—tangential axial view of the dorsal wrist, used to assess for fractures of the dorsal scaphoid, lunate, and triquetrum.
- Hand.
  - *Ball-catcher (Nørgaard) view*—helpful for detecting early erosive changes associated with an inflammatory arthritis; includes AP oblique views of both hands while the hands are internally rotated by approximately 45 degrees (similar to holding a ball).
  - *Coned-down views of the digits*—usually obtained in the posttraumatic setting to evaluate for subtle fractures.

MAGNETIC RESONANCE IMAGING

MRI is extremely useful for evaluation of the hand and wrist. Fluid-sensitive sequences are exquisitely sensitive for the detection of bone marrow edema, such as in the setting of acute fractures, osseous contusions, or subchondral changes related to osteoarthritis or inflammatory arthropathies. Additional osseous abnormalities, such as osteonecrosis or osseous erosions, are best evaluated by analyzing T1-weighted and fluid-sensitive sequences in combination. MRI can also detect myriad soft tissue abnormalities involving the tendons, ligaments, nerves, and muscles, and is also invaluable for the evaluation of soft tissue masses. Adequate evaluation of the small structures of the hand and wrist requires extremely high-quality imaging with a dedicated coil and a high-field-strength scanner (1.5 Tesla or greater). Imaging sequences for the wrist are a matter of personal preference but generally include:

- Coronal T1-weighted and fluid-sensitive (T2-weighted fat-suppressed or short tau inversion recovery [STIR]) images to assess the bone marrow for edema or fracture.
- Coronal high-resolution T2-weighted or gradient-echo (GRE) images to assess the interosseous ligaments and the TFCC.
- Axial T1 and fluid-sensitive images to assess the nerves and tendons, notably those in the carpal tunnel and extensor compartments.
- Sample wrist MRI protocol routinely used in our practices includes: coronal T1, coronal proton density (PD) fat-suppressed, coronal 2D or 3D gradient-echo (GRE)

T2*, axial PD or T2-weighted fat-suppressed, and sagittal STIR or T2 fat-suppressed sequences.

- The wrist should be imaged in a pronated position for optimal evaluation.
- The axial imaging plane is prescribed parallel to the distal radius, with image slices spanning the distal radial metaphysis through the proximal metacarpals.
- The coronal imaging plane is prescribed parallel to a line drawn from the ulnar styloid through the radial styloid, or to a line drawn from the volar tip of the hamate hook to the trapezial ridge.
- The sagittal imaging plane is prescribed perpendicular to the coronal imaging plane.
- Dynamic contrast-enhanced (DCE) MRI using intravenous gadolinium contrast may be requested for the evaluation of scaphoid proximal pole viability in the setting of scaphoid waist nonunion fracture; DCE MRI may also be requested to assess for synovitis in inflammatory conditions, such as rheumatoid arthritis.

MRI performed after intraarticular injection of gadolinium contrast solution (direct MR arthrography) is useful for the evaluation of interosseous ligament tears. Direct MR arthrography is achieved by injection of contrast into the radiocarpal joint, which can reveal tears of the LT and SL ligaments by visualizing contrast extension into the midcarpal joint. Similarly, full-thickness tears or perforations of the TFCC allow contrast extension from the radiocarpal joint into the DRUJ. Imaging principles for MR arthrography are similar to those discussed in the previous chapters.

- Sample wrist MR arthrogram protocol routinely used at our practices includes: coronal T1 fat-suppressed, coronal PD fat-suppressed, coronal 2D or 3D gradient-echo (GRE) T2*, axial PD fat-suppressed, axial T1, and sagittal PD fat-suppressed sequences.

The hand may be imaged in its entirety for evaluation of the joint spaces to aid in the diagnosis of various arthritides. Targeted MRI of a specific digit may be performed if there is clinical concern for an injury, such as a tear of the collateral ligaments, volar plate, extensor hood, tendons, or flexor pulleys. Targeted MRI of an injured digit should include adjacent normal digits for comparison.

- Sample hand/finger MRI protocol routinely used at our practices includes: coronal STIR, sagittal T1, axial T1, axial PD fat-suppressed, and sagittal T2 fat-suppressed sequences.

MRI of the thumb is most commonly performed for evaluation of the collateral ligaments of the MCP joint, and should be modified such that the imaging planes are performed with respect to the axis of the thumb.

- Sample thumb MRI protocol routinely used at our practices includes: coronal PD, coronal T2 fat-suppressed, axial T1, axial T1 fat-suppressed, and sagittal STIR sequences.

ULTRASOUND

- US of the hands and wrist is most commonly performed as part of a rheumatologic workup to assess for joint effusions, active synovitis, and osseous erosions.

- US can also be used for the assessment of treatment response in inflammatory arthropathies.
- US is also useful for assessing various tendon pathologies, including tenosynovitis, tendinopathy, and tendon tears; dynamic US may be particularly useful for evaluation of trigger finger and tendon pulley injuries.
- US can be used for localizing suspected retained foreign bodies, which occur commonly in the hand and wrist due to penetrating injury.
- US is useful for the evaluation of soft tissue masses in the hand and wrist, the two most common being ganglion cyst and tenosynovial giant cell tumor (giant cell tumor of tendon sheath).
- A small-footprint, high-frequency transducer (such as a 'hockey stock' probe) is mandatory for the evaluation of the small soft tissue structures and joints of the hand and wrist.

COMPUTED TOMOGRAPHY

- CT is useful for characterizing complex intraarticular fractures of the hand and wrist.
- CT can be used for assessment of fracture healing, in particular scaphoid waist fractures, and potential complications such as malunion, delayed union, or nonunion.
- Direct CT arthrography of the wrist may aid in detection of intrinsic ligament and TFCC tears, as well as articular cartilage abnormalities, when MRI is contraindicated.
- CT may be helpful for demonstrating the internal matrix of tumors.
- Dynamic CT may be performed for the evaluation of DRUJ instability by imaging the wrist in neutral, pronation, and supination positions.

FLUOROSCOPY

- Fluoroscopy may still be occasionally used for assessment of dynamic carpal instability, though dynamic fluoroscopic imaging has largely been supplanted by static imaging using modern advanced imaging modalities, namely MRI, which can reliably assess the ligamentous structures of the wrist.

Pathophysiology

CARPAL INSTABILITY

Understanding of carpal instability continues to evolve. A complete discussion of this complex topic is beyond the scope of this book but may be found in advanced textbooks and review articles. However, several of the more common and important instability patterns can be recognized on radiographs and are not difficult to learn (Fig. 4.11; features summarized in Box 4.2).

- Instability results from ligament injury and/or fractures of the distal radius or carpal bones.
- Wrist ligaments are most frequently injured by trauma, but inflammatory arthritis (usually rheumatoid arthritis) also may cause significant ligament damage.
- *Dissociation* is abnormal alignment and/or motion between bones within the same carpal row.

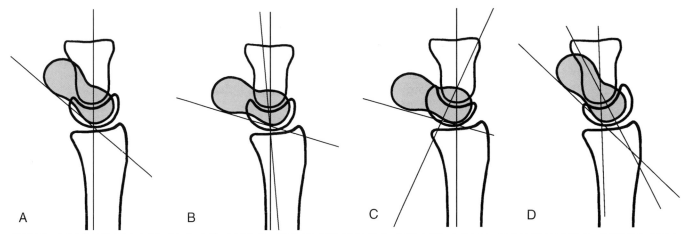

Fig. 4.11 Diagram of carpal instability patterns as seen on a lateral radiograph. All measurements require a well-positioned lateral view with the wrist in neutral alignment, not dorsiflexed. **(A)** Normal. Scapholunate angle is between 30 and 60 degrees, and the capitate and lunate are aligned. **(B)** Scapholunate dissociation. Scapholunate angle is greater than 60 degrees, but the capitate and lunate are approximately aligned. **(C)** Dorsal intercalated segment instability (DISI). Scapholunate angle is greater than 60 degrees and the lunate is tilted dorsally, with the capitolunate angle greater than 30 degrees. **(D)** Volar intercalated segment instability (VISI). Scapholunate angle is less than 30 degrees, and the lunate is tilted volar, with the capitolunate angle greater than 30 degrees. Note that neutral wrist alignment is essential for these measurements to be valid.

Box 4.2 Commonly Encountered Instability Patterns in the Wrist

Instability pattern	Features
Scapholunate dissociation	▪ Scapholunate interval widening (>4 mm) ▪ clenched-fist or ulnar deviation PA views may accentuate this finding
	▪ Increased scapholunate angle (>60 degrees)
	▪ Triangular appearance of the lunate on PA radiograph
	▪ Variable dorsal tilt of the lunate on lateral radiograph
	▪ May lead to SLAC
	▪ May be seen with DISI
Lunotriquetral Instability	▪ Often no obvious lunotriquetral interval widening
	▪ Possible subtle interruption of carpal arcs
	▪ Decreased scapholunate angle (<30 degrees) ▪ clenched-fist PA view may accentuate this finding due to increased volar flexion of the lunate
	▪ Often seen with VISI
DISI	▪ Increased capitolunate angle (>30 degrees)
	▪ Increased scapholunate angle (>60 degrees)
	▪ May be seen with scapholunate dissociation (ligamentous DISI)
	▪ May be seen with scaphoid fracture and SNAC
	▪ May be seen with distal radius fracture/malunion
VISI	▪ Increased capitolunate angle (>30 degrees)
	▪ Decreased scapholunate angle (<30 degrees)
	▪ Often seen with lunotriquetral instability

DISI, dorsal intercalated segmental instability; *PA*, posteroanterior; *SLAC*, scapholunate advanced collapse; *SNAC*, scaphoid nonunion advanced collapse; *VISI*, volar intercalated segmental instability.

- Some of the carpal instability patterns are dissociative, such as *SL dissociation*, and some have dissociation as an important (but not sole) feature, such as *dorsal intercalated segment instability (DISI)* and *volar intercalated segment instability (VISI)*, discussed later in this section.
- Because the proximal carpal row has no tendinous attachments, its position is determined by the position of the radius and the distal carpal row.
    - In the language of mechanical engineering, this makes the proximal carpal row an *intercalated segment*.
    - Intercalated segment instability patterns represent instability between carpal rows; thus, DISI and VISI refer to abnormal alignment between the carpal rows, with particular focus on alignment of the lunate and capitate.
- There are three carpal columns that run perpendicular to the carpal rows, which transmit forces from the hand to the forearm, primarily through the central column.
    - Central column: radius-lunate-capitate.
    - Ulnar column: ulna-triquetrum-hamate.
    - Radial column: radius-scaphoid-trapezoid and trapezium.
- Instability can be confined to one of the carpal columns.
- *Translocation* describes a shift of the entire carpus from its normal position relative to the radius.
- *Static* carpal instability produces abnormal carpal alignment that is visible on standard radiographs obtained with the wrist in neutral alignment.
- *Dynamic* carpal instability requires the patient to perform stress maneuvers during imaging, which may include wrist fluoroscopy or specialized radiographs (such as a clenched-fist view).
    - Real-time dynamic imaging with US, CT, or MRI has also been investigated but is infrequently used in clinical practice.

SL dissociation (SL instability, rotary subluxation, or rotatory subluxation of the scaphoid) is caused by disruption of the SL ligament and the capsular ligaments that stabilize this articulation (Fig. 4.12; see also Fig. 4.11). This is the most common carpal instability pattern.

- A normal lateral radiograph obtained with the wrist in neutral alignment shows the scaphoid in approximately 45 degrees of volar angulation (normal range, 30–60 degrees) and the lunate in neutral alignment.
- Compressive forces across the wrist created by both dorsal and volar muscle contraction tend to force the scaphoid into further volar flexion, which is normally prevented by ligamentous fixation.
- In SL dissociation, the scaphoid is released from the lunate and can rotate into greater volar flexion; thus, the key finding on the lateral radiograph is a SL angle >60 degrees.
- The lunate may tilt dorsally from its normal neutral alignment, although this is not always present.
    - Dorsal rotation of the lunate alters its appearance on a PA radiograph from the normal trapezoidal configuration into a triangular shape (see Fig. 4.12A).
- A PA radiograph may also reveal widening of the SL interval beyond its normal value of 2 mm; a SL interval measuring >4 mm is considered to be highly suggestive of SL dissociation (see Fig. 4.12A).
    - Abnormal gap between the scaphoid and lunate has been called the *Terry-Thomas sign* in reference to the late, gap-toothed British comedian.
    - A PA view obtained with a clenched fist or a PA view in ulnar deviation may elicit or increase this finding.
- In some cases of SL dissociation, PA and lateral radiographs are normal, and the abnormality becomes evident only with fluoroscopy or a stress series of radiographs that reproduces the range of motion examined with fluoroscopy.
- Abnormal motion and distribution of forces associated with SL dissociation can result in degeneration and collapse of the medial scaphoid and lateral lunate bones and radiocarpal joint, termed *scapholunate advanced collapse* (SLAC) or *SLAC wrist* (see Fig. 4.12).
    - A chronic united scaphoid waist fracture can cause a similar degenerative pattern, termed *scaphoid nonunion advanced collapse* (SNAC).

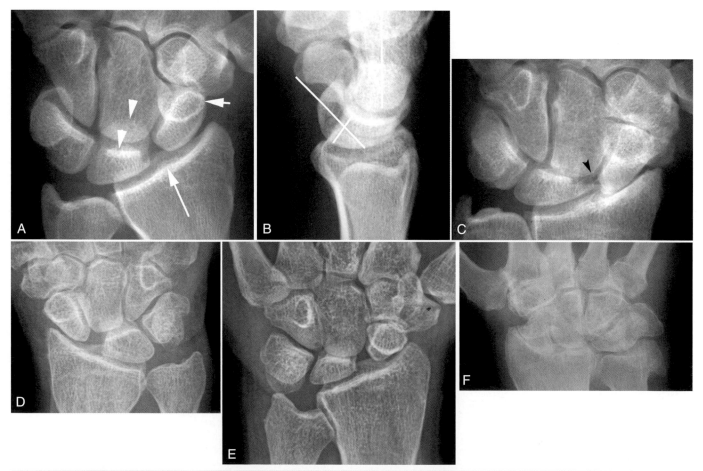

Fig. 4.12 Scapholunate dissociation, dorsal intercalated segment instability (DISI), and scapholunate advanced collapse (SLAC). (A) PA radiographic view shows a widened scapholunate interval *(long arrow)*. The *arrowheads* mark the dorsal and volar margins of the distal lunate, which should be superimposed on a PA view. They do not overlap because the lunate is rotated dorsally. The scaphoid is rotated volarly, causing it to appear shortened on this PA view *(short arrow)*. These findings suggest scapholunate dissociation. **(B)** Lateral view with the wrist in neutral alignment. Note that *lines* drawn through the long axes of the lunate, scaphoid, and capitate show the scapholunate angle to be greater than 60 degrees, indicating scapholunate dissociation. Additionally, the capitolunate angle is greater than 30 degrees, indicating DISI also is present. **(C)** Follow-up PA radiograph obtained 3 years later shows progression to SLAC, with collapse of the capitate into the lateral lunate and medial scaphoid *(arrowhead)* and secondary osteoarthritis. **(D)** Clenched-fist view in a different patient with scapholunate dissociation accentuates the wide scapholunate interval. **(E and F)** Additional examples of SLAC in different patients. F is severe.

DISI, also known as dorsiflexion instability, is usually but not necessarily associated with SL dissociation (ligamentous DISI). Other causes of DISI include scaphoid fracture, SNAC, and distal radius fracture or malunion. Like SL dissociation, DISI is a derangement of the radial side of the wrist and is often associated with radial-sided symptoms.

■ The lunate tilts dorsally, resulting in an increased capitolunate angle measuring >30 degrees.
■ SL dissociation is usually present, with an increased SL angle measuring >60 degrees (see Figs. 4.11 and 4.12).

LT instability results from disruption of the ligamentous fixation of the lunate and triquetrum. The condition is conceptually similar to SL dissociation, but LT instability does not typically result in internal widening.

■ Subtle interruption of the carpal arcs may be seen, and the SL angle may be decreased (<30 degrees).
■ A clenched-fist maneuver will roll the scaphoid and lunate into volar flexion.
■ LT instability is unusual as an isolated finding and usually occurs in association with VISI.

VISI, also known as volar flexion instability, is a consequence of ulnar-sided ligament derangement.

■ The lunate is angled volar and the capitolunate angle is greater than 30 degrees (Fig. 4.13; see also Fig. 4.11).
■ Comparing the alignment of the lunate and radius can also reduce false-positive diagnoses, because the lunate is usually volar flexed by at least 10 degrees relative to the radius.
■ LT instability is usually also present, so the SL angle is decreased (<30 degrees).
■ VISI is often seen in combination with LT instability and associated with ulnar-sided pain, though can occasionally be seen in asymptomatic patients due to ligamentous laxity.
■ VISI is much less common than DISI but can be seen from a fall onto the hypothenar eminence resulting in ulnar-sided ligamentous injury; VISI has also been reported to be the most frequent carpal instability pattern encountered in patients with rheumatoid arthritis.

Carpal translocation can occur in any direction. Ulnar translocation of the entire carpus is associated with rheumatoid arthritis. Radial and dorsal carpal translocation is associated with a prior Colles fracture. Volar carpal translocation is associated with a prior *reverse Barton fracture*.

Dynamic carpal instability is more difficult to diagnose because radiographs may not reveal the extent of abnormality or may even be normal. Terminology is less standardized than for static instabilities.

■ *Triquetrohamate instability* is one pattern of dynamic instability involving the medial column.
■ *Capitolunate instability* (capitolunate instability pattern, 'CLIP wrist') is a dynamic instability pattern of the central column centered at the capitolunate joint.

Disease Processes

DISTAL FOREARM FRACTURES

■ Distal forearm fractures are among the most common musculoskeletal injuries, and most are the result of a fall on an outstretched hand.
■ The age of the patient is an excellent predictor of the fracture pattern (Box 4.3).
  ■ Younger children usually sustain a transverse fracture of the metaphysis of the distal radius, and often a fracture of the distal ulna as well.
    ■ These fractures are frequently buckle (torus) fractures and are proximal to the physis (see Fig. 1.11).
  ■ Adolescents have stronger bones, so the fracture almost always extends partially through the comparatively weak physis, usually in a Salter–Harris II pattern.

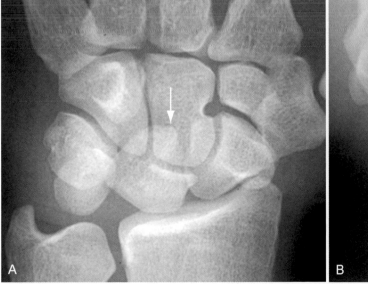 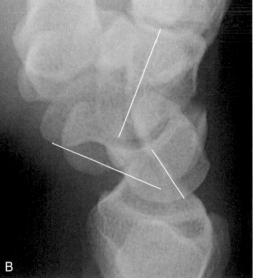

Fig. 4.13 Volar intercalated segment instability (VISI). (A) PA radiographic view shows disruption of the carpal arcs. Note the triangular or wedge shape of the lunate *(arrow)*, indicating that it is rotated. **(B)** Lateral view with lines drawn through the long axes of the lunate, scaphoid, and capitate shows VISI alignment, with the scapholunate angle less than 30 degrees and the capitolunate angle greater than 30 degrees.

- Also seen in preteens and adolescent gymnasts is a Salter–Harris I variant stress injury of the distal radius.
  - Radiographs in these children reveal widening of the physis with irregular, sclerotic margins (see Fig. 1.87).

- After closure of the physes in young adults, the scaphoid is the most commonly fractured bone in the wrist.
- As middle age approaches, the distal radius again becomes the most common site of fracture.
- Fractures seen in children and adolescents may be subtle but are usually straightforward to describe and treat, whereas fractures in adults are more variable in terms of comminution, alignment, intraarticular extension, and treatment.
- Several 'named' distal radius fracture patterns are so deeply ingrained in the orthopedic and radiology lexicon that radiologists should be familiar with these named injuries (Fig. 4.14).
  - *Colles fracture*—fracture of the distal radius with apex volar angulation and dorsal impaction; by far the most frequent wrist fracture in middle-aged and older adults (see Fig. 4.14A and B).
    - The clinical deformity that accompanies a Colles fracture is sometimes likened to an upside-down 'dinner fork'.

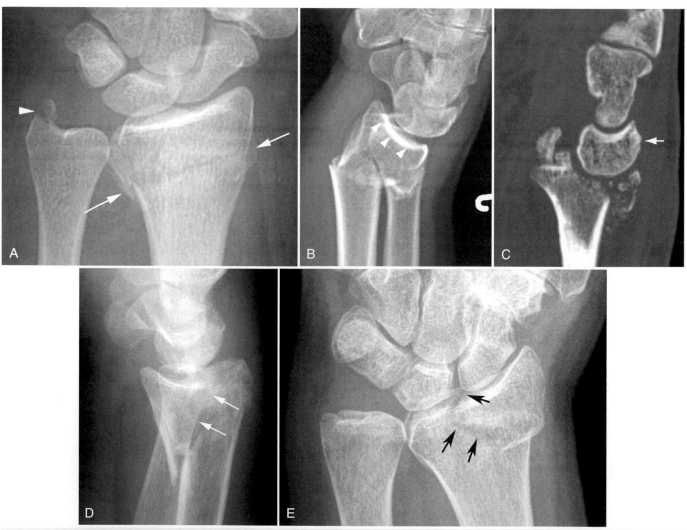

Fig. 4.14 Distal radius fractures. (A and B) Colles fracture: PA **(A)** and lateral **(B)** views in different patients show a dorsal impaction fracture of the distal radius that results in dorsal, rather than the normal volar, tilt of the articular surface of the distal radius. *Arrowheads* mark the distal radius articular surface in B. Also note the ulnar styloid fracture in A *(arrowhead)*. On the lateral view, the normal pronator fat pad is absent *(arrowheads* mark normal position of this fat pad). **(C)** Barton fracture. Sagittal CT reconstruction shows comminuted distal radius dorsal lip. Lunate *(arrow)* is displaced proximal and dorsal. **(D)** Reverse Barton fracture of the volar lip of the radius *(arrows)*, with volar subluxation of the carpus along with the radius fragment. This is an unstable fracture. **(E)** Hutchinson (chauffeur's) intraarticular fracture of the radial styloid *(arrows)*.

- Colles fracture is more common in women and is associated with hip and proximal humerus fractures in elderly patients.
- Dorsal impaction often worsens after casting because of compressive forces across the wrist from the dorsal and volar tendons.
- Posttraumatic complications include early osteoarthritis, acquired positive ulnar variance resulting in ulnar impaction syndrome, and complex regional pain syndrome (formerly known as reflex sympathetic dystrophy).
- Given the high rate of complications associated with Colles fractures, most are managed surgically with internal fixation using a plate and screw construct; volar plates cause less tendon irritation than dorsal plates and are therefore preferred.
- *Smith fracture*—reverse Colles fracture, with apex dorsal angular deformity resulting in volar tilt of the distal radius articular surface.
- *Barton fracture*—unstable intraarticular fracture of the dorsal lip of the radius, with dorsal subluxation of the carpus along with the dorsal radius fragment (see Fig. 4.14C).
  - Surgical reduction and fixation are required.
- *Reverse Barton fracture*—similar injury with volar displacement (see Fig. 4.14D).
- *Hutchinson fracture (chauffeur's fracture)*—intraarticular fracture of the radial styloid (see Fig. 4.14E).
  - Hutchinson fractures are caused by avulsion by the RCL or by a direct blow; the latter is often associated with a fracture-dislocation.
  - Hutchinson fractures are associated with SL ligament tears.
  - A fall on an outstretched hand is now the most frequent cause of this fracture.
  - The etymology of the term *chauffeur's fracture* dates back to before the introduction of electric car starters; a chauffeur was obliged to start a car by turning a crank inserted through the front grill into the engine. If the engine suddenly backfired or started during cranking, the crank would violently accelerate in the hand of the chauffeur, placing an enormous load across the radial styloid.
- Numerous classification systems of distal radius fractures have been described, each with advantages and disadvantages.
  - A radiologist may find it worthwhile to learn a system used by local orthopedic surgeons to enhance communication of abnormal findings.
  - Otherwise, it is suggested that the radiology report be limited to a clear description of the findings, with specific mention of the presence or absence of articular extension into the DRUJ or into the radiocarpal joint, as well as the presence or absence of an ulnar styloid fracture.
  - If intraarticular extension is present, articular step-off or diastasis should be measured, because defects of 2 mm or more are associated with development of posttraumatic osteoarthritis and thus serve as an indication for operative reduction.

DISTAL RADIOULNAR JOINT INSTABILITY

- Subluxation and instability of the DRUJ can occur as an isolated injury or as a component of a more complex injury such as a Colles fracture or a Galeazzi (see Fig. 3.18) or Essex-Lopresti fracture-dislocation (see Fig. 3.16).
- The distal ulna is normally slightly posterior relative to the radius; in most instances of DRUJ subluxation, the distal ulna subluxes further dorsally (Fig. 4.15).
- Diagnosis is suggested by physical examination, and axial CT or MRI can be used for confirmation.
  - A suggested protocol is to obtain limited axial CT or MR images through the DRUJ with the wrist in neutral position, in extreme pronation, and in extreme supination.
- The convex articular surface of the lateral distal ulna should be congruent with the sigmoid notch of the medial distal radius, regardless of wrist position.
- Wrist pronation (thumbs point medially and posteriorly) tends to accentuate any subluxation.
- Imaging the uninjured side for comparison purposes is helpful, because there may be some normal variation in joint laxity.

CARPAL FRACTURES AND DISLOCATIONS

Fractures

- The *scaphoid* is the most frequently fractured carpal bone (Fig. 4.16; see also Fig. 1.9).
  - Most scaphoid fractures occur through the waist (mid-portion) and are nondisplaced.
  - The distal pole has an excellent blood supply and usually heals promptly; however, the blood supply to the proximal pole enters the scaphoid at the distal waist and courses proximally within the bone.
    - A scaphoid waist or proximal pole fracture has a high likelihood of injuring the tenuous blood supply to the proximal pole.
    - Interruption of this blood supply due to fracture renders the proximal pole vulnerable to osteonecrosis, delayed union, or nonunion (Fig. 4.17; see also Fig. 1.28).

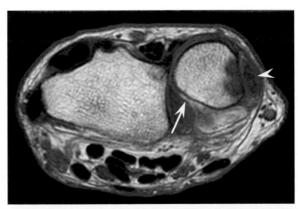

Fig. 4.15 **Distal radioulnar joint (DRUJ) instability.** Axial T1-weighted image of the wrist at the level of the DRUJ demonstrates dorsal subluxation of the distal ulna *(arrow)* related to tearing of the radioulnar ligaments (not shown). Extensor carpi ulnaris (ECU) tendinosis is also noted *(arrowhead)* with subtendinous cystic change in the ulna.

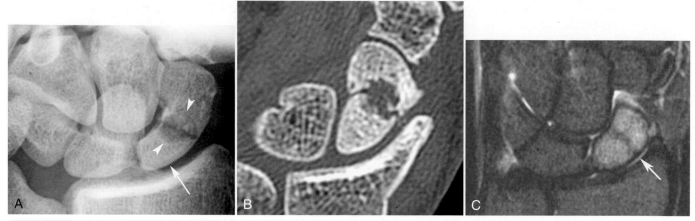

Fig. 4.16 Scaphoid fracture. (A) Subacute scaphoid fracture. Note the cyst-like bone resorption *(arrowheads)* around the fracture line and the diffusely increased density of the proximal pole *(arrow)*. Mild proximal pole sclerosis does not necessarily imply osteonecrosis and a poor prognosis. This case healed well with casting. **(B)** Oblique coronal CT reformat, oriented along the long axis of the scaphoid, shows similar findings. **(C)** Diagnosis by MRI. This patient had snuff box tenderness after a fall, but radiographs were negative, even in retrospect. Coronal STIR MR image shows diffuse scaphoid marrow edema. The fracture line is seen as a low-signal-intensity band traversing the scaphoid waist *(arrow)*. See also Fig. 1.9.

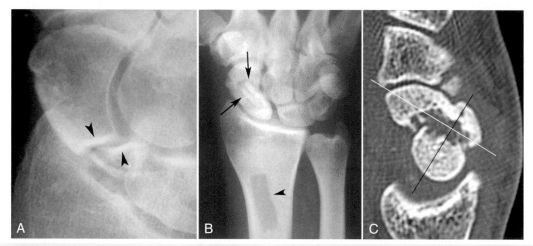

Fig. 4.17 Scaphoid fracture complications. (A) Nonunion. Note the sclerosis and smooth margins of the old fracture *(arrowheads)*, indicating that this is a chronic finding. **(B)** Delayed union, successfully treated with bone grafting. Note the graft fragments *(arrows)* and the graft donor site in the distal radius *(arrowhead)*. **(C)** Humpback deformity. Oblique coronal CT image aligned with the scaphoid shows dorsal tilt of the proximal fragment *(black line)* and volar tilt of the distal fragment *(white line)*, resulting in the 'humpback' deformity. Other images (not shown) showed that the fracture had healed in this position. Examples of scaphoid proximal pole osteonecrosis are shown in Fig. 1.28. Example of scaphoid nonunion advanced collapse (SNAC) is shown in Fig. 4.18.

- A delay in immobilization increases the risk of these complications; thus, prompt diagnosis and treatment are essential.
- Some scaphoid fractures are simply not visible on initial radiographs, even with dedicated views.
  - Negative radiographs in the presence of snuff box tenderness and a history of wrist trauma necessitate immobilization or further imaging with CT or MRI (see Fig. 4.16C).
  - If immobilization is selected, repeat radiographs obtained after 7–10 days usually reveal bone resorption or faint sclerosis around a fracture, though some fractures remain radiographically occult.
- Scaphoid waist and proximal pole fractures may take up to 2 years to fully heal.
- Cystic changes and fragmentation along the fracture margins can occur in delayed-healing fractures and in cases of nonunion (see Fig. 4.16).

- Screw fixation and bone grafting are occasionally required (see Fig. 4.17B).
- In addition to the complications of delayed union, nonunion, and osteonecrosis, a scaphoid fracture may heal with apex dorsal angular deformity, termed the *humpback deformity* (see Fig. 4.17C).
  - Thin-section CT images reconstructed parallel to the long axis of the scaphoid exquisitely demonstrate complications such as the humpback deformity and allow detailed assessment of the presence or absence of fracture healing (see Figs. 1.26 and 4.17C).
- A chronic united scaphoid waist fracture can result in DISI and *SNAC*, a degenerative pattern similar to SLAC (Fig. 4.18).
- Fracture of the *dorsal triquetrum* is the second most frequently encountered carpal bone fracture, representing an avulsion fracture of the dorsal joint capsule.

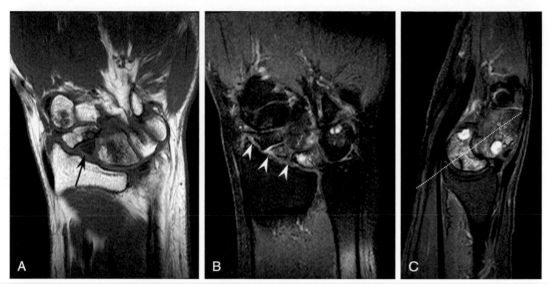

Fig. 4.18 Scaphoid nonunion advanced collapse (SNAC). (A) Coronal T1-weighted MR image of the wrist demonstrates a chronic ununited fracture of the scaphoid waist with avascular necrosis of the proximal pole, which is diminutive and T1-hypointense *(arrow)*. **(B)** Coronal proton density fat-suppressed MR image again shows the chronic ununited scaphoid fracture with secondary chondrosis along the radiocarpal joint *(arrowheads)*. **(C)** Sagittal STIR MR image shows marked dorsal tilt of the lunate *(dashed line)* with extensive subchondral marrow edema and cystic change in the lunate and capitate. Constellation of findings are consistent with SNAC.

- This fracture is usually visible only on a lateral or slightly off-lateral radiograph, where it is seen as a small cortical fragment displaced a few millimeters from the triquetrum (Fig. 4.19A).
- Point tenderness over the fracture is an important clue to this diagnosis.
- The *hook of the hamate* is another common site for fracture, typically due to a direct blow to the palm or as a stress fracture in carpenters or golfers.
  - The hook is seen 'on end' on PA radiographs as a dense "C" projecting over the mid-distal hamate; if the hook is displaced, this "C" may not be seen.
  - A carpal tunnel view radiograph or any other dedicated view may reveal the fracture; CT or MRI is usually definitive for diagnosis (Fig. 4.20).

- Main differential diagnosis is an *os hamuli proprium*, thought to represent an unfused hamulus ossification center, which has smooth, corticated margin (see Fig. 4.20A).
- *Pisiform fracture* can be seen following a direct blow, such as a fall on an outstretched hand (Fig. 4.21).
- *Trapezial ridge fractures* occur at the volar aspect of the trapezium and may likewise occur following a direct blow, but are often difficult to detect on radiographs (Fig. 4.22).
- Transverse fractures across the capitate and proximal hamate can be seen in isolation (Fig. 4.19B) or as part of complex fracture-dislocations.
- *Lunate fractures* are rare and usually result from high-impact trauma; however, the lunate is vulnerable to osteonecrosis (*Kienböck's disease*), which can progress

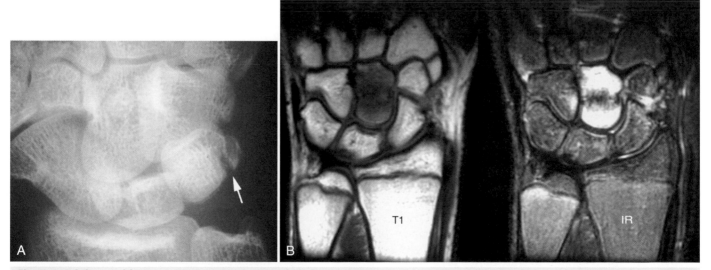

Fig. 4.19 Subtle carpal fractures. (A) Triquetral dorsal avulsion fracture *(arrow)*. These fractures may only be seen on an oblique view, as in this example. **(B)** Radiographically occult transverse capitate fracture easily detected with MRI. *IR*, inversion recovery; *T1*, T1-weighted.

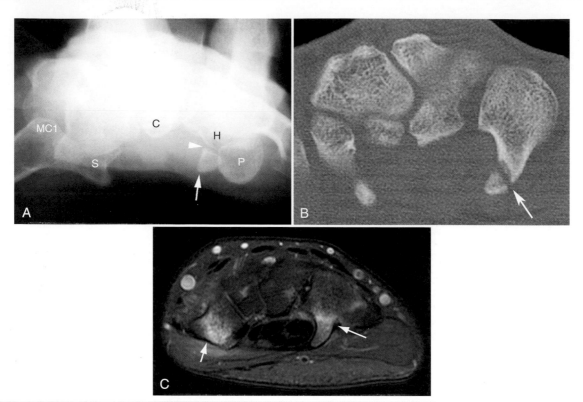

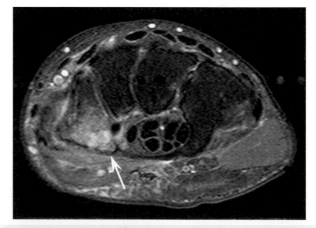

Fig. 4.20 Hamate hook fractures and os hamuli proprium. (A) Carpal tunnel view radiograph is obtained with the wrist dorsiflexed and the x-ray beam tangential to the wrist. *Arrow* indicates hook of hamate. This patient has an unfused hook of the hamate, or os hamuli proprium *(arrowhead)*. Note the straight, smooth, sclerotic margins, suggesting that this finding may be due to a developmental variant or a chronic ununited fracture. **(B)** CT image in a different patient shows an acute hamate hook fracture *(arrow)*. **(C)** Axial fat-suppressed T2-weighted MR image in a different patient shows nondisplaced fracture across the base of the hook *(long arrow)*. Also note intense bone marrow edema compatible with bone contusion in the trapezium *(short arrow)*. *C*, capitate; *H*, hamate; *MC1*, thumb metacarpal; *P*, pisiform; *S*, scaphoid and trapezium.

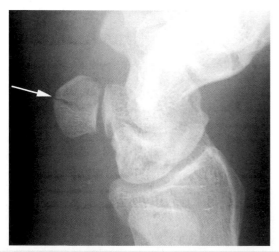

Fig. 4.21 Pisiform fracture. Acute fracture of the pisiform *(arrow)*, caused by a direct blow (a fall on the palm of the hand onto a hard surface).

Fig. 4.22 Trapezial ridge fracture. Axial T2-weighted fat-suppressed MR image of the wrist at the level of the distal carpal row demonstrates an acute nondisplaced fracture of the trapezial ridge *(arrow)* with associated intense marrow edema. This was not visible on preceding radiographs (not shown).

to lunate fragmentation and collapse, and should not be confused with acute fracture.

Dislocations

- Carpal trauma concentrates disruptive forces along arcs that run perpendicular to the Gilula arcs (Fig. 4.23), resulting in injury patterns known as *greater* and *lesser arc injuries*.

- *Greater arc injuries* extend across the radial styloid and scaphoid and across the proximal capitate, hamate, triquetrum, and ulnar styloid, or through the ligaments adjacent to these bones (Fig. 4.24).
  - This accounts for the relative frequency of scaphoid and radial and ulnar styloid fractures, as well as the ligamentous injuries that can accompany these fractures.

- A relatively common greater arc injury is the transscaphoid perilunate fracture-dislocation, in which the arc of injury passes through the scaphoid waist, across the ligaments fixing the distal carpal row and the triquetrum to the lunate, and through the ulnar styloid.
- Other greater arc injuries include the transscaphoid, transcapitate, perilunate fracture-dislocation, and the rare and severe transscaphoid, transcapitate, transhamate, transtriquetral fracture-dislocation.

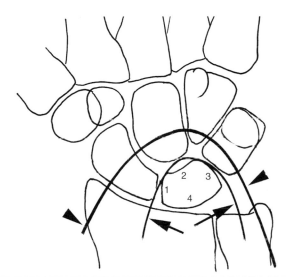

Fig. 4.23 Carpal arcs. Carpal trauma tends to concentrate disruptive forces along or close to these greater or lesser arcs. The greater arc *(arrowheads)* passes across the scaphoid waist; thus greater arc injuries are usually fracture-dislocations that include a scaphoid waist fracture. The lesser arc *(arrows)* surrounds the lunate. Lesser arc injuries cause a spectrum of ligamentous injuries and dislocations that involve the lunate in a predictable pattern of increasing severity. The mildest form (stage 1) disrupts only the scapholunate (SL) ligament, causing scapholunate dissociation (see Fig. 4.12). Stage 2 is more severe because it also disrupts the ligamentous fixation of the lunate to the capitate. Further ligamentous disruption continues around the lunate to stage 4, resulting in lunate dislocation (see Fig. 4.26).

- Restoration of normal function is difficult with any of these injuries.
- The bones can be restored to their proper positions, and the fractures can heal, but the extensive associated ligamentous damage often results in abnormal carpal motion with pain and loss of function.
- *Lesser arc injuries*, also termed *rotary subluxation of the lunate*, are confined to the ligaments surrounding the lunate.
  - Lesser arc injuries result from forced hyperextension (dorsiflexion) stress applied to the thenar eminence.
  - Ligamentous injury around the lunate occurs in a predictable pattern with increasing force (Figs. 4.25 and 4.26).
    - *Stage 1 injury* is interruption of the SL ligament and results in SL dissociation (discussed previously).
    - *Stage 2 injury* releases the fixation between the lunate and capitate (see Fig. 4.25); capitolunate instability or perilunate dislocation are the classic presentations of stage 2 rotary subluxation.
    - *Stage 3 injury* continues around the circumference of the lunate with interruption of ligamentous fixation of the lunate and triquetrum.
    - A stage 3 injury may present as a *midcarpal dislocation*, in which the lunate is tilted volarly and the other carpal bones are dislocated dorsally relative to the lunate and the radius.
    - In *stage 4 injury*, there is complete disruption of the ligamentous fixation of the lunate to the radius, resulting in volar lunate dislocation (see Fig. 4.26).
- The radiographic appearance of perilunate and midcarpal dislocations can overlap, blurring the distinction between some stage 2 and stage 3 injuries.
- Similarly, there can be overlap of the radiographic appearance of midcarpal and lunate dislocation, blurring the distinction between some stage 3 and stage 4 injuries; the distinction between these is not terribly important.

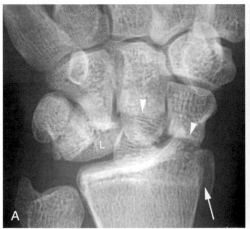
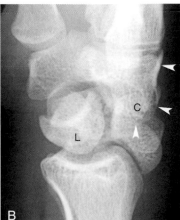
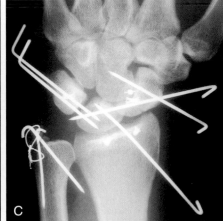

Fig. 4.24 Greater arc injuries. (A and B) Transradial, transscaphoid, transcapitate perilunate fracture-dislocation. PA view **(A)** shows fractures of the radial styloid *(arrow)* and the scaphoid waist and proximal capitate *(arrowheads)*, with ligamentous disruption medially completing the greater arc. Lateral view **(B)** shows the lunate has normal relation with the radius but the capitate is dislocated dorsally *(arrowheads* mark the proximal capitate in B). This pattern is termed *perilunate dislocation*. **(C)** Surgical reconstruction of the wrist after a transscaphoid perilunate fracture-dislocation in a different patient. The extensive fixation illustrates the severity of the ligamentous injuries associated with greater arc injuries. C, capitate; L, lunate.

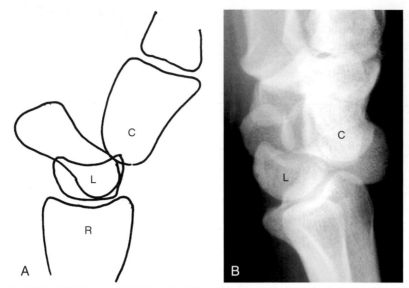

Fig. 4.25 Stage 2 lesser arc injury: perilunate dislocation. (A) Diagram shows alignment findings in perilunate dislocation. The lunate is not displaced volarly, although it is often tilted volarly. The capitate is displaced dorsally relative to the lunate and radius. Stage 3 lesser arc injury results in midcarpal dislocation (not shown), in which the lunate is volarly subluxed but not dislocated relative to the radius, and the capitate is dorsally dislocated relative to the lunate. **(B)** Lateral radiograph shows perilunate dislocation, with alignment similar to that seen in A. *C,* Capitate; *L,* lunate; *R,* radius.

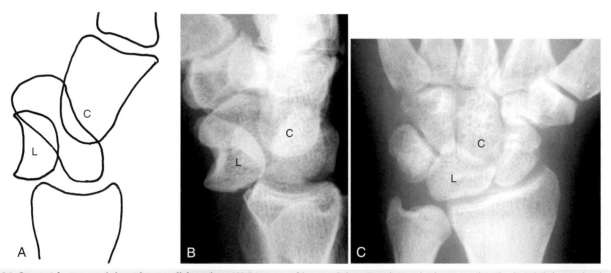

Fig. 4.26 Stage 4 lesser arc injury: lunate dislocation. (A) Diagram of lunate dislocation shows the lunate to be tilted and dislocated volarly. The capitate is colinear with the radius. **(B)** Lateral radiographic view shows the volar lunate dislocation, with alignment similar to that shown in A. In this dislocation pattern, there is true dislocation at both the radiolunate and capitolunate articulations. **(C)** PA radiographic view shows disruption of the carpal arcs and abnormal contour of the lunate due to the dislocation. *C,* Capitate; *L,* lunate.

FINGER FRACTURES AND DISLOCATIONS

Fractures

- Thumb injuries require dedicated radiographs because routine hand radiographs do not profile the thumb in true PA and lateral projections.
  - Extraarticular fractures of the first metacarpal tend to maintain anatomic alignment because the muscle attachments along the shaft resist displacement.
  - Intraarticular fractures at the base of the thumb can displace and are frequently unstable.
  - A *Bennett fracture* is an intraarticular two-part fracture of the first metacarpal base.

- The mechanism of injury is axial loading of a partially flexed first metacarpal, often sustained during a fistfight.
- The volar ligamentous fixation of the first metacarpal is very strong, so a small volar bone fragment known as the palmar beak fragment is avulsed from the first metacarpal and retains a normal position, while the larger fragment subluxes or dislocates dorsally (Fig. 4.27).
- A Bennett fracture is unstable and is treated surgically.
- A *Rolando fracture* is a comminuted Bennett fracture.
  - Restoration of anatomic alignment is often impossible because of the comminution, so Rolando

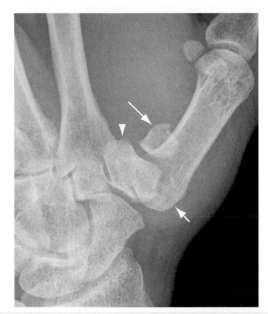

Fig. 4.27 Bennett fracture-dislocation. Note the oblique intraarticular fracture at the base of the thumb metacarpal. The volar medial fragment, known as the palmar beak fragment *(long arrow)*, is normally aligned with the trapezium *(arrowhead)*, but the main thumb metacarpal fragment *(short arrow)* is displaced lateral and proximal.

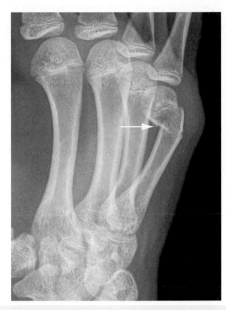

Fig. 4.28 Boxer's fracture. Fifth metacarpal neck fracture with apex dorsolateral angulation *(arrow)*.

fractures are frequently treated with casting or external fixation traction rather than internal fixation.

- Underlying first CMC joint osteoarthritis or ossicles adjacent to the first CMC joint are potential pitfalls on radiography that can simulate comminution.
- A *boxer's fracture* is a metacarpal fracture caused by abrupt axial loading, usually during delivery of a punch (Fig. 4.28).
  - The neck of the fifth metacarpal is the most frequent location, with the fourth metacarpal similarly fractured in many cases.
  - Apex dorsal angulation with volar comminution is common, and healing with this angular deformity is frequent.
  - A boxer's fracture can be complicated by infection due to contamination by the teeth of the recipient of the punch.
- Extraarticular fractures of the phalanges, particularly of the tufts, are often the result of blunt or sharp trauma (e.g., with a hammer, car door, or table saw).
  - Accurate assessment of fracture angulation requires a true lateral radiograph.
  - Rotational deformity is also important but may be assessed clinically.
- Intraarticular fractures of the phalanges can occur on the medial, lateral, volar, or dorsal surfaces.
  - Medial and lateral fractures are associated with collateral ligament avulsions (discussed later in this chapter).
  - An avulsion fracture of the proximal volar aspect of the middle phalanx is termed a *volar plate fracture.*
    - The volar plates are fibrocartilaginous structures that span the volar aspect of the PIP and MCP joints.

- Hyperextension can avulse the distal attachment of the volar plate at the PIP joint.
- A lateral radiograph reveals a small avulsion fragment displaced proximally from the donor site at the base of the middle phalanx (Fig. 4.29).
- A radiographically similar injury known as a *jersey finger* occurs at the distal interphalangeal (DIP) joint.

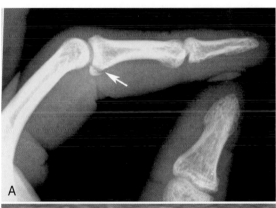
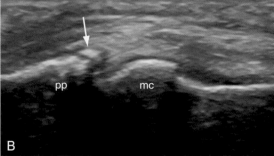

Fig. 4.29 Volar plate fracture. (A) Radiograph *(arrow* marks fracture). **(B)** US in a different patient shows a minimally displaced fragment *(arrow)* at the base of the proximal phalanx. The image is sagittal, with distal to the viewer's left and with the probe on the volar side of the finger. *mc,* Metacarpal head; *pp,* proximal phalanx.

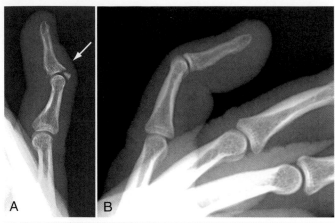

Fig. 4.30 **Extensor tendon avulsions. (A)** Mallet (baseball) finger fracture. Note the small avulsion from the dorsal base of the distal phalanx *(arrow)*. **(B)** Tendon injury without fracture. The patient was unable to extend his distal phalanx. Note that the proximal interphalangeal joint is extended. This is not a natural position and indicates a soft tissue mallet finger injury. Surgical repair of the extensor tendon was required.

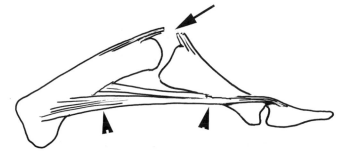

Fig. 4.31 **Diagram of boutonnière (buttonhole) deformity.** Lateral diagram demonstrates how interruption of the middle slip of the extensor tendon *(arrow)* allows the proximal interphalangeal (PIP) joint to flex while the distal interphalangeal joint is extended. The PIP joint has herniated between the lateral slips *(arrowheads)* (like a button through a buttonhole) and become fixed in this position. (Modified with permission from Manaster BJ. *Handbook of Skeletal Radiology.* 2nd ed. St. Louis: Mosby; 1997.)

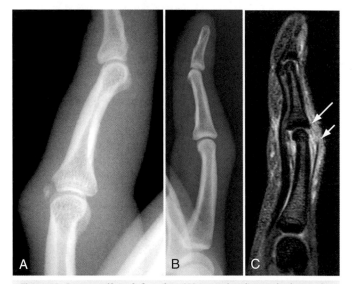

Fig. 4.32 **Boutonnière deformity. (A)** Lateral radiograph shows the dorsal avulsion fragment arising from the base of the middle phalanx. The proximal interphalangeal (PIP) joint is fixed in flexion while the distal interphalangeal joint is fixed in extension, causing the boutonnière deformity. **(B and C)** Boutonnière deformity in a different patient with ligament injury but no fracture. Radiograph **(B)** shows the abnormal alignment and soft tissue swelling dorsal to the PIP joint. Sagittal gradient-echo MR image **(C)** shows retracted short extensor tendon *(short arrow)* and normal insertion site *(long arrow).*

due to avulsion of the FDP tendon from its insertion onto the volar base of the distal phalanx.

- This injury is caused by forced extension while in flexion, such as when grabbing the jersey of an escaping football player.
- Physical examination reveals that the DIP joint cannot be flexed.
- Both volar plate and jersey finger injuries can result in loss of function if not treated appropriately.
- Similar injuries, with similar potential for disability if undiagnosed or improperly treated, occur on the *dorsal* margins of the middle and distal phalanges.
  - The extensor mechanism of the fingers consists of a middle tendon slip that inserts at the base of the middle phalanx and two lateral tendon slips that course around the middle phalanx and unite as the common extensor tendon to insert at the base of the distal phalanx (see Fig. 4.9).
  - A fracture of the dorsal base of the distal phalanx is caused by avulsion of the common extensor tendon and is termed a *baseball finger* or *mallet finger* (Fig. 4.30A).
  - This injury occurs when an extended DIP joint is forcibly flexed, as may occur when the finger is 'jammed' by a baseball striking the tip of the finger.
  - Most baseball finger injuries are confined to the extensor tendon; radiographs reveal no fracture but do reveal the DIP joint to be flexed (Fig. 4.30B); the combination of DIP flexion and PIP extension should suggest this diagnosis.
- A tear or avulsion of the middle slip of the extensor digitorum tendon with preservation of the remainder of the extensor mechanism can result in the *boutonnière (buttonhole) deformity* (Figs. 4.31 and 4.32).
  - The *boutonnière* deformity is flexion of the PIP joint with hyperextension of the DIP joint.
  - Middle slip interruption allows the PIP joint to flex while the DIP is extended.

- With time, the PIP can pass between the lateral tendon slips like a button through a buttonhole and become fixed in this position.

Dislocations

- Dislocations of the finger joints are associated with collateral ligament injuries and often with small avulsion fragments.
  - The PIP joints are the most frequently dislocated, usually dorsally (Fig. 4.33).
    - These dislocations often reduce spontaneously or are reduced by the patient or by nonmedical personnel before medical attention is reached.
    - Residual soft tissue swelling, mild subluxation, or small avulsion fragments may be the only radiographic evidence of the prior dislocation, though more severe associated fractures can occur.

- Dorsal dislocation of the PIP joint has been termed *coach finger.*
  - Less commonly, dislocations can be seen at the DIP or MCP joints.
- Hand and finger injuries can be surprisingly subtle on radiographs; commonly missed injuries that require a keen eye include:

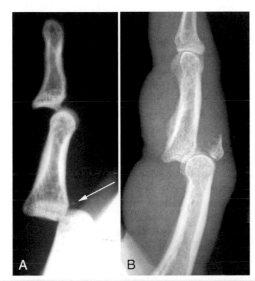

Fig. 4.33 Finger dislocations. (A) Dorsal dislocation of the thumb metacarpophalangeal (MCP) *(arrow)* and interphalangeal joints. A tiny avulsed fragment at the MCP joint is faintly visible at the tip of the *arrow.* **(B)** Second (index) finger proximal interphalangeal joint fracture-dislocation. This injury required surgical reduction and fixation.

- Carpometacarpal (CMC) joint dislocation.
- Palmar and dorsal avulsion fractures of the bases of the middle and distal phalanges.
- First metacarpal (thumb) base fracture (e.g., Bennett fracture).

SCAPHOLUNATE LIGAMENT TEAR

- Recall that the SL ligament has three components; the *dorsal component* is the thickest and functionally most important for SL stability.
- SL ligament tears may be complete (involving all three bundles) or partial.
- Traumatic SL ligament tears most commonly occur from fall onto the thenar eminence of the hand, with transmitted forces resulting in tear of the dorsal component or complete ligament rupture (Fig. 4.34).
- SL ligament tears are best evaluated by MRI or MR arthrography, though secondary findings may be seen on radiographs, including SL interval widening.
  - Recall that widening of the SL interval (>4 mm) has been called the *Terry-Thomas sign.*
- Complete tear of the SL ligament and supporting capsular ligaments results in carpal instability, namely SL dissociation and DISI (previously discussed; see Figs. 4.11 and 4.12).
- Degenerative tears or perforations commonly involve the membranous component of the SL ligament, which are likely clinically insignificant and do not result in carpal instability.

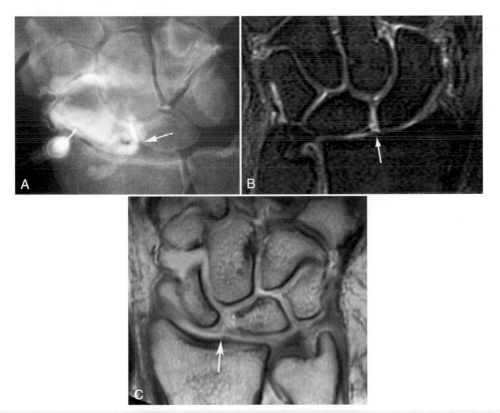

Fig. 4.34 Scapholunate (SL) ligament tears. (A) Radiocarpal injection shows contrast medium passing through an SL ligament tear *(arrow)* into the midcarpal joint. **(B)** Coronal fat-suppressed T2-weighted image in a different patient shows SL ligament tear *(arrow).* **(C)** Coronal T1-weighted MR arthrogram obtained after radiocarpal injection shows an SL ligament tear *(arrow)* with wide SL interval.

LUNOTRIQUETRAL LIGAMENT TEAR

- Recall that the LT ligament, similar to the SL ligament, has three components; the *volar component* of the LT ligament is thickest and functionally most important for LT stability, though the dorsal component also plays an important role as a rotational constraint.
- LT ligament tears are less commonly seen than SL ligament tears.
- Traumatic LT ligament tears most commonly occur from fall backward onto the hypothenar eminence of the hand, resulting in wrist hyperextension or radial deviation (Fig. 4.35).
- LT ligament tears may be seen on MRI but are best evaluated by MR or CT arthrography; LT interval widening is not a common feature on radiographs.
- Complete tear of the LT ligament results in carpal instability, namely LT instability and VISI (previously discussed; see Fig. 4.13).
- LT ligament injuries are frequently associated with TFCC injuries.

TRIANGULAR FIBROCARTILAGE COMPLEX TEAR

- Recall the anatomy of the TFCC, which is composed of the *central articular disc, peripheral foveal* and *styloid attachments, dorsal* and *volar radioulnar ligaments, ulnocarpal ligaments, ECU tendon sheath,* and *the meniscus homologue.*
- Many TFCC injuries occur during a wrist fracture and are not immediately apparent.
  - Traumatic tears of the TFCC often cause ulnar-sided wrist pain and weakness
  - An ulnar-sided click or pop with wrist motion may be present.
- Arthrography or MRI may reveal a defect in the central TFCC articular disc or communication between the radiocarpal joint and the DRUJ (Fig. 4.36; see also Fig. 4.35B).
- Patterns of TFCC tears are complex but generally occur as a perforation of the central articular disc or as a tear of the disc fixation to the radius, ulna, or dorsal or volar joint capsule.

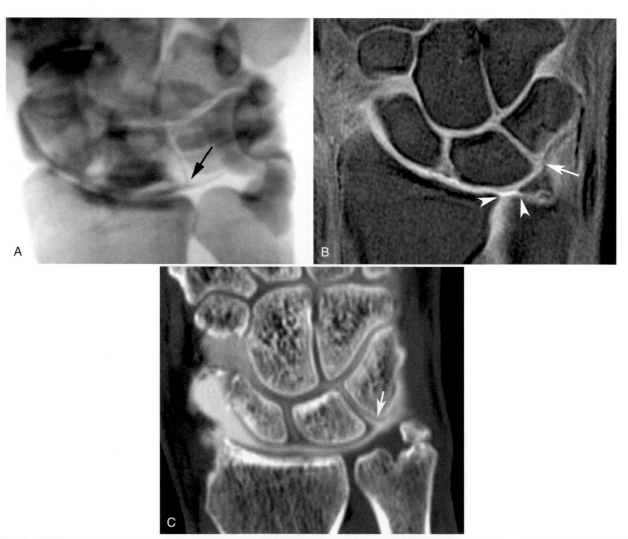

Fig. 4.35 Lunotriquetral (LT) ligament tears. (A) Ulnar deviation view obtained after radiocarpal injection shows an LT) ligament tear *(arrow)* with contrast medium filling the midcarpal compartment. **(B)** Coronal T1-weighted MR arthrogram image after radiocarpal injection shows LT ligament tear *(arrow)* and wide triangular fibrocartilage complex (TFCC) articular disc tear *(arrowheads)*. **(C)** CT arthrogram reformat in a different patient with LT ligament tear *(arrow)*. Note the intact scapholunate (SL) ligament and TFCC.

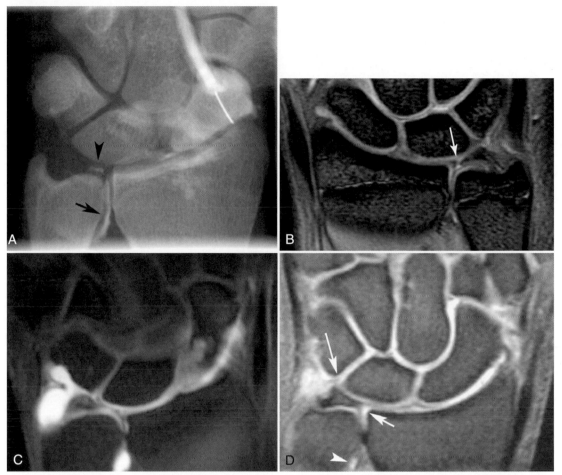

Fig. 4.36 Triangular fibrocartilage complex (TFCC) articular disc tears. (A) Spot image during radiocarpal joint injection shows contrast medium in the distal radioulnar joint *(arrow)*, indicating triangular fibrocartilage complex (TFCC) articular disc tear. The tear is visible as contrast medium in the expected position of the articular disc *(arrowhead)*. **(B)** Coronal fat-suppressed MR image in a different patient shows TFCC articular disc tear *(arrow)*. **(C)** Coronal fat-suppressed T1-weighted MR arthrogram obtained after radiocarpal injection in a different patient shows a TFCC articular disc tear. **(D)** MR arthrogram in another patient shows TFCC articular disc avulsion from its radial attachment *(short white arrow)*. Contrast medium has entered the distal radioulnar joint through this defect *(white arrowhead)*. Also note the high signal intensity within the midcarpal joint due to contrast medium passing through a lunotriquetral ligament tear *(long white arrow)*.

- TFCC tears may be seen as a consequence of positive ulnar variance, often seen in combination with *ulnar impaction syndrome*.
- Asymptomatic thinning or perforation of the central articular disc may be commonly observed in older individuals and thought to represent a consequence of age-related degeneration.

ULNAR VARIANCE

- *Ulnar variance* refers to the length of the distal ulna with respect to the distal radius, designated as *neutral, positive,* or *negative*.
- *Neutral ulnar variance*: the distal ulna is normally equal to (or a few millimeters shorter) than the adjacent radius.
- *Positive ulnar* (or *ulnar-plus*) *variance*: the distal ulna is longer or extends more distally than the radius.
  - An elongated ulna can impact against the TFCC and the proximal-ulnar aspect of the lunate, termed *ulnar impaction syndrome* (discussed later in this chapter).

- *Negative ulnar* (or *ulnar-minus*) *variance*: the distal ulna is more than a few millimeters shorter than the distal radius.
  - Negative ulnar variance is associated with an increased risk of *Kienböck's disease,* also termed *lunatomalacia* or osteonecrosis of the lunate (discussed in the subsequent section).
  - Negative ulnar variance can result in *ulnar impingement syndrome* in severe cases.
- Because ulnar variance is relative to the distal radius, causes of abnormal variance include prior fracture, growth plate insult, postsurgical change, or congenital abnormality affecting either of these two bones.
- Accurate identification of ulnar variance requires a properly positioned PA radiograph with the wrist and forearm in neutral alignment (see Fig. 4.1A).
  - If the PA radiograph is obtained with the wrist dorsiflexed and the hand flat on the x-ray detector plate, the dorsal ulna will project distally on the image, simulating positive ulnar variance (Fig. 4.37).
  - Wrist supination 'shortens' the ulna, and wrist pronation 'lengthens' the ulna relative to the distal radius (see Fig. 4.37).

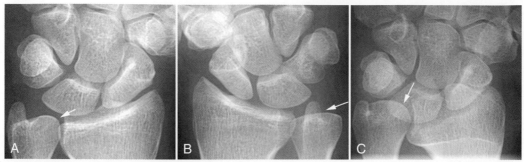

Fig. 4.37 Effect of wrist position on apparent ulnar variance. All images are of the same patient. A properly positioned PA radiograph is obtained with the wrist in neutral position (see Fig. 4.1A). Pronation **(A)** causes apparent lengthening of the ulna *(arrow)*. Supination **(B)** causes apparent shortening of the ulna *(arrow)*. Wrist dorsiflexion **(C)**, as can occur with the hand flat on the x-ray detector plate but with the elbow elevated, causes apparent lengthening of the ulna *(arrow)*.

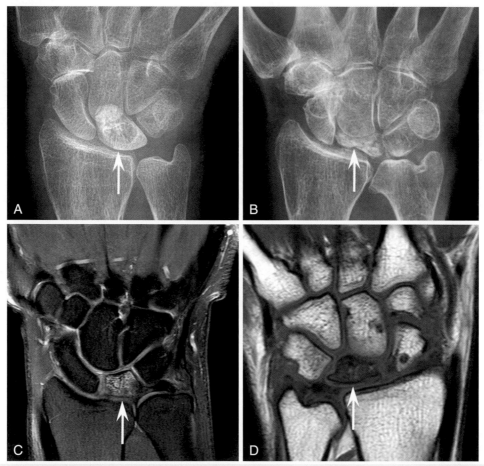

Fig. 4.38 Kienböck's disease in different patients. (A) PA radiograph of the wrist demonstrates sclerosis throughout the lunate *(arrow)* without morphologic collapse, consistent with stage II Kienböck's disease. **(B)** PA radiograph of the wrist demonstrates sclerosis and marked collapse of the lunate *(arrow)* with secondary degenerative changes in the wrist, consistent with stage IV Kienböck's disease. **(C)** Coronal T2-weighted fat-suppressed MR image of the wrist shows marrow edema throughout the lunate *(arrow)* without collapse, consistent with stage II Kienböck's disease. **(D)** Coronal T1-weighted MR image of the wrist shows diffuse hypointensity throughout the lunate *(arrow)* indicating osteonecrosis, with early collapse at the radial aspect, consistent with stage III Kienböck's disease.

KIENBÖCK'S DISEASE

- *Kienböck's disease* refers to osteonecrosis of the lunate (Fig. 4.38), which has a bimodal distribution in young men between 20–40 years of age and middle-aged women.
- Etiology remains unclear, though may be related to prior trauma or anatomic factors disturbing the vascular supply.

- Kienböck's disease is associated with negative ulnar variance, which increases biomechanical load on the lunate.
- The Lichtman staging system of Kienböck's disease (Stages I–IV) can be used to grade the severity of osteonecrosis, which ranges from marrow edema on MRI and normal radiographs to progressive lunate sclerosis,

morphologic collapse, and secondary osteoarthritis of the radiocarpal and/or midcarpal joints.

ULNAR IMPACTION SYNDROME

- *Ulnar impaction syndrome* (also called *ulnar abutment* or *ulnocarpal loading*) is impaction of the distal ulna against the TFCC and the proximal carpal row at the ulnar aspect.
- Positive variance transfers load at the wrist from the distal radius to the distal ulna.
- Chronic impaction causes degeneration and tearing of the TFCC, as well as cartilage injury typically at the proximal-ulnar lunate, distal ulna, and/or the proximal-radial triquetrum (Fig. 4.39).
- Radiographs may reveal positive ulnar variance and subchondral cysts, sclerosis, or osteophytes; MRI reveals similar findings, with the addition of subchondral marrow edema.
- Associated TFCC degeneration or tears are best seen by MRI or arthrography.

- Treatment is dependent on the degree of positive ulnar variance and clinical symptoms; cases that fail conservative therapy are managed surgically with ulnar shortening osteotomy, or resection of all or part of the distal ulna.

ULNAR IMPINGEMENT SYNDROME

- *Ulnar impingement syndrome* is mechanical impingement, often with pseudarthrosis, of a markedly shortened ulna against the distal metaphysis of the radius (Fig. 4.40).
- Clinical features may mimic those of ulnar impaction but are often more severe.
- Ulnar impingement is a potential complication of ulnar growth arrest, surgical ulnar shortening, or any traumatic or growth abnormality that reduces the length of the ulna resulting in negative ulnar variance.
- Radiographs in long-standing ulnar impingement demonstrate negative ulnar variance, radioulnar

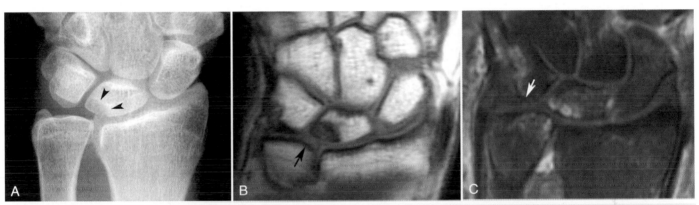

Fig. 4.39 Ulnar impaction syndrome. (A) PA radiograph shows mild positive ulnar variance. Note the small cystic lucencies in the proximal medial lunate *(arrowheads)* that are due to impaction against the ulna. Coronal T1-weighted **(B)** and STIR **(C)** MR images in a different patient show positive ulnar variance and cystlike lesions in the lunate and adjacent ulna, with adjacent marrow edema. The triangular fibrocartilage disc is torn *(arrow in B)*, with only a small residual, degenerated medial portion *(arrow in C)*.

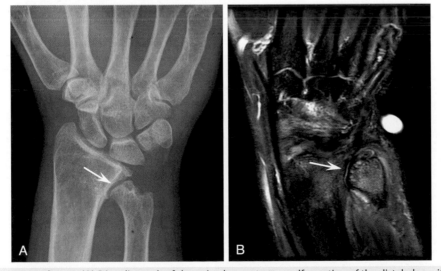

Fig. 4.40 Ulnar impingement syndrome. (A) PA radiograph of the wrist demonstrates malformation of the distal ulna with negative ulnar variance and scalloping of the adjacent distal radius *(arrow)*. **(B)** Coronal T2-weighted fat-suppressed MR image of the wrist in a different patient shows negative ulnar variance with remodeling of the sigmoid notch of the distal radius *(arrow)*, extensive marrow edema spanning the distal radioulnar joint (DRUJ) articulation, and cystic change in the distal ulna.

convergence, and sclerosis, scalloping, or pressure erosion of the distal radius.

■ MRI shows similar findings and may also demonstrate bone marrow edema at the pseudarthrosis.

HAMATOLUNATE IMPINGEMENT SYNDROME

■ In approximately 50% of individuals, the lunate has an accessory medial facet that articulates with the proximal hamate, termed a *type II lunate* (a type I lunate does not articulate with the hamate).

■ *Hamatolunate impingement* is a degenerative process that occurs at the articulation between a type II lunate and the proximal hamate, a cause of ulnar-sided wrist pain.

■ This normal variant carries a risk of symptomatic chondromalacia and subchondral marrow edema/cystic change at the proximal hamate or occasionally the lunate; findings are often subtle but characteristic on MRI (Fig. 4.41).

■ Surgical treatment is mainly by arthroscopic burring of the proximal hamate.

DE QUERVAIN'S SYNDROME

■ *De Quervain's syndrome* (or *De Quervain's tenosynovitis*) is an overuse syndrome involving the APL and EPB tendons of the first extensor compartment.

■ Patients typically present with radial-sided wrist pain, swelling, and limited thumb movement.

■ MRI and US can reveal tendinopathy, tenosynovitis, and sometimes even tendon tearing, which may affect one or both of the first extensor compartment tendons; occasionally, MRI may also show subtendinous bone marrow edema in the distal radius (Fig. 4.42).

CARPAL TUNNEL SYNDROME

■ *Carpal tunnel syndrome* (CTS) is median nerve dysfunction caused by increased pressure within the carpal tunnel.

■ Common symptoms include pain, weakness, and numbness/tingling in the thenar region and along the first through fourth digits; atrophy of the thenar musculature may be seen in advanced cases.

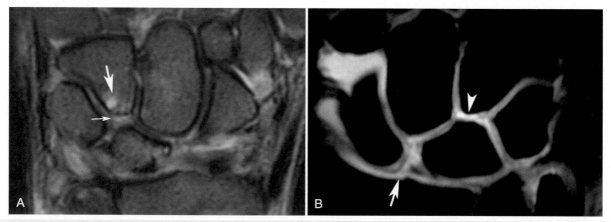

Fig. 4.41 Hamatolunate impingement. (A) Coronal STIR MR image shows a type II lunate, which articulates with the proximal hamate. There is subchondral edema and cystic change in the proximal hamate *(large arrow)* and high signal intensity in the overlying articular cartilage *(small arrow)*, indicating chondrosis. **(B)** Coronal fat-suppressed T1-weighted MR arthrogram image. The image is adjusted to display articular cartilage gray. Note high-signal-intensity contrast medium *(arrowhead)* abutting the subchondral bone plate of the hamate, indicating overlying articular cartilage loss. Also note scapholunate (SL) ligament tear *(arrow)*.

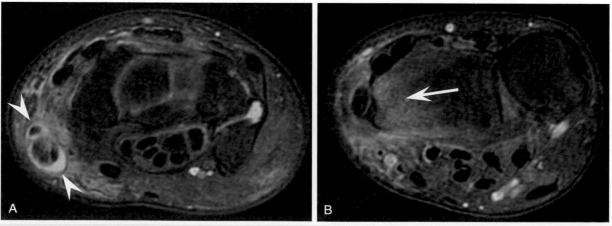

Fig. 4.42 De Quervain's syndrome. Axial T2-weighted fat-suppressed MR images at the level of the carpus **(A)** and distal radius **(B)** demonstrating first extensor tendon compartment tenosynovitis *(arrowheads* in A) with surrounding soft tissue edema. Subtendinous bone marrow edema is noted within distal radius *(arrow* in B).

- Many cases are idiopathic, but potential causes of CTS include fracture, tenosynovitis, rheumatoid arthritis, gout, amyloid, tuberculosis, tumors, pregnancy, diabetes, anomalous muscles and other anatomic variants, and repetitive stress and/or extrinsic compression.
- The role of MRI and US in making the diagnosis of CTS remains controversial.
  - Most studies promoting imaging diagnosis of CTS emphasize subtle volar bowing of the retinaculum and/or increased cross-sectional size of the median nerve as signs of CTS, but there is overlap between normal and abnormal.
- Both MRI and US can be useful in identifying or excluding a surgically correctable cause such as a mass lesion within the carpal tunnel (Fig. 4.43).

ULNAR TUNNEL (GUYON'S CANAL) SYNDROME

- Recall that *Guyon's canal* is a fibro-osseous tunnel at the volar-ulnar aspect of the wrist containing the ulnar nerve and vessels, located between the pisiform and the hook of the hamate (see Fig. 4.8B).
- *Ulnar tunnel syndrome* refers to compression of the ulnar nerve within Guyon's canal.
- Common symptoms include pain, weakness, and numbness/tingling in the hypothenar region and along the fifth and ulnar side of the fourth digits.
- Many of the same conditions that can cause median nerve impingement within the carpal tunnel can similarly afflict the ulnar nerve within the Guyon's canal.

INTERSECTION SYNDROMES

- Intersection syndromes occur at the decussation, or intersection, of various tendons related to mechanical friction and irritation, often seen in athletes or workers subjected to repetitive movements.
- Two intersection syndromes are encountered in the distal forearm and wrist, respectively: *intersection syndrome* and *distal intersection syndrome*.
- Both intersection syndromes are characterized on MRI or US by tenosynovitis and peritendinous edema.
- *Intersection syndrome* occurs at the crossover of the first and second extensor tendon compartments at the level of the distal forearm (Fig. 4.44).
  - This region may not be included on routine MRI of the wrist; concern for this condition warrants extending the field of view or a dedicated forearm MRI.
- *Distal intersection syndrome* occurs at the crossover of the second and third extensor tendon compartments at the level of the wrist (Fig. 4.45).

FLEXOR TENDON AND PULLEY INJURIES

- There are a range of abnormalities that may involve any of the flexor tendons, including tenosynovitis, tendinopathy, tendon tears, 'trigger finger', and flexor pulley injuries.
- *Tenosynovitis*, or inflammation of the tenosynovium, results in abnormal fluid accumulation within a tendon sheath, best diagnosed on imaging by US or fluid-sensitive MRI sequences.

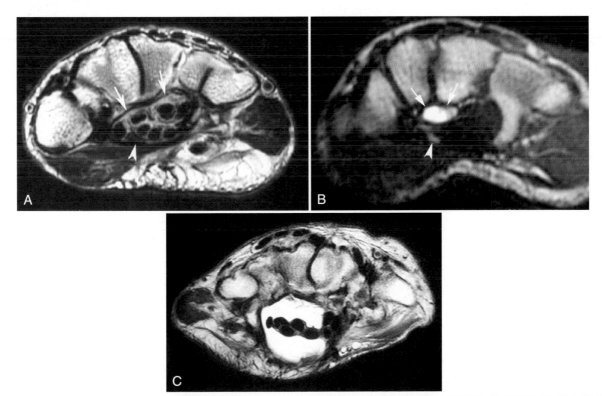

Fig. 4.43 Carpal tunnel syndrome due to mass lesions. All images were obtained with axial T2-weighted MRI. **(A)** Synovitis *(arrows)* in a patient with early rheumatoid arthritis. *Arrowhead* marks the median nerve. **(B)** Volar carpal ganglion. Note the round, sharply circumscribed mass with uniform high signal intensity in the dorsal portion of the carpal tunnel *(arrows)* typical of a ganglion cyst. Also note median nerve edema *(arrowhead)*, a finding that is associated with nerve dysfunction. Resection of the ganglion cured the carpal tunnel syndrome. **(C)** Massive ganglion simulating tenosynovitis in a different patient with carpal tunnel syndrome.

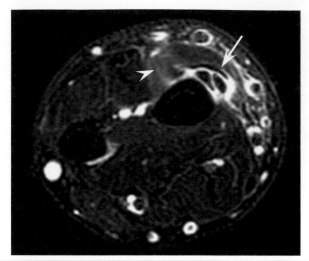

Fig. 4.44 Intersection syndrome (of the forearm). Axial STIR MR image demonstrates tenosynovitis at the decussation of the first and second extensor compartment tendons at the level of the dorsolateral distal forearm *(arrow)*. Reactive intramuscular edema versus low-grade muscle strain is noted within the abductor pollicis longus muscle near the distal myotendinous junction *(arrowhead)*.

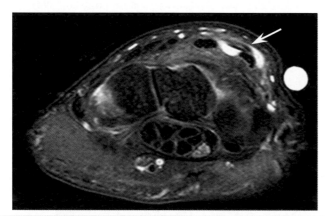

Fig. 4.45 Distal intersection syndrome (of the wrist). Axial T2-weighted fat-suppressed MR image demonstrates tenosynovitis at the decussation of the second and third extensor compartment tendons *(arrow)*. Linear hyperintense intrasubstance signal within the extensor pollicis longus (EPL) tendon represents interstitial tearing.

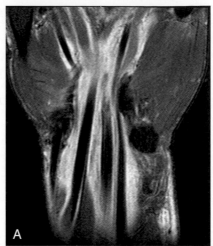

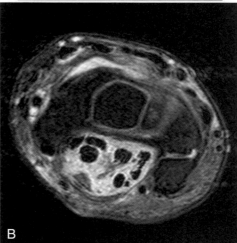

Fig. 4.46 Flexor compartment septic tenosynovitis. Coronal **(A)** and axial **(B)** T2-weighted fat-suppressed sequences of the wrist demonstrate extensive flexor compartment tenosynovitis within the carpal tunnel, extending proximally and distally into the forearm and hand. Fluid sampling revealed atypical mycobacterial infection, a complication of carpal tunnel surgery in this case.

- Tenosynovitis may be sterile, related to repetitive overuse or an underlying inflammatory condition (such as rheumatoid arthritis), or infectious (septic tenosynovitis).
- Septic tenosynovitis is most commonly bacterial in etiology and often associated with a history of penetrating trauma (Fig. 4.46).
- *Tendinopathy*, or *tendinosis*, represents a chronic degenerative process of the tendon that may occur with aging, chronic overuse, or repetitive microtrauma.
- *Tendon tears* are most commonly due to acute trauma or laceration (Fig. 4.47), though may be seen spontaneously in the setting of underlying tendinopathy.
  - As discussed previously, avulsion of the FDP tendon from its insertion on the volar base of the distal phalanx results in *jersey finger*, resulting in inability to actively flex the DIP joint; this may or may not be associated with an osseous avulsion fracture.

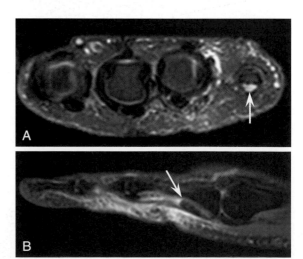

Fig. 4.47 Flexor digitorum profundus tendon rupture. (A) Axial T2-weighted fat-suppressed MR image of the hand demonstrates an empty, fluid-filled flexor digitorum profundus (FDP) tendon sheath at the fifth digit *(arrow)*. **(B)** Sagittal STIR MR image through the fifth digit shows the retracted tendon stump *(arrow)*.

- Complete tendon tears are characterized by tendon discontinuity, often with retraction and a tendon gap.
  - The empty tendon sheath between the tendon ends is often fluid-filled and conspicuously bright on T2-weighted images (see Fig. 4.47A).
  - Measurement of tendon gap or retraction is important to include in the report, as this information is critical for surgical repair.
  - Partial-thickness tendon tears demonstrate a focal change in the morphology, caliber, or signal within the tendon substance (Fig. 4.48).
- *Trigger finger* is characterized by the impedance of smooth tendon gliding during flexion and extension, often due to thickening of the A1 pulley; this condition is best diagnosed by dynamic US imaging.
- *Flexor pulley injuries* may be seen involving any of the digits; recall that the thumb has a different pulley system than the second through fifth digits.
  - As outlined previously, the flexor tendons of the fingers are held close to the volar surfaces of the proximal and middle phalanges by fibrous bands termed *flexor pulleys* (see Fig. 4.10A).
  - Repetitive flexion of the fingers while under extreme load (e.g., by rock climbers supporting their entire body weight by the flexed fingertips of one hand) can cause a pulley to tear.
  - Such injuries cause the flexor tendon to move away from the palmar surface of the phalanges during flexion like a bowstring of a violin, which can be seen on MRI or ultrasonography as abnormal palmar position of an affected flexor tendon (see Fig. 4.10B).
  - The A2 and A4 pulleys are most critical for providing normal digit flexion and preventing tendon bowstringing; the A2 pulley is the most frequently torn (Fig. 4.49), though multiple pulleys may be injured.

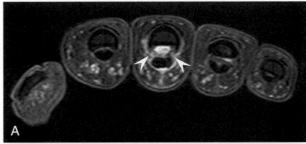
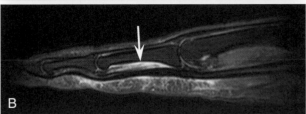

Fig. 4.49 **Annular A2 pulley tear.** Axial T2-weighted fat-suppressed MR image of the hand **(A)** and sagittal STIR MR image of the middle finger **(B)** demonstrate tear of the A2 pulley (*arrowheads* in A) with subtle tendon bowstringing. There is fluid/edema interposed between the flexor digitorum profundus (FDP) tendon and volar surface of the third proximal phalanx (*arrow* in B). See also Fig. 4.10.

EXTENSOR TENDON INJURY

- Extensor tendons of the wrist are vulnerable to overuse and traumatic injury, similar to the flexor tendons (see Fig. 4.48).
- As mentioned previously, *De Quervain's syndrome* is an overuse syndrome involving the tendons of the first extensor compartment, and *distal intersection syndrome* occurs at the decussation of the second and third extensor tendon compartments.
- Avulsions or tears of the extensor digitorum tendon can occur at the level of the DIP or PIP joints.
  - As mentioned previously, tear of the central (middle) slip of the extensor digitorum tendon results in a *boutonnière deformity* (see Figs. 4.31 and 4.32), whereas tear distal to the convergence of the lateral tendon slips at the DIP joint results in *mallet finger* (see Fig. 4.30).
  - Tendon avulsion may or may not be associated with an osseous avulsion fracture.
- Tear of a *sagittal band* (part of the extensor hood) at the MCP joint destabilizes the extensor digitorum tendon and allows abnormal tendon excursion.
  - Sagittal bands are best evaluated on axial MRI at the level of the MCP joint (Fig. 4.50).
- The *ECU tendon* can subluxate or dislocate from its groove in the distal ulna (Fig. 4.51).
  - The ECU is normally held in position in the ulnar groove by the ECU subsheath, which may tear due to acute trauma or chronic degeneration.

VOLAR PLATE INJURIES

- The volar plate is a capsular thickening that stabilizes the volar MCP and interphalangeal joints, preventing hyperextension.
- *Volar plate injuries* are usually seen in the setting of hyperextension injury or joint dislocation.

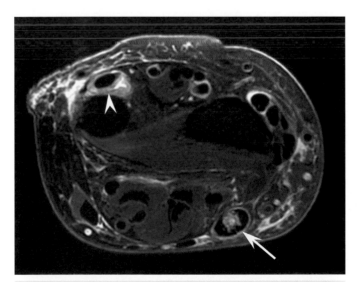

Fig. 4.48 **Flexor carpi radialis (FCR) tendinosis and partial tear.** Axial T2-weighted fat-suppressed MR image of the wrist demonstrates severe flexor carpi radialis (FCR) tendinosis (*arrow*) with high-grade interstitial tearing, denoted by near fluid-bright intrasubstance signal. Extensor carpi ulnaris (ECU) tenosynovitis is also noted (*arrowhead*).

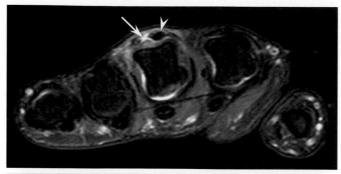

Fig. 4.50 Sagittal band tear. Axial T2-weighted fat-suppressed MR image of the hand demonstrates complete tear of the ulnar sagittal band *(arrow)* with subtle radial subluxation of the extensor digitorum tendon *(arrowhead)*.

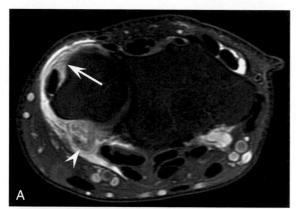

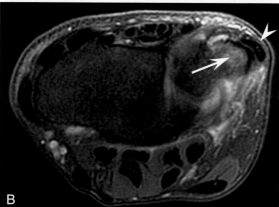

Fig. 4.51 Extensor carpi ulnaris (ECU) subsheath tears. (A) Axial T2-weighted fat-suppressed MR arthrogram image following intraarticular instillation of contrast into the radiocarpal joint demonstrates contrast extravasation into the ulnar-sided soft tissues and ECU tendon sheath. There is tearing of the ECU subsheath at its dorsoradial attachment site *(arrow)* and tearing of the volar radioulnar ligament *(arrowhead)*. **(B)** Axial T2-weighted fat-suppressed MR image in a different patient shows ulnar subluxation of the ECU tendon *(arrowhead)* due to tearing of the ECU subsheath. Subtendinous bone marrow edema is noted within the ulnar styloid process *(arrow)*.

- Injuries may be associated with an avulsion fracture, most common at the distal attachment site (see Fig. 4.29), and tear of the volar plate itself, which is more commonly seen at the proximal attachment site (Fig. 4.52).
  - Volar plate injuries may range from low-grade sprain to complete tear with displacement and entrapment within the joint, best evaluated on sagittal MRI.

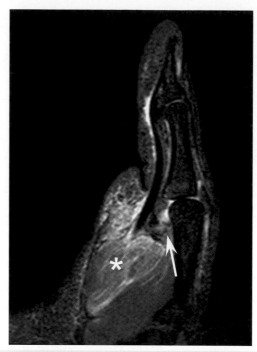

Fig. 4.52 Volar plate tear. Sagittal STIR MR image of the thumb demonstrates high-grade tearing of the first metacarpophalangeal (MCP) joint volar plate at the proximal attachment site *(arrow)*. There is also acute strain of the thenar musculature *(asterisk)*.

COLLATERAL LIGAMENT INJURIES

- The metacarpophalangeal (MCP) and interphalangeal joints are stabilized against valgus and varus stress by the ulnar (medial) and radial (lateral) collateral ligaments, respectively.
- Collateral ligament injuries can occur at any of these joints; injured ligaments may stretch, tear partially or completely, or avulse a small fragment.
- Historically, PA-view radiographs with valgus or varus stress were used for diagnosis of a collateral ligament injury, though this could theoretically worsen an already-existing partial tear.
  - Comparison with the uninjured side is helpful, because some laxity of the collateral ligaments is normal.
- Currently, MRI of the finger is the imaging study of choice for diagnosing collateral ligament injuries, although US may play a complimentary role.
  - Collateral ligaments are best evaluated in the coronal and axial imaging planes; high-resolution T2-weighted (or gradient-echo GRE) images are useful for evaluating these small structures.
  - Fluid-sensitive (T2-weighted fat-suppressed and STIR) sequences allow detection of soft tissue edema, which typically accompanies acute injuries.
  - T1-weighted sequences are helpful for detecting small avulsed osseous fragments; note that avulsed cortical fragments may contain no marrow component and appear entirely hypointense.
  - Imaging planes are prescribed with respect to the axis of the digit of interest; sagittal imaging should include adjacent 'normal' digits.

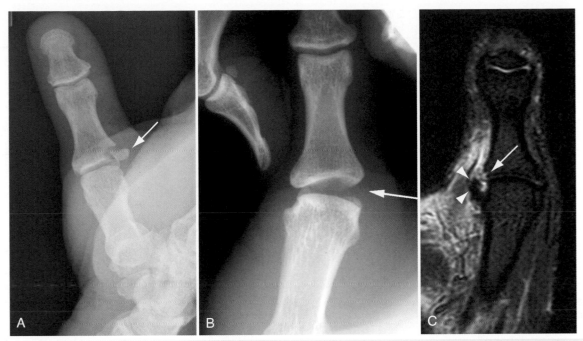

Fig. 4.53 Skier's (gamekeeper's) thumb. (A) Anteroposterior (AP) radiograph of the thumb shows an intraarticular avulsion fracture *(arrow)* at the distal insertion of the metacarpophalangeal (MCP) ulnar collateral ligament (UCL). **(B)** UCL injury without avulsion fracture in a different patient. The MCP joint has widened medially with stress *(arrow)*, indicating laxity or disruption of the UCL. **(C)** MR diagnosis. Coronal STIR MR image shows lax, retracted UCL *(arrowheads)*. Note the avulsion site on the proximal phalanx *(arrow)*.

- The most frequently injured collateral ligament in the hand is the ulnar collateral ligament (UCL) of the thumb MCP joint.
  - This injury, better known as *gamekeeper's thumb* or *skier's thumb*, is caused by valgus stress across the thumb, often combined with hyperextension (Fig. 4.53).
    - Gamekeeper's thumb was first recognized as an occupational hazard of British gamekeepers, whose method of killing wounded rabbits placed valgus stress across the thumb.
    - Today, an injury to the thumb MCP UCL is often sustained while falling on an outstretched hand while holding a ski pole, resulting in thumb valgus and hyperextension.
  - Most UCL sprains and partial tears, as well as some minimally displaced complete tears or avulsions, are managed by immobilization.
  - Complete tears often require surgical exploration to locate and reattach the free edges of the torn UCL.
  - The adductor pollicis brevis tendon aponeurosis can become interposed between the torn edges of the UCL, a situation termed the *Stener lesion* (Fig. 4.54).
    - Interposition of the adductor tendon aponeurosis or significant ligament displacement will prevent ligament healing and requires surgical reattachment.
    - High-resolution MRI of the thumb can help identify the position of the ligament.
    - Imaging planes should be prescribed relative to the axis of the thumb, not the hand; improper scan technique may render the MRI inadequate for interpretation and require reimaging.
  - RCL injuries are analogous to UCL injuries on imaging, occurring at the radial aspect of the joint (Fig. 4.55).

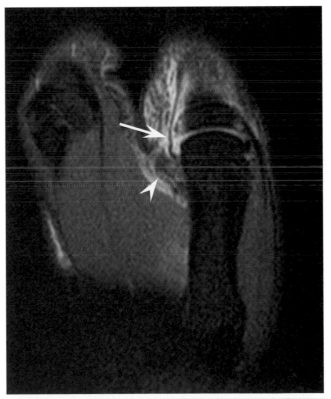

Fig. 4.54 Stener lesion. Coronal T2-weighted fat-suppressed MR image of the thumb demonstrates a complete tear of the first metacarpophalangeal (MCP) joint ulnar collateral ligament (UCL), which is proximally displaced *(arrowhead)*. The adductor pollicis brevis tendon aponeurosis *(arrow)* is interposed between the UCL and distal attachment site on the proximal phalanx base, which prevents ligament healing.

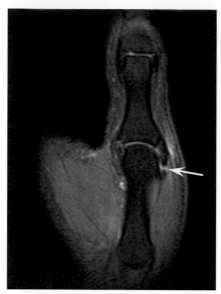

Fig. 4.55 Radial collateral ligament (RCL) tear. Coronal T2-weighted fat-suppressed MR image of the thumb demonstrates a full-thickness tear of the first metacarpophalangeal (MCP) joint radial collateral ligament (RCL) near its proximal attachment site *(arrow)*.

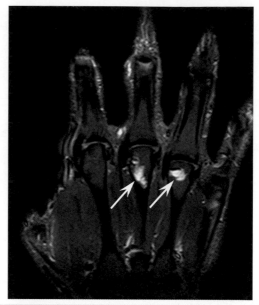

Fig. 4.56 Intraosseous ganglia. Coronal T2-weighted fat-suppressed MR image of the hand shows intraosseous ganglion cysts incidentally within the third and fourth metacarpal heads *(arrows)*, which emanate from the collateral ligament attachment sites.

ARTHROPATHIES

In addition to degenerative osteoarthritis, several arthropathies are commonly encountered in the hand and wrist. These include rheumatoid arthritis, erosive osteoarthritis, psoriatic arthritis, crystalline arthropathies (such as calcium pyrophosphate deposition [CPPD] arthropathy and gout), reactive arthritis, connective tissue disorder and metabolic-related arthropathies, and many others. Features that can help narrow the differential diagnosis on radiographs include the pattern of joint involvement and joint space narrowing, as well as the presence or absence of osteophytes, subchondral cysts, osseous erosions, periostitis, subluxations, juxtaarticular osteopenia, and soft tissue calcification or mineralization. These conditions are outlined in detail in Chapter 9—Arthritis.

OSSEOUS LESIONS

- *Intraosseous ganglion cysts* are frequently encountered in the hand and wrist, typically occurring at ligament attachment sites and most commonly seen in the carpal bones or metacarpal heads (Fig. 4.56).
  - Pathogenesis remains unclear, although these may form due to mucoid degeneration or intraosseous herniation of joint fluid.
  - Must distinguish intraosseous ganglia from osseous erosions, which can have a similar appearance; presence of adjacent synovitis, surrounding marrow edema, and multiplicity suggest the latter.
- *Enchondroma* is the most common benign osseous tumor to involve the small tubular bones of the digits (Fig. 4.57).
  - These are often found incidentally on radiographs but can present as a mass or with pathologic fracture due to weakening of the bone.
  - When encountered in the hand, radiographs often show a lucent, expansile lesion with endosteal

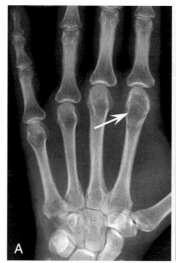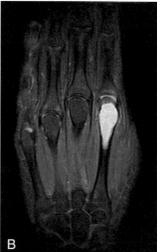

Fig. 4.57 Enchondroma. (A) PA radiograph of the hand demonstrates a lucent, expansile lesion within the distal second metacarpal *(arrow)*. No perceptible chondroid matrix is visible. Some enchondromas do not demonstrate chondroid matrix. **(B)** Coronal T2-weighted fat-suppressed MR image shows the lesion to be uniformly T2-hyperintense, with endosteal scalloping and cortical thinning. Imaging features and location are consistent with a benign enchondroma. No pathologic fracture was demonstrated in this case.

scalloping; only 30% of such lesions will show internal chondroid matrix.
  - Pathologic fracture may be obvious or seen as subtle periostitis with edema in the adjacent bone and soft tissues on MRI.
- *Bizarre parosteal osteochondromatous proliferation (BPOP, or Nora lesion)* is a rare osseous surface lesion that has a predilection for the hands (and to a lesser degree the feet), typically seen in patients 20–30 years of age.
  - Radiographic appearance is characterized by a mineralized exophytic growth arising from the cortex of the

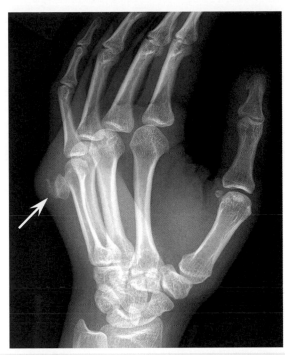

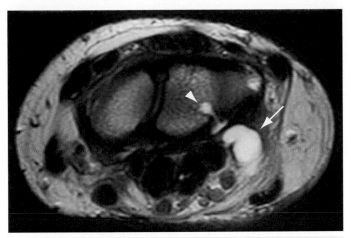

Fig. 4.59 **Ganglion cyst.** Axial T2-weighted fast spin-echo image shows bright signal ganglion with a small component in the lunate (*arrowhead*) and a larger component in the volar soft tissues (*arrow*). Intraosseous and soft tissue ganglia are both very common in the wrist. MRI demonstration of a combined lesion such as this case is uncommon.

Fig. 4.58 **Bizarre parosteal osteochondromatous proliferation (BPOP, or Nora lesion).** Oblique radiograph of the hand demonstrates a partially ossified exophytic lesion arising from the dorsal-ulnar aspect of the distal fifth metacarpal cortex (*arrow*).

metacarpals or phalanges (Fig. 4.58), which may enhance on postcontrast MRI.
- Histologically composed of bone, cartilage, and fibrous tissue with proliferative activity and 'bizarre' enlarged binucleate chondrocytes, which may mimic chondrosarcoma.
- This is a benign lesion without malignant potential, but has a high frequency of local recurrence.

SOFT TISSUE MASSES

- *Ganglion cysts* are the most commonly encountered 'masses' around the wrist and hand, usually diagnosed with US or MRI.
  - Most ganglion cysts are discovered incidentally, but some may be associated with wrist pain, and correlation of the imaging findings with clinical symptoms is necessary.
  - Lesions often develop at areas of relative weakness in the joint capsule, but some originate from tendon sheaths.
  - Imaging features are characteristic (Fig. 4.59; see also Figs. 4.43 and 12.1) and further discussed in Chapter 12—Soft tissue Tumors.
  - Resected ganglia tend to recur if the neck is not also removed, so identification of the source of the ganglion relative to the joint capsule is important information for the surgeon.
  - Proximity to neurovascular structures is particularly important when describing ganglion cysts in the wrist and hand.
- *Tenosynovial giant cell tumor* (TGCT; also termed *giant cell tumor of tendon sheath* [GCTTS]) represents the

second most commonly encountered soft tissue mass around the hand and wrist.
  - TGCT is identical to the localized form of pigmented villonodular synovitis (*PVNS*), a nonmalignant, likely neoplastic proliferation of synovium composed of variable components of villous, pigmented (hemosiderin-laden), fibrous, and inflammatory tissues.
  - Imaging features are characteristic and further discussed in Chapter 12—Soft Tissue Tumors (see Figs. 12.45 and 12.46).
  - Most common location of TGCT is along a flexor tendon sheath at the volar aspect of the hand or fingers.
- *Glomus tumor (glomangioma* or *neuromyoarterial glomus)* is a benign perivascular lesion consisting of neural, muscle, and arterial components similar to glomus body cells.
  - Most commonly occur at the dorsal aspect of the terminal phalanx of a digit, beneath the nail bed (subungual location).
  - Imaging features are characteristic and further discussed in Chapter 12—Soft Tissue Tumors (see Fig. 12.13).
  - Treatment is with surgical resection; role of MRI is to establish initial diagnosis and for postoperative follow-up, as incomplete excision will lead to recurrence.
- *Foreign bodies* may be seen on imaging following penetrating trauma (though the patient may not recall such history).
  - Foreign bodies may result in a granulomatous reaction, termed *foreign body granuloma*, typically identified on MRI as a small, ill-defined soft tissue mass with T2-hyperintensity and T1-hypointensity.
  - Radiographs are useful for detection of radiopaque foreign bodies (metal and glass), though most wood and certain plastics are radiolucent.
  - Foreign bodies may result in susceptibility artifact on MRI due to the presence of metal (metallic or additive-containing glass) or air (wood).
    - Main differential for susceptibility artifact overlying the subcutaneous tissues on MRI is debris on the skin surface.

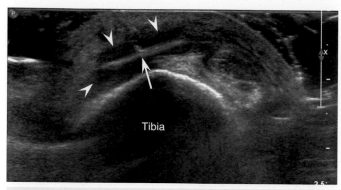

Fig. 4.60 Foreign body on ultrasound. Ultrasound image of the anterior shin demonstrates a linear, hyperechoic wood splinter *(arrow)*, with surrounding hypoechogenicity representing foreign body granuloma *(arrowheads)*. Tibia with posterior acoustic shadowing is labeled.

- US is exquisitely sensitive for the detection of retained superficial foreign bodies and can be performed to both identify and localize the retained foreign body to aid with retrieval (Fig. 4.60).
- As foreign bodies serve as a nidus for infection, additional findings such as cellulitis, abscesses, septic tenosynovitis, or osteomyelitis may be encountered; see Chapter 14—Musculoskeletal Infection for more details regarding infection.
- *Palmar fibromatosis*, also known as *Dupuytren's contracture*, is superficial fibromatosis of the palmar hand.
    - Fibrotic bands tether the hand flexor tendons, causing flexion contractures—most frequently of the medial fingers (see Fig. 12.21).
    - This is a common condition in older adults, particularly those of northern European descent.
- Other, less commonly encountered benign and malignant soft tissue masses of the hand and wrist are covered in Chapter 12—Soft Tissue Tumors.

Structured Report

REPORTING TIPS AND RECOMMENDATIONS

- Related findings may be separated in the body of the report due to template structure, but impression should tie findings together.
    - For example, in the setting of rheumatoid arthritis of the wrist, joint, osseous, tendon, and soft tissue, findings may all be related to the single underlying disease process.
- Mention findings clinically relevant to the clinician, such as degree of articular surface involvement for an intraarticular fracture, distance of retraction in the setting of tendon rupture, or ligament displacement for complete ligament tears.
- Organize impression points by order of importance.
- Directly answer any specific clinical questions in the impression.
- Ensure the study is technically adequate for evaluation of the structure(s) of interest.
    - MRI if targeted to a specific digit must include high-resolution imaging to adequately assess the small

ligamentous and capsular structures, with imaging planes prescribed with respect to the axis of the digit of interest.

Example Normal Wrist Report Template

Exam Type: MRI WRIST WITHOUT CONTRAST
Exam Date and Time: Date and Time
Indication: Clinical History
Comparison: Prior Studies

IMPRESSION: Impression

TECHNIQUE: MRI of the side wrist was performed on a scanner type system in three planes (axial, sagittal, and coronal) using a standard noncontrast protocol.

FINDINGS:

OSSEOUS STRUCTURES: No acute fracture or bone bruise. Carpal arc alignment is anatomic. Neutral ulnar variance.

JOINTS: No focal cartilage defects. No osseous erosions. No joint effusions.

LIGAMENTS: TFCC (Triangular fibrocartilage complex): Intact central TFCC articular disc. Intact peripheral TFCC foveal and styloid attachments.
Scapholunate: Intact scapholunate ligament with normal scapholunate interval.
Lunotriquetral: Intact lunotriquetral ligament with normal lunotriquetral interval.
Extrinsic ligaments: Intact.

TENDONS: Flexor tendons: No tendinosis or tear. No tenosynovitis.
Extensor tendons: No tendinosis or tear. No tenosynovitis.

CARPAL TUNNEL: No mass effect in the carpal tunnel. Median nerve is normal in morphology and signal intensity.

GUYON'S CANAL: No mass effect in Guyon's canal. Ulnar nerve is normal in morphology and signal intensity.

SOFT TISSUES: No soft tissue edema. No ganglion cyst, fluid collection, or soft tissue mass.

Example Normal Hand/Finger Report Template

Exam Type: MRI HAND (FINGER) WITHOUT CONTRAST
Exam Date and Time: Date and Time
Indication: Clinical History
Comparison: Prior Studies

IMPRESSION: Impression

TECHNIQUE: MRI of the side hand (target finger) was performed on a scanner type system in three planes (axial, sagittal, and coronal) using a standard noncontrast protocol.

FINDINGS:

JOINTS/BONES: No acute fracture or bone bruise. No focal cartilage defect or osteoarthritis. No joint effusions. No subluxation.

LIGAMENTS: Normal ulnar and radial collateral ligaments, sagittal bands, and volar plates. Intact joint capsules.

TENDONS: No flexor or extensor tendon tear. No tenosynovitis. Normal tendon pulleys.

MUSCLES: No atrophy or edema.

SOFT TISSUES: No soft tissue edema. No fluid collection or soft tissue mass.

Sources and Suggested Readings

Arnaiz J, Piedra T, Cerezal L, et al. Imaging of Kienböck disease. *AJR Am J Roentgenol.* 2014;203(1):131–139.

Bateni CP, Bartolotta RJ, Richardson ML, et al. Imaging key wrist ligaments: what the surgeon needs the radiologist to know. *AJR Am J Roentgenol.* 2013;200(5):1089–1095.

Beaty JH, Kasser JR, Shaggs DL, et al. eds. *Rockwood and Green's Fractures in Children.* Philadelphia: Lippincott-Raven; 2009.

Bucholz RW, Court-Brown CM, Heckman JD, Tornetta P, eds. *Rockwood and Green's Fractures in Adults.* Philadelphia: Lippincott-Raven; 2009.

Burns JE, Tanaka T, Ueno T, et al. Pitfalls that may mimic injuries of the triangular fibrocartilage and proximal intrinsic wrist ligaments at MR imaging. *Radiographics.* 2011;31(1):63–78.

Celik S, Bilge O, Pinar Y, et al. The anatomical variations of the extensor tendons to the dorsum of the hand. *Clin Anat.* 2008;21(7):652–659.

Cerezal L, de Dios Berná-Mestre J, Canga A, et al. MR and CT arthrography of the wrist. *Semin Musculoskelet Radiol.* 2012;16(1):27–41.

Cerezal L, del Piñal F, Abascal F, et al. Imaging findings in ulnar-sided wrist impaction syndromes. *Radiographics.* 2002;22(1):105–121.

Chiavaras MM, Jacobson JA, Yablon CM, et al. Pitfalls in wrist and hand ultrasound. *AJR Am J Roentgenol.* 2014;203(3):531–540.

Clavero JA, Alomar X, Monill JM, et al. MR imaging of ligament and tendon injuries of the fingers. *Radiographics.* 2002;22(2):237–256.

Clavero JA, Golanó P, Fariñas O, et al. Extensor mechanism of the fingers: MR imaging-anatomic correlation. *Radiographics.* 2003;23(3):593–611.

Goldfarb CA, Yin Y, Gilula LA, et al. Wrist fractures: what the clinician wants to know. *Radiology.* 2001;219:11–28.

Gupta P, Lenchik L, Wuertzer SD, et al. High-resolution 3-T MRI of the fingers: review of anatomy and common tendon and ligament injuries. *AJR Am J Roentgenol.* 2015;204(3):W314–W323.

Hirschmann A, Sutter R, Schweizer A, et al. MRI of the thumb: anatomy and spectrum of findings in asymptomatic volunteers. *AJR Am J Roentgenol.* 2014;202(4):819–827.

Jamadar DA, Robertson BL, Jacobson JA, et al. Musculoskeletal sonography: important imaging pitfalls. *AJR Am J Roentgenol.* 2010;194(1):216–225.

Lee CH, Tandon A. Focal hand lesions: review and radiological approach. *Insights Imaging.* 2014;5(3):301–319.

Manaster BJ, Roberts CC, Andrews CL, et al. *Expertddx: Musculoskeletal.* Salt Lake City: Amirsys; 2008.

Mohammadi A, Ghasemi-Rad M, Mladkova-Suchy N, et al. Correlation between the severity of carpal tunnel syndrome and color Doppler sonography findings. *AJR Am J Roentgenol.* 2012;198(2):W181–W184.

Moschilla G, Breidahl W. Sonography of the finger. *Am J Roentgenol.* 2002;178:1451–1457.

Nora FE, Dahlin DC, Beabout JW. Bizarre parosteal osteochondromatous proliferations of the hands and feet. *Am J Surg Pathol.* 1983;7(3):245–250.

Oneson SR, Scales LM, Timins ME, et al. MR imaging interpretation of the Palmer classification of triangular fibrocartilage complex lesions. *Radiographics.* 1996;16:97–106.

Rawat U, Pierce JL, Evans S, et al. High-resolution MR imaging and US anatomy of the thumb. *Radiographics.* 2016;36(6):1701–1716.

Resnick D. *Diagnosis of Bone and Joint Disorders.* 4th ed. Philadelphia: Saunders; 2002.

Robinson R. Sonography of common tendon injuries. *AJR Am J Roentgenol.* 2009;193(3):607–618.

Scalcione LR, Pathria MN, Chung CB. The athlete's hand: ligament and tendon injury. *Semin Musculoskelet Radiol.* 2012;16(4):338–349.

Smith DK. MR imaging of normal and injured wrist ligaments. *Magn Reson Imaging Clin N Am.* 1995;3:229–248.

Toms AP, Chojnowski A, Cahir JG. Midcarpal instability: a radiological perspective. *Skeletal Radiol.* 2011;40(5):533–541.

Vezeridis PS, Yoshioka H, Han R, et al. Ulnar-sided wrist pain. Part I: anatomy and physical examination. *Skeletal Radiol.* 2010;39(8):733–745.

Watanabe A, Souza F, Vezeridis PS, et al. Ulnar-sided wrist pain. II. Clinical imaging and treatment. *Skeletal Radiol.* 2010;39(9):837–857.

Wieschhoff GG, Sheehan SE, Wortman JR, et al. Traumatic finger injuries: what the orthopedic surgeon wants to know. *Radiographics.* 2016;36(4):1106–1128.

Wong SM, Griffith JF, Jui ACF, et al. Carpal tunnel syndrome: diagnostic usefulness of sonography. *Radiology.* 2004;232:93–99.

Yamabe E, Nakamura T, Pham P, et al. The athlete's wrist: ulnar-sided pain. *Semin Musculoskelet Radiol.* 2012;16(4):331–337.

5 *Pelvis and Hips*

Pelvis

ANATOMY

- The pelvis is a complex anatomic region created by three bones: the two innominate bones and the sacrum.
- Each innominate bone is formed by synostosis of the ilium, pubis, and ischium that join at the medial wall of the acetabulum, physically recognized in childhood as the triradiate or "Y" cartilage of the acetabulum.
  - In skeletally immature patients this region may be confused with fracture.
- Medially the innominate bones are adjoined at the symphysis pubis, which is a synchondrosis similar embryologically and morphologically to the discs of the spine.
- The sacrum and ilium are adjoined at the sacroiliac (SI) joints, which are a complex articulation consisting partly of synovial joint and partly of syndesmosis.
  - The true synovial joint is in the anterior third and inferior half of the articulation, whereas the strong ligamentous attachments of the syndesmosis are posterior superior.
- The pelvis is joined with the spine at the L5-S1 disc.
- The pelvis is attached at the lower extremity at the hip joints, two ball and socket synovial joints.
- The pelvis can be considered a ringlike structure formed by two dominant arches.

- The major arch is posterior and superior, formed by the iliac wings and sacrum, joined at the SI joints.
- The smaller arch is anterior and inferior, formed by the pubic and ischial bones, joined at the symphysis pubis.
- There are three rings in the pelvis.
  - The largest is the ring that connects the sacrum, SI joints, iliac and pubic bones, and symphysis pubis. The pelvic inlet is part of this ring.
  - The other two rings are the obturator foramina of the pubic bones and ischia.
  - As with any ring, a break in one portion of the ring is usually accompanied by a break in another portion of the ring.
  - Breaks may occur through a bone or an articulation (i.e. pubic symphysis or a sacroilliac joint).
  - When isolated fractures of the pelvis occur, they are usually in the form of an iliac wing–impacted fracture or an ischial tuberosity, iliac spine, or iliac crest avulsion fracture.
- The acetabulum resembles an inverted horseshoe, with a roof and anterior and posterior walls or rims. The open portion inferiorly is the acetabular notch. The central recess surrounded by the walls and roof is *cotyloid fossa*. The recessed medial wall of the cotyloid fossa is the *quadrilateral plate*.
- Any fracture involvement of the acetabulum requires detailed assessment to guide management.

Trauma Pathophysiology

- The bones of the pelvis are strong and are supported by strong ligaments.
  - It therefore requires a large force to cause a fracture of the pelvis or disrupt pelvic ligaments.
- The pelvis has a rich vascular supply and is therefore prone to life-threatening hemorrhage after trauma.
- Injury to the smaller nerves of the pelvis is common after pelvic trauma.
  - As an example, erectile dysfunction is a common complication after injury in males and results from a combination of neurologic and vascular injury.
  - The sciatic nerve, although only rarely transected, often is affected by adjacent hematoma, edema, or posttraumatic fibrosis that can result in a variable degree and duration of neurologic dysfunction.
- Urologic injury is also common after pelvic trauma with extraperitoneal and intraperitoneal bladder ruptures and, in males, urethral disruption.

Imaging

PELVIC FRACTURE

- Radiography is the first-line test for imaging of suspected fracture, although it may be omitted in patients proceeding directly to computed tomography (CT).
- Five major vertically oriented radiographic lines in each innominate bone require careful scrutiny on the anteroposterior (AP) pelvis radiograph (Fig. 5.1).
  - The iliopectineal (iliopubic) line. This line runs along the inner margin of the ilium and around the superior margin of the pubis.

- The *ilioischial line* runs along the inner margin of the ilium and then inferiorly along the medial margin of the ischium.
- The *teardrop* is a summation opacity related to the medial margin of the acetabulum and posterior acetabular wall.
- The other lines are the anterior and posterior rims of each acetabulum. These represent the lateral margins of the anterior and posterior walls of the acetabulum.
- Each of these five vertically oriented lines should be smoothly contoured. Any interruption or irregularity of the line should be viewed with suspicion for the presence of fracture, and absence suggests bone destruction (Fig. 5.2; see Fig. 11.127).
- Evaluation of the anterior and posterior acetabular rims is particularly difficult on frontal pelvis radiographs because isolated fractures are oriented in the coronal plane and thus may be obscured.
  - Presence of a posterior wall fracture on a frontal pelvis radiograph may be inferred by obscuration of visualization of the posterior rim; often there is a displaced fracture.
- The addition of Judet views (i.e., 45-degree bilateral oblique views) increases sensitivity and helps delineate fracture patterns in the pelvis. Judet views are obtained only rarely but are worth understanding.
  - The 45-degree oblique view allows better evaluation of the ischium and pubis in elongated projection.
  - Note that to many radiology technologists, an 'oblique pelvis view' means 30-degree oblique, so 'Judet' must be specified as the desired view.
  - The bilateral Judet views are complementary views: one view will show the ipsilateral posterior wall and ischium, and contralateral anterior wall and pubis (Fig. 5.3).
  - This is critical anatomy for assessment of acetabular fracture patterns.
  - Orthopedic surgeons use these landmarks when describing Judet views. For example, the left posterior oblique Judet view (i.e. the view with the left hip rolled onto the image receptor) is termed the *left iliac*

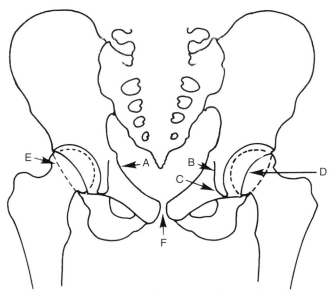

Fig. 5.1 Diagram of anteroposterior (AP) pelvis demonstrating anatomic landmarks to assess in the setting of trauma. **(A)** Iliopubic line; **(B)** ilioischial line; **(C)** teardrop; **(D)** anterior acetabular rim; **(E)** posterior acetabular rim; **(F)** symphysis pubis. (Reproduced with permission from Manaster BJ. *Handbook of Skeletal Radiology*. 2nd ed. St. Louis: Mosby; 1997.)

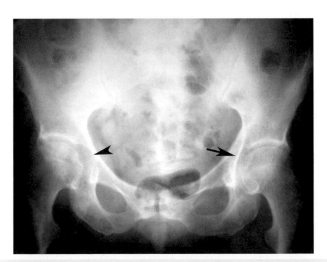

Fig. 5.2 Absent ilioischial line because of metastasis. AP radiograph shows normal left line *(arrow)* but absent right line *(arrowhead)* caused by a lytic bronchogenic carcinoma metastasis.

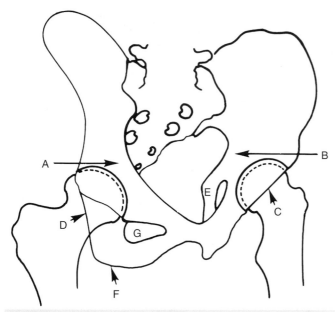

Fig. 5.3 Judet (45-degree oblique) view of the pelvis. Note that the anterior (obturator) oblique view shows the anterior column and posterior acetabular rim best, whereas the posterior (iliac) oblique view shows the posterior column and anterior acetabular rim best. **(A)** Anterior column and iliopubic line; **(B)** posterior column and ilioischial line; **(C)** anterior acetabular rim; **(D)** posterior acetabular rim; **(E)** ischial spine; **(F)** ischial tuberosity; **(G)** obturator foramen. (Reproduced with permission from Manaster BJ. *Handbook of Skeletal Radiology*. 2nd ed. St. Louis: Mosby; 1997.)

oblique view because it profiles the left iliac wing. This view is also termed the *right obturator oblique* view because it also profiles the right obturator foramen and acetabulum.

- CT is used frequently for detection and evaluation of pelvic fractures.
  - CT allows multiplanar and three-dimensional reformations for preoperative planning.
  - The soft tissues can be evaluated for hematoma and bladder injury.
- Magnetic resonance imaging (MRI) has a particularly useful role in the assessment of radiographically occult fracture, stress fracture, and muscle strain.
  - It is especially useful in patients with posttraumatic pain in the absence of radiographic or CT findings.
- Radionuclide bone scanning also can detect radiographically occult fractures, although it is less sensitive and specific than MRI and utilizes ionizing radiation.
  - Not useful in the acute setting in older adults because fractures do not accumulate radiotracer until the healing process progresses a few days after the injury.

SACRAL FRACTURE

- Many sacral fractures are subtle or simply invisible on radiographs.
  - The neural foraminal lines of the sacrum require careful evaluation because subtle irregularity will indicate a fracture.
  - L5 transverse process fracture suggests the presence of occult sacral fracture, because forces that produce this fracture are similar to those that produce a sacral fracture.

- The margins of the SI joints and symphysis pubis should be parallel and smoothly contoured.
  - SI joints are normally no greater than 4 mm wide in adults.
    - Any asymmetry should be viewed with suspicion for diastasis.
  - The symphysis pubis may be up to 5 mm wide in adults and 10 mm wide in skeletally immature patients. Superoinferior offset up to 2 mm is normal along the superior margin of the symphysis pubis. However, the inferior margins at the symphysis pubis should be aligned without any offset.
- Transverse sacral fractures may occur acutely caused by a direct blow.
- Insufficiency fractures are common in the sacrum (Fig. 5.4; see Fig. 1.39), most often in patients with osteoporosis, and are seen as vertical areas of mixed lucency and density along the sacral ala often with a horizontal portion through the mid-S2 or mid-S3 levels (like the letter "H").
  - More commonly, they are radiographically occult and are detected only with CT, MRI, or radionuclide bone scanning.

COCCYX INJURY

- Fractures are caused by direct trauma, and in some cases childbirth.
- F>M due to wider female pelvis with greater exposure of coccyx to direct trauma.
- Bruises and overuse injuries (e.g. in competitive rowers) also occur.
- Treatment is usually conservative and symptom driven, so imaging role is limited.
- Nonetheless radiographs are often obtained after acute trauma with "tailbone pain".
- Unless a fracture is clearly visible, diagnosis with radiographs is limited by normal highly variable coccyx orientation and relationship with the sacrum.
  - Coccyx may be subluxed anteriorly or posteriorly and variously angled as both normal and abnormal findings.
- CT is more sensitive.
- MRI is the best test, with edema in and around an injured coccyx.
- Remember to look for alternative diagnoses, e.g. a lytic lesion, mass, or sacroiliac joint pathology.

Pelvic Fractures: Biomechanical Classification

- Pelvic fractures can be caused by AP compression, lateral compression, or vertical shear forces. Each mechanism produces a unique fracture pattern.
- In *lateral compression*, which is the most common pattern, the essential forces result from lateral impaction injury.
  - This typically occurs in a 'T-bone' motor vehicle crash, in which one car strikes the door (and hence the occupant) of another at a 90-degree angle.

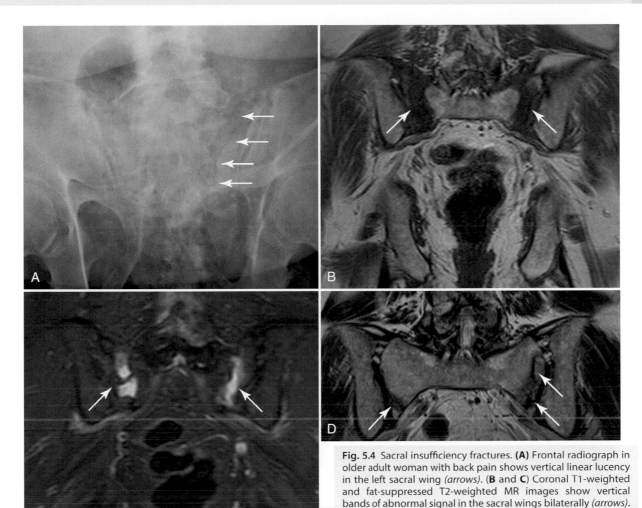

Fig. 5.4 Sacral insufficiency fractures. **(A)** Frontal radiograph in older adult woman with back pain shows vertical linear lucency in the left sacral wing *(arrows)*. **(B** and **C)** Coronal T1-weighted and fat-suppressed T2-weighted MR images show vertical bands of abnormal signal in the sacral wings bilaterally *(arrows)*. **(D)** Coronal T1-weighted MR image in another patient shows subtle bilateral linear sacral wing fracture lines *(arrows)*.

- A clue to lateral compression on radiographs is the presence of horizontal fractures of the superior and inferior pubic rami (Fig. 5.5).
- Type I injury also includes an impaction fracture of a sacral ala. Ligaments are intact. These are stable fractures.
- In type II fracture, the lateral compressive force is located more anteriorly, resulting in internal rotation of the ipsilateral iliac wing.
- This, in turn, causes not only pubic and ischial fractures but also disruption of the posterior SI joint ligaments (or a fracture through the posterior iliac wing or sacrum).
- A type III lateral compression involves a greater force in which there are internal rotation of the ipsilateral innominate bone and external rotation of the contralateral innominate bone.
- With the exception of type III injury, the incidence of substantial arterial hemorrhage is low with lateral compression.

Sample Report

History: Passenger in right-side T-bone automobile crash. CT pelvis without contrast.

Mildly impacted sagittal plane fracture left sacral ala.
Mildly impacted fractures of the left superior and inferior pubic rami.
Small hematomas noted around the fractures without mass effect.
No additional fracture is evident.
SI joints and symphysis pubis intact. Hip joints normally aligned.
No evidence of intrapelvic injury.
Increased density in subcutaneous fat lateral to the left hip, likely contusion. No soft tissue gas to suggest penetrating injury. No visible foreign body.
Impression: Lateral compression 1 pelvic fracture with mild fragment impaction.

- In *AP compression*, injury results from frontal or dorsal forces, usually in a motor vehicle crash.
  - With this injury pattern the identifying fractures are the vertical fractures of the superior and inferior pubic rami (Fig. 5.6).
  - A type I fracture shows vertical superior and inferior pubic rami fractures.
  - A type II fracture is an 'open-book' type of fracture with symphysis pubis diastasis and disruption of the anterior SI ligaments.

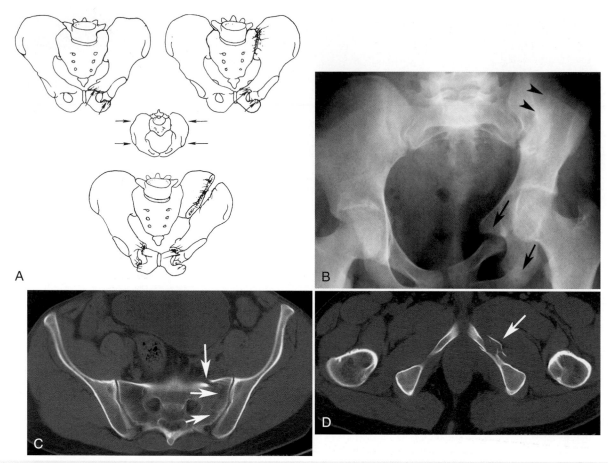

Fig. 5.5 (A) Diagram illustrating lateral compression injury. Center, figure demonstrates direction of force. Top left, type I injury. The impacted sacral ala fracture is not shown. Note the fractures of the superior and inferior pubic rami *(arrows)*. Greater degrees of force result in internal rotation of ipsilateral iliac wing with sacroiliac joint disruption or iliac wing fracture in the type 2 fracture (top right). Greater force will result in contralateral innominate bone external rotation in the type 3 fracture (bottom). Lower-force fractures tend to have more horizontal orientation in the pubic rami, and higher-force, more transverse relative to the bones. **(B)** Radiograph demonstrating features of lateral compression with horizontal fractures of superior and inferior pubic rami *(arrows)*, iliac wing fracture *(arrowheads)*, and internal rotation of ipsilateral innominate bone. **(C and D)** Axial CT scan in an automobile driver struck on the left side by another car. Note fractures *(arrows)* of the sacrum **(C)** and inferior pubic ramus/ischium **(D)**.

- Type III fracture is a 'sprung pelvis' involving diastasis of the symphysis pubis and SI joints with disruption of the anterior and posterior SI joint ligaments.
- Type II and III fractures are unstable and have a higher likelihood of associated arterial hemorrhage.
- Variations in AP compression injuries do occur. For example, in the bucket-handle fracture, there are ipsilateral vertical fractures of the superior and inferior pubic rami associated with contralateral SI joint diastasis or adjacent vertical fracture.
- Impact directly to the symphysis pubis may result in bilateral superior and inferior pubic rami fractures, called a straddle fracture.
- Posterior acetabular fractures often occur with AP pelvic compression fractures.
- In *vertical shear*, superior-inferior shear forces predominate, resulting in vertical displacement of a portion of the pelvis (Fig. 5.7).
  - The appearance of ipsilateral puboischial rami and SI disruptions is termed a *Malgaigne fracture.*
  - The site of displacement may be at the symphysis pubis and SI joint or the adjacent pubis, ilium, and sacrum.

- Unstable with the highest association with arterial hemorrhage.
- A straddle fracture also may result from a superiorly oriented blow to the symphysis region.
- Associated urethral injury is common in males with this injury.
- In general, disruption of an SI joint is associated with highly unstable injuries. In these injuries, the hemipelvis is no longer fixed to the axial skeleton, which allows for significant motion with associated vascular and nerve injury.
- Other findings associated with greater instability are L5 transverse process fractures and ischial spine avulsion fractures.
- In the acute setting the initial management of pelvic fractures is the control of life-threatening hemorrhage.
  - Hemorrhage is highly associated with type III lateral compression, types II and III AP compression, and vertical shear injuries.
- Initial orthopedic management is to stabilize the pelvis, most commonly with the placement of external fixation pins in the iliac wings.
  - SI joint diastasis or sacral distraction can be treated with placement of percutaneous or surgically placed

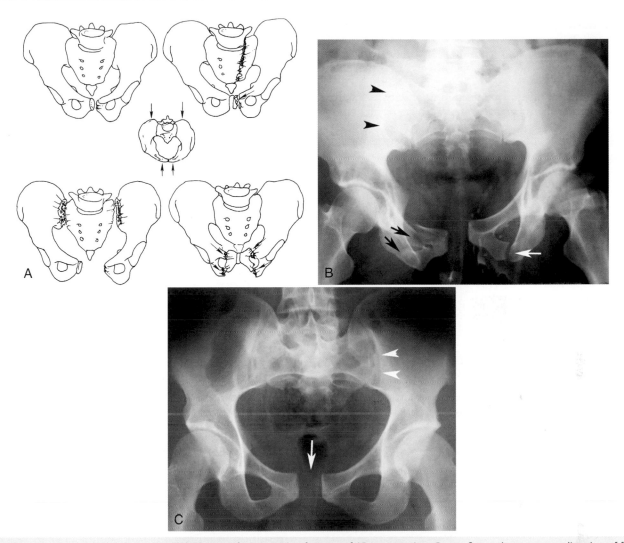

Fig. 5.6 Anteroposterior (AP) compression. **(A)** Diagram demonstrating features of AP compression. Center figure demonstrates direction of forces. Surrounding diagrams show various injury patterns with increasing severity from upper left clockwise to lower right. Signature fracture pattern is vertically oriented fractures of superior and inferior pubic rami *(arrows in the two figures on the right)* or symphysis pubis diastasis. With increasing force there is variable sacroiliac (SI) diastasis or sacral fracture. **(B)** Radiograph demonstrates features of AP compression with vertically oriented fractures of superior and inferior pubic rami *(arrows)*, symphysis pubis diastasis, and right SI joint diastasis *(arrowheads)*. **(C)** Radiograph demonstrating features of AP force with symphysis pubis *(arrow)* and left SI joint diastasis *(arrowheads)*.

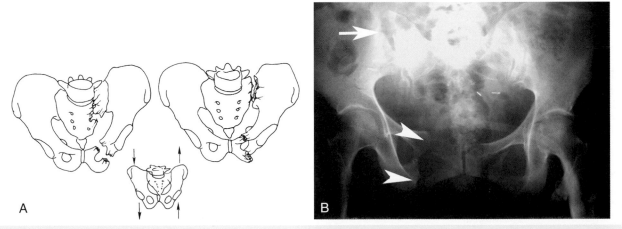

Fig. 5.7 Vertical shear. **(A)** Diagram demonstrating patterns of vertical shear fractures. Center lower figure demonstrates direction of forces. Signature feature is that of vertical malalignment of pelvis. **(B)** Malgaigne fracture. This pelvic fracture demonstrates ipsilateral fractures of the inferior and superior pubic rami *(arrowheads)* as well as the iliac wing adjacent to the sacroiliac joint *(arrow)*. Note the superior displacement of the right innominate bone relative to the sacrum and left side. This is an unstable fracture.

transverse lag screws, threaded hollow dowels, or other hardware.

- Symphysis pubis, pubic ramus, and iliac wing fractures may be fixated intraoperatively with malleable plates.
- External fixation may be used temporarily to stabilize the fragments and reduce the risk of arterial hemorrhage.
- Hemodynamically unstable patients, require immediate arteriography and embolization.
- Retrograde cystography and, in males, retrograde urethrography often are indicated, particularly when hematuria is present.

Key Concepts

Pelvic Fractures: Biomechanical Classification

Lateral Compression

Clue: Horizontal fractures of the superior and inferior pubic rami
Type I
- Medial acetabular wall without substantial associated innominate bone rotation
Type II
- Internal rotation of ipsilateral iliac wing
- Pubic and ischial fractures
- Disruption of the posterior SI joint ligaments or a fracture through the posterior iliac wing or sacrum
Type III
- Internal rotation of the ipsilateral innominate bone
- External rotation of the contralateral innominate bone
- Only lateral compression fracture with substantial risk for arterial hemorrhage

Anteroposterior Compression

Clue: Vertical fractures of the superior and inferior pubic rami
Type I
- Vertical pubic ramus fractures
Type II
- 'Open-book' type fracture
- Symphysis pubis diastasis
- Disruption of the anterior SI ligaments
Type III
- 'Sprung pelvis'
- Diastasis of the symphysis pubis and SI joints
- Disruption of the anterior and posterior SI joint ligaments
- Type II and III fractures are unstable and have a higher likelihood of associated arterial hemorrhage

Vertical Shear

Clue: Vertical displacement of a portion of the pelvis
- Malgaigne fracture
- Unstable injury most associated with arterial hemorrhage

Pelvic Fractures: Pelvic Ring Classification

- Pelvic fractures can also be classified by the degree of disruption of the pelvic ring.
- Class I fractures (Fig. 5.8) are isolated fractures that do not disrupt the pelvic ring (e.g., avulsion fractures).
- Class II fractures disrupt the ring in one location. Because the pelvic ring is quite rigid, class II fractures are unusual.

- Class III fractures disrupt the ring in at least two locations.
- Class IV fractures disrupt the acetabulum.
- Class I and Class II Fractures.
  - Apophyseal avulsion injuries are one form of class I fracture (Fig. 5.8, see Fig. 1.18).
  - The pelvis is a common site of tendon origin avulsion fractures, especially in the skeletally immature, where strong muscles are attached to unfused apophyses.
  - There are five pelvic apophyses that appear by puberty and fuse by the middle of the third decade or earlier:
    - Iliac crest (origin of abdominal wall musculature, tensor fascia lata, and gluteus medius).
    - Anterior superior iliac spine (ASIS, part of the origin of the sartorius muscle; the muscle origin also includes an "indirect head" attached to the adjacent shallow fossa below the ASIS).
    - AIIS (the origin of the rectus femoris muscle).
    - Inferior pubic ramus (the origin of the adductor muscles).
    - Ischial tuberosity (the origin of the hamstring muscles).
- These are Salter–Harris I–equivalent fractures.
- May be invisible or only faintly seen on radiographs.
  - Unossified cartilage in younger patients.
  - Ossified apophysis may be nondisplaced.
- Radiographs: Subtle asymmetry in the width of the physes may be present at the time of injury.
- MRI and ultrasonography (US) can detect the injury.
- The hematoma associated with displaced apophysis converts to bone over time. During the healing process, the radiographic appearance can resemble the osteoid matrix of osteosarcoma. Characteristic locations and history usually clarify the true nature of the finding.
- After healing, the apophysis displacement may remain, resulting in an osseous excrescence of mature bone at the tendon origin. The involved tendon originates on this boney prominence. This usually is easily recognized on imaging studies obtained later in life as an incidental finding due to characteristic location, but sometimes is symptomatic due to impingement on adjacent tissues.

Key Concepts

Pelvic Fractures: Pelvic Ring Classification
- Class I: Isolated fractures that do not disrupt the pelvic ring. Includes apophyseal avulsion fractures
- Class II: Pelvic ring disrupted in one location
- Class III: Pelvic ring disrupted in at least two locations
- Class IV: Acetabular fractures

- Other forms of class I and II fractures are iliac wing fractures, isolated sacral fractures, and isolated ischial or pubic rami fractures.
  - An isolated pubic ramus fracture may also occur from a direct blow and, like the sacrum, the pubic bones are prone to insufficiency fracture among osteoporotic patients and patients after radiation therapy.
  - These fractures may assume bizarre appearances during healing on radiographs, with bone expansion

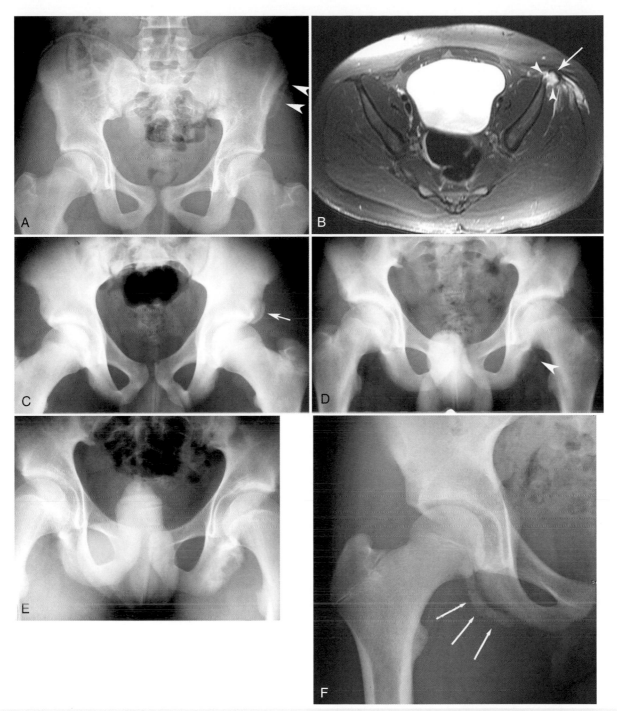

Fig. 5.8 Pelvic avulsion fractures. **(A)** Frontal radiograph of pelvis demonstrates avulsion of left anterior superior iliac spine (ASIS; part of the sartorius origin, *arrowheads*). **(B)** MRI of ASIS avulsion. Axial fat-suppressed T2-weighted image shows bright edema signal *(arrowheads)* between the avulsed low-signal ASIS cortex *(arrow)* and the ilium. **(C)** Avulsion of the anterior inferior iliac spine (rectus femoris origin, *arrow*). **(D and E)** Left ischial tuberosity avulsion (hamstring origin, *arrowhead* in **D**). Follow-up radiograph **(E)** obtained 13 months later shows new bone formation in a chronic avulsion, mimicking osteosarcoma. **(F)** Nonacute ischial tuberosity avulsion fracture in a different patient. Note the cloud-like calcification *(arrows)*.

and aggressive-appearing new bone formation mimicking osteosarcoma.
- Sacral fractures were previously discussed.
- The pubic bones are also common locations for pseudofractures of osteomalacia (Looser zones) and stress fractures in bones with normal mineralization.
- Pubic stress fractures are common adjacent to the pubic symphysis and at the junction of the pubis and ischium.

- The latter site is also the location of the developmental ischiopubic synostosis, which has a variable appearance in the skeletally immature patient that can simulate a healing fracture.
- Class III Fractures.
  - Involve pelvic disruption in two or more locations and can assume any of the patterns as described in the biomechanics section.

- Unstable.
- Significant risk for visceral injury and internal hemorrhage.

ACETABULAR FRACTURES

- Class IV fractures in the pelvic ring classification system.
- Occur with force directed to the acetabulum through the femoral head.
- Fracture patterns are varied and can be complex.
- Detailed assessment is needed for treatment planning.
- The most commonly used classification system is *Judet and Letournel* (Figs. 5.9 and 5.10).
  - This classification system is based on the concept of anterior and posterior column load bearing.
  - The *anterior column* consists of the iliopectineal line, the anterior acetabular wall, and the superior and inferior pubic rami.
    - The anterior column is the anterior portion of the pelvis that allows load bearing from the spine to the lower extremity.
  - The *posterior column* consists of the sciatic notch region of the hemipelvis, the posterior acetabular wall, and the ischium.
    - The posterior column is the posterior portion of the pelvis that allows load bearing from the spine to the lower extremity.

Acetabular Fracture Patterns

- The Judet and Letournel classification includes five *elemental* (or *elementary, primary,* or *simple*) and five associated fracture patterns.

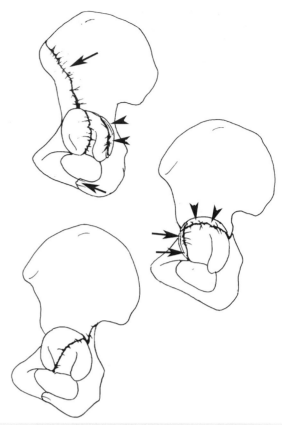

Fig. 5.10 Diagram demonstrating fracture patterns of the acetabulum. Top: anterior column *(arrows)* and posterior wall *(arrowheads)* patterns. Middle: anterior wall *(arrows)* and transverse *(arrowheads)* patterns. Bottom: posterior column pattern.

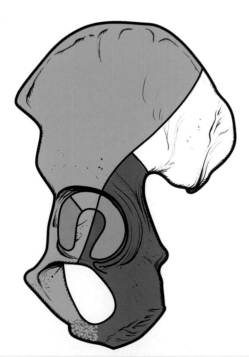

Fig. 5.9 Diagram demonstrating acetabular anatomy pertinent to acetabular fracture description and classification. Red: posterior column; Green: anterior column; Blue: posterior wall; Orange: anterior wall. Mixed red and green in the inferior pubic ramus and ischium may be fractured in both posterior and anterior column fractures.

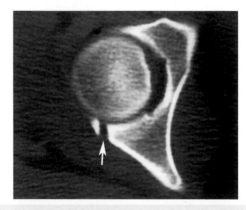

Fig. 5.11 Posterior wall fracture. Axial CT performed after relocation of a posterior hip dislocation demonstrates fracture of posterior wall *(arrow)* with only minimal displacement.

- There are five primary or elemental fracture patterns of the acetabulum:
  - Anterior wall.
  - Posterior wall.
  - Transverse.
  - Anterior column.
  - Posterior column.
- The most common primary fracture of the acetabulum is a posterior wall fracture, occurring in 17% of all acetabular fractures (Fig. 5.11).

- Wall fractures refer to fracture lines in the non–weight-bearing lips or rims of the anterior and posterior acetabulum.
- Column fractures refer to separation of the anterior or posterior weight-bearing portions of the pelvis from the remainder of the pelvis.
  - For example, in the posterior column fracture, the fracture line extends from the sciatic notch through the medial wall of the acetabulum, the acetabular floor, and the ischiopubic junction.
  - Thus the ischium, posterior acetabulum, and sciatic notch region are separated from the remainder of the hemipelvis.
- Anterior column fractures appear as fracture lines extending through the iliac wing, the medial wall of the acetabulum, the acetabular floor, and the ischiopubic junction (Fig. 5.12).
  - Thus an anterior column fracture separates the anterior weight-bearing portion of the hemipelvis from the remainder of the hemipelvis.
- A transverse fracture (Fig. 5.13) separates the upper hemipelvis from the lower hemipelvis and can occur above, at, or inferior to the roof of the acetabulum.
  - Transverse fractures occur in 10% of acetabular fractures.
- Associated, or combination, fractures are those in which more than one elemental fracture is present.
  - The five major associated fracture patterns:
    - Transverse–posterior wall (Fig. 5.14).
    - T-shaped (Fig. 5.15).
    - Both-column.
    - Posterior column–posterior wall.
    - Anterior wall–posterior hemitransverse fractures.
  - Of these associated fracture patterns, the transverse–posterior wall fracture is most common, occurring in 19% of acetabular fractures.
- Some generalizations: Most common fractures in younger patients are posterior all and transverse fractures. Most common fractures in older patients are anterior column and both-column fractures.

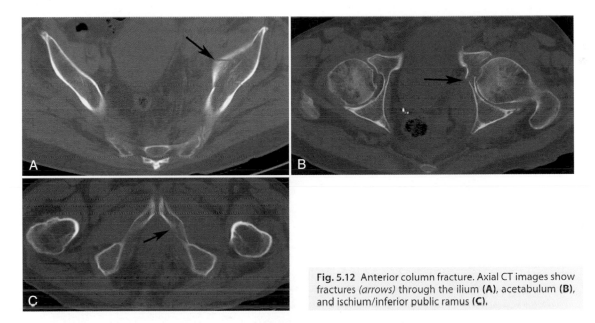

Fig. 5.12 Anterior column fracture. Axial CT images show fractures *(arrows)* through the ilium **(A)**, acetabulum **(B)**, and ischium/inferior public ramus **(C)**.

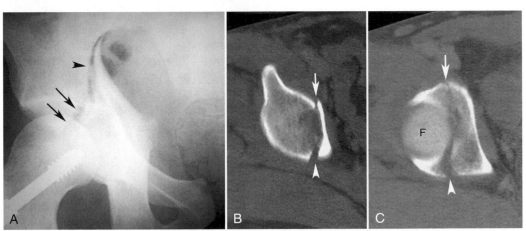

Fig. 5.13 Transverse fracture of acetabulum. **(A)** Frontal radiograph demonstrates fracture line through the superior acetabulum with extension across the ilioischial line *(arrowhead)*. Note transverse orientation of fracture line through the acetabulum *(arrows)*. **(B** and **C)** Consecutive axial CT images obtained through the acetabular roof demonstrate transverse fracture line. Note sagittal orientation of fracture with involvement of anterior *(arrow)* and posterior *(arrowhead)* walls. *F,* Top of the femoral head.

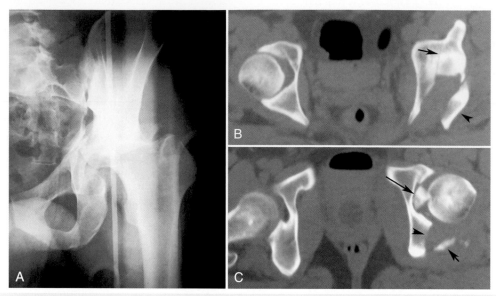

Fig. 5.14 Transverse–posterior wall fractures. This is a transverse fracture through the superior acetabulum and a posterior wall fracture. **(A)** Frontal radiograph demonstrates posterior dislocation of hip and complex fracture pattern at acetabulum. **(B)** Axial CT image obtained after hip relocation demonstrates transverse fracture line *(arrow)* and displaced posterior wall fragments *(arrowhead)*. **(C)** Axial CT image caudal to image shown in B demonstrates posterior wall fracture *(short arrow)* with blunted posterior wall margin *(arrowhead)* and displaced intraarticular fracture fragment *(long arrow)* preventing complete femoral head reduction.

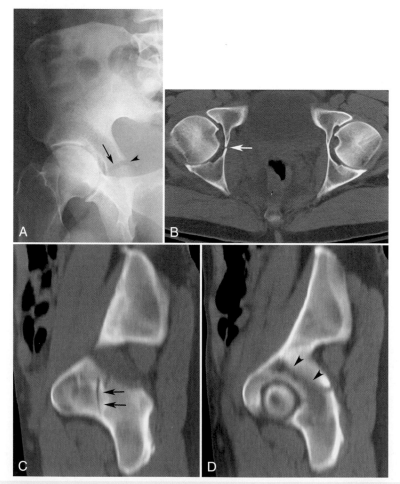

Fig. 5.15 T-shaped acetabular fracture. This is a transverse fracture through the acetabulum and a coronal fracture extending inferiorly. **(A)** Iliac Judet radiographic view demonstrates transverse fracture line *(arrow)* extending to ilioischial line *(arrowhead)*. **(B)** Axial CT image demonstrates the vertical component of T-shaped fracture in medial wall of acetabulum *(arrow)*. **(C and D)** Sagittal CT reformations at the medial acetabulum (C medial to D) demonstrate vertical *(arrows* in C) and transverse *(arrowheads* in D) components of T-shaped fracture in medial wall and roof of acetabulum.

Imaging Tips for Acetabular Fracture Classification

- CT with multiplanar reformats is the standard test. 3D reformats can be very helpful.
  - The following are quick clues to the elemental fracture pattern:
    - If an acetabular fracture plane is sagittal (directed anteroposteriorly), it is a transverse fracture.
    - If the fracture plane is coronal and through the medial wall, it is either an anterior or posterior column fracture.
    - Sagittally oriented or oblique fractures isolated to the anterior or posterior rim are wall fractures.
- Radiography:
  - Judet views are useful in evaluating acetabular fractures because these oblique views allow assessment of the acetabular cortical margins both anteriorly and posteriorly.
  - A fracture line extending anteroposteriorly involving iliopectineal and ilioischial lines must be a transverse fracture.
  - Vertical fractures arising from the sciatic notch must be posterior column fractures.
  - Vertically oriented fractures through the iliac wing and acetabulum must be anterior column fractures. Fractures isolated to the rims of the acetabulum must be anterior or posterior wall fractures.
  - If the obturator ring is disrupted, the acetabular fracture must be either a T-shaped fracture or a column fracture.
  - If there is a 'spur' sign, representing a spur of bone located superior and posterior to the acetabulum on the obturator oblique view, there must be a posterior column or both-column fracture.

Additional Injuries

STRESS FRACTURES

- Runners, soccer and hockey players, among other athletes, are particularly vulnerable to pubic stress fractures (Fig. 5.16). The symptoms of pubic stress fracture overlap with various groin soft tissue injuries. Stress injuries about the hip are further discussed later in this chapter.

OSTEITIS CONDENSANS ILII

- Osteitis condensans ilii (OCI) is dense sclerosis of the medial iliac bones adjacent to the SI joints (Fig. 5.17).
- This condition is most frequent in young multiparous women, but can be seen in men and women without children.
- The hypothesized mechanism is postpartum laxity of the symphysis pubis and SI joints that incites a sclerotic response, but the exact cause is not known.
- Can be considered as a type of stress injury.
- OCI is often asymptomatic but can be a cause of low back pain.
- The primary differential diagnosis in ankylosing spondylitis or other causes of sacroiliitis, which are further discuss in Chapter 9 - Arthritis.
  - OCI: no erosions or fusion.

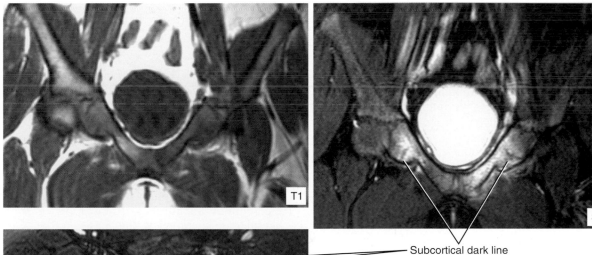

Subcortical dark line

Bilateral stress fractures of the superior pubic rami

Fig. 5.16 Stress fracture of the superior pubic rami bilaterally in an adolescent athlete with pain. Note subcortical dark line with surrounding bone marrow edema on MRI. Stress fractures around the hip in young patients often occur at the pubic rami. Whenever a fracture is seen at the pelvic ring, other fractures of the ring should be sought, whether the cause is acute trauma or stress. In older patients, they are seen more frequently at the sacrum and supraacetabular region; in this older population, they may be mistaken for tumor. The MRI finding of a dark line with surrounding edema is highly specific. (From Morrison W. *Problem Solving in Musculoskeletal Imaging*. Philadelphia: Elsevier; 2010.)

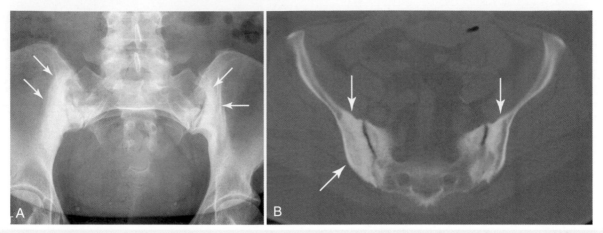

Fig. 5.17 Osteitis condensans ilii. Radiograph **(A)** and CT scan **(B)** show dense sclerosis of the medial iliac bones *(arrows)* in this multiparous 30-year-old woman. Sacroiliac joint osteoarthritis is present, which is not uncommon.

Hip and Femur

ANATOMY

- The hip is a ball-and-socket joint surrounded by a strong capsule and the iliofemoral, pubofemoral, and ischiofemoral capsular ligaments, with further support from the acetabular labrum, the transverse acetabular ligament, and ligamentum teres.
- The vascular supply to the femoral head is tenuous. Although the artery of the ligamentum teres contributes to the vascular supply of the femoral head, most of the arterial supply is from the medial and lateral circumflex femoral arteries, which are branches of the profunda femoris artery.
- In the frontal plane, the normal angle between the femoral neck and shaft averages 135 degrees (range, 115 to 140 degrees).
  - *Coxa valga* is an abnormally increased femoral neckshaft angle.
    - Internal or external rotation of the femur can falsely simulate coxa valga on radiographs.
  - *Coxa vara* is an abnormally decreased femoral neckshaft angle.
    - Hip flexion and internal rotation can falsely simulate coxa vara on radiographs.
- *Femoral anteversion*: The femoral neck is normally anteverted relative to the femoral shaft by approximately 15 degrees. In other words, if a femur were placed horizontally on a flat surface, resting on the posterior aspect of both condyles and the posterior intertrochanteric femur, the femoral neck would angle anteriorly away from the flat surface. Stated yet another way, the femoral condyles are internally rotated relative to the femoral neck. Femoral anteversion is discussed further in Chapter 15-Congenital and Developmental Conditions.
- The greater trochanter and lesser trochanter are both posterior structures. The lesser trochanter is posteromedial in location and the greater trochanter is posterolateral. Thus when the femur is internally rotated, the greater trochanter is shown in profile and the lesser trochanter is hidden from view. When the femur

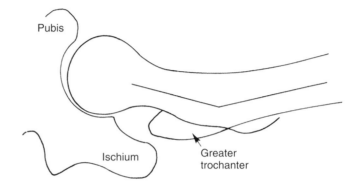

Fig. 5.18 Diagram of groin lateral radiographic view of the hip, demonstrating the normal anatomy and normal neck-shaft angle. Note that the trochanters project posterior to the femoral neck, allowing radiographic assessment of femoral neck fracture without superimposition of the trochanters. (Reproduced with permission from Manaster BJ. *Handbook of Skeletal Radiology.* 2nd ed. St. Louis: Mosby; 1997.)

is externally rotated, the lesser trochanter is in profile and the greater trochanter is obliqued.
  - Furthermore, the posterior positions of the greater and lesser trochanters obscure visualization of portions of the femoral neck on both externally rotated and frog-leg lateral radiographic views of the hip. These two views also foreshorten the radiographic appearance of the femoral neck. Because of these limitations, radiographic assessment of trauma to the hip requires an internally rotated AP or surgical lateral (true lateral) view (Fig. 5.18).
- Acetabular version: The acetabulum is normally *anteverted* (open anteriorly). *Retroversion* of the acetabular cup is associated with femoroacetabular impingement (FAI, discussed later). Acetabular anteversion can be measured at the widest part of the cup, but in clinical practice it sometimes is measured at the superior aspect because this is the usual site of impingement.
  - Acetabular retroversion is easily detectable on axial CT or MRI.
  - Radiographic evaluation of acetabular version is much less reliable. One popular radiographic sign of acetabular retroversion is the 'crossover' or 'figure of

eight' or 'infinity' sign: On a well-positioned AP radiograph (centered so that the coccyx and pubic symphysis are lined up, the coccyx about 2 cm above the top of the symphysis), the anterior and posterior acetabular margins should not overlap. In retroversion the lines at the upper margin of the joint cross over forming a 'figure of eight' or 'infinity' symbol). However, this sign has been shown to be less reliable than initially thought.

Hip Joint Capsule

- The hip joint capsule extends over the femoral neck to insert on the basicervical region.
    - On radiographs, fat planes around the hip may bulge away from the hip joint in the presence of a large hip joint effusion. However, this finding lacks sensitivity and specificity for the detection of effusion, especially in adults.
- In children, a more specific radiographic indicator is measurement of the distance between the teardrop of the acetabulum and the medial femoral head on a well-positioned AP view, with asymmetric increase indicating the side of effusion.
- US or MRI is the best imaging method for detection of a hip joint effusion. Sagittal plane US imaging using an anterior approach is a fast and reliable technique in infants and children.
- A constriction of the capsule is created at its mid portion by a capsular ligament around the proximal femoral neck (the *zona orbicularis* or annular ligament).

HIP DISLOCATION

- *Posterior hip dislocation:*
    - Approximately 90% of hip dislocations are posterior.
    - Posterior dislocations are especially common after motor vehicle accidents in which the flexed knee strikes the dashboard, driving the flexed hip posteriorly.
    - Posterior hip dislocation is commonly associated with fracture of the posterior wall of the acetabulum.
    - With posterior dislocation, the femoral head is typically not only posteriorly positioned relative to the acetabulum but also superiorly positioned, and the femur is in internal rotation with the greater trochanter in profile and the lesser trochanter obscured (Fig. 5.19).
    - On clinical observation of the patient, the lower extremity appears adducted, extended, internally rotated, and shortened because of superior femoral head displacement.
    - Radiographically, dislocations are easy to recognize if the femoral head is superior in position relative to the acetabulum.
    - In some posterior dislocations, the degree of superior displacement may be minimal.
        - In these situations dislocation may be difficult to recognize on a frontal radiograph.
        - Look for lack of congruence of the femoral head and the acetabulum.

In addition, a dislocated femoral head appears smaller than the contralateral femoral head because the dislocated femoral head is posterior in position and closer to the image receptor thereby less magnified.

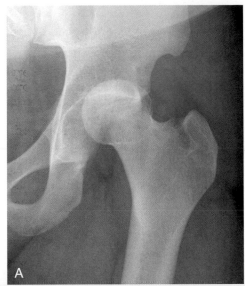
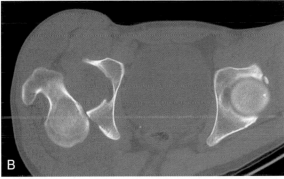

Fig. 5.19 Posterior hip dislocation. **(A)** AP radiograph demonstrates superior position of the left femoral head and internal rotation of the femur (lesser trochanter projects over the femoral shaft). Note also the smaller appearance of the left femoral head compared to the acetabulum. This is a result of the closer positioning of the femoral head to the x-ray cassette, with less radiographic magnification. **(B)** CT shows posterior femoral head dislocation in a different patient. Note the extreme internal rotation of the femur, with no visualization of the lesser trochanter.

Key Concepts

Hip Dislocation

- **Posterior:** Most common by far. Femoral head posterior and superior to acetabulum, femur in internal rotation
- **Anterior:**
    - Flexed thigh = obturator anterior dislocation. Femoral head medial and inferior, overlying the obturator foramen
    - Extended thigh = iliac dislocation. Femoral head superior to the acetabulum, like a posterior dislocation, but the femur is in external rotation

- *Anterior hip dislocation:*
    - Uncommon. Occur in the externally rotated and abducted thigh.
    - May present with the femur in either a flexed or extended position.
    - If the hip is flexed, the dislocation is known as an *obturator anterior dislocation* because the femoral head is positioned medially and inferiorly, overlying the obturator foramen (Fig. 5.20).

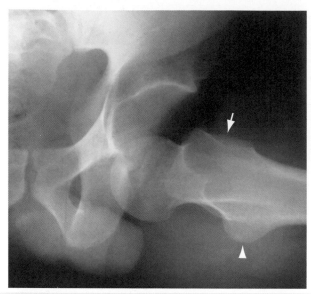

Fig. 5.20 Anterior hip dislocation. AP radiograph shows obturator anterior dislocation with inferomedial displacement of the femoral head and external rotation of the femur with profile view of lesser trochanter *(arrowhead)* and obscured greater trochanter *(arrow)*.

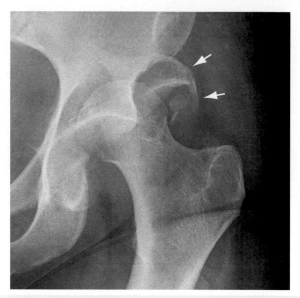

Fig. 5.21 Posterior dislocation with shear fracture of posterior acetabulum *(arrows)*. Note internal rotation of femur with obscuration of lesser trochanter and profile view of greater trochanter.

- If the hip is extended, the dislocated femoral head projects superior to the acetabulum over the iliac wing. This is known as *iliac dislocation*.
- Note that both posterior dislocation and iliac anterior dislocation both show superior femoral head displacement on radiographs. However, iliac dislocation can be discriminated from a posterior dislocation because the femur is in external rotation with the lesser trochanter in profile and the greater trochanter obscured, in contrast with posterior dislocation which internally rotates the femur.
- With both anterior and posterior dislocations, there is risk for fracture of the femoral head.
  - This can result from impaction injury with compression of a portion of the femoral head, similar to Hill–Sachs and trough fractures associated with shoulder dislocations.
- Another form of fracture-dislocation is shear fracture of the femoral head.
  - Intraarticular fragments may result from such fractures.
- Intraarticular fragments may also result from acetabular fracture (Fig. 5.21).
- Avulsion fractures related to tension of the ligamentum teres insertion on the femur are an additional cause of intraarticular bone fragments.
- Intraarticular loose bodies can be suspected on radiographs with demonstration of widening and incongruence of the femoral head and acetabulum and can cause increased distance between the acetabular teardrop and the medial femoral head.
  - Posttraumatic intraarticular bone fragments can cause difficulty in reducing hip dislocation; such cases may require open surgical reduction.
  - CT is usually definitive in detecting bone fragments.
- Another common complication after hip dislocation is femoral head osteonecrosis (avascular necrosis [AVN]),

which markedly increases in likelihood if a dislocation is not reduced within 24 hours.
- Approximately 50% of hip reductions delayed after 24 hours undergo subsequent osteonecrosis.

FEMORAL NECK FRACTURES

- Femur fractures are divided into those involving the femoral head, the femoral neck, the intertrochanteric region, the shaft, and distally, the femoral condyles at the knee.
- As noted previously, femoral head fractures can occur during dislocations and appear as impaction or shear injuries. CT is useful for searching for intraarticular fracture fragments, which require surgical removal.
- Femoral neck and intertrochanteric fractures are rare in young adults and middle-aged patients but common in older adults.
  - This high prevalence corresponds to the high prevalence of osteoporosis in older adults.
  - By age 80, 10% of white women and 5% of white men sustain a hip fracture. By age 90, the rates increase to 20% and 10%, respectively.
  - High associated mortality in the elderly within 1 year of injury.

Key Concepts

Proximal Femur Fractures
Head, neck, intertrochanteric, or shaft
Neck: Subcapital, midcervical, or basicervical
Subcapital fractures: Garden classification

- Femoral neck fractures are divided into *subcapital, midcervical (transcervical)*, and *basicervical* types.
- Femoral neck fractures have high risk for nonunion and femoral head osteonecrosis, especially subcapital

fractures (superior femoral neck, just under the femoral head).

■ In general, the more proximal the fracture line and the more displaced the fracture, the higher the risk for osteonecrosis and nonunion.

■ The *Garden classification* categorizes subcapital fractures into four types. An important clue to identifying the correct type on radiographs is the relative orientation of the trabeculae of the femoral neck, femoral head, and acetabulum.

■ *Type I:* incomplete fractures with valgus impaction. This is identified by the valgus orientation of the femoral head and neck trabeculae (i.e., the angle formed by the head and neck trabeculae is apex medial). Head trabeculae are more vertically oriented than normal (Fig. 5.22).

■ *Type II:* complete but nondisplaced or minimally displaced. Femoral head and neck trabeculae normally aligned or with mild valgus.

■ *Type III:* complete with partial displacement. The femoral shaft is externally rotated (look for prominent lesser trochanter), with mild varus. Head trabeculae are more horizontally oriented than normal (Fig. 5.23).

■ *Type IV:* complete fractures with obvious proximal displacement of the shaft relative to the head. The femoral shaft is externally rotated. The trabeculae of the femoral head and the acetabulum are parallel. Femoral head trabeculae are normally aligned (Fig. 5.24).

■ Simplified Garden classification:
   ■ *Nondisplaced* (types I and II).
   ■ *Displaced* (types III and IV).

■ The Garden staging system is used because it indicates the higher degree of complication with higher-stage fractures and therefore guides therapy.

■ Major complications after subcapital fracture are nonunion and osteonecrosis.

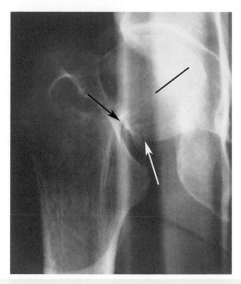

Fig. 5.23 Garden stage III subcapital femoral fracture. Note medial orientation of femoral head trabecular lines *(line)* and mild superior displacement of medial femoral neck *(black arrow)* compared with medial femoral head margin *(white arrow)*.

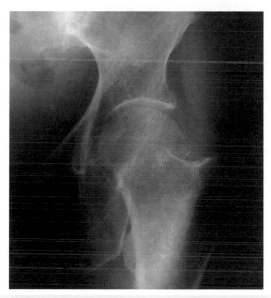

Fig. 5.24 Garden stage IV fracture. Femoral neck is completely displaced. Note substantial shortening of femoral neck and anatomic femoral head alignment.

■ The occurrence of both complications increases substantially with higher stages.
■ Hemiarthroplasty or total hip arthroplasty (THA) is used for surgical treatment of higher stages.

FEMORAL NECK FRACTURE DETECTION

■ Detection of a femoral neck fracture in osteoporotic patients may be extremely difficult. The bones are demineralized and hence poorly seen on radiographs. Cortical and trabecular disruption may be minimal.

■ Ringlike femoral head osteophytes in the setting of osteoarthritis may yield linear increased density overlying the femoral neck and give a false impression of fracture.

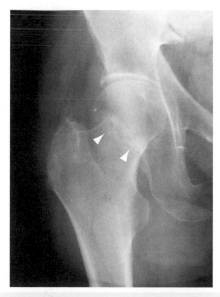

Fig. 5.22 Garden stage I subcapital fracture. Note fracture line *(arrowheads)* and impaction of the superior lateral head. The femoral head trabecular lines are oriented relatively craniocaudad.

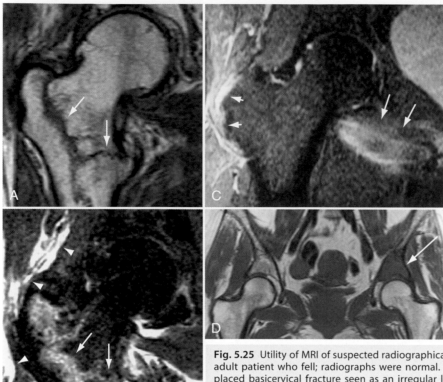

Fig. 5.25 Utility of MRI of suspected radiographically occult hip fracture. (A and B) MR images in older adult patient who fell; radiographs were normal. Coronal T1-weighted MR image **(A)** shows nondisplaced basicervical fracture seen as an irregular low-signal-intensity line *(arrows)*. Coronal inversion recovery MR image **(B)** shows high signal along the fracture *(arrows)* because of edema. Also note high-signal contusion and bursal fluid lateral to the hip *(arrowheads)*. **(C)** Coronal inversion recovery MR image in a different patient shows use of MRI for the exclusion of fracture and demonstration of the cause of the patient's symptoms. Marrow signal was normal on all sequences, excluding a fracture. Note high signal in obturator externus *(long arrows)* indicating strain, and tear of the gluteus medius insertion *(short arrows)* on the greater trochanter. **(D)** In another patient with severe hip pain, MRI shows a metastasis of the supraacetabular ilium *(arrow)*.

- When the diagnosis is unclear, CT with reformats usually is adequate. CT may also reveal fractures at other sites, contusions, and hematoma.
- The most sensitive test is MRI, which has extremely high accuracy, even with low-field scanners, and is not affected by patient age or osteoporosis (Fig. 5.25). The evaluation can be abbreviated to T1-weighted spin-echo and inversion recovery sequences, with total scan times of less than 10 minutes.
  - MRI also will demonstrate other fractures, such as fractures of the pelvic ring, soft tissue contusions, muscle strains/tendon tears (see Fig. 5.25C), and sometimes unexpected causes of pain such as metastatic disease (see Fig. 5.25D).
- Radionuclide bone scan (Fig. 5.26) is insensitive among older adults for fracture detection in the first 72 hours. After 72 hours the sensitivity is about 90%.

FEMORAL NECK FRACTURE TREATMENT

- Garden stage I subcapital fractures can be adequately treated with cannulated screw fixation.
- Hemiarthroplasty or THA is commonly used for subcapital and some lower femoral neck fractures. This avoids any issues with femoral head osteonecrosis and allows rapid return to mobility.
- Neck fractures more distal than subcapital may be internally fixed with sliding screw hardware that allows the

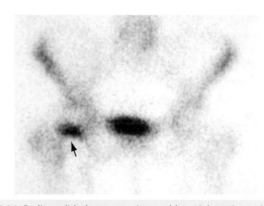

Fig. 5.26 Radionuclide bone scan in an older adult patient who fell 3 days previously and had continued hip pain and negative radiographs. Diphosphonate bone scan shows intense, linear tracer uptake *(arrow)* crossing the femoral neck, indicating fracture.

fragment impaction along a femoral neck fracture, enhancing healing potential.

INTERTROCHANTERIC FRACTURES

- Fracture in the region between the greater and lesser trochanters (Fig. 5.27).
- Key issue is fracture stability. Fractures with disrupted posteromedial cortex are unstable and always require internal fixation.

- Generally, intertrochanteric fractures have a good prognosis without compromise of blood supply. Osteonecrosis or nonunion as a result of such fractures is uncommon.
- Treatment is usually with internal fixation (Fig. 5.28).
  - Intramedullary hardware is commonly used.
  - Any type of femoral neck hardware has some potential to erode superiorly through the articular surface (see Fig. 5.28C).

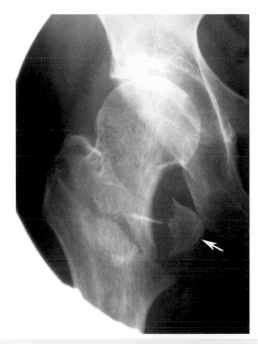

Fig. 5.27 Intertrochanteric fracture. Frontal radiograph demonstrates fracture with displaced lesser trochanter fragment *(arrow)*. Traction by the iliopsoas tendon tends to displace lesser trochanter fragments superiorly and anteriorly.

AVULSION FRACTURE OF THE LESSER TROCHANTER

- Nonpathologic lesser trochanteric avulsion is a common component of the fracture pattern in intertrochanteric fractures (see Fig. 5.27).
- However, isolated avulsion fracture of the lesser trochanter deserves special consideration.
  - Benign avulsion fractures related to iliopsoas tendon attachment can be seen in adolescents or in older, osteoporotic patients.
  - Isolated avulsion fracture of the lesser trochanter in an adult has a very high likelihood of representing a pathologic fracture related to an underlying lesion, and thus should raise concern for a metastatic lesion or myeloma. If a lesion is not visualized on radiographs or CT, MRI is recommended (Fig. 5.29).

SLIPPED CAPITAL FEMORAL EPIPHYSIS

- Slipped capital femoral epiphysis (SCFE) is seen during periods of rapid skeletal growth, at 10 to 16 years of age, during a period in which body weight and muscle strength increase rapidly and the femoral neck develops greater varus.
  - This results in increased shear loading on the capital femoral physis and predisposes the child to Salter–Harris I fracture with displacement.
  - The injury is probably a result of repetitive minor trauma.
  - More common in males, African Americans, Latinos, with obesity (single greatest risk factor), children with delayed skeletal maturation, hypothyroidism, deficient growth factor, and acetabular retroversion.
- The disorder occurs bilaterally in 25% of children but when bilateral is usually asymmetric.

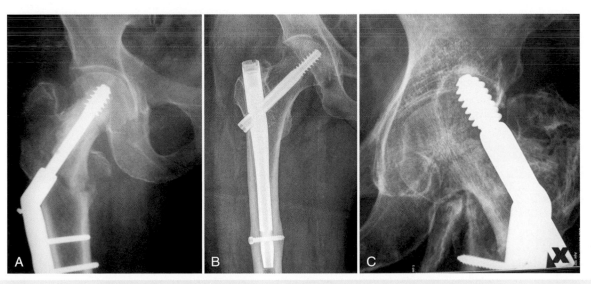

Fig. 5.28 Hip fixation hardware. **(A)** This patient with an intertrochanteric fracture has been stabilized with a dynamic screw and plate system, which allows settling at the fracture site without the screw cutting out through the osteoporotic bone of the femoral head. **(B)** Intramedullary fixation with a "gamma nail" or similar hardware is currently more widely used. **(C)** Dynamic hip screw failure in a different patient. The screw head has migrated through the top of the femoral head and neck and eroded into the acetabular roof. Note how the screw has backed out of the hollow cylindrical shaft (marked with an 'x').

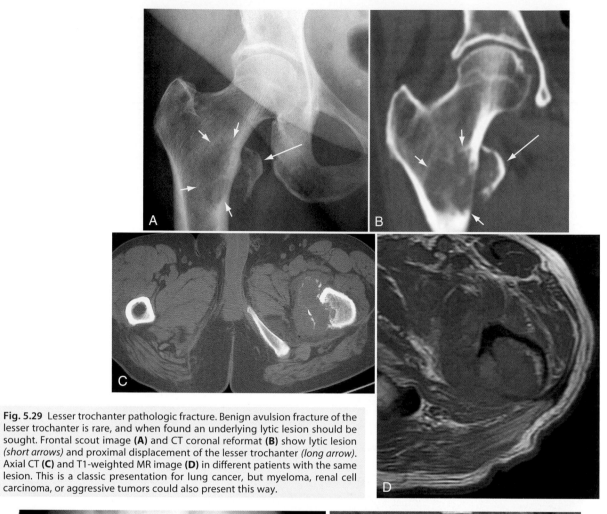

Fig. 5.29 Lesser trochanter pathologic fracture. Benign avulsion fracture of the lesser trochanter is rare, and when found an underlying lytic lesion should be sought. Frontal scout image **(A)** and CT coronal reformat **(B)** show lytic lesion *(short arrows)* and proximal displacement of the lesser trochanter *(long arrow)*. Axial CT **(C)** and T1-weighted MR image **(D)** in different patients with the same lesion. This is a classic presentation for lung cancer, but myeloma, renal cell carcinoma, or aggressive tumors could also present this way.

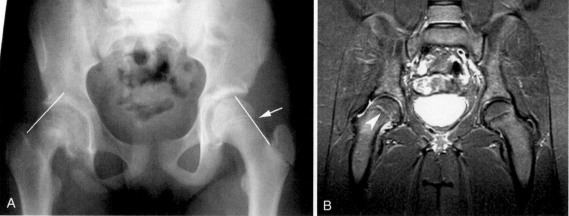

Fig. 5.30 Slipped capital femoral epiphysis (SCFE). **(A)** AP radiograph shows normal left side. Line drawn along superior cortex of the left femoral neck *(arrow)* crosses the capital femoral epiphysis. Right side is abnormal: this line fails to intersect femoral capital epiphysis. Note the wider physis on the right, which is another clue to the diagnosis. **(B)** Coronal inversion recovery MR image in a different child with right SCFE shows medial displacement of the right capital femoral epiphysis, a joint effusion, and edema in the physis *(arrowhead)*.

- Bilateral is becoming more frequent with increasing childhood obesity.
- The capital epiphysis displaces posteromedially relative to the neck.
- Radiographs:
  - The physis appears wider and with indistinct margins (Fig. 5.30).

- The most helpful sign of SCFE on a frontal radiograph is demonstrated by drawing a line tangent to the lateral cortex of the femoral neck, the *"line of Klein"*. Ordinarily this line should intersect a portion of the capital epiphysis. If the tangent line is superior and lateral to the capital epiphysis, SCFE is present. However, a mild slip will not show this finding.

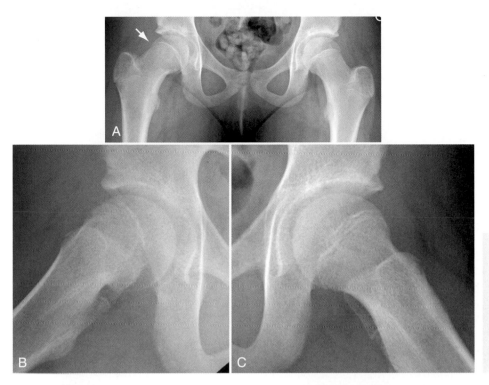

Fig. 5.31 Subtle slipped capital femoral epiphysis (SCFE). Left side is normal. **(A)** AP radiograph shows only minimal displacement of the right capital femoral epiphysis *(arrow)*, which could easily be overlooked. (B and C) Frog-leg lateral views of the right **(B)** and left **(C)** hips show more obvious medial and posterior displacement of the right capital femoral epiphysis. This example illustrates the need for a lateral radiograph when evaluating for suspected SCFE.

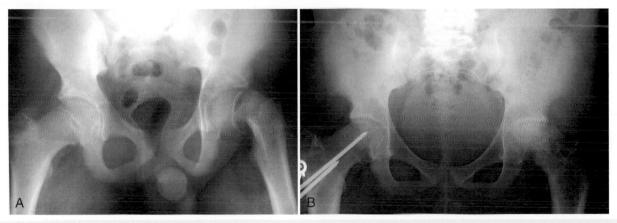

Fig. 5.32 Bilateral slipped capital femoral epiphyses. **(A)** Note severely displaced fracture on the left. **(B)** Same patient 3 years later shows collapsed left femoral head because of complication of osteonecrosis.

- It is very important to note that malalignment may be evident only on a frog-leg lateral radiograph, where the head is seen to be posterior relative to the femoral neck (Fig. 5.31).
- MRI shows the displacement and adjacent marrow edema, and may detect osteonecrosis when present.
  - Metaphyseal edema without displacement may progress to SCFE ('pre-SCFE').
- SCFE complications:
  - Early osteoarthritis, usually occurring after 30 years of age.
  - Osteonecrosis occurs in roughly 10%, more commonly with greater displacement and especially after attempts at reduction (Fig. 5.32).
  - Rarely, acute chondrolysis can occur.
- Most cases of SCFE are treated with cannulated screw fixation through the femoral neck into the head. Attempts at reduction are usually avoided due to risk of

osteonecrosis. This results in varus deformity with a short and broad femoral neck.
- The surgeon may elect to fix the contralateral hip in younger and high-risk children to prevent an SCFE from developing and to maintain symmetric growth.
- Severe deformity may later require a proximal femoral osteotomy.

FEMORAL SHAFT FRACTURE

- Fracture of the femoral shaft typically occurs from major trauma such as falls and motor vehicle collisions; it is often associated with other injuries.
  - Often the fracture is comminuted with butterfly or segmental fragments.
- Fractures in young children are usually treated with casting.

- Fractures in adults are usually fixed internally with an interlocking intramedullary nail (rod).
    - Side plate fixation is less desirable because placement of a plate requires disturbing too much of the numerous muscle attachments that cover much of the femoral shaft cortex; in addition, a side plate is not mechanically strong enough in this location.
    - The surgeon must check for rotational deformity so that appropriate reduction may be achieved.
    - CT can help assess for the degree of rotation (version) when only a few CT sections at the femoral neck and at the femoral condyles are obtained (Fig. 5.33).
    - The degree of version can be measured by summing the angles of the femoral neck and condyles. This is done at each location by drawing a line parallel to the bottom edge of the window, a second line through the middle of the femoral neck, and another line at the knee tangent to the posterior margin of the femoral condyles. The two angles are summed and can be compared with the contralateral side. The surgeon's goal is to be within 5 degrees of the uninjured side (see Fig. 5.34).

STRESS FRACTURES ABOUT THE HIP

- Bimodal peak: older, osteoporotic patients and adolescent/young adult athletes.
- *Sacral stress fracture* (see Fig. 5.4, see Fig. 1.39).
    - Older patients, predisposing factors as described earlier; often bilateral.
- *Pubic rami stress fracture.*
    - Younger patients, athletes.
    - Both superior and inferior pubic ramus, often bilateral. May occur adjacent to the symphysis.

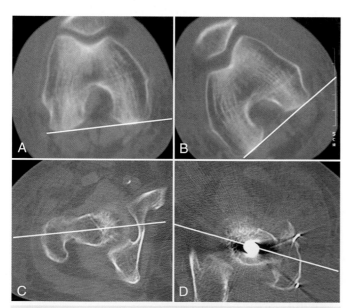

Fig. 5.33 Abnormal femoral torsion after fracture fixation. Adult patient who had a left femur fracture fixed with an intramedullary rod (nail). Limited CT sections were obtained through the knees; the table was then moved without moving the patient, and limited sections were obtained through the proximal femurs. Representative images are shown. The uninjured right side has 0 degrees of anteversion. On the left, the fragments had twisted around the rod, resulting in 55 degrees of femoral anteversion. Corrective surgery was required. **(A)** Right knee. **(B)** Left knee. **(C)** Right femoral neck. **(D)** Left femoral neck.

- *Supraacetabular fracture.*
    - Just above hip joint.
    - Transverse orientation.
    - Can simulate tumor (look for fracture line on T1-weighted images).
    - Older patients, predisposing factors.
- Femoral head subchondral fracture (Fig. 5.34).
    - Can overlap with *transient osteoporosis of the hip,* discussed in Chapter 13.
    - Can result in articular surface collapse and secondary osteoarthritis.
    - DDx: osteonecrosis.
        - Dynamic contrast-enhanced MRI (DCEMRI) can help differentiate (TOH is hyperemic).
- *Femoral neck stress fracture* (Fig. 5.34).
    - Younger patients, athletes, military recruits.
    - Medial more common than lateral.
    - Medial: usually base of femoral neck near lesser trochanter; stable (compressive side), treated with limited weight-bearing.
    - Lateral: uncommon, unstable (tensile side—fracture tends to propagate and complete); treated with fixation of the femoral neck.
- *Proximal femoral shaft stress fracture.*
    - Lateral femoral shaft (Fig. 5.34D).
        - Older, osteoporotic patients.
        - Associated with bisphosphonate therapy (drug for osteoporosis).
        - Aggressively treated with fixation.
        - Must be recognized early: look for a lateral 'bump' or beak at the proximal lateral femoral shaft cortex on radiographs.
        - Often bilateral.
- *Adductor insertion stress injury ('thigh splints')* (Fig. 5.35, see Fig. 1.36).
    - Medial femoral shaft, proximal to mid portion.
    - Young athletes, especially runners.
    - Periosteal reaction on radiographs, periosteal/subcortical edema on MRI.

SNAPPING HIP ('COXA SALTANS')

The sensation of snapping with pain may have many causes. These include:
- *Internal snapping hip:* Iliopsoas tendon snapping over the pubic tubercle.
    - The tendinous causes of snapping can be diagnosed clinically and directly visualized with dynamic US (observe the tendon as the patient reproduces the motion that causes the snapping).
- *External snapping hip:* Tensor fascia lata snapping over the greater trochanter, often with an associated bursitis.
    - Bursitis, when present, can be seen on US or MRI with bursal effusion.
    - Can be diagnosed clinically because this snapping sensation is more lateral than the anterior snapping sensation arising from the iliopsoas tendon or a torn labrum.
    - Can cause *'greater trochanteric pain syndrome'.*
- Acetabular labral tear or detachment, see next section.
- Intraarticular body (chondral or osteochondral fragment or synovial chondromatosis).

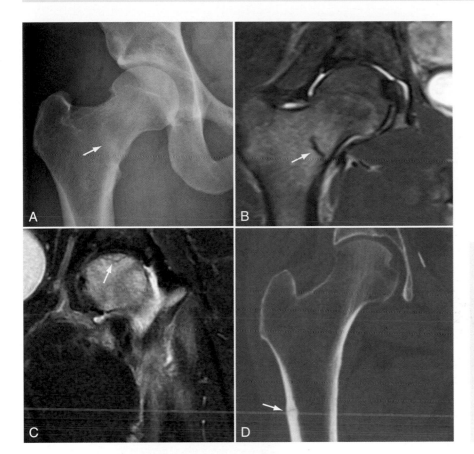

Fig. 5.34 Stress fractures. **(A)** AP radiographs shows subtle sclerosis of the medial femoral neck *(arrow)*. **(B)** Coronal inversion recovery MR image in the same patient as A shows incomplete, low-signal-intensity linear fracture line at medial femoral neck cortex *(arrow)* with surrounding bone marrow edema. **(C)** Fat-suppressed T2-weighted MR image in a different patient shows a subtle subchondral fracture line in the femoral head *(arrow)* surrounded by marked marrow edema. This is part of the process called 'transient osteoporosis of the hip'. **(D)** Coronal reformatted CT shows a subtle cortical fracture line in the lateral cortex of the subtrochanteric femur *(arrow)* in a patient with history of bisphosphonate treatment for osteoporosis.

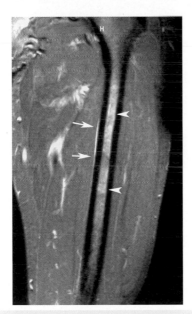

Fig. 5.35 Femoral shaft stress reaction in a 25-year-old female runner with left thigh pain. Coronal fat-suppressed T2-weighted MR image shows marrow edema *(arrowheads)* and periosteal edema *(arrows)* along the medial midshaft. This is also known as 'thigh splints'. These findings were unilateral and resolved with cessation of running. The findings are usually milder than in this example and may be only medial.

- Intraarticular bodies can be diagnosed with MRI or CT arthrography.
- Femoroacetabular impingement (FAI).
- Osteoarthritis.

ACETABULAR LABRAL TEAR

- The labrum is a fibocartilagenous structure analogous to the glenoid labrum in the shoulder and the menisci in the knee, which surrounds the majority of the acetabular rim (Fig. 5.36).
    - It is triangular in shape in cross section, and extends 270 degrees along the anterior, superior, and posterior acetabulum.
- The inferior aspect of the joint has no labral coverage; the labrum continues as the *transverse ligament* passing inferior to the femoral head at the medial joint margin.
- The labrum contributes to joint stability by providing increased surface area of articular contact, and providing a suction effect.
- Labral tear can result in pain and mechanical symptoms, such as locking or snapping.
- Labral tears can occur from injury, but most commonly morphologic variations of femoral head and/or acetabular anatomy predispose to tears—notably femoroacetabular impingement (FAI) and acetabular dysplasia.
- Tear or detachment of the acetabular labrum is best diagnosed with MR arthrography, which demonstrates contrast undermining a portion of the acetabular labrum (Fig. 5.37).
- The most frequent location of a labral tear is anterosuperior.
    - Often best seen on sagittal or oblique sagittal images.
- A normal variant sulcus may be seen between the posterior labrum and the acetabulum, which may simulate a tear.

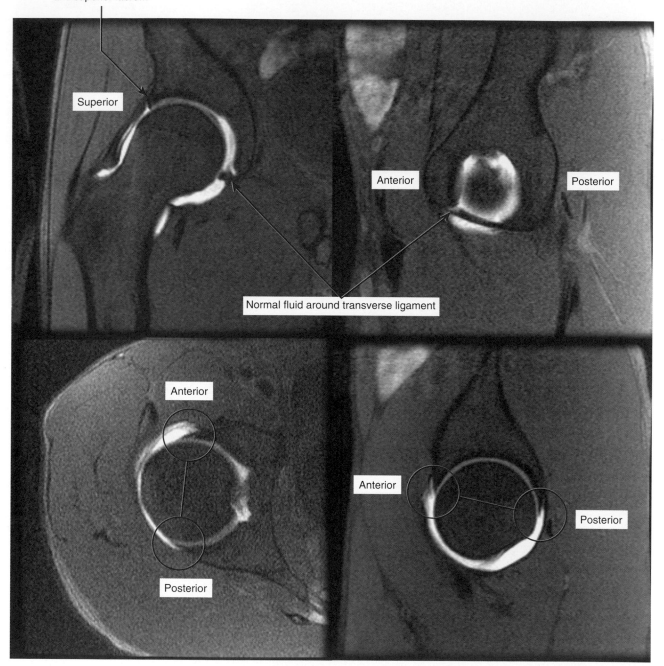

Normal recess between capsule and superior labrum

Superior

Anterior

Posterior

Normal fluid around transverse ligament

Anterior

Posterior

Anterior

Posterior

Normal: Sharp, dark triangle
Size and shape: anterior = posterior

Fig. 5.36 Normal labral anatomy on an MR arthrogram. Unlike the glenoid labrum, the acetabular labrum is not a complete ring but extends across the inferior acetabulum as a transverse ligament. Also, unlike the glenoid labrum, the hip labrum is fairly uniform in size and shape in different regions. There is a recess around the transverse ligament and between the labrum and capsule. Like the glenoid labrum, the dark signal of fibrocartilaginous labrum blends with the intermediate signal hyaline cartilage. (From Morrison W. *Problem Solving in Musculoskeletal Imaging*. Philadelphia: Elsevier; 2010.)

- The normal variant sulcus is smooth and does not extend to the edge of the capsular margin with an otherwise intact, dark triangle of labral tissue, whereas a tear is irregular, with contrast or fluid extending to the capsular margin, and/or contrast/fluid penetrating the labral substance.
- Presence of a paralabral cyst (lobulated fluid adjacent to the acetabular rim with a 'neck' communicating with the labrum) virtually confirms presence of an underlying labral tear, the same principle as a cyst at the glenoid labrum, and parameniscal cysts at the knee associated with fibrocartilage tears in those locations (Fig. 5.38).
- MR arthrography is also the most reliable test for detection of hip joint articular cartilage defects (Fig. 5.39).

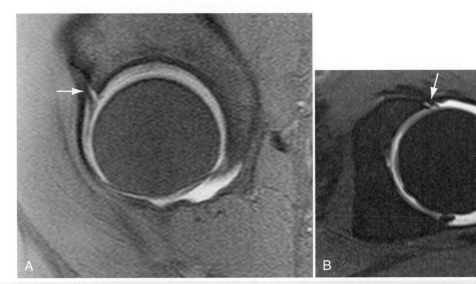

Fig. 5.37 Acetabular labral tears. **(A)** Sagittal fat-suppressed T1-weighted MR arthrogram shows high signal intensity *(arrow)* extending into a tear in the anterosuperior labrum. This is the most common labral tear location and is usually best seen on sagittal and oblique sagittal images. **(B)** Oblique sagittal T1-weighted MR arthrogram in another patient demonstrates the location of an anterosuperior labral tear *(arrow)* on this sequence. Oblique sagittal images are generated tangential to the femoral neck on coronal images.

Paralabral
cyst

Neck extending
to labrum

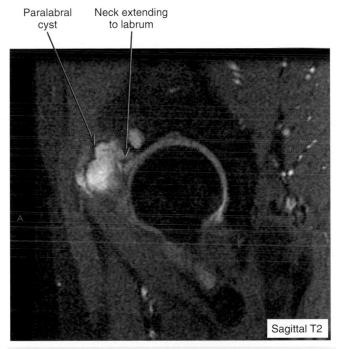

Sagittal T2

Fig. 5.38 Labral tear with paralabral cyst. Sagittal T2-weighted MR image shows lobulated fluid adjacent to the anterior acetabular rim, with a neck extending to the torn anterior labrum. This communication helps differentiate a paralabral cyst from iliopsoas bursitis or a ganglion cyst originating from the joint capsule. Paralabral cysts are almost invariably associated with labral tear and usually are lobulated if large. (From Morrison W. *Problem Solving in Musculoskeletal Imaging.* Philadelphia: Elsevier; 2010.)

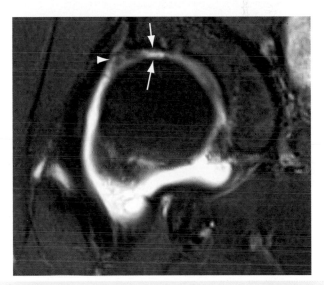

Fig. 5.39 Hip joint articular cartilage defects. Coronal fat-suppressed T1-weighted MR arthrogram shows matching chondral defects in the acetabulum and femoral head *(arrows)*. Note adjacent labral tear *(arrowhead).*

FEMOROACETABULAR IMPINGEMENT

- Femoroacetabular Impingement (FAI) is impingement of the acetabular labrum and adjacent articular cartilage between the femur head–neck junction and the acetabular rim. The impingement leads to labral tear and degeneration of adjacent articular cartilage (Fig. 5.40), eventually leading to osteoarthritis.
- Clinically: hip pain especially during leg flexion and internal rotation; sitting for long periods.
- Caused by a mismatch in the ball/cup morphology of the hip joint: a nonspherical femoral head or a deep acetabular cup.
- Nonspherical femoral head can be caused by *cam* morphology: osseous prominence at the femoral head–neck junction, typically lateral or anterolateral.
    - Referred to as *cam-type FAI.*
        - 'Cam' refers to the asymmetric shape of lobes on a camshaft of a motor vehicle engine (Fig. 5.41).

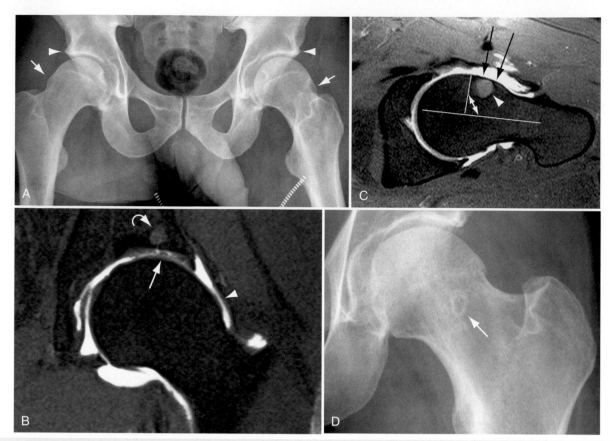

Fig. 5.40 Femoroacetabular impingement (FAI). **(A)** AP radiograph shows dysmorphic overgrowth of both anterior superior femoral head–neck junctions *(arrows)*. These act like the lobe (bulge) of a cam when the hip is flexed or internally rotated. Also note the upsloping lateral acetabular margins *(arrowheads)*, a finding that has been reported to be associated with FAI, although this is controversial. **(B)** Coronal fat-suppressed T1-weighted MR arthrogram shows obvious lateral osseous prominence of the femoral head *(arrowhead)* in a patient with cam impingement. Note the chondral defect of the acetabular roof *(straight arrow)* and the acetabular subchondral cyst *(curved arrow)*. There was a large anterosuperior labral tear (not shown). **(C)** Oblique axial fat-suppressed T1-weighted MR arthrogram in a different patient. The image is parallel to the femoral neck. Note the anterior cam-like bulge *(arrows)*. Other images (not shown) found an anterior superior labral tear. Also note the intermediate-signal-intensity synovial herniation pit *(arrowhead)*, which some authors believe is associated with FAI. **(D)** Herniation pit in a different patient with cam-type FAI. AP hip radiograph shows small lucent region surrounded by a thin sclerotic rim in the anterior femoral neck *(arrow)*.

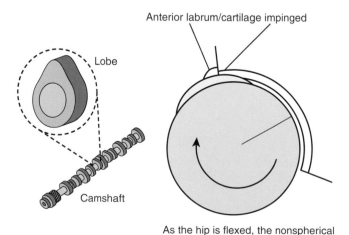

Fig. 5.41 Mechanism of cam impingement. A nonspherical femoral head with focal osseous prominence at the head–neck junction can compress the anterosuperior labrum during hip flexion. The shape of the femoral head in this situation resembles the lobe of a camshaft in a car engine. (From Morrison W. *Problem Solving in Musculoskeletal Imaging*. Philadelphia: Elsevier; 2010.)

- Can occur with displacement of the femoral head relative to the femoral neck similar to deformity resulting from SCFE.
  - Also called *gun type* since proximal femur looks like an old flintlock gun (Fig. 5.42).
- Can occur without femoral head displacement.
- Note that these 'bumps' are not osteophytes—cartilage is intact initially.
  - An osteophyte acquired later in life can act as a cam.
- Loss of normal concavity at the lateral femoral neck.
- Osseous prominence can be best seen on frog lateral radiographs and cross-sectional imaging.
- 'Bump' contacts anterior acetabular rim on hip flexion (i.e., sitting) (Fig. 5.43).
- Can occur as sequala of childhood disease.
  - *Legg–Calve–Perthes disease* (also known as *Legg-Perthes*, osteonecrosis of the femoral head during childhood) can lead to deformity and a nonspherical femoral head (Fig. 5.44) Legg-Perthes is discussed further in Chapter 15.
  - *SCFE* (previously discussed).

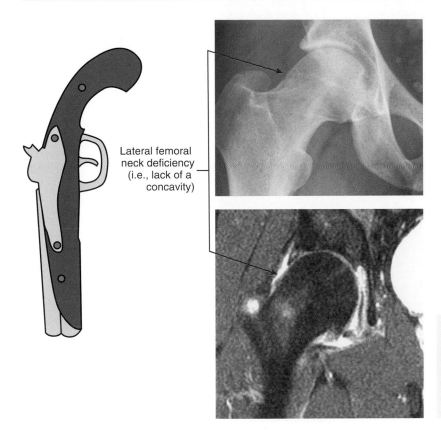

Lateral femoral neck deficiency (i.e., lack of a concavity)

Fig. 5.42 'Gun type' cam impingement. This morphology is medial offset of the femoral head relative to the neck, leading to straightening or convexity of the lateral femoral neck. The appearance has been likened to the shape of an old flintlock gun handle. The shape can predispose to femoral-acetabular impingement. (From Morrison W. *Problem Solving in Musculoskeletal Imaging*. Philadelphia: Elsevier; 2010.)

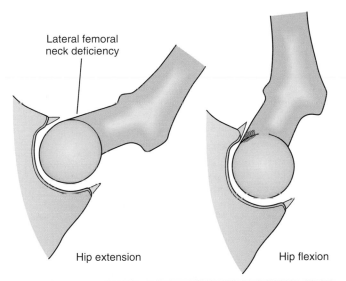

Lateral femoral neck deficiency

Hip extension   Hip flexion

Fig. 5.43 Gun-shaped cam impingement. Offset of the femoral head relative to the neck leads to 'deficiency' of the normal femoral head–neck concavity anteriorly and laterally. On hip flexion this can lead to impingement on the acetabular rim and labrum. (From Morrison W. *Problem Solving in Musculoskeletal Imaging*. Philadelphia: Elsevier; 2010.)

- Treated by surgically shaving down the osseous prominence (called femoroacetabular osteotomy, cheilectomy, or 'bumpectomy') (Fig. 5.45).
- 'Alpha angle' has been used to measure osseous deformity in cam-type FAI (Fig. 5.46).
    - Oblique axial MRI or CT (axial image prescribed along femoral neck).
    - Draw a circle exactly covering the femoral head.
- Draw a line through the center of the femoral neck to the center of the femoral head.
- Draw a line from the center of the femoral head to the point where bone leaves the femoral head circle.
- Measure angle between the two lines = alpha angle.
- Symptomatic FAI: average approximately 70 degrees.
- Normal is considered to be less than 55 degrees*.
    - *High level of measurement variability and location of osseous prominence has made measurement of alpha angle very controversial—limited usefulness.
- FAI can also be caused by a developmentally deep acetabular cup (increased center-edge angle).
    - Also called *pincer impingement* or *pincer-type FAI*.
    - Can lead to labral tear, anterior and posterior cartilage damage, and eventual osteoarthritis.
    - Deep acetabular cup represents a spectrum.
        - *Coxa profunda*: On an AP pelvis radiograph the medial wall of the acetabulum extends medial to the ilioischial line (Figs. 5.47 and 5.48).
        - Protrusio acetabulae: On an AP pelvis radiograph the medial wall of the acetabulum extends medial to the iliopectineal line; may be developmental or related to bone softening disorders such as osteomalacia, or chronic inflammatory arthropathies such as rheumatoid arthritis (Fig. 5.49).
- Retroversion of the acetabulum can also cause FAI (Figs. 5.50 and 5.51).
    - Anterior border of the acetabulum contacts the femoral neck during hip flexion.
    - Potentially as 'figure of eight' or 'infinity' sign on AP pelvis radiograph (crossover of the anterior and posterior acetabular lines), discussed earlier.

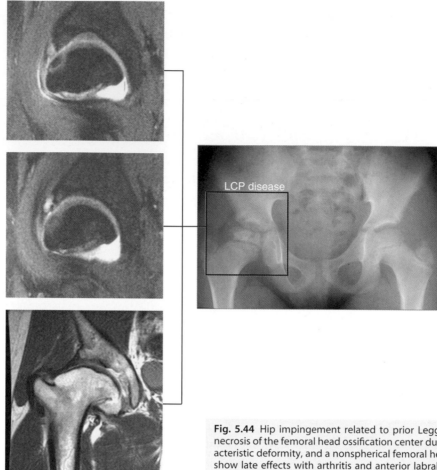

Fig. 5.44 Hip impingement related to prior Legg–Perthes (LCP) disease. Avascular necrosis of the femoral head ossification center during development resulted in characteristic deformity, and a nonspherical femoral head in adulthood. MRI (left images) show late effects with arthritis and anterior labral tear. A different, younger patient with Perthes disease is shown on an AP radiograph on the right. (From Morrison W. *Problem Solving in Musculoskeletal Imaging.* Philadelphia: Elsevier; 2010.)

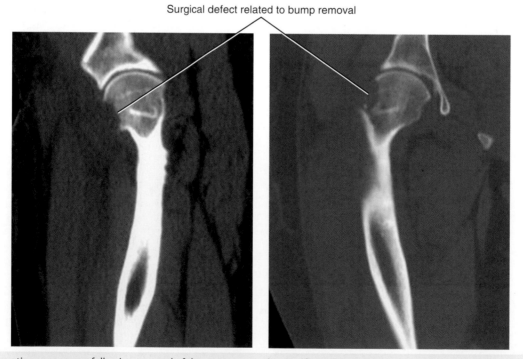

Fig. 5.45 Postoperative appearance following removal of the osseous prominence ('bump') at the anterolateral femoral head–neck junction that has been implicated in impingement. (From Morrison W. *Problem Solving in Musculoskeletal Imaging.* Philadelphia: Elsevier; 2010.)

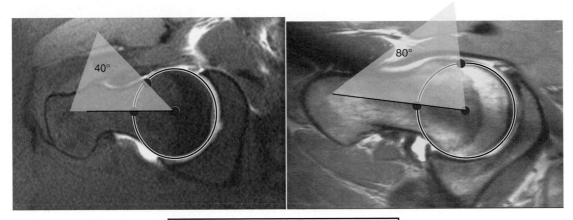

Normal and abnormal values
Control group (no FAI):   avg 42 ±2.2 degrees
FAI group: avg 74 ±5.4 degrees

Fig. 5.46 Alpha angle: Examples of normal and abnormal measurement. Usually the bump is easily seen, but surgeons may request reporting of the angle. The alpha angle is measured off an oblique axial image oriented along the femoral neck. A circle is drawn around the femoral head and a point is marked where the cortex leaves the circle anteriorly. The angle between this point and the center of the femoral neck is the alpha angle. *FAI*, femoral-acetabular impingement. (Data from Nötzli HP, Wyss TF, Stoecklin CH, et al. The contour of the femoral head-neck junction as a predictor for the risk of anterior impingement. *J Bone Joint Surg Br.* 2002;84:556-560.) (From Morrison W. *Problem Solving in Musculoskeletal Imaging.* Philadelphia: Elsevier; 2010.)

AP pelvis hip detail

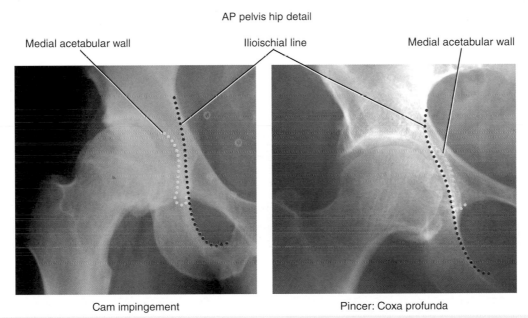

Fig. 5.47 Coxa profunda (deep acetabulum). The hip in the left image shows osseous prominence at the femoral head–neck junction which is associated with cam-type femoroacetabular impingement. Note that on a well-positioned AP view of the pelvis, the medial acetabular wall *(yellow line)* lies lateral to the ilioischial line *(red line)*. The hip in the right image shows acetabular over-coverage with a deep acetabular socket, referred to as coxa profunda. In coxa profunda the medial acetabular wall *(yellow line)* lies medial to the ilioischial line *(red line)*. Coxa profunda is associated with pincer-type femoroacetabular impingement. In more severe cases, protrusio acetabuli (inward bowing of the iliopectineal line) is seen. (From Morrison W. *Problem Solving in Musculoskeletal Imaging.* Philadelphia: Elsevier; 2010.)

- Acetabular causes for FAI can be treated surgically with acetabular osteotomy and labral repair with suture anchors.
- Findings that can be associated with FAI:
  - *Synovial herniation pits* ('Pitt's pits') at the anterior femoral neck (see Fig. 5.40).
  - *Os acetabuli:* ossification, usually at the anterolateral acetabulum.
  - Upsloping of lateral acetabular roof.

- All of these findings may be seen in asymptomatic individuals.

Key Points—*Differences in cam- and pincer-type FAI*

Cam-type FAI.
- Males >> females = 13:1.
- Age of presentation: 20s–30s.
- Anterosuperior labral and cartilage damage.

Deep acetabulum
(coxa profunda)

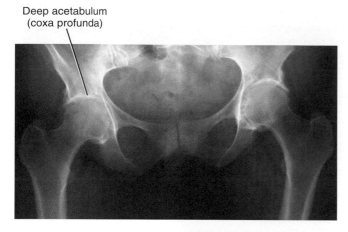

Pincer effect: Overhanging
edges of acetabular rim can
impinge on femoral neck

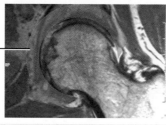

Fig. 5.48 Coxa profunda resulting in pincer-type femoroacetabular impingement. (From Morrison W. *Problem Solving in Musculoskeletal Imaging*. Philadelphia: Elsevier; 2010.)

Protrusio
acetabuli

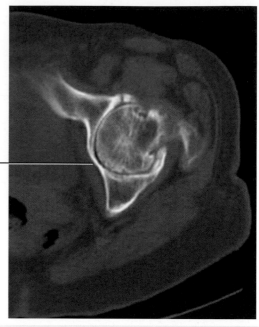

Fig. 5.49 Protrusio acetabuli. On this axial CT of the hip. Note convexity of the medial wall related to a deep acetabular socket, referred to as protrusio acetabuli (basically a more extreme form of coxa profunda). This can be associated with pincer-type femoroacetabular impingement. Secondary osteoarthritis is present with diffuse joint narrowing and overhanging marginal osteophytes. Protrusio acetabuli can be developmental, but is occasionally acquired, related to bone softening disorders such as Paget disease, renal osteodystrophy/osteomalacia, and chronic inflammatory arthropathies such as rheumatoid arthritis. (From Morrison W. *Problem Solving in Musculoskeletal Imaging*. Philadelphia: Elsevier; 2010.)

Acetabular retroversion
AP view of the pelvis:
Anterior (red) and posterior (blue)
acetabular lines make a figure-of-eight

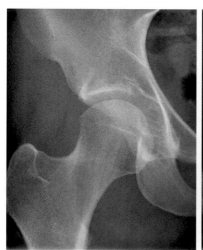
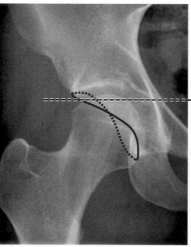
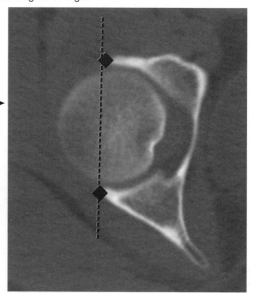

Relative retroversion of acetabulum

Fig. 5.50 Acetabular retroversion on anteroposterior (AP) pelvis radiograph and CT. The normal acetabulum 'opens' anteriorly; axial CT image (on right) shows relative retroversion, as the anterior acetabular rim *(red diamond)* is not medial to the posterior rim *(blue diamond)*. Right hip detail from an AP pelvis radiograph shows an 'infinity' sign or 'figure of eight' sign, with the anterior acetabular wall *(red line)* and posterior wall *(blue line)* crossing over each other. This finding is associated with abnormal acetabular retroversion but is not highly reliable. (From Morrison W. *Problem Solving in Musculoskeletal Imaging*. Philadelphia: Elsevier; 2010.)

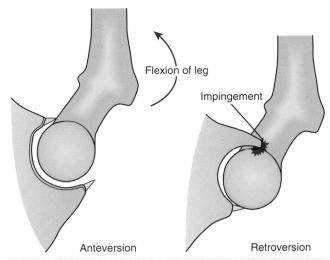

Fig. 5.51 How acetabular retroversion is associated with impingement. An overhanging edge anteriorly or bone deficiency posteriorly results in relative posterior tilt of the acetabular cup (retroversion). This prominence anteriorly can impinge on the femoral neck during flexion of the hip. (From Morrison W. *Problem Solving in Musculoskeletal Imaging.* Philadelphia: Elsevier; 2010.)

Pincer-type FAI.

- Females > males = 3:1.
- Age of presentation: 40s.
- Anterosuperior labral degeneration and tear.
- Anterior and posterior cartilage damage (contra-coup effect; during flexion acetabulum impinges on anterior femoral neck, head is driven posteriorly).

Other Causes of FAI.

- Other mechanical issues can accentuate effects of FAI:
  - Excess lordosis tilts pelvis anteriorly.
  - Coxa valga/vara.
  - Abnormal femoral torsion.
  - Activity with excess hip flexion/internal rotation.

Acetabular Dysplasia.

- Acetabular dysplasia refers to a developmentally small or shallow acetabulum.
- Can be a sequela of childhood developmental dysplasia, discussed in Chapter 15. Also commonly seen in ballet dancers.
- Seen on radiographs as:
  - Uncovering of the lateral femoral head (decreased center-edge angle).
  - Upturn of the lateral acetabular roof on a frontal radiograph.
- Dysplasia results in altered mechanics with excess stress at the lateral acetabular rim.
  - Early superior labral degeneration and tearing (Fig. 5.52).
  - Articular cartilage damage and joint space narrowing superolaterally.
- Secondary osteoarthritis is common and can occur in early adulthood (Fig. 5.53).
- Variations include isolated anterior acetabular dysplasia and isolated posterior dysplasia (retroversion).
- Anterior acetabular dysplasia can be diagnosed on false-profile hip radiographs (Fig. 5.54).

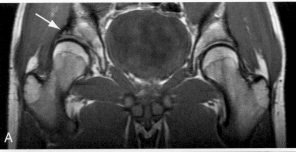
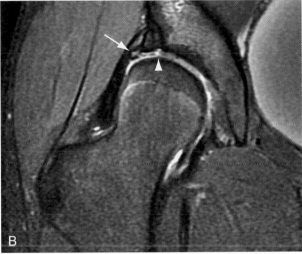

Fig. 5.52 Hip dysplasia with labral tear and cartilage damage. **(A)** Coronal T1-weighted MR image shows acetabular dysplasia with uncovering of the lateral femoral articular surface and coxa valga. Note cystic changes in the lateral acetabular rim *(arrow)*. **(B)** Coronal fat-suppressed intermediate-weighted MR image in same patient shows superior labral tear *(arrow)* and adjacent chondral defect *(arrowhead)*.

- Dysplasia can coexist with cam morphology to cause combined pathology.

Key Concepts—*Findings Associated With Femoroacetabular Impingement*

Cam-type FAI.

- Osseous prominence at the anterolateral femoral head–neck junction (best seen on frog lateral view).
- Lack of concavity at the lateral femoral neck junction.
- Anterosuperior labral tear and articular cartilage damage.

Pincer-type FAI.

- Medial wall of acetabulum extends beyond ilioischial line (coxa profunda) or iliopectineal line (protrusio acetabuli).

Acetabular retroversion

- Crossover of anterior and posterior acetabular lines on radiography ('figure of eight' or 'infinity' sign, not highly reliable).
- More reliably diagnosed with CT or MRI.

General associated findings:

- Anterosuperior labral tear.
- Anterior and posterior cartilage damage.
- Os acetabuli.
- Synovial herniation pit.

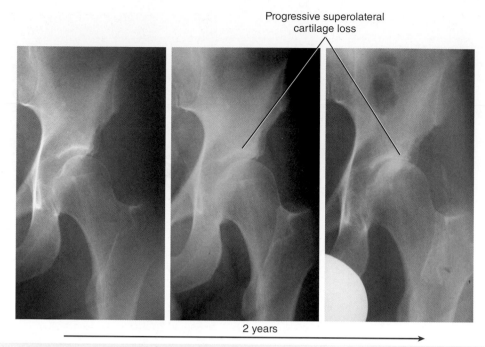

Progressive superolateral
cartilage loss

2 years

Fig. 5.53 Hip dysplasia in a young adult patient with development of osteoarthritis over a 2-year follow-up period. Note cartilage loss is superolateral, related to altered mechanics from acetabular undercoverage. (Courtesy of Javad Parvizi, MD, Philadelphia. From Morrison W. *Problem Solving in Musculoskeletal Imaging*. Philadelphia: Elsevier; 2010.)

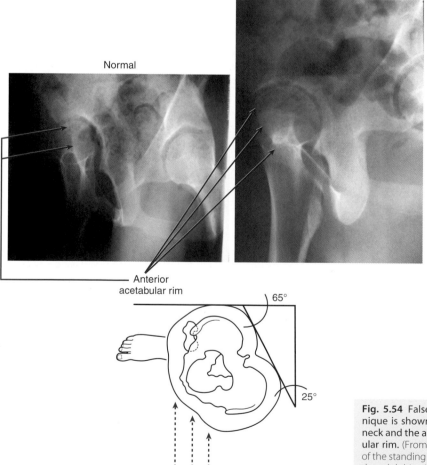

Retroversion

Normal

Anterior
acetabular rim

65°

25°

Fig. 5.54 False-profile view (faux profile). Proper radiographic technique is shown below. This special view profiles the anterior femoral neck and the anterior acetabular rim. *Red arrows* show anterior acetabular rim. (From Lequesne MG, Laredo JD. The faux profile [oblique view] of the standing position. Contribution to the evaluation of osteoarthritis of the adult hip. *Ann Rheum Dis*. 1998;57[11]:676-681. Reproduced with permission from BMJ Publishing Group.) From Morrison W. *Problem Solving in Musculoskeletal Imaging*. Philadelphia: Elsevier; 2010.

Findings Associated With Acetabular Dysplasia

- Uncovering of the lateral femoral head.
- Upturn of the lateral acetabular rim.
- Lateral joint space narrowing.
- Superior labral degeneration and tear.

*Note that many of these morphologic findings associated with FAI and are often seen in asymptomatic individuals.

AIIS AND SUBSPINE IMPINGEMENT

- Anterior inferior iliac spine (AIIS) impingement occurs when a low-lying or enlarged anterior inferior iliac spine contacts the femoral neck with hip flexion; it is a type of extraarticular hip impingement.
  - The AIIS is immediately superior to the anterior acetabular rim.
  - The rectus femoris (direct head) and the iliocapsularis muscle of the hip joint capsule attach in this location.
  - Healed avulsion of the rectus femoris tendon can lead to enlargement of the AIIS (see Fig. 5.8C).
  - Bony prominence can also occur at the attachment of the iliocapsularis muscle.
- Subspine impingement may coexist with AIIS impingement, but some authors consider it a separate pathology from true AIIS impingement.
  - Bony ridging between the acetabular rim and the caudad border of the AIIS, resulting in soft tissue and/or bony impingement on hip flexion.
  - Subspine location is the attachment site of the anterior fibers of the hip joint capsule.
  - Bony prominence may develop from excessive and recurrent tension of the iliofemoral ligament and the anterior hip capsule during athletic activity.
- Symptoms of AIIS and subspine impingement can simulate cam- or pincer-type FAI.
- As with FAI, predisposing anatomy occurs frequently in asymptomatic individuals.
- Cross-sectional imaging (MRI, CT) is helpful for definition of anatomy, as well as false-profile radiographic view (a 25-degree shallow oblique lateral view).

ISCHIOFEMORAL IMPINGEMENT

- Another form of extraarticular impingement at the hip, ischiofemoral impingement occurs when the ischium is in close proximity to the lesser trochanter; edema and bursitis can be seen in the intervening soft tissues, as well as adjacent muscle edema (Fig. 5.55).
- In more chronic cases bone proliferation and sclerosis can be seen, with bone remodeling, creating a 'facet' between the two bones, (similar to a pseudarthrosis).
- MRI is the test of choice to show the soft tissue changes. MRI, radiographs, and CT can detect the osseous production present in advanced cases.
- Radiologists should have a high index of suspicion for this condition when the patient has hip pain, especially during internal/external rotation with the leg in adduction.

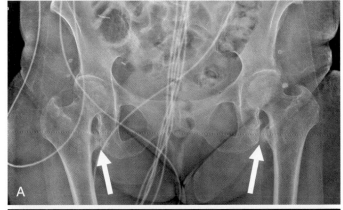

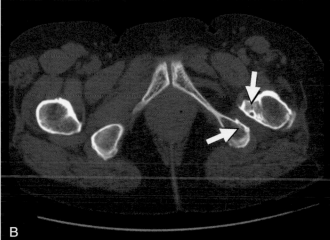

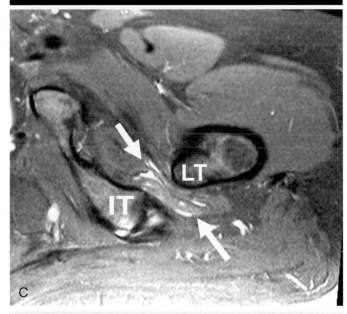

Fig. 5.55 Ischiofemoral impingement. **(A)** Frontal radiograph of the pelvis shows bony prominence at the lesser trochanter and ischial tuberosity bilaterally *(arrows)* with sclerosis in a patient with ischiofemoral impingement. **(B)** Axial CT of the lower pelvis in a different patient showing bony prominence, sclerosis, and cystic changes associated with close proximity of the lesser trochanter and ischial tuberosity *(arrows)* on the left. **(C)** Axial T2-weighted fat-suppressed MR image in a different patient shows less severe involvement without bone production, but with edema and fluid signal *(arrows)* between the lesser trochanter (LT) and ischial tuberosity (IT).

Muscle/Tendon Injury

- The musculotendinous complexes of the pelvic girdle are frequent sites of strain and tear (see Figs. 1.53 and 1.54).
- The thigh is a frequent site of muscle hematoma and myositis ossificans owing to the large size of thigh muscles and the frequent occurrence of blunt trauma to this region (see Figs. 1.56 and 1.57).

HAMSTRING INJURY

- The hamstring muscles (semitendinosus, semimembranosus, and biceps femoris) originate from two attachments at the ischial tuberosity (biceps and semitendinosus from a conjoined origin inferomedially, and the semimembranosus from a separate origin superolaterally).
    - Distally the biceps femoris joins with the fibular collateral ligament of the knee to form the 'conjoined tendon', inserting on the fibular head.
    - The semimembranosus inserts on the posteromedial aspect of the proximal tibia near the joint line.
    - The semitendinosus extends around the medial knee, inserting on the pes anserinus along with the sartorius, gracilis, and medial collateral ligament.
- The hamstring muscles often undergo eccentric contraction (contraction during elongation) during sports (especially with rapid stopping and starting). Eccentric contraction increases the risk of strain in athletes (Fig. 5.56).

- In adolescents the attachment at the growing ischial apophysis can avulse leading to osseous irregularity or overgrowth and prominence of the ischium upon healing (see Fig. 5.8).
- Hamstring injuries can occur at the origin, ranging from interstitial tears and partial tears to complete tears with retraction and hematoma.
- The sciatic nerve courses by the proximal hamstring tendons and muscles which can lead to nerve-related symptoms.
- The myotendinous junction proximally or distally is another common site for injury.
- Tears can also occur within the muscle belly, or at the distal attachments.
- The variety of injures and locations results in difficulty of clinical diagnosis; MRI is the test of choice for assessing extent of injury and for predicting return to play for an athlete.

ADDUCTOR ORIGIN INJURY (ATHLETIC PUBALGIA/CORE MUSCLE INJURY)

- Formerly called 'sports hernia', 'sportsman's hernia', and 'Gilmore's groin'.
- Injury is much more common in males (male:female = 10:1).
- Pubalgia is a sports injury, seen in a variety of contact and noncontact activities, especially football, hockey, baseball, and soccer.

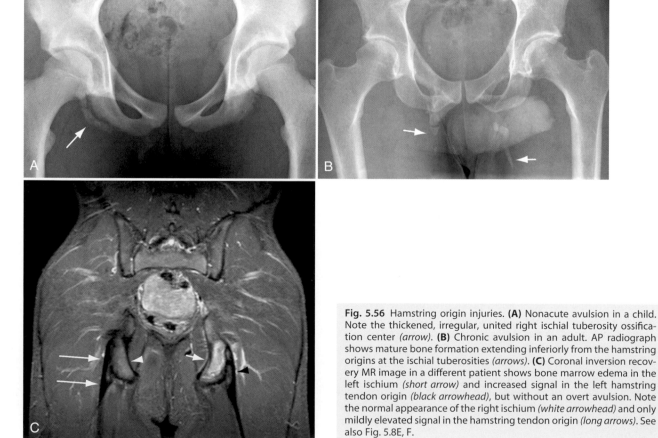

Fig. 5.56 Hamstring origin injuries. **(A)** Nonacute avulsion in a child. Note the thickened, irregular, united right ischial tuberosity ossification center *(arrow)*. **(B)** Chronic avulsion in an adult. AP radiograph shows mature bone formation extending inferiorly from the hamstring origins at the ischial tuberosities *(arrows)*. **(C)** Coronal inversion recovery MR image in a different patient shows bone marrow edema in the left ischium *(short arrow)* and increased signal in the left hamstring tendon origin *(black arrowhead)*, but without an overt avulsion. Note the normal appearance of the right ischium *(white arrowhead)* and only mildly elevated signal in the hamstring tendon origin *(long arrows)*. See also Fig. 5.8E, F.

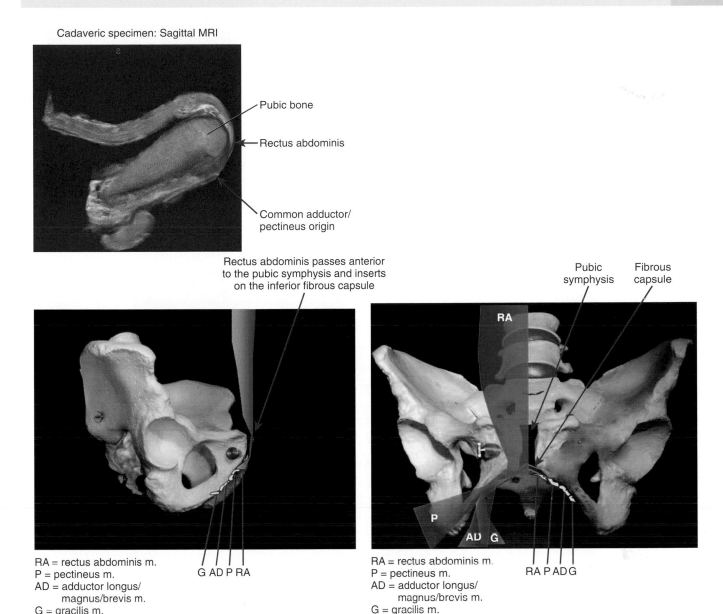

Cadaveric specimen: Sagittal MRI

Pubic bone

Rectus abdominis

Common adductor/
pectineus origin

Rectus abdominis passes anterior
to the pubic symphysis and inserts
on the inferior fibrous capsule

Pubic symphysis   Fibrous capsule

RA = rectus abdominis m.
P = pectineus m.
AD = adductor longus/
  magnus/brevis m.
G = gracilis m.

G AD P RA

RA = rectus abdominis m.
P = pectineus m.
AD = adductor longus/
  magnus/brevis m.
G = gracilis m.

RA P AD G

Fig. 5.57 Anatomy of the common rectus/adductor aponeurosis. *AD*, adductor longus/magnus/brevis muscles. Corresponding MRI of a cadaveric specimen shown at the top, with rectus abdominis muscle reflected back. (From Morrison W. *Problem Solving in Musculoskeletal Imaging*. Philadelphia: Elsevier; 2010.)

- Clinically, pubalgia can simulate a hernia; pain radiates to external inguinal ring, and pressure on the inguinal ring elicits pain. However, no hernia is palpable.
- The injury is centered at the rectus abdominis tendon and adductor tendon origin (the adductor longus, magnus, and brevis share a common origin) which together form an aponeurosis (the rectus-adductor aponeurosis) that attaches to the anterior capsule-ligamentous complex of the pubic symphysis (Fig. 5.57).
- Injury typically begins as a separation of the rectus-adductor aponeurosis from the anterior capsule of the pubic symphysis (Fig. 5.58).
  - Tear causes fluid to extend out of the pubic symphysis into the aponeurosis (the 'cleft sign', discussed below).
  - With more severe injury, the tear extends into the adductor origin and rectus abdominis attachment.

- Adductor origin can pull off from the pubis completely with retraction (Fig. 5.59).
- Injury is often bilateral (Fig. 5.60).
- Variation of injury: strain of the adductor longus muscle belly ('hockey goalie—baseball catcher syndrome').
- Chronic injury can lead to muscle atrophy, best seen on T1-weighted MRI with decreased muscle size and/or fatty infiltration.
- The pubic symphysis can be a source of athletic pubalgia pain.
  - Acute presentation: '*osteitis pubis*'—diffuse bone marrow edema on both sides of the joint; bone resorption; associated with injury to the capsule-ligamentous complex and the rectus-adductor aponeurosis. May represent a subchondral stress injury (Fig. 5.61). Sagittally oriented low-signal stress fracture lines are seen in some advanced cases.

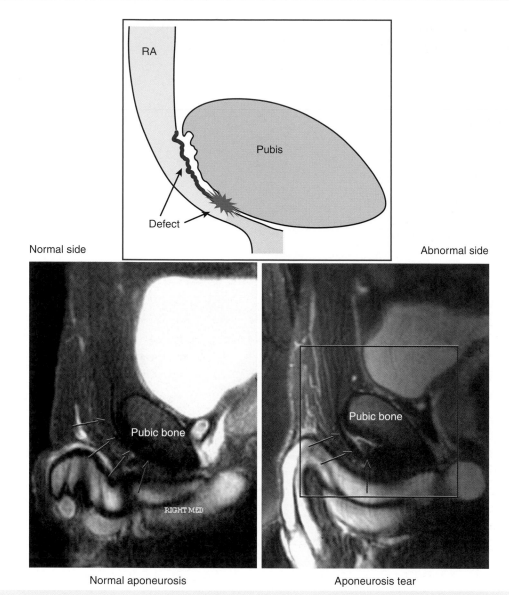

Normal side   Abnormal side

Normal aponeurosis   Aponeurosis tear

Fig. 5.58 Athletic pubalgia (core injury). The rectus abdominis tendon *(red arrows)* passes anteriorly over the pubic bone, joining with the common adductor tendon origin. This common rectus-adductor aponeurosis *(red arrows)* is invested into the ligamentous capsule of the anterior pubic symphysis. Injury can manifest as stripping of the aponeurosis from the pubis (shown on MRI on the right, and diagrammatically above) and eventually avulsion from the bone and capsule. *RA*, rectus abdominis. (From Morrison W. *Problem Solving in Musculoskeletal Imaging*. Philadelphia: Elsevier; 2010.)

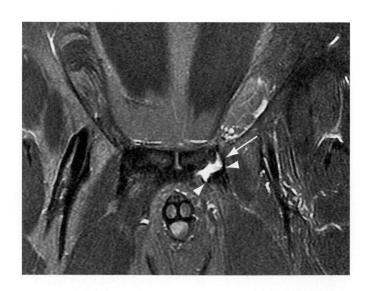

Fig. 5.59 Athletic pubalgia in an elite soccer player. Coronal fat-suppressed T2-weighted MR image centered at the symphysis pubis shows large left adductor origin tear. The *arrow* indicates a small hematoma in the tendon gap, and the *arrowheads* indicate the free margin of the retracted tendon.

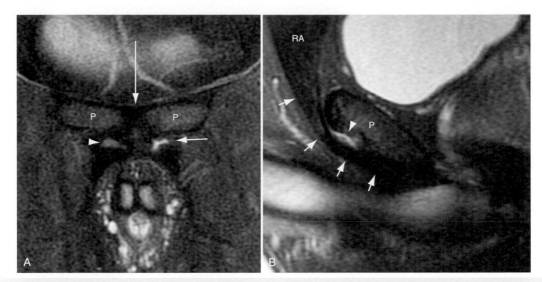

Fig. 5.60 Bilateral adductor longus origin tears. (A) Coronal fat-suppressed T2-weighted image shows transverse high-signal clefts at the bilateral adductor longus origins, milder on the right *(arrowhead)* than the left *(short arrow)*. *Long arrow* marks the symphysis pubis. *P,* Medial superior right and left pubic bones. (B) Sagittal image through the left tear *(arrowhead)*. Note how the low-signal rectus abdominis tendon and the adductor origin tendons blend in a continuous band draped over the anterior pubic bone cortex *(short arrows)*. *P,* Medial left pubic bone; *RA,* distal rectus abdominis muscle.

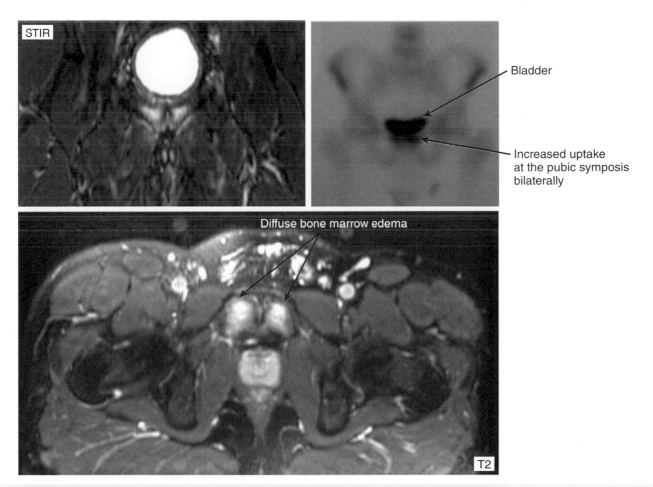

Fig. 5.61 Osteitis pubis. Diffuse bone marrow edema on MRI (and uptake of radiotracer on bone scan, upper right) is often associated with core injury; findings can represent stress response at the joint, or in later stages, osteoarthritis. (From Morrison W. *Problem Solving in Musculoskeletal Imaging.* Philadelphia: Elsevier; 2010.)

- Chronic: osteoarthritis (spurs, sclerosis at the pubic symphysis).

ABDUCTOR INJURY

- The major abductors of the hip are the gluteus medius and minimus muscles. The tensor fasciae latae muscles also play a minor role in hip abduction.
- The gluteus minimus and medius muscles originate from the superior lateral iliac bone, with the medius muscle more superficial than the minimus. Both insert on the greater trochanter of the femur, minimus more anterior and lateral and medius more posterior and medial.
- The tensor fasciae latae is superficial to both, passing over the greater trochanter, extending down the lateral thigh as the iliotibial band, past the knee joint to insert on Gerdy's tubercle at the anterolateral tibia.
- Tendinosis and tears of the gluteus medius and minimus tendons are especially common on older individuals (as opposed to most other tendon injuries at the hip/pelvis which are mainly seen in athletes).
  - Clinically, this is a common cause of 'greater trochanteric pain syndrome'.
  - Partial and complete tears are associated with adjacent edema and fluid in adjacent greater trochanteric or subguteal bursae on US and MRI (Fig. 5.62).

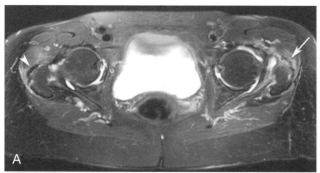

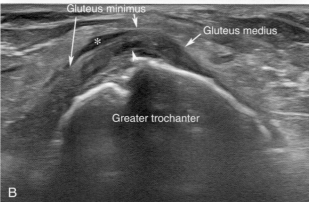

Fig. 5.62 Abductor tendinopathy. **(A)** Gluteus minimus partial tear. Axial T2-weighted MR image with fat suppression. Note the edema in the distal left gluteus minimus tendon *(arrow)* and adjacent soft tissue edema. Contrast with the normal right tendon *(arrowhead)*. **(B)** Ultrasound in a different patient. Axial image. Anterior is to the viewer's left, posterior to the right, and lateral is at the top of the image. The gluteus minimus tendon is thickened and hyperechoic, with a hypoechoic interstitial tear *(arrowhead)*, and adjacent fluid *(asterisk)*. The gluteus medius shows much milder tendinopathy and is mildly hyperechoic.

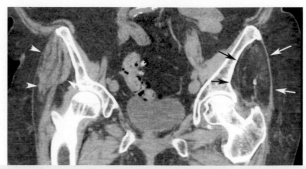

Fig. 5.63 Chronic adductor injuries. CT coronal reconstruction. Note the fatty atrophy of the left gluteus medius and minimus muscles *(arrows)* due to chronic tendon tears. Contrast with the normal muscles on the right *(arrowheads)*.

- Chronic tears can lead to muscle atrophy (Fig. 5.63).
- These muscles are needed to stand on one leg, and to balance the body during walking. Atrophy results in weakness, Trendelenburg gait, and predispose to falls in the elderly.
- Abductor tears can also be a complication of hip replacement surgery (especially using a lateral approach).
- Abductor tendon tear can be suspected if the patient presents with sudden onset of lateral hip pain and weakness when standing on one foot.
- In athletes with tightening of the tensor fasciae latae, a friction syndrome can occur at the grater trochanteric bursa. This is associated with iliotibial band friction syndrome at the knee.
  - Especially common in runners and cyclists.
  - Edema and fluid are present in the greater trochanteric bursa.

HIP FLEXOR INJURY

- The major hip flexors include the rectus femoris, the sartorius, and the iliopsoas.
  - The rectus femoris has two origins:
    - The direct head originates from the AIIS, just above the hip joint.
    - The indirect head originates more posterolaterally and joins with the direct head as it passes in front of the hip.
    - The muscle courses along the anterior thigh, and along with the vastus medialis, intermedius and lateralis form the quadriceps tendon, attaching to the superior patella.
  - Injury can occur in adults but is most common in adolescent athletes presenting as avulsion of the AIIS (See Figs. 1.18B and 5.8C).
- The sartorius originates from the ASIS and the shallow concavity below the ASIS and courses along the medial thigh to insert on the pes anserinus at the knee.
  - Injury can present in adolescence as an avulsion of the ASIS (see Fig. 5.8A, B), or as a tear of the tendon or muscle in adulthood.
  - Injury to the tendon or proximal muscle can lead to damage to the adjacent lateral femoral cutaneous nerve, leading to a clinical syndrome called *meralgia paresthetica* (anterior thigh skin numbness).

- The iliacus and psoas muscles form the iliopsoas, inserting on the lesser trochanter.
  - As earlier, avulsion from this attachment is highly associated with an underlying bone lesion including metastasis or myeloma.

BURSITIS

- Tendons around the hip and pelvis have bursae that cushion the attachment and to allow smooth gliding of adjacent tissues. They are named for their associated tendon or location. Most are not associated with symptoms. However, focal fluid signal around a tendon attachment should suggest bursitis, typically a secondary findings of adjacent tendon pathology.
- Bursitis may be a primary process or secondary to adjacent tendon or other pathology.
- Bursal anatomy around the hip is variable. Some patients have several bursae, and some have none. Bursae are more common in older patients.
- Some bursae around the hip/pelvis are recognized as a source of symptoms:
  - *Greater trochanteric bursitis* (Fig. 5.64).
    - The greater trochanteric bursa lies superficial to the gluteus medius attachment on the greater trochanter, deep to the tensor fasciae latae muscle.
    - Inflammation of the bursa is associated with localized pain over the lateral hip, presenting clinically as *greater trochanteric pain syndrome*.

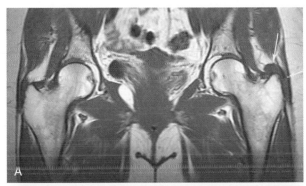
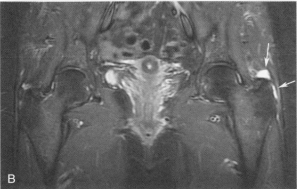

Fig. 5.64 Trochanteric bursitis. Coronal T1-weighted **(A)** and STIR **(B)** images show a fluid collection adjacent to the proximal left greater trochanter *(arrows)*. Gluteus medius and/or minimus tendinopathy is a potential cause of fluid accumulation at this site, which warrants careful evaluation of these tendons. In this case the tendons appeared normal and the presumptive diagnosis was bursitis, perhaps due to mechanical irritation.

- As noted earlier, fluid in the bursa can be a sign of adjacent tendon pathology. In older patients there is usually a partial or complete tear of the gluteus medius and/or gluteus minimus tendon at their greater trochanteric attachment. Fluid may track proximally along the involved tendon, beyond the expected confines of the bursa.
- In younger patients with lateral hip pain, fluid in the bursa can be due to friction from the overlying tensor fasciae latae. This is seen in patients with tight lateral fascia and is associated with iliotibial band friction syndrome at the knee as well as excessive lateral pressure syndrome that can result in lateral patellar maltracking.
- Between the gluteus medius and minimus tendons there are subgluteal bursae. These can also exhibit fluid due inflammation or underlying tendon tear.
  - *Iliopsoas bursitis* (Fig. 5.65).
    - The iliopsoas bursa almost completely surrounds the iliopsoas tendon from above the hip joint to the insertion on the lesser trochanter.
    - Bursitis can result from friction of the tendon across the anterior acetabulum.
    - Fluid in the bursa can also be seen with hip joint effusion, since the bursa has been reported to communicate with the joint in 15% of individuals. Therefore, visualizing fluid in the bursa (like a Baker cyst at the knee) should prompt review of the hip joint for underlying pathology.
  - *Obturator externus bursitis.*
    - Fluid in this bursa, located between the lesser trochanter and the ischium, has been associated with ischiofemoral impingement.

PIRIFORMIS SYNDROME

- Piriformis syndrome is gluteal pain that radiates in an L5 or S1 distribution caused by irritation of the sciatic nerve as it courses between the small hip external rotator muscles posterior to the femoral neck.
- Causes are numerous and include mass, piriformis muscle hypertrophy, trauma, and aberrant course of the sciatic nerve through or around the piriformis. CT or MRI may show a mass, asymmetric muscle atrophy, or subtle inflammatory changes around the sciatic nerve.

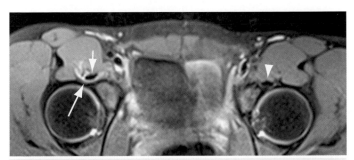

Fig. 5.65 Iliopsoas bursitis. Axial fat-suppressed MR image shows small U-shaped right iliopsoas effusion *(long arrow)*. Note the normal right *(short arrow)* and left *(arrowhead)* iliopsoas tendons. Bursal effusions vary in size and can be significantly larger than in this example.

MOREL-LAVALLEE LESION (FASCIAL DEGLOVING INJURY)

- Discussed in more detail in Chapter 1.
- Closed degloving injury in which subcutaneous fat is detached from the underlying muscle fascia.
- Shear injury, with the lateral hip and thigh being a common site (Fig. 5.66, see also Fig. 1.64).
- Potentially huge collections of blood, lymph, and debris can develop over time, as well as a secondary inflammatory reaction and capsule formation.
- Usually (but not always) shows acute angles at the fascial margin of the lesion, unlike a mass that exhibits rounded margins.

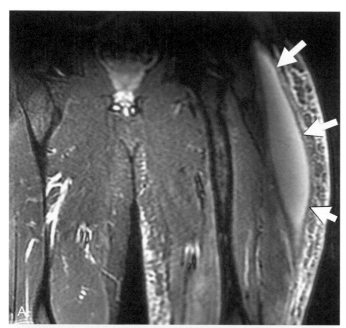

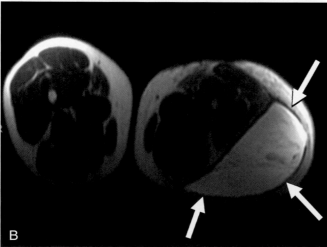

Fig. 5.66 Morel-Lavallée (closed fascial degloving) lesion in a patient with history of fall onto the side. **(A)** Coronal STIR MR image of the upper thigh shows a large, flat fluid collection *(arrows)* along the fascia of the vastus lateralis musculature. **(B)** Axial T2-weighted image of the same patient shows the large fluid collection *(arrows)* along the muscular fascia. See also Fig. 1.64.

Example Normal Hip Report Template

Exam Type: MRI HIP WITHOUT CONTRAST
Exam Date and Time: Date and Time
Indication: Clinical History
Comparison: Prior Studies

IMPRESSION: Impression

TECHNIQUE: MRI dedicated to the side hip was performed on a scanner-type system using a standard noncontrast protocol, including small field-of-view imaging of the affected hip in three planes (axial oblique, sagittal, and coronal), as well as large field-of-view imaging of the bony pelvis in two planes (axial and coronal).

FINDINGS:
SIDE HIP JOINT: Labrum: No labral tear by nonarthrogram MRI.
Cartilage: No chondrosis or focal cartilage defect.
Effusion: No hip joint effusion.
Femoroacetabular impingement (FAI): No cam- or pincer-type femoroacetabular impingement morphology. No acetabular dysplasia.

OSSEOUS STRUCTURES: Alignment is anatomic. No acute fracture or osseous stress response. No avascular necrosis in either femoral head. Background marrow signal is normal without infiltrative marrow process. No suspicious osseous lesions.

TENDONS and BURSAE: Common adductor tendon origins: Intact without tendinosis or tear.
Rectus femoris tendon origins: Intact without tendinosis or tear.
Iliopsoas tendons: Intact without tendinosis or tear.
Hamstring tendon origins: Intact without tendinosis or tear.
Gluteal tendons: Intact without tendinosis or tear.
Bursae: No greater trochanteric bursitis. No iliopsoas bursitis.

MUSCLES: No asymmetric muscle atrophy or acute muscle strains.

OTHER: Contralateral side hip joint: No joint effusion, secondary findings of labral tear, or osteoarthritis.
Sacroiliac joints: No sacroiliitis or joint effusion.
Pubic symphysis: No osteitis pubis.
Sciatic nerves: Symmetric in size and signal. Preserved perineural fat planes.
Ischiofemoral fossae: No narrowing of the ischiofemoral spaces. No edema in the quadratus femoris muscles.
Lower lumbar spine (only partially imaged): Unremarkable.
Pelvic viscera (only partially imaged): Unremarkable.

Appendix: Measurements of Acetabular Dysplasia and Femoroacetabular Impingement in Adolescents and Adults

Acetabular dysplasia and femoroacetabular impingement are common, underdiagnosed conditions that predispose young patients to premature osteoarthritis. Dysplastic acetabulae are often shallower, cover less of the femoral head, and have roofs that are less steep compared with normal hips. Femoracetabular impingement often occurs when there is incongruity between the femoral head and the acetabulum. In particular, cam-type femoroacetabular dysplasia refers to a developmental protruberance arising from the femoral head and neck junction that causes labral tears in predictable locations. Radiologists and clinicians have sought reliable radiographic signs and measurements to accurately characterize acetabular dysplasia and femoroacetabular impingement. Below are descriptions of the most commonly used measurements used to diagnose acetabular dysplasia and cam-type femoroacetabular impingement. Many of the measurements to assess dysplastic acetabulae utilize the position and orientation of the acetabular "sourcil" (acetabular roof) relative to the femoral head to establish the degree of dysplasia. (*Sourcil* or *acetabular roof* refers to the convex superior sclerotic curve of superior acetabular subchondral bone as seen on an AP radiograph. *Sourcil* is French for eyebrow.)

ACETABULAR INDEX OF THE SOURCIL (FIG. 5 APPENDIX 1)

- Steepness of acetabular roof.
- How to measure:
    - *Draw a horizontal line intersecting the medial margin of the sourcil.*
    - *Draw a line from the medial sourcil to lateral acetabular rim.*
- *Normal is less than 10 degrees.*

FEMORAL HEAD EXTRUSION INDEX (FIG. 5 APPENDIX 2)

- Percentage of femoral head *uncovered* by acetabulum.
- How to measure:
    - *Draw a vertical line from the medial femoral head; measure to:*
    - *Vertical line from lowest point at the lateral acetabular roof (line A).*

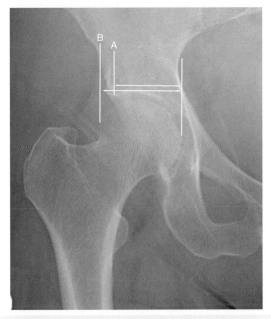

Fig. 5 Appendix 2 Femoral head extrusion index.

- *Vertical line from the lateral femoral head (line B).*
- $\% = (B-A / B) \times 100$.
- *Normal is less than 25%.*

ACETABULAR INDEX OF DEPTH TO WIDTH (FIG. 5 APPENDIX 3)

- Measures acetabular shallowness.
- Predictor of development of osteoarthritis before age 65.
- How to measure:
    - *Draw a line connecting the medial and lateral margins of the acetabular rim. This represents the acetabular width (W).*

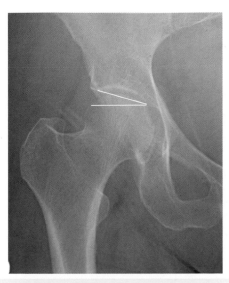

Fig. 5 Appendix 1 Acetabular index.

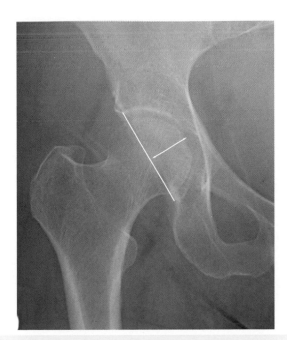

Fig. 5 Appendix 3 Acetabular index of depth to width.

■ *Draw a perpendicular line from W to the deepest point of the acetabulum. This represents the depth (D).*
   ■ *% = (D/W) × 100%.*
■ *Normal is greater than 48%.*
■ *Borderline is 32 to 47%.*
■ *Abnormal is less than 31%.*

LATERAL CENTER-EDGE ANGLE OF WIBERG (FIG. 5 APPENDIX 4)

■ Degree of lateral coverage.
■ How to measure:
   ■ *Determine the center point of the femoral head.*
   ■ *Draw a vertical line through this point.*
   ■ *Draw a second line from the center point to the lateral acetabular margin.*
■ *Normal is greater than or equal to 25 degrees.*
■ *Borderline is 20–24 degrees.*
■ *Abnormal is less than 20 degrees.*

CONGRUENCE (FIG. 5 APPENDIX 5)

■ Evaluates the position of the femoral head to the sourcil.
■ How to assess:
   ■ *Draw a best-fit circle of the femoral head and determine the center point of this circle.*
   ■ *Draw a best-fit circle of the acetabulum and determine the center point of this circle. If the acetabulum is not circular, the drawn circle should most closely parallel the sourcil.*
■ The hip is *congruent* if the center points for the two circles are the same.
■ The hip is *incongruent* if the center points do not overlie one another.

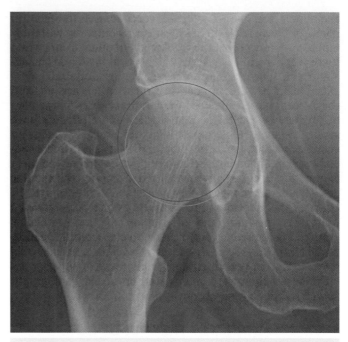

Fig. 5 Appendix 5 Congruence. The lack of congruence in this case is due to osteoarthritis with axial migration of the femoral head.

ANTERIOR CENTER-EDGE ANGLE OF LEQUESNE (FIG. 5 APPENDIX 6)

■ Determines the degree of anterior femoral head coverage by the acetabulum.
■ Assessed on the false-profile view (standing 65 degree anterior oblique view); lateral view of the acetabulum.
■ How to assess:
   ■ *Determine the center of the femoral head.*

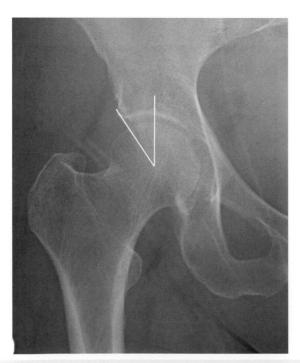

Fig. 5 Appendix 4 Lateral center-edge angle of Wiberg.

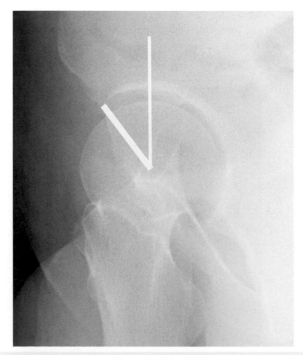

Fig. 5 Appendix 6 Anterior center-edge angle of Lequesne.

- *Draw a vertical line through the femoral head center point.*
- *Draw a second line connecting the center point with the anterior acetabular rim.*
- *The angle between the two lines represents the anterior center-edge angle.*
- *Normal is greater than or equal to 25 degrees.*
- *Borderline is between 20 and 25 degrees.*
- *Abnormal is 20 degrees or less.*

ACETABULAR VERSION (SEE FIG. 5.53)

- Refers to the relative position of the anterior and posterior acetabular lines on a standard AP radiograph of the pelvis.
- Definitions:
  - Anteversion: *The anterior acetabular line is medial to the posterior acetabular line along its entire course.*
  - Neutral version: *The anterior acetabular line overlies the posterior acetabular line.*
  - Retroversion: *The upper one-third of the anterior acetabular line is lateral to the posterior acetabular, and crosses over inferiorly to have a more normal inferior course.*
- On CT, the normal degree of acetabular anteversion in adults is 17 ± 6 degrees.

Fig. 5 Appendix 7 Alpha and beta angles. Sagittal oblique MR image, parallel to the femoral neck. Anterior is to the viewer's left. Alpha angle a, beta angle b.

ALPHA ANGLE OF CAM-TYPE FEMOROACETABULAR DYSPLASIA (FIG. 5 APPENDIX 7 AND FIG. 5.49)

- Assesses the sphericity of the femoral head and posterior concavity of the femoral head–neck junction to determine the degree of cam-type impingement.
- How to assess:
  - *Measured from a mid-sagittal oblique MR image as assessed on a mid-coronal image.*
  - *Draw a circle matching the femoral head contour.*
  - *Draw a line along the long axis of the femoral neck and bisecting the femoral head.*
  - *Draw a second line from the center of the femoral head to the point where the anterior femoral neck diverges from the circle.*
- Normal is less than 55 degrees.

BETA ANGLE OF CAM-TYPE FEMOROACETABULAR DYSPLASIA (FIG. 5 APPENDIX 7)

- Assesses the sphericity of the femoral head and posterior concavity of the femoral head–neck junction to determine the degree of cam-type impingement.
- How to assess:
  - *Measured from a mid-sagittal oblique sequence as assessed on a mid-coronal image.*
  - *Draw a circle matching the femoral head contour.*
  - *Draw a line along the long axis of the femoral neck and bisecting the femoral head.*
  - *Draw a second line from the center of the femoral head to the point where the posterior femoral neck diverges from the circle.*

Sources and Suggested Readings

Affram P. An epidemiologic study of cervical and trochanteric fractures of the femur in an urban population: analysis of 1664 cases with special reference to etiologic factors. *Acta Orthop Scand Suppl.* 1964;64:11.

Badillo K, Pacheco JA, Padua SO, et al. Multidetector CT evaluation of calcaneal fractures. *Radiographics.* 2011;31(1):81–92.

Beltran LS, Rosenberg ZS, Mayo JD, et al. Imaging evaluation of developmental hip dysplasia in the young adult. *AJR Am J Roentgenol.* 2013;200:1077–1088.

Bencardino JT, Beltran J, Feldman MI, Rose DJ. MR imaging of complications of anterior cruciate ligament graft reconstruction. *Radiographics.* 2009;29(7):2115–2126.

Bowden DJ, Byrne CA, Alkhayat A, et al. Injectable viscoelastic supplements: a review for radiologists. *AJR Am J Roentgenol.* 2017;209:883–888.

Chan SS, Rosenberg ZS, Chan K, Capeci C. Subtrochanteric femoral fractures in patients receiving long-term alendronate therapy: imaging features. *AJR Am J Roentgenol.* 2010;194(6):1581–1586.

Chaturvedi A, Mann L, Cain U, et al. Acute fractures and dislocations of the ankle and foot in children. *Radiographics.* 2020; online article. https://doi.org/10.1148/rg.2020190154.

Chhabra A, Subhawong TK, Carrino JA. A systematised MRI approach to evaluating the patellofemoral joint. *Skeletal Radiol.* 2011;40(4):375–387.

Costa CR, Morrison WB, Carrino JA. Medial meniscus extrusion on knee MRI: is extent associated with severity of degeneration or type of tear? *AJR Am J Roentgenol.* 2004;183:17–23.

Crema MD, Roemer FW, Marra MD, et al. Articular cartilage in the knee: current MR imaging techniques and applications in clinical practice and research. *Radiographics.* 2011;31(1):37–61.

Delfaut EM, Demondion X, Dieganski A, et al. Imaging of foot and ankle nerve entrapment syndromes: from well-demonstrated to unfamiliar sites. *Radiographics.* 2003;23:613–623.

De Smet AA. How I diagnose meniscal tears on knee MR. *AJR Am J Roentgenol.* 2012;199(3):481–499.

De Smet AA, Blankenbaker DG, Alsheik NH, Lindstrom MJ. MRI appearance of the proximal hamstring tendons in patients with and without symptomatic proximal hamstring tendinopathy. *AJR Am J Roentgenol.* 2012;198(2):418–422.

De Smet AA, Nathan DH, Graf BK, et al. Clinical and MRI findings associated with false-positive knee MR diagnoses of medial meniscal tears. *AJR Am J Roentgenol.* 2008;191(1):93–99.

Diederichs G, Issever AS, Scheffler S. MR imaging of patellar instability: injury patterns and assessment of risk factors [published correction appears in *Radiographics.* 2011;31(2):624]. *Radiographics.* 2010;30(4):961–981.

Disler DG. Fat-suppressed 3-D spoiled gradient-recalled MR imaging: assessment of articular and physeal hyaline cartilage. *AJR Am J Roentgenol.* 1997;169:1117–1123.

Flores DV, Gomez M, Fernandez HM, et al. Adult acquired flatfoot deformity: anatomy, biomechanics, staging, and imagings. *Radiographics.* 2019;39:1437–1460.

Flores DV, Gomez CM, Pathria MN. Layered approach to the anterior knee: normal anatomy and disorders associated with anterior knee pain. *Radiographics.* 2018;38:2069–2101.

Ganz R, Parvizi J, Beck M, et al. Femoroacetabular impingement: a cause for osteoarthritis of the hip. *Clin Orthop Relat Res.* 2003;417:112–120.

Garden RS. Stability and union of subcapital fractures of the femur. *J Bone Joint Surg.* 1964;46B:630–712.

Greif DN, Baraga MG, Rizzo MG, et al. MRI appearance of the different meniscal ramp lesion types, with clinical and arthroscopic correlation. *Skeletal Radiology.* 2020;49:677–689.

Hegazi TM, Belair JA, McCarthy EJ, et al. Sports injuries about the hip: what the radiologist should know. *Radiographics.* 2016;36:1717–1745.

Judet R, Judet J, Letournel E. Fractures of the acetabulum: classification and surgical approaches to reduction. *J Bone Joint Surg.* 1964;46A:1615–1646.

Kamel SI, Belair JA†, Hegazi TM, Halpern EJ, Desai V, Morrison WB, Zoga AC. Painful type II os naviculare: introduction of a standardized, reproducible classification system. Skeletal Radiol. 2020 Dec;49(12):1977–1985.

Khan I, Ashraf T, Saifuddin A. Magnetic resonance imaging of impingement and friction syndromes around the knee. *Skeletal Radiology.* 2020;49:823–836.

Khurana B, Sheehan SE, Sodickson AD, et al. Pelvic ring fractures: what the orthopedic surgeon wants to know. *Radiographics.* 2014;34:1317–1333.

Kijowski R, Rosas HG, Lee KS, et al. MRI characteristics of healed and unhealed peripheral vertical meniscal tears. *AJR Am J Roentgenol.* 2014;202:585–592.

Kijowski R, Blankenbaker DG, Shinki K, et al. Juvenile versus adult osteochondritis dissecans of the knee: appropriate MR imaging criteria for instability. *Radiology.* 2008;248(2):571–578.

Kraus C, Ayyala RS, Kazam JK, et al. Imaging of juvenile hip conditions predisposing to premature osteoarthritis. *Radiographics.* 2017;37:2204–2205.

Laborie LB, Lehmann TG, Engesæter IØ, et al. Prevalence of radiographic findings thought to be associated with femoroacetabular impingement in a population-based cohort of 2081 healthy young adults. *Radiology.* 2011;260:494–502.

Lauge-Hansen N. Fractures of the ankle: genetic roentgenologic diagnosis of fractures of the ankle. *AJR Am J Roentgenol.* 1954;71:456–471.

Li AE, Jawetz ST, Greditzer HG, et al. MRI Evaluation of femoroacetabular impingement after hip preservation surgery. *AJR Am J Roentgenol.* 2016;207:392–400.

Lungu E, Michaud J, Bureau NJ. US assessment of sports-related hip injuries. *Radiographics.* 2018;38:867–889.

Mainwaring B, Daffner R, Reiner B. Pylon fractures of the ankle: a distinct clinical and radiographic entity. *Radiology.* 1998;168:215–218.

Manganaro MS, Morag Y, Weadock WJ, et al. Creating three-dimensional printed models of acetabular fractures for use as educational tools. *Radiographics.* 2017;37:871–880.

Matcuk GR, Cen SY, Keyfes V, et al. Superolateral hoffa fat-pad edema and patellofemoral maltracking: predictive modeling. *AJR Am J Roentgenol.* 2014;203:W207–W212.

Markhardt BK, Gross JM, Monu JU. Schatzker classification of tibial plateau fractures: use of CT and MR imaging improves assessment. *Radiographics.* 2009;29(2):585–597.

Mellado JM, Bencardino JT. Morel-Lavallée lesion: review with emphasis on MR imaging. *Magn Reson Imaging Clin N Am.* 2005;13(4):775–782.

Meyers AB, Haims AH, Menn K, Moukaddam H. Imaging of anterior cruciate ligament repair and its complications. *AJR Am J Roentgenol.* 2010;194(2):476–484.

Mohankumar R, Palisch A, Khan W, et al. Meniscal ossicle: posttraumatic origin and association with posterior meniscal root tears. *AJR Am J Roentgenol.* 2014;203:1040–1046.

Mullens FE, Mullens FE, Zoga AC, et al. Review of MRI technique and imaging findings in athletic pubalgia and the "sports hernia". *Eur J Radiol.* 2012;81(12):3780–3792.

Naraghi A, White LM. MRI of labral and chondral lesions of the hip. *AJR Am J Roentgenol.* 2015;205:479–490.

Stacy GS, Lo R, Motang A. Infarct-associated bone sarcomas: multimodality imaging findings. *AJR Am J Roentgenol.* 2015;205:W432–W441.

Omar IM, Zoga AC, Kavanagh EC, et al. Athletic pubalgia and "sports hernia": optimal MR imaging technique and findings. *Radiographics.* 2008;28(5):1415–1438.

Perrich KD, Goodwin DW, Hecht PJ, Cheung Y. Ankle ligaments on MRI: appearance of normal and injured ligaments. *AJR Am J Roentgenol.* 2009;193(3):687–695.

Prince J, Laor T, Bean J. MRI of ACL injuries and associated findings in the pediatric knee: changes with skeletal maturation. *AJR Am J Roentgenol.* 2005;185:756–762.

Robinson R. Sonography of common tendon injuries. *AJR Am J Roentgenol.* 2009;193(3):607–618.

Rosas HG. Unraveling the posterolateral corner of the knee. *Radiographics.* 2016;36:1776–1791.

Rowe CR, Sakellarides HT, Freeman PA, Sorbie C. Fractures of the os calcis: a long term follow-up study of 146 patients. *JAMA.* 1963;184:920.

Samim M, Walter W, Gyftopoulos S, et al. MRI assessment of subspine impingement: features beyond the anterior inferior iliac spine morphology. *Radiology.* 2019;293:412–421.

Schwappach J, Murphey M, Kokmayer S, et al. Subcapital fractures of the femoral neck: prevalence and cause of radiographic appearance simulating pathologic fractures. *AJR Am J Roentgenol.* 1994;162:651–654.

Scheinfeld MH, Dym AA, Spektor M, et al. Acetabular fractures: what radiologists should know and how 3D CT can aid. *Radiographics.* 2015;35:555–577.

Sharif B, Ashraf T, Saifuddin A. Magnetic resonance imaging of the meniscal roots. *Skeletal Radiology.* 2020;49:661–676.

Sheehan SE, Shyu JY, Weaver MJ, et al. Proximal femoral fractures: what the orthopedic surgeon wants to know. *Radiographics.* 2015;35:1563-1584.

Silva MS. Radiography, CT, and MRI of hip and lower limb disorders in children and adolescents. *Radiographics.* 2019;39:779–794.

Subhawong TY, Eng J, Carrino JA, Chhabra A. Superolateral Hoffa's fat pad edema: association with patellofemoral maltracking and impingement. *AJR Am J Roentgenol.* 2010;195(6):1367–1373.

Yamada AF, Crema MD, Nery C, et al. Second and third metatarsophalangeal plantar plate tears: diagnostic performance of direct and indirect MRI features using surgical findings as the reference standard. *AJR Am J Roentgenol.* 2017;209:W100–W108.

Zoga AC, Kavanagh EC, Omar IM, et al. Athletic pubalgia and the "sports hernia": MR imaging findings. *Radiology.* 2008;247(3):797–807.

6   Knee

Radiographic Anatomy

- The knee joint is composed of three articulations: the medial and lateral femorotibial and the patellofemoral articulations. Although they share a common joint capsule, these articulations are often referred to separately as the medial, lateral, and patellofemoral compartments or joints.
  - Each femoral condyle has an anterior weight-bearing surface distally, a posterior weight-bearing surface posteriorly, and a mid–weight-bearing surface in between.
  - An anteroposterior (AP) knee radiograph shows the femoral condyles and tibial plateaus (Fig. 6.1). The medial and lateral compartment radiolucent 'joint spaces' represent the summated thickness of the tibial plateau and anterior weight-bearing articular cartilage surfaces; normally the medial compartment is slightly narrower.
  - Standing views often better demonstrate the true extent of cartilage loss in the medial and lateral compartments.
  - A standing view with the knees flexed (*Rosenberg view* or *notch view*) can demonstrate cartilage loss on the mid and posterior weight-bearing surfaces depending on the degree of flexion.
  - Shallow oblique AP views may demonstrate a subtle fracture not visible on AP or lateral views. Thus a four-view series is used in acute trauma (AP, lateral, both obliques).
- There is normally about 5 degrees of valgus in the adult knee, slightly greater in women because of a wider pelvis.
- Infants and toddlers frequently have physiologic bowlegs, with genu varum (knee varus) and lateral tibial bowing.

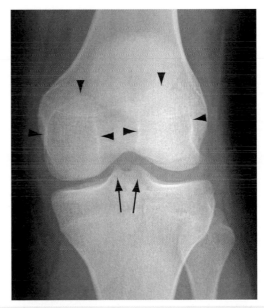

Fig. 6.1 Normal knee radiographic anatomy: AP view. Note the medial and lateral tibial eminences *(arrows)* and femoral condyles *(arrowheads).*

  - This situation reverses by age 3 to 4 years, when genu valgum ('knock knees', i.e., knee valgus) may be seen as a normal variant.
- A lateral radiograph profiles the anterior weight-bearing, mid–weight-bearing, and posterior weight-bearing surfaces of the femoral condyles and also reveals differences between the condyles and medial/lateral tibial plateau (Fig. 6.2).

213

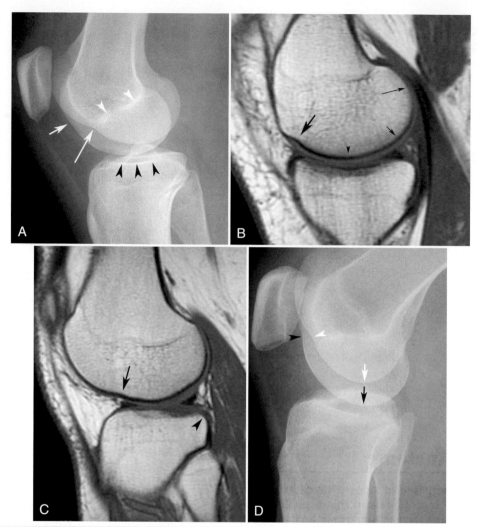

Fig. 6.2 Normal knee radiographic anatomy: lateral view. **(A)** This example is slightly oblique in the coronal plane, with the medial compartment projecting slightly lower, to better demonstrate the subtle differences between compartments. Note the concave medial tibial plateau *(black arrowheads)* projecting just below the straight lateral tibial plateau. Each femoral condyle has a flat or concave region termed the *condylar sulcus*, which is located on the anterior weight-bearing surface of the lateral condyle *(long arrow)*, but more anteriorly on the medial condyle *(short arrow)*. Also note the roof of the intercondylar notch *(white arrowheads)*. **(B)** Sagittal T1-weighted MR image in the medial compartment shows the concave medial condylar sulcus anteriorly *(large arrow)*, and concave contour of the medial tibial plateau and matching contour of the medial femoral condyle. The articular surface of each femoral condyle may be subdivided into trochlea (anteriorly, articulates with patella) and anterior *(small arrowhead)*, mid *(short small arrow)*, and posterior *(long small arrow)* surfaces. **(C)** Sagittal T1-weighted MR image in the lateral compartment in the same patient as in B shows the concave lateral condylar sulcus more posterior in position, at the anterior weight-bearing surface *(arrow)*, and flat contour of the lateral tibial plateau. Also note the convex contour of the posterior margin of the lateral plateau *(arrowhead)*, which is also visible on radiographs. **(D)** Slightly oblique lateral radiograph with the knee flexed 40 degrees shows the mid–weight-bearing surfaces of the femoral condyles *(arrows)* in contact with the tibial plateaus. Note that the articular contact is centered somewhat posteriorly, and the articular contact area of the condyles, especially the lateral condyle *(white arrow)*, is smaller than at extension. This view also shows the femoral condylar sulci *(black arrowhead,* medial; *white arrowhead,* lateral).

- Some pathologic conditions may be visible only on a lateral radiograph, so awareness of these differences can be useful for localizing a lesion.
- The lateral femoral condyle has a slight flattening at its anterior weight-bearing surface (condylar sulcus). This is important because it is the impaction point during *pivot-shift injury*; a deep indentation can be a radiographic sign of anterior cruciate ligament (ACL) tear. The medial femoral condyle has a rounder contour of the distal surface.
- Similarly, the lateral tibial plateau has a slightly convex surface, whereas the medial plateau has a slightly concave surface.

- The knee joint capsule extends several centimeters above the upper pole of the patella.
  - A joint effusion or synovitis can be seen on a lateral radiograph as thickening of the suprapatellar joint recess shadow (Fig. 6.3).
  - A cross-table lateral radiograph can be used to identify fluid-fluid levels within a knee joint. Hemarthrosis after knee trauma usually indicates the presence of a fracture, severe osseous contusion, or other internal derangement, such as an ACL tear. A lipohemarthrosis indicates an intraarticular fracture, with leakage of marrow fat into the joint. (see Fig. 1.15).

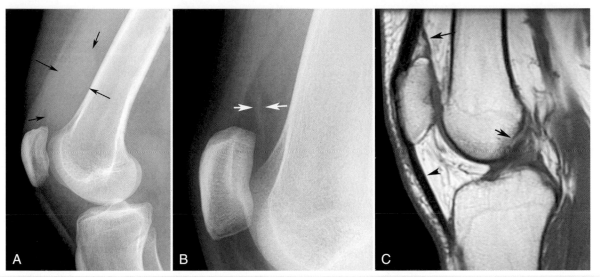

Fig. 6.3 Knee joint effusion. **(A)** Lateral radiograph shows distention of the superior joint capsule seen as soft tissue density *(arrows)*. **(B and C)** Normal superior joint *(arrows)* shown for comparison. C is sagittal T1-weighted MR image. Also note roof of intercondylar notch *(short arrow)* and patellar tendon *(arrowhead)* in C. (See also Fig. 1.15.)

- A lateral radiograph also demonstrates the distal quadriceps tendon, which inserts into the anterior patellar upper pole. Quadriceps tendon fibers continue anteriorly along patella as the "quadriceps continuation", blending with the patellar tendon, which connects the anterior patellar lower pole and the tibial tubercle.
  - The patellar tendon, patella, and quadriceps tendon are collectively termed the *extensor mechanism*.
  - On lateral radiographs the quadriceps and patellar tendons should be well seen; if indistinct and surrounded by soft tissue edema, a tendon tear should be considered, especially if there is alteration of patellar position: patella alta (high) with patellar tendon tear; patella baja (low) with quadriceps tendon tear.
- Hoffa's fat pad is located posterior to the patellar lower pole and patellar tendon and anterior to the knee joint and proximal tibia.
- The fabella is a variably present small sesamoid in the head of the lateral gastrocnemius that is often best seen on the lateral view. When seen on an AP view, a fabella usually projects over the lateral femoral condyle. It is usually smooth and fairly round.
- A notch or tunnel view is a frontal view with the knee flexed 45 degrees and the x-ray beam parallel to the tibial plateau (Fig. 6.4). This view is useful for detection of calcified intraarticular bodies, which often settle within the intercondylar notch.
- A sunrise (or axial) view is useful for assessing patellar alignment in patients with anterior knee pain. Optimally the knee is flexed only about 20 to 25 degrees when this view is obtained (Merchant technique) because clinically significant patellofemoral malalignment may not be evident with greater flexion (Fig. 6.5).
  - The posterior articular surface of the patella has three relatively flat surfaces called facets: the lateral, medial, and odd facets. The lateral facet is usually the widest. The lateral and medial facets meet at the median ridge. The odd facet is the most medial, may be devoid of cartilage, and is sagittal in orientation.

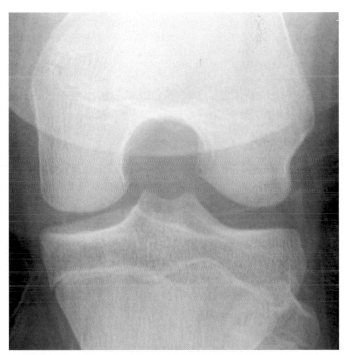

Fig. 6.4 Normal knee radiographic anatomy: notch (tunnel) view.

- The trochlea (trochlear groove or sulcus) is the femoral articular surface of the patellofemoral joint, in which the patella glides during flexion and extension.

Fractures and Dislocations

- A common trauma radiographic protocol includes AP, cross-table lateral, and bilateral oblique views. Notch views are often obtained for chronic knee pain or if an intraarticular body is suspected. Sunrise views are often obtained when anterior knee pain is present.

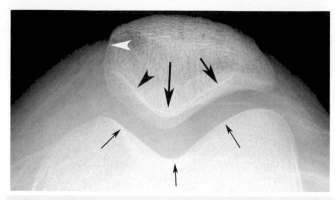

Fig. 6.5 Normal knee radiographic anatomy: axial (sunrise) view. This view is optimally obtained with knee flexed about 20 degrees. Note the medial patellar facet *(black arrowhead)* separated from the wider lateral facet *(short black arrow)* by the median ridge *(long black arrow)*, odd facet *(white arrowhead)*, and femoral trochlea (groove, *small arrows*).

- Computed tomography (CT) with coronal and sagittal reformats is frequently used in preoperative assessment of a tibial plateau fracture.
- The main role of magnetic resonance imaging (MRI) of the knee is soft tissue assessment, but it is also the most sensitive technique for fracture detection and is therefore useful when traumatic knee pain is not explained with radiographs or CT.
- Bone scan can also depict occult fractures but is inferior to MRI and rarely used for this indication.

INTERCONDYLAR FRACTURES

- Transcondylar fractures of the distal femur usually involve metaphyseal and condylar components (Fig. 6.6).
  - The metaphyseal component is usually transverse in orientation.
  - The condylar component may be in sagittal or coronal planes.
- Coronal intraarticular fractures place the patient at risk for osteonecrosis of the condylar fragments.

- Coronally oriented intraarticular condylar fractures also have a worse prognosis than sagittal fractures because of the risk for displacement and joint incongruity when the patient begins weight-bearing, despite internal fixation.

TIBIAL PLATEAU FRACTURE

- Tibial plateau fractures are classically seen in high-energy trauma such as pedestrian-automobile accidents in younger patients and following minor trauma in elderly patients, usually women with osteoporosis.
- Most (80%) are localized to the lateral tibial plateau because most fractures result from a valgus load with impaction at the lateral tibial condyle.
- Tibial plateau fractures are intraarticular fractures that typically produce large hemarthroses, often lipohemarthroses.
- These fractures are classified by the location of fracture lines, articular depression, and metaphyseal extension.

Key Concepts

Tibial Plateau Fracture

- 80% are localized to the lateral tibial plateau
- Large hemarthrosis, often lipohemarthrosis with fat-fluid level
- CT with reformats for presurgical planning
- Describe any articular depression and diastasis

- Although not a reflection of the severity of injury, the Schatzker classification is useful for communication of the findings and surgical planning (Fig. 6.7; see Fig. 1.14).
- The classification is as follows:
  - *Type I:* cleavage fracture of the lateral tibial plateau.
  - *Type II:* combined cleavage and depressed fracture of the lateral tibial plateau.
  - *Type III:* purely depressed fracture of the lateral tibial plateau.
  - *Type IV:* lateral condylar tibial cleavage fracture that extends to the medial tibial condyle.

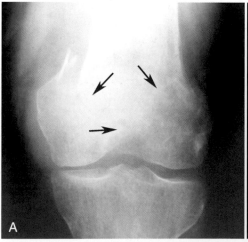
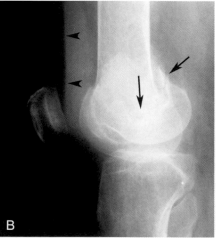

Fig. 6.6 Comminuted intercondylar fracture of the distal femur. **(A)** Frontal radiograph shows Y-shaped fracture *(arrows)*. **(B)** Lateral view demonstrates fracture line *(arrows)* and fat-fluid level of lipohemarthrosis *(arrowheads)*.

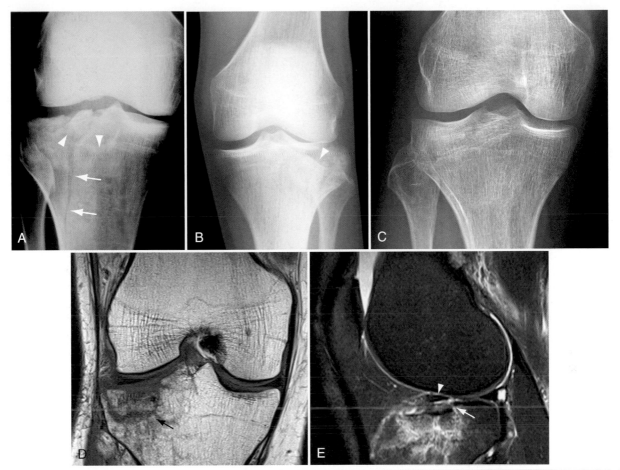

Fig. 6.7 Tibial plateau fractures in different patients. **(A)** Schatzker II fracture with sagittal cleavage line *(arrows)* and depressed lateral plateau fracture *(arrowheads).* **(B)** Schatzker III fracture with depressed lateral tibial plateau *(arrowhead).* **(C)** Frontal radiograph showing just how obscure a tibial plateau fracture can be. This radiograph appears essentially normal. **(D)** Coronal T1-weighted image in same patient as C shows a Schatzker III fracture with depression of lateral tibial plateau *(arrow).* **(E)** Same patient as shown in C and D; sagittal fat-suppressed T2-weighted MR image shows depressed lateral tibial plateau fracture with surrounding osseous edema and incongruent articular margin *(arrow).* Any articular incongruence is considered undesirable. Note anterior horn of the lateral meniscus *(arrowhead).*

- *Type V:* bicondylar fracture.
- *Type VI:* any fracture with a transmetaphyseal component.
- Imaging is important in the assessment of tibial plateau fractures because the goal of surgery is restoration of congruence of the articular margin to decrease the risk for eventual posttraumatic osteoarthritis (OA).
- CT with reformats is the standard imaging modality for fracture characterization and surgical planning.
- Radiographs are the first-line test for knee trauma. The presence of a tibial plateau fracture can be subtle.
  - The fracture line is often in an oblique plane, therefore AP and lateral views may completely miss a tibial plateau fracture (see Fig. 6.7C).
  - The lateral tibial plateau normally down-slopes slightly and thus its margins are not tangential to the knee joint on AP radiographs. A *plateau view* radiograph with the beam angled 10 degrees caudal better profiles the lateral tibial plateau articular surface.
  - Fragment depression is easily overlooked anteriorly and exaggerated posteriorly.
  - Subtle fractures in osteoporotic patients often show a fuzzy transverse band 1 cm or so below the plateau, representing impacted trabecular bone.
  - Cross-table lateral can show fluid levels within an effusion.

- MRI is sometimes requested, for example when evaluation of associated soft tissue injuries is needed.
- Management decisions are complex. Generally, articular surface depression greater than 3 mm or distraction/diastasis greater than 3 mm benefits from surgical reduction (to the extent possible) with internal fixation.
- Various forms of fixation are used in tibial plateau fractures. In addition to internal fixation hardware, bone cement may be placed to support elevated fragments and fill voids. This is seen as an amorphous area of increased density in the operated bone.
- The main complication of tibial plateau fracture is OA. Coexisting ACL and meniscal tears also occur. Compartment syndrome and vascular injury can occur with Schatzker VI fractures.

PATELLAR FRACTURE

- Patellar fractures in adults may be caused either by direct impaction (falling on the patella), resulting in a comminuted fracture, or by sudden tension of the extensor mechanism of the thigh, resulting in transverse and often distracted fractures (Figs. 1.3 and 6.8A).

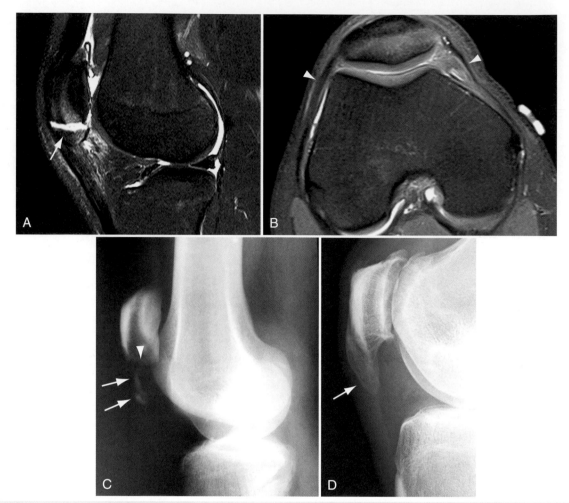

Fig. 6.8 Patellar fractures. **(A)** Sagittal fat-suppressed T2-weighted MR image and **(B)** axial fat-suppressed T2-weighted MR image show a transverse fracture of the patellar lower pole (*arrow* in A), which occurred following a sudden eccentric contraction of the extensor mechanism of the knee. Note that the fracture is only mildly distracted. Intact anterior longitudinal fibers from the extensor mechanism and intact medial and lateral patellofemoral ligaments (*arrowheads* in B) were strong enough in this injury to maintain alignment. Contrast with Fig. 1.3. **(C)** Acute patellar sleeve fracture. Note patella alta (high position of the patella), avulsion of the lower pole of the patella (*arrowhead*), and small fragments more distally (*arrows*). These fractures are extraarticular, and thus this fracture had no hemarthrosis. **(D)** Patellar sleeve fracture, untreated, late appearance. The inferiorly displaced patellar periosteum over time formed new bone, resulting in an elongated patella with a cone-shaped excrescence extending distally from the lower pole *(arrow)*. The articular portion of the patella is permanently shifted higher, which can cause patellofemoral instability and osteoarthritis. Osteoarthritis is present in this case. Note the ostephytes at the upper and lower portions of the patellar articular surface.

- Often both mechanisms are present, usually resulting in a transverse fracture.
  - 60% of patellar fractures are transverse.
  - The degree of distraction depends on the integrity of the soft tissue supporting structures medial, lateral, and across the anterior patella (Fig. 6.8B). Transverse fibers from the medial and lateral patellofemoral retinacula and longitudinal fibers from the rectus femoris cross the anterior patella (the "quadriceps continuation") provide support during distracting stress.
- *Patellar sleeve avulsion* is a fracture at the inferior margin of the patella in adolescent patients.
  - The avulsed patellar tendon insertion includes unossified cartilage and often a curvilinear calcification next to the inferior pole with surrounding swelling (Fig. 6.8C).
  - The gap between the patellar lower pole and avulsed fragment ultimately ossifies, resulting in an elongated, tapering patellar lower pole (Fig. 6.8D).

- Osteochondral fractures of the patella and avulsion of the medial patellar border may occur in association with transient lateral patellar dislocation (see following section).
- Osteochondritis dissecans can involve the patella, usually the lateral facet.
- Patellar normal variants:
  - *Bipartite* and *multipartite patella* represents fragmentation of the patella with well-corticated margins (Fig. 6.9). Fibrocartilage fixes the ossicle or ossicles to the remainder of the patella. Normally MRI shows intact overlying articular cartilage bridging the gap.
  - May be mistaken for a fracture, but in contradistinction has well-corticated margins.
  - Bipartite patella is often bilateral (50%).
  - Type III bipartite patella is most common (75%, superolateral location); Type I (<1%, inferior pole) and Type II (25%, lateral location) are less common superolateral location.

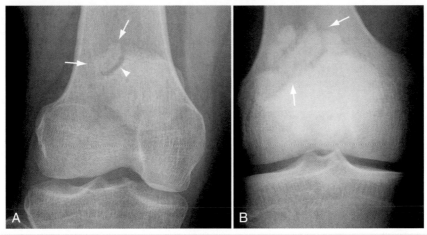

Fig. 6.9 Normal variant patellar fragmentation. **(A)** Bipartite patella. Note the typical superolateral location of fragment *(arrows)* and smooth cleft *(arrowhead).* **(B)** Multipartite patella *(arrows).*

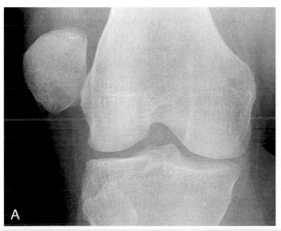

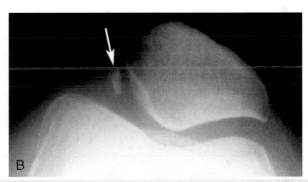

Fig. 6.10 Patellar dislocation. **(A)** Note lateral position of the patella. This is an unusual radiographic finding, because most patellar dislocations are transient. **(B)** Axial view of patella in a different patient after transient patellar dislocation demonstrates medial pole patellar osseous fragment *(arrow)* caused by transient dislocation.

- Rarely symptomatic. Edema or a fluid-filled cleft in the fibrocartilage and/or adjacent bone marrow edema suggests abnormal mechanics or pseudarthrosis formation; this can be a source of pain.
- *Dorsal defect of the patella* is a rounded lucency at the superolateral dorsal (articular) margin of the patella. CT or MRI shows a focal concave contour defect of subchondral bone filled with intact articular cartilage.

PATELLAR DISLOCATION

- Lateral patellar dislocation is almost always transient and is a commonly overlooked injury.
- In transient patellar dislocation, the patella briefly dislocates laterally and then relocates.
- Dislocations are almost always lateral because of the normal valgus alignment of the knee and 'Q angle' (see following section) and the weaker mechanical properties of the medial supporting structures.
- Impaction occurs between the medial pole of the patella and the anterolateral margin of the lateral femoral condyle.

- Bone bruises (osseous contusions) or fractures occur at the sites of impaction at the medial patella and the lateral femoral condyle. An osteochondral fracture of the lateral trochlear ridge or far anterior weight-bearing lateral femoral condyle may occur. Fracture location depends on the degree of knee flexion during dislocation and relocation (Fig. 6.10).
- Medial soft tissue supporting structures become stretched or torn (Figs. 6.11 and 6.12).
    - The *medial patellar retinaculum.*
        - At the level of the patella on axial images.
        - A minor stabilizer.
        - Tears at the patellar attachment.
        - Can avulse bone from the medial patella.
    - The *medial patellofemoral ligament (MPFL).*
        - Arises from the medial femoral condyle near the adductor tubercle.
        - Extends anteroinferiorly to the superomedial patella.
        - Tears at the adductor tubercle attachment.
        - Visualized best on sagittal MR images, just below the vastus medialis obliquus (VMO).
        - Look for soft tissue edema at the VMO, extending superiorly along the adductor magnus.

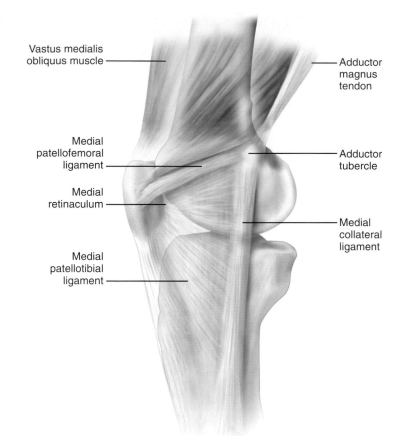

A

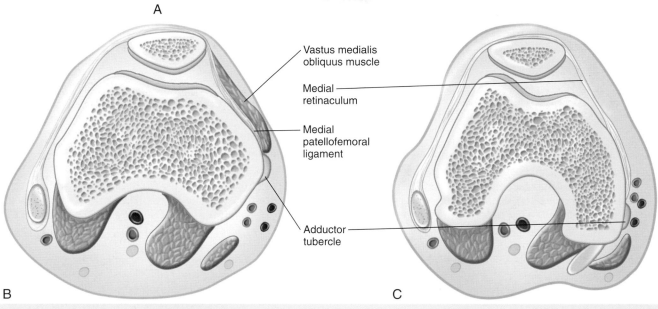

B

C

Fig. 6.11 Artwork shows the medial patellofemoral ligament (MPFL) and the medial retinaculum and its association with the overlying vastus medialis obliquus (VMO) muscle. **(A)** Medial side of the knee. Note the MPFL arising from the medial aspect of the superior pole of the patella and inserting onto the adductor tubercle. The MPFL is located deep into the VMO muscle. **(B)** Axial image through the level of the VMO muscle shows the MPFL extending from the superior pole of the patellar to insert onto the adductor tubercle. **(C)** Axial image below the level of the VMO muscle shows the medial retinaculum rather than the MPFL. The VMO muscle acts as a landmark on axial images to determine whether the structure arising along the medial aspect of the patella represents the MPFL or the medial retinaculum. (From Morrison W. *Problem Solving in Musculoskeletal Imaging*. Philadelphia: Elsevier; 2010.)

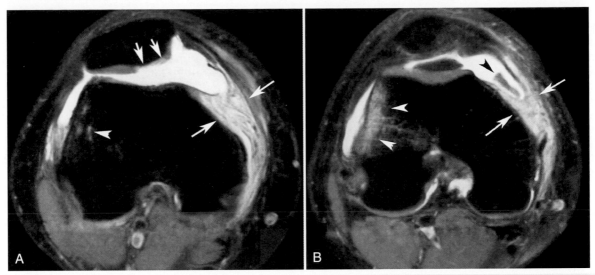

Fig. 6.12 MRI after transient dislocation of the patella. (**A** and **B**) Two contiguous axial fat suppressed proton density weighted MR images show lateral femoral bone bruise *(white arrowheads)*, chondral delamination defect at medial pole of patella *(short arrows)*, and medial patellofemoral ligament tear with substantial edema *(long arrows)*. Note displaced chondral body surrounded by joint fluid *(black arrowhead in B)*.

- Can simulate medial collateral ligament (MCL) tear both clinically and on MRI (the MCL originates near the adductor tubercle close to the MPFL attachment). However, coexisting MCL injury is in fact rare and easily overcalled on MRI.
- MRI is the ideal modality with which to evaluate transient patellar dislocation (see Fig. 6.12).
  - Bone bruises of the inferomedial patella and anterolateral femoral condyle are pathognomonic.
  - The medial retinaculum and MPFL should be assessed for tear.
  - Chondral and osteochondral injuries can be extremely subtle and require careful review of the medial patella and lateral femoral trochlear ridge. Look for cartilage delamination defects and displaced cartilage fragments.
  - MRI report should also include anatomic findings that increase the risk of lateral dislocation: shallow femoral trochlear groove, patella alta, increased tibial tubercle–trochlear groove (TT–TG) distance. These are discussed in the following section.
  - Edema and hemorrhage often track posteriorly around the MCL, simulating MCL injury. Be careful not to overcall MCL injury.

PATELLAR MALTRACKING

- *Patellar maltracking* and the similar term, *patellar instability*, refer to a tendency for lateral patellar subluxation and/or lateral patellar tilting with quadriceps contraction that can contribute to lateral dislocation, impingement of Hoffa's fat and anterior knee pain, and/or chronic patellofemoral cartilage damage.
  - Related terms are *lateral patellar compression syndrome* and *excessive lateral patellar pressure syndrome* (ELPS).
- Clinical: Anterior or anterolateral pain with climbing stairs or prolonged sitting. Grinding or clicking with knee extension may be present.

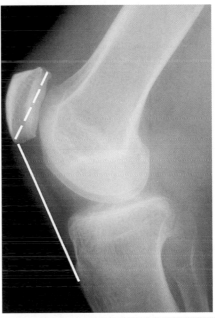

Fig. 6.13 Patella alta. Note substantially greater length of patellar tendon *(solid line)* compared with length of patella *(dashed line)*.

- Biomechanical causes for patellar maltracking:
  - Shallow femoral trochlear groove or sulcus (*femoral trochlear dysplasia*). A deep groove keeps the patella normally aligned, but a shallow groove allows lateral subluxation.
  - *Patella alta* is the high position of the patella relative to the distal femur.
    - There are numerous methods to measure patellar height, both subjective and objective.
    - The widely used *Insall–Salvati ratio* is measured on a lateral radiograph or sagittal MR or CT image. The length of the patellar tendon is divided by the length of the patella (Fig. 6.13). Greater than 1.2 is considered patella alta.

- If there is no overlap of the patellar and trochlear articular surfaces at full extension, this also represents patella alta.
- Prominent *Q angle*.
  - Q angle is the angle between the quadriceps mechanism and a line drawn along the patellar tendon continued proximally.
  - Quadriceps muscle contraction during knee extension draws the patella laterally, with greater force if the angle is large.
  - Q angle is usually greater in females due to knee valgus and wider pelvic architecture.
    - Also increased by genu valgum, external tibial torsion ("penguin feet"), and foot pronation.
  - The surrogate for measuring Q angle on axial imaging (CT or MRI) is the *tibial tuberosity–trochlear groove (TT-TG) distance or offset* (Fig. 6.14):
    - Measured best on axial MR or CT images.

- Increased TT-TG distance.
  - Normal TT-TG measurement range varies widely and can be altered by patient positioning.
  - Over 20 mm is generally considered to be abnormal, although lower values can be seen in patients with maltracking, usually 15-20 mm, occasionally less.
  - Weak vastus medialis muscle.
  - Medial ligamentous laxity; usually from prior dislocation.
  - Tight lateral fascia. Can be associated with a tight iliotibial band.
- When present, actual lateral patellar displacement (translation) or tilting primarily occurs in the first 20 degrees of knee flexion.
  - Greater flexion usually forces the patella into the groove, but lateral pressure can still cause symptoms and cartilage damage.

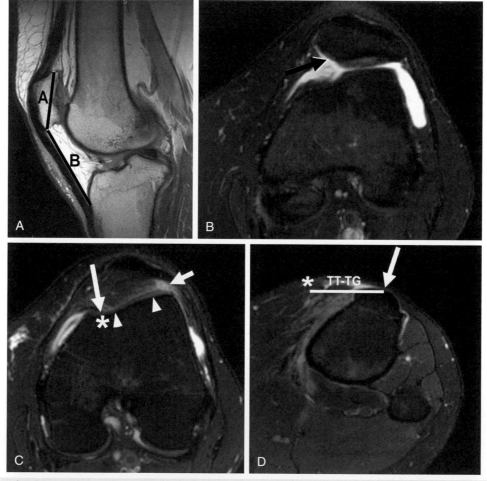

Fig. 6.14 Patellar maltracking on MRI in a 26-year-old woman. **(A)** Sagittal T1-weighted image shows patella alta (high position of the patella relative to the trochlear groove). A common method for measurement is the Insall–Salvati method, in which the length of the patellar tendon (labeled B) is divided by the length of the patella **(A)**; a ratio 1.2 or greater is considered to represent patella alta. In this situation on extension the patella does not track in the trochlear sulcus, leading to predisposition to subluxation and dislocation. **(B)** Axial T2-weighted fat-suppressed image at the level of the patella shows lateral subluxation of the patella as well as cartilage thinning and irregularity *(black arrow)*. **(C)** Axial T2-weighted fat-suppressed image at the level of the trochlear groove shows a shallow sulcus *(arrowheads)*; the center of the groove is identified with a *long arrow* and an *asterisk*. There is soft tissue edema at the lateral aspect of Hoffa's fat pad *(short arrow)* which is a common finding in patella maltracking often referred to as patello-femoral friction. **(D)** Axial T2-weighted fat-suppressed image at the level of the tibial tuberosity shows method for measurement of the TT–TG (tibial tuberosity–trochlear groove distance). In a single axial image, the distance *(line)* is measured between the center of the tibial tuberosity *(arrow)* and the extrapolated location of the center of the trochlear groove *(asterisk in C and D)*. The TT–TG measures a portion of the Q angle, the angle between the course of the quadriceps mechanism and the patellar tendon; a high Q angle and a TT–TG over 20 mm is associated with patellar maltracking.

- The patellar position can be visualized on radiographs using the lateral view (for patella alta) and the sunrise view (for lateral subluxation/tilt and trochlear sulcus depth). As noted previously, shallow knee flexion (Merchant technique) best demonstrates patellar subluxation.
- MRI is best for evaluation of patellar position, the trochlear sulcus, ligament injury, and cartilage damage.
  - Maltracking can impinge fat in the superolateral aspect of Hoffa's fat pad. Edema at this site is evidence of an underlying patellar tracking disorder.
- CT can be performed in different degrees of knee flexion to demonstrate patellar subluxation (Fig. 6.15).
- A pathologically thickened medial plica can produce symptoms overlapping with maltracking (discussed later in this chapter).
- Management options for patellofemoral maltracking:
  - Vastus medialis strengthening.
  - Arthroscopic lateral release—surgically divide the lateral retinaculum.
  - Surgical relocation of the tibial tubercle (tibial tubercle transfer osteotomy)—move the patellar tendon insertion medially, anteriorly, or both.

ILIOTIBIAL BAND FRICTION SYNDROME

- Iliotibial band (ITB) anatomy:
  - Originates from the deep fascia of the thigh, the gluteus maximus, and the distal tensor fascial lata (TFL) and inserts on Gerdy's tubercle at the anterolateral knee. The TFL originates from the iliac crest.
- The IT band crosses both the hip and knee joints.
- ITB friction syndrome clinical: pain over the lateral femoral condyle, greatest at 30 degrees flexion.
- Especially common in runners and cyclists.

- Friction between the IT band and lateral distal femur can result in bursitis that is visible on MRI as a band of fluid medial to the distal IT band and separate from the knee joint (Fig. 6.16).
- A similar friction syndrome can occur at the greater trochanter (presenting clinically as greater trochanter pain syndrome).

PATELLA BAJA

- Low-lying patella.
- Usually a normal variation or simulated by the measurement technique (only the articular surface contact is important; if there is a prominent inferior patellar pole, for example, after patellar sleeve injury, the Insall–Salvati ratio can be artificially low).
- Quadriceps tendon rupture (see "Tendon Pathology", discussed later).
- Can be seen following total knee arthroplasty (TKA).

AVULSION INJURY

- There are numerous avulsion sites at the knee (Fig. 6.17).
- Common locations include:
  - The ACL insertion on the intercondylar eminence of the tibia (tibial spine) (Fig. 6.18).
  - The posterior cruciate ligament insertion at the posterior tibia.
  - The lateral capsular ligaments at the lateral margin of the tibia (Fig. 6.19), also termed a *Segond fracture*. This fracture is highly associated with ACL injury. The specific minor ligament associated with this fracture is debated. The variably present *anterolateral ligament* (ALL) is a top candidate, though is inconsistently visualized on MRI. The ALL connects the

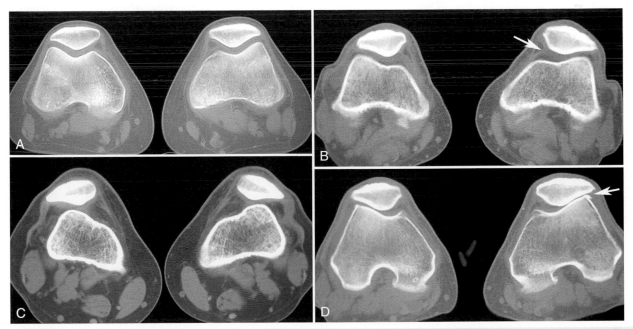

Fig. 6.15 Patellofemoral maltracking in different patients. All images are axial CT images with the knees flexed 15 to 20 degrees. **(A)** Normal. **(B)** Lateralized left patella *(arrow)*. **(C)** More severe, bilateral subluxation in a patient with patella alta. Note that the patella is above the trochlear sulcus (i.e., not tracking in the groove on knee extension). **(D)** Chronic bilateral tracking error with early osteoarthritis with joint space narrowing and osteophyte formation, more advanced on the left *(arrow)* in a patient with chronic excessive lateral pressure syndrome (ELPS). See also Fig. 6.77.

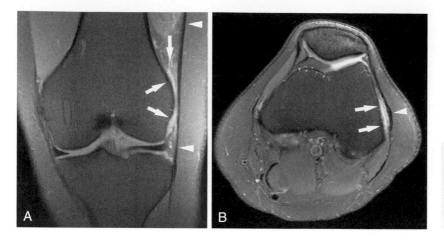

Fig. 6.16 Iliotibial band friction syndrome. **(A)** Coronal proton density fat-suppressed MR image shows edema and fluid accumulation *(arrows)* between the low-signal distal IT band *(arrowheads)* and the lateral distal femur. **(B)** Axial T2-weighted fat-suppressed MR image shows the same finding, and also shows the fluid to be separate from the knee joint.

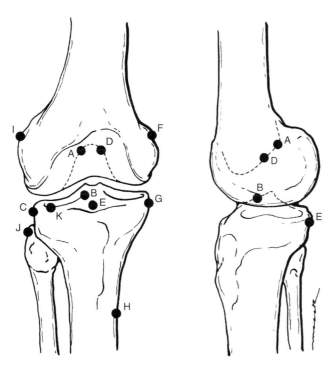

Fig. 6.17 Avulsion sites around the knee. **(A)** Anterior cruciate ligament (ACL) proximal attachment; **(B)** ACL distal attachment; **(C)** lateral capsular attachment (Segond); **(D)** posterior cruciate ligament (PCL) proximal attachment; **(E)** PCL distal attachment; **(F)** medial collateral ligament (MCL) proximal attachment; **(G)** MCL deep fiber (meniscotibial) distal attachment; **(H)** MCL superficial fiber distal attachment; **(I)** lateral collateral ligament (LCL) proximal attachment; **(J)** common attachment of distal LCL and biceps femoris tendon; **(K)** Gerdy's tubercle, insertion of iliotibial band. (Reproduced with permission from Manaster BJ. *Handbook of Skeletal Radiology*. 2nd ed. St. Louis: Mosby; 1997.)

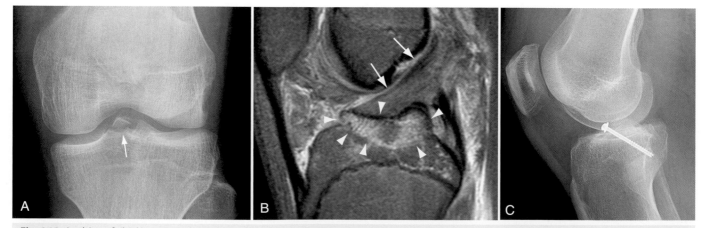

Fig. 6.18 Avulsion of tibial insertion of anterior cruciate ligament. **(A)** Frontal radiograph demonstrates fracture at medial tibial intercondylar eminence (tibial spine) *(arrow)*. **(B)** Sagittal fat-suppressed T2-weighted MR image shows the slightly elevated, edematous avulsion fracture fragment *(arrowheads)* with adjacent marrow edema. The intact anterior cruciate ligament *(arrows)* inserts onto the fragment. **(C)** Lateral radiograph following surgical repair with arthroscopic reduction and screw fixation of the fragment.

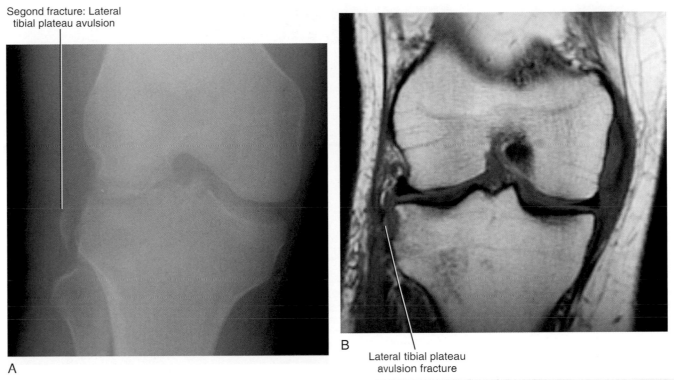

Fig. 6.19 Segond fracture. Frontal radiograph **(A)** and coronal T1-weighted image **(B)** demonstrate a small cortical avulsion fracture of the lateral tibial plateau resulting from avulsion of the lateral capsule structures. This sign is specific for anterior cruciate ligament disruption. (From Morrison W. *Problem Solving in Musculoskeletal Imaging*. Philadelphia. Elsevier, 2010.)

Segond fracture: Lateral tibial plateau avulsion

Lateral tibial plateau avulsion fracture

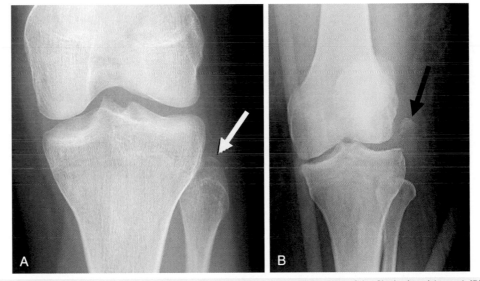

Fig. 6.20 Arcuate fracture. **(A)** Frontal radiographic view of the knee shows a nondisplaced fracture of the fibular head *(arrow)*. **(B)** Frontal radiographic view of the knee shows a superiorly displaced fracture *(arrow)* from the fibular head, at the site of insertion of the conjoined tendon (combination of the biceps femoris and fibular collateral ligament).

lateral femoral condyle and proximal lateral collateral ligament to the proximal lateral tibia between the fibular head and Gerdy's tubercle.
■ The anterior lateral tibial margin (Gerdy's tubercle) at the site of the iliotibial band insertion; often associated with lateral tibial plateau fracture.
■ The lateral collateral ligament/biceps femoris insertion at the proximal fibula (the 'conjoined tendon'), also called an *arcuate fracture* (Fig. 6.20).

■ The proximal and distal MCL attachment sites on the medial femoral condyle and medial tibia, respectively.
■ The anterior tibial tuberosity is another site prone to tension injury of the patellar tendon, which is commonly seen in children and young adolescents (Fig. 6.21).
    ■ With repetitive stress, the anterior tibial tubercle may become chronically fragmented, and if

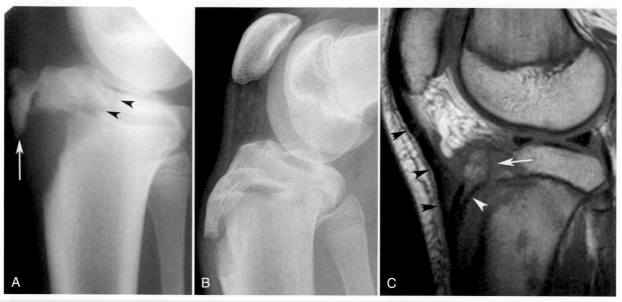

Fig. 6.21 Tibial tubercle avulsion. **(A)** Complete avulsion *(arrow)*. Also note Salter–Harris III fracture of the proximal tibial epiphysis *(arrowheads)*. **(B)** In an older child the tibial tubercle ossification center fuses to the proximal tibial epiphysis, and traction injury may result in a Salter–Harris I injury, as in this example. **(C)** Salter–Harris III fracture in an older child with fused tibial tubercle and proximal tibial epiphysis *(white arrowhead)*. Sagittal T1-weighted MR image shows the epiphyseal fracture line *(arrow)* and intact patellar tendon *(black arrowheads)*.

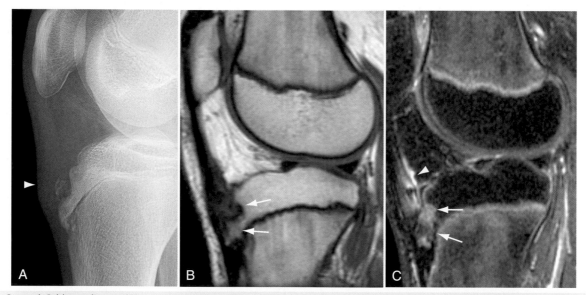

Fig. 6.22 Osgood–Schlatter disease. **(A)** Lateral radiograph of proximal tibia shows the typical osseous irregularity and soft tissue swelling at the patellar tendon insertion *(arrowhead)*. The child was tender at the tibial tubercle, making the diagnosis. Sagittal T1-weighted **(B)** and fat-suppressed T2-weighted **(C)** MR images in a different child with Osgood–Schlatter disease show similar findings at the tibial tubercle *(arrows)* and edema within and adjacent to the distal patellar tendon *(arrowhead in C)*.

associated with tenderness and swelling, the disorder is termed *Osgood–Schlatter disease* (Fig. 6.22).

- Most cases are associated with overuse and rapid growth and are self-limited.
- It is rarely complicated by either nonunion of the tibial tubercle or premature closure of the tibial tubercle physis with secondary development of genu recurvatum (posterior bowing of the knee).
- Adults with old Osgood–Schlatter disease often have asymptomatic or minimally symptomatic ossicles in the posterior distal patellar tendon.

- *Sinding–Larsen–Johansson syndrome* is a process similar to Osgood–Schlatter disease that occurs at the lower pole of the patella in the same age group (Fig. 6.23).

PHYSEAL INJURY

- Growth plate injuries at the knee are uncommon, but they are highly associated with complications, particularly growth disturbance (see discussion in Chapter 1).
- Proximal tibial epiphyseal fractures often occur in association with patellar tendon traction (see Fig. 6.21).

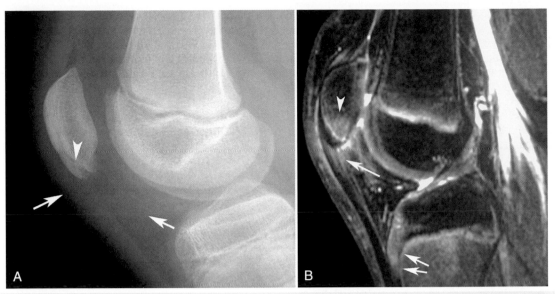

Fig. 6.23 Sinding–Larsen–Johansson disease. Lateral radiograph **(A)** and sagittal fat-suppressed T2-weighted MR image **(B)** in a 12-year-old soccer player show fragmentation of the patellar lower pole *(arrowhead)* and adjacent soft tissue edema *(arrows)*. Also note mild marrow edema in the tibial tubercle *(short arrows* in B) that was not symptomatic. This is a benign stress reaction.

- In the distal femur, Salter–Harris II fractures predominate, occurring in 70% of injuries; the next most common pattern is Salter–Harris III fractures, occurring in 15% of children.
- Most Salter–Harris III fractures of the distal femur involve the medial femoral condyle and are caused by valgus stress. They usually are nondisplaced and occult radiographically but can be demonstrated at MRI.
- Sagittal plane Salter–Harris IV distal femur fractures through the intercondylar notch are easily displaced proximally. Just a few millimeter displacement results in metaphysis of one fragment apposed to epiphysis in the other. Healing in this position creates a bone bar across the physis with potential for severe growth disturbance in younger patients.
- The knee is the most common site for Salter–Harris V fractures, which occur at the proximal tibia and have a high frequency of localized growth plate arrest with angular deformity or limb shortening.
- Salter–Harris I fractures can be subtle, seen only as asymmetry of the physis (Fig. 6.24).

STRESS INJURY

- *Stress fractures* are common in the tibia.
  - Especially common in long-distance runners; anterior cortex of the mid-tibia is most common in this group.
  - The imaging findings were reviewed in Chapter 1 (see Figs. 1.33, 1.34, and 1.38). Briefly, initial findings are periosteal reaction, with progression to visible fracture or fractures, which may manifest in the tibia with one or more small transverse lucencies (the '*dreaded black line*') in the anterior cortex.
  - MRI and nuclide bone scan play an important role in the early detection of these injuries. MRI has almost completely replaced bone scan in most clinical practices due to lack of ionizing radiation and evaluation of adjacent soft tissues.

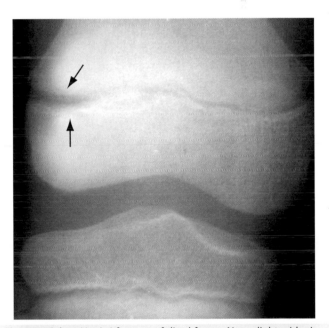

Fig. 6.24 Salter–Harris I fracture of distal femur. Note slight widening of lateral distal femoral physis *(arrows)*.

- Most stress fractures in the body are oriented perpendicular to the cortex. Tibial stress fractures can be an exception; occasionally the fracture line is oriented longitudinally along the tibial shaft. In this setting periosteal reaction without an obvious transverse line can erroneously raise concern for malignancy. The vertical line can be subtle and should be sought.
- Tibial shaft stress fractures are often best detected and characterized on MRI on axial fluid-sensitive sequences (Short tau inversion recovery [STIR] or fat-suppressed T2-weighted) (see Figs. 1.34 and 1.37).
- Main differential diagnosis is exertional compartment syndrome.

- *Shin splints* is a milder stress injury centered at the mid and distal tibia shaft characterized by medial/posteromedial and less commonly anterior pain.
  - Also termed *medial (or posteromedial) tibial stress syndrome (MTSS)* and *anterior tibial stress syndrome (ATSS)*.
  - Overuse injury with osseous stress response, which precedes fracture.
  - Radiographs initially are normal, but mild periosteal reaction (new bone formation) may be visible.
    - No visible fracture on radiographs.
  - MRI shows longitudinal, typically mild periosteal edema. More advanced cases show endosteal marrow edema adjacent to the tibial cortex.
- In addition to the above findings, a stress fracture is diagnosed on MRI when intracortical signal abnormality is observed. Accompanying marrow edema is often intense.
  - Bone scan is similar to MRI, with cortical tracer uptake without a focal hot spot in milder cases and superimposed intense focal tracer uptake at the site of a stress fracture.
- Multiple stress injuries, especially in a young female athlete, should raise suspicion for *RED-S syndrome* (relative energy deficiency in sport) (Fig. 6.25).
  - Associated with bulimia/anorexia nervosa.
  - Occurs by far most often in women but sometimes in men.
  - Earlier term is *female athletic triad* of eating disorder, amenorrhea, and osteoporosis.
  - RED-S nomenclature reflects the systemic involvement of the disease, affecting metabolism and multiple organ systems around the body in addition to the psychiatric features.

KNEE DISLOCATION

- Knee dislocations (i.e., femorotibial dislocations) can occur in any direction.

- Often spontaneously reduces and alignment on radiographs may be normal or near normal.
  - High index of suspicion with appropriate history.
  - Extensive soft tissue swelling.
  - Look for subtle alignment abnormality, joint space widening, and avulsion fractures, for example, Segond, tibial eminence, tibial tubercle.
  - May occur with tibial plateau fracture.
- Multiple ligament tears are invariably encountered.
  - If both the anterior and posterior cruciate ligaments are torn, it is safe to assume that the knee was dislocated. Note that some dislocations tear only the ACL or the posterior cruciate ligament (PCL).
- Associated popliteal arterial injury is common and requires emergent evaluation.
  - Any question of arterial injury requires CT or catheter arteriography for detection of intimal arterial disruption or pseudoaneurysm (Fig. 6.26).
- Peroneal nerve injury is also common in dislocation because of the tenuous course of the nerve around the knee, where it runs posterior to the margin of the fibular head and lateral to the margin of the fibular neck.

Menisci

MENISCAL ANATOMY AND MECHANICS

- The menisci of the knee are semicircular bands of fibrocartilage that line the peripheral aspects of the medial and lateral compartments and function to increase the tibiofemoral contact area, thus allowing a more evenly distributed load across the knee joint.
- Each meniscus as an upper or femoral surface and a lower or tibial surface.
- Each meniscus has three sections: anterior horn, body, and posterior horn. Each meniscus anterior and

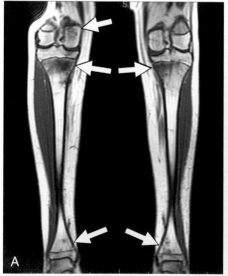
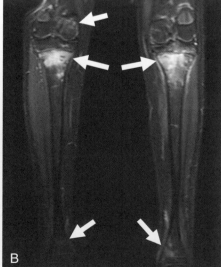

Fig. 6.25 Relative energy deficiency in sport (RED-S) in a 16-year-old girl. (**A** and **B**) Coronal T1 (**A**) and STIR (**B**) MR images of the lower legs show multiple areas of stress response and stress fracture *(arrows)* in a young long-distance runner with anorexia and bulimia. This diagnosis and its protean metabolic consequences should be considered when multiple areas of stress are seen in a young patient. In later stages the marrow can undergo serous atrophy, also known as gelatinous transformation.

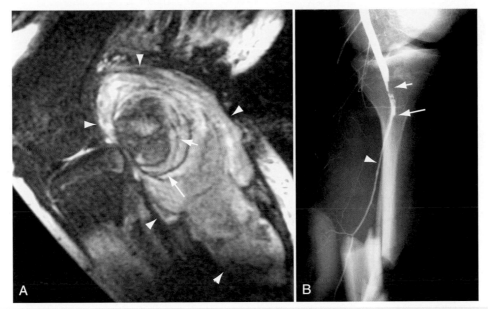

Fig. 6.26 Posttraumatic popliteal artery injury. **(A)** Sagittal inversion recovery MR image shows large pseudoaneurysm *(arrowheads)*. Note concentric rings of clot *(arrows)*. **(B)** AP angiogram in a different patient with comminuted tibial fracture and knee dislocation (after reduction) shows popliteal artery intimal injury with in situ thrombosis *(short arrow)* and occlusion at popliteal trifurcation *(long arrow)*. Distal runoff is limited to the peroneal artery *(arrowhead)*.

posterior horn is attached to the tibia with a fibrous root. These roots are essential for meniscal stability.

- The medial tibial plateau is larger and longer anteroposterior. Consequently, the medial meniscus is larger and slightly more C-shaped than the smaller and more circular lateral meniscus (Fig. 6.27).
- The menisci taper from a height of 3 to 5 mm at the periphery to a thin, sharp, central free margin.
- The menisci appear triangular in shape when viewed in cross-section on coronal and sagittal MRI (Fig. 6.28).
- The anterior and posterior horns of the lateral meniscus are similar in size; however, the posterior horn of the medial meniscus is larger than its anterior horn.
- On sagittal imaging the lateral meniscus shows a bow tie configuration with closely apposed anterior and posterior horns.
- Because the medial meniscus is larger, the horns are spaced farther apart, and on some images the medial meniscus does not resemble a bow tie (see Fig. 6.28).
- The menisci function not only as shock absorbers but also as passive stabilizers of the knee.
- Meniscofemoral ligaments course from the posterior horn of the lateral meniscus to the medial femoral condyle (Fig. 6.29).
  - *Anterior meniscofemoral ligament* or *meniscofemoral ligament of Humphry* is anterior to the PCL.
  - *Posterior meniscofemoral ligament* or *meniscofemoral ligament of Wrisberg* is posterior to the PCL.
  - The eponyms are not particularly important. These ligaments are variably present.
- The periphery of the medial meniscus is firmly attached to the joint capsule and has limited mobility except at the anterior and posterior tibial root insertion sites where it is fixed.
  - The firm attachment of the periphery of the medial meniscus makes the medial meniscus less mobile and thus at greater risk for tear.

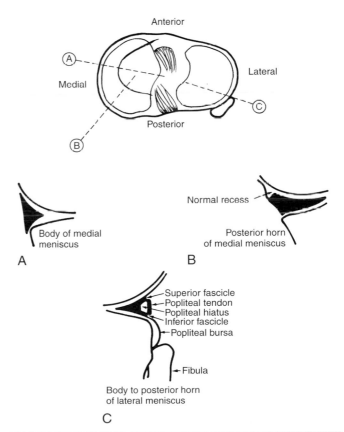

Fig. 6.27 Meniscal anatomy. *Top:* Diagram of the medial and lateral menisci, looking down on the tibial plateau. The labeled lines represent the various planes in which MR sequences are commonly obtained. **(A and B)** Radial planes through the body and posterior horn, respectively, of the medial meniscus. **(C)** Radial cut through the posterior body of the lateral meniscus. (Reproduced with permission from Manaster BJ. *Handbook of Skeletal Radiology.* 2nd ed. St. Louis: Mosby; 1997.)

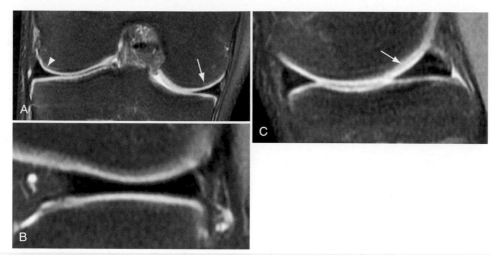

Fig. 6.28 MR images showing normal meniscal morphology. **(A)** Coronal fat-suppressed proton density MR image shows triangular appearance of medial *(arrow)* and lateral *(arrowhead)* menisci. Note that height is greatest peripherally and that height tapers to a sharp central free margin. (B and C) Sagittal fat-suppressed proton density MR images of lateral **(B)** and medial **(C)** menisci demonstrate uniform dark signal intensity of the menisci. Note equal size of anterior and posterior horns of lateral meniscus in B compared with larger size of posterior horn of medial meniscus in C *(arrow in C)*.

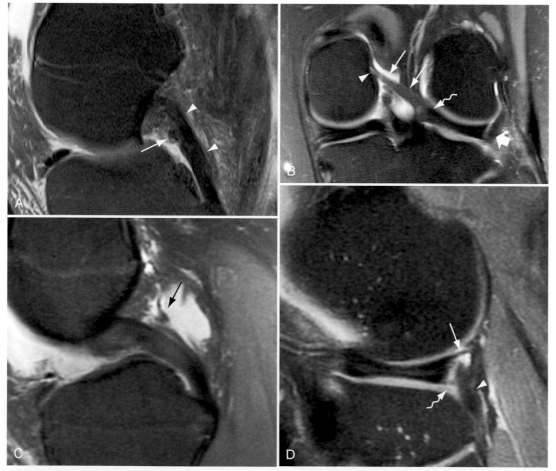

Fig. 6.29 Meniscofemoral ligaments and lateral meniscus retinacula. (A and B) Anterior meniscofemoral ligament (Humphry). Sagittal **(A)** and coronal **(B)** fat-suppressed proton density–weighted MR images show the obliquely oriented ligament of Humphry *(straight thin arrows)* connecting the posterior horn of lateral meniscus *(curved arrow in B)* to lateral margin of medial femoral condyle *(arrowhead in B)*. The ligament is anterior to posterior cruciate ligament (PCL) *(arrowheads in A)*. Also note popliteus tendon *(thick arrow)* adjacent to the lateral meniscus in B. Normal fluid between this tendon and the peripheral margin of the meniscus can be confused with a meniscal tear. Knowledge of this anatomy allows discrimination between the popliteus tendon and a meniscal tear. **(C)** Posterior meniscofemoral ligament (Wrisberg). Sagittal fat-suppressed proton density–weighted MR image shows ligament in cross section *(arrow)*, located posterior to the PCL. **(D)** Lateral meniscus superior retinaculum and meniscopopliteal ligament. Sagittal fat-suppressed proton density MR image shows superior retinaculum *(straight arrow)* between the posterior horn and the joint capsule, and the meniscopopliteal ligament *(curved arrow)* between the posterior horn and the popliteus tendon *(arrowhead)*.

- In contrast, the lateral meniscus is less tightly attached to the joint capsule than is the medial meniscus to allow greater motion in the lateral compartment that is needed to 'lock' the knee in full extension during standing.
- The lateral meniscus is loosely attached to the joint capsule and popliteus tendon by retinacula which are variably present posteriorly (Fig. 6.29D).
- Posterolaterally the popliteus tendon courses peripheral to the meniscus from the lateral femoral condyle to its musculotendinous junction posterior to the proximal tibial metaphysis (region is called the *popliteal hiatus*); normal joint fluid around the popliteal tendon can be confused for a meniscal tear.
- Microscopically the menisci consist of circumferential horizontal bundles of collagen fibers interspersed with fibers extending radially from the periphery toward the free margin. The unique collagen fiber orientation results in remarkable stabilization of menisci against centripetal loading, called *hoop strain*, which occurs with weight-bearing.
- The peripheral 10–20% of the menisci (called the *pink* or *red zone*) has some vascularity and potential for healing. The rest of the meniscus is avascular tissue with low capacity for healing.
- The anisotropic structure of menisci results in uniform low signal intensity on MR images. Normal vascularity in young people and degeneration in older individuals leads to intermediate intrasubstance signal on T1- and T2-weighted MR images (Fig. 6.30). The periphery (pink zone or red zone) normally exhibits intermediate signal.

MENISCAL TEAR

- Disruptions of menisci are called meniscal tears.
- Best imaging studies: MRI, MRI arthrography, and CT arthrography.
- MRI has high accuracy for the detection of meniscal tear as well as for determination of its location.
    - Proton density–weighted images have best sensitivity.
    - T2-weighted images are highly specific but have lower sensitivity.
- The MR signal within the normal meniscus is uniformly dark at the femoral and tibial articular surfaces.
- Meniscal tear is seen as linear or occasionally hazy signal <u>extending to the tibial or femoral surface</u> (not peripheral) on at least two consecutive images.
    - This finding on a single image is highly sensitive for tear but has poor sensitivity
- Tears most commonly occur at the body and posterior horn of the medial meniscus but can occur anywhere.
- Meniscal tears can occur in various configurations that can be broken down into radial and longitudinal types (Figs. 6.31 through 6.33).
    - **Radial**: A *radial tear* extends perpendicular to the circumference (cutting across the meniscal C shape).
        - Tear cuts across collagen fibrils inside the meniscus that normally provide resistance to hoop stress.
        - This can be the most destabilizing type of meniscal tear.
        - If complete, causes the meniscus to split into separate parts; the meniscus 'extrudes' or squeezes out

Nonsurfacing intrasubstance signal in an adult representing intrasubstance degeneration

Nonsurfacing intrasubstance signal in a pediatric meniscus representing prominent residual vascularity

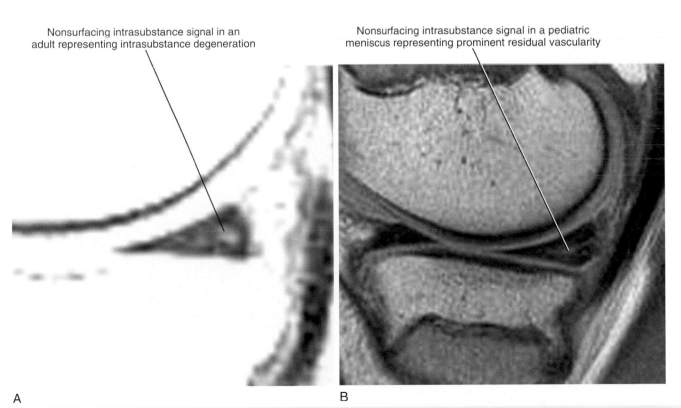

A

B

Fig. 6.30 Intrasubstance signal of the meniscus. **(A)** Nonsurfacing intrasubstance signal in the posterior horn of the medial meniscus in this adult patient represents intrasubstance degeneration and not a tear. **(B)** Nonsurfacing intrasubstance signal in the meniscus of a child represents prominent vascularity of the meniscus and should not be interpreted as intrasubstance degeneration. (From Morrison W. *Problem Solving in Musculoskeletal Imaging.* Philadelphia: Elsevier; 2010.)

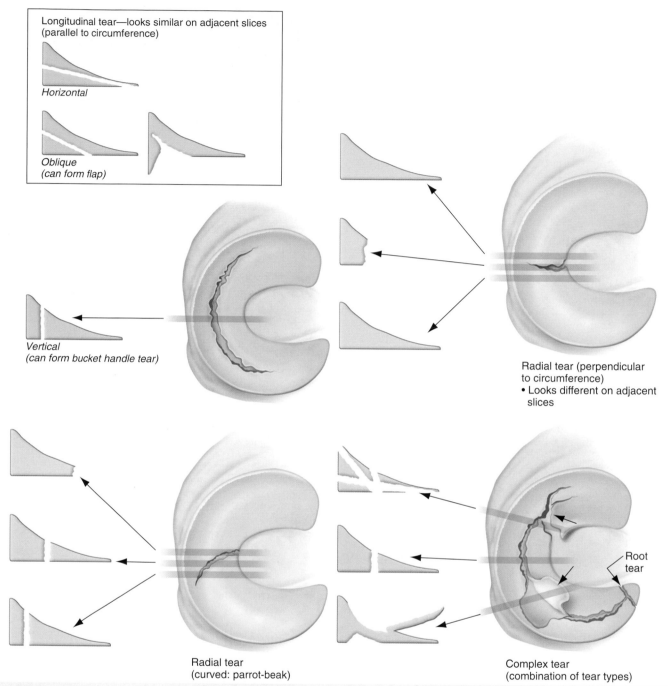

Fig. 6.31 MRI appearance of various meniscal tear patterns. (From Morrison W. *Problem Solving in Musculoskeletal Imaging*. Philadelphia: Elsevier; 2010.)

of the joint margin, which can lead to rapid development of chondrosis and eventually OA.

- Obliquely oriented incomplete radial tears have been called *parrot beak* tears due to their beak-like configuration on axial images; these can displace and cause locking.
- Radial tear often occurs at the posterior root attachment of the medial meniscus; look closely at the root attachments for fluid signal (Fig. 6.34).
- **Longitudinal**: A *longitudinal* tear extends along the circumference of the meniscal C shape. Orientation can be horizontal, oblique, or vertical (see Fig. 6.32).

- A *horizontal cleavage tear* consists of a longitudinal tear in the axial plane splitting the meniscus into superior and inferior portions.
  - More common in older patients.
  - Associated parameniscal cysts are frequent (discussed in the following text).
- A *longitudinal oblique* tear is like a horizontal tear but the oblique orientation results in the tear typically extending to the undersurface of the meniscus.
  - Also termed a *flap tear*.
  - Mechanical locking.
  - Usually medial meniscus.

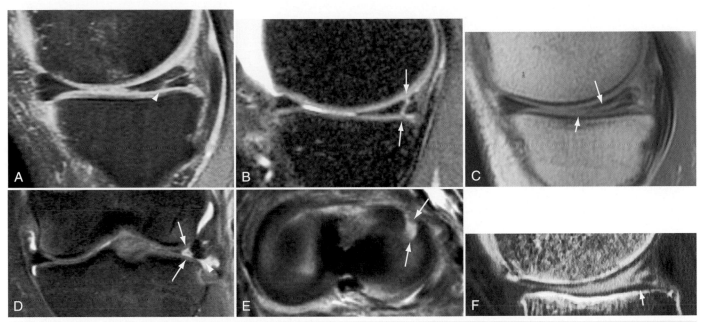

Fig. 6.32 Meniscal tears. **(A)** Sagittal fat-suppressed proton density fast spin-echo MR image showing a longitudinal oblique tear to the undersurface (tibial surface) at the medial meniscus posterior horn *(arrowhead)*. **(B)** Vertical longitudinal tear of the medial meniscus posterior horn. Sagittal fat-suppressed T2-weighted fast spin-echo MR image shows vertical linear fluidlike signal in meniscus *(arrows)*. T2-weighted images are less sensitive in detection of meniscal tear than T1-weighted and proton density–weighted images, but are highly specific. **(C)** Sagittal T1-weighted MR image showing a horizontal tear of the medial meniscus posterior horn *(long arrow)* extending to the inner margin (free edge *short arrow*). This pattern is often seen as degenerative tears in older patients. (D and E) Radial tear of the lateral meniscus at the junction of the anterior horn and body *(arrows)*. Coronal **(D)** and axial **(E)** fat-suppressed proton density–weighted fast spin-echo MR images show a radially oriented defect in the meniscus *(arrows)*, resulting in a fluid-filled gap and meniscal extrusion *(arrowhead)*. Extrusion is due to the loss of capacity of the meniscus to resist hoop strain. **(F)** Meniscus tear diagnosed with CT arthrogram in patient with pacemaker. Sagittal CT reformation shows horizontal tear of the posterior horn of the medial meniscus *(arrow)*.

- Flap fragments can displace:
  - Inferiorly into the inferior meniscotibial recess, a small potential space between the proximal tibia and the joint capsule. *Inferior meniscotibial gutter, inferior medial gutter,* or simply *medial gutter* are alternative terms for this space.
  - Superiorly between the distal femur and joint capsule (i.e., into the *superior meniscofemoral recess* or *superior medial recess* or *gutter*).
  - Toward or into the intercondylar notch.
- A *vertical longitudinal tear* extends vertically around the circumference, often involving the peripheral aspect (the pink zone).
  - If the tear is long enough, the central fragment can displace, called *bucket handle* tears (see Fig. 6.33).
  - Bucket handle tears are more common at the medial meniscus (90–95%).
  - Classic displacement patterns include posterior horn central fragment located adjacent to the anterior horn, and central fragment displaced into the intercondylar notch, called a *flipped bucket handle tear*.
  - A displaced bucket handle fragment identified on sagittal imaging through the intercondylar notch has been termed the "double PCL sign" (see Fig. 6.33E–F).
- *Meniscocapsular separation* or *meniscotibial ligament tear* is disruption of the capsular attachments (Fig. 6.35A).

- Mainly an injury of the medial meniscus, which is extensively fixed to the joint capsule, most commonly posterior horn and may involve the body.
- MRI sensitivity is lower than for other meniscal injuries. A fluid-filled gap between the peripheral medial meniscus and the capsule is the classic appearance but may not be present. (Knee flexion shows this finding better, but knees are imaged in extension.)
- MRI pitfalls (potential overcalls):
  - Edema signal between the medial meniscus and capsule does not necessarily imply tear but should be viewed with suspicion.
  - A cleft between the *superior* peripheral medial meniscus and capsule is a frequent normal variant.
- Due to peripheral location, meniscocapsular separation injuries have good potential to heal but may be unstable and may require surgery.
- Some peripheral injuries are a combination of meniscal tear and meniscocapsular separation ligament tear (Fig. 6.35B and C).
- *Ramp lesion* is a type of medial meniscus posterior horn meniscocapsular separation, peripheral longitudinal tear, or a combination of the two. The term is usually used only when an ACL tear is also present.
  - 'Ramp' refers to appearance of the normal medial meniscus posterior horn at arthroscopy, where it resembles a ramp rising from the tibial plateau to the posterior capsule.
  - Can be unstable.

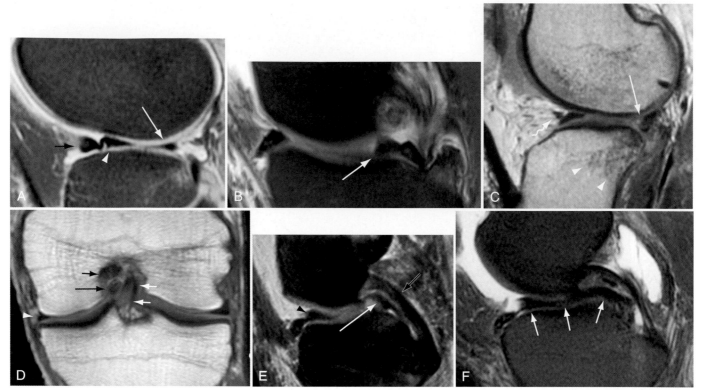

Fig. 6.33 Displaced meniscal tears. **(A)** Flipped posterior horn lateral meniscus tear. Sagittal fat-suppressed proton density–weighted fast spin-echo MR image shows attenuated-sized posterior horn *(long arrow)* and displaced posterior horn *(arrowhead)* adjacent to anterior horn *(arrow)*. **(B)** Sagittal fat-suppressed proton density–weighted MR image showing a medial meniscal tear with flipped fragment *(arrow)* adjacent to posterior horn. **(C)** Displaced tear of the lateral meniscus posterior horn. Sagittal proton density–weighted spin-echo MR image shows a blunted free edge *(arrow)*. Note indirect evidence of anterior cruciate ligament (ACL) tear (discussed later in text) with posterior lateral tibial bone bruise *(arrowheads)* and substantial anterior tibial subluxation. **(D and E)** Bucket handle medial meniscus tear with double posterior cruciate ligament (PCL) sign. Coronal T1-weighted spin-echo MR image **(D)** shows small body of medial meniscus *(white arrowhead)*. Note normal ACL *(short white arrows)* and PCL *(short black arrow)*. The displaced meniscal fragment *(long black arrow)* represents a third intercondylar region structure, and thus is a clue to the presence of bucket handle meniscal tear. Sagittal fat-suppressed T2-weighted MR image **(E)** shows the normal PCL *(black arrow)* and displaced meniscal fragment *(white arrow)* creating the 'double PCL sign'. Note the portion of the displaced meniscus *(arrowhead)* attached to the anterior horn. **(F)** Another medial meniscus bucket handle fragment *(arrows)*, in this example flipped far into the center of the notch.

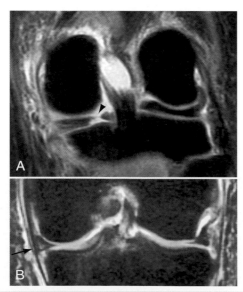

Fig. 6.34 Meniscal root tear. Coronal fat-suppressed proton density–weighted MR images. **(A)** Posterior image shows a radial tear *(arrowhead)* separating the posterior root and the posterior horn of the medial meniscus. **(B)** More anterior image shows extrusion of the medial meniscus body *(arrow)*.

- Ramp lesions occur at a potential blind spot at arthroscopy. Suggesting that a ramp lesion *might* be present can be helpful to the surgeon.
- Ramp lesions can be very subtle at MRI. If an ACL tear is present, extra scrutiny of the medial meniscus posterior horn and adjacent capsule is needed. Look for edema at the meniscocapsular junction and subchondral marrow edema in the adjacent tibia.
- *Complex meniscal tears* have multiple orientations. Any unstable components (radial tears, root tears, or displaced fragments) should be described.
- *Meniscal roots*, as noted earlier, fix the anterior and posterior horns of both menisci to the tibia. A complete root tear is functionally similar to a complete meniscectomy or a complete radial tear, as all hoop strength is essentially lost (see Fig. 6.34).
  - Root tears usually occur at the posterior horns, medial > lateral.
- *Displaced tears* often fit one of these patterns:
  - Bucket handle.
  - Flap.
  - Parrot beak.
  - Complex.

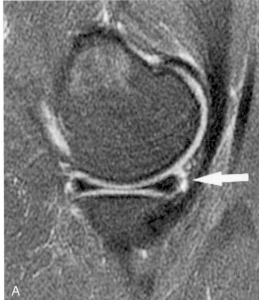

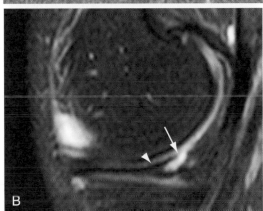

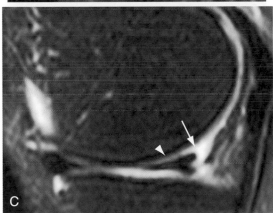

Fig. 6.35 (A) Meniscocapsular ligament tear (mensicocapsular separation). Sagittal fat-suppressed T2-weighted MR image shows fluid signal between the medial meniscus posterior horn and the joint capsule *(arrow)*. **(B** and **C)** Combination of meniscocapsular separation and peripheral meniscal tear. Note the tear *(arrow)* is partially between the meniscus and capsule and partially within the peripheral meniscus *(arrowhead)*.

- Meniscal extrusion is peripheral displacement, usually of the body (see Fig. 6.34).
    - Measure the displacement of the peripheral edge of the meniscal body compared to the peripheral margin of the tibial plateau.

- > 3 mm is definitely abnormal.
- Associations:
    - Often related to meniscal tear, especially complete radial tears, complex tears, and root tears.
    - Subchondral insufficiency fracture in older patients.
    - Highly associated with development and progression of OA in that compartment.
- Medial meniscal extrusion is more common than lateral meniscal extrusion.
- Meniscal degeneration can also result in mild extrusion.
- A *meniscal flounce* is a normal variant buckled, zig zag, or crenulated appearance of the meniscal body free edge, usually medial, as seen on a sagittal MR image.
- Menisci can also be evaluated for indirect evidence of meniscal tear (see Figs. 6.33 and 6.34).
    - Meniscal morphology; if the free edge appears blunted or meniscal margins are irregular, tear is likely (in the absence of prior surgery). Free edge blunting or abnormal morphology of a nonoperated meniscus should prompt additional review for flipped or otherwise displaced fragments.
    - *Parameniscal cyst* is a ganglion-like cyst originating from a meniscus.
        - Usually multiloculated.
        - Often track around the periphery of a meniscus.
        - Parameniscal cysts have a high association with meniscal tears (see Fig. 6.36).
            - Approximately 7% of meniscal tears exhibit a parameniscal cyst. Presence is virtually

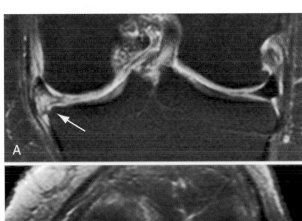

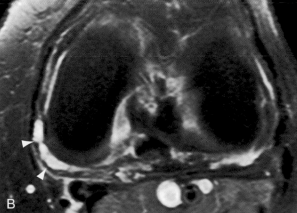

Fig. 6.36 Parameniscal cyst. **(A)** Coronal fat-suppressed proton density–weighted MR image shows a highly degenerated and partly extruded meniscus containing fluid signal *(arrow)*. **(B)** Axial fat-suppressed proton density–weighted MR image shows parameniscal cyst *(arrowheads)* wrapping around posterior joint line.

pathognomonic for tear. Therefore, the finding is very specific but not very sensitive.
- Potential overcall pitfalls: prominent or distended joint recesses, geniculate vessels, periarticular fluid collections, and ganglion cysts of a nonmeniscal origin can simulate parameniscal cysts.
- In order to diagnose a parameniscal cyst, the fluid collection should abut the peripheral margin of the meniscus and be associated with altered meniscal signal.
- Parameniscal cysts usually are multiloculated whereas normal recesses usually are not.
- Meniscal extrusion > 3 mm has a high association with tear, especially radial tears, complex tears, and posterior root tears.
- Meniscal tear is often associated with articular cartilage damage in the same compartment. Therefore, when a meniscal finding is borderline for tear, adjacent chondrosis suggests that it represents a tear.
  - Also, when a meniscal tear is identified, careful evaluation of articular cartilage in the same compartment should be sought.
- Subchondral bone marrow edema adjacent to a borderline meniscal finding suggests a tear. Marrow edema can be linear, oriented along the articular surface, or flame-shaped, related to cartilage damage.

- Perimeniscal soft tissue edema represents hyperemia and is associated with joint line tenderness on clinical exam. However, this finding has low specificity.
- *Discoid meniscus* is a developmental variant in which the meniscus is disc-shaped rather than semicircular and in which a portion of meniscus extends to the central portion of the tibial plateau (Fig. 6.37).
  - Discoid meniscus is seen almost exclusively in the lateral meniscus and is clinically significant for two reasons.
    - First, a discoid meniscus may itself be symptomatic, causing locking and joint line pain.
    - Second, a discoid meniscus is prone to tear because of its aberrant morphology and suboptimal biomechanical properties.
  - Suspected when children and young adolescents present with knee pain, swelling, locking, or snapping.
  - Can be a complete discoid meniscus, which covers nearly the entire articular surface, or a partial (incomplete) discoid meniscus, which is wider than normal.
  - Well seen on coronal MR images when the horizontal measurement between the free margin and periphery of the body of the meniscus is greater than or equal to 1.5 cm.
  - In addition, on sagittal images obtained at 3- to 4-mm section thickness with 1-mm interslice sections, the

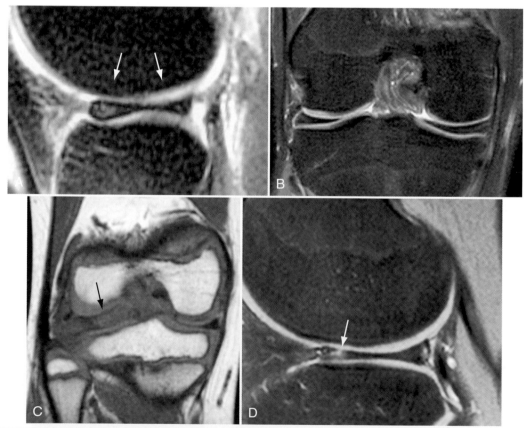

Fig. 6.37 Discoid meniscus. **(A)** Sagittal fat-suppressed T2-weighted MR image shows discoid lateral meniscus *(arrows)*. **(B)** Coronal fat-suppressed proton density–weighted MR image through the center of the knee joint shows a rare discoid medial meniscus. At the center of the compartment if the meniscus extends farther than the midpoint of the femoral condyle, it is suspicious for a discoid meniscus. **(C)** Degenerated and torn discoid lateral meniscus. Coronal T1-weighted MR image demonstrates a discoid meniscus with surfacing signal *(arrow)*. The meniscus was found to be highly degenerated and torn at arthroscopy. **(D)** Sagittal fat-suppressed proton density–weighted MR image shows a discoid lateral meniscus with vertical longitudinal tear of anterior horn *(arrow)*.

body of the meniscus (i.e., bowtie configuration) should not be shown on more than three sequential images. If it is shown on more than three images, a discoid meniscus is diagnosed.

- "Wrisberg variant" refers to a hypermobile discoid lateral meniscus characterized by an absent posterior meniscocapsular/meniscopopliteal ligament, and can present clinically with a snapping sensation in the knee.
- A meniscal ossicle is ossification of a portion of the meniscus (Fig. 6.38).
  - Most common at the posterior horn of the medial meniscus.
  - Associated with prior meniscal tear, especially at the root attachment.
  - Not a normal variant.
- There are numerous **pitfalls** on MRI in diagnosing meniscal tears. Most are due to the presence of normal structures that are in close proximity to the periphery of the meniscus and which cause signal that can be confused with surfacing meniscal signal.
  - One example is the popliteus tendon within the popliteal hiatus. The popliteus tendon courses through the posterolateral joint space, adjacent to the lateral meniscus at the junction of the body and posterior horn. Fluid around the tendon can simulate a peripheral tear in the lateral meniscus.
  - The junction of the lateral meniscus posterior horn and the meniscofemoral ligaments also may produce an appearance that mimics meniscal tear.
    - Conversely, posterior horn lateral meniscus is a frequent site of undercalling meniscal tear in the

setting of an acute ACL tear, and these tears can occur at the meniscofemoral ligament attachment (such as the "Wrisberg rip" tear).
- The *transverse anterior meniscal ligament* extends from the anterior horn of the medial and lateral menisci; attachment sites can simulate anterior horn tear.
- Additional potential pitfalls include striations at the root attachments, fluid in normal recesses, and MRI artifact.
- Chondrocalcinosis (meniscal calcification due to calcium phosphate deposition), usually seen in older patients, can appear as increased signal and be mistaken for a tear.
- **Postoperative meniscus.**
  - Can be very challenging to evaluate.
  - A successfully surgically treated tear without resection heals with fibrosis than can resemble and acute tear on all MR sequences. High rather than intermediate T2 signal (fluid signal) can indicate joint fluid entering a tear rather than fibrosis. Thus when reviewing a postoperative meniscus, emphasize findings on T2W images.
  - Alteration of anatomy is also important. Partial meniscectomy usually results in a smooth, blunted appearance due to free edge resection, or a normal-appearing but smaller triangular-shaped meniscus (Fig. 6.39). If the postoperative meniscus has irregular margins, a recurrent tear is more likely.
  - Accuracy of detection of recurrent tears is enhanced with MR or CT arthrography by demonstration of contrast extending into a true meniscal tear.
    - MR and CT arthrography have a high accuracy in the diagnosis of a recurrent tear—approximately

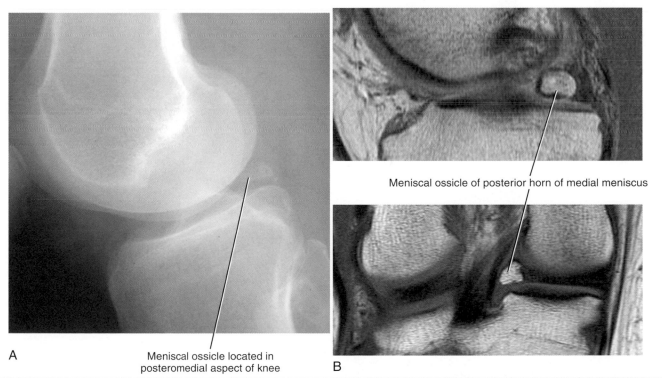

A   Meniscal ossicle located in posteromedial aspect of knee

B

Meniscal ossicle of posterior horn of medial meniscus

Fig. 6.38 Meniscal ossicle. **(A)** Lateral radiograph shows an ossicle at the posterior joint margin. **(B)** Sagittal and coronal T1-weighted MR images show fat signal within the ossicle reflecting fatty marrow. Although radiographs might suggest a loose body, MRI shows that the ossification is located within the posterior horn of the medial meniscus, at the site of a previous meniscal root tear. (From Morrison W. *Problem Solving in Musculoskeletal Imaging.* Philadelphia: Elsevier; 2010.)

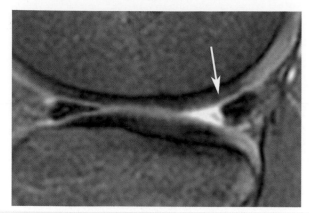

Fig. 6.39 Postoperative meniscus. Fat-suppressed sagittal T2-weighted MR image shows resected free edge of the lateral meniscus posterior horn *(arrow)*. Knowledge of the surgical history is necessary to avoid mistaking this finding for a tear. Note the similarity of the appearance of the free margin with the meniscal tear in Fig. 6.33C.

90%, compared with about 80% for unenhanced MRI. Some authors advocate MR arthrography in all postoperative knees; others recommend MR arthrography only if the meniscus has indeterminate signal.

WHAT THE CLINICIAN WANTS TO KNOW

Meniscal Tears

- Location: Medial versus lateral; anterior horn/body/posterior horn/root attachment; superior/inferior surface; peripheral versus central (inner margin/free edge).
- Configuration: Horizontal, oblique, vertical, bucket handle, radial, parrot beak, complex.
- Displacement; flipped fragments; extrusion.
- Discoid meniscus.

Key Concepts

Pitfalls in Overdiagnosing Meniscal Tears on MRI

Popliteus tendon crossing the lateral meniscus at the popliteal hiatus	Junction PH/Body LM
Meniscofemoral ligaments arising from the lateral meniscus	PHLM near posterior root
Transverse meniscal ligament (anterior horns)	AH MM and AH LM near anterior root
Normal striations at root attachment	AH LM
Normal fluid in meniscocapsular recesses	Lateral meniscus
Previous repair or partial meniscectomy	Anywhere
Artifact (i.e., motion)	Anywhere
Chondrocalcinosis	Anywhere

PH = posterior horn, AH = anterior horn, LM = lateral meniscus, MM = medial meniscus.

Ligaments

CRUCIATE LIGAMENTS

- The cruciate ligaments are major stabilizing ligaments of the knee that are intracapsular yet extrasynovial in location (i.e., they are covered by the joint synovium).
- **ACL:**
  - The ACL is the primary stabilizer of the knee against anterior tibial translation (subluxation).
  - The ACL originates from the medial margin of the lateral femoral condyle at the intercondylar notch and courses anteriorly, medially, and inferiorly to insert at the anterior aspect of the intercondylar eminence (Figs. 6.40 and 6.41).
  - The ACL consists of two discrete bundles, the more dominant *anteromedial bundle* and less dominant *posterolateral bundle*. Bundles are best seen individually on coronal MR images.
  - The ACL remains taut throughout the range of knee motion. The anteromedial bundle resists anterior tibial subluxation in knee flexion, and the posterolateral bundle does so in knee extension.
- **PCL:**
  - The PCL is the primary restraint against posterior tibial translation (subluxation).
  - It originates from the lateral margin of the medial femoral condyle at the intercondylar notch to course in a posterior, lateral, and inferior direction to insert in a depression behind the intercondylar region of the tibia.
  - The PCL is round in cross section, and is taut only in knee flexion (assuming that the ACL is intact).
  - On sagittal MR images with the knee in extension, the PCL appears thick, black, and curved, with its apex (called the *genu*) posterior (Fig. 6.42).

ANTERIOR CRUCIATE LIGAMENT INJURY

- The ACL is the most commonly completely torn ligament of the knee, and a search for ACL tear is a frequent indication for MRI.
- ACL tear typically occurs from pivot-shift or hyperextension mechanism.
  - *Pivot-shift injury* is the most common mechanism for ACL tear (Fig. 6.43).
    - The body (and femur) rotate externally on the planted leg.
    - The MCL is the center of rotation creating shear injury at the medial meniscus attachment to the posterior capsule (resulting in a peripheral vertical meniscal tear or ramp lesion).
    - At the lateral compartment the femur slides posteriorly over the tibia (ACL failure).
    - The lateral femoral condylar surface near the sulcus terminalis impacts on the posterolateral tibia (bone bruises, impaction injury at the far posterior lateral tibial plateau, posterior horn lateral meniscal tear). Similar injury can also occur in the medial compartment.
    - There may be additional distraction medially (valgus—MCL injury).

Roof of the intercondylar notch

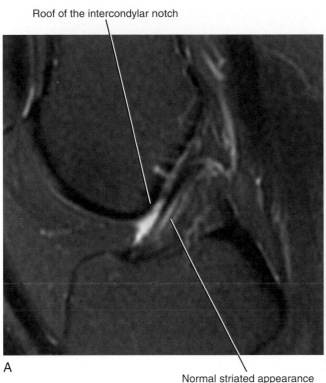

A

Normal striated appearance
of distal ACL

Normal oval appearance of the ACL
at level of femoral attachment

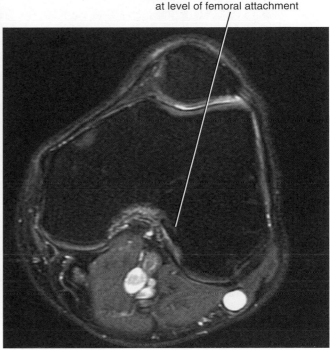

B

Anteromedial bundle of the ACL

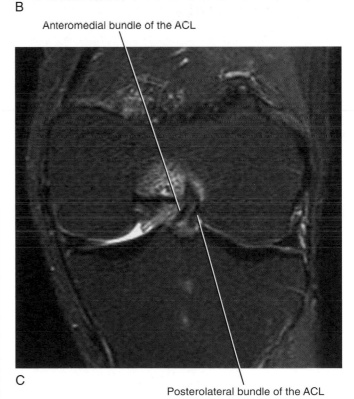

C

Posterolateral bundle of the ACL

Fig. 6.40 Normal anterior cruciate ligament (ACL). T2-weighted sagittal images. **(A)** The normal ACL appears as a dark bandlike structure 3 to 4 mm thick that parallels but does not touch the roof of the intercondylar notch (Blumensaat's line). The normal striated appearance of the distal ACL results from fluid, fat, and synovium tracking between the two bundles of the ACL and should not be misinterpreted as a tear. **(B)** The axial imaging plane is excellent for demonstrating the femoral attachment of the ACL. At this level, the ACL is a low-signal-intensity oval-appearing structure located immediately adjacent to the intercondylar notch portion of the lateral femoral condyle. **(C)** Coronal images clearly demonstrate the two separate bundles of the ACL and depict the normal proximal and distal ACL attachments. (From Morrison W. *Problem Solving in Musculoskeletal Imaging*. Philadelphia: Elsevier; 2010.)

- Hyperextension injury may occur upon landing from a jump (Fig. 6.44).
  - The anterior femoral condyle impacts on the anterior tibial plateau (bone bruises/fracture).
  - Distraction occurs at the posterior joint (ACL and/or PCL tear, posterior capsular tear).
  - Can result in tibiofemoral dislocation (with injury to popliteal vascular structures).
    - There may be additional varus distraction (posterolateral corner injury).
- There are three primary signs of ACL tear on MRI: ligament edema, fiber discontinuity, and change in the expected ligament course (Fig. 6.45). These signs apply for any ligament and are highly accurate for the assessment of the ACL. For ACL evaluation, these primary signs have accuracy in excess of 90%.

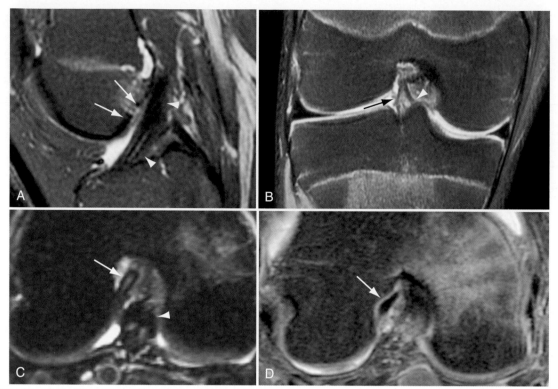

Fig. 6.41 Normal anterior cruciate ligament (ACL). **(A)** Sagittal fat-suppressed proton density MR image shows the posterior margin of the ACL denoted by *arrowheads*. Note the roof of the intercondylar notch *(arrows)*. Also note the normal orientation of the ACL, which is more vertical than the roof of the femoral intercondylar notch. **(B)** Coronal fat-suppressed proton density MR image shows normal fanlike appearance of ACL with the anteromedial *(arrowhead)* and posterolateral *(arrow)* bands of the ligament. **(C and D)** Axial fat-suppressed T2-weighted MR images with normal ACLs show normal ovoid cross section of the ACL *(arrows)*. The periphery of the ligament should have low signal intensity, although the central portion may have high T2 signal (as in **C**) or low signal (as in **D**). Also note the posterior cruciate ligament *(arrowhead)*.

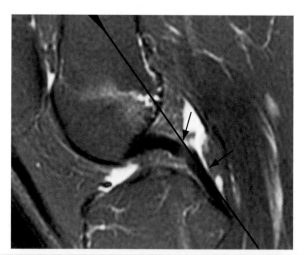

Fig. 6.42 Normal posterior cruciate ligament (PCL). Sagittal fat-suppressed proton density–weighted MR image shows a normal PCL *(arrows)*. Note that a line drawn tangent to the posterior margin of the descending limb intersects the distal femur. If this line was more vertical and did not intersect the distal femur ('buckled PCL'), that would be an indirect sign of a torn anterior cruciate ligament.

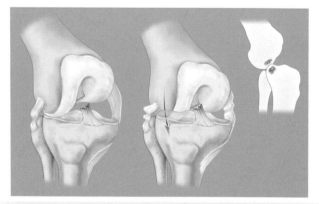

Fig. 6.43 Pivot-shift injury, a noncontact injury commonly seen in American football players and skiers. With the foot planted, a combination of valgus stress applied to the knee and internal rotation of the femur results in disruption of the anterior cruciate ligament. The tibia then translates anteriorly relative to the distal femur, allowing impaction of the lateral femoral condyle against the posterolateral tibial plateau and resulting in the pivot-shift bone contusion pattern (far right image). Increasing degrees of flexion at the time of injury result in a more posteriorly located contusion on the femur. (From Morrison W. *Problem Solving in Musculoskeletal Imaging*. Philadelphia: Elsevier; 2010.)

- Normally the ACL fibers are aligned parallel to or steeper than the roof of the intercondylar notch (called *Blumensaat's line*). In the setting of ACL disruption, the ligament fibers may fall to a more horizontal position; ligament fibers may also be displaced or flipped anteriorly in the intercondylar notch.

- The most common location of ACL tear is at the midportion ('midsubstance'). Second most common location is at the femoral attachment.
- Distal ACL injuries are rare, and usually consist of avulsion fractures from the tibial spines, typically seen in skeletally immature patients.

- The most useful imaging sequences for the evaluation of the ACL are fat-suppressed intermediate or T2-weighted fast spin-echo sequences. These allow the best demonstration of edema-like signal while still allowing clear visualization of soft tissue anatomy.
- The ACL should be evaluated in all three planes on MRI. Be aware that sagittal images can miss ligament detachment from the femur, and volume averaging of joint fluid between ACL bundles in some patients can suggest ligament edema and tear when none is present. The authors find the coronal plane to be the most reliable for detection of an ACL tear.
- The demonstration of a normal ACL without swelling or edema-like signal in any imaging plane generally excludes an ACL tear. An exception is some cases of

ligament detachment from the femur, which may be seen only on coronal or axial images.

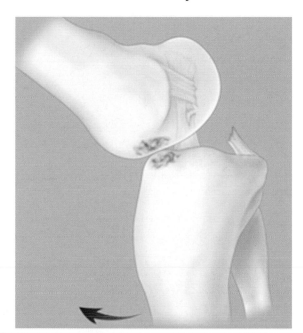

Fig. 6.44 Hyperextension injury. A kissing contusion bone edema pattern occurs from impaction of the anterior tibia against the anterior femur. This injury can occur from a forceful kicking motion, but the most severe injuries often occur as the result of the bumper of a car making impact against the anterior tibia. (From Morrison W. *Problem Solving in Musculoskeletal Imaging*. Philadelphia: Elsevier; 2010.)

Key Concepts

Anterior Cruciate Ligament Injury

- Pivot-shift or hyperextension mechanism
- If the ACL appears intact on any sequence, it usually is intact
- Primary signs of tear: fiber disruption, abnormal orientation
- Secondary signs include characteristic bone bruises and signs associated with anterior tibial displacement (PCL buckling, lateral meniscal uncovering, lateral collateral ligament [LCL] sign)
- Associated findings: bone bruises, meniscal tear, MCL injury

- Several secondary signs of ACL tear independently show high accuracy in assessment of ACL disruption (Fig. 6.46). However, these signs are only occasionally helpful in diagnosing an ACL tear because they usually are present only when the ACL is obviously torn. Secondary signs include:
  - *Bone bruises.* The most specific of these secondary signs is a pattern of 'pivot shift' subchondral bone bruises at the lateral femoral condyle and the posterior lateral tibial plateau (representing impaction from a pivot-shift mechanism). Often there is also a bone bruise at the posterior margin of the medial tibial plateau. An exception to this association is among pediatric patients, in whom this bone bruise pattern may occur in the absence of an ACL tear. This is due to greater laxity of the ACL in children.
  - *Hemarthrosis.* Another secondary sign of ACL tear is the presence of a hemarthrosis (Fig. 6.46B). In fact, as many as 75% of acute knee hemarthroses are the result of ACL rupture. The other causes of hemarthrosis in the setting of trauma are intraarticular fractures and large bone bruises.
  - The other signs are all '*anterior drawer sign*' related—measurements that become abnormal as the tibia translates anteriorly related to ACL insufficiency:
    - Buckling of the PCL: In the setting of ACL injury, the PCL can appear hyperangulated ('buckled').

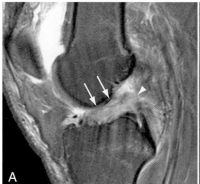
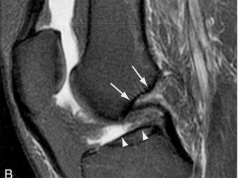
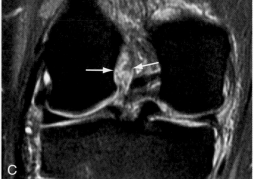

Fig. 6.45 Anterior cruciate ligament (ACL) tear. **(A)** Sagittal fat-suppressed T2-weighted MR image shows fiber discontinuity and edema of a torn ACL *(arrows)*. The ACL is lax, wavy, and horizontally oriented. Note the torn ligament margin proximally *(arrowhead)*. **(B)** Sagittal fat-suppressed proton density–weighted MR image in another patient shows abnormal course of ACL. The ACL *(arrowheads)* remnant is oriented more horizontally than the notch roof *(arrows)*. Note lack of edema compatible with chronic ACL tear. **(C)** Coronal fat-suppressed proton density MR image shows localized increased signal *(arrows)* in the lateral intercondylar notch at expected location of the proximal ACL. This is called an 'empty sulcus' or 'empty notch' sign.

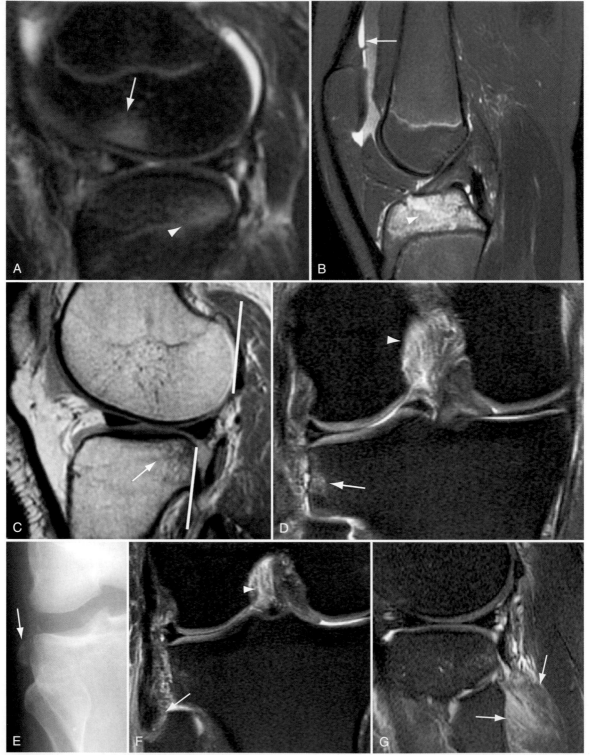

Fig. 6.46 Secondary signs of anterior cruciate ligament (ACL) tear. **(A)** Bone bruises. Sagittal fat-suppressed T2-weighted MR image shows marrow edema in the anterior lateral femoral condyle *(arrow)* and posterior lateral tibia *(arrowhead)*. **(B)** Hemarthrosis in the setting of ACL insertional avulsion. Sagittal fat-suppressed proton density MR image shows a hemarthrosis with a fluid-fluid level *(arrow)*. Note the nondisplaced fracture of the intercondylar eminence *(arrowhead)* and normal-appearing ACL. **(C)** Anterior tibial subluxation. Sagittal proton density spin-echo MR image with vertical *lines* drawn along the posterior margin of the lateral femoral and tibial condyles illustrating substantial anterior tibial subluxation. Also note the posterolateral tibial condyle bone bruise *(arrow)* and the posterior subluxation of the posterior horn of the lateral meniscus. **(D)** Segond fracture. Coronal fat-suppressed proton density MR image shows edema and capsular disruption at midlateral tibial condyle *(arrow)*. Note increased signal *(arrowhead)* at location where a normal ACL should be expected. **(E)** Segond fracture *(arrow)*. **(F)** Lateral collateral ligament avulsion. Coronal fat-suppressed proton density MR image shows avulsion of the lateral collateral ligament insertion *(arrow)*. Note increased signal at location where the ACL is expected *(arrowhead)*. Failure of recognition and repair of posterolateral corner injury will result in persistent rotational instability of the knee and failure of ACL repair. **(G)** Popliteus tendon strain. Note high signal throughout the musculotendinous junction *(arrows)*. Posterolateral corner injury such as this has a high association with ACL tear. See also Fig. 6.42.

Normally a line drawn tangent to the posterior margin of the PCL should intersect the femur (see Fig. 6.42). When this line fails to intersect the femur, this usually means the tibia is translated anteriorly.

- Direct measurement of anterior drawer (Fig. 6.46C): Vertical lines are drawn along the posterior margin of the lateral tibial plateau and the posterior margin of the lateral femoral condyle. ACL tear is likely if the tibia is subluxed more than 5 mm anteriorly relative to the femoral condyle.
- Uncovering of the lateral meniscus: The peripheral margin of the posterior horn of the lateral meniscus is posteriorly displaced relative to the posterior margin of the lateral tibial plateau, and loses contact with the tibia.
- LCL sign: Normally the lateral collateral ligament (fibular collateral ligament) courses obliquely on coronal images and is seen on more than one coronal image; if it is visualized on just one slice, this can mean the tibia is translated anteriorly.

- An ACL injury can be associated with MCL injury and medial meniscal tear. This association is known as *O'Donoghue's unhappy triad*, the unhappy medial triad, or O'Donoghue's terrible triad.
- Note that MCL injury frequently occurs without ACL tear. MCL injury is seen with valgus mechanism.
- Medial meniscal tears reflect anatomy and mechanism. The medial meniscus has tight capsular attachments. Twisting results in a shear injury that preferentially causes peripheral vertical tears including the ramp lesion and bucket handle tears.
- Lateral meniscus tears also reflect the mechanism. Pivot-shift injury results in impaction of the posterior horn between the femoral condyle and tibial plateau, causing complex and radial tears in this location. Lateral meniscus posterior horn tears are one of the most frequently overlooked findings in MRI studies with ACL tear.
- Another associated injury is the *Segond fracture*, which is a lateral capsular/ALL avulsion fracture at the lateral tibial plateau due to rotational injury (Figs. 6.19 and 6.46D,E). Segond fractures are nearly always associated with an ACL tear.

Sample Report

MRI left knee
Standard noncontrast protocol
No comparison studies
Major ligaments: The ACL is lax, with wavy, edematous fibers. MCL, LCL, and PCL are intact.
Menisci: Vertical longitudinal linear signal in the peripheral medial meniscus posterior horn, extends to upper and lower surfaces (or femoral and tibial surfaces if you prefer). No additional meniscal tear. Lateral meniscus intact.
Tendons: No tendinopathy
Articular Cartilage: Normal. No defect.
Bone Marrow: Subchondral marrow edema deep to far posterior margin lateral tibial plateau without deformity. Subchondral marrow edema also noted deep to the far anterior weight-bearing lateral femoral condyle, also without deformity. Marrow signal otherwise normal.

Joint fluid: Moderate joint effusion with increased T1 signal compatible with hemarthosis. No Baker cyst.
Impression:
Complete ACL tear
MCL intact
Peripheral longitudinal tear medial meniscus posterior horn.
Pivot-shift pattern lateral compartment bone bruises without deformity.

- *Posterolateral corner injuries* may occur with ACL or PCL tears.
  - Posterolateral corner structures include the LCL (fibular collateral ligament) (Fig. 6.46F), the biceps femoris tendon, the lateral capsule, the popliteus tendon (Fig. 6.46G), as well as some smaller structures: the popliteofibular ligament, the arcuate ligament, and the fabellofibular ligament.
  - The occurrence of posterolateral corner injuries at MRI implies ACL and/or PCL tear.
  - Unstable injuries of the posterolateral corner are considered an indication for repair in addition to cruciate reconstruction because of concern for delayed instability and failure of the cruciate graft.
  - Other signs of posterolateral corner injury are the Segond fracture and avulsion fracture of the fibular head (called an '*arcuate fracture*'; see Fig. 6.20A).
  - Posterolateral corner injuries are further discussed below.
- Partial ACL tear.
  - Partial ACL tear is uncommon compared to complete tear.
  - Partial tear can be diagnosed when one bundle is torn and one remains intact (Fig. 6.47).
  - Partial tears are best depicted on coronal images.
  - On MRI, look for the typical bone bruises and edema within the ligament. Follow the individual bundles - if only one is disrupted, this represents a partial tear.
- ACL degeneration can also occur, with diffuse intermediate signal on T1- and T2-weighted images (also called *mucoid degeneration*). This is associated with ACL ganglion cyst formation (Figs. 6.48 and 6.49).
  - ACL ganglion cysts may be intra- or peri-ligamentous, and can extend posteriorly or anteriorly from the tendon substance. They can cause limited range of motion on flexion/extension and pain.
  - To differentiate an ACL ganglion cyst from a normal recess, look for lobulation, mass effect, and fluid disproportionate to joint fluid.
- **ACL reconstruction**.
  - ACL tears may be managed nonoperatively with muscle strengthening, especially in older and/or less-active patients. Early OA is the main complication.
  - The only surgical option is ligament reconstruction.
    - Successful reconstruction improves function (e.g., necessary for many athletes) and reduces but does not eliminate risk of early OA.
  - Reconstruction of the ACL can be performed arthroscopically either with tendon autografts or with cadaveric allografts.
    - Goal is to reproduce normal anatomy with a viable graft.
    - Proper graft placement is essential to success (Fig. 6.50).

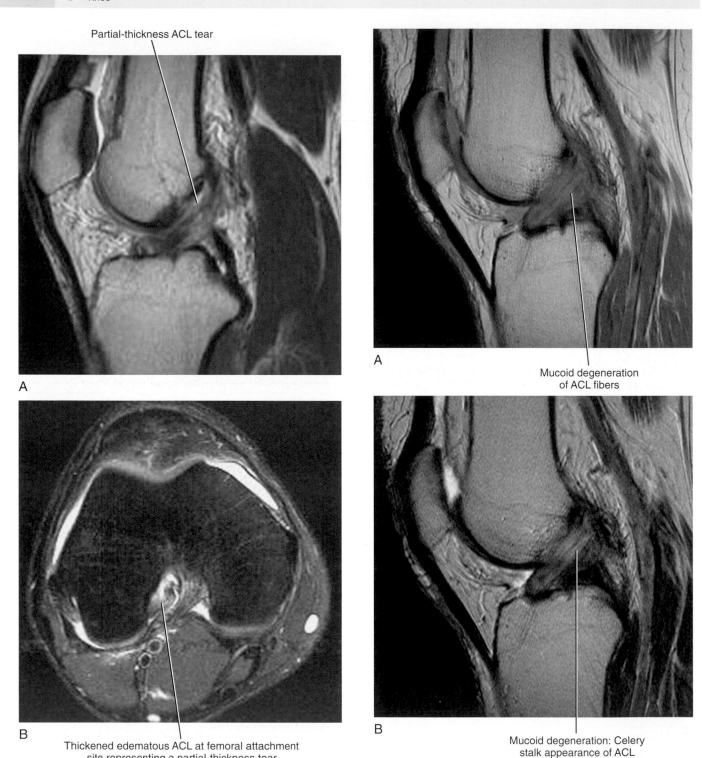

Partial-thickness ACL tear

A

B

Thickened edematous ACL at femoral attachment
site representing a partial-thickness tear

Fig. 6.47 Partial-thickness anterior cruciate ligament (ACL) tear. Sagittal T2-weighted **(A)** and axial **(B)** images demonstrate a partial-thickness tear of the proximal ACL. High signal and thickening of the proximal fibers of the ACL are seen. However, some fibers do remain intact, and on the basis of the clinical exam the patient had a competent ACL. (From Morrison W. *Problem Solving in Musculoskeletal Imaging*. Philadelphia: Elsevier; 2010.)

A

Mucoid degeneration
of ACL fibers

B

Mucoid degeneration: Celery
stalk appearance of ACL

Fig. 6.48 Mucoid degeneration of the anterior cruciate ligament (ACL). Sagittal proton density **(A)** and T2-weighted **(B)** images demonstrate a thickened ACL with splaying of its fibers and intermediate signal abnormality described as a celery stalk appearance. (From Morrison W. *Problem Solving in Musculoskeletal Imaging*. Philadelphia: Elsevier; 2010.)

Intracruciate ACL ganglion

Pericruciate ganglion arising from
proximal ACL fibers

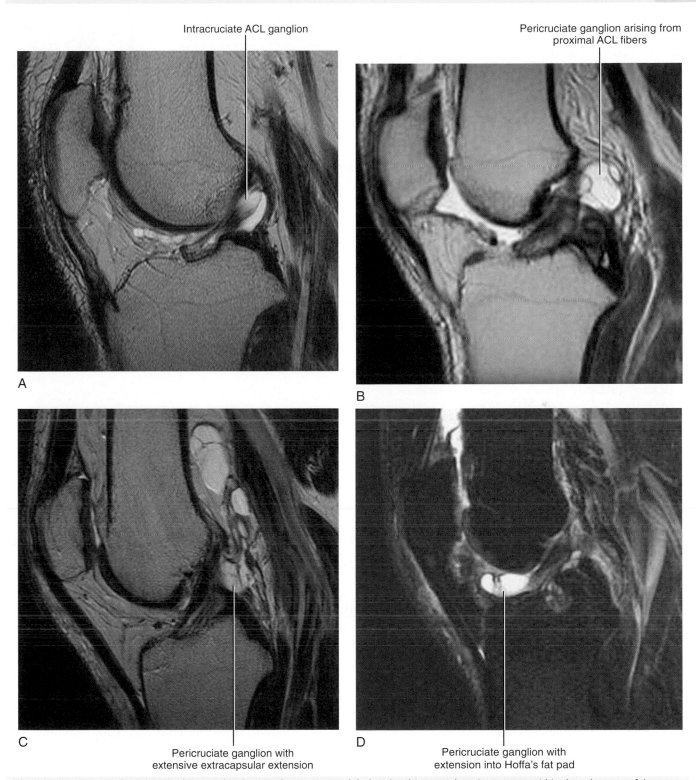

A

B

C

D

Pericruciate ganglion with
extensive extracapsular extension

Pericruciate ganglion with
extension into Hoffa's fat pad

Fig. 6.49 Cruciate ganglia. **(A)** Sagittal T2-weighted image demonstrates a lobulated multiseptated cystic structure within the substance of the anterior cruciate ligament (ACL) consistent with an intracruciate ganglion. **(B)** A pericruciate ganglion arising along the posterior margin of the ACL. **(C)** A large pericruciate ganglion that has penetrated the posterior joint capsule and has dissected into the posterior soft tissues of the knee. **(D)** A large pericruciate ganglion arising from the distal ACL fibers and dissecting into Hoffa's fat pad anteriorly. (From Morrison W. *Problem Solving in Musculoskeletal Imaging.* Philadelphia: Elsevier; 2010.)

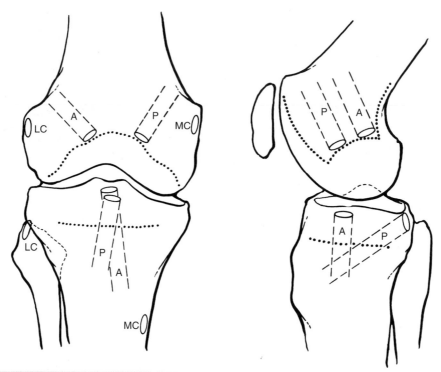

Fig. 6.50 Diagrams show anatomic sites for anterior and posterior cruciate ligament reconstructions, as well as isometric points for attachments of the lateral and medial collateral ligaments. Optimal tunnel positioning or ligament attachment should roughly match the sites shown on these diagrams. *A*, Anterior cruciate ligament; *LC*, lateral collateral ligament; *MC*, medial collateral ligament; *P*, posterior cruciate ligament. (Reproduced with permission from Manaster BJ. *Handbook of Skeletal Radiology*. 2nd ed. St. Louis: Mosby; 1997.)

- *Patellar bone–tendon–bone (BTB) autograft*: The central third of the patellar tendon is harvested longitudinally, along with a piece of bone from the attachment sites at the inferior patella and the tibial tuberosity.
  - The graft is placed along the course of the ACL and may be secured within femoral and tibial tunnels by wedging an interference screw next to the bony portion of the graft within the tunnel.
  - The bony portions of the graft heal well to the femur and tibia, resulting in a very strong construct.
  - Currently this is the most common technique.
- *Hamstring autograft*: The semitendinosus and gracilis tendons are harvested.
  - The tendons are folded over, forming a four-bundle construct; this is placed through femoral and tibial tunnels with fixation via washers to the outer cortices.
- *Cadaveric allograft*: Graft acquired via various sources. Placed via tunnels and fixated.
- Extraarticular reconstructions using the hamstring tendons have been performed, but the practice is uncommon currently.
- Improper tunnel placement can lead to graft impingement or excess laxity.
- MRI is useful after ACL graft reconstruction for evaluating the integrity of the graft. The graft revascularizes during the first 6 months (more or less) after surgery and consequently may initially contain increased T2 signal. Fiber continuity, dark signal, and normal tendon orientation should be expected thereafter.

- Long-term complications after ACL reconstruction:
  - Graft failure, including degeneration and tear.
  - Tunnel expansion and graft laxity: The femoral and/or tibial tunnels can undergo widening with fibrous or fluid signal (often with a ganglion cyst); this sign is associated with graft laxity and mobility and is a harbinger of graft failure (Fig. 6.51).
  - *Graft impingement*: Seen as posterior bowing or 'S' shaped curvature of the graft on sagittal images, the intercondylar notch roof can impinge upon the graft resulting in degeneration and tear (Fig. 6.52).
  - *Arthrofibrosis lesion (cyclops lesion)*: Fibrous proliferation can occur anterior to the distal graft, known as anterior arthrofibrosis or a 'cyclops' lesion (because it is round and whitish on arthroscopy, looking like an eye). A cyclops lesion will interfere with terminal knee extension (see Fig. 6.52A).
  - Pain and accelerated OA with suboptimal tunnel placement.
  - Rarely the patellar tendon can rupture or the patella can fracture at the bone-tendon graft harvest site.

POSTERIOR CRUCIATE LIGAMENT INJURY

- Ruptures of the PCL are uncommon because of the large size and strength of the PCL.
- The majority of PCL tears are partial tears, occurring at the midportion (the 'genu'). This contrasts with ACL tears, which are usually complete.

ACL graft normal in region of intercondylar notch

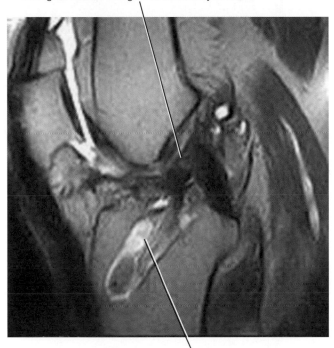

Tibial tunnel expansion with granulation tissue

Fig. 6.51 Tunnel lysis (expansion). Sagittal T2-weighted image shows marked expansion of the tunnel and high-signal granulation tissue surrounding the anterior cruciate ligament (ACL) graft fibers within the osseous tunnel. (From Morrison W. *Problem Solving in Musculoskeletal Imaging.* Philadelphia: Elsevier; 2010.)

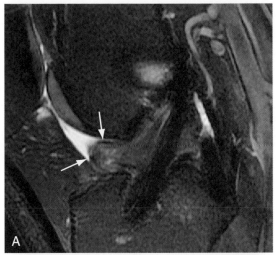

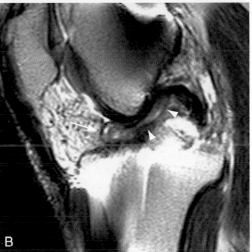

Fig. 6.52 Arthrofibrosis (cyclops) lesion and anterior cruciate ligament (ACL) impingement. **(A)** Sagittal fat-suppressed T2-weighted MR image obtained parallel to an ACL graft shows a low/intermediate signal mass *(arrows)* originating from the anterior distal graft, occluding the anterior joint recess representing a cyclops lesion (anterior arthrofibrosis). **(B)** Sagittal T2-weighted MR image in a different patient shows an attenuated ACL graft *(arrowheads)* with posterior bowing resulting in an 'S' shape; this is a sign of graft impingement and pending failure.

- PCL injury can occur from hyperextension and varus stress, or from blunt trauma to the anterior proximal tibia with the knee in flexion resulting in direct posterior tibial translation (dashboard injury) (Fig. 6.53).
- PCL tear can occur with severe injury in association with other ligament tears, such as in combination with ACL tear in tibiofemoral dislocation.
  - In particular, PCL tear is classically associated with injury to the posterolateral corner structures.
  - A '*reverse Segond*' fracture may be seen, that is, an avulsion of the deep MCL insertion on the proximal medial tibia.
- MRI criteria for PCL rupture are the same as for other ligaments and include swelling, increased signal intensity, fiber discontinuity, and abnormal course (Fig. 6.54).
  - Normally, in the extended knee position, the PCL is slightly curved with its apex posteriorly directed and is easily shown on at least two contiguous sagittal cuts. Sharp bowing of the PCL indicates laxity of the tendon either from a tear of the PCL or as a secondary sign of ACL disruption.
  - Avulsions of the PCL rarely occur and are located either at the medial femoral origin or at the posterior tibial insertion.
  - PCL reconstructions are uncommon. Most PCL tears are partial tears, and an isolated PCL injury is not felt to be associated with substantial instability.

Key Concepts

Cruciate injury comparison

ACL tear
- Pivot-shift or hyperextension mechanism
- Common (95% of cruciate tears)
- Usually complete tear
- Associated with MCL sprain and meniscal tears in the acute setting, and early OA chronically
- Reconstruction is the only surgical option

PCL tear
- Tibia driven posteriorly (dashboard injury)
- Uncommon (5% of cruciate tears)
- Usually partial tear
- Rarely reconstructed

Combined ACL and PCL tear
- Usually seen with tibiofemoral dislocation
- Associated with vascular injury in the popliteal fossa

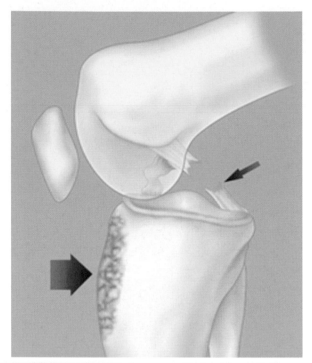

Fig. 6.53 Dashboard injury. The bone contusion results from the application of an external force to the proximal anterior tibia of the flexed knee. The impact results in the posterior translation of the tibia relative to the femur. With the knee in 90 degrees of flexion, the posterior cruciate ligament is taut and at risk for disruption, whereas the anterior cruciate ligament is lax and usually spared injury. (From Morrison W. *Problem Solving in Musculoskeletal Imaging.* Philadelphia: Elsevier; 2010.)

COLLATERAL LIGAMENTS

- The medial and lateral collateral ligaments are the primary restraints to valgus and varus loads, respectively.

Medial Collateral Ligament

- The MCL is a large, complex structure. It is composed of three layers.
  - The most superficial layer is comprised of superficial fascia.
  - The middle layer is the true ligament, which originates just distal to the adductor tubercle of the femur, coursing inferiorly to the medial tibial tubercle, and attaches approximately 5 cm below the joint line near the pes anserinus tendon insertion (Fig. 6.55).
  - The deep layer represents the capsular attachments (the coronary ligament extending from the superior border of the meniscus and the meniscotibial ligament extending from the inferior border).

Key Concepts

Pes anserinus components

- Medial collateral ligament
- Sartorius tendon
- Gracilis tendon
- Semitendinosus tendon
- Bursa (extension of the gastrocnemius/semitendinosus bursa from the knee joint)

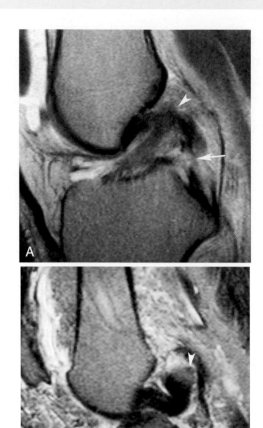

Fig. 6.54 Posterior cruciate ligament (PCL) tears. **(A)** Sagittal fat-suppressed T2-weighted MR image shows complete tears of the distal PCL *(arrow)* and proximal anterior cruciate ligament *(arrowhead)* after a knee dislocation. **(B)** Avulsion fracture of the PCL tibial insertion. Sagittal fat-suppressed T2-weighted MR image shows avulsed tibial insertion *(arrowhead)* with superior displacement. Note edema at the fracture donor site *(arrow)*.

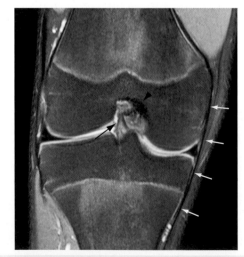

Fig. 6.55 Normal medial collateral ligament. Coronal fat-suppressed proton density MR image shows normal medial collateral ligament *(small white arrows)*. This is the middle layer of the ligament. The deep layer is the joint capsule. Also note the anterior cruciate ligament *(black arrow)* with its fan-shaped appearance of anteromedial and posterolateral bundles, and the posterior cruciate ligament origin *(arrowhead)*.

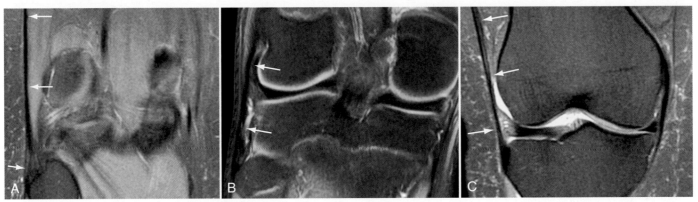

Fig. 6.56 Lateral landmarks. Coronal fat-suppressed proton density–weighted MR images from posterior to anterior in three different patients. **(A)** Biceps femoris tendon *(arrows)*. **(B)** Lateral collateral ligament *(arrows)*. This ligament courses obliquely and tends not to be seen in its entirety on a single image. **(C)** Iliotibial band *(arrows)*.

- The LCL (Fig. 6.56) is also called the fibular collateral ligament (FCL); it is part of the lateral complex of the knee and originates from the lateral femoral condyle (immediately superior to the popliteus tendon origin), extending distally and posteriorly to insert on the fibular head as a 'conjoined tendon' along with the biceps femoris tendon. It is a major contributor to posterolateral stability.
- Injuries of the MCL and LCL often occur in combination with other injuries.
- MCL injury is commonly associated with ACL tears and meniscal tears.
  - Injuries of the MCL are associated with valgus injuries and, like other ligament injuries, range from stretching injury (grade 1 sprain: intact ligament with surrounding edema), to partial tear (grade 2 sprain: disruption of some fibers) to complete disruption (grade 3 sprain). Proximal tears are most common (Fig. 6.57). Distal tears are unusual (Fig. 6.58A).
  - Higher-grade injuries are associated with surrounding edema and hemorrhage in the acute phase.
  - Edema around an otherwise intact MCL can be seen from nontraumatic causes:
    - Ruptured Baker cyst with fluid extending anteriorly along the MCL fascia.
    - Medial meniscal tear.
    - Medial compartment OA.
    - Subchondral stress fracture.
    - History should be reviewed for injury; if there is edema surrounding the MCL without history of trauma, one of these etiologies may be the cause.
  - Lateral patellar dislocation can cause edema around the MCL, simulating MCL injury. (Be careful not to overcall MCL injury when a patellar dislocation is evident.) If called an MCL sprain, the actual injury can be overlooked.
  - *Pellegrini–Stieda* represents posttraumatic ossification at the MCL origin related to previous trauma (Fig. 6.58B). It is of no clinical significance.

LATERAL COLLATERAL COMPLEX AND THE POSTEROLATERAL CORNER

- The *lateral collateral complex* is a combination of tendons and ligaments that stabilize the lateral knee. They include major supporting structures (the iliotibial band, LCL [FCL], and the biceps femoris tendon) and minor structures including the popliteus, the popliteofibular ligament, the arcuate ligament, and the fabellofibular ligament.
- The *iliotibial (IT) band* is the tendinous extension of the tensor fasciae latae which arises from the iliac crest. The IT band inserts onto a bony prominence at the anterolateral tibia (Gerdy's tubercle).
- Collectively the other structures are referred to as the posterolateral corner.
  - The FCL arises from the lateral femoral condyle and attaches distally onto the fibular head (Fig. 6.59).
  - The biceps femoris is one of the hamstring muscles; the tendon distally combines with the FCL to form the *conjoined tendon*, inserting on the fibular head.
    - Distraction injury can cause the conjoined tendon to avulse a curved fragment from the fibular head; this is called an *arcuate fracture*. Recognition of this *arcuate sign* on radiographs implies cruciate injury and posterolateral corner instability (see Fig. 6.20).
  - The *popliteus tendon* arises from the lateral femoral condyle from a sulcus just inferior to the FCL origin; it courses obliquely around the posterolateral joint and down the calf deep to the gastrocnemius muscles.
    - Injury to the muscle or proximal myotendinous junction is very common, seen as intramuscular edema and/or tearing of muscle fibers just below the knee joint. Isolated popliteus muscle strain is not associated with posterolateral instability.
  - The *popliteofibular ligament* is a small but important ligament that extends from the popliteus tendon sheath to insert on the fibular head next to the conjoined tendon. It can be seen on sagittal or coronal images. Injury can result in posterolateral instability (Fig. 6.60).
  - The *arcuate ligament* is a triangular fascial plane draping over the popliteus and popliteofibular ligament; it is not easily or consistently seen on MRI.

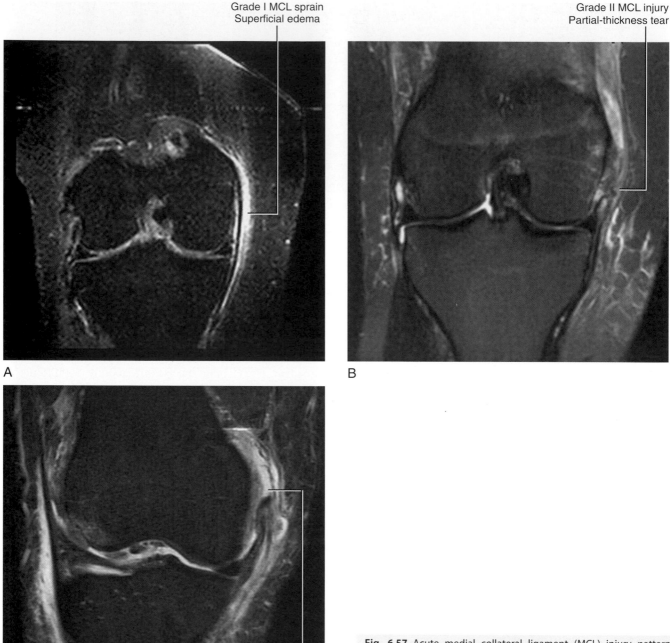

Grade I MCL sprain
Superficial edema

Grade II MCL injury
Partial-thickness tear

Grade III MCL injury
Full-thickness tear

Fig. 6.57 Acute medial collateral ligament (MCL) injury patterns. **(A)** Grade I injury. Edema superficial to the MCL represents a mild sprain but no partial- or full-thickness tear. The MCL fibers appear intact. **(B)** Grade II injury. Mild thickening and edema are seen within the substance of the MCL and superficial soft tissue edema consistent with a partial-thickness tear. **(C)** Grade III injury. There is a complete tear of the proximal MCL fibers with mild retraction of the more distal fibers and adjacent soft tissue edema. (From Morrison W. *Problem Solving in Musculoskeletal Imaging*. Philadelphia: Elsevier; 2010.)

- The fabella is an ovoid ossicle that articulates with the posterior lateral femoral condyle and is actually a sesamoid of the gastrocnemius. It is only present in about 25% of knees; the prevalence and significance is disputed. If a fabella is present, a thin ligament extends from the ossicle to the fibula called the *fabellofibular ligament*.
- Injury to the posterolateral corner is important and rarely occurs in isolation (see Fig. 6.58C).

- Mechanism includes posterolateral twisting and/or distraction, which can occur from pivot-shift, hyperextension, direct posterior tibial translation (dashboard injury), and varus overload.
  - Therefore, injury is typically associated with ACL and/or PCL injury.
- Injury can result in posterolateral instability which can lead to failure of ACL reconstruction and acceleration of patellofemoral OA.

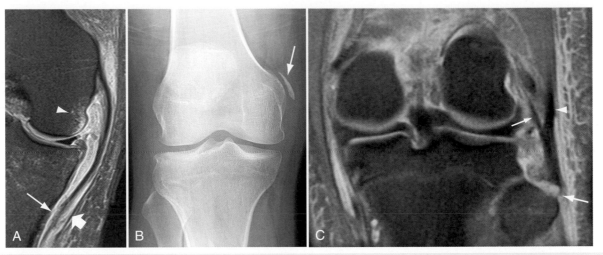

Fig. 6.58 Collateral ligament injuries. **(A)** Coronal fat-suppressed proton density MR image shows edema around the MCL with disruption of the deep layer, with adjacent bone bruise *(arrowhead)*. The deep layer is actually the joint capsule. The middle layer, which is the true ligament, is intact proximally although torn distally *(thin arrow)*. The most superficial layer, which is the superficial fascia, is diffusely torn as well, with some intact fibers distally *(thick arrow)*. **(B)** Pellegrini–Stieda syndrome. Note curvilinear calcification medial to the medial femoral condyle *(arrow)*. This is the typical location and configuration. In many cases the proximal margin of the calcification is continuous with the femur rather than separate as in this example. **(C)** Coronal fat-suppressed proton density MR image shows a fibular avulsion *(large arrow)* of the conjoint insertion of the biceps femoris tendon *(arrowhead)* and lateral collateral ligament *(small arrow)*. In contrast with the conspicuous marrow edema associated with traumatic impaction bone injuries, the marrow edema associated with ligament and capsular avulsion injuries can be extremely subtle.

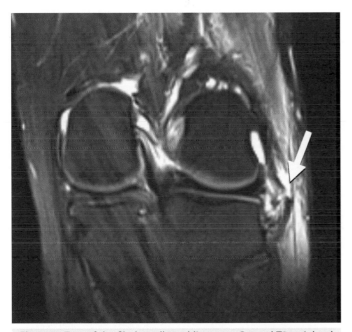

Fig. 6.59 Tear of the fibular collateral ligament. Coronal T2-weighted fat-suppressed MR image through the posterior knee shows edema and disruption of the fibular collateral ligament *(arrow)*.

- Posterolateral corner injury can also be associated with peroneal nerve injury because of the nerve's proximity to the fibular head and LCL insertion (Fig. 6.61).

Tendon Pathology

- Knee injury may be isolated to tendon pathology.
- In the popliteal fossa (excluding the gastrocnemius and soleus muscles), there is only one major muscle laterally (the biceps femoris) but four medially (semimembranosus, semitendinosus, sartorius, and gracilis) (Fig. 6.62).
  - The semimembranosus inserts on the posteromedial tibia near the plateau with a large footprint. The other medial tendons insert on the pes anserinus further distally.
  - The plantaris arises from the lateral fascia above the knee and extends down the calf posterolaterally between the gastrocnemius and popliteus. It crosses the calf obliquely and inserts on the calcaneus, medial to the Achilles.
    - The tendon is of variable size; if robust it can be used as tendon graft material during tendon reconstructions at other sites such as in the wrist.
    - An intact plantaris can result in a false-negative Thompson test on physical exam for Achilles tendon tear. (Thompson test: Squeeze the gastrocnemius and soleus muscles. A positive test is absent foot plantar flexion which implies complete Achilles tendon disruption).
    - The tendon can tear near the knee resulting in posterolateral pain; fluid is seen on MRI between the gastrocnemius and popliteus muscles, appearing like a ruptured Baker cyst—but lateral instead of medial.
- The gastrocnemius is also prone to injury and can cause neurovascular impingement.
  - The gastrocnemius has medial and lateral heads that arise from the superolateral femoral condyles. They course down the calf and join with the soleus muscle to form the Achilles' tendon.
  - Variant anatomy can occur, with altered course of the muscles around the popliteal neurovascular bundle, leading to entrapment and ischemic or neurologic effects in certain positions or with exercise. This is called *popliteal entrapment syndrome.*
  - Tears of the tendon origins are rare.

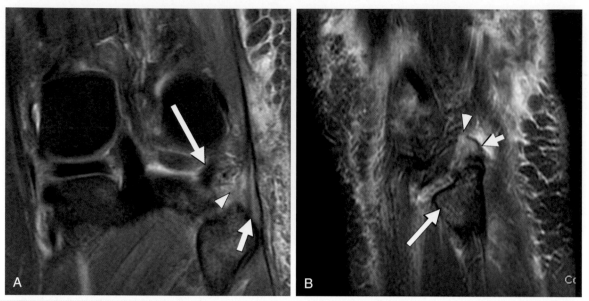

Fig. 6.60 Posterolateral corner injury. **(A)** Coronal T2-weighted fat-suppressed MR image through the posterior knee shows a partial tear of the biceps femoris *(short arrow)* at the insertion on the fibular head. There is a complete tear of the popliteofibular ligament *(arrowhead)* with edema and disrupted fibers in the expected location. The adjacent popliteus tendon *(long arrow)* can be used as a guide to find the popliteofibular ligament. **(B)** Sagittal T2-weighted fat-suppressed MR image of the same patient shows the popliteofibular ligament *(short arrow)* with disruption proximally *(arrowhead)*. Note bone bruise within the fibular head *(long arrow)*.

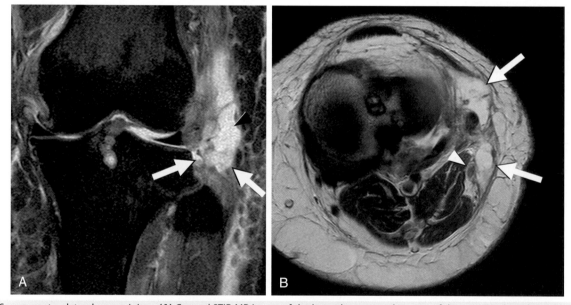

Fig. 6.61 Severe posterolateral corner injury. **(A)** Coronal STIR MR image of the knee shows complete tear of the conjoined tendon *(arrows)* near the insertion on the fibular head, with hematoma *(arrowhead)* at the tear site. **(B)** Axial T2-weighted image in the same patient shows hematoma *(arrows)*. Note close proximity of the posterolateral stabilizing structures with the common peroneal nerve *(arrowhead)*. Severe posterolateral corner injury can result in nerve damage and foot drop.

- Muscle strains are common, especially in athletes. These usually occur at the myotendinous junction, presenting on MRI as V-shaped fluid signal resulting from the tear and hematoma extension along the fascia (Fig. 6.63).
    - *Tennis leg* is a strain at the medial head medial myotendinous junction, typically in older patients. This term is also sometimes used to describe a plantaris tear.
- Small bursae are located between the proximal heads and the posterior femur. Ganglia frequently arise from these bursae, usually small but occasionally large, can be confused for a Baker cyst.
- In children and adolescents, a cortical lucency can appear on lateral radiographs at the gastrocnemius origin, usually medially (Fig. 6.64). This finding represents delayed ossification at the muscle origin and is called an *avulsive cortical irregularity*. It is of no clinical significance but can simulate an aggressive process. An older term for this finding is cortical desmoid. That term has fallen out of favor, since it incorrectly implies a neoplastic etiology.

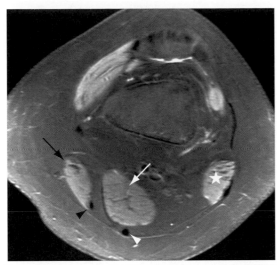

Fig. 6.62 Axial fat-suppressed proton density MR image showing the normal muscle anatomy of the popliteal fossa. On the medial side there are four muscles and/or tendons: the sartorius *(black arrow)*, gracilis *(black arrowhead)*, semimembranosus *(white arrow)*, and semi-tendinosus *(white arrowhead)*. On the lateral side, there is only the biceps femoris muscle and tendon *(white star)*.

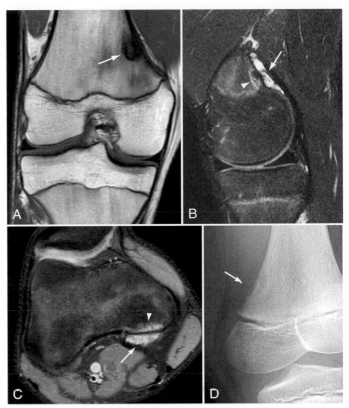

Fig. 6.64 Avulsive cortical irregularity (cortical desmoid) in a 15-year-old boy. **(A)** Coronal T1-weighted MR image shows an eccentrically located geographic low-signal-intensity lesion *(arrow)* at the postero-medial distal femoral metaphysis. **(B)** Sagittal fat-suppressed T2-weighted MR image shows high signal intensity of the adductor magnus enthesis *(arrow)* and subtle underlying bone edema *(arrow-head)*. These lesions will progress to lower signal intensity as they os-sify. **(C)** Axial fat-suppressed T2-weighted MR image shows adductor insertional enthesitis *(arrow)* and reactive bone edema *(arrowhead)*. **(D)** Radiograph in a different child shows typical appearance with concave defect, with subtle calcification in the defect that simulates a bone-forming tumor *(arrow)*.

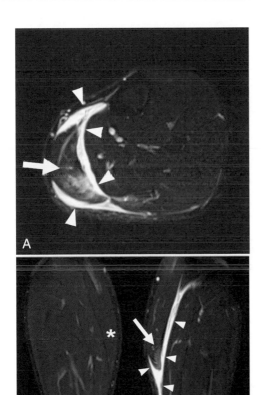

Fig. 6.63 Gastrocnemius tear. **(A)** Axial T2-weighted fat-suppressed MR image of the calf shows edema of the medial head of the gastrocnemius muscle *(arrow)*. Fluid signal *(arrowheads)* surrounds the muscle near the myotendinous junction. **(B)** Coronal STIR image of the same patient shows retraction of the torn medial gastrocnemius *(arrow)* with surrounding fluid *(arrowheads)* in a 'V' shaped pattern. Note normal contralateral muscle *(asterisk)*.

- Anteriorly, the quadriceps muscles (rectus femoris, vastus lateralis, vastus intermedius, vastus medialis, and VMO) join to form the quadriceps tendon.
  - Sagittal MRI images almost always show multiple layers in the quadriceps tendon.
  - The classic arrangement is: superficial layer is the rectus femoris, the middle layer is the conjoined vastus lateralis and medialis, and the deep layer is the vastus intermedius. Variations from this pattern are common.
  - Fascial extensions of the quadriceps aponeurosis form a hood over the anterior half of the knee, known as the retinacula. It is the medial retinaculum and MPFL that can stretch and tear during transient patellar dislocation.
  - Partial tears of the quadriceps tendon are common, affecting one or more of the separate layers (see Fig. 6.65C).
  - Risk factors for quadriceps tendon tear:
    - Age - tears of the distal quadriceps tendon are fairly common in older athletes; typically there is significant underlying tendinosis (Fig. 6.65).
    - Corticosteroid use (including inhaled and knee joint injections).

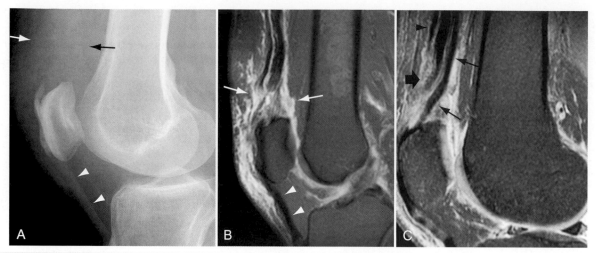

Fig. 6.65 Quadriceps tendon tears. (A and B) Complete rupture. Lateral radiograph **(A)** and sagittal fat-suppressed T2-weighted MR image **(B)** show edema *(arrows)* and interrupted distal tendon. Contrast with normal patellar tendon *(arrowheads)*. **(C)** Incomplete tear. Sagittal fat-suppressed proton density–weighted MR image in a patient with weak knee extension. The superficial layer (rectus femoris, *arrowhead*) and middle layer (vastus medialis and lateralis, *thick arrow*) are ruptured, but the deepest layer (vastus intermedius, *arrows*) is intact.

- Chronic renal failure.
- Diabetes.
- Ciprofloxacin and other fluoroquinolone antibiotics (the Achilles is the most commonly torn tendon with these drugs).
- Patellar tendinosis and tears are common in athletes and nonathletes.
  - Predisposing factors include repetitive injury and overuse, as well as steroid treatment and underlying metabolic conditions such as renal failure and diabetes.
  - *Jumper's knee* is an overuse injury associated with certain sports such as basketball.
    - In jumper's knee, findings predominate in the proximal patellar tendon and appear at MRI as increased transverse dimension and increased signal on T2-weighted images, particularly in the posterior midline fibers.
    - Marrow edema may be present in the adjacent patella.
  - Tendinosis is more commonly seen in the posterior proximal tendon, with thickening and intermediate T2 signal within the tendon. Focal fluid signal represents a tear (Fig. 6.66). Edema may be seen in adjacent Hoffa's fat pad.
  - The childhood conditions *Sinding–Larsen–Johansson disease* and *Osgood–Schlatter disease* also include varying degrees of adjacent patellar tendinosis (Fig. 6.67).
  - Patellar tendon disorders are prone to healing with heterotopic ossification within the substance of the patellar tendon and at the attachment sites.
  - Prior ACL graft harvesting can result in tendon thickening, which may represent a combination of normal postoperative change and/or tendinopathy.

Fluid Collections: Cysts and Bursitis

- *Baker cyst*: Also known as a popliteal cyst, this represents distension of the gastrocnemius-semimembranosus

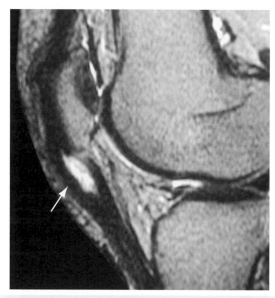

Fig. 6.66 Patellar tendinosis and tear. Sagittal T2-weighted spin-echo MR image shows thickening of the proximal patellar tendon representing tendinosis; fluid signal is present within the tendon extending to the patellar attachment *(arrow)* consistent with a large interstitial tear. This is a common appearance in basketball players and other 'jumping' athletes.

bursa, which becomes a synovial cyst that extends from the joint between the medial gastrocnemius and semimembranosus tendons (Fig. 6.68).
- The Baker cyst deserves special mention because it is so common.
- The narrow opening between the medial gastrocnemius and semimembranosus creates a one-way valve effect, leading to accumulation of fluid.
- May become multiloculated, large, and filled with osteochondral bodies and synovial proliferation (Fig. 6.69).
- May become very large and dissect distally within the gastrocnemius fascia creating painful mass effect on the muscle.

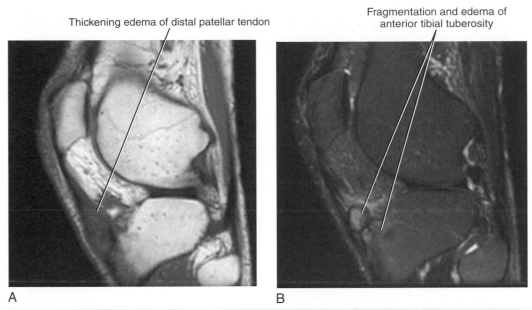

Thickening edema of distal patellar tendon

Fragmentation and edema of anterior tibial tuberosity

A

B

Fig. 6.67 Osgood–Schlatter disease. **(A)** Sagittal T1-weighted image shows marked thickening and signal alteration involving the distal attachment of the patellar tendon. **(B)** Sagittal T2-weighted image shows marked thickening of the distal patellar tendon, fragmentation, and marrow edema of the anterior tibial tuberosity. The marrow edema within the area of fragmentation indicates acute Osgood–Schlatter disease. (From Morrison W. *Problem Solving in Musculoskeletal Imaging.* Philadelphia: Elsevier; 2010.)

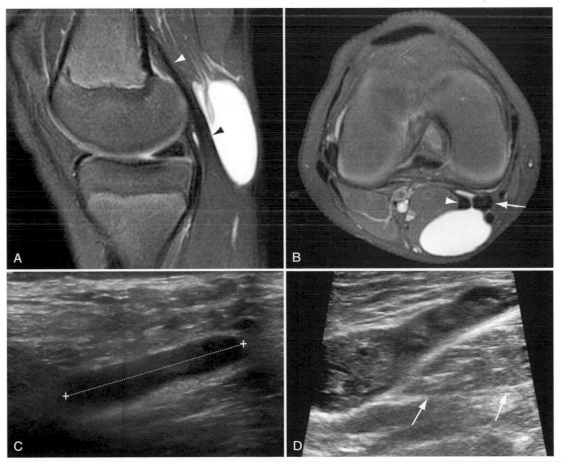

A

B

C

D

Fig. 6.68 Baker cyst. Sagittal **(A)** and axial **(B)** fat-suppressed T2-weighted MR images of an uncomplicated Baker cyst show the distended gastrocnemius-semimembranosus bursa. Note tendons of the gastrocnemius medial head *(arrowheads)* and semimembranosus *(arrow* in B). **(C)** Baker cyst on ultrasound. This uncomplicated cyst contains anechoic fluid. **(D)** Sagittal ultrasonogram in a different patient with a complex Baker cyst (with superior at the left of the image) shows a hypoechoic collection with internal echoes representing hemorrhage and synovitis. Aspiration yielded chronic hemorrhage. Note the medial gastrocnemius muscle *(arrows).*

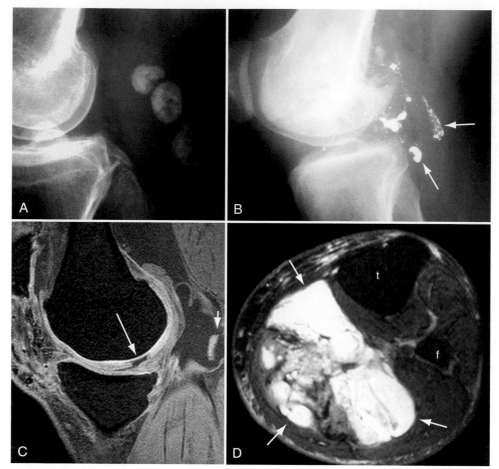

Fig. 6.69 **(A)** Lateral radiograph of the knee showing osteochondral bodies in a Baker cyst, which may be seen in the setting of osteoarthritis. **(B)** Lateral radiograph of the knee showing bullet fragments *(arrows)* in the location of the posterior joint recesses and a Baker cyst. **(C)** Sagittal fat-suppressed spoiled gradient-echo MR image shows an articular cartilage fragment in a Baker cyst *(short arrow)*. Note the medial femoral condyle donor site *(long arrow)*. **(D)** Axial fat-suppressed T2-weighted MR image in the proximal left leg shows a complex-appearing mass *(arrows)* with mixed signal intensity; more superior images showed the mass was continuous with the gastrocnemius-semimembranosus bursa. Large Baker cysts complicated by synovitis and hemorrhage can attain bizarre appearances. Surgical biopsy yielded old blood. *f*, Fibula; *t*, tibia.

- Mass effect on the popliteal vessels and nerves can also occur.
- May rupture, leading to diffuse soft tissue edema posteromedially, often with pain in the popliteal fossa and/or calf.
- Baker cysts are a sign of persistent or recurrent joint effusion. Therefore, a Baker cyst can be a sign of chronic inflammatory arthropathy or chronic internal derangement.
- Gastrocnemius medial and lateral head bursae are located between the proximal muscles and the posterior distal femur. Like the gastrocnemius-semimembranosus bursa, these ganglia may communicate with the knee joint. Ganglia arising from these bursae are common but usually are small.
- A bursa located anterior to the popliteus tendon that also can communicate with the knee joint.
- The *prepatellar bursa* (see Fig. 1.51) is located anterior to the patella can be filled with fluid or synovial tissue in the setting of acute injury (i.e., falling directly on the knee) or from chronic injury from kneeling (previously called *housemaid's knee*). In acute injury the bursa can contain hemorrhage (with hyperintensity on T1-weighted images).

- The *deep* and *superficial infrapatellar bursae* are located posterior and anterior to the distal patellar tendon, respectively. They can become inflamed and filled with fluid in patients with acute injuries, chronic kneeling, or in patients with Osgood–Schlatter disease.
- The *pes anserinus bursa*. Patients may present with pain at the pes anserinus insertion related to a bursitis, which can be documented at MRI with the demonstration of a fluid collection surrounding the tendons as they insert on the medial aspect of the proximal tibia (Fig. 6.70). Fluid can extend proximally and simulate a Baker cyst. However, fluid in this location is often fluid extending inferiorly from a Baker cyst along the semitendinosus tendon.
- *Ganglion cysts* are common around the knee. As noted earlier, similar cysts may originate from meniscal tears (parameniscal cysts).
- Ganglia may develop within or around the ACL or PCL (Fig. 6.71) and may cause mechanical symptoms of impingement on flexion/extension.
- Cruciate ligament ganglion cysts are usually associated with mucoid degeneration of the ligament, usually the ACL.

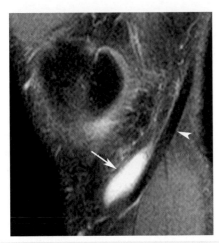

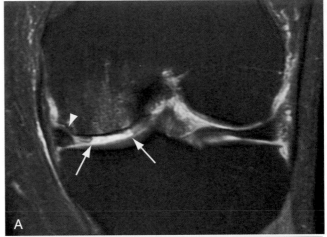

Fig. 6.70 Pes anserinus bursitis. Sagittal fat-suppressed T2-weighted MR image obtained through the medial knee shows well-circumscribed bursal fluid collection *(arrow)* adjacent to the semitendinosus tendon *(arrowhead)*

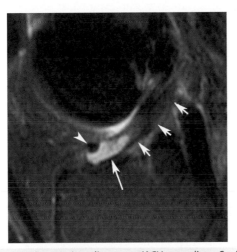

Fig. 6.71 Anterior cruciate ligament (ACL) ganglion. Sagittal fat-suppressed T2-weighted MR image shows well-circumscribed ganglion *(long arrow)* in the distal ACL *(short arrows)*. Note the transverse meniscal ligament *(arrowhead)* that connects the anterior horns of the menisci.

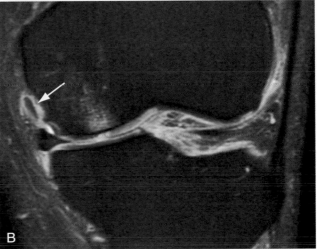

Fig. 6.72 (A) Coronal fat-suppressed proton density MR image shows a large chondral delamination defect *(arrows)* of the medial femoral condyle. Note the adjacent meniscal tear *(arrowhead)*. **(B)** Coronal fat-suppressed proton density MR image in the same patient shows a chondral loose body *(arrow)* in coronary (meniscofemoral) recess of the medial compartment. Note meniscal extrusion associated with underlying tear.

Articular Cartilage Injury

- Descriptors for cartilage damage are presented in Chapter 1 and again in Chapter 9 - Arthritis.
- Knee articular cartilage defects are most common at the patellar and medial tibiofemoral surfaces (see Fig. 6.69C; see also Fig. 1.67).
- Abnormalities of articular cartilage range from chondral to osteochondral damage, and associated pathology is common (Fig. 6.72).
- Associations:
  - Patellofemoral is more prevalent with underlying patellar maltracking disorder.
  - Medial or lateral adjacent to meniscal tear and/or meniscal extrusion (displacement of the meniscus away from the joint).
    - As previously discussed, meniscal body extrusion greater than 3 mm is associated with complete, radial tears, complex tears, and tears at the root attachment.
    - Articular surface deformity (i.e., prior fracture) and/or mechanical abnormality.
- The knee is the most common site for osteochondritis dissecans, a distinctive type of osteochondral lesion in adolescents, with other common sites including the talar dome at the ankle and the capitellum at the elbow. This lesion is discussed in Chapter 1.

Miscellaneous Knee Conditions

SUBCHONDRAL FRACTURE

- Subchondral trabecular insufficiency fractures are common around the knee, especially in older, osteoporotic patients.
- Painful condition usually related to altered joint mechanics. Clinical presentation is sudden onset of severe pain and difficulty weight-bearing.

- Initial radiographs and CT may be normal or show a subtle thin band of sclerosis a few mm deep to and +/- parallel to subchondral bone representing the fracture.
- MRI shows the fracture as a thin low signal line. Adjacent marrow edema may be intense.
- Bone scan: tracer uptake at the site of fracture.
- Some subchondral fractures have a high risk of progression to fragmentation, collapse, and disability often requiring arthroplasty. These almost always occur in the anterior weight bearing medial femoral condyle in association with medial meniscus failure due to posterior root tear.
  - Pathomechanics: An intact meniscus spreads compressive forces across a wide area. Meniscal insufficiency results in all forces concentrated on a small area, especially in the medial femoral condyle due to its convex contours.
  - Approximately 50% heal, 50% progress to articular surface collapse.
  - MRI: test of choice for diagnosis / evaluation (Fig. 6.73).
  - Later imaging findings with collapse: Sclerosis, articular surface collapse; intense bone marrow edema with black subchondral signal / fragmentation on T1 and T2-weighted images representing necrosis.
  - Typically seen in an older population, over 55 years; females > males. There is a higher risk with underlying osteoporosis.
  - There is a negative association with pre-existing osteoarthritis (the bone is already buttressed against altered mechanics).

- Initial management is pain control and strict non-weightbearing. If collapse occurs, arthroplasty is often needed to regain function.
- The imaging appearance of the initial injury and propensity for collapse bear some similarities to osteonecrosis at other sites, hence the original term for this condition, SONK, spontaneous osteonecrosis of the knee. Osteonecrosis does occur within the fragmented bone, but trauma rather than osteonecrosis is the initiating injury. Therefore the term SONK is therefore no longer preferred, but perhaps because it so easily said and remembered, it remains in usage.
- The disease represents a perfect storm of altered mechanics and stress, accelerated by a predisposition for fracture (osteoporosis). These conditions occur in other areas and may represent a similar pathoetiology.
  - Other potential sites/conditions associated with subchondral fracture:
    - *Transient osteoporosis of the hip.*
    - *Clavicular osteolysis* (Seen in weightlifers and/or after grade 1 AC separation).
    - *Osteitis pubis* (seen in athletes with injury to the capsule of the pubic symphysis and/or rectus-adductor aponeurosis.
    - Various bones of the ankle / hindfoot (no specific names for condition).
  - MRI appearance in these locations is similar to that described for subchondral fracture at the knee.
- At the knee, partial meniscectomy can also alter mechanics and can be associated with development of subchondral fracture (Fig. 6.74).

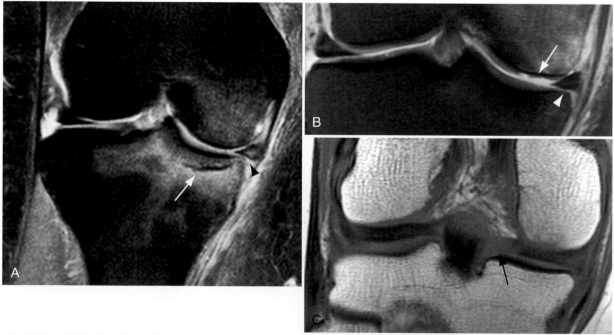

Fig. 6.73 Subchondral insufficiency fracture. **(A)** Coronal fat-suppressed T2-weighted MR image shows intense bone marrow edema in the medial femoral condyle and tibial with low signal line *(arrow)* surrounded by marrow edema. Note medial compartment joint space narrowing and medial meniscal extrusion *(arrowhead)*. Extrusion is commonly associated with subchondral insufficiency fracture because it results in the transmission of excessive loads to the subchondral bone. **(B)** Coronal fat-suppressed proton density–weighted MR image in a different patient shows femoral subchondral stress reaction with overlying high-grade chondral defect *(arrow)* and medial meniscal extrusion *(arrowhead)*. **(C)** Coronal T1-weighted MR image in same patient as B shows the cause for medial meniscal extrusion, namely posterior root tear of the meniscus *(arrow)*.

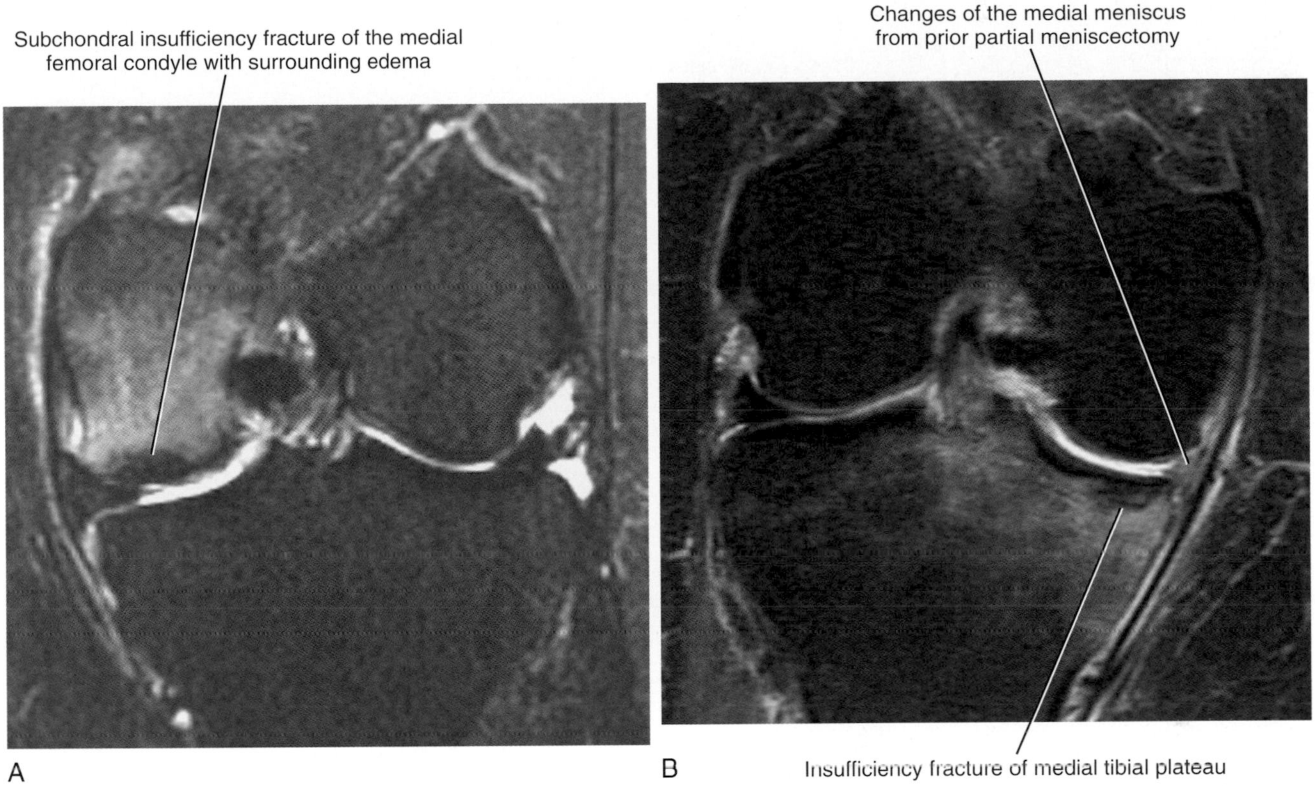

Subchondral insufficiency fracture of the medial
femoral condyle with surrounding edema

Changes of the medial meniscus
from prior partial meniscectomy

A

B   Insufficiency fracture of medial tibial plateau

Fig. 6.74 Insufficiency fracture as a source of pain after partial meniscectomy. **(A)** Coronal T2-weighted image shows a subchondral insufficiency fracture of the medial femoral condyle with extensive surrounding edema following meniscal surgery. **(B)** Coronal T2-weighted image from a different patient shows an insufficiency fracture involving the medial tibial plateau with extensive surrounding edema following partial medial meniscectomy. (From Morrison W. *Problem Solving in Musculoskeletal Imaging*. Philadelphia: Elsevier; 2010.)

Key Concepts

Subchondral Insufficiency Fracture

- Previously called spontaneous osteonecrosis of the knee (SONK)
- *NOT* osteonecrosis, at least not initially
- Often seen with acute complete radial/posterior root tear of the medial meniscus
- Most common in older individuals, especially female
- Medial femoral condyle most common
- Initial MRI appearance: intense bone marrow edema, subchondral crescent or line of low signal
- 50% heal, 50% progress to collapse, necrosis

POPLITEAL ARTERY ENTRAPMENT

- Popliteal artery entrapment occurs as the result of an anomalous course of the popliteal artery relative to the proximal gastrocnemius muscle, most often with the artery coursing through or around the medial head. It can also be seen with normal variation in gastrocnemius anatomy.
  - Patients present in their 20s or 30s with a syndrome of calf claudication when standing or exercising. Definitive diagnosis can be made with MR angiography, angiography, or ultrasonography.

PERONEAL NERVE IMPINGEMENT/INJURY

- The *common peroneal* nerve is vulnerable to injury below the knee as it courses superficially around the fibular neck.

- Mass effect from a lesion such as a ganglion cyst from the proximal tibiofibular joint or an osteochondroma, or trauma to this region (including fibular head fracture and posterolateral corner injury) can result in peroneal nerve dysfunction with foot drop and evidence of denervation of the anterior and lateral leg musculature on MR images.
  - Look for edema (early finding) or fatty infiltration (later finding) in leg anterior and lateral compartment muscles.

PLICAS

- The suprapatellar, medial patellar, and infrapatellar plicae are variably present synovial infoldings of the knee joint capsule that are remnants of normal embryologic development (Fig. 6.75).
  - *Medial:*
    - The most commonly identified on imaging studies is the medial plica, which is a coronally oriented band at the level of the patella that can extend into the joint.
    - Most medial plicae are incidental, but, occasionally, a thickened medial plica can cause joint effusion, anteromedial knee pain, snapping, and eventual patellofemoral articular cartilage damage (Fig. 6.76).
    - Anterior knee snapping in a young patient should prompt close inspection for a medial plica.

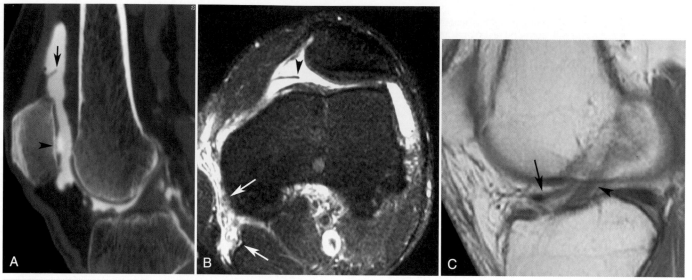

Fig. 6.75 Normal knee plicae. **(A)** Suprapatellar plica *(arrow)* oriented transversely in the superior joint recess. Sagittal reformation of a CT arthrogram. Also note high-grade patellar chondral defect *(arrowhead)*. **(B)** Axial fat-suppressed T2-weighted MR image shows a medial plica *(arrowhead)* oriented coronally in the medial joint. Also note the ruptured Baker cyst *(arrows)*. **(C)** Oblique sagittal T1-weighted MR image shows an infrapatellar plica *(arrow)* extending from the anterior intercondylar notch anteriorly into Hoffa's fat pad. Also note normal anterior cruciate ligament *(arrowhead)*.

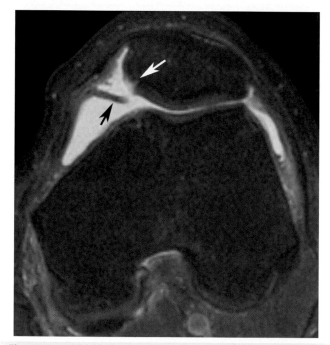

Fig. 6.76 Axial fat-suppressed T2-weighted MR image in a 22-year-old woman with anterior knee pain shows a thick medial plica *(black arrow)* with an associated chondral defect in the medial patellar facet *(white arrow)*.

- *Suprapatellar:*
  - The suprapatellar plica extends horizontally across the suprapatellar recess. Usually it is asymptomatic.
  - Rarely a suprapatellar plica can have a small fenestration (hole) that can obstruct flow of synovial fluid creating a one-way valve effect. Synovial proliferation occurs in the compartmentalized recess.

- This is called an 'obstructing plica' and can present clinically as a mass above the patella, or as a 'chronic effusion'.
- *Infrapatellar plica:*
  - The infrapatellar plica (also termed the *ligamentum mucosum*) is the most common plica in the knee and is also the least likely to be a source of symptoms.
  - The plica extends in the sagittal plane through the middle and lower portion of Hoffa's infrapatellar fat pad to the intercondylar notch, where it may attach to the ACL.

HOFFA'S FAT PAD

- The infrapatellar fat pad is a triangular region, commonly referred to as *Hoffa's fat pad*. It lies between the patellar tendon, the anterior joint recess, and the proximal tibia.
- MRI findings and symptoms in Hoffa's fat pad have been referred to as Hoffa's disease. This is a nonspecific term without a well-defined pathoetiology. There are a number of conditions that can affect the fat pad which can be a source of symptoms, including:
  - Irritation or impingement of the fat pad or fat necrosis presenting as edema.
  - Synovial cyst, parameniscal cyst, or ACL cyst extending into the fat pad.
  - Synovial proliferation with extension into the anterior recesses.
  - Edema in the superolateral fat pad due to impingement or friction from lateral patellar maltracking (Fig. 6.77).
  - Reactive edema adjacent to the patellar tendon secondary to patellar tendinosis or tear.

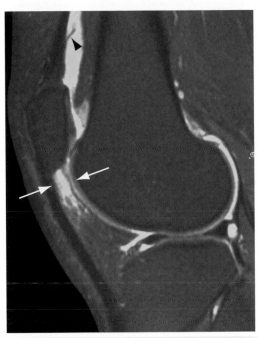

Fig. 6.77 Edema in superior lateral Hoffa's fat pad associated with patellar maltracking and anterior knee pain. A 29-year-old woman with patella alta and anterior knee pain. Sagittal fat-suppressed T2-weighted MR image shows focal edema *(arrows)* in lateral superior Hoffa's fat pad. Also note incidental superior plica *(arrowhead)*.

Knee MRI Report Template

Exam Type: MRI KNEE WO CONTRAST
Exam Date and Time:
Indication:
Comparison:

IMPRESSION: Normal exam.

TECHNIQUE: MRI of the right or left knee was performed on an x Tesla system using standard noncontrast protocol in three planes (axial, sagittal, and coronal).

FINDINGS:
Fluid: There is no significant joint effusion or Baker cyst. No loose intraarticular bodies are seen.
Soft tissues: Surrounding soft tissues are normal.
Menisci
Medial: Intact.
Lateral: Intact.
Cruciate ligaments: The anterior and posterior cruciate ligaments are intact.
Collateral structures: The medial collateral ligament and lateral collateral ligament complex are intact.
Extensor mechanism: The quadriceps and patellar tendon are normal. There is no patellar subluxation.
Cartilage/subchondral bone
Patellofemoral: Intact.
Medial tibiofemoral compartment: Intact.
Lateral tibiofemoral compartment: Intact.
Marrow: Bone marrow signal is normal.

Sources and Suggested Readings

Affram P. An epidemiologic study of cervical and trochanteric fractures of the femur in an urban population: analysis of 1664 cases with special reference to etiologic factors. *Acta Orthop Scand Suppl.* 1964;64:11.

Badillo K, Pacheco JA, Padua SO, et al. Multidetector CT evaluation of calcaneal fractures. *Radiographics.* 2011;31(1):81–92.

Beltran LS, Rosenberg ZS, Mayo JD, et al. Imaging evaluation of developmental hip dysplasia in the young adult. *AJR Am J Roentgenol.* 2013; 200:1077–1088.

Bencardino JT, Beltran J, Feldman MI, Rose DJ. MR imaging of complications of anterior cruciate ligament graft reconstruction. *Radiographics.* 2009;29(7):2115–2126.

Bowden DJ, Byrne CA, Alkhayat A, et al. Injectable viscoelastic supplements: a review for radiologists. *AJR Am J Roentgenol.* 2017;209:883–888.

Chan SS, Rosenberg ZS, Chan K, Capeci C. Subtrochanteric femoral fractures in patients receiving long-term alendronate therapy: imaging features. *AJR Am J Roentgenol.* 2010;194(6):1581–1586.

Chaturvedi A, Mann L, Cain U, et al. Acute fractures and dislocations of the ankle and foot in children. *Radiographics.* 2020; online article. https://doi.org/10.1148/rg.2020190154.

Chhabra A, Subhawong TK, Carrino JA. A systematised MRI approach to evaluating the patellofemoral joint. *Skeletal Radiol.* 2011;40(4):375–387.

Costa CR, Morrison WB, Carrino JA. Medial meniscus extrusion on knee MRI: is extent associated with severity of degeneration or type of tear? *AJR Am J Roentgenol.* 2004;183:17–23.

Crema MD, Roemer FW, Marra MD, et al. Articular cartilage in the knee: current MR imaging techniques and applications in clinical practice and research. *Radiographics.* 2011;31(1):37–61.

Delfaut EM, Demondion X, Dieganski A, et al. Imaging of foot and ankle nerve entrapment syndromes: from well-demonstrated to unfamiliar sites. *Radiographics.* 2003;23:613–623.

De Smet AA. How I diagnose meniscal tears on knee MR. *AJR Am J Roentgenol.* 2012;199(3):481–499.

De Smet AA, Blankenbaker DG, Alsheik NH, Lindstrom MJ. MRI appearance of the proximal hamstring tendons in patients with and without symptomatic proximal hamstring tendinopathy. *AJR Am J Roentgenol.* 2012;198(2):418–422.

De Smet AA, Nathan DH, Graf BK, et al. Clinical and MRI findings associated with false-positive knee MR diagnoses of medial meniscal tears. *AJR Am J Roentgenol.* 2008;191(1):93–99.

Diederichs G, Issever AS, Scheffler S. MR imaging of patellar instability: injury patterns and assessment of risk factors [published correction appears in *Radiographics.* 2011:31(2):624]. *Radiographics.* 2010;30(4):961–981.

Disler DG. Fat-suppressed 3-D spoiled gradient-recalled MR imaging: assessment of articular and physeal hyaline cartilage. *AJR Am J Roentgenol.* 1997;169:1117–1123.

Flores DV, Gomez M, Fernandez HM, et al. Adult acquired flatfoot deformity: anatomy, biomechanics, staging, and imagings. *Radiographics.* 2019;39:1437–1460.

Flores DV, Gomez CM, Pathria MN. Layered approach to the anterior knee: normal anatomy and disorders associated with anterior knee pain. *Radiographics.* 2018;38:2069–2101.

Ganz R, Parvizi J, Beck M, et al. Femoroacetabular impingement: a cause for osteoarthritis of the hip. *Clin Orthop Relat Res.* 2003;417:112–120.

Garden RS. Stability and union of subcapital fractures of the femur. *J Bone Joint Surg.* 1964;46B:630–712.

Greif DN, Baraga MG, Rizzo MG, et al. MRI appearance of the different meniscal ramp lesion types, with clinical and arthroscopic correlation. *Skeletal Radiology.* 2020;49:677–689.

Hegazi TM, Belair JA, McCarthy EJ, et al. Sports injuries about the hip: what the radiologist should know. *Radiographics.* 2016;36:1717–1745.

Judet R, Judet J, Letournel E. Fractures of the acetabulum: classification and surgical approaches to reduction. *J Bone Joint Surg.* 1964;46A:1615–1646.

Kamel SI, Belair JA†, Hegazi TM, Halpern EJ, Desai V, Morrison WB, Zoga AC. Painful type II os naviculare: introduction of a standardized, reproducible classification system. Skeletal Radiol. 2020 Dec;49(12): 1977–1985.

Khan I, Ashraf T, Saifuddin A. Magnetic resonance imaging of impingement and friction syndromes around the knee. *Skeletal Radiology.* 2020;49:823–836.

Khurana B, Sheehan SE, Sodickson AD, et al. Pelvic ring fractures: what the orthopedic surgeon wants to know. *Radiographics.* 2014;34:1317–1333.

Kijowski R, Rosas HG, Lee KS, et al. MRI characteristics of healed and unhealed peripheral vertical meniscal tears. *AJR Am J Roentgenol.* 2014;202:585–592.

Kijowski R, Blankenbaker DG, Shinki K, et al. Juvenile versus adult osteochondritis dissecans of the knee: appropriate MR imaging criteria for instability. *Radiology.* 2008;248(2):571–578.

Kraus C, Ayyala RS, Kazam JK, et al. Imaging of juvenile hip conditions predisposing to premature osteoarthritis. *Radiographics.* 2017;37:2204–2205.

Laborie LB, Lehmann TG, Engesæter IØ, et al. Prevalence of radiographic findings thought to be associated with femoroacetabular impingement in a population-based cohort of 2081 healthy young adults. *Radiology.* 2011;260:494–502.

Lauge-Hansen N. Fractures of the ankle: genetic roentgenologic diagnosis of fractures of the ankle. *AJR Am J Roentgenol.* 1954;71:456–471.

Li AE, Jawetz ST, Greditzer HG, et al. MRI Evaluation of femoroacetabular impingement after hip preservation surgery. *AJR Am J Roentgenol.* 2016;207:392–400.

Lungu E, Michaud J, Bureau NJ. US assessment of sports-related hip injuries. *Radiographics.* 2018;38:867–889.

Mainwaring B, Daffner R, Reiner B. Pylon fractures of the ankle: a distinct clinical and radiographic entity. *Radiology.* 1998;168:215–218.

Manganaro MS, Morag Y, Weadock WJ, et al. Creating three-dimensional printed models of acetabular fractures for use as educational tools. *Radiographics.* 2017;37:871–880.

Matcuk GR, Cen SY, Keyfes V, et al. Superolateral hoffa fat-pad edema and patellofemoral maltracking: predictive modeling. *AJR Am J Roentgenol.* 2014;203:W207–W212.

Markhardt BK, Gross JM, Monu JU. Schatzker classification of tibial plateau fractures: use of CT and MR imaging improves assessment. *Radiographics.* 2009;29(2):585–597.

Mellado JM, Bencardino JT. Morel-Lavallée lesion: review with emphasis on MR imaging. *Magn Reson Imaging Clin N Am.* 2005;13(4):775–782.

Meyers AB, Haims AH, Menn K, Moukaddam H. Imaging of anterior cruciate ligament repair and its complications. *AJR Am J Roentgenol.* 2010;194(2):476–484.

Mohankumar R, Palisch A, Khan W, et al. Meniscal ossicle: posttraumatic origin and association with posterior meniscal root tears. *AJR Am J Roentgenol.* 2014;203:1040–1046.

Mullens FE, Mullens FE, Zoga AC, et al. Review of MRI technique and imaging findings in athletic pubalgia and the "sports hernia". *Eur J Radiol.* 2012;81(12):3780–3792.

Naraghi A, White LM. MRI of labral and chondral lesions of the hip. *AJR Am J Roentgenol.* 2015;205:479–490.

Stacy GS, Lo R, Motang A. Infarct-associated bone sarcomas: multimodality imaging findings. *AJR Am J Roentgenol.* 2015;205:W432–W441.

Omar IM, Zoga AC, Kavanagh EC, et al. Athletic pubalgia and "sports hernia": optimal MR imaging technique and findings. *Radiographics.* 2008;28(5):1415–1438.

Perrich KD, Goodwin DW, Hecht PJ, Cheung Y. Ankle ligaments on MRI: appearance of normal and injured ligaments. *AJR Am J Roentgenol.* 2009;193(3):687–695.

Prince J, Laor T, Bean J. MRI of ACL injuries and associated findings in the pediatric knee: changes with skeletal maturation. *AJR Am J Roentgenol.* 2005;185:756–762.

Robinson R. Sonography of common tendon injuries. *AJR Am J Roentgenol.* 2009;193(3):607–618.

Rosas HG. Unraveling the posterolateral corner of the knee. *Radiographics.* 2016;36:1776–1791.

Rowe CR, Sakellarides HT, Freeman PA, Sorbie C. Fractures of the os calcis: a long term follow-up study of 146 patients. *JAMA.* 1963;184:920.

Samim M, Walter W, Gyftopoulos S, et al. MRI assessment of subspine impingement: features beyond the anterior inferior iliac spine morphology. *Radiology.* 2019;293:412–421.

Schwappach J, Murphey M, Kokmayer S, et al. Subcapital fractures of the femoral neck: prevalence and cause of radiographic appearance simulating pathologic fractures. *AJR Am J Roentgenol.* 1994;162:651–654.

Scheinfeld MH, Dym AA, Spektor M, et al. Acetabular fractures: what radiologists should know and how 3D CT can aid. *Radiographics.* 2015;35:555–577.

Sharif B, Ashraf T, Saifuddin A. Magnetic resonance imaging of the meniscal roots. *Skeletal Radiology.* 2020;49:661–676.

Sheehan SE, Shyu JY, Weaver MJ, et al. Proximal femoral fractures: what the orthopedic surgeon wants to know. *Radiographics.* 2015;35:1563–1584.

Silva MS. Radiography, CT, and MRI of hip and lower limb disorders in children and adolescents. *Radiographics.* 2019;39:779–794.

Subhawong TY, Eng J, Carrino JA, Chhabra A. Superolateral Hoffa's fat pad edema: association with patellofemoral maltracking and impingement. *AJR Am J Roentgenol.* 2010;195(6):1367–1373.

Yamada AF, Crema MD, Nery C, et al. Second and third metatarsophalangeal plantar plate tears: diagnostic performance of direct and indirect MRI features using surgical findings as the reference standard. *AJR Am J Roentgenol.* 2017;209:W100–W108.

Zoga AC, Kavanagh EC, Omar IM, et al. Athletic pubalgia and the "sports hernia": MR imaging findings. *Radiology.* 2008;247(3):797–807.

7 Ankle and Foot

Ankle

BONES

- The ankle (tibiotalar) joint is formed by the tibia, the fibula, and the talus, which form a hinge joint.
- The tibial articular margin is called the *tibial plafond* (ceiling).
- The lateral malleolus is positioned 1 cm distal and posterior to the medial malleolus (Fig. 7.1A and B).
- The medial and lateral articular margins of the ankle joint are formed by the talus and medial malleolus, and by the talus and lateral malleolus, which are obliquely oriented such that a 15- to 20-degree internal oblique view (*mortise view*) allows visualization of the articular margins in profile (Fig. 7.1B and C).
- The talar dome has a complex shape: semicircular when viewed from the side but saddle-shaped when viewed anteriorly (Fig. 7.1D). It fits snugly within the articulation formed by the tibia and fibula so that there is a uniform 3- to 4-mm space between the entire talar surface and the plafond and malleolar margins.

LIGAMENTS

The ankle is supported by a complex array of ligaments (Figs. 7.2 and 7.3).

The Tibiofibular Syndesmosis

- A syndesmosis is present between the tibia and fibula along its entire craniocaudal course, the distal aspect of which forms the strong anterior and posterior distal tibiofibular ligaments.
- The anterior and posterior distal tibiofibular (syndesmotic) ligaments (also called the anterior inferior talofibular ligament [AITFL] and posterior inferior talofibular ligament [PITFL], respectively) are the most superior set of ankle ligaments and are seen on axial magnetic resonance imaging (MRI) immediately above the ankle joint.
- These appear on all MRI sequences as uniform, thin, low-signal-intensity structures that pass between the anterior and posterior margins of the tibia and the apposing fibula.
- The medial margin of the fibula is convex or straight at this level and appears concave below this level.

Below the anterior and posterior distal tibiofibular ligaments, the lateral collateral ligaments are found.

The Lower Lateral Ligament Complex

This ligament complex is composed of three structures (see Figs. 7.2 and 7.3).

Anterior Talofibular Ligament

- The *anterior talofibular ligament* (ATFL) extends from the anterior fibula to the lateral talar neck and is shown best on the axial plane at the level where the medial aspect of the fibula is concave.
- The ATFL is the most frequently torn ankle ligament.

Posterior Talofibular Ligament

- The *posterior talofibular ligament* (PTFL) is a large fan-shaped ligament that extends from the distal aspect of

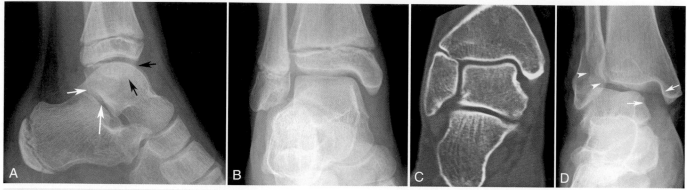

Fig. 7.1 Ankle radiographic anatomy. **(A)** Lateral radiograph. Note that the lateral malleolus *(white arrows)* is posterior to the medial malleolus *(black arrows)*. **(B)** Mortise view. Note uniform thickness of the joint space. **(C)** Obliquely reformatted CT image showing uniformity of the joint space around the ankle mortise. **(D)** Mortise view of fracture subluxation shows the saddle shape of the talar dome and matching contour of the tibial plafond. Note the oblique fracture *(arrowheads)* in the distal fibula at the level of the tibiotalar joint and the widened medial ankle joint space *(arrows)* indicating deltoid ligament tear. This represents a Weber B or Lauge-Hansen pronation injury pattern (see later in text).

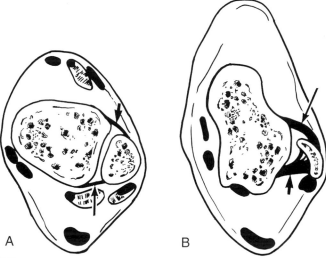

Fig. 7.2 Lateral ligaments at the ankle. **(A)** Axial diagram immediately superior to the ankle joint demonstrates the anterior and posterior tibiofibular ligaments *(short and long arrows,* respectively). Note the convex medial fibular shape and matching concave lateral tibial shape at this level. **(B)** Axial diagram demonstrating the anterior talofibular *(long arrow)* and posterior talofibular *(short arrow)* ligaments. Note that the fibular shape is concave at its medial aspect at this level. (Reproduced with permission from Manaster BJ. *Handbook of Skeletal Radiology.* 2nd ed. St. Louis: Mosby; 1997.)

the concave lateral malleolar fossa to the lateral tubercle of the posterior talar process.

■ The ligament is seen at the same level on axial MR images as the ATFL but appears more inhomogeneous because of its fan-shaped ligament fibers.

Calcaneofibular Ligament

■ The third ligament of the lateral collateral ligaments is the *calcaneofibular ligament* (CFL; see Fig. 7.3C), which extends from the inferior tip of the lateral malleolus to the lateral aspect of the calcaneus.

■ This is the most difficult of the lateral ankle ligaments to see at MRI; it can be seen partially on either coronal or axial images but is best shown on oblique axial images with the foot in plantar flexion.

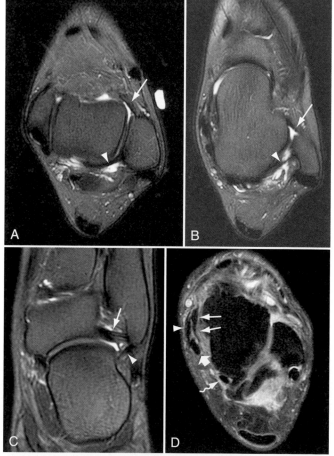

Fig. 7.3 Lateral collateral ligament complex. **(A)** Axial fat-suppressed T2-weighted MR image shows the anterior *(arrow)* and posterior *(arrowhead)* distal tibiofibular (syndesmotic) ligaments. **(B)** Axial fat-suppressed T2-weighted MR image shows anterior talofibular ligament *(arrow)* and posterior talofibular ligament *(arrowhead)*. **(C)** Coronal fat-suppressed T2-weighted MR image shows posterior talofibular ligament *(arrow)* and calcaneofibular ligament *(arrowhead)*. **(D)** Axial fat-suppressed T2-weighted MR image shows the deltoid ligament *(thin arrows)*, deep to the tibialis posterior tendon *(arrowhead)*. Note the flexor digitorum longus *(wide arrow)* and flexor hallucis longus *(wavy arrow)* tendons.

The Medial (Deltoid) Ligament

- The medial collateral ligament is also known as the *deltoid ligament or deltoid complex* and consists of five overlapping parts.
- The medial collateral ligament is a much stronger ligament complex than the lateral collateral ligaments and is less commonly torn.
- The deltoid ligament, located deep to the flexor tendons, consists of superficial and deep components.
- The superficial components are the *tibiocalcaneal, tibiospring, and tibionavicular* (see Fig. 7.3D) *ligaments*, which course from the tibia to the calcaneus, spring ligament, and navicular bone.
- The deep components are the *anterior and posterior tibiotalar ligaments*. Of all the deltoid ligaments, the tibionavicular ligament is the weakest.

Key Concepts

Ankle Ligaments

Distal tibiofibular syndesmosis: Strong anterior and posterior distal tibiofibular ligaments
Lateral:
- ATFL (most frequently torn ankle ligament)
- CFL (most difficult to see at MRI)
- PTFL (strongest lateral ligament)

Medial:
- Deltoid complex, with deep and superficial components

TENDONS

Achilles Tendon

- The largest of the tendons found at the ankle is the *Achilles tendon*; it is formed by the gastrocnemius and soleus muscles, which merge to form a thick tendon (Fig. 7.4) that inserts on the posterior calcaneus.

Medial Tendons

- The flexor tendons of the ankle are found posteromedially at the ankle and are, from medial to lateral, the tibialis posterior *(posterior tibial)*, the flexor digitorum longus, and the flexor hallucis longus tendons (see Fig. 7.4).
- These three tendons course through the tarsal tunnel, which is a fibro-osseous space confined by the flexor retinaculum, in which are also found the posterior tibial nerve and its branches, and the posterior tibial artery, veins, and lymphatics.
- The *posterior tibial tendon* (PTT) is found in a groove along the posterior margin of the medial malleolus and continues through the tarsal tunnel to insert primarily on the navicular bone, with continuation of the tendon to the plantar aspect of the medial and middle cuneiform bones and the second through fourth metatarsal bases.
  - The PTT is the principal inverter of the foot and helps maintain the longitudinal arch.
  - As a rule of thumb, the normal PTT should be no greater than twice the cross-sectional area of the adjacent flexor digitorum longus.
- The *flexor digitorum longus (FDL) tendon* also courses in the groove found in the medial malleolus, continuing through the tarsal tunnel to insert on the second to fifth distal phalanges.
- The flexor hallucis longus passes beneath the sustentaculum tali of the calcaneus, using its groove as a pulley, and continues between the two sesamoid bones of the hallux to insert on the base of the first distal phalanx.
- The muscle and musculotendinous junction of the flexor hallucis longus extends further distally than the other

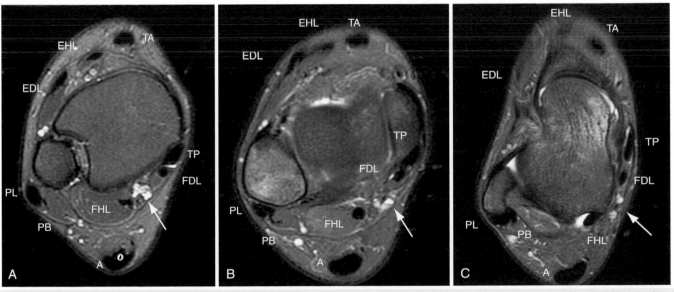

Fig. 7.4 Tendon anatomy at the ankle. (A–C) Axial fat-suppressed T2-weighted MR images of the ankle, at three progressively more caudal levels, show the tibialis posterior (TP) and flexor digitorum longus (FDL), and flexor hallucis longus (FHL) musculotendinous unit of the posterior compartment. The anterior compartment tendons are the tibialis anterior (TA), extensor hallucis longus (EHL), and extensor digitorum longus (EDL) tendons. Note also peroneus brevis (PB) musculotendinous unit, peroneus longus (PL) tendon, and Achilles tendon (A). The FHL and PB musculotendinous junctions are typically found more caudally than the others. Note the medial and lateral plantar vessels and nerves (arrows).

flexor tendons and can usually be found at the level of the ankle joint line.

Mnemonic for Contents of the Tarsal Tunnel (Covered by the Flexor Retinaculum)

Tom	posterior **T**ibialis tendon	Anterior
Dick	flexor **D**igitorum longus tendon	
And **V**ery **N**ervous	posterior tibial **A**rtery, **V**ein, and **N**erve	
Harry	flexor **H**allucis longus tendon	Posterior

Lateral Tendons

- The *peroneal longus and brevis tendons* are found postero-laterally at the ankle (see Fig. 7.4).
- Both tendons pass behind the lateral malleolus within a groove, where they are confined by the peroneal retinaculum.
- The peroneus brevis is found anterior to the peroneus longus at the distal fibula and below.
- The peroneus brevis inserts on the fifth metatarsal base, and the peroneus longus extends beneath the midfoot to insert on the first metatarsal base.
- The peroneus longus contributes to maintaining the longitudinal arch of the foot.

Anterior (Extensor) Tendons

- The extensor tendons (see Fig. 7.4) are found anteriorly at the ankle, and from medial to lateral consist of the anterior tibialis, extensor hallucis longus, and extensor digitorum longus (mnemonic: Tom, Harry, and Dick) and peroneus tertius tendon when this accessory muscle is present.
- These tendons are confined by the anterior extensor retinaculum.
- The *tibialis anterior* (anterior tibial) inserts on the medial and inferomedial base of the first metatarsal bone.

- The *extensor hallucis longus* inserts on the dorsal base of the distal phalanx of the hallux.
- The *extensor digitorum longus* inserts on the dorsal bases of the second through fifth distal phalanges, and the variably present peroneus tertius inserts on the dorsal base of the fifth metatarsal.

FRACTURE PATTERNS

- Ankle injuries are common and are the among most common indications for trauma-associated radiographic evaluation in emergency departments.
- In general, the presence of an ankle joint effusion or soft tissue swelling should prompt a search for a fracture, particularly if the patient is unable to bear weight. In the ankle, effusion is seen on the lateral film as an anteriorly convex soft tissue density at the ankle joint (Fig. 7.5).
- Soft tissue swelling may be evident over the medial and lateral malleoli as well as in the fat posterior to the ankle.
    - This posterior fat is known as the *pre-Achilles triangle, pre-Achilles fat pad,* or *Kager's fat pad* and is usually sharply circumscribed at its margin with the Achilles tendon.
    - Obscuration of the margins of the fat triangle in the setting of trauma indicates soft tissue swelling.

Classification of Ankle Fracture: Weber

- Several classifications are used in the assessment of ankle fractures.
- The *Weber (AO) classification* is a simple anatomic classification scheme that correlates well with treatment and prognosis.
- It is based on determining the level of fibular fracture to deduce the injury to the tibiofibular ligaments.
- A *Weber A injury* is a transverse avulsion fracture of the lateral malleolus at or distal to the ankle joint (see Fig. 1.18A). There may be associated fracture of the medial malleolus.
    - In type A injury, the tibiofibular ligaments and syndesmosis are intact.

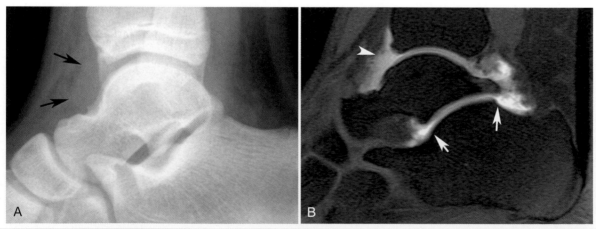

Fig. 7.5 Ankle joint capsule. **(A)** Lateral radiograph shows soft tissue density in the shape of a teardrop *(arrows)* anterior to ankle joint, indicating an ankle effusion. This may be the only finding of an intraarticular fracture. **(B)** MR arthrogram shows similar findings, with ankle joint distention. Sagittal fat-suppressed T1-weighted MR image shows that contrast medium injected into the ankle joint *(arrowhead)* communicates freely with the posterior subtalar facet joint *(arrows)*. This is a common normal variant.

- This fracture is caused by ankle supination (inversion), with avulsion of the tip of the lateral malleolus.
- *Weber B injury* represents oblique fractures of the lateral malleolus beginning at the level of the ankle joint.
  - This injury pattern is usually caused by supination–external rotation or pronation.
  - The important point with type B injury is that the tibiofibular ligaments are partially disrupted.
  - These injuries may be associated with fractures of the medial malleolus below the ankle joint or with deltoid ligament rupture (see Fig. 7.1D).
- *Weber C injury* represents fibular fracture proximal to the level of the ankle joint.
  - This involves tear of the tibiofibular ligaments and tibiofibular syndesmosis.
  - This injury is usually due to pronation–external rotation.
  - A proximal fibular fracture indicates a *Maisonneuve* fracture with syndesmosis tear to the level of the fracture (Fig. 7.6).

Key Concepts

Ankle Fractures: Weber (AO) Classification
Based on location of distal fibular fracture relative to tibiotalar joint
WEBER A
  - Transverse fracture distal to the ankle joint
  - Usual mechanism: supination
  - Major ligaments usually intact
WEBER B
  - Oblique fracture at the level of ankle joint
  - Usual mechanism: supination–external rotation or pronation
  - Partial disruption of the tibiofibular ligaments
  - May require surgery
WEBER C
  - Proximal to the level of ankle joint
  - Usual mechanism: pronation–external rotation
  - More extensive ligament and often syndesmotic disruption
  - Usually requires surgery

Note: AO stands for the Arbeitsgemeinschaft für Osteosynthesefragen, an orthopedic study group formed in 1958 that focuses on research in fracture healing.

Classification of Ankle Trauma: Lauge-Hansen

- The more complex *Lauge-Hansen classification* is based on the mechanism of the ankle injury.
- Memorization is not required for a practicing radiologist, but familiarity may help one conceptualize common fracture patterns.
- This system is useful because an understanding of the forces that produce a specific injury indicates the direction of forces required for fracture reduction. (Recall that fracture reduction applies forces reverse of the mechanism of injury.)
- Five basic patterns of force can result in ankle fracture: supination, supination–external rotation, pronation, pronation–external rotation, and axial loading.
  - Supination refers to plantar flexion of the ankle, inversion of the hindfoot, and adduction of the foot, whereas pronation refers to dorsiflexion of the ankle, eversion of the hindfoot, and abduction of the foot.
  - Either supination or pronation may be isolated or associated with external rotation.
- It is useful to be mindful of the fracture pattern in the fibula in each of these injury patterns, because the fibular fracture pattern in each injury will be unique.
- For each fracture pattern, the ankle mortise is carefully assessed for any evidence of loss of parallel margins.
- Such loss of joint-space uniformity implies extensive ligament and osseous disruption resulting in ankle instability.
- In considering the Lauge-Hansen classification, injury stages are sequential with lowest-stage injury patterns occurring before higher-stage injuries; with a higher-stage of injury, there is increasing severity of bone and/or ligament injury, along with a greater likelihood of instability.
  - In supination, tension is placed on the fibula, resulting in either a tear of the lateral collateral ligament or a low transverse avulsion fracture of the lateral malleolus (see Fig. 1.18A). This is considered a stage 1 injury.

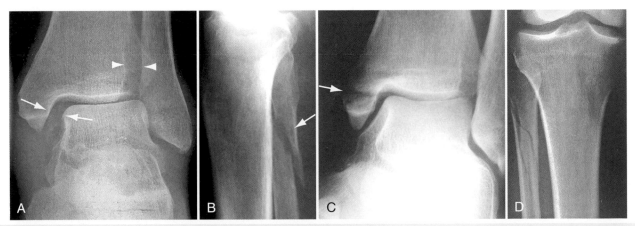

Fig. 7.6 Maisonneuve fractures. **(A)** Frontal radiograph demonstrates widening of ankle joint space at medial ankle mortise *(arrows)*, indicating deltoid ligament tear. Also note widened tibia-fibula syndesmosis (between *arrowheads*). **(B)** Lateral view of proximal leg demonstrates oblique fracture of proximal fibular diametaphysis *(arrow)*. (C and D) Another patient with a slightly different pattern of Maisonneuve fracture, with transverse fracture of the medial malleolus *(arrow in C)*, but still showing characteristic widening of the distal tibia-fibula syndesmosis and proximal fibular shaft fracture (shown in D).

- Stage 2 supination injury includes the findings at stage 1, with the addition of a vertically oriented fracture of the medial malleolus.
- Supination–external rotation is the most common injury pattern in the ankle, accounting for nearly three-fourth of all ankle injuries.
  - In supination–external rotation, the lateral wall of the distal talar pole rotates and impacts against the anterior wall of the lateral malleolus, driving it posteriorly.
  - This results in an oblique fibular fracture oriented in the coronal plane that is best seen on the lateral view of the ankle (Fig. 7.7).
- Stage 1 supination–external rotation injury represents disruption of the anterior distal tibiofibular ligament.
- Stage 2 injury includes stage 1 findings plus the distal fibular fracture.
- Stage 3 injury includes findings from stages 1 and 2 plus a tear of the posterior distal tibiofibular ligament or fracture of the posterior malleolus (avulsion of posterior distal tibiofibular ligament attachment).
- Stage 4 injury represents findings of stages 1 through 3 with the addition of a transverse fracture of the medial malleolus. Thus the presence of a transverse malleolar fracture indicates the most severe stage of supination–external rotation injury.
- In pronation, the lateral wall of the proximal talar pole impacts against the medial wall of the lateral malleolus, driving it laterally.
  - This results in an oblique fracture of the lateral malleolus oriented in the sagittal plane, which is best seen on the frontal view of the ankle (see Fig. 7.1D).
- There are three stages of pronation injury.
  - Stage 1 represents an avulsion of the medial malleolus or a tear of the deltoid ligaments.
  - Stage 2 represents stage 1 findings plus rupture of the anterior and posterior distal tibiofibular ligaments.

- Stage 3 represents stage 1 and 2 findings plus the fibular fracture. Thus, demonstration of a sagittally oriented oblique fracture of the fibula indicates the most severe form of pronation injury.
- In pronation–external rotation, talar impaction at both the medial and anterior fibular surfaces results in a spiraling force through the tibiofibular syndesmosis with forces exiting through the fibula at a point more proximal to the ankle joint (see Fig. 7.6).
- There are four stages of pronation–external rotation injury.
  - Stage 1 injury involves avulsion of the medial malleolus or a deltoid ligament tear.
  - Stage 2 represents stage 1 findings plus tear of the anterior distal tibiofibular ligament and the tibiofibular syndesmosis.
  - Stage 3 represents stage 1 and 2 findings plus the fibular fracture.
  - Stage 4 injury represents the findings from stages 1 to 3 plus a tear of the posterior distal tibiofibular ligament or posterior malleolar fracture. Therefore if medial malleolar swelling is demonstrated and there is a posterior malleolar fracture, absence of a fibular fracture on an ankle radiograph implies a more proximal fibular fracture and should prompt further radiographic assessment with imaging of the entire tibia/fibula.

Fractures in Skeletally Immature Patients

- In the skeletally immature, fusion of the distal tibial epiphysis begins at 12 to 13 years of age, beginning at a superior convexity in the growth plate known as the *Kump bump* (or Kump hump) (Fig. 7.8), which is located in the anterior-medial quadrant of the physis.
- Children in this age range are prone to lateral Salter–Harris fractures.
- One such fracture, known as the juvenile *Tillaux fracture*, is a Salter–Harris III fracture of the anterior lateral

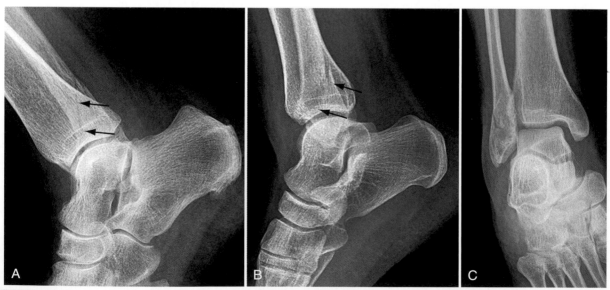

Fig. 7.7 Supination–external rotation injury at ankle. (A and B) Lateral views in two different patients demonstrate coronally oriented oblique fractures of distal fibula *(arrows)*. The lateral view is the best for detecting these fractures because the coronal orientation of the fracture line projects in profile on this view. **(C)** AP view shows how difficult these fractures can be to detect because the fracture line projects en face on this view.

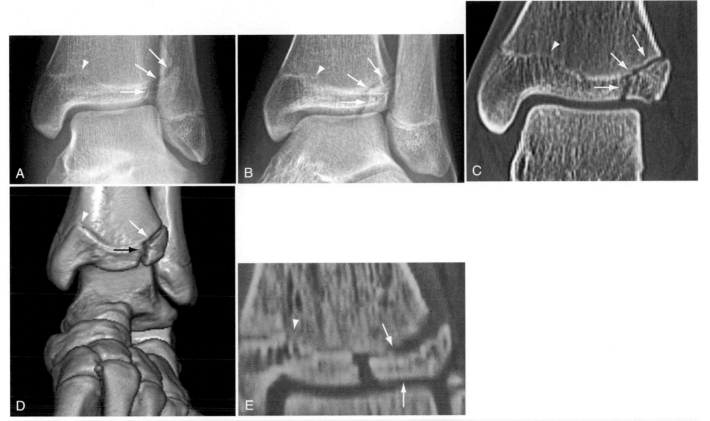

Fig. 7.8 Tillaux fracture. **(A and B)** Frontal **(A)** and mortise view **(B)** radiographs demonstrate Salter–Harris III (epiphyseal) fracture of lateral tibial plafond *(arrows)*. **(C and D)** Coronal **(C)** and three-dimensional **(D)** CT reformations show same fracture *(arrows)*. **(E)** Coronal CT reformation in another patient shows a similar fracture but with articular surface diastasis, which requires surgical reduction. In all images, note a Kump bump medially *(arrowhead)*, a proximal undulation of the distal tibial physis that fuses before the remainder of the physis.

portion of the distal tibial epiphysis, sparing the fused medial portion of the epiphysis (see Fig. 7.8).

- Tillaux fracture results from avulsion of the anterior syndesmotic ligament.
- Fracture displacement of more than 2 mm or articular incongruence indicates the need for surgical intervention.
- A *triplane fracture* is another growth plate fracture of the ankle, and includes the lateral half of the distal tibial epiphysis and a triangular posterior metaphyseal component.
  - The term *triplane* indicates the three planes of the fracture—coronal-oblique through the posterior distal tibial metaphysis, horizontal through the tibial growth plate, and sagittal through the tibial epiphysis (Fig. 7.9).
  - There are two types. If a triplane fracture occurs after the medial portion of the epiphysis has fused, the medial malleolus remains intact and a two-fragment triplane fracture results.
  - If the triplane fracture occurs before the epiphysis begins to fuse, there may be a three-fragment fracture.
  - With either type, the appearance of a triplane fracture consists of a combination of a Tillaux fracture and a Salter–Harris II fracture.
- Other growth plate injury patterns occur at the ankle, including Salter–Harris II and Salter–Harris IV fractures of the distal tibia and fibula (Fig. 7.10).

- Salter–Harris V fractures are uncommon and result from axial loading.

Other Fractures: Fifth Metatarsal Base

- It is important to include the base of the fifth metatarsal on images of the ankle because fracture in this location is common and may clinically mimic ankle fracture (Fig. 7.11). Lateral and frontal views are both useful for detection.
- Proximal fifth metatarsal fractures are distinguished by their location relative to the articulation between the proximal fourth and fifth metatarsals (intermetatarsal joint), specifically either proximal to, in, or distal to this articulation. The distinction has important implications for fracture etiology and management.
- Fractures proximal to the intermetatarsal joint are avulsion fractures due to pull from the insertion of the peroneus brevis tendon. These fractures may extend into the articulation with the cuboid (cubometatarsal joint). These fractures are also called *pseudo-Jones* fractures. There is variable distraction of the avulsed fracture fragment, with retraction usually mild but occasionally extending to the level of the ankle, with lateral ankle pain.
  - Good blood supply. Usually heal well with immobilization.
- A *Jones fracture* is a fracture of the fifth metatarsal proximal metaphysis-metadiaphyseal junction, with extension into the intermetatarsal joint.

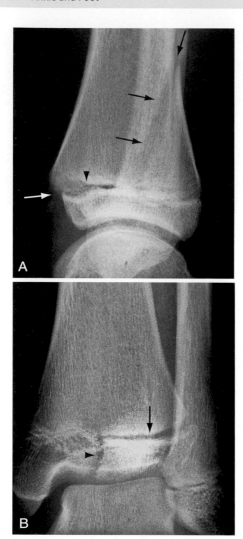

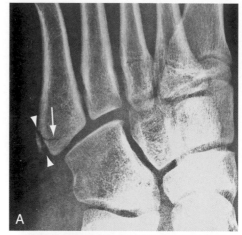

Fig. 7.11 Fracture at base of fifth metatarsal. **(A)** Oblique foot radiograph demonstrates transverse fracture *(arrow)*. Fractures at this site are transverse and are not to be confused with the sagittally oriented physis for the lateral apophysis *(arrowheads)*, which is a normal finding. **(B)** Normal apophysis and associated growth plate *(arrow)* for comparison.

Fig. 7.9 Triplane fracture. **(A)** Lateral ankle radiograph shows coronally oriented fracture of posterior aspect of distal tibial metaphysis *(black arrows)* and transverse fracture through anterior growth plate *(arrowhead)*. Note posterior displacement of the distal fragment, seen as a step-off anteriorly at the physeal fracture line *(white arrow)*. **(B)** Frontal radiograph demonstrates sagittally oriented epiphyseal fracture *(arrowhead)* and transversely oriented physeal fracture *(arrow)*.

- ■ This part of the bone has a poor blood supply. Slow healing and nonunion are common.
  - ■ Internal fixation sometimes used.
- ■ Proximal fifth metatarsal fractures distal to the intermetatarsal joint are often stress fractures in athletes, especially basketball players. These also heal poorly and often require internal fixation (Fig 7.12).
- ■ Commonly missed fractures after an ankle injury (look harder, computed tomography [CT] if in doubt).
  - ■ Anterior process of the calcaneus.
  - ■ Lateral process of the talus ('snowboarder's fracture').
  - ■ Dorsal capsular avulsion fractures at the talonavicular joint.
  - ■ Avulsion of the extensor digitorum brevis from the anterolateral calcaneus.

Other Fractures: Pilon Fracture

- ■ Axial loading results in intraarticular fractures of the tibial plafond, called *pilon fractures*.
- ■ In this setting, the talar dome acts as a wedge, splitting the tibial plafond and pushing fragments apart (Fig. 7.13).
- ■ Severe distal tibial comminution may result, while the malleoli usually maintain an anatomic relationship with the talus.

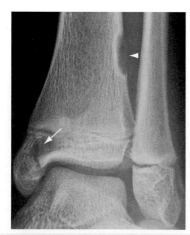

Fig. 7.10 Salter–Harris fracture. Salter–Harris III fracture of medial malleolus *(arrow)*. Note the incidental well-circumscribed lytic lesion at the lateral tibial cortex *(arrowhead)*. This is an incidental fibrous cortical defect, also termed a fibroxanthoma or nonossifying fibroma (see Chapter 11-Bone Tumors for further discussion of this lesion).

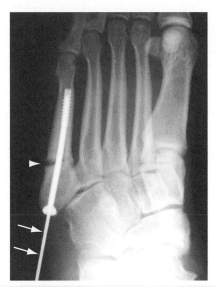

Fig. 7.12 Proximal 5th metatarsal stress fracture *(arrowhead)* in a collegiate basketball player. Note cannulated screw placed over a guide pin *(arrows)* in this intraoperative image.

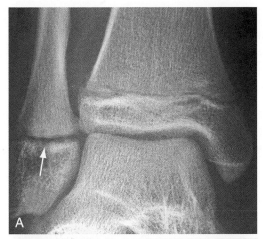

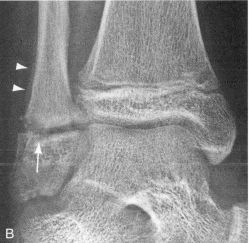

Fig. 7.14 Stress fracture of distal fibular physis. **(A)** Initial radiograph demonstrates only minimal widening of distal fibular growth plate *(arrow)*. **(B)** Radiograph obtained 3 weeks later demonstrates interval irregularity of growth plate of distal fibula *(arrow)*, indicating partial healing. Note periosteal new bone along distal fibular shaft *(arrowheads)*.

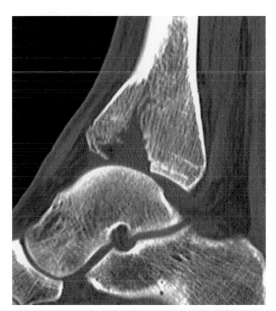

Fig. 7.13 Pilon fracture. Sagittal CT reconstruction shows coronally oriented intraarticular fracture of the distal tibia with diastasis.

- Pilon fractures are classified as type 1 (nondisplaced), type 2 (moderately displaced), and type 3 (severely displaced and impacted).
- Talar fractures may coexist.

Stress Fractures at the Ankle

- Stress fractures may occur around the ankle, especially among skeletally immature runners, and are seen occasionally as Salter I injuries with widening and irregular contour of the distal fibular growth plate (Fig. 7.14).
- In adults, stress fractures are seen as linear bands of lucency or sclerosis (depending on the stage of healing) in the distal tibial metaphysis 3–4 cm proximal to the level of the tibial plafond (Fig. 7.15) or in the distal fibula

3–7 cm from the tip of the lateral malleolus (Fig. 7.16). Stress fractures may simultaneously occur in the distal tibia and fibula.

ANKLE TRAUMA COMPLICATIONS

Instability

- Common complication of ankle injury.
- Stress radiographic views, with varus and valgus force applied to the calcaneus and with anterior drawer stress (anterior force applied to the posterior calcaneus), are useful for determining laxity in the ankle joint.
- Medial talar tilt (varus) on stress radiographs is normally less than 10–12 degrees, and anterior drawer is usually less than 1 cm.
- However, it is important to compare these views with the contralateral side because congenital laxity is sometimes present. In general, varus greater than 15 degrees represents lateral collateral ligament injury, and anterior talar displacement greater than 1 cm indicates injury to the ATFL.
- Pain and early osteoarthritis may result.

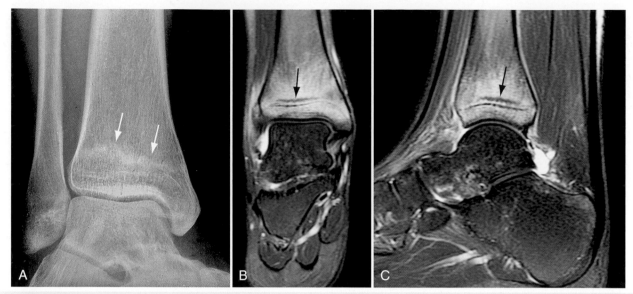

Fig. 7.15 Distal tibial stress fracture. **(A)** Oblique radiograph of ankle demonstrates linear sclerotic band *(arrows)* related to healing stress fracture. **(B and C)** Coronal **(B)** and sagittal **(C)** fat-suppressed T2-weighted MR images demonstrate linear band of low signal intensity representing fracture line *(arrows)*, surrounded by high-signal-intensity edema.

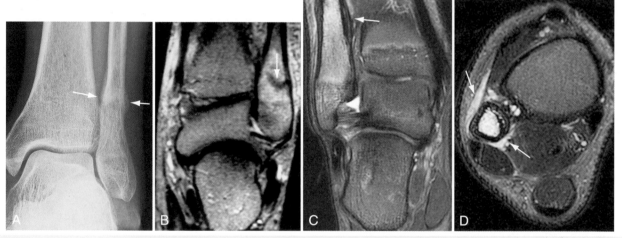

Fig. 7.16 Distal fibular stress fractures. **(A)** AP radiograph shows transverse sclerosis of the distal fibular diaphysis with solid periosteal reaction *(arrows)*. **(B)** Coronal T2-weighted spin-echo MR image in another patient demonstrates incomplete, curved, low-signal-intensity stress fracture *(arrow)* with surrounding marrow edema. **(C)** Coronal fat-suppressed T2-weighted MR image in another patient with edema throughout distal fibula and dark-signal periosteal reaction *(arrow)*. **(D)** Axial fat-suppressed T2-weighted MR image in same patient as C, showing fibular marrow and periosteal *(arrows)* edema.

Posttraumatic Subluxation

- The distal tibiofibular joint may be widened by syndesmotic ligament injuries, fractures, or both. The talus should maintain an anatomic relation with the lateral margin of the tibial plafond. Because of the saddle shape of the talar dome, even minimal lateral subluxation of the talus relative to the tibial plafond can significantly reduce the articular contact area of the tibiotalar joint, resulting in pain and early osteoarthritis.

Osteochondral Lesions

- The talar dome is a frequent site of osteochondral lesions (OCL, formerly called osteochondral defects), termed *osteochondral lesion of the talus* (OLT).

- OLT is a focal lesion involving talar dome articular cartilage and subchondral bone.
- Frequently posttraumatic due to shearing force during ankle trauma.
  - Some lesions are due to repetitive microtrauma.
    - Osteochondritis dissecans (OCD) likely is an example of this mechanism.
    - OCD is a distinctive form of OCL in adolescents, with repetitive trauma and other factors resulting in abnormal enchondral ossification that can progress to fragmentation.
    - The knee is the most common site, but also occurs in the talar dome and other sites.
    - OCD is discussed in more detail in Chapter 1.

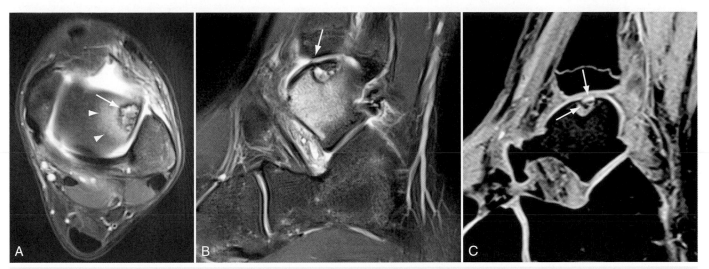

Fig. 7.17 Unstable osteochondral lesion of the talar dome. **(A)** Axial fat-suppressed proton density MR image shows an osteochondral defect *(arrow)* in the medial talar dome, surrounded by abundant osseous edema *(arrowheads).* **(B)** Sagittal fat-suppressed T2-weighted MR image shows the osteochondral defect with surrounding edema. Note the slight irregularity of the articular margin *(arrow).* **(C)** Sagittal water-excitation three-dimensional gradient-echo MR image clearly shows the small in situ osteochondral fragment *(upper arrow,* chondral component; *lower arrow,* osseous component).

- Imaging features of talar dome OCL (Fig. 7.17; see alsoFig. 1.17C).
  - Radiographs/CT: Abnormal subchondral bone: absent, sclerotic, and cystlike changes may coexist.
  - CT arthrography can be very useful to detect overlying cartilage fissuring and fluid extending around the lesion that can indicate instability.
- MRI is the preferred imaging technique, as it can display injury to both cartilage and bone. Important findings to search for:
  - Intact cartilage over a bone injury at the articular surface can help heal the lesion (like a cast over a fracture, immobilizing it).
  - Overlying cartilage fissuring, flap, or defect is associated with lesion progression.
  - Dark T1 signal/collapse of the articular surface often represents osteonecrosis.
  - Fluid signal extending under a bone fragment usually indicates that the osteochondral fragment is unstable.
  - Cystic changes under the osteochondral lesion also can be associated with instability but are less specific.
  - Large cysts can also complicate management techniques of microfracture or grafting.
  - Adjacent bone marrow edema is associated with pain; it can be seen early or late in the process.
- End stage of the disease is displacement of the osteochondral fragment into the joint as a loose body, with eventual secondary osteoarthritis.

Key Concepts

OCL of the talar dome (and other sites): factors associated with instability and tendency to progress

- Overlying cartilage damage
- Articular surface collapse
- Fluid undermining the fragment
- Cystic changes under the lesion

TENDON INJURY

- Tendon abnormalities at the ankle and foot are primarily degenerative disorders of multifactorial origin.
- Age, chronic repetitive overuse injury, arthropathies, and metabolic disorders can all play a role.
- With repetitive injury and repair, tendons undergo mucoid degeneration, which eventually can result in tendon rupture.

Key Concepts

Factors predisposing to tendon pathology

- Age
- Injury, overuse
- Obesity
- Diabetes
- Renal failure
- Medication (steroids, fluoroquinolones)
- Gout, amyloid infiltration
- Rheumatoid arthritis
- Altered mechanics/deformity
- Hyperlipidemia

Achilles Tendon

- The tendon is formed from a combination of the gastrocnemius and soleus muscles (Achilles tendon = the tendon of the 'gastrosoleus' musculature).
- Normally the anteroposterior (AP) dimension is no more than 8 mm, and its anterior margins are concave or flat on axial images.
- Achilles tendinosis is common among runners and jumpers.
- On radiography, acute injury results in increased density of fat in the adjacent *pre-Achilles fat (Kager's fat pad).*
- The Achilles tendon does not have a tendon sheath. The surface of the tendon is covered with a thin membrane

called the *paratenon*, which may become inflamed if the tendon is injured. Irritation of the paratenon is referred to as *paratenonitis or peritendinitis*.

- The vascular paratenon supplies the Achilles tendon with nutrients.
- On MRI, peritendinitis is seen as edema in the peritendinous region (Fig. 7.18A).

- Recurrent bouts of tendinosis and peritendinitis result in thickening of the tendon (Fig. 7.18B to H), referred to as chronic tendinosis.
- Acute ruptures are nearly always superimposed on chronic tendinosis and occur most commonly in middle-aged men who are involved in sporadic exercise (the weekend warrior) or in sports involving running or jumping.
- Rupture also may be seen in individuals with weakened tendons as a result of systemic diseases such as rheumatoid arthritis, renal disease, and diabetes, as a result of long-term steroid use, and with fluoroquinolone (ciprofloxacin) usage, among other causes.
- Tears should be described in terms of location, extent (i.e., percent of cross-sectional area), and gap, if any.

- Achilles tendon tears usually occur in one of three locations:
  - Soleus myotendinous junction (Fig. 7.19).
    - Related to acute injury, often in athletes.
    - *Note*: Soleus myotendinous junction is somewhat variable in location—in some individuals it is closer to the calcaneal insertion than in others.
  - Midportion.
    - Usually about 5 cm from the calcaneal insertion, halfway between the myotendinous junction and the calcaneus.
    - Also called the *watershed zone*: a relatively hypovascular region (vascular supply of the tendon is via the muscle proximally, the bone distally, and the paratenon at the midportion).
    - Thickening occurs from repetitive injury, causing the tendon to look round, with a convex anterior border (instead of concave).
    - Initially the tendon is dark (*hypoxic tendinosis*).
    - Later mucoid degeneration can occur with intermediate signal on T1- and T2-weighted images. This predisposes to tear.
    - Fluid signal in the tendon represents a tear.

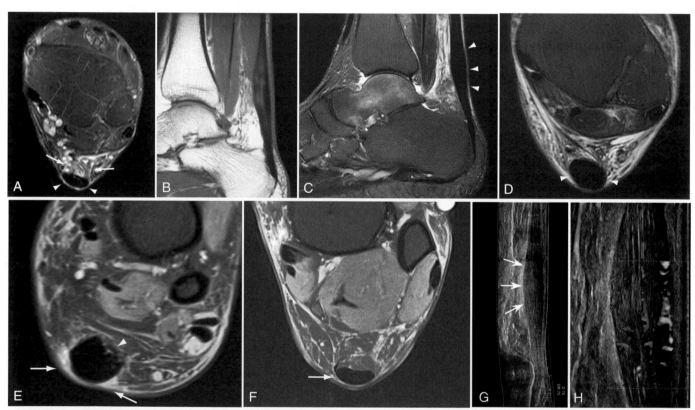

Fig. 7.18 Achilles tendinosis (tendinopathy). **(A)** Axial fat-suppressed T2-weighted MR image shows normal-sized Achilles tendon with high signal intensity *(arrowheads)* surrounding tendon due to peritendinitis. Note abundant edema in pre-Achilles fat pad *(arrows)*. **(B)** Sagittal T1-weighted MR image shows fusiform thickening of Achilles tendon with central vertically oriented increased signal, indicating tendinosis and longitudinal interstitial tearing. **(C)** Sagittal fat-suppressed T2-weighted MR image shows fusiform thickening of Achilles tendon *(arrowheads)* with peritendinitis and pre-Achilles fat pad edema. **(D)** Axial fat-suppressed T2-weighted MR image shows substantial thickening of the tendon *(arrowheads)*, with a convex anterior tendon margin and abundant surrounding peritendinous and fat pad edema. **(E)** Axial fat-suppressed T2-weighted MR image at a more superior level shows tendon thickening with anterior increased signal *(arrowhead)* indicating cross-sectional appearance of interstitial tear. Note peritendinitis *(arrows)*. **(F)** Axial fat-suppressed T2-weighted MR image shows a normal Achilles tendon for comparison. Note the narrow anteroposterior dimension, concave anterior margin, and uniformly dark signal of the normal tendon *(arrow)*. **(G)** Ultrasound findings of severe Achilles hypoxic tendinopathy. Sagittal composite image oriented to match sagittal MRI orientation, with anterior to the viewer's left, shows marked fusiform thickening of the Achilles tendon centered at the critical/watershed zone *(arrows)* with tendon hypoechogenicity. **(H)** Sagittal color Doppler image in the same patient demonstrating associated tendon hyperemia.

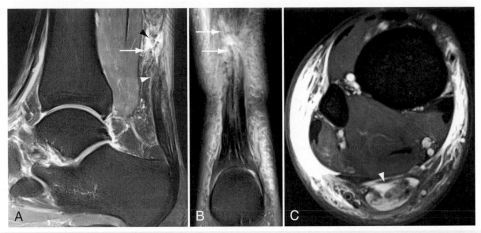

Fig. 7.19 Achilles tendon rupture: myotendinous junction. **(A)** Sagittal fat-suppressed T2-weighted MR image shows an acute Achilles rupture *(arrowheads)* at the myotendinous junction. Note the hematoma at the site of tendon rupture *(arrow)*, and note the marked thickening indicative of chronic tendinopathy in the remnant distal tendon. **(B)** Coronal fat-suppressed T2-weighted MR image shows the ruptured tendon ends *(arrows)*. **(C)** Axial fat-suppressed T2-weighted MR image through the site of rupture shows an expanded paratenon *(arrowhead)* with complex internal signal indicating hematoma and remnant tendon substance.

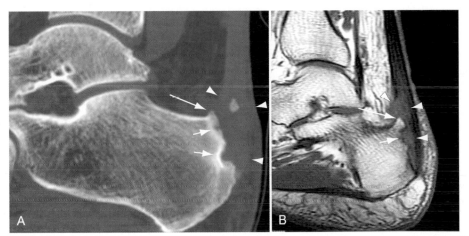

Fig. 7.20 Achilles insertional pathology; Haglund syndrome. **(A)** Sagittal CT reconstruction shows spurring at the posterosuperior calcaneus (the Haglund deformity, *long arrow*), erosions on the posterior calcaneus *(short arrows)*, and thickened distal Achilles tendon (between *arrowheads*). **(B)** Sagittal T1-weighted MR image in a different patient shows similar findings with Haglund deformity *(long arrow)* and erosion *(short arrow)*. Note the abnormal intermediate signal in the distal anterior Achilles tendon *(arrowheads)*.

- Insertional (Fig. 7.20).
  - Associated with Haglund deformity (bony prominence and upturn of the posterior calcaneal tubercle).
  - Commonly combined with bursitis (retrocalcaneal— in front of the tendon) and/or retro-Achilles (subcutaneous, also called a 'pump bump' related to wearing of fashionable women's high-heeled shoes).
  - Combination of a Haglund deformity, bursitis, and Achilles insertional pathology is referred to as *Haglund syndrome*.
  - Calcification and ossification may occur within the tendon at the site of a previous tendinopathy and tear.
- After surgery, the Achilles tendon may continue to appear thickened and retain areas of high signal.
- Nontraumatic causes of thickening of the Achilles tendon may also occur.
  - A thickened Achilles tendon may also be seen with *xanthomatosis*, which occurs in the setting of familial hyperlipidemias. Radiographs show severe tendon thickening (Fig. 7.21). MRI also shows marked tendon enlargement, and also heterogeneously mixed low- and intermediate-signal masses and stippled or linear areas of low signal intensity). Multiple tendons may be affected with this disorder, although the Achilles is the most common.
  - Achilles tendon infiltration can also occur in gout and with amyloid deposition.
- An accessory soleus muscle may mimic Achilles tendon thickening on radiographs, although this is easily recognized at MRI.

Plantaris Tendon

- The plantaris when present, originates from the lateral femoral condyle and inserts anteromedial to the Achilles tendon on the calcaneal tuberosity.
- The muscle is short and the tendon is the longest in the human body.

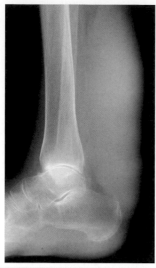

Fig. 7.21 Xanthomatosis. Xanthomatosis of the Achilles tendon due to familial hyperlipidemia. Note the extraordinary tendon enlargement.

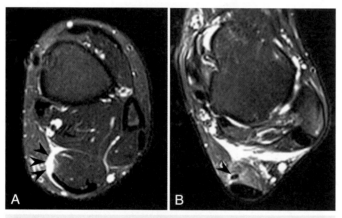

Fig. 7.22 Plantaris tendon complete tear. Sequential axial T2-weighted fat-suppressed MR images of ankle show fluid and edema in the expected location of the ruptured plantaris tendon (arrowheads in A), with reconstitution of the tendon more distally (arrowhead in B).

■ The plantaris tendon is highly variable in size. If large enough, it is sometimes harvested for tendon repair/ augmentation at other sites.
■ An intact plantaris tendon in the setting of a complete Achilles tear may mimic a partially intact Achilles tendon on physical exam.
  ■ The patient may still be able to plantar flex the ankle.
  ■ The Thompson test evaluates the Achilles tendon by squeezing the gastrosoleus muscle to elicit ankle plantar flexion. An intact plantaris can result in a false-negative test in a patient with a complete Achilles tear.
■ Plantaris muscle or tendon tear may result in edema between the gastrocnemius medial head and the medial soleus (Fig. 7.22).

Posterior Tibialis Tendon

■ The PTT is a dynamic stabilizer of the medial longitudinal arch and transverse arch of the foot. (The *spring ligament* deep to the PTT is a major static stabilizer.)

■ Posterior tibial tendinopathy is most common among women older than 50 years of age, usually with a clinical picture of an acquired painful flatfoot that progressively worsens. It is also associated with diabetes and obesity.
■ As with tendinopathies in general, other predisposing factors include rheumatoid arthritis, renal failure, steroid treatment, and chronic overuse.
■ The pathologic process is slow stretching of the PTT due to accumulated microtears. This is referred to as *posterior tibialis tendon dysfunction.*
■ Constellation of findings in PTT dysfunction include:
  ■ Pes planus (loss of 'calcaneal inclination').
  ■ Hindfoot valgus (increase in the talocalcaneal angle on all views).
  ■ Lateral rotation of the forefoot.
  ■ Depression of the medial longitudinal arch (*Meary's angle*—the angle between the talus and the first metatarsal, normally zero, becomes positive).
  ■ The encompassing term for the aforementioned findings is *planovalgus*. PTT dysfunction is basically the opposite of clubfoot (equinovarus).
■ A clinician standing behind the patient can observe the 'too many toes' sign, which is seeing most of the patient's toes due to lateral rotation of the navicular and forefoot. The patient may have difficulty when standing and raising onto their toes, or go into valgus due to PTT weakness.
■ Unlike most tendons, the abnormal PTT rarely tears completely; it generally thickens (hypertrophic tendinosis) or thins (atrophic tendinosis, discussed below).
■ Ultrasonography (US) may show abnormal tendon thickness, tendon sheath fluid, and loss of the normal tendon echogenicity. It is often tender when pressed on with the probe.
■ The equivalent MRI findings are abnormal tendon thickness, tendon sheath fluid, and increased tendon signal on T2-weighted images.
■ As noted previously, the PTT should not have more than twice the cross-sectional area of the adjacent flexor digitorum longus tendon (Figs. 7.23 through 7.25). Thicker than 2× the flexor digitorum longus (FDL) represents 'hypertrophic tendinosis'.
■ Diffuse thinning of the PTT can occur; if the PTT is the same cross-sectional size as the FDL or smaller, the PTT is referred to as exhibiting 'atrophic' or 'attritional' tendinosis.

Pitfalls in PTT Diagnosis

■ There are several pitfalls in diagnosis of PTT tendinosis. The tendon normally broadens at the PTT insertion at the navicular bone, where it may normally be larger than the guidelines noted earlier.
■ Additionally, the tendon normally divides into multiple fascicles distally, inserting in part on the cuneiforms and other sites. Occasionally the tendon nearly completely misses the navicular bone, inserting preferentially on the undersurface of the cuneiforms.
■ Magic angle effect can cause increased signal within any tendon on short echo time sequences (e.g., gradient-echo, T1, and proton density) at the locations where the tendon is aligned at approximately 55 degrees relative to

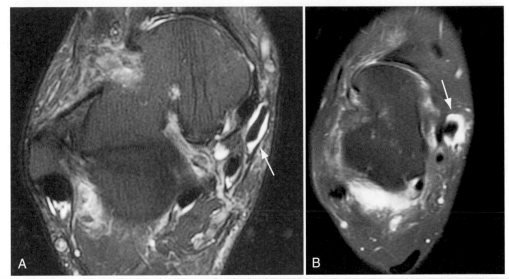

Fig. 7.23 Posterior tibialis tenosynovitis and mild tendinosis. **(A)** Axial fat-suppressed T2-weighted MR image shows enlargement of inframalleolar posterior tibialis tendon sheath *(arrow)* containing fluid, with mild tendon enlargement but normal tendon signal. **(B)** Axial fat-suppressed T2-weighted MR image in another patient shows distended posterior tibialis tendon sheath *(arrow)* with tendon sheath fluid and thickened tendon. The tendon in this example is somewhat irregular in contour and signal.

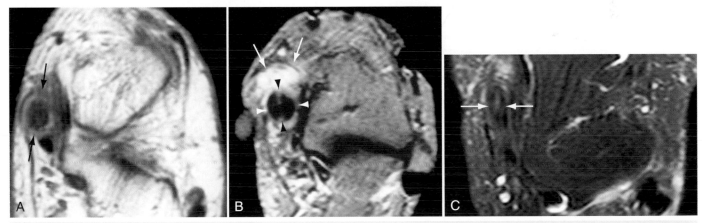

Fig. 7.24 Posterior tibialis: hypertrophic tendinosis. **(A)** Axial proton density MR image shows marked thickening of tendon *(arrows)*. **(B)** T2-weighted MR image in the same patient shows that much of the appearance of the tendon thickening in A is actually due to tendon sheath fluid *(arrows)*. However, substantial tendon thickening *(white arrowheads)* is still shown. Also note the cleft *(black arrowheads)* in the tendon, indicating a longitudinal tear. **(C)** Axial fat-suppressed T2-weighted MR image in another patient shows moderate posterior tibialis tendon thickening *(arrows)* with intratendinous signal indicative of a longitudinal tear.

the main magnetic field. This often occurs where ankle tendons curve around the ankle malleoli. Thus, when one is unsure of magic angle versus tendinopathy on a T1-weighted or a proton density–weighted sequence, one should rely on a T2-weighted sequence or change the angle of the foot in the scanner.

- Likewise, the echogenicity of the tendon on US is highly dependent on transducer position due to normal tendon anisotropy, and subtle changes in transducer position can falsely suggest tendinosis where the tendon curves around the medial malleolus.

Accessory Navicular Ossicle

- Anomalies of the navicular bone can predispose to posterior tibial tendinosis.
- There are three types of *accessory navicular ossicle* (also called *os tibiale externum* or *os naviculare*).

- Type 1 accessory navicular is a tiny ossicle near the medial pole of the navicular bone—functionally a sesamoid bone—and is typically asymptomatic.
- Type 2 accessory navicular is larger with a flat articulation with the parent navicular bone, connected by a low-signal fibrous synchondrosis. With this type the PTT at least partially inserts on the ossicle. This can result in altered mechanics with separation of the synchondrosis and pseudarthrosis formation.
  - The synchondrosis can become destabilized from direct trauma or repetitive microtrauma due to traction forces from the PTT
  - Instability across the synchondrosis can result in medial foot pain, termed 'painful accessory navicular syndrome'
  - MRI features include marrow edema indicating osseous stress response; eventually degenerative

change may develop across the synchondrosis, characterized by osseous irregularity and cystic change.

- Painful accessory navicular syndrome is also associated with PTT tenosynovitis and accelerated tendinosis.

- Type 3 accessory navicular is also called a *cornuate navicular*. This is a navicular bone with an enlarged navicular tuberosity. This is essentially a fused os naviculare with synostosis rather than synchondrosis.

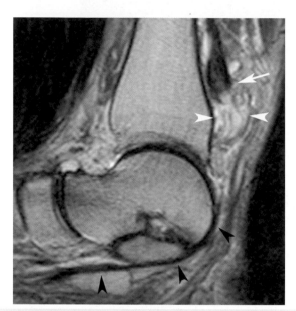

Fig. 7.25 Posterior tibialis tendon: complete tear. Sagittal T2-weighted MR image shows retracted torn tendon posterior to the distal tibial metaphysis *(arrow)*. Note fluid around the tendon margin *(white arrowheads)*. Also note normal flexor hallucis longus coursing below the sustentaculum tali *(black arrowheads)*. Complete tear of the PTT is very uncommon.

- Can be symptomatic due to compression of the overlying soft tissues against the bony prominence by footwear or associated PTT insertional tendinopathy.

Flexor Hallucis Longus

- Among the other flexors of the ankle, injury is rare with the exception of the flexor hallucis longus (Fig. 7.27), where occasionally injury may be seen in ballet dancers as a result of the repetitive push-off from the forefoot or from impingement against the os trigonum.

- Fluid within the tendon sheath of the flexor hallucis longus does not necessarily indicate the presence of tenosynovitis, because in 20% of the population there is normally free communication of fluid between the ankle joint and the flexor hallucis longus tendon sheath. However, disproportionately increased fluid within the tendon sheath or complexity of fluid in the sheath indicating synovitis is suggestive tendon pathology.

Peroneal Tendons

- The peroneus brevis and longus tendons course along the lateral ankle posterior to the distal fibula, held in place by the peroneal retinaculum, with the peroneus brevis tendon anterior to the longus. The brevis inserts on the fifth metatarsal base. The longus extends under the cuboid (assisted by the *os peroneum* when present) and inserts on the first metatarsal base.

- The peroneal tendon sheath is intimately associated with the lateral ligamentous complex, especially the calcaneofibular ligament.

- Peroneal tendon pathology is commonly seen in patients with previous lateral ankle ligament injury.

- Tendinopathy is more common in the peroneus brevis; it is most commonly affected with a pattern known as *split*

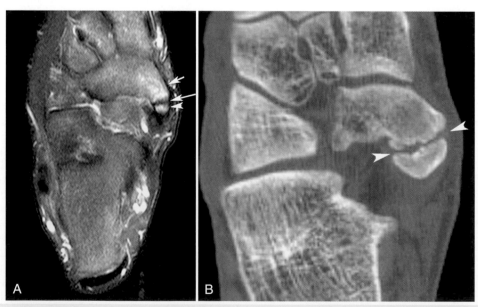

Fig. 7.26 Symptomatic accessory navicular. **(A)** Axial inversion recovery MR image shows marrow edema in an os naviculare *(arrowhead)* and adjacent navicular bone *(short arrow)*, with irregular margin between the two *(long arrow)*. **(B)** Axial CT image in a different patient shows irregular margin *(arrowheads)* between the os and the navicular.

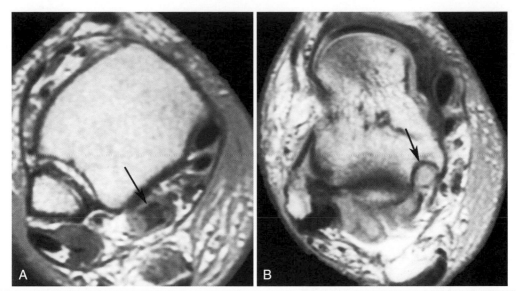

Fig. 7.27 Flexor hallucis longus tendon tear. **(A)** Axial proton density MR image shows marked thickening at the level of distal tibial epiphysis *(arrow)*. **(B)** More distal image shows only fluid signal intensity and absence of tendon in expected groove in the posterolateral talus *(arrow)*. Findings indicate tendon rupture.

peroneus brevis syndrome, which refers to longitudinal tearing of this tendon.

- With this disorder, the peroneus brevis, which is normally the more anteriorly located tendon, is compressed between the peroneus longus and the fibula (Figs. 7.28 through 7.30).
- In extreme cases, the peroneus brevis splits longitudinally, with the peroneus longus interposed between the split halves of the peroneus brevis (sometimes called *intrasubstance subluxation*).
- In milder cases, the peroneus brevis tendon may assume a boomerang or U-shaped cross-sectional contour. Anatomic variants that predispose to peroneus brevis tendinopathy include a tight compartment resulting from an accessory muscle, an abnormally distal position of the peroneus longus or brevis muscle bellies, dysplasia of the adjacent fibula, and peroneal intrasheath subluxation.

- Dynamic subluxation (subluxation that may only occur with certain positioning of the foot) is best evaluated with dynamic ultrasound (Fig. 7.31) An important example is *intrasheath subluxation*, where the tendons flip over each other within the sheath.
  - While monitoring the peroneal tendons posterior to the fibula in the transverse plane, the patient circumducts the foot (spins the forefoot around in a circle while holding the ankle still).

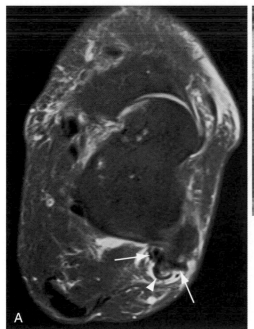

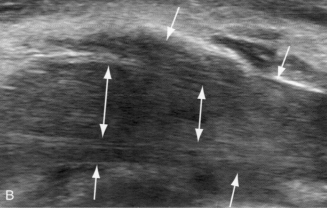

Fig. 7.28 Peroneus brevis split tears. **(A)** Axial fat-suppressed proton density MR image at the level of the inferior tip of the lateral malleolus shows a split peroneus brevis tendon *(arrows)* with the peroneus longus tendon *(arrowhead)* interposed between the two components of the torn tendon. Note thickened and heterogeneous signal in the peroneus longus tendon, indicating substantial peroneus longus tendinosis. **(B)** Longitudinal US image distal to the lateral malleolus in a different patient. Note the thickened peroneus longus tendon (spanned by *double arrows*) between the split peroneus brevis tendon fragments *(arrows)*.

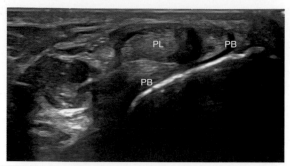

Fig. 7.29 Peroneus brevis split tear. Axial US image at the lateral malleolus in a different patient. The peroneus longus tendon (PL) is located between the split peroneus brevis tendon (PB).

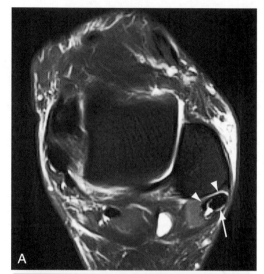

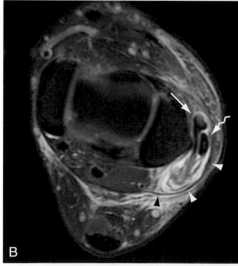

Fig. 7.30 Peroneus brevis tendon dislocation and tear. **(A)** Axial fat-suppressed T2-weighted MR image at the level of the lateral malleolus shows a U-shaped split peroneus brevis tendon *(arrowheads)*, and a mildly thickened peroneus longus tendon *(arrow)*. Note that the peroneal tendons are laterally subluxed and the posterior margin of the lateral malleolus is convex in shape. **(B)** Axial fat-suppressed proton density MR image in another patient shows lateral dislocation of the peroneus longus *(wavy arrow)* and brevis *(straight arrow)* tendons. The peroneus brevis tendon shows a bizarre shape. Note marked enlargement of peroneal tendon sheath *(arrowheads)* with internal complex signal representing synovitis and fluid. Also note the convex contour of the posterior margin of the lateral malleolus with a lateral hooked appearance.

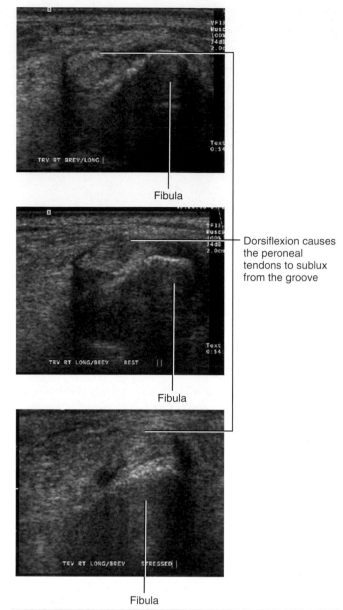

Fig. 7.31 Ultrasound examination demonstrating subluxation of the peroneal tendons. Dynamic scan of the ankle demonstrates peroneal tendon subluxation only during dorsiflexion of the ankle. (From Morrison W. *Problem Solving in Musculoskeletal Imaging.* Philadelphia: Elsevier; 2010.)

- The peroneus longus and brevis tendons should glide smoothly past each other.
- With intrasheath subluxation, the peroneus brevis snaps around the longus. Often the patient will report that this snapping is part of their symptomatology.
- Normally, the posterior margin of the fibula is concave and forms a *retromalleolar groove* where it contacts the peroneal tendons. If the posterior margin is convex, the tendons are prone to subluxing laterally during plantar flexion of the ankle. The overlying peroneal retinaculum may avulse during forced plantar flexion, further leading to tendon subluxation or dislocation (Fig. 7.32).
- The peroneal tendons are prone to *stenosing tenosynovitis*, which is difficult to diagnose radiologically unless

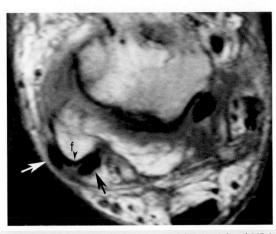

Fig. 7.32 Peroneus tendon dislocation. Axial T1-weighted MR image shows dislocated peroneus longus *(white arrow)* tendon lateral to the lateral malleolus and peroneus brevis *(black arrow)* tendon. The normal peroneus longus tendon should be located posterior to the peroneus brevis at this level. Note that the distal fibula has a rounded contour *(arrowhead)*, a finding that can be associated with peroneal subluxation. *f,* Fibula.

tendon sheath contrast medium is administered. In this disorder, contrast within the tendon sheath appears cut off or beaded rather than continuous.

- The *peroneus quartus* is an accessory muscle that originates from the muscular portion of the peroneus brevis, from the peroneus longus or from the fibula, and inserts onto the peroneal tubercle of the calcaneus, which is a bony prominence located laterally along the calcaneus. It is present in about 1–5% of ankles.
    - This muscle and its tendon can be confused for a peroneus brevis split tear because it lies adjacent to the normal peroneus tendons giving the appearance of three tendons instead of two.
    - It can be recognized by following the course of the accessory tendon to where it inserts on the lateral calcaneus rather than continuing on to the midfoot.
    - The peroneus quartus may be responsible for peroneus longus and brevis tendinopathy, because the accessory muscle and tendon can cause encroachment of the tight compartment encased by the peroneal retinaculum. However, it is more significant as a potential imaging pitfall rather than a symptomatic variant.

Painful Os Peroneum Syndrome

- The *os peroneum* is a normal sesamoid within the peroneus longus tendon adjacent to the cuboid. Rarely it can be a source of symptoms.
    - The ossicle is normally smooth and oval.
    - Sesamoids, in general, assist tendons in going around corners (like the patella and the extensor mechanism of the knee); the os peroneum guides the peroneus longus as it changes direction around the cuboid.
    - Pathology in the distal peroneus longus can alter the appearance of the ossicle.
    - The ossicle can appear sclerotic and fragmented. Bone marrow edema can be seen on MRI.
    - This is associated with lateral pain at the hindfoot with tenderness over the cuboid. This is referred to as *painful os peroneum syndrome (POPS)*.

- If the peroneus longus tears completely, the ossicle becomes displaced. Displacement proximal to the calcaneocuboid joint is associated with a distal complete peroneus longus tendon tear.
- Displacement of a sesamoid (such as the os peroneum and patella) can be used to help diagnose tendon tear on radiographs.

Extensor Tendons

- Extensor tendon injury is uncommon and may be confusing clinically.
- The anterior tibialis tendon (ATT) injury occurs in two populations: athletes who participate in kicking sports, and older individuals.
- Unlike the PTT, the ATT more commonly tears completely and retracts, often above the ankle joint. It may be perceived clinically as a painful soft tissue mass at the anterior ankle.
    - On ultrasound or MRI, diagnosis is straightforward as the painful lump is demonstrated to represent the retracted ATT.
- The ATT is primarily used to lift the foot during the swing phase of gait. However, because other extensor tendons can take over this function, there is generally no noticeable effect on gait.

ACCESSORY MUSCLES AT THE ANKLE

- Accessory muscles around the ankle are very common. They may cause confusion on imaging, but more commonly they are overlooked. Accessory muscles may cause mass effect and impingement within compartments, friction against adjacent structures, or have other mechanical effects. These include:
    - *Peroneus quartus*: adjacent to the peroneus longus and brevis at the fibula; usually inserts on the lateral calcaneus. Can cause mass effect under the peroneal retinaculum.
    - *Peroneus tertius*: lateral to the extensor tendons; inserts on the dorsal aspect of the proximal fifth metatarsal base. Can rarely cause snapping across the talus.
    - *Accessory soleus*: anterior to the Achilles tendon; inserts on the dorsal-medial aspect of the posterior calcaneus. Can cause mechanical effects and exertional posterior pain.
    - *Flexor digitorum accessories longus*: present medially within the tarsal tunnel between the FDL and the flexor hallucis longus (FHL); inserts on the musculature (FDL, quadratus plantae) distally. Can cause mass effect and impingement on the posterior tibial nerve.
    - *Peroneocalcaneus internus*: posteromedial location at the posterior tarsal tunnel; inserts on the medial calcaneus. Can cause mass effect on the posterior tibial nerve.

LIGAMENT INJURY

- Ligament injury at the ankle is typically a result of acute trauma, unlike tendon injury, which is usually a result of chronic repetitive microtrauma.
- Because inversion (supination–external rotation) is the most common injury at the ankle, the lateral ligaments are most commonly injured.

Anterior Talofibular Ligament Injury

- The ATFL is generally the first and most severely injured ligament (Fig. 7.33). In fact, if the ATFL is normal, then the other lateral ligaments are almost always intact as well.
- The ATFL is the best seen on axial MR images and US. It normally appears on MRI as a thin, black, taut ligament with joint fluid extending to its inner margin.
- Surrounding edema or disruption of fibers indicates sprain or tear.
- As the ligament starts to heal, it may look markedly thickened with diffuse edema.
- Eventually, healing restores the ligament to a relatively normal appearance, with some residual thickening (see Fig. 7.33A).
- About 10% of ATFL tears will heal abnormally:
  - Diffuse thickening with scar tissue occupying the anterolateral joint 'gutter'. As described in more detail later in this chapter, this can result in *anterolateral ankle impingement*.
  - Resorption of the ligament; the ATFL appears absent, thinned, and bowed. This can result in ankle instability and acceleration of tibiotalar osteoarthritis.

Calcaneofibular Ligament Injury

- The CFL is second most commonly injured after the ATFL.
- MRI shows edema/disruption of fibers; later changes include ligament thickening with scarring of the peroneal sheath and retinaculum in more severe cases.
- Because of the intimate association of the CFL and the peroneal complex, delayed effects of CFL injury can include:
  - Peroneal tendinosis and tenosynovitis.
  - Scarring of the sheath and retinaculum with stenosing tenosynovitis.
  - Peroneal tendon tear, especially longitudinal tear of the peroneus brevis (peroneal split syndrome).

- Ossification at the peroneal retinaculum insertion at the fibula.
- Because the CFL resists ankle inversion, patients can present later with instability and accelerated osteoarthritis.

Posterior Talofibular Ligament

- The PTFL is almost never injured in routine ankle trauma. It can be torn with severe injury such as ankle or subtalar dislocation.
- The striated nature of the ligament can be a pitfall for overcalling tear.

Syndesmosis Injury

- The distal tibiofibular ligaments and the syndesmosis stabilize the distal tibiofibular joint.
- Syndesmosis sprains, also called *high ankle sprains*, range from mild distal tibiofibular ligament injuries to syndesmotic diastasis, as, for example, in a Maisonneuve fracture.
- The mechanism of injury is usually pronation and external rotation. These mechanisms cause the talus to pry apart the malleoli.
- Nondisplaced sprains may show only edema between the distal tibial and fibula or isolated tears of the anterior distal tibiofibular ligament and may be easily overlooked on MRI (Fig. 7.34).
- If the syndesmosis is torn, the surgeon will place screws or a stabilizer band across the tibiofibular joint or just above.
- Untreated tear of the syndesmosis can lead to severe accelerated osteoarthritis of the ankle joint.

Deltoid Ligament Injury

- The deltoid ligament is a fan-shaped set of ligamentous bundles extending between the medial malleolus and the talus/calcaneus, deep to the PTT.
- Anatomy is complex but can be simplified into deep and superficial layers.

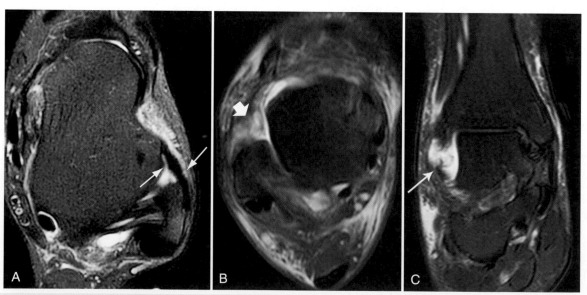

Fig. 7.33 Lateral ankle ligament injury. **(A)** Chronic injury with scarring. Axial fat-suppressed proton density MR image shows irregularly thickened anterior talofibular ligament (between *arrows*) with adjacent edema representing scarring from previous tear. (B and C) Acute sprain in another patient. Axial fat-suppressed proton density–weighted MR image **(B)** shows complete tear of anterior talofibular ligament *(thick arrow)*. Coronal fat-suppressed T2-weighted MR image **(C)** shows complete tear of calcaneofibular ligament *(thin arrow)*.

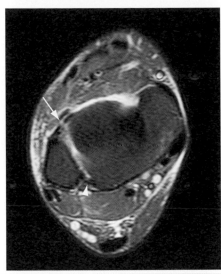

Fig. 7.34 Syndesmosis sprain (high ankle sprain). Axial fat-suppressed T2-weighted MR image shows interrupted anterior distal tibiofibular ligament *(arrow)*. Note the intact posterior distal tibiofibular ligament *(arrowhead)*.

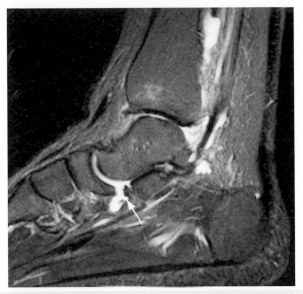

Fig. 7.35 Spring ligament tear. Sagittal fat-suppressed T2-weighted MR image shows torn ligament *(arrow)*. Tears of the spring ligament can result in collapse of the longitudinal arch of the foot.

- The deltoid can become injured from inversion or eversion injury mechanism.
- Inversion mechanism compresses the ligament between the bones, resulting in edema and/or partial tearing.
- Eversion mechanism can tear the deltoid ligament; however, more commonly (because of its strength) the ligament 'wins' and avulses the medial malleolus.

Spring Ligament Injury

- The spring ligament, also termed the *plantar calcaneonavicular ligament*, is perhaps the most important ligament in the hindfoot because it helps to support the medial longitudinal arch, along with the PTT.
- The spring ligament is located between the talus, medial calcaneus, and navicular bone, anterior to the deltoid ligament.
- A spring ligament tear (Fig. 7.35) is a serious injury and can result in collapse of the medial longitudinal arch of the foot.
- More commonly the spring ligament stretches and fails in association with chronic posterior tibialis tendinosis. This results in a constellation of findings including:
  - Collapse of the medial longitudinal arch.
  - Hindfoot valgus.
  - Overpronation.
  - Pes planus.

ANKLE IMPINGEMENT SYNDROMES

- Anterior ankle impingement with dorsiflexion may be caused by bone production at the dorsal talar neck and anteromedial distal tibia (Fig. 7.36).
  - Often referred to as *anteromedial impingement*.
  - Seen in young adults, especially athletes in kicking sports (i.e., soccer).
  - Treated with spur removal (called *cheilectomy*).
- *Anterolateral impingement*, also termed *anterolateral gutter impingement*, is anterolateral ankle pain exacerbated by

Synovitis with loose body   Anterior spur distal tibia

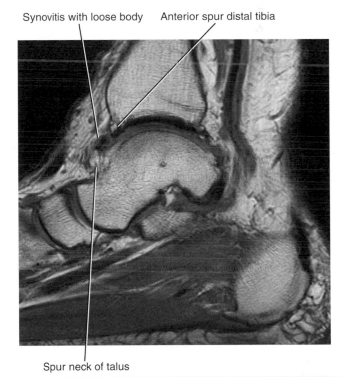

Spur neck of talus

Fig. 7.36 Anterior impingement. Sagittal T1-weighted image shows anterior osteophyte formation involving the anterior aspect of the distal tibia and the adjacent talar neck. There is also adjacent synovitis and loose body formation. (From Morrison W. *Problem Solving in Musculoskeletal Imaging.* Philadelphia: Elsevier; 2010.)

dorsiflexion because of soft tissue fibrosis, synovitis, and cartilage injury at the anterolateral margin of the ankle joint (Fig. 7.37).

- The condition is initiated by trauma, typically preceded by lateral ligament injury.
- A subset of patients develop firm, triangular scar tissue, hence the term *meniscoid syndrome*.

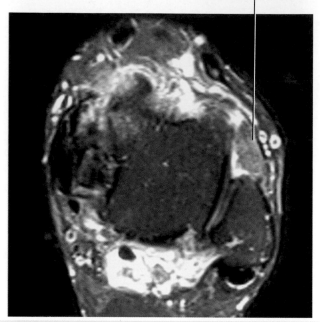

Meniscoid lesion (scarring and fibrosis) within the anterolateral gutter

Fig. 7.37 Anterolateral impingement syndrome. Axial T2-weighted image with fat saturation shows thinning and attenuation of the anterior talofibular ligament consistent with a partial-thickness tear from an old inversion injury. A moderate-sized joint effusion outlines the discoid lesion in the anterolateral gutter. (From Morrison W. *Problem Solving in Musculoskeletal Imaging.* Philadelphia: Elsevier; 2010.)

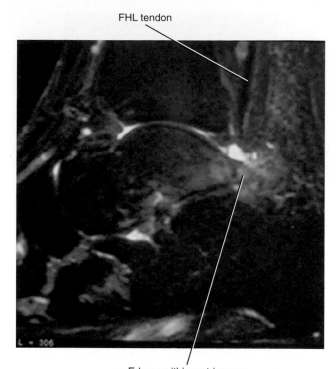

FHL tendon

Edema within os trigonum

Fig. 7.38 Os trigonum syndrome (posterior impingement). Sagittal T2-weighted image with fat saturation shows extensive edema within a prominent os trigonum and extensive adjacent soft tissue edema. There is also moderate tendinosis of the flexor hallucis ligament (FHL) tendon at this level (not seen on this image) in this patient with posterior ankle pain. (From Morrison W. *Problem Solving in Musculoskeletal Imaging.* Philadelphia: Elsevier; 2010.)

- ■ MRI shows soft tissue filling the anterolateral ankle joint under the ATFL and/or anterior syndesmosis.
- ■ *Posterior ankle impingement* during plantar flexion may occur with a large posterior talar process or in association with an os trigonum (Fig. 7.38).
  - ■ The os trigonum is a classic example of a normal variant that may be symptomatic. In this case posterior impingement is also called *os trigonum syndrome.*
  - ■ The os trigonum usually is an unfused apophysis attached to the posterior talus by a fibrous synchondrosis.
  - ■ During skeletal growth, the apophysis usually fuses with the talus as part of the talus posterior process; however, in approximately 10–14% of individuals, it remains as a separate ossicle.
  - ■ In some cases an os trigonum may be a chronic ununited fracture.
  - ■ An asymptomatic os trigonum is likely to have the following features: a smooth contour, a uniform cortical margin, and a gap of no more than a few millimeters between the ossicle and the talus.
  - ■ A painful os trigonum is likely to have the following features: irregular contour, sclerosis, and subcortical cysts at the junction with the talus; marrow edema; fluid between the ossicle and talus (pseudarthrosis); and synovitis in the posterior tibiotalar or subtalar joint recesses.
  - ■ *Talus partitus* is an extreme form of os trigonum, with a large ossicle that includes part of the posterior talus articular surface. Pain, instability, and ankle joint degeneration are often associated.

- ■ Symptomatic os trigonum is more common in ballet dancers and soccer players. These activities involve repetitive, forceful plantar flexion.
- ■ MRI shows marrow edema.
- ■ Bone scan demonstrates intensely increased activity in the posterior talus.
- ■ Potential mimics:
  - ▪ Ganglion cysts off the posterior joint recesses can also result in posterior pain on plantar flexion.
  - ▪ The FHL tendon lies medial to the os trigonum; tenosynovitis may produce symptoms in this region. As noted earlier, some fluid in the FHL tendon sheath may be seen as a normal finding, since it normally communicates with the ankle joint.

TARSAL TUNNEL SYNDROME

- ■ The tarsal tunnel is a fibro-osseous tunnel at the medial ankle; the talus and calcaneus are the base and the flexor retinaculum is the covering.
- ■ Structures that pass through this space including, from anterior to posterior:
  - ■ PTT.
  - ■ FDL tendon.
  - ■ Posterior tibialis artery and vein.
  - ■ Posterior tibial nerve and branches:
    - ▪ Medial plantar nerve (supplies the medial sole).
    - ▪ Lateral plantar nerve (supplies the lateral sole).
    - ▪ Baxter's nerve (supplies the heel/plantar fascia).

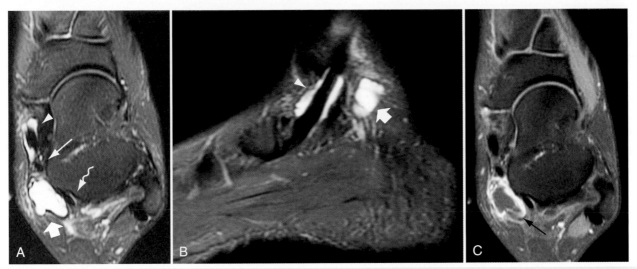

Fig. 7.39 Tarsal tunnel syndrome. **(A and B)** Axial and sagittal fat-suppressed T2-weighted MR images show a ganglion cyst *(thick arrows)* in tarsal tunnel. Note fluid within the posterior tibialis tendon sheath *(arrowheads)* representing tenosynovitis. Also note flexor digitorum longus *(thin arrow)* and flexor hallucis longus *(wavy arrow)*. **(C)** Axial fat-suppressed T1-weighted MR image after intravenous gadolinium contrast administration confirms the cystic nature of the lesion *(arrow)*.

- FHL tendon (see Fig. 7.4).
- Mass effect on the posterior tibial nerve and its branches results in the syndrome that is analogous to carpal tunnel syndrome that consists of tingling, pain, and burning in the sole extending to the toes.
- Common causes include flexor tenosynovitis, anomalous musculature, scarring related to injury, and ganglion cysts (Fig. 7.39). Uncommon causes include neurogenic tumors, lymphangiomas or hemangiomas, varices, or other masses.

Hindfoot, Midfoot, and Forefoot

ANATOMY

- The foot is divided into the hindfoot (calcaneus and talus), midfoot (cuboid, navicular, and cuneiforms), and forefoot (metatarsals and phalanges). The articulation between the hindfoot and midfoot is termed the *Chopart joint*. The articulation between the midfoot and forefoot is termed the *Lisfranc joint*.
- In addition to the 28 bones in the foot, accessory ossicles are extremely common and are often bilateral in occurrence.
  - Accessory ossicles normally are corticated and smoothly contoured, which helps differentiate them from fracture fragments.
  - The most common accessory ossicles are the os trigonum (posterior to the talus on a lateral view of the foot), os peroneum (lateral to the cuboid), and accessory navicular bone (adjacent to the navicular bone medially on a frontal radiograph of the foot).
  - Not all accessory ossicles are always incidental. Some, including the os trigonum and accessory navicular, can be associated with pain syndromes, as previously discussed.

Key Concepts

Foot Anatomy

Hindfoot (calcaneus and talus)
Midfoot (cuboid, navicular, and cuneiforms)
Forefoot (metatarsals and phalanges)
Hindfoot and midfoot articulation: *Chopart joint*
Midfoot and forefoot articulation: *Lisfranc joint*

HINDFOOT

Anatomy

- The calcaneus is the largest bone of the foot and is a tent-shaped bone that consists of a nonarticulating tuberosity posteriorly and an articulating body and anterior process.
- The talus articulates with the calcaneus at the *posterior*, *middle*, and *anterior facets*, which in combination form the calcaneal side of the subtalar joint create a tripod-like support for the talus (Fig. 7.40).
  - The anterior facet is small and communicates with the middle facet.
  - The *sustentaculum tali* at the medial calcaneus forms the middle facet as it articulates with the talus; it is best seen on an oblique frontal radiograph known as a *Harris or skier's view* (see Fig. 7.40B).
  - The posterior facet is the largest of the subtalar joint facets. It does not communicate with the anterior or medial facet.
- The cone-shaped *sinus tarsi* is interposed between the talus and calcaneus, and between the middle and posterior subtalar facets. Its apex is medial, and its broad opening is lateral.
- The cuboid articulates with the calcaneus at the calcaneocuboid joint, and it spans the midfoot between two rows of tarsals.

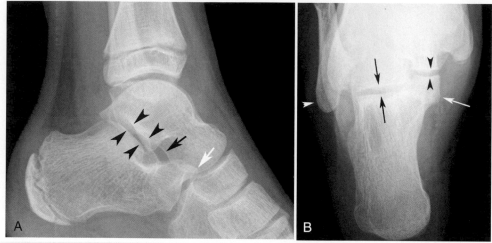

Fig. 7.40 Subtalar (talocalcaneal) radiographic anatomy. **(A)** Lateral radiograph shows the posterior *(black arrowheads)* and middle *(black arrow)* subtalar joints and the anterior process of the calcaneus *(white arrow)*. **(B)** Harris (skier's) view of the right hindfoot shows the posterior *(black arrows)* and middle *(black arrowheads)* subtalar joints, sustentaculum tali *(white arrow)*, and base of fifth metatarsal *(white arrowhead)*.

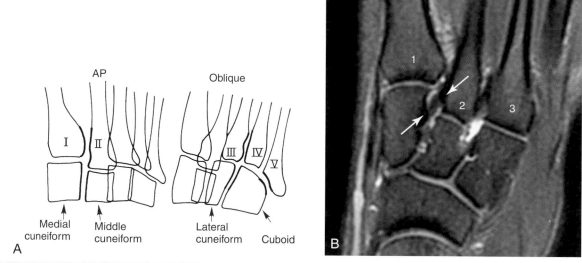

Fig. 7.41 Tarsometatarsal joints. **(A)** Diagram of normal alignment. The first and second metatarsals are evaluated on the AP view. The third, fourth, and fifth metatarsals are evaluated on the oblique view. The bold lines indicate which surfaces of the tarsals and metatarsals must align with one another on each view. The alignment must be precise. **(B)** Lisfranc ligament. Oblique axial fat-suppressed T2-weighted MR image shows the obliquely oriented Lisfranc ligament *(arrows)* between the medial cuneiform and the base of the second metatarsal. There is no ligament between the proximal first and second metatarsals, so the Lisfranc ligament is an essential midfoot-forefoot stabilizer. ([A] Reproduced with permission from Manaster BJ. *Handbook of Skeletal Radiology.* 2nd ed. St. Louis: Mosby; 1997.)

- The first row consists of the navicular bone, and the second row consists of the medial, middle (or intermediate), and lateral cuneiform bones.
- The cuboid articulates with the fourth and fifth metatarsals, whereas the medial, middle, and lateral cuneiforms articulate with the first, second, and third metatarsals, respectively.
- It is extremely important to study the tarsometatarsal articulations carefully on frontal, oblique, and lateral radiographs because subtle malalignment may indicate the presence of midfoot-forefoot (Lisfranc) fracture-dislocation, which is discussed later.
  - A normal AP foot radiograph will show the medial border of the second metatarsal aligning with the medial margin of the middle cuneiform (Fig. 7.41).

- The second metatarsal base is inset compared to the bases of the other metatarsal bones. Its morphology (trapezoidal) and location (at the superior margin of the transverse arch) function like that of a keystone in a Roman arch.
- The second metatarsal base is supported by a strong ligament, named the *Lisfranc ligament*, which connects the lateral-distal margin of the medial cuneiform bone with the adjacent medial-proximal margin of the second metatarsal bone (see Fig. 7.41B).

Apophyseal Development

- It is important to be aware of two secondary centers of ossification in the skeletally immature. The first is at the apophysis of the posterior calcaneal tuberosity. In the skeletally immature, the apophysis is normally dense and frequently fragmented. This was previously referred to as *Sever's disease* but is a normal appearance and does not represent avascular necrosis (AVN) or fracture.

■ The second ossification center of which one should be aware is the apophysis at the lateral base of the fifth metatarsal, which is longitudinally oriented (see Fig. 7.11). This must not be mistaken for an avulsion fracture. Avulsion fractures are transverse in orientation.

Tarsal Coalition

■ Coalitions (anomalous connection of two or more bones) occur in many areas of the body including the hindfoot, wrist, and spine. The two most common hindfoot coalitions are: (Fig. 7.42):

    ■ Calcaneonavicular.

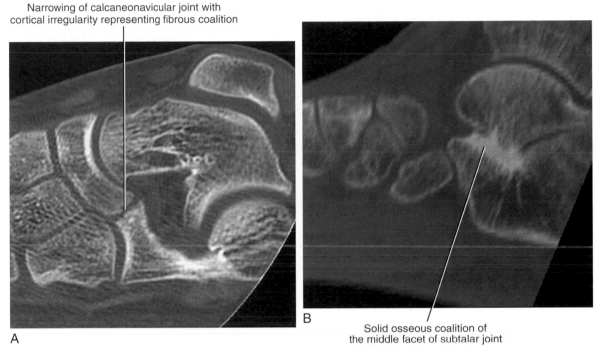

Narrowing of calcaneonavicular joint with cortical irregularity representing fibrous coalition

A

B

Solid osseous coalition of the middle facet of subtalar joint

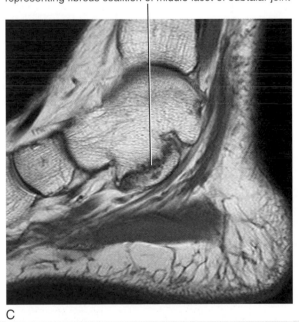

Joint space narrowing and cortical irregularity representing fibrous coalition of middle facet of subtalar joint

C

Fig. 7.42 Tarsal coalition. **(A)** Sagittal reconstruction CT image of the midfoot demonstrates narrowing of the calcaneonavicular joint with cortical irregularity, minimal subchondral cyst formation, and sclerosis consistent with a fibrous coalition. **(B)** Sagittal reconstruction CT image shows extensive sclerosis across the middle facet of the subtalar joint consistent with an osseous coalition. **(C)** Sagittal T1-weighted image of the subtalar joint shows marked narrowing of the subtalar joint with cortical irregularity and subchondral marrow signal changes consistent with a fibrous coalition. (From Morrison W. *Problem Solving in Musculoskeletal Imaging.* Philadelphia: Elsevier; 2010.)

- Subtalar (most commonly involves the middle facet, but can be extensive).
- Cuboid-navicular coalition has been reported but is very rare.
- The connection between the bones can be cartilaginous, fibrous, osseous, or a combination thereof.
  - Cartilaginous: flat articulation, increased T2 signal at the interval.
  - Fibrous: low signal at the interval; usually associated with bone production at the joint.
  - Osseous: medullary continuity.
- Marrow edema often seen in adjacent bones in adults, arthritis at adjacent joints due to altered mechanics.
- The coalition and adjacent bone production can cause classic radiographic signs including:
  - *'Talar beak'*: triangular spur at the superior talar head/neck.
  - *'C sign'*: bone production at the sustentaculum tali looks like a complete 'C' connected with the ankle joint, seen on lateral radiographs (only with subtalar coalition).
  - *'Anteater sign'*: anterior process of the calcaneus blends with the navicular bone on lateral radiographs (seen only in calcaneonavicular coalitions).
  - These radiographic signs are discussed further an illustrated in Chapter 15 - Congenital and Developmental Conditions.
- Coalitions typically present clinically in adolescence; prior to this the tarsal bones are partially composed of flexible cartilage. As the bones ossify and become less flexible, the patient presents with pain and stiffness.

Calcaneus Fracture

- Calcaneus fractures usually occur after falls from heights. Because a jump from a balcony to escape the unexpected arrival of a spouse can cause these fractures, they are known as 'lover's' fractures or 'Don Juan' fractures.
- 10% are bilateral.
- In patients with calcaneus fractures and a history of falling from a height, evaluation of the thoracic and lumbar spine is indicated to assess for associated axial skeletal fractures.
- The most common method for classifying these fractures is the *Rowe classification scheme*, with five types.
  - Type I fractures occur in 21% of cases and are fractures of the calcaneal tuberosity, sustentaculum tali, or anterior process (Fig. 7.43).
  - Type II fractures occur in approximately 4% of cases and are horizontal fractures of the calcaneal tuberosity.
  - Type III fractures occur in approximately 20% of cases and are oblique fractures without extension to the subtalar joint.
  - Type IV fractures occur in approximately 25% of cases and extend to the subtalar joints.
  - Type V fractures occur in 31% of cases and are intraarticular fractures with depression of the posterior subtalar joint or substantial comminution.
- A simpler way to characterize calcaneus fractures that is useful for management decisions is first to make the distinction between fractures with a displaced posterosuperior fracture parallel to the sole of the foot that extends through the posterior margin of the bone—termed *tongue-type* (see Fig. 7.43C and D)—and all others, the majority of which are referred to as *joint depression type*; and second to characterize articular involvement, especially of the posterior subtalar facet.
- The *Bohler angle* is a measure of the degree of depression of the central calcaneus.

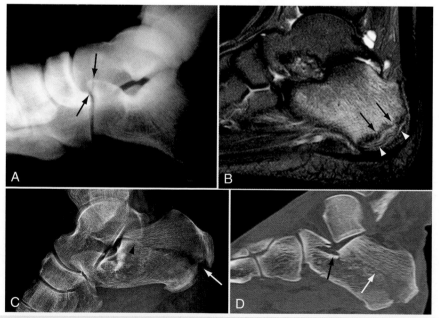

Fig. 7.43 Calcaneus fractures. **(A)** Anterior process fracture of the calcaneus *(arrows)* shown on lateral radiograph. **(B)** Stress fracture in an older child. Sagittal fat-suppressed T2-weighted MR image shows diffuse marrow edema in the calcaneus and a low-signal fracture line *(arrows)* in typical orientation, orthogonal to the major trabecular lines of the calcaneus. The location is also typical, in the tuberosity anterior to the physis *(arrowheads)*. **(C)** (radiograph) and **(D)** (sagittal CT reformation), Tongue-type tuberosity fracture. Note the tuberosity fracture parallel to the sole of the foot that extends to the posterior calcaneus *(white arrows)*. Also note extension to posterior subtalar joint *(arrowhead in C)*. CT reformation **(D)** better demonstrates articular step-off at the posterior facet with anterior rotation of the facet *(black arrow)*.

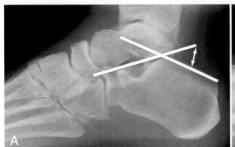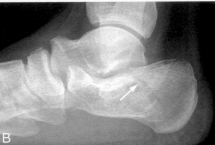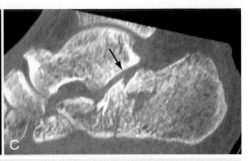

Fig. 7.44 Calcaneus fracture and Bohler angle. **(A)** Lateral radiograph of normal foot demonstrates the Bohler angle, with a line drawn along superior-anterior margin of anterior process and superior-posterior margin of posterior facet and another line drawn between posterior-superior margin of posterior facet and posterior-superior margin of calcaneal tuberosity. The angle subtended by these two lines should be between 28 and 48 degrees. A decreased Bohler angle is associated with fracture of the posterior facet. **(B)** Lateral radiograph demonstrates comminution of calcaneus with flattened Bohler angle. Note fracture extension to posterior subtalar joint *(arrow)*. **(C)** Sagittal CT reconstruction better demonstrates the fractures. Note articular step-off at the posterior facet *(arrow)*.

- It is measured from two lines off the lateral radiograph (Fig. 7.44).
- One line connects the superior margin of the anterior process with the posterior margin of the posterior articular facet of the calcaneus.
- The other line connects the posterior margin of the posterior articular facet of the calcaneus with the posterosuperior margin of the calcaneal tuberosity.
- The angles subtended by these two lines should be between 28 and 48 degrees.
- With depression of the posterior articular facet in Rowe type V fractures, the angle can diminish substantially.
- Both articular depression and the degree of comminution of the lateral margin of the calcaneus are important to assess on radiographs; plate fixation is usually placed along the lateral calcaneus.
- Excessive comminution of the lateral calcaneus limits placement of hardware plates.
- CT is extremely useful for evaluation of calcaneal fractures.
- Stress fractures of the calcaneus are often seen within the calcaneal tuberosity and appear by 10–14 days after the onset of symptoms.
- They usually run perpendicular to the major trabeculae of the calcaneal tuberosity and are seen as curved, vertically oriented linear densities on the lateral radiographic view (see Fig. 1.35 C to E) with a low-signal line and surrounding bone marrow edema on MRI (see Fig. 7.43B).
- MRI is the study of choice to assess for radiographically or clinically suspected calcaneal stress fractures.
- An avulsion at the Achilles insertion can occur as an insufficiency fracture, especially among diabetic patients (see Fig. 7.2B) or patients with chronic renal failure. Aside from these populations, Achilles tendon insertion avulsion fractures are extremely rare.

TALUS FRACTURE

- Talar neck fractures may be associated with talar dislocations (Fig. 7.45).
- Owing to the precarious vascular supply of the talus, talar neck fractures are associated with osteonecrosis within the talar body and talar dome (Fig. 7.46).

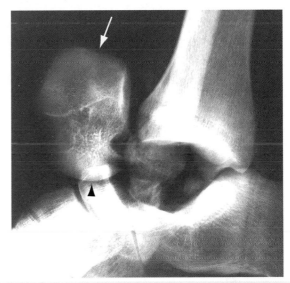

Fig. 7.45 Lateral radiograph demonstrates anterior talar dislocation. The talar dome is denoted by the *arrow* and the talar head (navicular articular margin) by the *arrowhead*.

- Osteonecrosis risk is increased with fracture-dislocation; risk is increased further with more than one joint (subtalar, tibiotalar, talonavicular) dislocated.
- Lucency is expected in the subchondral bone related to resorption a week or more after the fracture, indicating normal blood flow (it takes blood flow to resorb bone). This is called *Hawkins sign*. Lack of subchondral resorption is associated with AVN (see Fig. 7.46).
- Avulsion fractures are most common in the anterior-superior talus, at the ankle joint and talonavicular joint capsule attachment site.
- Chip fractures are seen along the lateral process of the talus ('snowboarder's fracture').
- Osteochondral fractures of the talar dome can be seen laterally or medially following trauma (see Figs. 1.17 and 7.17).
- Fracture of the lateral tubercle of the posterior process (*Stieda process*), called a *Shepherd fracture*, or the medial tubercle of the posterior process, called a Cedell fracture, may resemble an os trigonum.

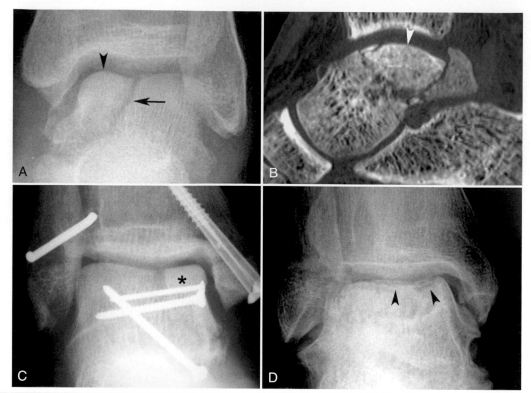

Fig. 7.46 Talus fracture and posttraumatic talar dome osteonecrosis. (A and B) AP radiograph **(A)** and sagittal reformatted CT **(B)** show an intraarticular talus fracture *(arrow in A)* that occurred 6 weeks previously. Note the sclerosis and lack of subchondral bone resorption in the medial fragment *(arrowhead)*. **(C)** Frontal radiograph of ankle in a different patient shows medial malleolar, lateral malleolar, and talar fixation. Osteonecrosis of medial talar bone fragment *(asterisk)* is shown by increased density, which relates to lack of a hyperemic healing response. **(D)** AP radiograph of the ankle in a different patient, who sustained a talar neck fracture several months previously, shows late-stage findings of osteonecrosis. The talar dome is sclerotic and the subchondral bone has fragmented and collapsed *(arrowheads)*.

- Stress and insufficiency fractures also can occur in the talus (Fig. 7.47).

SINUS TARSI SYNDROME

- The sinus tarsi is a cone-shaped space between the talus and the calcaneus that narrows medially and opens at the lateral hindfoot. It is directly anterior to the posterior facet of the subtalar joint.
- This space is occupied by fat, a neurovascular bundle, roots of the inferior extensor retinaculum, and the talocalcaneal ligaments, which provide stability to the lateral ankle.
- Sinus tarsi syndrome results from scarring or mass effect within the space. Patients present with lateral foot pain and a feeling of instability.
- Causes include ankle inversion injury, plantar arch collapse due to PTT dysfunction, and rheumatoid arthritis.
- On MR images, the abnormal sinus tarsi shows replacement of the normal fat signal on T1-weighted images (Fig. 7.48).
- T2-weighted images may show signal consistent with edema, fibrosis, or synovial cysts arising from the adjacent subtalar joint.
- Because this disorder usually arises after inversion injury, many patients have sequalae of lateral ligament injury.

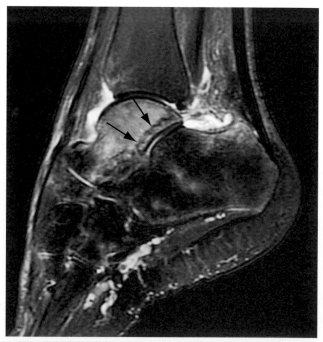

Fig. 7.47 Talus stress fracture. Sagittal fat-suppressed T2-weighted MR image shows diffuse talar edema with low signal subchondral fracture *(arrows)* adjacent to posterior articular facet.

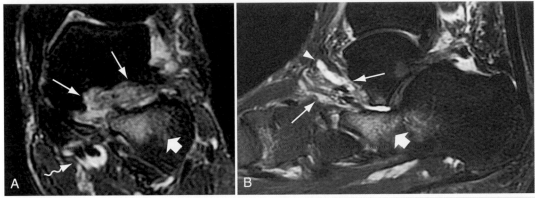

Fig. 7.48 Sinus tarsi syndrome. Short-axis **(A)** and sagittal **(B)** fat-suppressed T2-weighted MR images demonstrate pronounced sinus tarsi edema *(thin straight arrows)* with ganglion cyst *(arrowhead)* and stress reaction *(thick arrows)* in underlying anterior process of the calcaneus. Note flexor digitorum longus and flexor hallucis longus tenosynovitis *(wavy arrow)*.

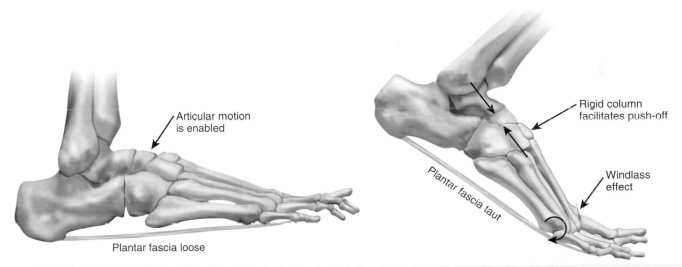

Fig. 7.49 The windlass mechanism and function of the plantar fascia. When the foot is at rest, there is some mobility between the bones of the midfoot, allowing flexibility. During the push-off phase of gait, this flexibility would be detrimental. The plantar fascia, which inserts distal to the metatarsophalangeal (MTP) joints, tightens as the toes are dorsiflexed, which pulls the tarsal bones together and 'locks' them into a rigid column. This effect has been likened to a windlass, which is a rope or chain extending over a drum used to raise and lower sails and anchors on a ship. (From Morrison W. *Problem Solving in Musculoskeletal Imaging.* Philadelphia: Elsevier; 2010.)

MIDFOOT ANATOMY AND BIO MECHANICS

- The midfoot is superbly constructed for ambulation; the tarsal bone articulations have capability for motion that allows for twisting of the foot and pronation/supination.
- However, during the push-off phase of walking, a stable midfoot column is more important than flexibility. This goal is achieved via the 'windlass mechanism' (Fig. 7.49).
  - A windlass is a mechanism commonly used on boats, referring to a cylinder that, when cranked, tightens a rope attached to a sail, anchor, etc.
  - The plantar fascia acts as a windlass of the foot. The plantar fascia is connected to the calcaneus and the digits; during the push-off phase of ambulation, dorsiflexion of the toes causes the plantar fascia to wrap around the metatarsal heads (i.e., the cylinder), which tightens the fascia, pulling the tarsal bones together and creating a stable column across the midfoot.

- Deformity of the arch or forefoot, or plantar fascia disruption prevents this from working and can lead to pain with walking.
- The Lisfranc joint is very important in stabilization of the midfoot and longitudinal arch.
  - The second metatarsal base is inset compared to the other tarsometatarsal joints, and this and the middle cuneiform are shaped like a keystone in the coronal (short axis) plane (Fig. 7.50).
  - The Lisfranc joint is shaped like a Roman arch, which is well known for its stability. (Many arches constructed by the ancient Romans remain intact today.).
  - There are intercuneiform and intermetatarsal ligaments (Figs. 7.51 and 7.52); however, the Lisfranc ligament running obliquely from the medial cuneiform to the second metatarsal base (Fig. 7.53) is the

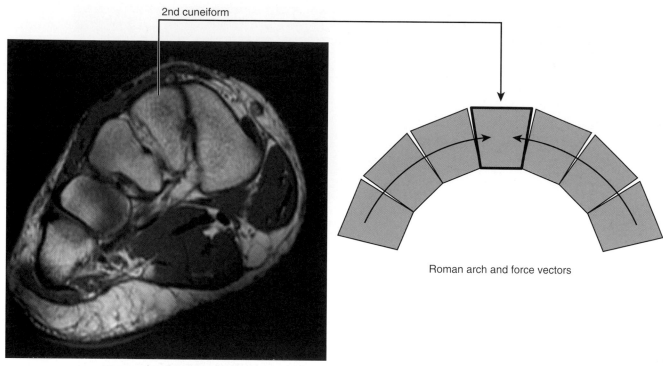

2nd cuneiform

Roman arch and force vectors

Transverse arch of the midfoot

Fig. 7.50 The second (middle) cuneiform and second metatarsal base are shaped like a keystone in the coronal plane. The Lisfranc joint is shaped like a Roman arch. This anatomy, and stabilization by the Lisfranc ligament, is important for support of the arch of the foot. (From Morrison W. *Problem Solving in Musculoskeletal Imaging.* Philadelphia: Elsevier; 2010.)

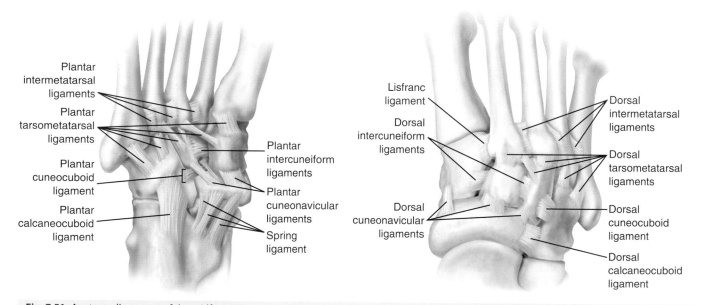

Plantar intermetatarsal ligaments
Plantar tarsometatarsal ligaments
Plantar cuneocuboid ligament
Plantar calcaneocuboid ligament
Plantar intercuneiform ligaments
Plantar cuneonavicular ligaments
Spring ligament

Lisfranc ligament
Dorsal intercuneiform ligaments
Dorsal cuneonavicular ligaments
Dorsal intermetatarsal ligaments
Dorsal tarsometatarsal ligaments
Dorsal cuneocuboid ligament
Dorsal calcaneocuboid ligament

Fig. 7.51 Anatomy: ligaments of the midfoot. (From Morrison W. *Problem Solving in Musculoskeletal Imaging.* Philadelphia: Elsevier; 2010.)

main structure keeping the midfoot congruent—it is the 'cement' of the Roman arch.

- There is no intermetatarsal ligament between the first and second metatarsals. Therefore fracture of the second metatarsal base or disruption of the Lisfranc ligament creates instability of the entire tarsometatarsal axis and destabilizes the midfoot, resulting in collapse of the longitudinal arch.

NAVICULAR BONE FRACTURE

- Stress fractures of the navicular bone are one of the more common types of stress fractures in basketball players.
  - The middle third of this bone has a relatively poor blood supply and thus is the usual site.
  - Patients present with pain that is usually poorly localized in the medial arch of the foot.

Lisfranc ligament   Intermetatarsal ligaments

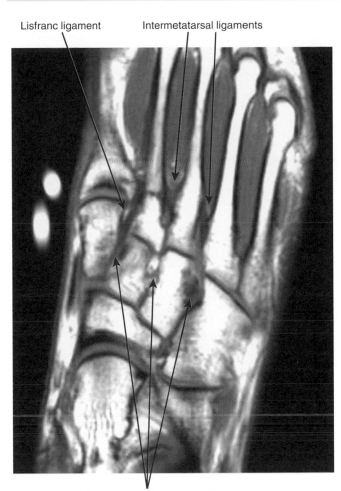

Intercuneiform ligaments and
cuneocuboid ligament

Fig. 7.52 Ligaments of the midfoot, seen on long-axis proton density MR image. (From Morrison W. *Problem Solving in Musculoskeletal Imaging.* Philadelphia: Elsevier; 2010.)

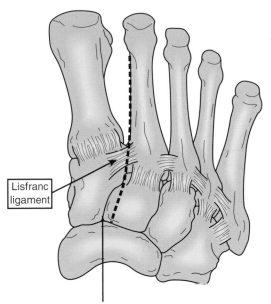

Lisfranc
ligament

With intact Lisfranc ligament there should be an unbroken line from the 2nd MT to 2nd cuneiform medially

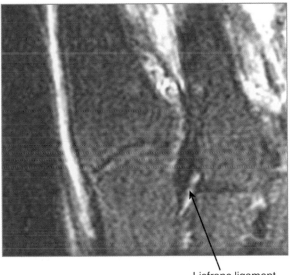

Lisfranc ligament
• Extends from 1st cuneiform to 2nd MT base

Fig. 7.53 The Lisfranc ligament extends obliquely from the medial cuneiform to the second metatarsal base. On a longitudinal image of the foot, the medial margin of the second metatarsal should align exactly with the medial border of the middle cuneiform. If these are malaligned, tear of the Lisfranc ligament should be suspected. (From Morrison W. *Problem Solving in Musculoskeletal Imaging.* Philadelphia: Elsevier; 2010.)

- Most are sagittally oriented at the junction of the middle and lateral thirds of the navicular bone (Fig. 7.54).
  - Acute navicular fractures also may present with this orientation, but the history will distinguish between acute and stress fractures.
- Although they are usually occult on radiographs, navicular fractures are well shown on CT and MRI.
- Radionuclide bone scanning will show localized activity in the navicular bone and is thus sensitive but not specific.
- Osteonecrosis of the lateral fracture fragment is a potential complication of navicular fracture.
- Avulsion fractures of the navicular bone also occur, at the dorsal talonavicular capsule insertion. They present as a dorsal bone fragment at the proximal navicular margin.
  - Smoothly corticated ossicles—usually incidental—are frequently seen at this site as well. These may represent remote capsular avulsions.
- Rarely fractures of the medial tuberosity of the navicular bone may occur at the insertion site of the PTT and the tibionavicular bundle of the deltoid ligament complex.
- Navicular tuberosity fractures may also occur from a direct blow, such as when a hockey puck strikes the medial foot. Fractures can be differentiated from an accessory navicular os by sharp, non-corticated margins.

CUBOID AND CUNEIFORM FRACTURE

- These fractures are usually related to complex fractures involving multiple bones, such as Lisfranc fracture/dislocation.
- Cuboid fractures can be seen in association with calcaneal fractures. Isolated cuboid fractures can be seen with twisting injuries.

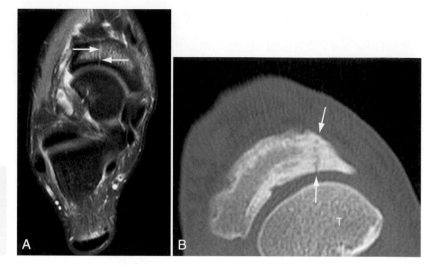

Fig. 7.54 Navicular fractures. **(A)** Obliquely oriented long-axis fat-suppressed T2-weighted MR image shows diffuse navicular edema with a nondisplaced sagittally oriented fracture of navicular bone *(arrows)*. **(B)** Chronic fracture. Axial CT image shows nondisplaced fracture *(arrows)* with adjacent sclerosis. T marks the talar head. This could be a normally healing fracture or a stress fracture.

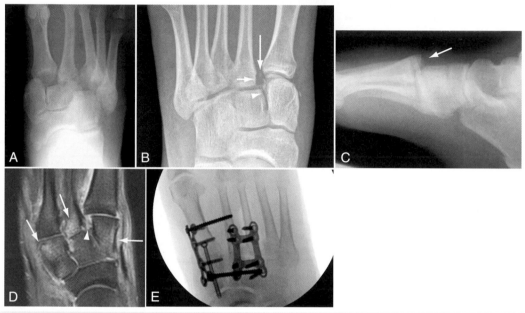

Fig. 7.55 Lisfranc fracture-dislocations. **(A)** Convergent (homolateral) pattern. AP radiograph shows lateral displacement of all five metatarsal bones, including first metatarsal. **(B)** Divergent pattern in which the first metatarsal is not displaced. Oblique foot radiograph shows widening of interspace between first and second metatarsals associated with subluxation of the second metatarsal base. The medial margins of the middle sesamoid *(arrowhead)* and proximal second metatarsal *(short arrow)* should be aligned. Note the small avulsion fragment *(long arrow)* between the metatarsal bases. **(C)** Lateral view of patient with Lisfranc fracture-dislocation demonstrates superior metatarsal subluxation at tarsometatarsal joints *(arrow)*. **(D)** Obliquely oriented long-axis fat-suppressed T2-weighted MR image shows interruption of the Lisfranc ligament *(arrowhead)*. Note fracture edema of the second metatarsal base and the lateral cuneiform bone *(arrows)*. **(E)** Intraoperative spot radiograph in a different patient with a Lisfranc fracture shows internal fixation of the tarsometatarsal and intercuneiform articulations.

LISFRANC FRACTURE-DISLOCATION

- A Lisfranc fracture-dislocation typically occurs in the setting of axial loading of the plantar-flexed foot.
- This can occur with twisting injury at the midfoot (e.g., misstepping when coming down stairs or falling from a bike with foot entrapment in an enclosed pedal).
- These injuries involve rupture of the major supporting ligaments of the tarsometatarsal articulations, especially the Lisfranc ligament.
- Alternatively, the Lisfranc ligament may remain intact even though an avulsion occurs at either the medial cuneiform or second metatarsal base insertions.

- With this injury, stability of the tarsometatarsal articulations is disrupted and lateral subluxation of the second through fifth metatarsals ensues (Fig. 7.55).
- There is usually dorsal subluxation or dislocation of the tarsometatarsal joints, which may appear quite subtle on the lateral views.
- Two types of subluxation occur.
    - *Homolateral (convergent) subluxation*: all five metatarsal bones are subluxed laterally (see Fig. 7.55A).
    - *Divergent subluxation*: lateral subluxation of the second through fifth metatarsals and variable medial subluxation of the first metatarsal (see Fig. 7.55B).

- Regardless of type, dorsal subluxation of the metatarsal bases is typical.
- There are usually associated fractures of the metatarsal bones, although these may be radiographically occult.
- A Lisfranc fracture-dislocation also is a common complication of diabetic neuropathic arthropathy.
- The degree of subluxation may be extremely subtle and, in suspected cases, CT or MRI will prove useful for detecting radiographically occult fracture, ligament disruption, and subluxation at the tarsometatarsal articulations.
- Diagnosis on radiographs:
  - Slight widening of the interspace between the first and second metatarsals may be the only clue to the appropriate diagnosis on radiographs and should prompt additional imaging. Widening may be accentuated by weightbearing views.
  - Similarly, the medial margin of the second metatarsal bone should line up exactly with the medial margin of the second cuneiform. Any offset in the setting of injury or diabetes should prompt additional evaluation (usually with MRI).
- If the diagnosis is questionable on imaging, the patient may undergo 'exam under anesthesia': the patient is sedated and the surgeon squeezes the midfoot to see if the bones separate.
- Lisfranc fracture-dislocations have a poor prognosis. The likelihood of eventual osteoarthritis is high, with progressive deformity (arch collapse). For this reason, such injuries typically undergo surgical reduction and fixation.
- Lisfranc disruption may be seen after acute injury or in the setting of neuropathic disease; in both cases there is usually superior migration of the metatarsal bases and inferior excursion of the tarsal bones. This can create a 'rocker-bottom' deformity with reversal of the longitudinal arch curvature (Fig. 7.56).

Key Concepts

Lisfranc Fracture-Dislocation

- **Homolateral (convergent):** All five metatarsal bones subluxed laterally
- **Divergent:** Lateral subluxation of the second through fifth metatarsals away from first metatarsal
- Radiographs: Widening of interspace between first and second metatarsals and/or offset of the second metatarsal and middle cuneiform
- Test of choice for confirmation: MRI
- Common in diabetic neuropathic arthropathy

LISFRANC JOINT LIGAMENTOUS INJURY

- Lisfranc injuries occur from twisting at the midfoot; the classic mechanism of falling from a horse with the foot twisted in the stirrup is not seen frequently; more commonly the patient twists their foot in a pothole or lands wrong after a jump; more extensive injuries may be seen in multitrauma patients.
- Lisfranc injuries are common in athletes and may be seen in sports that require pivoting, or when another player steps on their foot immobilizing the forefoot as the body rotates around the midfoot.
- Clinically, the injury is very painful and patients cannot bear weight on the affected extremity, so the diagnosis is usually suspected before imaging.
- If imaging is indeterminate, patients may undergo examination under anesthesia to demonstrate abnormal motion at the Lisfranc joint and widening of the ligament interval under stress.

Imaging of Lisfranc Injury

- When Lisfranc injury is suspected, radiographs are the best initial examination.

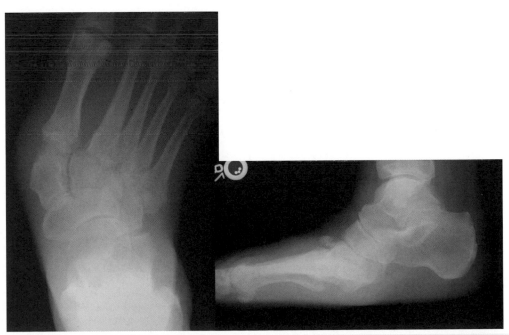

Fig. 7.56 Chronic untreated Lisfranc injury seen here in a patient with diabetic neuropathy results in deformity with collapse of the arch and a rocker-bottom configuration. (From Morrison W. *Problem Solving in Musculoskeletal Imaging.* Philadelphia: Elsevier; 2010.)

- On the AP view of the foot the medial margin of the second metatarsal (MT) should line up exactly with the medial margin of the second cuneiform (see Fig. 7.53 and Fig. 7.55).
- The first tarsometatarsal joint should also be congruent.
- Distance between the first and second MT bases is of less importance, and can vary.
- Presence of an ossicle, the os intermetatarseum, can result in false-positive diagnosis. Unlike true Lisfranc ligament avulsions, this ossicle is rounded and projects superiorly on the lateral view.
- Avulsions are very thin, linear, and positioned between the first cuneiform and second MT base. CT may be needed to confirm the finding (Fig. 7.57).
- CT is typically required to evaluate the extent of fractures, which is characteristically underestimated on radiographs.
- MRI is an excellent test to directly evaluate the Lisfranc ligament (and other ligaments of the midfoot) as well as to diagnose associated fractures and bone bruises, often obviating the need for exam under anesthesia.
  - The best plane is axial (long-axis) in the plane of the metatarsals; the best sequence is T2-weighted with fat suppression (see Fig. 7.55D).
  - An important concept in interpreting MRI of suspected Lisfranc ligament injury is that a ligament with a mechanically significant injury may still appear intact on MRI.
    - First, small avulsions can be very hard to detect on MRI.

- Second, the ligament may be stretched and insufficient without appearing discontinuous.
- In the setting of injury, any edema in or around the ligament should be considered suspicious for a significant injury; a T2-weighted fat-suppressed sequence is recommended.
- Secondary signs are also very useful. A very common association is bone bruise or fracture of the inferior aspect of the middle cuneiform or second metatarsal base (Fig. 7.58). In more severe injuries bone bruises or fractures are also observed in various other tarsal bones and metatarsal bases.
- Another secondary sign is soft tissue edema extending distally along the second metatarsal shaft, frequently with strain of the first interosseous muscle between the first and second metatarsals. Resultant feathery edema in the muscle is not significant by itself but is a sign of traumatic separation of the metatarsals.
- It is helpful to the surgeons to identify other ligaments that are injured, such as the intercuneiform ligaments, intermetatarsal ligaments, and deep plantar ligaments of the midfoot. The intercuneiform ligaments and intermetatarsal ligaments are somewhat variable in presence and are not consistently seen on routine MRI but are best evaluated on axial (long-axis) images (see Fig. 7.52).
- The deep plantar ligaments are best seen on coronal (short-axis) images (Fig. 7.59), just inferior to the tarsal bones, and just deep to the peroneus longus tendon as it courses toward the first metatarsal base.

Fracture fragment

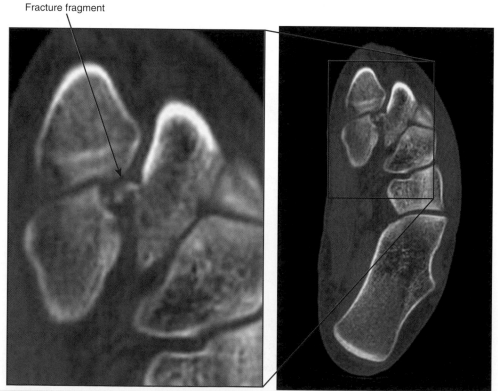

Fig. 7.57 Lisfranc injury on CT. CT is very useful for confirming a fracture suspected clinically, especially if radiographs are negative. CT is also useful for identifying additional fractures. However, a significant Lisfranc injury may exist in the absence of fracture. MRI is the test of choice for evaluation of the ligament itself as well as bone bruises and muscle tears indicative of a more severe injury. Still, CT serves a complementary role, since small fracture fragments may not be visible on MRI. (From Morrison W. *Problem Solving in Musculoskeletal Imaging.* Philadelphia: Elsevier; 2010.)

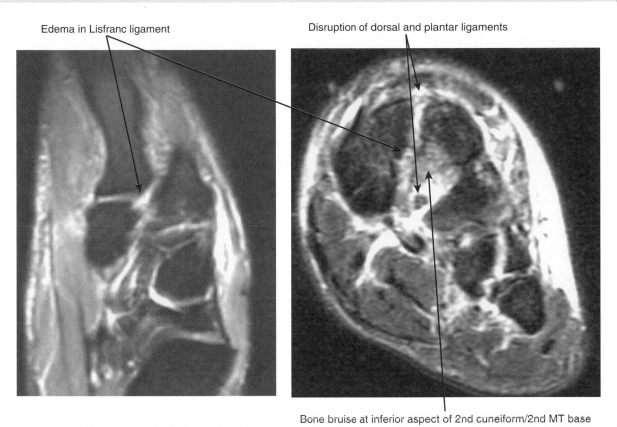

Edema in Lisfranc ligament

Disruption of dorsal and plantar ligaments

Bone bruise at inferior aspect of 2nd cuneiform/2nd MT base

Fig. 7.58 Lisfranc ligament tear. Axial (left) and coronal (right) fluid-sensitive MR images show edema in the Lisfranc ligament with disruption of fibers. Soft tissue edema and bone bruise or fracture of the second metatarsal base is commonly associated. (From Morrison W. *Problem Solving in Musculoskeletal Imaging.* Philadelphia: Elsevier; 2010.)

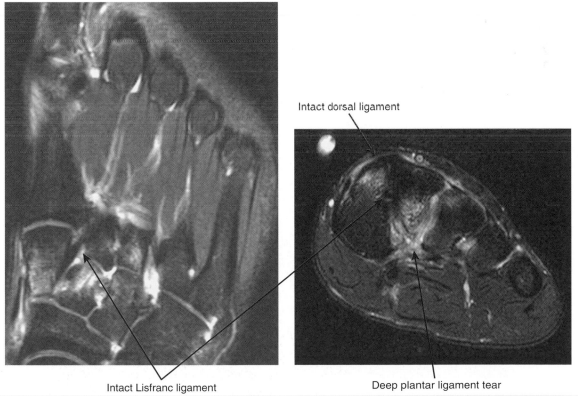

Intact dorsal ligament

Intact Lisfranc ligament

Deep plantar ligament tear

Fig. 7.59 Lisfranc injury without ligament tear. Professional football player with twisting injury during a game. Bone bruises are present; there is disruption of the deep plantar ligament, but the main Lisfranc ligament remains intact. The foot was stable on exam under anesthesia. (From Morrison W. *Problem Solving in Musculoskeletal Imaging.* Philadelphia: Elsevier; 2010.)

However, prominent veins in this region make it difficult to detect soft tissue edema.

FOREFOOT FRACTURES

- Proximal fifth metatarsal fractures were discussed previously.
- Metatarsal stress fractures are common, usually occurring in the second or third metatarsal shafts (Fig. 7.60; see also Fig. 1.35A), which are the longest and exposed to disproportionate stress.
    - The synonym *march fracture* refers to the classic etiology of extended marches by new military recruits.
    - These fractures are usually nondisplaced and become radiographically apparent 7 to 10 days after the onset of symptoms, with the appearance of ill-defined periosteal new bone formation at the site of fracture.
    - Eventually a sclerotic healed fracture line will appear.
- Stress injury can also occur at the metatarsal head (most commonly the second—the longest, exposed to the most stress); this can occur during adolescence and result in necrosis, collapse, and flattening of the metatarsal head superiorly, referred to as *Freiberg infraction* (Fig. 7.61).
- As discussed previously, fractures of the proximal fifth metatarsal distal to the intermetatarsal joint are often stress fractures (See Fig. 7.12).

Forefoot Anatomy (Figs. 7.62 and 7.63)

- The medial (tibial) and lateral (fibular) sesamoid bones that articulate on facets at the inferior aspect of the first metatarsal head; facets are separated by a bony prominence called the *crista*.
- Articular cartilage is present on the metatarsal head and the sesamoids (the metatarsal sesamoid, or MTS joint) and synovial fluid communicates with the rest of the first metatarsophalangeal (MTP) joint.
- Processes that alter the position or tracking of the sesamoids, or result in cartilage loss, can cause pain and secondary osteoarthritis; also, any articular disease affecting the first MTP joint will also affect the MTS joint.
- The sesamoid bones are stabilized by their capsular location and metatarsal articulation. Additional stabilization is provided by an intersesamoid ligament that extends between them as well as sesamoid-phalangeal ligaments distally. However, this stable position under the first metatarsal head also makes the sesamoid bones (especially the tibial sesamoid) susceptible to compressive force.
- Loss or migration of the plantar fat pad from callus, from diseases such as rheumatoid arthritis and diabetes or from excessive dorsiflexion (i.e., high-heeled shoes), can leave the sesamoid bones relatively unprotected.
- The sesamoid bones are also part of the flexor complex of the first ray; the FHL tendon passes between the sesamoids, superficial to the intersesamoid ligament.
- Separate slips of the flexor hallucis brevis tendon insert on the tibial and fibular sesamoid bones.
- The sesamoid bones are also intimately associated with the capsule near the attachment of the tendons of the abductor hallucis (adjacent to the tibial sesamoid), and adductor hallucis (adjacent to the fibular sesamoid).
- The structures described previously comprise the plantar plate of the first MTP joint. The 'lesser' MTP joints (second through fifth) also have plantar plates, composed of thickening of the inferior joint capsule.
    - This thickened, fibrous capsule makes a dark 'U-shaped' structure on coronal (short-axis) MR images when intact (Fig. 7.64). Flexor and extensor tendons pass by the MTP joints inferiorly and superiorly, on course to insert on the phalanges.
- Between the metatarsal heads there is an anatomic bursa called the intermetatarsal bursa, which can be filled with fluid; on coronal T2-weighted images it is seen as a third 'line' of fluid between the bones (joint, bursa, joint), separated by the adjacent joint capsules (Fig. 7.64).
    - Immediately inferior to this bursa is a fascial arch that extends between the metatarsal heads.

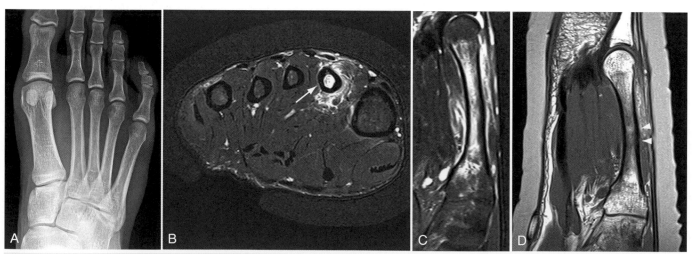

Fig. 7.60 Fatigue fracture of second metatarsal bone. **(A)** Frontal radiograph shows a normal appearance. Stress fractures can be radiographically occult during the first 1 to 2 weeks of symptoms. **(B)** Short-axis fat-suppressed T2-weighted MR image shows marked endosteal and periosteal edema-like signal of the second metatarsal *(arrow)*. **(C)** Sagittal fat-suppressed T2-weighted MR image shows the extent of second metatarsal edema. **(D)** Sagittal T1-weighted MR image shows marrow edema and subtle periosteal new bone formation *(arrowheads)*.

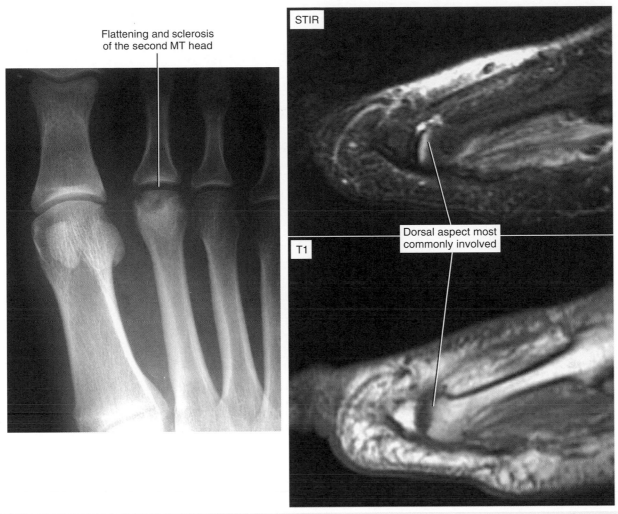

Flattening and sclerosis
of the second MT head

STIR

T1

Dorsal aspect most
commonly involved

Fig. 7.61 Freiberg infraction. Osteonecrosis of the metatarsal head (typically the second, especially in the setting of a long second toe). Dorsal articular surface is most commonly involved and may be related to chronic repetitive stress. (From Morrison W. *Problem Solving in Musculoskeletal Imaging*. Philadelphia: Elsevier; 2010.)

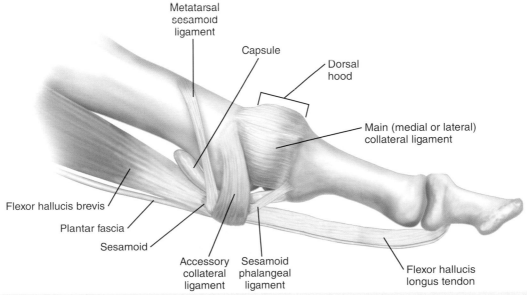

Metatarsal
sesamoid
ligament

Capsule

Dorsal
hood

Main (medial or lateral)
collateral ligament

Flexor hallucis brevis

Plantar fascia

Sesamoid

Accessory
collateral
ligament

Sesamoid
phalangeal
ligament

Flexor hallucis
longus tendon

Fig. 7.62 Anatomy: the great toe and first metatarsophalangeal joint. (From Morrison W. *Problem Solving in Musculoskeletal Imaging*. Philadelphia: Elsevier; 2010.)

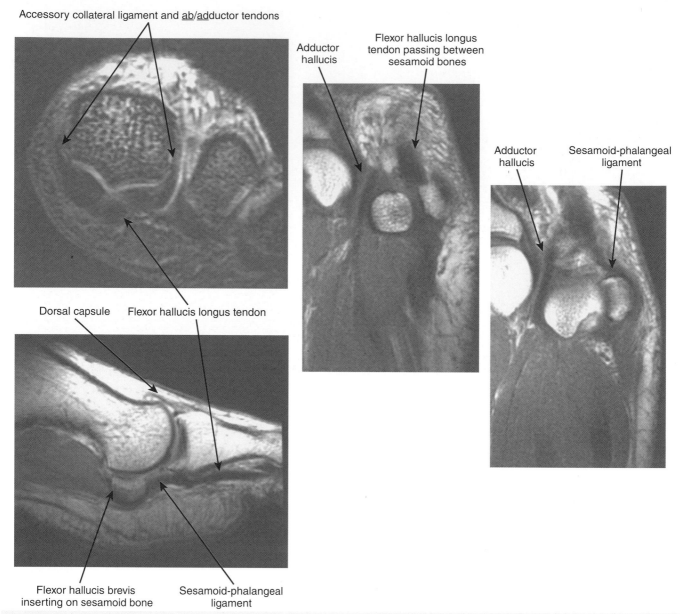

Accessory collateral ligament and ab/adductor tendons

Adductor hallucis

Flexor hallucis longus tendon passing between sesamoid bones

Adductor hallucis

Sesamoid-phalangeal ligament

Dorsal capsule   Flexor hallucis longus tendon

Flexor hallucis brevis inserting on sesamoid bone   Sesamoid-phalangeal ligament

Fig. 7.63 Anatomy of the first metatarsophalangeal joint and sesamoids on MRI. (From Morrison W. *Problem Solving in Musculoskeletal Imaging*. Philadelphia: Elsevier; 2010.)

- Inferior to this courses the interdigital nerve; using standard protocols at or below 1.5T this nerve is not routinely seen unless pathologically enlarged due to perineural fibrosis (e.g., Morton neuroma).
- Interosseous muscles extend between the metatarsal shafts, thinning distally as they insert on the MTP joint capsules.
- The flexor muscles are separated into three compartments (medial, central, and lateral) between which are two neurovascular bundles, containing the medial and lateral plantar calcaneal branches of the posterior tibial nerve from the tarsal tunnel.
- The plantar fascia originates from the inferior calcaneus and inserts onto the superficial fascia and the flexor tendons of the toes. It is also intimately associated with fascial arches that bridge the gap between the metatarsal heads inferior to which the neurovascular bundles run.

BURSITIS IN THE FOREFOOT

- Bursitis generally appears on imaging as a focal, flattened fluid collection. In the foot there are *anatomic* bursae (i.e., those present in all individuals, in place to cushion areas prone to friction due to natural activities ike walking) and *adventitial (acquired) bursae* (bursae that arise as an adaptive response to atypical friction, such as from wearing tight shoes or a foot deformity).
  - An example of an anatomic bursa is the intermetatarsal bursa between metatarsal heads (see Figs. 7.62 and 7.64).
  - Adventitial bursae can occur at a variety of locations. Common locations are inferior to the metatarsal heads (Fig. 7.65), medial to the first metatarsal head (over the bunion in hallux valgus; Fig. 7.66)

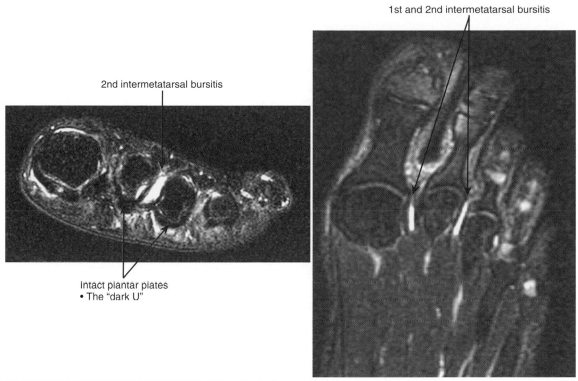

1st and 2nd intermetatarsal bursitis

2nd intermetatarsal bursitis

Intact plantar plates
• The "dark U"

Fig. 7.64 Intermetatarsal bursitis on MRI. Coronal (left) and axial (right) fluid-sensitive images show focal fluid between the metatarsal heads representing bursitis. Note intact low-signal plantar plates, forming dark, 'U-shaped' structures at the inferior border of the MTP joint capsules. (From Morrison W. *Problem Solving in Musculoskeletal Imaging.* Philadelphia: Elsevier; 2010.)

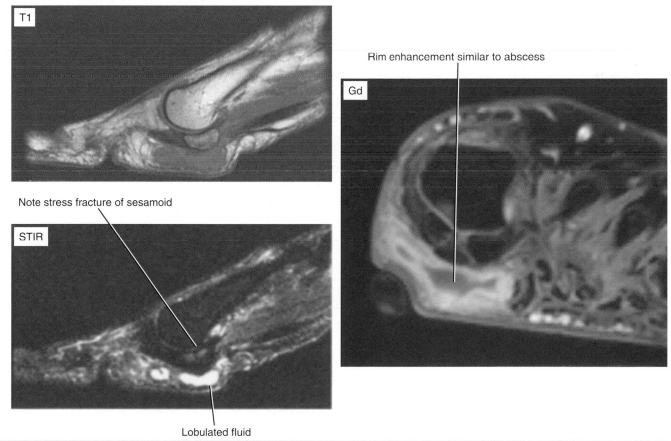

T1

Rim enhancement similar to abscess

Gd

Note stress fracture of sesamoid

STIR

Lobulated fluid

Fig. 7.65 Altered stresses in a ballerina. Friction may induce mechanical bursitis. (From Morrison W. *Problem Solving in Musculoskeletal Imaging.* Philadelphia: Elsevier; 2010.)

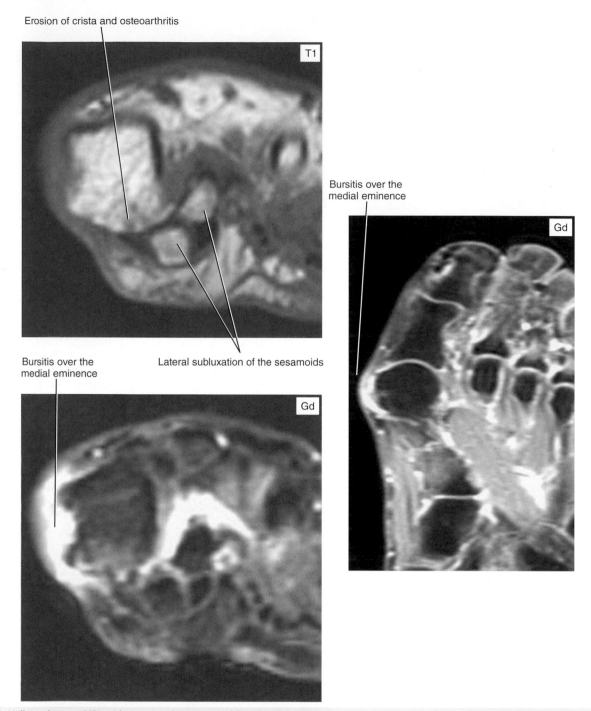

Erosion of crista and osteoarthritis

T1

Bursitis over the
medial eminence

Gd

Bursitis over the
medial eminence

Lateral subluxation of the sesamoids

Gd

Fig. 7.66 Hallux valgus on MRI, with associated osseous proliferation (bunion) at the medial aspect of the first metatarsal head and overlying bursitis. (From Morrison W. *Problem Solving in Musculoskeletal Imaging.* Philadelphia: Elsevier; 2010.)

and lateral to the fifth metatarsal head (over a bunionette deformity).

■ As mentioned earlier, whether on MRI or ultrasound, a flat subcutaneous fluid collection in the foot should be considered suspicious for bursitis.

■ Even in anatomic bursae, any fluid should be considered pathologic and potentially a source of the patient's pain.

■ Contrast enhanced CT and MRI images of an inflamed bursa will reveal thick rim enhancement resembling an abscess, but without clinical suspicion of infection and in the absence of adjacent soft tissue findings of cellulitis, abscess can usually be excluded.

■ The morphology and classic location usually helps differentiate bursal fluid collections from tumor.

■ Ganglion cysts can occasionally appear like bursal fluid collections, but communication with a joint or tendon sheath helps make the diagnosis of a ganglion.

■ Bursitis associations:

   ■ Although most cases of bursitis in the foot are mechanical, it may also be seen in various inflammatory arthropathies, such as gout and rheumatoid arthritis.

- These conditions will also show involvement of joints or tendon sheaths.
- Bursitis under the first metatarsal head (submetatarsal bursitis) is commonly seen in association with sesamoid pathology (see Fig. 7.65), and also can be seen with plantar plate injuries.
- Bursitis is common in diabetic patients with foot deformity or decreased sensation, making them vulnerable to repetitive trauma.
- Intermetatarsal bursitis has a high association with Morton neuroma, discussed later.

PLANTAR PLATE INJURY

- The *plantar plate* is a fibrocartilaginous structure on the plantar aspect of the MTP and proximal interphalangeal joints, analogous to the volar plate in the hand.
- Plantar plate injury at the first MTP joint is also referred to as *turf toe*.
  - Occurs in athletes, especially American football.
  - Toe is caught under the weight of the body, hyperdorsiflexed.
  - Plantar structures torn, including: sesamoid-phalangeal ligaments, intersesamoid ligament, joint capsule, and adjacent musculature.
  - Sesamoids may appear separated from each other, subluxed from their facets or proximally displaced.
  - MRI best for diagnosis of specific structures injured.
- Plantar plate injury is more common at the *lesser MTP joints* (second through fifth). While the first MTP plantar plate typically is acutely injured in athletic patients, the lesser MTP joints (especially the second, occasionally the third) are typically an indolent problem due to chronic, repetitive injury.
  - The second MTP is the most distal and exposed to disproportionate stress during push-off phase of gait.
  - Most commonly seen in people wearing high-heeled shoes; this adds additional stress on the plantar plate. Additionally, with the toes dorsiflexed, the inferior fat pad shifts anteriorly away from the plantar plates leaving them exposed.
  - May start as a small tear that propagates over time.
  - Disruption of the plantar plate at the phalangeal attachment with focal T2 signal on MRI; hypoechogenicity on US.
  - Associated joint effusion, synovitis, and/or pericapsular edema (often referred to as *capsulitis*).
  - Granulation tissue forms and extends into the adjacent intermetatarsal space.
  - Can be confused for a Morton neuroma.
- Similar to chronic plantar fasciitis: as the capsule scars, it is recurrently injured before it heals completely, leading to chronic pain especially during the push-off phase of ambulation.
- On MRI the normal lesser MTP plantar plate has a dark, thick, linear 'U-shaped' pattern that is easily identified on T2-weighted short-axis (coronal) images (see Fig. 7.64).
  - An important clue that there is a plantar plate injury is effusion and synovitis at a single MTP joint (Fig. 7.67), usually the second.
  - Like turf toe, synovitis is ubiquitous in chronic lesser MTP plantar plate injury. This monoarticular pattern

would be uncommon in the setting of an inflammatory arthropathy, and osteoarthritis is also relatively uncommon in the second to fifth MTP joints. Therefore, this finding alone should prompt one to carefully inspect the plantar plate.
- If the dark 'U' is discontinuous, thickened, or edematous, the diagnosis of plantar plate injury can be made.
- On MRI it is helpful to compare with the other normal MTP joints.
- Frequently, disruption of the plantar plate results in synovitis extending beyond the normal joint confines into the adjacent intermetatarsal space, which can simulate a Morton neuroma (Figs. 7.67 and 7.68).
- In more advanced cases there can be dorsal subluxation of the proximal phalanx, with an appearance suggestive of neuropathic arthropathy (see Fig. 7.68). Associated marrow edema related to instability can simulate septic or other inflammatory arthritis.
- Associated joint instability eventually leads to development of osteoarthritis.

MORTON NEUROMA

- A *Morton neuroma* is not a neoplasm but rather perineural fibrosis caused by compression and irritation, which occurs at the interdigital nerve as it passes beyond the metatarsal (MT) heads.
- The presumptive etiology is repetitive injury to or pressure on the nerve, which is in a susceptible location and can become impinged during walking or running, especially if there is dorsiflexion of the toes, for example in people who wear high-heeled shoes.
- There is a close association with intermetatarsal bursitis, which may be causal (mass effect from the bursa above the nerve can place added pressure on the nerve) or due to a common etiology (footwear with a narrow toebox may cause pinching of the MT heads, inciting bursitis between them). In any case, both intermetatarsal bursitis and Morton neuroma can be a source of pain and should be sought and reported if absent or present.
- Bursitis has high T2 signal that is often best seen on short-axis images. Neuroma T2 signal is more variable, as it may be bright or intermediate. Short-axis T1-weighted sequence sometimes best shows neuromas with intermediate signal replacing normal fat signal.
- Absence of bursitis, however, does not exclude the presence of a Morton neuroma.
- Intermetatarsal bursitis hurts when wearing tight shoes or when squeezing the forefoot and MT heads together. Morton neuroma hurts during the push-off phase of ambulation or when pressing focally over the lesion at the plantar aspect of the foot. It is also helpful to place a vitamin E marker at the site of pain, which, in the case of Morton neuroma, the patient can usually localize precisely (but place it at the dorsal aspect to avoid soft tissue distortion in the area of concern).
- Morton neuroma is most common at the third greater than second intermetatarsal spaces; fourth is uncommon, and first is extremely rare.
  - It is common to have two lesions, which may result in recurrent or persistent pain if only one is resected.

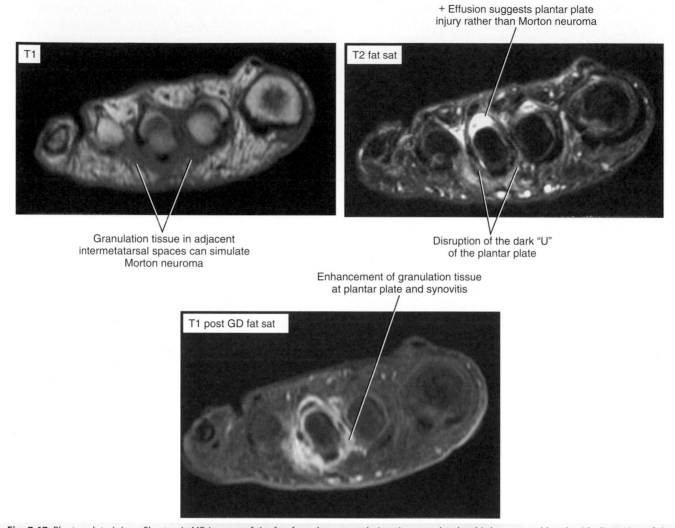

+ Effusion suggests plantar plate
injury rather than Morton neuroma

T1

T2 fat sat

Granulation tissue in adjacent
intermetatarsal spaces can simulate
Morton neuroma

Disruption of the dark "U"
of the plantar plate

Enhancement of granulation tissue
at plantar plate and synovitis

T1 post GD fat sat

Fig. 7.67 Plantar plate injury. Short-axis MR images of the forefoot show granulation tissue under the third metatarsal head, with disruption of the plantar plate. Associated synovitis is present in the third MTP joint. Intravenous gadolinium contrast (lower image) makes the granulation tissue and synovitis even more apparent. (From Morrison W. *Problem Solving in Musculoskeletal Imaging*. Philadelphia: Elsevier; 2010.)

■ Size of the lesion is important to describe, since larger lesions are more likely to be a source of pain and are more likely to be treated interventionally. Measure the medial-to-lateral dimension; the superior-to-inferior dimension is often difficult to measure due to volume averaging effects.

■ If open surgery is performed, the approach is dorsal (as is most surgery of the forefoot, in order to avoid scarring and pain at the plantar surface). Recently, more lesions are being treated with percutaneous thermal or alcohol ablation.

■ On MRI, Morton neuroma is best seen on short-axis (coronal) images.

■ As mentioned earlier, first look at the fluid sensitive images and search for vertically oriented, linear or bulbous fluid signal between the joint capsules of adjacent MT heads, representing intermetatarsal bursitis.

■ At that same location look at the short-axis T1-weighted images, paying attention to the plantar fat. Follow the images distally, and a Morton neuroma will appear as a rounded focus of low to intermediate signal at the distal margin of the MT heads, with mass effect on the adjacent fat (Figs. 7.69 and 7.70).

■ Refer back to the T2-weighted images; a Morton neuroma will appear intermediate to low in signal, helping to differentiate it from prominent bursitis or a ganglion cyst which will appear as fluid signal.

■ Most but not all Morton neuromas enhance with intravenous contrast; the authors feel that contrast is not necessary to make the diagnosis in most cases.

■ While not often used in practice, imaging the foot in plantarflexion can help visualize the lesion. This position pushes the neuroma further into plantar fat, increasing conspicuity.

■ Ultrasound can also effectively visualize a Morton neuroma as a focal hypoechoic mass in the characteristic location (Fig. 7.71), with tenderness elicited upon increased pressure.

■ Mass effect between the MT heads may be caused by bursitis or a ganglion cyst, as mentioned earlier. However, a very common mimicker is a plantar plate injury of the adjacent MTP joint.

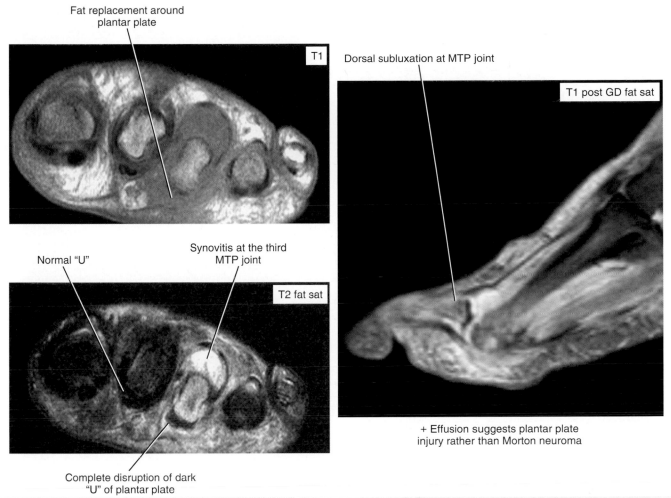

Fat replacement around plantar plate

T1

Dorsal subluxation at MTP joint

T1 post GD fat sat

Synovitis at the third MTP joint

Normal "U"

T2 fat sat

Complete disruption of dark "U" of plantar plate

+ Effusion suggests plantar plate injury rather than Morton neuroma

Fig. 7.68 Chronic plantar plate injury. With more long-standing injury the proximal phalanx subluxes dorsally; osteoarthritis often ensues. Differential diagnosis includes inflammatory arthropathy, septic arthritis, or neuropathic joint. (From Morrison W. *Problem Solving in Musculoskeletal Imaging.* Philadelphia: Elsevier; 2010.)

- As discussed, chronic injury of the lesser MTP plantar plates (especially common in patients who wear high-heeled shoes) can result in synovial proliferation extending into the adjacent soft tissues, the very location where Morton neuromas occur.
- This synovial proliferation will also appear intermediate in signal and will enhance brightly.
- The key is to look at the adjacent joints; if one of the adjacent MTP joints (usually the second) has effusion and synovitis, the correct diagnosis may very well be plantar plate injury rather than Morton neuroma.
- Look closely at the plantar plate of the joint in question on short-axis T2-weighted images. An intact plantar plate will appear as an unbroken low-signal 'U-shaped' line.

HALLUX VALGUS/BUNION

- Hallux valgus is angulation of the first MTP joint, usually associated with medial angulation of the first metatarsal shaft (*metatarsus primus adductus*).
- This angulation results in poor fitting of shoes and soft tissue friction at the medial eminence of the first MT head, eventually causing bursitis and callus in the soft tissues (which may be exquisitely painful) and proliferation and cystic change of adjacent bone (see Fig. 7.66). Therefore a clinically perceived 'bunion deformity' can be composed of soft tissue, bone, or a combination of pathology; in the report it is helpful to be specific about the tissue involved.
- Bursitis can be treated conservatively whereas bone proliferation may be resected (medial eminence resection, or bunionectomy).
- Bursitis coexisting with hallux valgus is usually mechanical but can also be seen in rheumatoid arthritis or gout. It is also common in the setting of diabetes, in which case ulceration may also occur over the medial eminence.
- The valgus deformity causes the flexor and extensor tendons to displace laterally, likened to a bow string.
  - The FHL forces the sesamoids laterally as well, and they rotate so that the metatarsal sesamoid joints become incongruent.
  - The bony prominence (the *crista*) between the facets erodes, facilitating lateral sesamoid subluxation and propagation of osteoarthritis with edema and cyst formation on both sides of the joint (see Fig. 7.66).

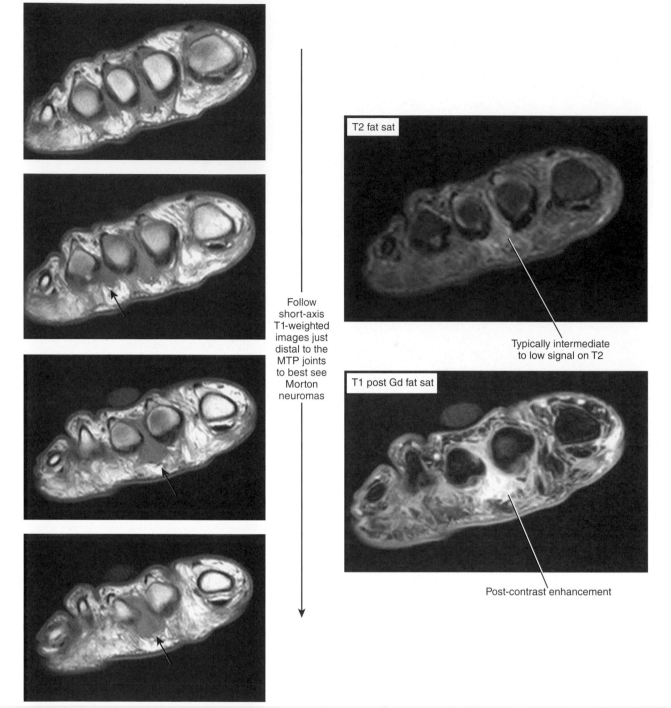

Follow
short-axis
T1-weighted
images just
distal to the
MTP joints
to best see
Morton
neuromas

Typically intermediate
to low signal on T2

T2 fat sat

T1 post Gd fat sat

Post-contrast enhancement

Fig. 7.69 Morton neuroma—detection and characteristic features on MRI. MTP, metatarsophalangeal. (From Morrison W. *Problem Solving in Musculoskeletal Imaging.* Philadelphia: Elsevier; 2010.)

- As the sesamoids sublux further laterally, they may abut the second metatarsal head with intervening bursitis.
- The laterally deviated great toe may displace the second toe dorsally (*crossover toe deformity*).
- Surgical management: If the first intermetatarsal angle is greater than 12 degrees (metatarsus primus adductus), generally a first metatarsal rotational or shifting (*chevron*) osteotomy is performed in addition to the bunionectomy (Fig. 7.72).

BUNIONETTE

- A *bunionette* is bony prominence of the lateral aspect of the fifth metatarsal head (Fig. 7.73) caused by friction (with or without bursitis); this is also called a *tailor's bunion* because tailors would cross their legs placing weight on the fifth metatarsal head.
- The condition may be due to a laterally curving fifth metatarsal or a 'splay foot' in which the metatarsal angles are all widened with widening of the forefoot.

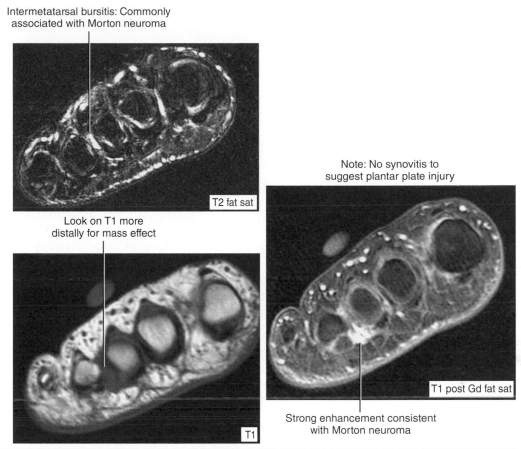

Intermetatarsal bursitis: Commonly associated with Morton neuroma

T2 fat sat

Look on T1 more distally for mass effect

Note: No synovitis to suggest plantar plate injury

T1

T1 post Gd fat sat

Strong enhancement consistent with Morton neuroma

Fig. 7.70 Morton neuroma on MRI. Mass effect is present at the plantar aspect of the intermetatarsal space, with adjacent bursitis. The neuroma (actually representing perineural fibrosis) is low-signal on T1- and T2-weighted images, with strong enhancement on postcontrast images. (From Morrison W. *Problem Solving in Musculoskeletal Imaging.* Philadelphia: Elsevier; 2010.)

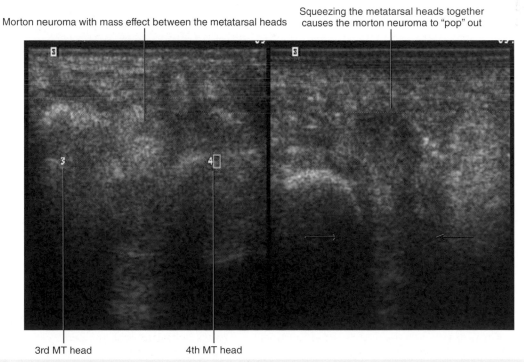

Morton neuroma with mass effect between the metatarsal heads

Squeezing the metatarsal heads together causes the morton neuroma to "pop" out

3rd MT head   4th MT head

Fig. 7.71 Morton neuroma on ultrasound. Mass effect with echotexture of a solid lesion is present at the plantar foot between the third and fourth metatarsal heads representing a Morton neuroma. Diagnosis is assisted by dynamic exam, with displacement of the mass upon squeezing the metatarsal heads together. (From Morrison W. *Problem Solving in Musculoskeletal Imaging.* Philadelphia: Elsevier; 2010.)

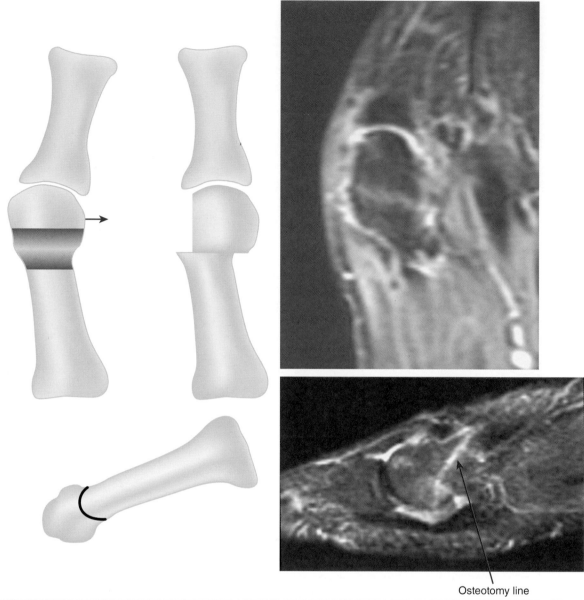

Osteotomy line

Fig. 7.72 Medial eminence (bunion) resection and distal metatarsal shaft chevron osteotomy. Alternatively, osteotomy can be performed at the proximal shaft. Osteotomy is performed when there is an increase in the first intermetatarsal angle (metatarsus primus adductus). (From Morrison W. *Problem Solving in Musculoskeletal Imaging*. Philadelphia: Elsevier; 2010.)

HALLUX SESAMOID PATHOLOGY

- In evaluating the sesamoid bones on MRI one should review their location, cartilage, and marrow signal as well as signal of the adjacent first metatarsal head and subcutaneous tissues.
- If there is malalignment, it is usually due to hallux valgus, in which case there is likely to be osteoarthritis.
- Equivalent involvement of the metatarsal head also suggests arthritis, which can be degenerative or inflammatory.
- The capsule and separate ligaments should be inspected in the setting of trauma.
- If a marrow abnormality is observed that is isolated to a sesamoid, consider a bipartite sesamoid (with or without superimposed injury), fracture/stress fracture/stress response, or osteonecrosis.

- Associated signal abnormality in adjacent subcutaneous tissues could represent bursitis, callus, various manifestations of arthropathy or metabolic disease (e.g., rheumatoid pannus or gouty tophus), or transcutaneous spread of infection.

Acute fracture, Stress fracture, and 'Sesamoiditis'

- Acute sesamoid fracture can generally be detected radiographically, like other acute fractures (Fig. 7.74). Fractures can be overlooked on initial inspection because of the high incidence of bipartite sesamoids, which can have a similar appearance.
    - The bipartite sesamoid has rounded edges and smooth margins whereas an acute fracture has sharp, irregular edges.

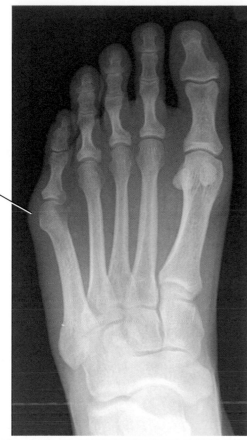

Lateral bowing of the fifth metatarsal bone with resultant osseous prominence

Fig. 7.73 Bunionette deformity (Tailor's bunion). Lateral bowing of the fifth metatarsal bone distally. (From Morrison W. *Problem Solving in Musculoskeletal Imaging*. Philadelphia: Elsevier; 2010.)

- The fragments of a bipartite are larger in total than the other sesamoid.
- Bipartite sesamoids should not change over time. A short follow-up period of 5–7 days will show evolution of a fracture; review of previous exams can be helpful.
- Because sesamoid fractures are often overlooked on initial radiographs, patients are occasionally referred for MRI to explain the persistent pain.
  - Because of the delay in referral to MRI, the injury is nearly always subacute when imaging is performed.
  - As noted earlier, the MR appearance of subacute sesamoid fracture is virtually indistinguishable from stress fracture (Fig. 7.75), except for history of a single traumatic episode.
- *Sesamoiditis* is a painful condition of the hallux sesamoid complex and surrounding soft tissues. The term *sesamoiditis* is a nonspecific clinical term (like 'metatarsalgia'); sesamoid pain has a differential, the underlying pathology of which can be distinguished on MRI.
  - Most cases of clinical sesamoiditis are likely in the spectrum of stress response. Radiographs and CT are generally normal.
  - On MRI, sesamoiditis is seen as diffuse high signal on T2-weighted or STIR images. Diffuse enhancement may be seen in the same distribution; this can be useful to distinguish sesamoiditis from osteonecrosis, which would show little to no enhancement. On T1-weighted images, sesamoiditis may show intermediate to low signal, but if signal is black, consider osteonecrosis.
  - Stress changes can also occur at a bipartite sesamoid; these normal variants can thereby be a source of pain.

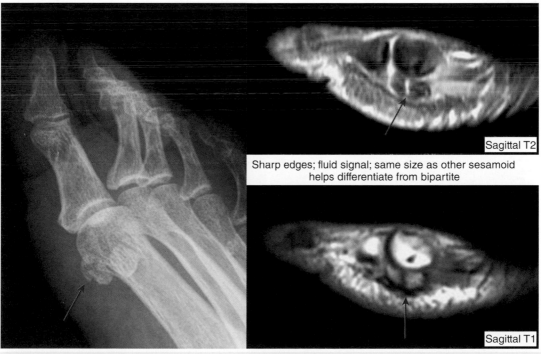

Sharp edges; fluid signal; same size as other sesamoid helps differentiate from bipartite

Sagittal T2

Sagittal T1

Fig. 7.74 Acute fracture of the tibial (medial) sesamoid bone. Oblique radiograph (left) shows a lucent line through the sesamoid; MRI (right images) shows linear fluid signal representing recent fracture. Sharp edges help differentiate fracture from a bipartite sesamoid; also, a bipartite sesamoid bone is typically larger than the other sesamoid. (From Morrison W. *Problem Solving in Musculoskeletal Imaging*. Philadelphia: Elsevier; 2010.)

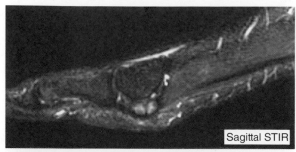

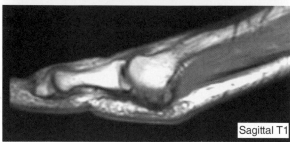

Fig. 7.75 Subacute fracture versus stress fracture of the sesamoid on MRI. There is bone marrow edema in the sesamoid diffusely, with a low-signal line. Subacute fracture and stress fracture can both have this appearance. History of injury versus change in activity helps differentiate these entities. (From Morrison W. *Problem Solving in Musculoskeletal Imaging.* Philadelphia: Elsevier; 2010.)

Nonunion and Pseudoarthrosis

- Occasionally a sesamoid fracture does not heal; on radiographs, there is persistence of the fracture line. The edges may become rounded and sclerotic like a bipartite.
- A similar situation can occur at a developmentally bipartite sesamoid, where acute trauma or chronic stress ruptures the normal fibrous connection: this is undetectable on radiographs apart from presence of an apparently innocuous bipartite.
- On MRI, fluid signal between the fragments can indicate a pseudarthrosis with *synovial nonunion.*
- Low signal on fluid sensitive sequences may represent a fibrous union of a prior fracture or a normal developmental bipartite sesamoid. If there is edema in the adjacent marrow, there is likely ongoing stress response.

Osteonecrosis

- On radiography and CT, osteonecrosis is seen as increased sesamoid density; typically only one sesamoid bone is involved (Fig. 7.76). The sclerosis is generally more extensive than would be expected from osteoarthritis and is not present on the metatarsal side of the joint.

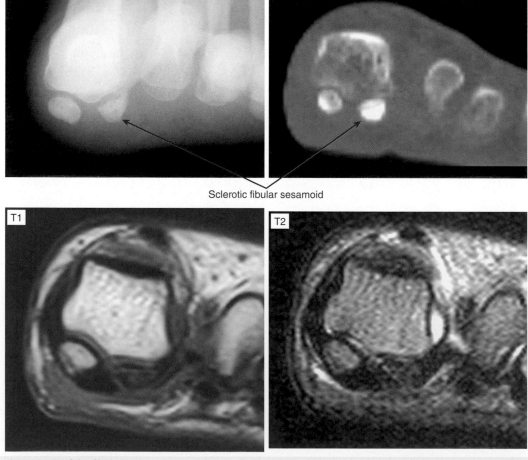

Sclerotic fibular sesamoid

Fig. 7.76 Avascular necrosis of the fibular sesamoid. Note sclerosis on CT with low signal on T1- and T2-weighted images. (From Morrison W. *Problem Solving in Musculoskeletal Imaging.* Philadelphia: Elsevier; 2010.)

- On MR images, T2 signal can vary from low to high; the T1-weighted images help confirm the diagnosis; the T1 signal of the affected sesamoid is diffusely low in osteonecrosis with replacement of the normal marrow fat (a black sesamoid on T1 is compatible with osteonecrosis; if T1 signal is not black, consider other pathology).
- Osteonecrosis chronically may result in collapse and fragmentation of the sesamoid, and secondary osteoarthritis of the MTS joint.

PLANTAR FASCIA INJURY

- Plantar fascia injury, referred to as plantar fasciitis, is an extremely common cause of plantar heel pain (Figs. 7.77 and 7.78).
- The plantar fascia is divided into three bundles: medial, central, and lateral.
    - The medial bundle is most commonly injured, followed by the central bundle. The lateral bundle is rarely injured.
    - The lateral bundle originates from the central bundle just distal to the calcaneal attachment; therefore

at the origin the plantar fascia can be described as having medial or lateral attachments, the lateral attachment being the conjoined central and lateral bundle.

- On physical exam, patients have focal tenderness at the plantar fascia calcaneal attachment; patients have pain on weight-bearing and push-off phase of gait. Pain is greatest in the morning (the first step out of bed they may feel a tearing sensation).
- Overnight the fascial injury begins healing, with the foot in plantar flexion. The first step out of bed, the fascia stretches and tears again; repeated injury and partial healing continues. The result is thickening of the fascia proximally.
- Diffuse thickening of the proximal fascia without edema is referred to as *chronic plantar fasciitis*. Thickening with edema is referred to as *acute-on-chronic plantar fasciitis*.
- A variety of findings can be seen with active plantar fasciitis, including:
    - Interstitial tearing (longitudinal fluid-bright T2 signal) of the fascia at the origin.

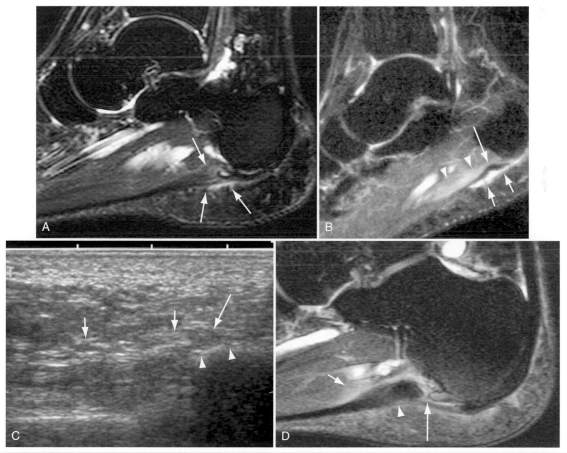

Fig. 7.77 Plantar fasciitis. **(A)** Sagittal fat-suppressed T2-weighted MR image shows thickening and increased signal in the proximal middle cord of the plantar aponeurosis *(arrows)* with surrounding edema. **(B)** Partial tear. Sagittal inversion recovery MR image in a different patient shows thickened and wavy middle cord of plantar aponeurosis *(long arrow)* with adjacent fluid *(short arrows)*, and edema *(arrowheads)* in the flexor digitorum brevis muscle. **(C)** Proximal tear. US in a different patient shows thickened proximal plantar fascia *(short arrows)* and low echogenicity of surgically proven proximal tear *(long arrow)*. Note shadowing plantar calcaneal spur *(arrowheads)*. The transducer is in the sagittal plane, with distal to the viewer's left and the plantar surface of the foot at the top of the image. **(D)** Surgical release. Sagittal fat-suppressed T2-weighted MR image in a different patient shows marked thickening of the plantar fascia *(arrowhead)* with abundant surrounding edema, including within flexor digitorum brevis muscle *(short arrow)*. Note interruption of the aponeurosis *(long arrow)*, which was surgically created in an effort to provide pain relief. This expected post-operative appearance could be confused with a plantar fascia tear on imaging. (B courtesy of Michael Recht, MD.)

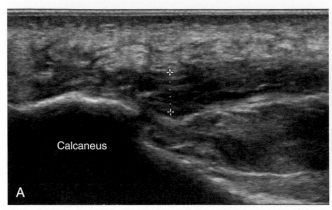
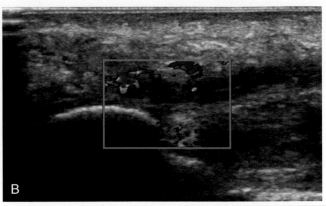

Fig. 7.78 Severe acute plantar fasciitis. Sagittal US images, posterior is to the viewer's left and plantar is at the top of the image. **(A)** Grayscale and **(B)** color Doppler US images show thickened, edematous proximal plantar fascia (marked with caliper in A), with wavy fibers. Note hyperemia around the fascia in B with subtle intrasubstance blood flow in B.

- ■ Partial or complete tearing of one or more bundles.
- ■ Surrounding perifascial soft tissue edema.
- ■ Underlying muscle edema (quadratus plantae/ flexor digitorum brevis).
- ■ Bone marrow edema at the calcaneal attachment.
- ■ Bone marrow edema indicates more severe involvement and symptoms; may clinically simulate a stress fracture.
- ■ Spurring at the inferior calcaneal attachment is generally incidental and does not correlate with symptoms.
- ■ Differential diagnosis.
  - ■ Plantar fibromatosis (Ledderhose disease) is one of the superficial fibromatoses (including Peyronie's disease and Duypuytren's contracture) and affects the plantar fascia, typically at the medial midfoot. This is discussed in detail in the Chapter 12, Soft Tissue Tumors.
  - ■ Differential features:
    - ■ Plantar fasciitis: proximal at the calcaneal attachment; diffuse thickening; surrounding edema.
    - ■ Plantar fibroma: centered at the midfoot; masslike, focal; often multiple.
    - ■ A traumatic plantar fascia rupture (i.e., a laceration) can occur distal to the calcaneal attachment resulting in focal thickening upon healing, simulating a plantar fibroma.

THE POSTOPERATIVE FOOT

At the midfoot and forefoot, the preferred location for incision and access for most operations is dorsal. Plantar incisions are associated with increased pain and longer healing/rehabilitation.

Key Concepts

Common forefoot surgeries

Medial first metatarsal—bunionectomy
Distal first metatarsal shaft—hallux valgus repair
Dorsal first metatarsal—cheilectomy (spur removal)
Distal aspect of proximal phalanges—hammertoe repair
Between metatarsal heads—Morton neuroma resection
Plantar foot—plantar fibroma resection

Imaging Evaluation of the Postop Foot

Postop Resection of a Mass

- ■ For mass and masslike surgery (e.g., Morton neuroma, plantar fibroma, sarcoma), the radiologist should look through the postoperative artifact and scar for any mass effect that could indicate recurrence.
- ■ Granulation tissue can appear masslike within a few months after surgery but should become flattened over time; it is very helpful to acquire a baseline postoperative exam a month or two after surgery for surveillance, particularly in cases of sarcoma resection.
- ■ Contrast is useful to delineate recurrent masses, but scar also enhances; again, focal mass effect on adjacent structures is the important finding. Ultrasound is also useful for detection of recurrent mass.

Amputation/Osteotomy/Fixation

- ■ Amputation-type surgeries such as hammertoe repair (resection of the distal aspect of the proximal phalanx) and amputations related to osteomyelitis generally leave little artifact, and even shortly after surgery the marrow signal should be normal.
  - ■ In the setting of infection/wound breakdown, any abnormal marrow signal on MRI in the amputated bone should be considered suspicious. However, amputation can also alter weight-bearing resulting in stress response with marrow edema in adjacent bones.
- ■ Fixation with plates and/or screws may be performed for fractures, fusions, or osteotomies. This makes it very challenging to interpret on MRI, even with metal artifact-suppression techniques, and other modalities such as CT may be needed to evaluate the bone next to the metal or to look for fusion under the hardware.
  - ■ Always look for lucency around the screws or screws 'backing out', indicating loosening and motion. Look for aberrant placement of screws inadvertently into joints.
- ■ One commonly seen osteotomy of the forefoot is hallux valgus repair (see Figs. 7.72 and 7.79). This is performed as a proximal or distal first metatarsal osteotomy, either rotating (with a curved osteotomy) or shifting (with a

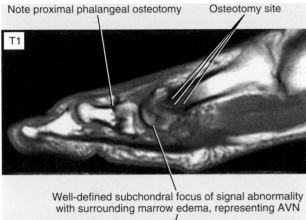

Note proximal phalangeal osteotomy   Osteotomy site

T1

Well-defined subchondral focus of signal abnormality with surrounding marrow edema, representing AVN

STIR

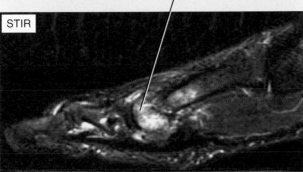

Fig. 7.79 Distal first metatarsal osteotomy (chevron osteotomy) with secondary avascular necrosis. Note well-defined subchondral signal abnormality with surrounding marrow edema. Areas of devascularized bone often exhibit entrapped, or mummified fat. *AVN*, avascular necrosis. (From Morrison W. *Problem Solving in Musculoskeletal Imaging*. Philadelphia: Elsevier; 2010.)

V-shaped 'chevron' osteotomy) the distal aspect of the first MT laterally.

- Osteotomy lines may remain for years on T1-weighted images, but there should not be fluid signal at the interval after healing. Soft tissue edema and mass effect may be a sign of complication such as infection. Bone proliferation on radiographs or CT is also a sign of motion or infection.
- With hallux valgus repair, another potentially devastating complication is AVN of the first metatarsal head; this is especially common in distal osteotomies due to cutoff of the blood supply which enters through the metaphysis.
  - Look for dark/black signal on T1-weighted images and lack of enhancement; increased density and later fragmentation may be seen on radiographs or CT.

INFLAMMATORY CONDITIONS

- Inflammatory arthropathies such as rheumatoid arthritis, psoriatic arthritis, reactive arthritis, and gout may involve the forefoot.
- All can cause synovitis, with complex effusion and thick, hyperemic synovium, the appearance of which is similar to that of septic arthritis.
- Inflammatory bursitis can result in formation of complex fluid collections and rim enhancement that can simulate abscess.
- Inflammatory tenosynovitis is also common.

- Synovial inflammation can cause marginal erosions and reactive edema on MRI.
- Although the pattern of disease and differential diagnosis is facilitated by radiographs, subtle erosion may be more apparent on CT or MR images.
- Of the inflammatory arthropathies, gout can have a distinct appearance on MR images; intraarticular tophi produce masslike foci of low-to-intermediate signal on T1- and T2-weighted images. Extraarticular tophi are also common adjacent to the first MTP joint, and can cause extrinsic erosion (periarticular erosion).
- Rheumatoid arthritis in particular causes capsular and ligamentous laxity resulting in joint deformity.
- Manifestations of inflammatory arthropathies will be discussed in detail in Chapter 9 - Arthritis.
- Infection of the foot is discussed in Chapter 14 - Musculoskeletal Infection.

Standard Report Templates

Exam Type: MRI ANKLE W/O CONTRAST
Exam Date and Time:
Indication:
Comparison:

IMPRESSION:
Normal exam.

TECHNIQUE:
MRI of the ankle was performed on an x Tesla system in three planes (axial, sagittal, and coronal) using a standard noncontrast protocol.

FINDINGS:
JOINTS/BONES:
No acute fracture, bone bruise, or osseous stress response. No osteochondral lesion. No cartilage defects or osteoarthritis. No joint effusions. No coalition. Normal hindfoot alignment on this non–weight-bearing examination.

LATERAL LIGAMENTS:
Anterior talofibular (ATFL): Intact.
Calcaneofibular (CFL): Intact.
Posterior talofibular (PTFL): Intact.
Anterior/posterior syndesmosis: Intact.

MEDIAL LIGAMENTS:
Deltoid: Intact.
Spring: Intact.

LISFRANC LIGAMENT: Intact.
FLEXOR TENDONS:
Posterior tibialis: No tendinosis or tear.
Flexor digitorum longus: No tendinosis or tear.
Flexor hallucis longus: No tendinosis or tear.

PERONEAL TENDONS:
Peroneus longus: No tendinosis or tear.
Peroneus brevis: No tendinosis or tear.

EXTENSOR TENDONS:
Anterior tibialis: No tendinosis or tear.
Extensor hallucis longus: No tendinosis or tear.
Extensor digitorum longus: No tendinosis or tear.

ACHILLES TENDON: No tendinosis or tear.
PLANTAR FASCIA: No thickening or perifascial edema.
SINUS TARSI: Sinus tarsi fat preserved.
TARSAL TUNNEL: Unimpinged; no mass effect.
MUSCLES: No atrophy or edema.
SOFT TISSUES: No soft tissue edema. No fluid collection or soft tissue mass.

Exam Type: MRI FOOT W/O CONTRAST
Exam Date and Time:
Indication:
Comparison:

IMPRESSION:
Normal exam.

TECHNIQUE:
MRI of the foot was performed on an x Tesla scanner in three planes (axial, sagittal, and coronal) using a standard non-contrast protocol.

FINDINGS:
JOINTS/BONES:
No acute fracture, bone bruise, or osseous stress response. Alignment is anatomic. No focal cartilage defects or osteoarthritis. No joint effusions. Hallux sesamoid interval is normal.

PLANTAR PLATES:
Intact plantar plates without tear.

INTERMETATARSAL SPACES:
No intermetatarsal neuroma. No intermetatarsal bursitis.

TENDONS:
Visualized portions of the flexor, extensor, and peroneal tendons are intact without tendinosis or tear. No tenosynovitis.

LISFRANC LIGAMENT:
Intact.

MUSCLES:
No atrophy or edema of the intrinsic musculature.

SOFT TISSUES:
No soft tissue edema. No fluid collection or soft tissue mass.

Sources and Suggested Readings

Affram P. An epidemiologic study of cervical and trochanteric fractures of the femur in an urban population: analysis of 1664 cases with special reference to etiologic factors. *Acta Orthop Scand Suppl.* 1964;64:11.

Badillo K, Pacheco JA, Padua SO, et al. Multidetector CT evaluation of calcaneal fractures. *Radiographics.* 2011;31(1):81–92.

Beltran LS, Rosenberg ZS, Mayo JD, et al. Imaging evaluation of developmental hip dysplasia in the young adult. *AJR Am J Roentgenol.* 2013; 200:1077–1088.

Bencardino JT, Beltran J, Feldman MI, Rose DJ. MR imaging of complications of anterior cruciate ligament graft reconstruction. *Radiographics.* 2009;29(7):2115–2126.

Bowden DJ, Byrne CA, Alkhayat A, et al. Injectable viscoelastic supplements: a review for radiologists. *AJR Am J Roentgenol.* 2017;209:883–888.

Chan SS, Rosenberg ZS, Chan K, Capeci C. Subtrochanteric femoral fractures in patients receiving long-term alendronate therapy: imaging features. *AJR Am J Roentgenol.* 2010;194(6):1581–1586.

Chaturvedi A, Mann L, Cain U, et al. Acute fractures and dislocations of the ankle and foot in children. *Radiographics.* 2020; online article. https://doi.org/10.1148/rg.2020190154.

Chhabra A, Subhawong TK, Carrino JA. A systematised MRI approach to evaluating the patellofemoral joint. *Skeletal Radiol.* 2011;40(4): 375–387.

Costa CR, Morrison WB, Carrino JA. Medial meniscus extrusion on knee MRI: is extent associated with severity of degeneration or type of tear? *AJR Am J Roentgenol.* 2004;183:17–23.

Crema MD, Roemer FW, Marra MD, et al. Articular cartilage in the knee: current MR imaging techniques and applications in clinical practice and research. *Radiographics.* 2011;31(1):37–61.

Delfaut EM, Demondion X, Dieganski A, et al. Imaging of foot and ankle nerve entrapment syndromes: from well-demonstrated to unfamiliar sites. *Radiographics.* 2003;23:613–623.

De Smet AA. How I diagnose meniscal tears on knee MR. *AJR Am J Roentgenol.* 2012;199(3):481–499.

De Smet AA, Blankenbaker DG, Alsheik NH, Lindstrom MJ. MRI appearance of the proximal hamstring tendons in patients with and without symptomatic proximal hamstring tendinopathy. *AJR Am J Roentgenol.* 2012;198(2):418–422.

De Smet AA, Nathan DH, Graf BK, et al. Clinical and MRI findings associated with false-positive knee MR diagnoses of medial meniscal tears. *AJR Am J Roentgenol.* 2008;191(1):93–99.

Diederichs G, Issever AS, Scheffler S. MR imaging of patellar instability: injury patterns and assessment of risk factors [published correction appears in *Radiographics.* 2011;31(2):624]. *Radiographics.* 2010;30(4): 961–981.

Disler DG. Fat-suppressed 3-D spoiled gradient-recalled MR imaging: assessment of articular and physeal hyaline cartilage. *AJR Am J Roentgenol.* 1997;169:1117–1123.

Flores DV, Gomez M, Fernandez HM, et al. Adult acquired flatfoot deformity: anatomy, biomechanics, staging, and imagings. *Radiographics.* 2019;39:1437–1460.

Flores DV, Gomez CM, Pathria MN. Layered approach to the anterior knee: normal anatomy and disorders associated with anterior knee pain. *Radiographics.* 2018;38:2069–2101.

Ganz R, Parvizi J, Beck M, et al. Femoroacetabular impingement: a cause for osteoarthritis of the hip. *Clin Orthop Relat Res.* 2003;417:112–120.

Garden RS. Stability and union of subcapital fractures of the femur. *J Bone Joint Surg.* 1964;46B:630–712.

Greif DN, Baraga MG, Rizzo MG, et al. MRI appearance of the different meniscal ramp lesion types, with clinical and arthroscopic correlation. *Skeletal Radiology.* 2020;49:677–689.

Hegazi TM, Belair JA, McCarthy EJ, et al. Sports injuries about the hip: what the radiologist should know. *Radiographics.* 2016;36:1717–1745.

Judet R, Judet J, Letournel E. Fractures of the acetabulum: classification and surgical approaches to reduction. *J Bone Joint Surg.* 1964;46A:1615–1646.

Kamel SI, Belair JA†, Hegazi TM, Halpern EJ, Desai V, Morrison WB, Zoga AC. Painful type II os naviculare: introduction of a standardized, reproducible classification system. Skeletal Radiol. 2020 Dec;49(12): 1977–1985.

Khan I, Ashraf T, Saifuddin A. Magnetic resonance imaging of impingement and friction syndromes around the knee. *Skeletal Radiology.* 2020;49:823–836.

Khurana B, Sheehan SE, Sodickson AD, et al. Pelvic ring fractures: what the orthopedic surgeon wants to know. *Radiographics.* 2014;34:1317–1333.

Kijowski R, Rosas HG, Lee KS, et al. MRI characteristics of healed and unhealed peripheral vertical meniscal tears. *AJR Am J Roentgenol.* 2014;202:585–592.

Kijowski R, Blankenbaker DG, Shinki K, et al. Juvenile versus adult osteochondritis dissecans of the knee: appropriate MR imaging criteria for instability. *Radiology.* 2008;248(2):571–578.

Kraus C, Ayyala RS, Kazam JK, et al. Imaging of juvenile hip conditions predisposing to premature osteoarthritis. *Radiographics.* 2017;37: 2204–2205.

Laborie LB, Lehmann TG, Engesæter IØ, et al. Prevalence of radiographic findings thought to be associated with femoroacetabular impingement in a population-based cohort of 2081 healthy young adults. *Radiology.* 2011;260:494–502.

Lauge-Hansen N. Fractures of the ankle: genetic roentgenologic diagnosis of fractures of the ankle. *AJR Am J Roentgenol.* 1954;71:456–471.

Li AE, Jawetz ST, Greditzer HG, et al. MRI Evaluation of femoroacetabular impingement after hip preservation surgery. *AJR Am J Roentgenol.* 2016;207:392–400.

Lungu E, Michaud J, Bureau NJ. US assessment of sports-related hip injuries. *Radiographics.* 2018;38:867–889.

Mainwaring B, Daffner R, Reiner B. Pylon fractures of the ankle: a distinct clinical and radiographic entity. *Radiology.* 1998;168:215–218.

Manganaro MS, Morag Y, Weadock WJ, et al. Creating three-dimensional printed models of acetabular fractures for use as educational tools. *Radiographics.* 2017;37:871–880.

Matcuk GR, Cen SY, Keyfes V, et al. Superolateral hoffa fat-pad edema and patellofemoral maltracking: predictive modeling. *AJR Am J Roentgenol.* 2014;203:W207–W212.

Markhardt BK, Gross JM, Monu JU. Schatzker classification of tibial plateau fractures: use of CT and MR imaging improves assessment. *Radiographics.* 2009;29(2):585–597.

Mellado JM, Bencardino JT. Morel-Lavallée lesion: review with emphasis on MR imaging. *Magn Reson Imaging Clin N Am.* 2005;13(4):775–782.

Meyers AB, Haims AH, Menn K, Moukaddam H. Imaging of anterior cruciate ligament repair and its complications. *AJR Am J Roentgenol.* 2010;194(2):476–484.

Mohankumar R, Palisch A, Khan W, et al. Meniscal ossicle: posttraumatic origin and association with posterior meniscal root tears. *AJR Am J Roentgenol.* 2014;203:1040–1046.

Mullens FE, Mullens FE, Zoga AC, et al. Review of MRI technique and imaging findings in athletic pubalgia and the "sports hernia". *Eur J Radiol.* 2012;81(12):3780–3792.

Naraghi A, White LM. MRI of labral and chondral lesions of the hip. *AJR Am J Roentgenol.* 2015;205:479–490.

Stacy GS, Lo R, Motang A. Infarct-associated bone sarcomas: multimodality imaging findings. *AJR Am J Roentgenol.* 2015;205:W432–W441.

Omar IM, Zoga AC, Kavanagh EC, et al. Athletic pubalgia and "sports hernia": optimal MR imaging technique and findings. *Radiographics.* 2008;28(5):1415–1438.

Perrich KD, Goodwin DW, Hecht PJ, Cheung Y. Ankle ligaments on MRI: appearance of normal and injured ligaments. *AJR Am J Roentgenol.* 2009;193(3):687–695.

Prince J, Laor T, Bean J. MRI of ACL injuries and associated findings in the pediatric knee: changes with skeletal maturation. *AJR Am J Roentgenol.* 2005;185:756–762.

Robinson R. Sonography of common tendon injuries. *AJR Am J Roentgenol.* 2009;193(3):607–618.

Rosas HG. Unraveling the posterolateral corner of the knee. *Radiographics.* 2016;36:1776–1791.

Rowe CR, Sakellarides HT, Freeman PA, Sorbie C. Fractures of the os calcis: a long term follow-up study of 146 patients. *JAMA.* 1963;184:920.

Samim M, Walter W, Gyftopoulos S, et al. MRI assessment of subspine impingement: features beyond the anterior inferior iliac spine morphology. *Radiology.* 2019;293:412–421.

Schwappach J, Murphey M, Kokmayer S, et al. Subcapital fractures of the femoral neck: prevalence and cause of radiographic appearance simulating pathologic fractures. *AJR Am J Roentgenol.* 1994;162:651–654.

Scheinfeld MH, Dym AA, Spektor M, et al. Acetabular fractures: what radiologists should know and how 3D CT can aid. *Radiographics.* 2015;35:555–577.

Sharif B, Ashraf T, Saifuddin A. Magnetic resonance imaging of the meniscal roots. *Skeletal Radiology.* 2020;49:661–676.

Sheehan SE, Shyu JY, Weaver MJ, et al. Proximal femoral fractures: what the orthopedic surgeon wants to know. *Radiographics.* 2015;35:1563-1584.

Silva MS. Radiography, CT, and MRI of hip and lower limb disorders in children and adolescents. *Radiographics.* 2019;39:779–794.

Subhawong TY, Eng J, Carrino JA, Chhabra A. Superolateral Hoffa's fat pad edema: association with patellofemoral maltracking and impingement. *AJR Am J Roentgenol.* 2010;195(6):1367–1373.

Yamada AF, Crema MD, Nery C, et al. Second and third metatarsophalangeal plantar plate tears: diagnostic performance of direct and indirect MRI features using surgical findings as the reference standard. *AJR Am J Roentgenol.* 2017;209:W100–W108.

Zoga AC, Kavanagh EC, Omar IM, et al. Athletic pubalgia and the "sports hernia": MR imaging findings. *Radiology.* 2008;247(3):797–807.

8 *Spine*

Introduction

This chapter reviews imaging of acute spine trauma. Spine infection is discussed in Chapter 14 (Musculoskeletal Infection) and pediatric spine conditions are reviewed in Chapter 15 (Congenital and Developmental Conditions.) Degenerative disease of the spine is covered in Chapter 9 - Arthritis.

Anatomy

CERVICAL SPINE

- There are normally seven cervical vertebrae, C1 through C7.
- C1 (the *atlas*) has a ringlike configuration, joining the skullbase to the cervical spine.
  - Anatomically divided into the anterior arch, posterior arch, paired lateral masses (which include superior and inferior articular facets), and paired transverse processes (which contain the foramina transversarium).
    - Posterior arch may be incomplete as a normal variant, and rarely the anterior arch may be incomplete at the midline.
  - *Atlanto-occipital joint* consists of the paired condyloid synovial joints between the lateral masses of C1 and the occipital condyles, which primarily allow for head flexion and extension.
- C2 (the *axis*) has a unique configuration.
  - Anatomically divided into the body, the conical-shaped odontoid process (*dens*), paired lateral masses, paired transverse processes, paired superior and inferior articular facets, and posterior elements (including the lamina, pedicles, and a bifid spinous process).
  - *Atlantoaxial joint* is a pivot joint consisting of the median atlantoaxial (*atlantodental*) articulation between the anterior arch of C1 and the dens, and two paired lateral atlantoaxial articulations between the lateral masses of C1 and C2.

- *Facet joints* (or *zygapophyseal joints*) are paired synovial joints located posteriorly, beginning at C2-C3 and at each subsequent level of the spine to the lumbosacral junction.
  - Formed by the inferior articular process (from the level above) articulating with the superior articular process (from the level below).
- *Uncovertebral joints* (or *Luschka's joints*) are small paired posterolateral synovial joints from C2-C3 through C6-C7 (and sometimes at C7-T1).
  - Articulation formed by the hook-shaped uncinate processes at the superior margin of the level below with corresponding grooves at the inferior margin of the level above.
- C7 (*vertebra prominens*) is characterized by a long spinous process, to which the nuchal ligament and several muscles attach.
  - The prominent C7 spinous process is a clinically palpable anatomic landmark, hence the term *vertebra prominens*; occasionally the T1 spinous process may be larger than C7.
- *Cervical ribs* may occasionally be present at C7, which are typically asymptomatic but can be a cause of thoracic outlet syndrome.

Familiarity with normal anatomy and subtle signs of injury is essential. The following checklist pertains specifically to radiographs, but the concepts translate to computed tomography (CT). Most of the relevant information can be found on the lateral radiograph. An adequate lateral radiograph must show the anatomy from the *clivus* (at the skullbase) to the top of the T1 vertebral body. A lateral swimmer's view is often necessary to demonstrate the lower cervical spine. The following items must be evaluated on the lateral view:

1. Prevertebral soft tissues
   - Normal width in adults: *6 mm* at C2 and *20 mm* at C6.
   - Normal width in children: no more than *2/3 the width of the C2 body* at the level of *C3 and C4* and no more than *14 mm* at C6 (less if younger).

2. Cervical alignment
   - Normal cervical alignment is lordotic (approximately 20–40 degrees).
   - Loss of lordosis may represent muscle spasm or be attributable to patient positioning, as loss of lordosis is noted in 70% of uninjured persons when the chin is depressed.
   - Loss of lordosis is expected in patients on a backboard or in a cervical collar.
3. Four continuous curves (Fig. 8.1)
   - These curves describe the normal position of the bony elements:
     - *Anterior vertebral body line.*
     - *Posterior vertebral body line.*
     - *Spinal laminar line.*
     - *Posterior spinous process line.*
   - Spinal laminar line should form a continuous line, regardless of the degree of flexion or extension.
   - Exception of alignment of the three other curves is found in children.
     - There may be physiologic offset of 2–3 mm at the C2-C3 and C3-C4 levels with flexion and extension.
4. Distance between adjacent posterior vertebral bodies
   - Should be uniform at all levels in the absence of degenerative disc disease.
   - Gap at one level suggests posterior ligamentous injury.
   - Finding can be supported by distraction of the associated spinous processes.
   - Note: normal 'fanning' of the spinous processes is not uniform because it is greater for the proximal and distal cervical levels than for the middle levels.

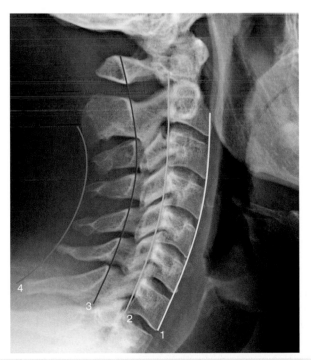

Fig. 8.1 Four continuous curves on the normal lateral cervical spine radiograph. *1 (yellow line),* anterior vertebral line; *2 (green line),* posterior vertebral line; *3 (purple line),* spinal laminar line; *4 (blue line),* posterior spinous line.

5. Superimposition of the right and left facet joints
   - Degree of overlap should be uniform at all levels in the absence of rotation.
   - A slightly off-lateral radiograph will show partial overlap of the right and left facet joints.
   - An abrupt change in the amount of overlap in adjacent levels indicates abnormal rotation along the longitudinal axis of the spine.
   - Additionally, the articular surfaces of each facet must be congruent; absence of such congruence indicates a subluxed, perched, or dislocated facet.
6. Odontoid process tilt
   - Odontoid process normally tilted posteriorly on the body of C2.
   - If posterior tilt is not seen, consider a fracture of the odontoid at its waist, which allows anterior subluxation of the odontoid process.
     - This can be confirmed by spinal laminar line disruption.
7. *Atlantoaxial interval (Atlantodental interval, ADI)*
   - Distance between the posterior cortex of the C1 anterior arch and anterior cortex of the dens, measured at the base of the dens.
   - In adults, this distance is not more than 2.5 mm and does not change with flexion.
   - In children, the distance may be as great as 5 mm and may change by 1–2 mm with flexion.
   - Abnormal ADI may be seen in injuries that destabilize the atlantoaxial (C1-C2) articulation.
     - Note: abnormal ADI can also be seen with rheumatoid arthritis in adults and various congenital conditions in children.
8. Spinous process alignment (on anteroposterior [AP] radiograph)
   - Spinous processes should form a fairly continuous, often slightly irregular line.
   - A fractured spinous process may be obviously displaced from this line, or there may appear to be two spinous processes (one representing the nondisplaced base of the fractured process and the other representing the displaced fragment).
9. Atlantoaxial alignment (on open-mouth odontoid view)
   - The open-mouth odontoid view is used to detect odontoid process fractures and the integrity of the ring of C1.
   - In neutral position, there is alignment of the lateral margins of the lateral masses of C1 and C2.
   - With rotation, the atlas normally moves as a unit with lateral facet offset on one side and medial offset on the contralateral side.
   - Lateral offset of the lateral margins of both C1 lateral masses indicates a C1 ring fracture in adults.
     - In children, bilateral offset may be a normal variant as a result of discrepant growth of C1 and C2.
10. Evaluation of the posterior elements on oblique view radiographs
    - Oblique views provide better visualization of the posterior elements and facet joints.
    - Facets should line up like roof shingles, with the articular process from the level above positioned posterior to the articular process from the level below.

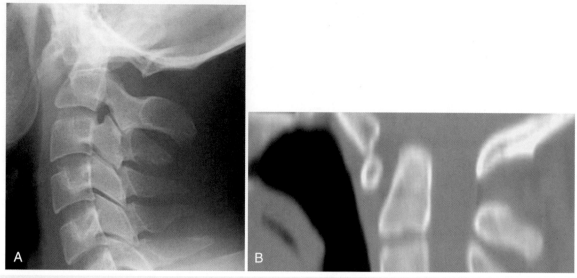

Fig. 8.2 Occipitalization of the atlas. **(A)** Lateral radiograph demonstrating no significant separation between the occiput and the atlas. **(B)** CT image demonstrates that the anterior arch and the hypoplastic posterior arch of the atlas are fused to the occiput. The odontoid moves independently of the occipitalized atlas, hence the abnormal atlantoaxial distance.

Several developmental variants can simulate an upper cervical spine fracture.

- *Occipitalization of the atlas (atlanto-occipital assimilation)* is lack of segmentation (congenital fusion) at the atlanto-occipital junction, which may be complete or incomplete.
    - Characterized on imaging by an abnormally large gap between the spinous processes of C1 and C2, and the atlas located unusually close to the occiput (Fig. 8.2).
    - Flexion lateral radiograph demonstrates fixation of the atlas to the occiput; CT may also be used to establish the diagnosis.
- Congenital ossification center fusion anomalies of the atlas (C1) and axis (C2).
    - C1 has three primary ossification centers: one body anteriorly and two neural arches posteriorly.
        - Most common anomaly of C1 is fusion anomaly of the posterior arch, which may range from a small cleft to complete aplasia.
        - Rarely, C1 may be bifid, with interruption of the anterior and posterior arches.
        - Fusion anomaly margins are smooth and corticated, in contrast with acute fractures.
    - C2 has four primary ossification centers: one body (which occasionally may be bifid), two neural arches, and one odontoid.
        - Body-neural arch synchondroses fuse asymmetrically between the ages of 3 and 6 years, and the body-odontoid synchondrosis also fuses at this time.
        - A lucent synchondrosis may persist into adult life, located well below the level of the apparent 'base' of the odontoid, seen as a thin, straight, well-defined transverse lucency in the body of C2 below the base of the dens (Fig. 8.3); this must be differentiated from an odontoid fracture, which usually occurs at the true base of the odontoid.

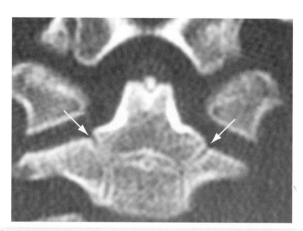

Fig. 8.3 Normal synchondroses of C2. Coronal CT image shows the multiple synchondroses of C2. The body of C2 is seen with the adjacent ossification centers of the posterior arches. The odontoid is a large structure that extends below the level of the apparent 'base of the odontoid'. This synchondrosis *(arrows)* normally fuses between the ages of 3 and 6 years but may remain unfused throughout life, potentially simulating a type 3 dens fracture. Finally, there is a small os terminale, which is located at the superior tip of the odontoid process. Before its ossification the tip may be seen as a V-shaped defect. The os terminale normally fuses by age 12 but may also persist unfused, simulating a tip of odontoid fracture. (Image used with permission from B.J. Manaster, MD, from the American College of Radiology Learning File.)

- A transverse dens fracture may also be simulated on odontoid view radiographs by a *Mach band*, due to the superimposed bottom teeth incisors or the arch of the atlas.
- *Ossiculum terminale* is a secondary ossification center located at the superior tip of the odontoid process.
    - Before it ossifies, the tip of the dens may be seen as a V-shaped defect on radiographs or CT.
    - Normally fuses by age 12 but may stay unfused, termed a persistent *ossiculum terminale* or *Bergmann's ossicle*, which can simulate a fracture of the odontoid tip.

- *Os odontoideum* is an anatomic variant, characterized by a large ossicle that occupies the space normally occupied by the odontoid process.
  - Thought to represent congenital failed fusion of the body-odontoid synchondrosis or prior trauma through the growth plate during development.
  - May be symptomatic due to instability.
    - The os odontoideum (i.e., the dens) is fixed to the anterior arch of the atlas, moving with C1 on flexion and extension, resulting in abnormal motion between the dens and C2.
  - May appear quite bizarre and may simulate a fracture (Fig. 8.4).

THORACIC SPINE

- There are normally 12 thoracic vertebrae, T1 through T12.
- Thoracic vertebrae progressively increase in size from cranial to caudal.
- Anatomically comprised of the vertebral body, paired laminae, pedicles, superior and inferior articular processes, transverse processes, and a single spinous process.
- Facets (and demifacets) exist at the posterolateral aspects of the thoracic vertebral bodies, which articulate with the ribs.
- Thoracic spine above T11 is the least mobile spine segment.
- Normal thoracic alignment is kyphotic (approximately 20–40 degrees).

LUMBAR SPINE

- There are normally five lumbar vertebrae, L1 through L5.
  - Variations are common at the lumbosacral junction, aptly termed *transitional lumbosacral anatomy*.
  - Variations include four or six non–rib-bearing lumbar-type vertebrae, partial or complete sacralization of L5, and partial or complete lumbarization of S1.
  - Small, partially formed ribs may be seen at the L1 level.
- Lumbar vertebrae are the largest segments in the spine.
- Anatomically comprised of the vertebral body, paired laminae, pedicles, superior and inferior articular processes, transverse processes, and a single spinous process.

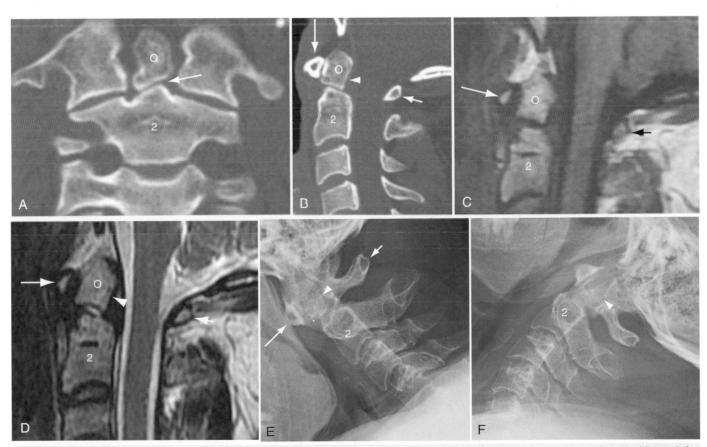

Fig. 8.4 Os odontoideum. **(A)** CT image shows os odontoideum *(O)* separated from the remainder of C2 *(2)* by a smoothly corticated, oblique cleft *(arrow)*. **(B)** Sagittal CT image also shows the os. Note that the os is displaced anterior relative to C2 *(arrowhead)* along with the anterior *(long arrow)* and posterior *(short arrow)* arches of C1. Malalignment is frequent with os odontoideum. T1-weighted **(C)** and T2-weighted **(D)** MR images show findings similar to B. Note the high signal between the os and C2 on the T2 (D), representing fluid in a false joint. Also note the anterior subluxation of the os *(arrowhead in D)* relative to C2. As in B, the *long arrow* marks the anterior arch of C1 and the *short arrow* marks the posterior arch of C1. Flexion **(E)** and extension **(F)** lateral radiographs show the os *(arrowhead)* changes position relative to C2 but maintain unchanged relation with C1 *(arrows)*.

- There is gradual widening of the interpediculate distances from L1 to L5 as seen on the AP radiograph.
- On the lateral view the disc spaces gradually increase in height from the L1-L2 level to L4-L5, with L5-S1 being slightly narrower.
- Normal lumbar alignment is lordotic (approximately 40–70 degrees).
- *Limbus vertebra* is a well-corticated ossific fragment at the anterosuperior (or occasionally anteroinferior) corner of a vertebral body, separated by an oblique radiolucent cleft.
  - Limbus vertebra is thought to represent an unfused ring apophysis or the result of an intravertebral disc herniation.
  - Generally considered an incidental finding that could simulate a fracture (Fig. 8.5).

Imaging Techniques

RADIOGRAPHY

- Routine radiographic projections of the *cervical spine* typically include AP, lateral, and odontoid views, with additional specialized views as needed.
  - *AP*—demonstrates vertebral bodies, disc spaces, alignment in coronal plane.
  - *Lateral*—demonstrates vertebral bodies, disc spaces, alignment in sagittal plane, prevertebral soft tissues.
  - *Odontoid*—obtained as a coned-down AP view of the C1-C2 (atlantoaxial) articulation and odontoid process (or dens).

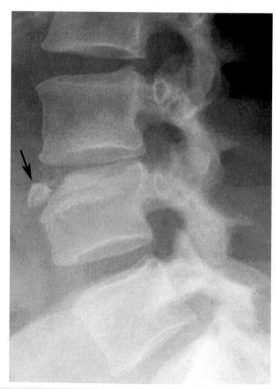

Fig. 8.5 Limbus vertebra *(arrow).*

- *Oblique*—typically obtained as two frontal oblique projections to assess the left and right posterior elements and bony neural foramina.
- *Swimmer's lateral*—helps visualize the C7-T1 level when obscured; obtained with the arm closest to the detector above the head to move the humeral heads off the cervical spine.
- *Flexion/extension lateral*—obtained to assess for spinal instability on dynamic maneuvers, which can be seen in the setting of ligament laxity or injury (should not be performed for known unstable fractures).
- Routine radiographic projections of the *thoracic spine* typically include AP and lateral views.
  - *AP*—demonstrates vertebral bodies, disc spaces, alignment in coronal plane.
  - *Lateral*—demonstrates vertebral bodies, disc spaces, alignment in sagittal plane.
- Routine radiographic projections of the *lumbar spine* typically include AP and lateral views, with additional specialized views as needed.
  - *AP*—demonstrates vertebral bodies, disc spaces, alignment in coronal plane.
  - *Lateral*—demonstrates vertebral bodies, disc spaces, alignment in sagittal plane.
  - *L5-S1 spot projection*—coned-down view to better visualize the lumbosacral junction.
  - *Oblique*—typically obtained as two frontal oblique projections to assess the left and right facet joints and pars interarticularis.
  - *Flexion/extension lateral*—obtained to assess for spinal instability on dynamic maneuvers.

COMPUTED TOMOGRAPHY

- CT with multiplanar reformations plays a critical role in spine imaging following acute trauma.
- Imaging of acute spine trauma, especially cervical spine trauma now usually begins with CT, supplanting radiographs as the first-line imaging study.
- CT is significantly more sensitive for detection and characterization of spinal fractures compared to radiographs.
- CT has superior spatial and contrast resolution of bones and fracture fragments than magnetic resonance imaging (MRI).
- CT angiography is an excellent test for suspected vertebral artery injury.

MAGNETIC RESONANCE IMAGING

- MRI is the study of choice to evaluate for critical soft tissue injuries, such as epidural hematoma or injury to the spinal cord, conus medullaris, or nerve roots.
- MRI can demonstrate many vertebral artery injuries and some fractures not visible on CT.

Pathophysiology

- Same basic forces that cause fractures in the appendicular skeleton cause spine fractures: compression, tension, and shear.

- Rotational forces, which combine the basic forces, frequently come into play with spine trauma.
- A useful concept in spine trauma is the *three-column model* of spine stability.
  - *Anterior column* consists of the anterior longitudinal ligament and the anterior half of the vertebral bodies, intervertebral discs and supporting soft tissues.
  - *Middle column* consists of the posterior longitudinal ligament and the posterior half of the vertebral bodies, intervertebral discs and supporting soft tissues.
  - *Posterior column* consists of the posterior elements, the facet joints, and the numerous associated ligaments.
- Three-column model helps predict whether a spine injury is stable or unstable.
  - Disruption of only one column generally does not result in spine instability, whereas disruption of two or three columns does.
  - Because a column disruption may involve only the soft tissues, spine instability may be present even in the absence of a fracture.
- Radiographic signs of instability include abnormal spinous process fanning, widening of the intervertebral disc space, horizontal displacement of one body on another more than 3.5 mm, angulation greater than 11 degrees, disruption of facets, or severe injury, such as multiple fractures at one segment.

CERVICAL SPINE

- Cervical spine injuries usually occur in predictable patterns based on the mechanism of injury.
- Knowledge of these patterns can help the radiologist to avoid missing an important injury.
- *Flexion injuries* result in compression forces anteriorly and tensile forces posteriorly.

- May range from the innocuous anterior wedge compression to the devastating flexion teardrop (burst) fracture.
- Severe flexion injuries often disrupt the posterior longitudinal ligament, in which case there may be localized increased height of the intervertebral disc space, associated with fanning of spinous processes and a focal kyphotic angulation (Fig. 8.6).
- These findings are accentuated on lateral flexion images and may allow facet subluxation or even locking; however, cervical stability may be temporarily maintained by surrounding soft tissue swelling and muscle spasm.
  - Delayed instability is found in 20% of these patients.
  - MRI can demonstrate facet joint capsular disruption.
- *Extension injuries* result in tensile forces anteriorly and compression forces posteriorly.
  - Some extension injuries have extremely subtle radiographic signs.
    - Facet compression fractures can result from hyperextension with rotation and may be occult on radiographs and subtle on CT or MRI.
  - Hyperextension injuries can cause spinal cord injury even without fracture or dislocation.
    - When hyperextension injury is suspected, MRI should be considered to delineate the soft tissue injury and to determine the likelihood of instability.
    - MRI may demonstrate spinal cord contusion or hemorrhage, epidural hematoma, and traumatic disc herniation.
  - There may be a tear or stretch of the anterior longitudinal ligament and disruption of the anterior anulus fibrosus (anterior column injury).
    - This can result in avulsion of the adjacent anterior vertebral body endplate (Fig. 8.7).

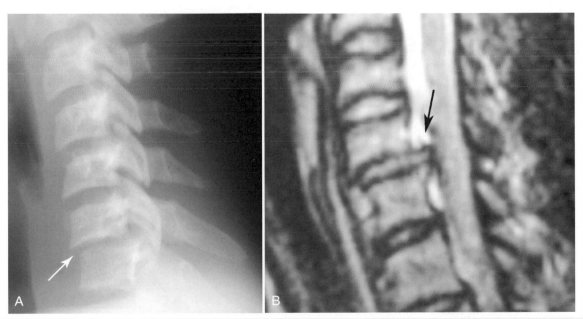

Fig. 8.6 Hyperflexion injury. **(A)** Lateral flexion radiograph of the cervical spine in a patient who sustained a neck injury in a motor vehicle accident. Although the neutral view (not shown) showed no abnormality, the flexion view shows anterolisthesis of C6 on C7 *(arrow)*, as well as narrowing of the disc space. This is not normal in a 14-year-old. **(B)** T2-weighted sagittal MR image demonstrates the anterolisthesis of C6 on C7, along with the disc herniation and posterior longitudinal ligament disruption *(arrow)*.

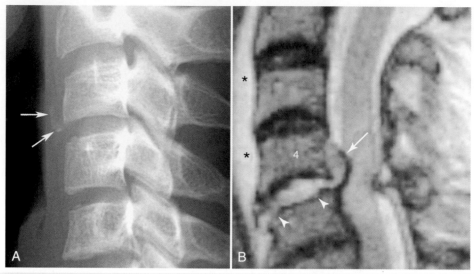

Fig. 8.7 Hyperextension injury. (A) Lateral radiograph shows no prevertebral soft tissue swelling. However, there is a subtle avulsion fracture of the anteroinferior C3 vertebral body end plate *(arrows)*. This is an indicator of a hyperextension injury, and MRI should be performed for evaluation of possible spinal cord injury. **(B)** Sagittal T2-weighted MR image of a different patient with hyperextension injury shows disruption of the C4-C5 disc *(arrowheads)* and epidural *(arrow)* and prevertebral *(asterisks)* hematomas. (Image courtesy of W. Smoker, MD)

- More severe extension injuries may also involve the middle and posterior columns and result in profound instability.
  - Despite the serious soft tissue disruptions, these injuries can spontaneously reduce, so radiographs may not reveal the true extent of injury.
  - Prevertebral soft tissue swelling is an important clue.
  - There may be posterior body displacement or a widened intervertebral disc space, especially anteriorly.
- In the absence of degenerative disc disease, a vacuum phenomenon at the anulus fibrosus is highly suggestive of an extension injury.
  - When present, anteroinferior vertebral body avulsion usually may suggest the diagnosis of hyperextension injury.
- Some injuries may have both hyperflexion and hyperextension features (Fig. 8.8).
- Vertebral artery injury can be seen in patients with both hyperflexion and hyperextension injuries.
  - Must be suspected in patients with facet fractures or dislocations or fractures traversing the course of the vertebral arteries (such as the foramina transversarium).
  - Best evaluated by CT angiogram (CTA) (Fig. 8.9).

THORACIC AND LUMBAR SPINE

As with the cervical spine, thoracic and lumbar injuries usually occur in predictable patterns based on the mechanism of injury.

- Traumatic injuries in the thoracic and lumbar spine are easier to understand than injuries in the cervical spine because the anatomy is less complex.
- The thoracic and lumbar spine differ biomechanically from the cervical spine because of the generally larger, stronger discs, supporting ligaments, and muscles.

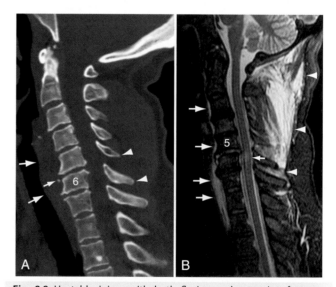

Fig. 8.8 Unstable injury with both flexion and extension features. **(A)** CT image shows prevertebral soft tissue swelling *(large arrows)*, widened interspinous distance at C5-C6 *(arrowheads)*, and small fragment anterior to C5-C6 *(small arrow)* that might be an avulsion fragment or degenerative calcification of the ALL displaced by ligament disruption. **(B)** STIR MR image shows prevertebral edema *(arrows)*, edema throughout the disrupted C5-C6 disc, cord contusion *(small arrow)*, and edema in sprained interspinous ligaments and ligamentum nuchae *(arrowheads)*.

- Compression and flexion injuries tend to overlap in the thoracic and lumbar spine, because the strong posterior and middle columns can convert flexion force into vertebral body compression in a nutcracker-like mechanism.
  - Compression and flexion account for 75% of injuries.
- The rib cage and the orientation of the thoracic facets above T11 help to stabilize the thoracic spine, and the exceptionally strong ligaments and muscular support help to stabilize the lower lumbar spine.

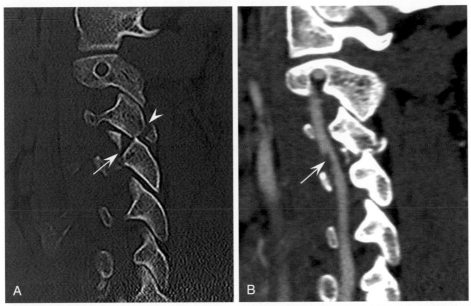

Fig. 8.9 Posterior element fractures with traumatic vertebral artery dissection. **(A)** Sagittal reconstruction CT image of the cervical spine shows acute displaced fractures of the left C3 inferior articular process *(arrowhead)* and left C4 superior articular process *(arrow)*. **(B)** Curved planar reformation CTA image of the left vertebral artery shows a luminal filling defect consistent with a dissection flap *(arrow)*.

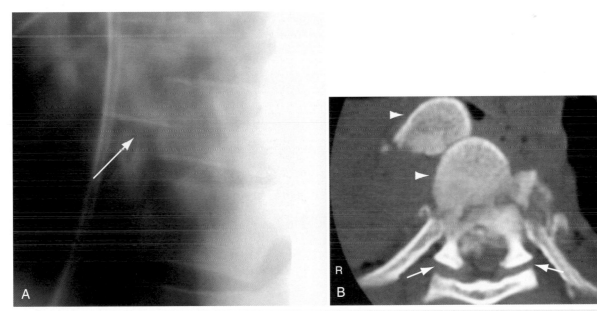

Fig. 8.10 Unstable upper thoracic spine injury. **(A)** Lateral radiograph shows severe anterolisthesis in the midthoracic spine *(arrow)*. This degree of displacement implies sternal and probably multiple rib fractures. **(B)** CT image at the level of anterolisthesis shows the two vertebral bodies as they overlap *(arrowheads)*, as well as retropulsed fragments narrowing the spinal canal and diastasis of the facets *(arrows)*. (Image used with permission from B.J. Manaster, MD, from the American College of Radiology Learning File.)

- As a result, forces acting on the thoracic and lumbar spine are focused at the thoracolumbar junction, with 60% of fractures occurring from the T12 through L2 levels and 90% between T11 and L4
- Hyperextension injuries of the thoracic and lumbar spine are unusual but can disrupt the anterior longitudinal ligament and cause posterior element and facet compression injuries.
- On the AP radiograph, careful attention should be given to the interpediculate distances because widening at a single level suggests a burst fracture.

- Widening of the paraspinous soft tissues on x-ray may be caused by a hematoma.
- A midthoracic or upper thoracic fracture is more likely to be unstable if multiple rib fractures or a sternal fracture is present (Fig. 8.10).
- Presence of a calcaneus fracture after a fall from a height (the so-called *lover's fracture* or *Don Juan fracture*) is associated with a significantly increased risk for a thoracic or lumbar spine fracture (and vice versa).
  - Thus, if a calcaneus fracture is found, imaging of the thoracic and lumbar spine should be considered.

Disease Processes

CERVICAL SPINE

Occipital Condyle Fracture

- Uncommon injury that typically occurs from high-impact trauma and often requires CT for diagnosis (Fig. 8.11).
- These fractures may involve the hypoglossal canal or jugular foramen, so clinical features of injury to cranial nerves IX to XII may be found.

Craniocervical Dissociation (Atlanto-Occipital Dislocation)

- Can be a surprisingly easy injury to miss radiographically but is clinically devastating.
- Normal occipital–vertebral relationship is maintained by ligaments extending from the axis (C2) to the clivus and occipital condyles via the tectorial membrane and alar ligaments, respectively.
- A true dislocation is often fatal and obvious on a lateral image (Fig. 8.12).
- Subluxation is rare and may not have a neurologic deficit or obvious radiographic findings; in such cases, the following measurements are useful for detection of such injuries:
  - *Basion-axial interval*—the distance from the inferior tip of the clivus (the basion) to the posterior body of C2 normally measures less than 12 mm.
  - *Basion-dens interval*—the distance from the basion to the top of the odontoid process (dens) normally measures less than 10 mm.
  - *Atlantodental interval*—the distance between the posterior cortex of the C1 anterior arch and anterior cortex of the dens normally measures less than 3 mm.
- One should maintain a high level of suspicion for craniocervical junction injuries in patients with severe facial and/or head trauma.

Jefferson Fracture

- Axial loading burst fracture of the atlas (C1) that involves both the anterior and posterior arches (Fig. 8.13).
- May be a four-part fracture (bilateral anterior and posterior arch fractures) as traditionally described, or three-part or two-part fracture.

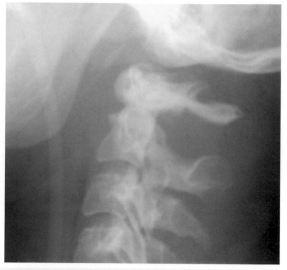

Fig. 8.12 Craniocervical dissociation (atlanto-occipital dislocation). This lateral radiograph demonstrates a critical injury. Note the tremendous prevertebral soft tissue swelling and complete dissociation of the occiput from the atlas. Also note the wide interval between the posterior margin of the mandible and the cervical spine.

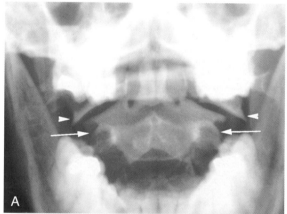

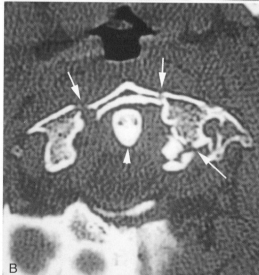

Fig. 8.13 Burst fracture of C1. **(A)** Open-mouth odontoid view shows lateral translocation of the lateral masses of C1 *(arrowheads)* relative to C2 *(arrows)*. **(B)** Axial CT image shows multiple breaks in the ring of C1 *(arrows)*. *Arrowhead* marks the dens. (Image courtesy of W. Smoker, MD)

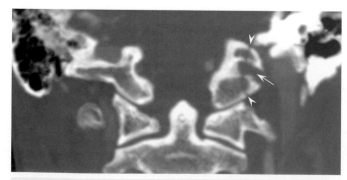

Fig. 8.11 Occipital condyle fracture. Coronal reconstruction CT image demonstrates a nondisplaced left occipital condyle fracture *(arrowheads)*, which traverses the left hypoglossal canal *(arrow)*.

- Must be differentiated from congenital defects of the atlas.
- Normal angulation of the C1 facets tends to drive the C1 fragments laterally with axial loading.
- Surprisingly, this may be a stable fracture with minimal displacement and no neurologic deficit unless there is displaced fragment into the canal or disruption of the transverse ligament of the atlas, which normally fixes the odontoid to the anterior arch of the atlas.
- MRI is useful for characterizing associated soft tissue injuries.

Atlantoaxial Rotatory Displacement

- Rotation injury with locking of the facets of C1 and C2, more common in children and presenting with impaired rotation of the head (torticollis).
- Radiographs of this condition can be difficult to interpret owing to the alteration of familiar landmarks by the cervical rotation.
    - On the open-mouth odontoid view radiograph, one lateral mass of C1 appears wider and closer to the midline, with the opposite appearing narrower and laterally offset.
    - Overlapping osseous and soft tissue structures may obscure the facets.
- CT is usually needed to diagnose this condition (Fig. 8.14). 3D reformats are often helpful.

Odontoid Fracture

- Odontoid fractures are typically classified by the location of the fracture (Fig. 8.15).
    - *Type I*—fracture involving the tip of the dens; rarely encountered, usually (but not always) a stable injury.
    - *Type II*—fracture through the waist or base of the dens; most common pattern, unstable fracture, high risk of nonunion.
    - *Type III*—fracture extending below the base of the dens through the body of C2; may be unstable or partially stable, best prognosis for healing.
- Frequently missed with radiographs. CT is diagnostic (Fig. 8.16).

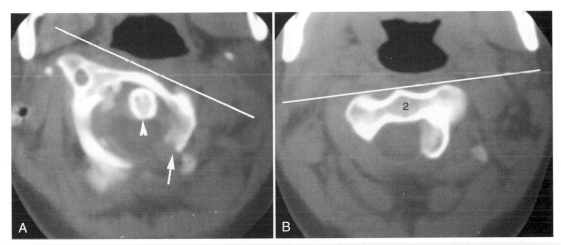

Fig. 8.14 Rotatory subluxation of C1 on C2. Axial CT images obtained through the ring of C1 and the body of C2 show rotation of C1 **(A)** relative to C2 **(B)**. Also note the fracture of C1 (*arrow* in A). *Arrowhead* marks the dens in A. (Image courtesy of W. Smoker, MD)

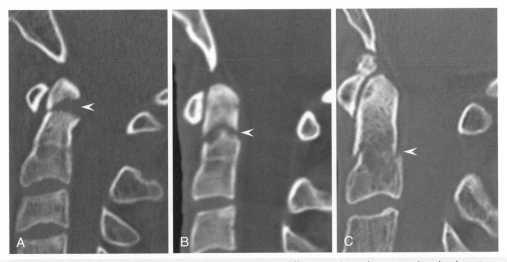

Fig. 8.15 Types of odontoid (dens) fractures. Sagittal reconstruction CT images in different patients demonstrating the three types of odontoid (dens) fractures *(arrowheads)*. **(A)** Type I fracture. **(B)** Type II fracture. **(C)** Type III fracture.

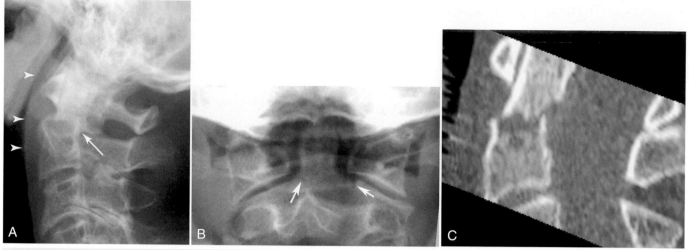

Fig. 8.16 Odontoid (dens) fracture. **(A)** Lateral radiograph shows that this patient has only mild prevertebral swelling, which is centered at the odontoid *(arrowheads)*. The odontoid is displaced posteriorly relative to the C2 body *(arrow)* and is angled posteriorly. These findings indicate a fracture. **(B)** The fracture is extremely subtle on the open-mouth odontoid radiograph *(arrows)*. **(C)** Sagittal CT reconstruction shows the fracture.

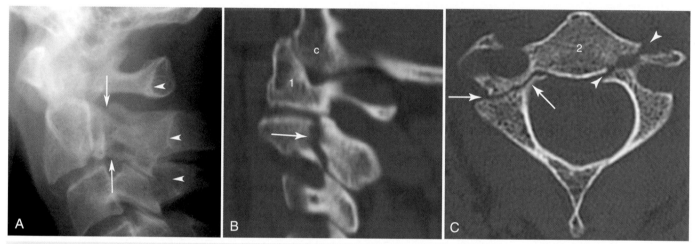

Fig. 8.17 Hangman's fracture. **(A)** Lateral radiograph shows the bilateral neural arch fractures at C2 that constitute a hangman's fracture *(arrows)*. The fracture extends into the posterior body of C2, and there is anterior subluxation of C2 on C3, making this a type III injury. Note the disruption of the normally straight spinal laminar line at C1-C3 *(arrowheads)*. **(B)** Sagittal paramedian CT scan in a different patient with hangman's fracture. Note the occipital condyle *(c)*, C1 lateral mass *(1)*, and C2 fracture *(arrow)*. **(C)** Axial CT in a different patient shows coronal plane fractures across the right neural arch *(arrows)* and anterior to the left foramen transversarium in the body *(arrowheads)*. A key finding is that neither fracture crosses the foramen transversarium, which would indicate high risk for vertebral artery injury.

Hangman's Fracture

- Most frequently seen at C2 but can be seen at other levels.
- Typically occurs from a hyperextension injury that results in bilateral neural arch fractures (*traumatic spondylolysis* of C2).
- Interruption of the spinal laminar line is the radiographic hallmark of this injury (Fig. 8.17).
- Unstable fracture, but cord injury is uncommon owing to the usual absence of spinal canal narrowing.
- Odontoid process and its ligament attachments are usually intact.
- Hangman's fractures can be classified by the degree of displacement of C2 on C3.
  - *Type I*—most common type, involves the posterior part of the body of C2 (or any part of the ring) with less than 3 mm translation, no angulation, intact

C2-C3 disc, relatively stable, and often treated by external immobilization or surgical stabilization.
  - *Type II*—greater than 3 mm translation of C2 on C3, greater than 11 degrees angulation, disruption of the C2-C3 disc, may be treated surgically or by external immobilization depending on degree of instability.
  - *Type III*—severe translation and angulation with locked facets, unstable and often fatal, treated surgically.

Anterior Wedge Compression Fracture

- Flexion injury generally affecting only the anterior column, thus a stable injury.
- However, if the posterior ligamentous complex is disrupted, then this is a potentially unstable two-column injury (Fig. 8.18).

Teardrop Burst Fracture (Flexion Teardrop Fracture)

- Most severe flexion injury compatible with life, with 80% of patients sustaining neurologic injury (Fig. 8.19).
- Mechanism of a teardrop burst fracture is combined flexion and compression, with diving injuries and motor vehicle accidents being the most frequent causes.

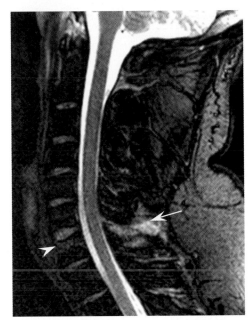

Fig. 8.18 Cervical anterior wedge compression fracture with posterior ligamentous injury. Sagittal fluid-sensitive MR image of the cervical spine demonstrates a subtle C7 anterior wedge compression fracture with mild marrow edema *(arrowhead)*. There is associated disruption of the posterior ligamentous complex *(arrow)*, making this a two-column injury.

- Comminuted vertebral body fractures with coronal and sagittal fracture planes and a triangular fragment at the anteroinferior border of the vertebral body (teardrop fragment).
- Posterior body is often displaced into the spinal canal, with a high probability of neural damage.
- Classic associated neurologic presentation is that of an anterior cord syndrome including diminished motor function and loss of pain and temperature sensation, with intact vibration and proprioception, caused by injury of the anterior spinal cord.
- Extent of injury is often underestimated on radiographs but is well demonstrated on CT.
- Spinal cord injury, ligamentous injury, and epidural hematoma are best shown by MRI.

Unilateral Locked Facet (Unilateral Interfacetal Dislocation)

- Results from flexion, distraction, and rotation forces.
- On lateral radiographs, there is an abrupt change in the amount of facet overlap (Fig. 8.20).
- Most common locations for a unilateral locked facet are C4-C5 and C5-C6.
- 35% of these cases are associated with fracture, most frequently of the facet.
- Vertebral body subluxation may be mild with a unilateral locked facet.
- A variant is a *perched facet* in which the facet is not fully dislocated or locked.

Bilateral Locked Facets (Bilateral Interfacetal Dislocation)

- Result from flexion, but with enough distraction for both facets to become dislocated.
- Vertebral body is displaced, usually 50% of the body length as seen on the lateral radiograph (Fig. 8.21).

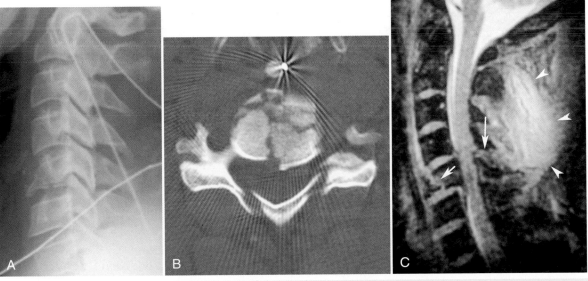

Fig. 8.19 Flexion teardrop burst fracture. **(A)** Lateral radiograph shows a comminuted teardrop type of fracture at the anterior-inferior aspect of the body of C5. There is no obvious retropulsed fragment, and the extent of this injury is easily underestimated on this radiograph. **(B)** CT image better shows the severity of the injury, with three-column disruption. **(C)** Sagittal fluid-sensitive MR image shows not only the fracture *(short arrow)* but also C4-C5 interspinous ligament edema due to disruption *(long arrow)*, diffuse high signal in the posterior ligamentous structures *(arrowheads)*, and retropulsion of the C5 vertebral body with cord compression.

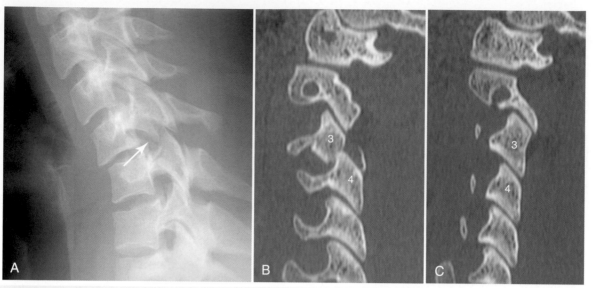

Fig. 8.20 Unilateral locked facet (unilateral interfacetal dislocation). **(A)** Lateral radiograph shows an abrupt transition in alignment at C5-C6, where there is mild anterolisthesis of C5 on C6, splaying of the spinous processes, and a change in alignment of the facets *(arrow)*. The facets at C3, C4, and C5 are in a bow-tie configuration; at C6 and C7 they are in a pure lateral configuration. There is a lock of the more anterior-inferior C5 facet on the superior facet of C6. (B and C) Sagittal CT reformats in a different patient with unilateral interfacetal dislocation show fracture-dislocation **(B)** at C3-C4 and normal side **(C)**.

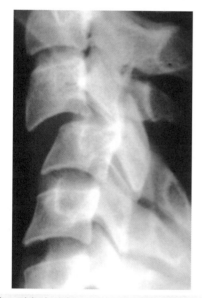

Fig. 8.21 Bilateral locked facets. Lateral radiograph shows bilateral locked facet of C3-C4 with near-complete anterolisthesis of C3 on C4 and abnormal alignment of the posterior facets.

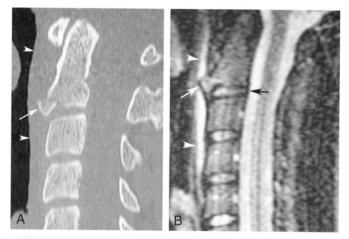

Fig. 8.22 Hyperextension teardrop fracture of C2 with intact posterior ligaments. Sagittal CT reformat **(A)** and inversion recovery MR image **(B)** show anterior-inferior C2 corner fracture *(arrow)* with anterior soft tissue swelling and edema *(white arrowheads)*. The posterior longitudinal ligament *(black arrow)* is intact, and there is no posterior element fracture or ligament injury. Because this fracture can occur in conjunction with a hangman's fracture, it is essential to evaluate the neural arch of C2 before diagnosing a hyperextension teardrop fracture of C2.

- Both lateral and oblique images show the locked ('jumped') facets.
- High incidence of cord injury with bilateral locked facets.

Extension Teardrop Fracture

- Results from forced hyperextension, resulting in avulsion of the anteroinferior corner of the vertebral body at the anterior longitudinal ligament (ALL) attachment site.
- May see additional fractures in the cervical spine, but overall extension teardrop fractures are considered less severe than teardrop burst fractures.
- Hyperextension teardrop fracture of C2 is a common variant and can occur with relatively minor force in older patients with osteoporosis and degeneration-related limited cervical spine mobility.
  - Cardinal feature is a triangular fragment at the anteroinferior C2 body (Fig. 8.22).

Clay Shoveler's Fracture

- Isolated avulsion of the C7 spinous process (may also occur at other lower cervical or upper thoracic levels) caused by abrupt contraction of the trapezius and other muscles that attach to the spinous process (Fig. 8.23).
- Usually occurs in isolation and is a stable injury treated by immobilization with excellent outcomes.

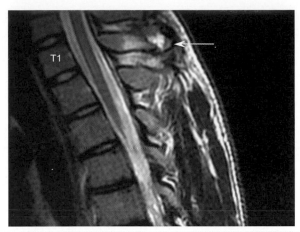

Fig. 8.23 Clay shoveler's fracture. Sagittal T2-weighted MR image of the upper thoracic spine demonstrates an acute avulsion fracture of the T1 spinous process *(arrow)*. The patient reported a recent injury accompanied by a 'pop'.

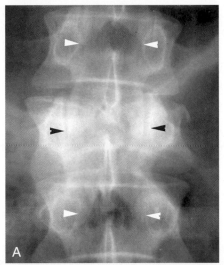

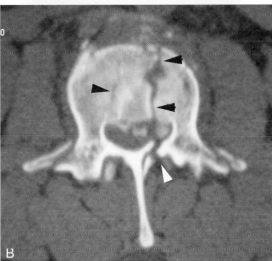

Fig. 8.25 Burst fracture. **(A)** AP radiograph shows widened interpediculate distance at L2 *(arrowheads)*. This indicates the 'burst' nature of the fracture. **(B)** CT image confirms fractures through the posterior vertebral body and posterior elements *(arrowheads)*. Note the severe spinal canal narrowing.

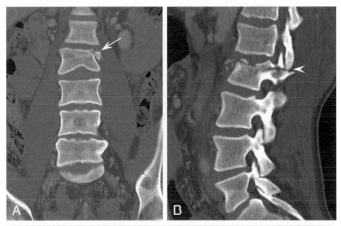

Fig. 8.24 Lateral compression fracture. Coronal **(A)** and sagittal **(B)** reconstruction CT images of the lumbar spine show an acute compression fracture involving the left lateral aspect of L2 *(arrow, A)*, which extends into the left posterior elements *(arrowhead, B)*.

THORACIC AND LUMBAR SPINE

Vertebral Body Compression Fracture

- Most acute vertebral body compression fractures demonstrate anterior wedging or depression of the superior endplate with intact posterior elements.
  - These fractures are generally stable, one-column injuries.
- Lateral compression fractures are caused by lateral flexion injuries (Fig. 8.24).
  - An AP radiograph or coronal CT or MR images reveals a vertebral body compression that is asymmetrically greater on the right or left side, often with associated scoliosis.
- Osteoporotic compression fractures are a particular subset of vertebral body compression fractures seen in patients without major trauma, as discussed later.

Burst Fracture

- Unstable three-column fracture due to high-force axial loading.

- Disruption of the vertebral body posterior cortex with retropulsion into the spinal canal.
- Requires CT to evaluate for retropulsed bony fragments in the spinal canal and to guide surgical approach.
- MRI is often also obtained to evaluate for spinal cord or conus medullaris injury and epidural hematoma.
- Facets may be fractured, subluxed, perched, dislocated, or locked (Fig. 8.25).
- Presence of a burst fracture is associated with a 40% chance that another spine fracture is present.
  - If a burst fracture is found, imaging of the entire spine is usually appropriate.

Osteoporotic Compression Fracture

- Especially common in older adults and a common cause of disabling pain (Fig. 8.26).
- Insufficiency fracture due to underlying osteoporosis, often occurring with normal activities or minor trauma.

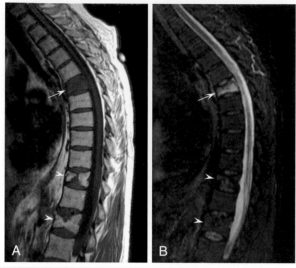

Fig. 8.26 Osteoporotic compression fractures. Sagittal T1-weighted **(A)** and STIR **(B)** MR images demonstrate an acute T7 osteoporotic compression fracture *(arrows)*. Associated marrow hypointensity on T1-weighted imaging **(A)** is due to the intense marrow edema **(B)**. Chronic healed osteoporotic compression fractures are seen at T12 and L2 *(arrowheads)* without associated marrow edema.

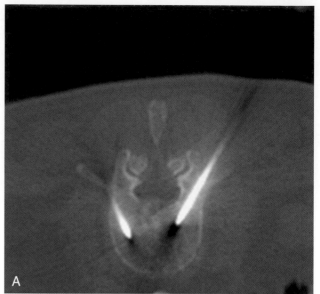

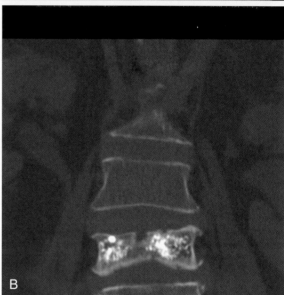

Fig. 8.27 CT-guided vertebroplasty. Intraprocedure CT image **(A)** demonstrates placement of vertebral access cannulas for percutaneous vertebroplasty. Immediate postprocedure coronal reconstruction CT image **(B)** demonstrates excellent fill of the compressed vertebral body with composite bone cement filling material.

- Pain is often severe and disabling, which can be mitigated via percutaneous intervention.
    - *Vertebroplasty* (i.e., image-guided injection of polymethylmethacrylate or other composite bone cement filling material into the fractured vertebral body) is a safe, effective treatment method (Fig. 8.27).
    - *Kyphoplasty* is a similar technique in which a balloon is inflated within a compressed vertebral body followed by injection of the filling material.
    - Vertebroplasty and kyphoplasty are equally effective for pain reduction.
        - Kyphoplasty has been shown to have decreased risk for cement leakage but requires longer procedure time and is more expensive.
        - A recent meta-analysis suggests that patients treated with vertebral augmentation (vertebroplasty or balloon kyphoplasty) have a 22% less mortality rate at 10 years post-treatment compared to those patients treated nonsurgically.
    - Recently fractured vertebral bodies with marrow edema (acute or subacute fractures) are most likely to benefit from these techniques.
    - MRI including a sagittal inversion recovery sequence (which can reliably depict marrow edema) is often performed as a screening examination before vertebroplasty or kyphoplasty (see Fig. 8.27).
- Vertebral body compression fracture may progress to osteonecrosis, or *Kümmell disease*, characterized by further compression and intraosseous vacuum phenomenon or a fluid filled cleft (Fig. 8.28).

Chance Fracture (Seat Belt Fracture)

- Flexion-distraction injury of the spine.
- Historically, a frequent cause was a lap-type of seat belt, which acts as a fulcrum during rapid deceleration in a motor vehicle crash.

- Unstable fracture that may be subtle and nondisplaced on radiographs and CT because of spontaneous reduction.
- Characterized by a transverse fracture extending through the posterior elements and the vertebral body or disc space with little or no vertebral body compression (Fig. 8.29).
- Associated with solid organ and visceral injuries in the abdomen/pelvis.
- Chance fractures are seen less commonly since the introduction of shoulder belts and air bags.
    - Now, they are most frequently encountered after a fall from a height, with hyperflexion occurring as the patient's feet strike the ground while the waist is flexed.

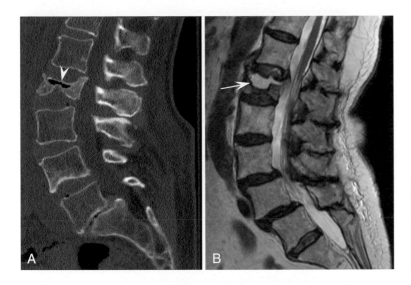

Fig. 8.28 Vertebral body osteonecrosis (Kümmell disease). **(A)** Sagittal reconstruction CT image demonstrates a compression fracture of the L2 vertebral body with intravertebral gas, consistent with osteonecrosis *(arrowhead)*. **(B)** Sagittal T2-weighted MR image demonstrates compression fracture of the L1 vertebral body in a different patient, with a large fluid-filled cleft *(arrow)* indicating osteonecrosis.

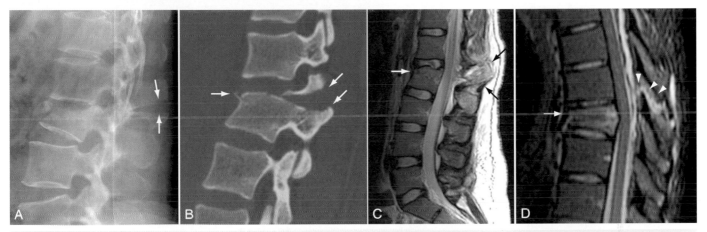

Fig. 8.29 Chance fractures. **(A)** Lateral radiograph shows upper end plate compression of the L2 body and distracted axial plane fracture through the L1 spinous process *(arrows)*. Sagittal CT image **(B)** and T2-weighted MR image **(C)** in a different patient show mild L2 compression *(anterior arrow)* and distracted posterior element fracture *(posterior arrows)*, seen as complex mostly high signal in C due to edema and hemorrhage. **(D)** Thoracic chance fracture. Note the compressed T11 vertebral body *(arrow)*. The injury extends posteriorly through the T10-T11 interspinous ligament *(arrowheads)*. These are all unstable injuries.

- Also occurs in spines fused by ankylosing spondylitis and other causes of multilevel fusion such as diffuse idiopathic skeletal hyperostosis (DISH). Chance fractures in these patients can be extremely subtle on CT but neurologically devastating if missed.

Transverse Process Fracture

- Can occur as an isolated finding or as part of a more extensive spine injury (Fig. 8.30).
- A finding of multiple lumbar transverse process fractures is associated with an increased risk for significant intraabdominal injury.
- L5 transverse process fractures are associated with sacral fractures.
- The combined use of a lap and shoulder belt without an air bag concentrates forces in a motor vehicle crash at the cervicothoracic junction, often with a twisting component because only one shoulder is braced by the shoulder belt.
  - Cervicothoracic transverse process fractures may be seen.

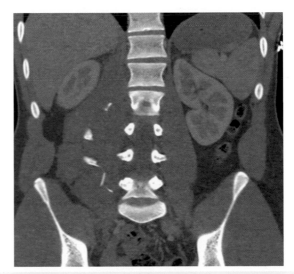

Fig. 8.30 Multiple transverse process fractures. Coronal reconstruction CT image demonstrates multiple right-sided lumbar transverse process fractures with extensive paraspinal hematoma.

Spondylolysis (Pars Fracture or Pars Defect)

- Disruption of the pars interarticularis (portion of the posterior arch that connects the superior and inferior articular processes).
- Stress fracture that typically develops over time with repetitive microtrauma, (Fig. 8.31).
  - Less likely due to acute trauma, particularly in the lumbar spine.
- May be unilateral or bilateral, most commonly seen at the L5 level (90% of cases).
- Can result in anterolisthesis in the chronic setting.
- Spondylolysis is discussed further in Chapter 15—Congenital and Developmental Conditions.

Reporting Tips and Recommendations

- Compile succinct impression points and address high-acuity findings first.
- Expeditiously communicate urgent findings to the emergency medicine physician, and appropriately document communication in the report.
- Make appropriate imaging recommendations if warranted, such as follow-up MRI, CTA, or complete imaging of the spine.
- Scrutinize CT images carefully for soft tissue findings in addition to acute fractures or malalignment.
- Recognize and address normal variants in the body of the report to avoid confusion with acute injuries.

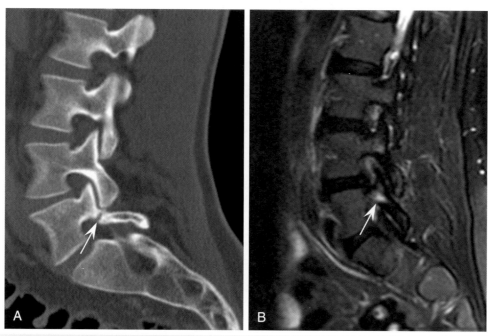

Fig. 8.31 Spondylolysis (pars interarticularis defect). **(A)** Sagittal reconstruction CT image demonstrates a unilateral pars interarticularis defect in a young adult. **(B)** Sagittal STIR image in another patient demonstrates marrow edema in the pars interarticularis *(arrow)* consistent with osseous stress response, which has not progressed to a stress fracture.

Sources and Suggested Readings

Benedetti PF, Fahr LM, Kuhns LR, et al. MR imaging findings in spinal ligamentous injury. *AJR Am J Roentgenol.* 2000;175(3):661–665.

Bernstein MP, Mirvis SE, Shanmuganathan K. Chance-type fractures of the thoracolumbar spine: imaging analysis in 53 patients. *AJR Am J Roentgenol.* 2006;187(4):859–868.

Dreizin D, Letzing M, Sliker CW, et al. Multidetector CT of blunt cervical spine trauma in adults. *Radiology.* 2014;34(7):1842–1865.

Gu CN, Brinjikji W, Evans AJ, et al. Outcomes of vertebroplasty compared with kyphoplasty: a systematic review and meta-analysis. *J Neurointerv Surg.* 2016;8(6):636–642.

Guarnieri G, Izzo R, Muto M. The role of emergency radiology in spinal trauma. *Br J Radiol.* 2016;89(1061):20150833.

Helms CA, Major NA, Anderson MW, Kaplan PA. *Musculoskeletal MRI.* 2nd ed. Philadelphia: Saunders; 2008.

Hinde K, Maingard J, Hirsch JA, et al. Mortality outcomes of vertebral augmentation (vertebroplasty and/or balloon kyphoplasty) for osteoporotic vertebral compression fractures: a systematic review and meta-analysis. *Radiology.* 2020;18:191294.

Jinkins JR, Matthes JC, Sener RN, et al. Spondylolysis, spondylolisthesis, and associated nerve root entrapment in the lumbosacral spine: MR evaluation. *AJR Am J Roentgenol.* 1992;159(4):799–803.

Khurana B, Sheehan SE, Sodickson A, et al. Traumatic thoracolumbar spine injuries: what the spine surgeon wants to know. *Radiographics.* 2013;33(7):2031–2046.

Kim KS, Chen HH, Russell EJ, et al. Flexion teardrop fracture of the cervical spine: radiographic characteristics. *AJR Am J Roentgenol.* 1989;152(2):319–326.

Konin GP, Walz DM. Lumbosacral transitional vertebrae: classification, imaging findings, and clinical relevance. *AJNR Am J Neuroradiol.* 2010;31(10):1778–1786.

Kumar Y, Hayashi D. Role of magnetic resonance imaging in acute spinal trauma: a pictorial review. *BMC Musculoskelet Disord.* 2016;17:310.

Lenchik L, Rogers LF, Delmas PD, Genant HK. Diagnosis of osteoporotic vertebral fractures: importance of recognition and description by radiologists. *AJR Am J Roentgenol.* 2004;183(4):949–958.

Leone A, Cerase A, Colosimo C, et al. Occipital condylar fractures: a review. *Radiology.* 2000;216(3):635–644.

Lustrin ES, Karakas SP, Ortiz AO, et al. Pediatric cervical spine: normal anatomy, variants, and trauma. *Radiographics.* 2003;23(3):539–560.

Munera F, Rivas LA, Nunez DB Jr, et al. Imaging evaluation of adult spinal injuries: emphasis on multidetector CT in cervical spine trauma. *Radiology*. 2012;263(3):645–660.

Nuñez DB Jr, Zuluaga A, Fuentes-Bernardo DA, et al. Cervical spine trauma: how much more do we learn by routinely using helical CT? *Radiographics*. 1996;16(6):1307–1318; discussion 1318–1321.

Patten RM, Gunberg SR, Brandenburger DK. Frequency and importance of transverse process fractures in the lumbar vertebrae at helical abdominal CT in patients with trauma. *Radiology*. 2000;215(3):831–834.

Raniga SB, Skalski MR, Kirwadi A, et al. Thoracolumbar spine injury at CT: trauma/emergency radiology. *Radiographics*. 2016;36(7):2234–2235.

Rao S, Wasyliw C, Nunex D. Spectrum of imaging findings in hyperextension injuries of the neck. *Radiographics*. 2005;25:1239–1254.

Rao SK, Wasyliw C, Nunez DB Jr. Spectrum of imaging findings in hyperextension injuries of the neck. *Radiographics*. 2005;25(5):1239–1254.

Riascos R, Bonfante E, Cotes C, et al. Imaging of atlanto-occipital and atlantoaxial traumatic injuries: what the radiologist needs to know. *Radiographics*. 2015;35(7):2121–2134.

Rojas CA, Bertozzi JC, Martinez CR, et al. Reassessment of the craniocervical junction: normal values on CT. *AJNR Am J Neuroradiol*. 2007;28(9):1819–1823.

Rojas CA, Hayes A, Bertozzi JC, et al. Evaluation of the C1-C2 articulation on MDCT in healthy children and young adults. *AJR Am J Roentgenol*. 2009;193(5):1388–1392.

Sonin A, Manaster BJ, Andrews CL, et al. *Diagnostic Imaging: Musculoskeletal: Trauma*. Salt Lake City: Amirsys; 2010.

Wang B, Zhao CP, Song LX, et al. Balloon kyphoplasty versus percutaneous vertebroplasty for osteoporotic vertebral compression fracture: a meta-analysis and systematic review. *J Orthop Surg Res*. 2018;13(1):264.

9 Arthritis

Introduction

This chapter reviews an approach to diagnosis of arthritis based on specific imaging findings and discusses some of the arthropathies most relevant to the practicing radiologist. Many of the examples in this chapter are of advanced disease, with characteristic findings.

Joint anatomy and embryology are discussed in general in Chapter 1. Anatomy specific to each joint was reviewed in the previous chapters.

Arthropathies affect joints by a variety of mechanisms, notably autoimmune synovial inflammation in rheumatoid arthritis (RA), or by mechanical and biochemical mechanisms in osteoarthritis (OA). Mechanisms are further discussed in detail in the specific sections that follow.

Imaging Modalities

Radiographs are the primary modality for the initial assessment of a clinically suspected arthropathy. Radiographs for evaluation of arthritis typically involve multiple orthogonal and oblique views for detection of effusion and erosions. Standing views are acquired to assess alignment and joint narrowing in the weight-bearing joints.

Key Concepts

Uses of Cross-Sectional Imaging in Arthritis

Ultrasonography (US): Synovium, effusion, tendon sheaths, small joint erosions

Computed tomography (CT): Large and small joint erosions and productive change, synovium, effusion, cartilage (with arthrography)

Magnetic resonance imaging: Cartilage, synovium, tendon sheaths, effusion, erosions, earliest changes of inflammatory arthritis (including marrow edema)

The advent of more effective medications for inflammatory arthritis and advanced surgical techniques for cartilage repair often requires more detailed assessment of bone, cartilage, and synovium than can be provided by radiographs. Cross-sectional imaging, especially with ultrasound (US) and magnetic resonance imaging (MRI), is now commonly used in making a definitive diagnosis and planning and monitoring therapy.

- US and MRI can detect effusion, synovial proliferation, erosions, and periarticular disease such as tenosynovitis.
- MRI assesses articular cartilage degeneration and loss, intraarticular bodies, ligament and fibrocartilage tear, marrow signal alteration, and periarticular disease.
- US can assess articular cartilage at some sites, for example, metacarpal heads.
- Power and color Doppler US and MRI with IV contrast can roughly gauge the degree of synovial inflammation. This is useful both for initial diagnosis and monitoring of drug efficacy.
  - Disease-modifying antirheumatic drugs (DMARDs) including immune-modifying 'biologic' medications are often started before any imaging is obtained, with the goal of articular cartilage preservation. Because articular cartilage damage can continue even with an apparent good clinical response, sensitive disease monitoring is needed to optimize dosage of these potentially toxic drugs. US and MRI are more sensitive than radiographs and clinical exam, and thus can help to optimize dosage.
- US is used along with radiography for initial evaluation in some specialized centers.

CT is used less frequently. CT can detect and evaluate erosions, joint effusions, and soft tissue abnormalities with greater precision than radiography, but is inferior to MRI. CT can also depict articular cartilage defects and intraarticular bodies with high special resolution when using CT arthrography. Similarly, tomosynthesis can provide high-resolution images of joints in the hands and feet.

Nuclear medicine can be used to evaluate the distribution of multifocal disease. Special tracers have been developed that have some specificity for certain conditions, but are not widely used. Use of nuclear medicine to help distinguish infectious from noninfectious arthritis is discussed in Chapter 14 – Musculoskeletal Infection.

Approach to Radiographic Assessment of Arthritis

Regardless of the modality used, the first decision is whether the imaging findings in question actually represent arthritis, or some other pathology. Imaging findings suggesting a joint-centered process include effusion, synovitis, and, on MRI, adjacent marrow edema. However, these findings are not specific for arthritis and can be due to other etiologies, such as trauma.

Important considerations in evaluation of arthritis include:

- Clinical history.
- Demographics, notably age and gender of the patient.
- Location: As with both real-estate and tumor evaluation, 'location' is of prime importance in distinguishing among the arthritides. Throughout this chapter, you will find that 'location' (i.e., distribution) is stressed as a vital piece of information.
- Joint deformities.
- An important parameter in radiographic evaluation of an arthritic process is the determination of whether it is primarily erosive, productive of bone, or mixed.
  - In general, erosive arthropathies have an initial inflammatory stage that produces pannus (inflammatory granulation tissue). The pannus destroys cartilage and bone by means of lytic enzymes and by direct interference with movement of nutrients across the joint surface. Rheumatoid arthritis (RA) is an example of a purely erosive arthritic process. As shown in Fig. 9.1, the early erosions may be extremely subtle.

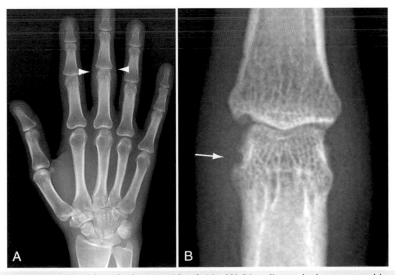

Fig. 9.1 Purely erosive arthritis: young woman with early rheumatoid arthritis. **(A)** PA radiograph shows normal bone density. The only hint of an abnormality is fusiform soft tissue swelling around the proximal interphalangeal joint of the third finger (between *arrowheads*). **(B)** Magnified view of the third proximal interphalangeal joint shows a marginal erosion *(arrow)*; the erosion is within the joint capsule, but this portion of bone is not protected by articular cartilage, thus making the erosion 'marginal'. Note that the cartilage width is not yet lost. This was the only site of erosion in this patient with early disease.

- Osteoarthritis (OA, or degenerative joint disease) is at the other end of the spectrum, with predominantly productive rather than erosive manifestations. OA also involves cartilage and subchondral bone destruction, but by a different mechanism than RA: abnormal mechanical forces combine with host reactive processes produce these changes, which include osteophyte formation, subchondral sclerosis, subchondral cysts, and cortical buttressing (Fig. 9.2).
- Most of the other arthropathies generally fall between the erosive and productive ends of the spectrum, often demonstrating both erosive and productive changes (Fig. 9.3).

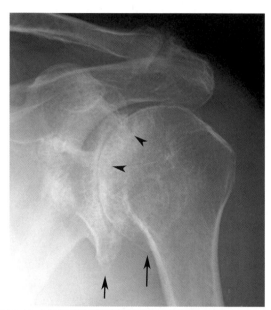

Fig. 9.2 Purely productive arthritis: osteoarthritis. AP shoulder radiograph shows osteophytes *(arrows)* and subchondral sclerosis *(arrowheads)*.

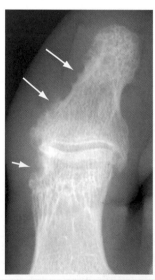

Fig. 9.3 Mixed erosive and destructive arthritis. AP radiograph of the great toe in a patient with psoriatic arthritis demonstrates erosion at the interphalangeal joint *(short arrow)* and new bone production, seen as periostitis along the shaft of the distal phalanx *(long arrows)*.

- Labs:
  - *Rheumatoid factor* (RF) refers to the presence of serum antibodies that are anti–immunoglobulin G. RF is not specific for RA but is strongly associated, especially with more severe active disease.
  - *Seronegative* specifically means normal serum RF, but the term is used more generally to refer to inflammatory arthritides that usually do not cause elevated RF, such as reactive arthritis, psoriasis, and ankylosing spondylitis (AS).
  - Specific antinuclear antibodies (ANA) are associated with lupus, scleroderma and related conditions, and mixed connective-tissue disease.

RADIOGRAPHIC ASSESSMENT OF ARTHRITIS: THE ABCDE'S

The 'ABCDE'S stand for alignment, bone, cartilage, distribution, erosions, and soft tissues. This approach dissects the often complex radiographic findings into individual components, which can make interpretation much easier. You may choose to evaluate these features in any order, as long as all are covered.

Key Concepts

Radiographic Assessment of Arthritis: The ABCDEs

Alignment: Subluxation, angulation, translocation
Bone: Density (diffuse or periarticular changes), new bone production
Cartilage: Focal defects or diffuse thinning
Distribution: Specific involved joints; region affected within a joint
Erosions: Presence and location within or around a joint
Soft tissues: Focal swelling, calcification

Alignment

Alignment deformities can occur secondary to ligamentous laxity without erosion, as in lupus or Jaccoud arthropathy. Deformities related to osteoarthritis include varus or valgus caused by asymmetric cartilage wear. Classic alignment deformities of RA include the *swan neck* and *boutonnière* deformities of the fingers, volar subluxation and ulnar deviation at the metacarpophalangeal (MCP) joints, and deformities related to severe erosion (see Table 9.1).

Bone

This refers to bone density. Inflammation and associated hyperemia induce osteoclast activation with bone resorption, which can be periarticular or regional (Fig. 9.4A). The pattern of osteopenia reflects the pattern of active inflammation in inflammatory arthropathies. Periarticular osteopenia can be extremely subtle and may not be observable in the earliest disease process (see Fig. 9.1A). Remember also that osteopenia must be interpreted in the context of the patient age, gender, and general condition. Thus the osteopenia seen in Fig. 9.4A would not be surprising in a 70-year-old woman but is distinctly abnormal in a 45-year-old man.

Bone density may become locally increased in reactive, reparative processes. Classic examples are subchondral sclerosis and osteophyte formation in osteoarthritis.

Table 9.1 Joint Deformity Associations

Joint Deformity	Main Differential Diagnosis
Windswept digits	RA
Ulnar translocation	RA
Carpal collapse	RA, SLAC
Boutonnière	RA
Swan neck	RA
Arthritis mutilans	RA, gout, psoriatic, reactive arthritis, neuropathic
Talar (tibial) tilt	Hemophilia
Protrusio acetabuli	RA, particle disease, bone softening disorders (e.g., osteomalacia, Paget's)
Arch collapse at the foot (rocker bottom)	Neuropathic, PTT dysfunction
Atlantoaxial instability	RA, ankylosing spondylitis, spondyloepiphyseal dysplasias, Down syndrome
Segmental instability of the spine	Paralysis, fusion above or below, interspinous ligament injury, facet arthropathy, amyloid, prior discitis, pars defect, neuropathic
Varus/valgus in extremities	RA, severe OA
Subluxation in extremities	RA, severe OA, SLE, miscellaneous inflammatory arthropathies, neuropathic

Abbreviations: OA, osteoarthritis; PTT, posterior tibial tendon; RA, rheumatoid arthritis; SLAC, scapholunate advanced collapse; SLE, systemic lupus erythematosus.

Enthesophyte, a late consequence of enthesial inflammation, refers to new bone formation at an enthesis (site of tendon or ligament attachment to bone). Large, bulky enthesophytes are associated with reactive arthritis, psoriasis, and diffuse idiopathic skeletal hyperostosis. Delicate ossifications of annular disc and spinal ligament fibers are termed *syndesmophytes* and are a classic finding in AS.

Cartilage

Hyaline (articular) cartilage destruction causes joint space narrowing (Fig. 9.5) (Table 9.2). In inflammatory arthritis, pannus produces proteolytic enzymes and interferes with nutrient diffusion, causing uniform cartilage loss throughout the joint. In noninflammatory arthritis, especially osteoarthritis, cartilage loss occurs along lines of force and thus tends to be asymmetrically greater at load-bearing surfaces.

Some arthritides are associated with preservation of articular cartilage, at least until late in the disease (Table 9.3).

Ankylosis is fibrous, cartilaginous, or osseous fusion across a joint (Table 9.4). Ankylosis is associated with AS (sacroiliac [SI] joints and spine), late-stage juvenile idiopathic arthritis (wrists and cervical facet joints), reactive arthritis and psoriasis (hand), end-stage RA (wrist), and can be seen following any process that completely destroys a joint's cartilage. Ankylosis in the hand is most often caused by trauma, infection, or seronegative spondyloarthropathy.

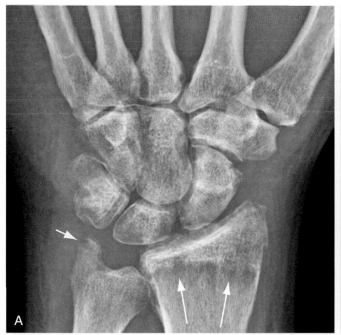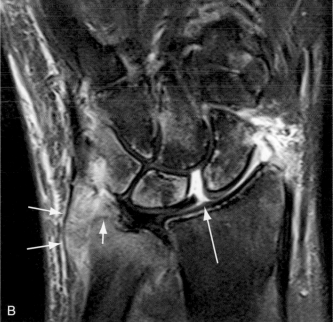

Fig. 9.4 Early changes of rheumatoid arthritis in a young adult, confirmed by MRI. **(A)** PA view of the wrist shows soft tissue swelling over the ulnar styloid *(short arrow)*. There is demineralization of the ulnar styloid (loss of the normally sharp cortex), as well as multiple other bones of the carpus. Note demineralization along the distal radial physeal scar *(long arrows)*. **(B)** Coronal fat-saturated T2-weighted MR image, same wrist, shows marrow edema in multiple carpal bones, particularly the lunate and triquetrum, as well as the distal ulna. There is pannus overlying the ulnar styloid *(midlength arrows)*. There is a true erosion at the ulnar styloid *(short arrow)*. The scapholunate ligament is disrupted *(long arrow)*. Despite minimal erosive change, the MR appearance is typical of (and was proven to be) rheumatoid arthritis.

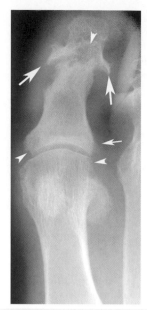

Fig. 9.5 Cartilage destruction in mixed erosive and destructive disease. AP radiograph of the great toe in a middle-aged man with psoriatic arthritis shows multiple erosions *(arrowheads)*, new bone production *(arrows)*, and complete cartilage destruction in the interphalangeal joint.

Table 9.2   Typical Patterns of Joint Narrowing and Main Differential Diagnosis

Pattern	Main Differential Diagnosis
Diffuse within joint	Rheumatoid arthritis
	Septic arthritis
	Psoriatic arthritis/reactive arthritis
	Gout
	Hemophilia
	Neuropathic disease
	OA (small joints)
	PVNS
	Synovial osteochondromatosis (late)
	Thermal injury
Asymmetric within joint	OA (weight-bearing joints or due to injury)

Abbreviations: OA, osteoarthritis; PVNS, pigmented villonodular synovitis.

Table 9.3   Arthritis With Preserved Joint Space

Amyloid
Gout
Infection with low-virulence organisms (fungus, tuberculosis)
Early bacterial infection
Any arthritis in early stages

Distribution

Distribution of disease is an essential factor when considering the differential diagnosis of an uncharacterized arthropathy (Table 9.5). Arthritis may be *monoarticular* (one joint involved), *oligoarticular* (just a few joints), or *polyarticular* (multiple joints). Polyarticular disease virtually excludes infection because septic arthritis usually is a monoarticular disease and only rarely is oligoarticular.

Table 9.4   Causes of Ankylosis

Developmental fusion (coalition)
Surgical fusion
Ankylosing spondylitis/IBD (spine, SI joints)
Juvenile idiopathic arthritis
Rheumatoid arthritis (uncommon)
Psoriatic arthritis/reactive arthritis
Erosive osteoarthritis (digits)
Severe degenerative disc disease (spine)
DISH (spine)
Thermal/electrical injury
Septic arthritis (end stage)
Heterotopic ossification/fibrodysplasia ossificans progressiva

Abbreviations: DISH, diffuse idiopathic skeletal hyperostosis; IBD, inflammatory bowel disease; SI, sacroiliac.

Table 9.5   Distribution of Common Arthropathies

Primary OA: First CMC, STT, IPs, weight-bearing joints, first MTP, spine
Bilateral asymmetric
RA: Carpus, MCPs, MTPs (esp. fifth), elbow, shoulders, C-spine, knees, hips, ankles
Bilateral symmetric
Psoriatic arthritis: IPs, MCPs, MTPs, SI joints
Bilateral asymmetric
Reactive arthritis: IPs (feet), MTPs, SI joints
Bilateral asymmetric
Ankylosing spondylitis: L > T > C-spine, SI joints, hips
Bilateral symmetric
Gout: First IP (foot), first MTP, Lisfranc, various hand/wrist joints
Bilateral asymmetric
Neuropathic osteoarthropathy (related to diabetes):
Lisfranc, hindfoot, MTPs
Unilateral or bilateral asymmetric
Hemophilia:
weight-bearing joints; ankles, knees
Bilateral symmetric
Scattered traumatized upper extremity joints
Unilateral or bilateral asymmetric
Juvenile idiopathic arthritis: knees, hips, ankles, wrists
Bilateral symmetric (if polyarticular)
Typically monoarticular
Septic arthritis
Secondary OA (e.g., post-traumatic)
Synovial osteochondromatosis
PVNS

Abbreviations: CMC, carpometacarpal; IP, interphalangeal; MCP, metacarpophalangeal; MTP, metatarsophalangeal; OA, osteoarthritis; PVNS, pigmented villonodular synovitis; RA, rheumatoid arthritis; SI, sacroiliac STT, scaphoid-trapezoid-trapezium.

Monoarticular and oligoarticular involvement are unusual for RA except in very early cases but are more typical of seronegative arthritis, infection, pigmented villonodular synovitis, synovial chondromatosis, crystal deposition disease, and hemophilic arthropathy.

Although it sometimes is important to provide a catalogue of specific joints involved in oligoarticular and polyarticular disease, more generalized terms are helpful in describing the pattern of distribution. Arthritis is judged to be *symmetric* versus *asymmetric* with regard to the contralateral side. (Note that it is not the specific interphalangeal [IP] or metacarpal joints that shows symmetry—i.e., not mirror image symmetry, but rather the set of joints on the right versus the left side.) Also, symmetry indicates involvement but not extent of disease. Symmetry favors RA and calcium pyrophosphate deposition disease (CPPD). Asymmetry can be seen in osteoarthritis, seronegative spondyloarthropathies, and gout, although these can be symmetric as well.

Arthritis in the hands and feet can occur in a *distal* (involves the distal interphalangeal [DIP] and proximal interphalangeal [PIP] joints) or *proximal* (MCP and wrist) distribution. Proximal disease favors RA. Distal and first-ray disease favors osteoarthritis (and gout in the foot). Either pattern can be seen with seronegative arthritis. Distal inflammatory disease favors seronegative arthritis.

Some arthritides may primarily involve the axial skeleton. *Spondyloarthropathy* means arthritis with spine involvement. Symmetric SI joint disease favors AS or inflammatory bowel disease (IBD) associated arthropathy. Reactive arthritis and psoriatic arthritis may have symmetric or asymmetric SI joint involvement. RA rarely involves the SI joints, in which case it is usually symmetric. AS tends to ascend the spine continuously, especially in males. Reactive arthritis and psoriatic arthritis often skip levels. Involvement of the vertebral body "corners" at the insertion of disc annular fibers indicates enthesitis, which excludes RA.

Within a particular joint, findings can be symmetric/uniform in distribution, or they can mainly involve one side of the joint (eccentric). Arthropathies associated with synovial proliferation (i.e., RA) usually result in uniform involvement (symmetric erosions, diffuse cartilage loss, diffuse soft tissue swelling), whereas degenerative arthritis typically involves one aspect of the joint more severely—especially in larger or weight-bearing joints. Extraarticular pathology, notably soft tissue tophi in gout, can also result in eccentric erosion and swelling at a joint.

Erosions

Erosion is focal cortical and subcortical bone loss. Erosions are classified as marginal, nonmarginal (or periarticular), and subchondral (Table 9.6).

Marginal erosions occur along the periphery of the joint space in 'bare areas' of bone that are within the joint capsule but are not protected by articular cartilage (see Fig. 9.1B). Marginal erosions occur in inflammatory arthritis. The borders of acute or active erosions are indistinct. One must look at the edges of erosions for evidence of bone proliferation because such production, as well as capsular enthesophytes and periostitis, is associated with seronegative arthropathy (see Fig. 9.3).

Nonmarginal or *periarticular erosions* are further removed from the joint margin and usually show sharp borders with overhanging edges. These erosions are associated with crystal deposition diseases.

Table 9.6 Erosion Location and DDx

Central	EOA
	Thermal injury
	Psoriasis (late)
	Reactive arthritis (late)
Marginal	Rheumatoid arthritis
	Psoriatic arthritis (proliferative)
	Reactive arthritis (proliferative)
	Gout
Periarticular	Gout

Abbreviation: DDx, differential diagnosis; EOA, erosive osteoarthritis.

Subchondral erosions occur in the central aspect of the joint and can overlap in appearance with subchondral cysts of osteoarthritis. Subchondral erosions can be caused by inflammatory or noninflammatory joint disease. Subchondral cysts caused by inflammatory joint disease are a result of pannus intrusion in subchondral bone. Subchondral cysts caused by noninflammatory joint disease are a result of liquefaction of subchondral bone following necrosis, or synovial intrusion at joint surfaces worn down to bone. (In general, subchondral cysts precede subsequent full-thickness loss of overlying articular cartilage.) Sharp, sclerotic borders suggest a noninflammatory process or an inactive chronic inflammatory process.

The *pencil-in-cup deformity* of psoriatic arthritis is an example of extreme bone erosion and remodeling. Note this deformity can be seen in other inflammatory arthritides.

Soft Tissues

Focal soft tissue swelling on X-ray is often the initial indicator of an early arthritis (see Figs. 9.1A and 9.4A) (Table 9.7). Fusiform swelling (diffuse swelling around a joint) is an indicator of inflammatory synovitis or effusion. This is the pattern most associated with RA and septic arthritis. Diffuse swelling (e.g., involving an entire digit) suggests inflammation beyond the joint, typically in a flexor tendon sheath, as can occur in psoriatic arthritis and reactive arthritis. Tophaceous deposits in gout tend to be eccentric and near, but not at, the joint. Thus soft tissue swelling caused by gout tends to be eccentric and 'lumpy-bumpy' in appearance rather than fusiform. This matches the nonmarginal pattern of erosions associated with gout.

Periarticular soft tissue calcification may be caused by crystals, enthesophytes, and dystrophic and vascular calcifications (Table 9.8). Tophaceous urate deposits in gout tend to be radiographically dense, though less dense than calcium. Calcium hydroxyapatite deposits (HADD,

Table 9.7 Causes of Soft Tissue Swelling in Arthritis on X-ray

Joint effusion
Synovial proliferation
Ganglion cyst
Soft tissue edema
Tenosynovitis
Bursitis
Deposition of amyloid, calcium, crystals, or other material

Table 9.8 Soft tissue Calcification/Ossification and Associations

Radiographic Finding	Disease/Association
Cloudlike calcification; calcific tendinosis/bursitis	HADD
Chondrocalcinosis; calcification in hyaline/fibrocartilage	CPPD arthropathy Gout Diabetes Renal failure Hemochromatosis Wilson's disease
Cloudlike calcification around joints	Renal failure; tumoral calcinosis Hypervitaminosis D
Vascular: arterial; linear calcification	Diabetes Renal failure
Vascular: round ossifications; venous	Phleboliths; hemangioma
Connective tissues; sharp soft tissue calcification	Scleroderma Dermatomyositis Mixed connective-tissue disease Hypervitaminosis D
Neural; linear calcification within nerves	Leprosy; neuropathic disease
Tumor: calcified mass	Synovial sarcoma, liposarcoma
Infection with calcification	Tuberculosis Cysticercosis (muscle) Echinococcus
Heterotopic ossification; soft tissue	Paralysis Injury Surgery
Myositis ossificans; muscle	Injury; hematoma
Tendon/ligament ossification	Healed tear Fibrodysplasia ossificans progressiva

Abbreviations: CPPD, calcium pyrophosphate deposition disease; HADD, hydroxyapatite deposition disease.

hydroxyapatite deposition disease) occur in tendons, bursae, and pericapsular locations. These tend to be uniformly dense and amorphous. Crystals of calcium pyrophosphate dihydrate (CPPD) are seen as fine linear or stippled deposits in articular cartilage, capsule, synovium, and entheses.

DEMOGRAPHICS

Gender and age are also important when considering a differential diagnosis for an arthropathy (Table 9.9). For example, RA is more common in females while AS, hemophilia, and reactive arthritis are male-dominated. Most inflammatory arthropathies are active in younger people in their 20s to 40s. In older age the arthritis often becomes quiescent, and secondary osteoarthritis develops. Pigmented villonodular synovitis (PVNS), hemophilia, and synovial osteochondromatosis are also diseases of young patients (discussed in more detail later in the chapter). Osteoarthritis and crystal-associated disorders are generally seen in older individuals.

Finally, be aware that a patient may have two types of arthritis. This can manifest as established osteoarthritis with superimposed new inflammatory arthritis, or chronic inflammatory arthritis with secondary osteoarthritis. Do not hesitate to offer two diagnoses in these cases.

Table 9.9 Gender and Age in Arthropathies

AGE	
Children	Juvenile idiopathic arthritis
Adults	Rheumatoid arthritis Psoriatic arthritis Reactive arthritis Pigmented villonodular synovitis Synovial osteochondromatosis
Older adults	Gout Osteoarthritis Erosive osteoarthritis CPPD
GENDER	
Male	Ankylosing spondylitis Gout Reactive arthritis
Female	Rheumatoid arthritis Connective-tissue disease

Abbreviation: CPPD, calcium pyrophosphate deposition disease.

Imaging Characteristics of Specific Diseases

For simplicity, diseases will be categorized into degenerative processes, inflammatory arthropathies, connective-tissue diseases, crystalline disorders, metabolic conditions, noninflammatory monoarticular diseases, and miscellaneous diseases affecting joints.

Degenerative Disease

OSTEOARTHRITIS

- Osteoarthritis (OA) is by far the most common arthropathy and the most common cause of disability among older adults in the United States.
- The condition may be primary or secondary.
  - *Secondary OA* can be caused by abnormal mechanical forces (joint deformity, obesity, instability, impingement, altered biomechanics) or as an end-stage consequence of a preceding joint insult, such as an trauma, chronic inflammatory arthritis, or infection.
  - *Primary OA* presents without such antecedent insult. Primary OA is less common and may be caused by a genetic defect in articular cartilage synthesis.
- Articular cartilage is one of the few tissues of the musculoskeletal system that is incapable of regeneration.
- Damaged cartilage inadequately cushions the subchondral bone, which results in adaptive changes including osteophyte formation with subchondral fibrosis, necrosis, and sclerosis.
- Subchondral cysts form, which are often associated with an overlying cartilage defect or fissuring.
- Adaptive remodeling of subchondral bone may lead to articular surface or joint alignment deformity; associated ligament damage contributes to instability further accelerating the degenerative process.

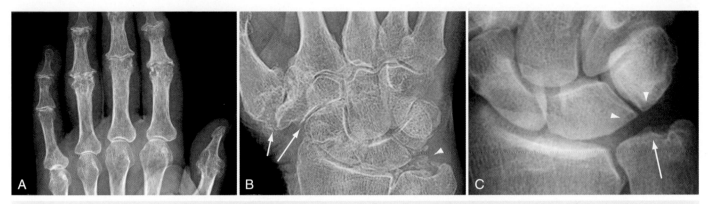

Fig. 9.6 Osteoarthritis: hand and wrist. **(A)** PA radiograph demonstrates the typical appearance of osteoarthritis of the hand, with normal bone density and loss of cartilage width in the presence of osteophyte formation in the distal interphalangeal and proximal interphalangeal joints. **(B)** Wrist in the same patient shows severe cartilage loss, osteophyte formation, and mild subluxation of the first carpometacarpal joint *(short arrow)*. In addition, the scapho-trapezio-trapezoid joint shows sclerosis and cartilage loss *(long arrow)*. These are the classic sites of involvement of osteoarthritis (OA) of the wrist. Note that there is chondrocalcinosis at the triangular fibrocartilage *(arrowhead)*; this may be seen in posttraumatic and OA cases and does not require consideration of the diagnosis of pyrophosphate arthropathy. **(C)** Secondary OA of the lunate and triquetrum, manifested as osteophytes *(arrowheads)*, caused by ulnar positive variance *(arrow)* and resultant ulnar abutment.

- In addition to these mechanisms of cartilage destruction, synovial fluid biochemistry is altered in OA, with elevated catabolic factors.
- Because OA is not primarily an inflammatory process, some authors use the synonymous term *osteoarthrosis*.

Imaging Characteristics

- On imaging, both primary and secondary osteoarthritis are defined by the hallmarks of *osteophytes*, *joint narrowing*, *subchondral cysts*, and *subchondral sclerosis* (Figs. 9.6 through 9.8).
  - However, these hallmarks individually are not specific for OA.
- In weight-bearing joints, distribution of joint narrowing typically reflects the line of force (e.g., superior joint narrowing at the hip [Figs. 9.8 and 9.9A,B], medial compartment narrowing at the knee).

- Patients with acromegaly experience premature primary osteoarthritis related to lack of nutrition of abnormally thickened cartilage. Similarly, paralyzed patients often acquire degenerated joints, which may result from chondrolysis or decreased diffusion of nutrient-supplying synovial fluid into the hyaline cartilage.
- Patients with joint deformity (e.g., related to epiphyseal dysplasia or Legg-Calvé-Perthes disease) are also more susceptible to hyaline cartilage wear.
- Secondary osteoarthritis is seen as a delayed consequence of some joint insult. This includes diverse mechanisms such as:
  - Altered biomechanics (e.g., acetabular dysplasia or femoroacetabular impingement [FAI] in the hip).
  - Instability (e.g., ACL or meniscal tear in the knee; glenoid labral tear in the shoulder) (Figs. 9.9 and 9.10).

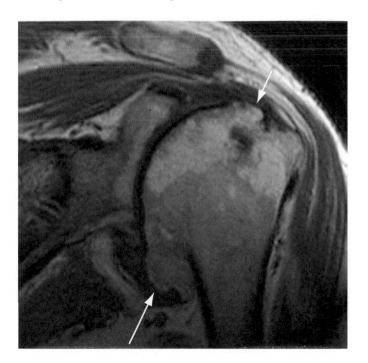

Fig. 9.7 Osteoarthritis: shoulder. T1-weighted MR image shows a huge ring osteophyte surrounding the margin of the humeral head, superiorly at the junction of the head with the tuberosities *(short arrow)* and inferiorly *(long arrow)*. In this example the arthritis is secondary to joint instability related to glenoid labral tear. The inferior osteophyte may act as a mass lesion within the quadrilateral space, with encroachment on the axillary nerve. Note also that the glenoid is enlarged and broadened, often seen in long-term osteoarthritis of the shoulder.

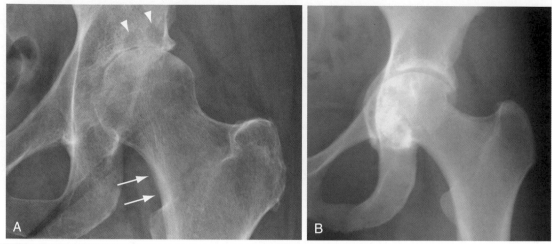

Fig. 9.8 Osteoarthritis: hip. **(A)** AP radiograph demonstrates typical osteoarthritis with loss of cartilage width at the superior, weight-bearing portion of the hip, osteophyte formation, normal bone density, and subchondral cysts in the acetabular roof *(arrowheads)*. Also note the calcar buttressing (thick cortex of the medial femoral neck cortex; *arrows*). Distribution of cartilage loss reflects OA secondary to a mechanical disturbance, in this case likely related to underlying acetabular labral tear. **(B)** Different patient with osteoarthritis. Osteophytes are present, but in this example there is diffuse joint narrowing. This is often secondary to underlying inflammatory arthropathy such as rheumatoid arthritis, resulting in uniform cartilage loss. Protrusio acetabuli develops in some of these cases because of bone remodeling. (Image used with permission from BJ Manaster, MD, from the American College of Radiology Learning File.)

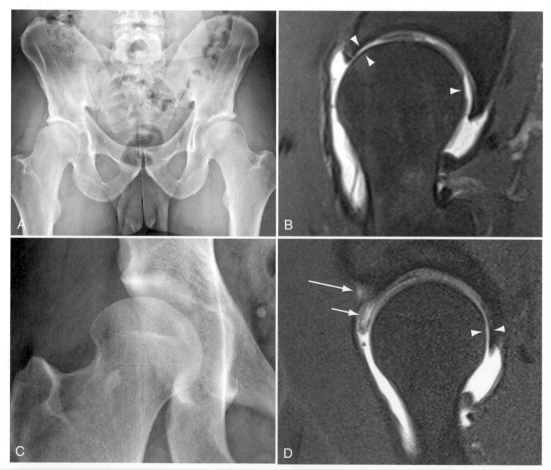

Fig. 9.9 Osteoarthritis: hip. **(A)** AP radiograph of the pelvis in a 41-year-old with right hip pain. There is mild superior joint narrowing at the right hip compared to the left. **(B)** Oblique sagittal T1-weighted fat-suppressed arthrogram image of the right hip in the same patient, showing regions of femoral head and acetabular high-grade cartilage loss *(arrowheads)* representing osteoarthritis. **(C)** AP radiograph of the right hip of a 22-year-old with right hip pain shows acetabular dysplasia, with undercovering of the lateral femoral head. Hip dysplasia is associated with hyperplasia of the acetabular labrum and tears associated with increased shear forces. **(D)** Sagittal T1-weighted fat-suppressed gadolinium arthrogram in the same patient shows the torn, hypertrophied labrum *(short arrow)* with a small paralabral cyst that is partially filled with gadolinium contrast *(long arrow)*. There is posterior cartilage thinning *(arrowheads)*; other planes showed other sites of cartilage destruction. Hip dysplasia (acetabular undercoverage) is a recognized cause of secondary, early-onset OA.

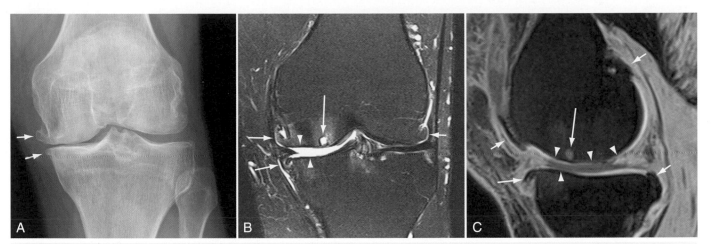

Fig. 9.10 Osteoarthritis: knee. **(A)** AP left knee radiograph shows osteophytes *(arrows)* and medial compartment joint narrowing. **(B and C)** MR images in the same knee. Coronal fat-suppressed proton density–weighted **(B)** and sagittal fat-suppressed spoiled gradient echo **(C)** images show low-signal osteophytes *(short arrows)*, large high-grade chondral defects *(arrowheads)*, and a subchondral cyst in the medial femoral condyle *(long arrow)*, related to chronic meniscal tear with extrusion.

- Articular incongruity (e.g., intraarticular fracture with malunion and articular step-off; osteonecrosis/avascular necrosis (AVN) with articular surface collapse; developmental deformity such as hip dysplasia; progressive deformity of bone such as with Paget disease; malalignment such as scapholunate advanced collapse of the wrist).
- Cartilage destruction (e.g., septic arthritis, RA, or hemophilia with primary chondrolysis and subsequent OA) (see Fig. 9.8B). Secondary OA due to cartilage destruction may cause confusion since there will be signs of the primary process as well as the hallmarks of osteoarthritis. A common example is chronic RA, with marginal erosions and diffuse joint narrowing due to hyaline cartilage destruction, with superimposed osteophytes.
- Ganglion cysts often arise from degenerated joints, especially at the knee. Lobulated fluid is seen with a narrow neck extending to the synovium or adjacent sheath.
  - Ganglion cysts may become complex if they contain synovial proliferation (e.g., in rheumatoid arthritis) or if they are traumatized (e.g., at the foot/ankle), and as a result may resemble a neoplasm. Ganglion cysts are usually lobulated and most tumors are not. Definitively demonstrating communication of a cyst with a joint or tendon sheath can help exclude tumor.

Treatment

- Management of osteoarthritis is based on conservative or invasive measures, depending on the degree of symptoms and exam findings.
- Medications including nonsteroidal anti-inflammatory drugs (NSAIDs).
- Injection of corticosteroid, stem cells, platelet-rich plasminogen (PRP), and viscosupplementation.
- Subchondral bone substitute material injection (subchondroplasty).
- Surgery:
  - Numerous options, including from arthroscopic surgery to trim fibrocartilage/remove bodies, to high

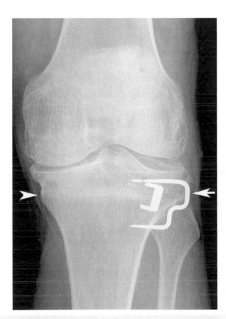

Fig. 9.11 High tibial osteotomy for knee osteoarthritis. This patient has severe medial compartment knee osteoarthritis. A wedge of bone was removed from the proximal tibia. The apex of the wedge was at the medial cortex *(arrowhead)*. After the wedge of bone was removed, the defect was closed, correcting varus malalignment. The osteotomy is fixed with two lateral staples. Note the Coventry staple *(arrow)*, which matches the step-off of the lateral tibial cortex created by the osteotomy. This procedure rebalances forces across the knee, delaying or sometimes avoiding the need for arthroplasty.

tibial osteotomy (in the knee), to joint fusion/removal/replacement (Fig. 9.11).
- Some advanced techniques such as osteochondral transfer are discussed in Chapter 1.
- Some painful, arthritic joints can be removed (e.g., the acromioclavicular joint).
- Large joints are typically replaced (i.e., hip, knee, shoulder, elbow).

Key Concepts

Causes of secondary OA

Joint incongruity/altered biomechanics
Internal derangement/instability (e.g., meniscal tear, ACL tear)
Intraarticular fracture
Paget disease
Developmental deformity
Osteonecrosis with collapse
Articular Cartilage destruction
    Septic arthritis
    Noninfectious inflammatory arthropathies (e.g., RA)
    Hemophilia
    Crystalline arthropathies (Gout, CPPD arthropathy)
    PVNS
    Synovial osteochondromatosis

MRI Protocol for Articular Cartilage

- Detecting hyaline cartilage defects can be a challenge in certain joints even with high-field MRI.
- Low-field scanners are at a great disadvantage due to low resolution, signal, and limited fat suppression.
- Cartilage is bright on fast spin-echo sequences with echo times (TEs) below 60 ms in which fat suppression is used. (Without fat suppression, or with high TEs, hyaline cartilage appears intermediate to dark). Optimized imaging uses sequences with high resolution and signal-to-noise ratio (SNR), with sufficient contrast between joint fluid and cartilage. Here are some techniques to help acquire diagnostic-quality cartilage imaging:
  - On high-field scanners the most common sequences used are proton density (PD) or T2-weighted sequences with fat suppression and 2D or 3D fat-suppressed T1-weighted spoiled gradient echo (GRE) sequences.
  - A cartilage-sensitive fat-suppressed PD or intermediate sequence should optimally have a TE of around 30–50 ms, in order to increase SNR while retaining high fluid conspicuity.
  - A GRE gradient echo sequence can be acquired with a flip angle of 40–60 degrees, using the same value for TR (40–60 ms) and minimum TE, combined with fat suppression; this yields a T1-weighted sequence in which cartilage is bright and fluid is dark.
  - Another popular gradient echo sequence is a fat-suppressed 3D gradient recalled with RF or gradient spoiling (called FSSPGR in GE scanners, FLASH in Siemens, FFE in Phillips, Field Echo in Toshiba).
  - Many sequences are sensitive for cartilage loss but the fat-suppressed PD sequence is the most versatile, also useful for ligaments, tendons, and marrow. GRE sequences can offer higher spatial resolution that is very useful in situations where cartilage is thin or the joint is small, for instance in the wrist and elbow.
  - Intraarticular contrast can be useful to demonstrate cartilage defects, using fat-suppressed T1-weighted images. Additionally, damaged cartilage may 'imbibe' (absorb) gadolinium.
- Various other MR sequences are useful in detection of cartilage defects. 3D acquisition techniques allow multiplanar reformats in a variety of planes, an advantage when evaluating curved joint surfaces. Other sequences that perform well in cartilage evaluation generally involve steady-state GRE and hybrid techniques; nomenclature is vendor specific.
- Physiological imaging techniques including T2-mapping, T1-rho imaging, spectroscopy, and delayed contrast-enhanced MRI of cartilage (dGEMRIC) can be used to map areas of dehydration and proteoglycan depletion indicative of early cartilage degeneration. T2 mapping is expanding slowly from the research realm into clinical imaging, but whether this will improve patient management or outcomes has not been determined.
- CT arthrography demonstrates defects with high contrast and spatial resolution.

Reporting Osteoarthritis and Articular Cartilage Findings

- The *Kellgren and Lawrence system* grades knee OA based on radiographic findings of joint space narrowing, osteophytes, and subchondral sclerosis.
  - This system was developed before MRI and is limited by imprecise terminology and the inherent limitations of radiographs in assessing cartilage defects.
  - Also, the radiographic severity of disease does not always correlate with the degree of pain.
  - Because of these limitations, more precise and reproducible MRI-based evaluation is preferred in current arthritis research as well as for clinical decision-making.
- The radiologist interpreting MRI should use a common language with referring clinicians, and strive to be accurate and precise in describing cartilage damage (Fig. 9.12). A commonly used grading system in the orthopedic nomenclature is the Outerbridge system, which dates back to the late 1950s, subsequently modified in 1975 (Table 9.10).
  - The system was based on probing of the cartilage surface at surgery: grade 1 is cartilage softening; grade 2 is a cartilage defect smaller than ½ inch wide (the width of the probe end); grade 3 is a defect greater than or equal to ½ inch wide; and grade 4 is a full-thickness defect with exposed bone.
  - This system is awkward to apply to MRI since there is usually a combination of grades present, and the surgical grading is based on surface analysis.
- Other classification systems have subsequently been developed (see Table 9.10).
- The commonly used term *chondromalacia* (meaning 'cartilage softening') is particularly vague and the authors do not use this term in MRI reports.
- The most useful method for characterizing cartilage loss is to describe the location, size, and depth of cartilage defects seen.
- Cartilage loss can be divided into diffuse and focal lesions (Fig. 9.13). Some useful descriptors are listed in the following text (Table 9.11).
- *Bone marrow edema lesions* (BMLs):
  - Areas of T2-hyperintensity in the subchondral bone related to cartilage damage and are thought to represent microtrabecular fracture (Fig. 9.14).

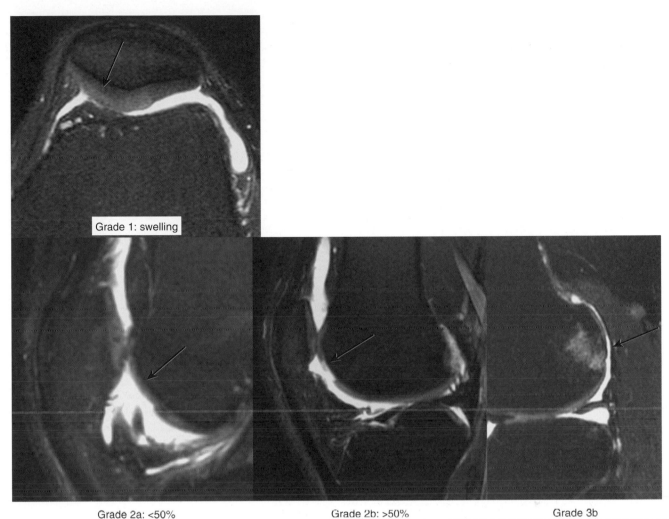

Fig. 9.12 Chondrosis of the knee. Examples of different grades of cartilage damage using the Noyes classification system (see Table 9.10) (From Morrison W. *Problem Solving in Musculoskeletal Imaging.* Philadelphia: Elsevier; 2010.)

Table 9.10 MRI Articular Cartilage Defect Classification Systems

MODIFIED NOYES

Grade 0: normal cartilage

Grade 1: increased T2 signal intensity of morphologically normal cartilage

Grade 2a: superficial partial-thickness cartilage defect <50% of total articular surface thickness

Grade 2b: deep partial-thickness cartilage defect >50% of total articular surface thickness

Grade 3: full-thickness cartilage defect

ICRS (INTERNATIONAL CARTILAGE REGENERATION AND JOINT PRESERVATION SOCIETY)

Grade 0: normal

Grade 1: Cartilage edema and superficial defects

Grade 2: Defects extending down to <50% of cartilage depth

Grade 3: Cartilage defects extending down >50% of cartilage depth but not full thickness

Grade 4: Full thickness defects with exposed subchondral bone

- BMLs generally correlate with pain.
- Should be included in the report.
- Cartilage flaps and delamination deserve special consideration. These represent unstable cartilage lesions and should be described separately.
  - A *cartilage flap* is an oblique linear defect (see Fig. 9.13), causing the fragment to be potentially mobile; this can result in pain and locking, and the fragment can break off to form a loose body.
  - *Delamination* is separation of the hyaline cartilage from underlying bone (Figs. 9.15 and 9.16). Fluid enters the gap, making it visible on T2-weighted images. These lesions may not be observed on arthroscopy. These lesions can progress to cartilage flaps and high-grade defects.
- Subchondral cyst formation, typically a progression from BMLs (Fig. 9.17).
- Cartilage lesions almost always progress but occasionally spontaneously fill in with dark fibrocartilage or bone, with the latter forming flat spurs on the articular surface termed *central osteophytes* or *subchondral* or *button osteophytes* (Fig. 9.18).

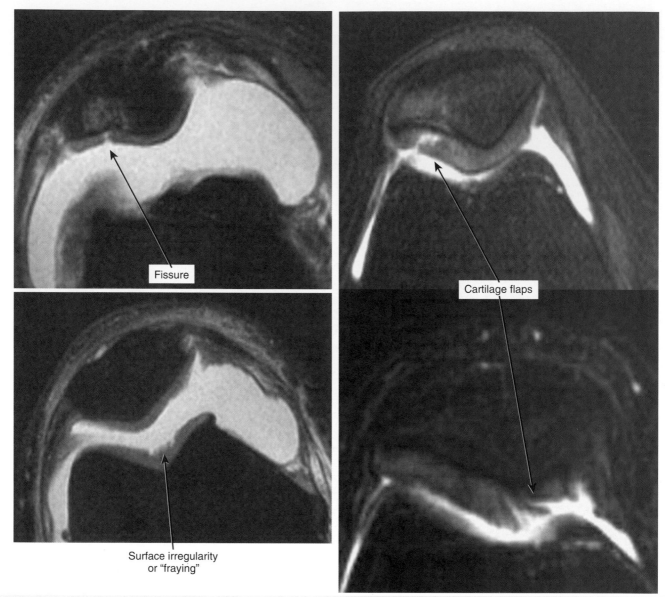

Fissure

Cartilage flaps

Surface irregularity
or "fraying"

Fig. 9.13 Cartilage abnormalities on MRI: Fissures, flaps and fraying (surface irregularity). (From Morrison W. *Problem Solving in Musculoskeletal Imaging.* Philadelphia: Elsevier; 2010.)

Table 9.11   Useful Cartilage Descriptors on MRI

DIFFUSE

Diffuse cartilage thinning

Diffuse surface irregularity/fraying

Diffuse low-grade partial-thickness cartilage loss

Diffuse high-grade partial-thickness cartilage loss

Full-thickness cartilage denudation

FOCAL

Fissuring (vertical linear defect)

Flap (oblique linear defect)

Delamination (fluid underneath cartilage; separation of cartilage from bone)

Partial-thickness defect (some cartilage remaining); measure size and determine low-grade (<50%) or high-grade (>50%)

Full-thickness defect (no cartilage remaining with exposed subchondral bone); measure size

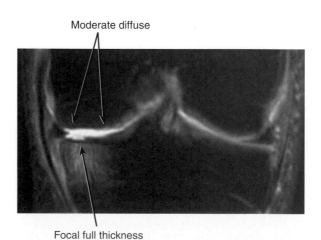

Moderate diffuse

Focal full thickness

Fig. 9.14 Cartilage descriptors. (From Morrison W. *Problem Solving in Musculoskeletal Imaging.* Philadelphia: Elsevier; 2010.)

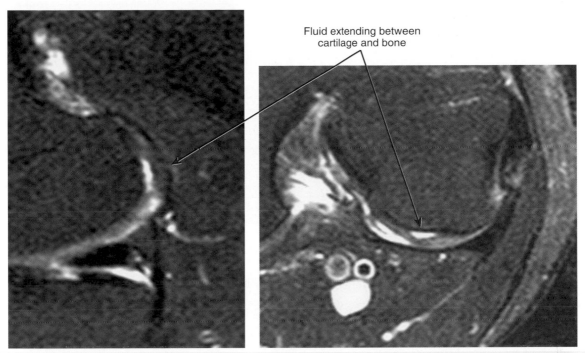

Fluid extending between
cartilage and bone

Fig. 9.15 Delamination is separation of the hyaline cartilage from underlying bone. Fluid undermines the cartilage, and although the lesion may not be observed on arthroscopy, the 'bubble' of fluid can propagate and form a flap. (From Morrison W. *Problem Solving in Musculoskeletal Imaging.* Philadelphia: Elsevier; 2010.)

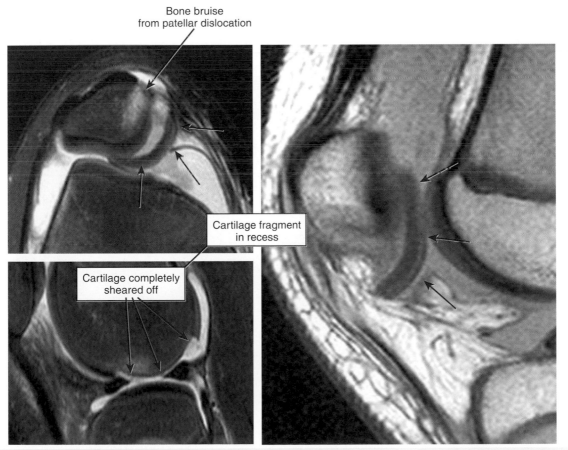

Bone bruise
from patellar dislocation

Cartilage fragment
in recess

Cartilage completely
sheared off

Fig. 9.16 Acute cartilage delamination in a 13-year-old boy following patellar dislocation. (From Morrison W. *Problem Solving in Musculoskeletal Imaging.* Philadelphia: Elsevier; 2010.)

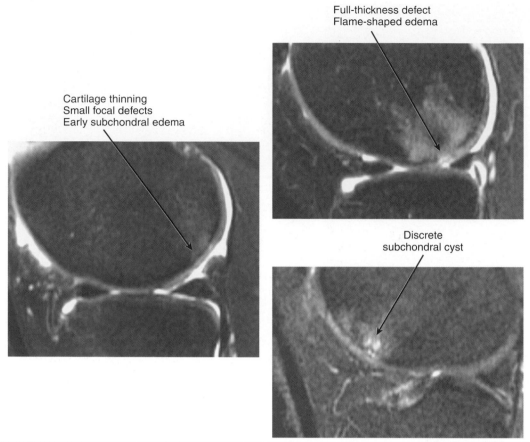

Fig. 9.17 Subchondral changes associated with cartilage lesions of different stages. (From Morrison W. *Problem Solving in Musculoskeletal Imaging.* Philadelphia: Elsevier; 2010.)

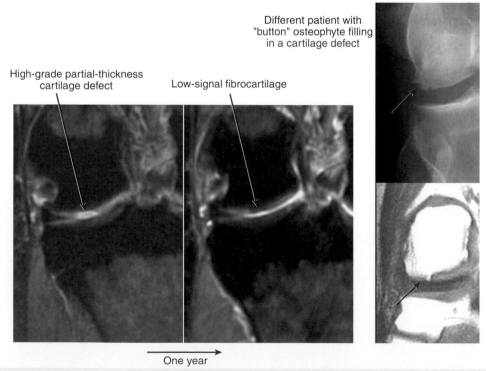

Fig. 9.18 Cartilage is avascular and has an intricate internal collagen architecture; therefore, it does not heal with the same structural makeup. However, cartilage defects can 'fill in' naturally, with disorganized dark signal fibrocartilage or with bone. A similar outcome is seen after surgical microfracture technique. (From Morrison W. *Problem Solving in Musculoskeletal Imaging.* Philadelphia: Elsevier; 2010.)

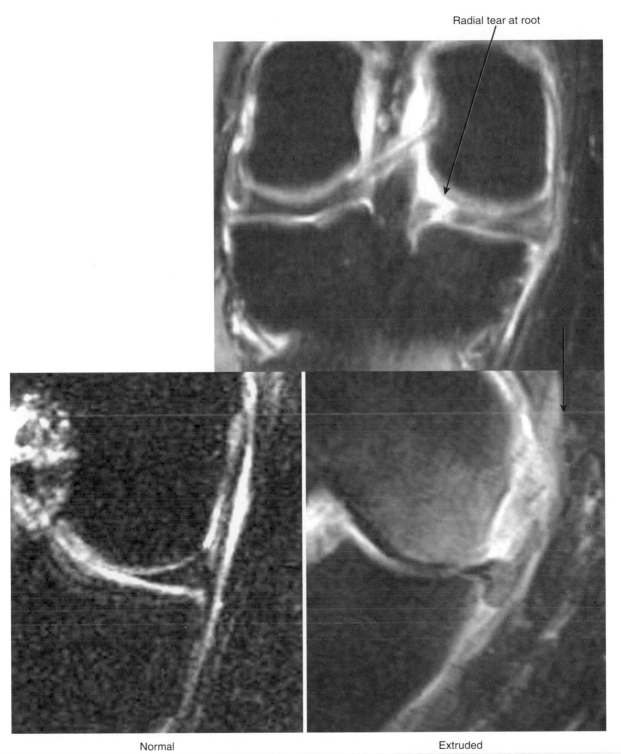

Radial tear at root

Normal   Extruded

Fig. 9.19 Meniscal extrusion. Disruption of circular central meniscal fibers destabilizes the meniscus and leads to extrusion. Complex tears, large radial tears, and tears at the root attachments are associated with major (>3 mm) meniscal extrusion. Extrusion leads to compartmental osteoarthritis. (From Morrison W. *Problem Solving in Musculoskeletal Imaging.* Philadelphia: Elsevier; 2010.)

- Meniscal extrusion and unstable meniscal tears (especially complex tears, complete radial tears, and root tears) can result in rapid compartmental cartilage loss (Figs. 9.19 and 9.20). Impingement and instability in other joints can also be associated with osteoarthritis.

DEGENERATIVE DISEASE OF THE SPINE

Degenerative disc disease is extremely common. It manifests on imaging as a constellation of findings:

- Disc desiccation.
  - Normally the central disc (nucleus pulposus) in adults is intermediate in signal on T2-weighted images.

Meniscal extrusion
following tear

⟵ 6 months ⟶

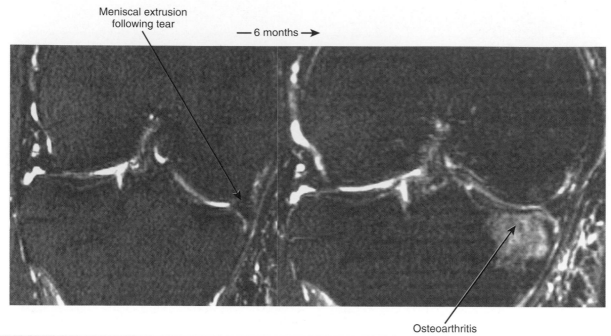

Osteoarthritis

Fig. 9.20 Rapid development of arthritis due to meniscal tear and extrusion. (From Morrison W. *Problem Solving in Musculoskeletal Imaging.* Philadelphia: Elsevier; 2010.)

- As discs undergo degeneration, T2 signal decreases.
- Decreased T2 signal in the discs diffusely is a normal part of the aging process.
- Annular fissure.
  - The nucleus pulposus is contained by a thick fibrous outer margin called the annulus fibrosus.
  - The annulus fibrosus is normally uniformly black in signal on T1- and T2-weighted images.
  - Focal (usually curvilinear) T2 hyperintensity can be seen within the annulus. This represents an *annular fissure*.
    - The MRI finding is also termed a *hyperintense zone (HIZ)*.
    - The term *annular tear* has fallen out of favor; this finding may not be traumatic.
    - Annular fissure can be a source of pain; it can also be a harbinger of disc disease progression, since it provides a route for herniation of the nucleus pulposus.
- Disc bulge.
  - By definition, diffuse (greater than 90 degrees around the circumference) extension of the disc beyond the endplate.
  - Can be a normal finding in the aging spine; may not be symptomatic.
  - Larger disc bulges can result in spinal stenosis and neural foraminal narrowing.
  - *Asymmetric bulge* is a bulge greater on one side.
- Disc herniation.
  - Extension of nucleus pulposus beyond the annulus involving less than 90% of the circumference.
  - Can cause spinal/foraminal stenosis and nerve impingement symptoms by mechanical compression and chemical irritation.
  - Descriptive terminology varies.

- Can be divided into protrusion, extrusion, and sequestered fragment, which are based on morphology.
  - *Protrusion:* Broad base at the disc margin; remains at the level of the disc.
  - *Extrusion:* Narrow base at the disc margin or disc material extends superior and/or inferiorly.
  - *Sequestered fragment:* A disc fragment detached from the parent disc; can migrate in the epidural space.
- Disc narrowing; as the disc degenerates, the disc space may narrow (Fig. 9.21B).
- Vacuum phenomenon; degenerated discs may contain gas, referred to as a vacuum phenomenon (Fig. 9.22C and 9.23). Disc vacuum is virtually pathognomonic for degeneration, excluding the presence of infection. A vacuum may appear in extension of the spine on flexion/extension views.
- *Spondylolisthesis:* displacement of one vertebral body compared to an adjacent body.
  - *Anterolisthesis:* upper body anterior to lower body; *retrolisthesis:* upper body posterior to lower body; *lateral listhesis:* upper body left or right compared to lower body.
  - Usually related to degenerative disc and facet disease.
  - In lower lumbar spine, anterolisthesis may be related to a complete fracture of the pars interarticularis (*pars defect*).
  - Seen in segmental instability: altered mechanics at a disc level (i.e., disc/facet disease, spinal fusion above or below, paralysis) resulting in abnormal motion and rapidly progressive disc/facet disease; can simulate infection or neuropathic disease.
- Endplate spurs: arise from annular attachments; can result in spinal canal and neural foraminal stenosis

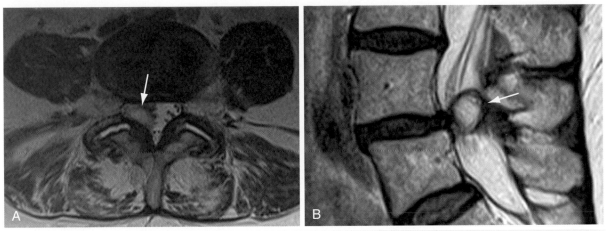

Fig. 9.21 Facet joint osteoarthritis. **(A)** Axial T2-weighted MR image at L4-5 shows degenerated, hypertrophic facet joints with mild thickening of the ligamenta flava. In addition, there is a synovial cyst extending from the right facet into the spinal canal *(arrow)* associated with severe lateral recess stenosis; this cyst compresses the traversing right L5 and S1 nerve roots. **(B)** Sagittal T2-weighted MR image shows disc desiccation, disc narrowing, and mild anterolisthesis; the large synovial cyst *(arrow)* displaces the traversing nerve roots.

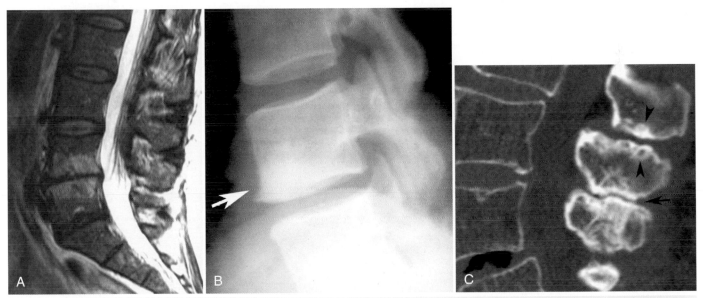

Fig. 9.22 Vertebral changes caused by disc degeneration. **(A)** Sagittal T2-weighted MR image shows disc narrowing and minimal retrolisthesis at L4-5. High signal intensity is present in the adjacent marrow representing Modic degenerative endplate changes. **(B)** Lateral radiograph of a different patient. MR imaging is more sensitive to vertebral changes related to disc degeneration, but reactive bone sclerosis and endplate spurs can be seen on radiographs. Note the disc space narrowing at L4-L5, with sclerosis seen at the anterior inferior endplate at L4 *(arrow)*. The triangular pattern of sclerosis is typical of discogenic sclerosis. **(C)** Another consequence of disc degeneration is impaction of adjacent spinous processes with secondary osteoarthritis-like degenerative changes, shown on this sagittal CT reconstruction of a different patient, known as Baastrup disease. Note subcortical 'cysts' *(arrowheads)*, cortical sclerosis, and impaction of adjacent spinous processes *(arrow)*. The disc level below shows anterolisthesis and a vacuum phenomenon.

in association with disc bulge ('disc osteophyte complex'). In the cervical spine the uncovertebral ('uncinate') joints at the posterolateral disc margin often hypertrophy in association with degenerative disc disease, leading to neural foraminal stenosis (Fig. 9.24).

■ Modic-type degenerative endplate changes (Fig. 9.25; see Figs. 9.20 and 9.21).

  ■ As the disc degenerates, marrow in the adjacent vertebral bodies undergo characteristic signal changes.

    ■ *Modic type 1:* edematous (low T1, high T2 signal) – can simulate disc infection.

    ■ *Modic type 2:* fatty (high T1, high T2 signal) – 'hemangioma-like'.

    ■ *Modic type 3:* sclerotic (low T1, low T2 signal) – may appear localized and rounded, may simulate blastic tumor ('hemispherical spondylosclerosis').

■ Schmorl nodes (see Fig. 9.25).

  ■ Invagination of disc material through the endplate into the vertebral body.

  ■ Appears rounded with adjacent Modic changes.

  ■ Typically seen with degenerative disc disease; however, other etiologies include:

    ■ Developmental: if seen at multiple levels, especially T-spine, associated with irregular endplates and loss of vertebral body height, called *Schuermann disease* or painful kyphosis of adolescence.

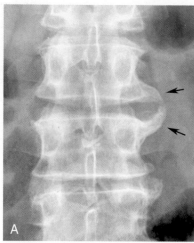

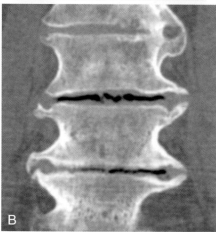

Fig. 9.23 Degenerative endplate spurs. **(A)** AP radiograph shows typical endplate spurs *(arrows)* caused by disc bulges with stretching of annular fibers. Note that the spurs initially extend horizontally away from the vertebral body. **(B)** Coronal CT reconstruction in a different patient shows similar findings. Other terms for these bony excrescences include 'traction spurs', and 'claw osteophytes'. Contrast this appearance with the nearly vertical fine marginal syndesmophytes of ankylosing spondylitis (see Fig. 9.77) and the syndesmophytes of psoriasis and reactive arthritis that do not extend horizontally (see Fig. 9.68).

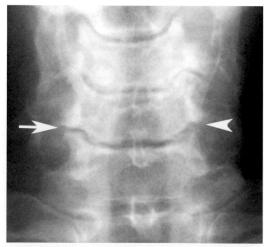

Fig. 9.24 Cervical spine uncovertebral joint osteoarthritis. AP cervical spine radiograph shows right side spurs and joint space narrowing at C6-C7 *(arrow)*, compared with the relatively normal left side *(arrowhead)*.

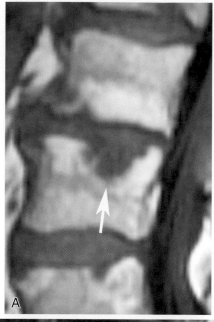

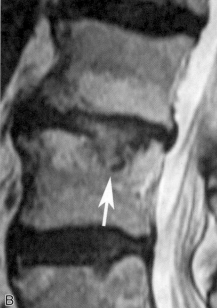

Fig. 9.25 Schmorl nodes. Sagittal T1-weighted **(A)** and T2-weighted **(B)** MR images show Modic type 2 changes (high signal on T1- and T2-weighted sequences) with disc extension into an adjacent endplate, termed a 'Schmorl node' *(arrow)*.

- Trauma: injury can result in Schmorl node formation.
- Bone softening: if the endplate is weakened (i.e., from osteomalacia, osteoporosis, tumor, or infection), Schmorl nodes can form.
- Inflammatory arthropathy: conditions leading to spinal fusion can lead to Schmorl node formation (i.e., AS).
- Invagination of disc material at the peripheral margin during development results in separation and displacement of the ring apophysis (endplate growth center), resulting in ossification referred to as a 'limbus vertebrae' (Fig. 9.26).

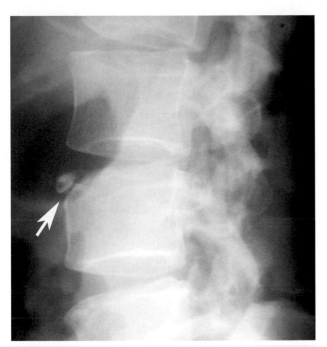

Fig. 9.26 Limbus vertebra. Note the normal variant limbus vertebra, with a separated triangular fragment from the anterior superior endplate of L4 *(arrow)*, resulting from anterior disc herniation through the ring apophysis while the patient was still skeletally immature.

EROSIVE OSTEOARTHRITIS

- Erosive osteoarthritis (EOA), also called *inflammatory osteoarthritis*, is seen in a subset of patients with underlying OA of the hands.
    - Patients are typically elderly and often female.
    - Arthritic IP joints (especially the DIP joints) become tender, painful, and swollen.
    - Central erosions occur leading to the classic 'gullwing' or 'seagull' pattern of the joint surface (Fig. 9.27).
    - Eventually the joint may undergo ankylosis.

NEUROPATHIC OSTEOARTHROPATHY

- Neuropathic osteoarthropathy, also known as *Charcot arthropathy*, can be considered as a severe, aggressive form of osteoarthritis with a component of instability typically associated with loss of sensation.
- Some features of osteoarthritis are often present, including sclerosis, osteophytes, and bodies. However, there is often subluxation, erosion, and joint destruction, which may be extreme and deforming.
- The arthropathy begins as a sensory neuropathy which may be from diabetes, syringomyelia, tabes dorsalis (neurosyphilis), leprosy, or other conditions (Table 9.12).

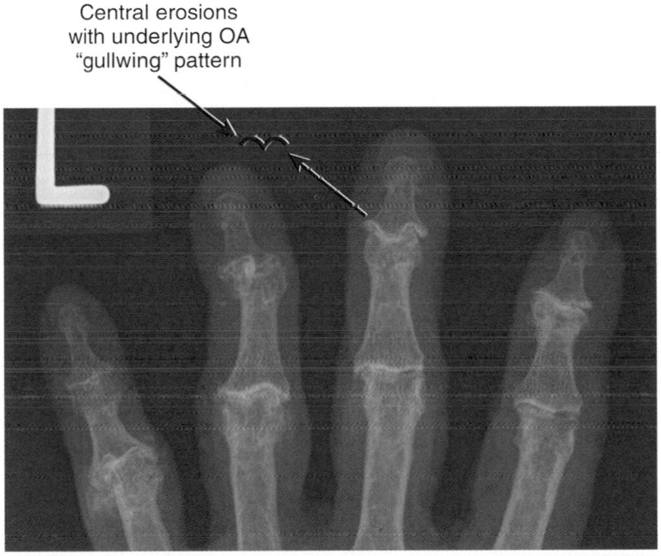

- Facet joint arthropathy (see Fig. 9.21).
    - The facet joints (zygoapophyseal joints) are synovial joints with a capsule, articular cartilage, and joint fluid.
    - As such, degeneration of the facet joints mirrors that of other joints: with cartilage damage, subchondral cysts, marginal spurs, sclerosis, and thickening of the collateral ligaments (in the case of the facet joint, the ligamentum flavum).
    - Ganglion cysts can extend from the anterior or posterior margin of the joint, called 'facet cysts'. These can impinge upon the spinal canal or neural foramen.
    - Facet and ligamentum flavum hypertrophy contributes to spinal canal (especially lateral recess) stenosis and neural foraminal narrowing.
- Posterior spinous process abutment (*Baastrup disease*, or 'kissing spines', (see Fig. 9.22C): loss of disc height and facet disease in older patients can result in abutment of the posterior spinous processes. This can lead to intervening bursitis (fluid signal between the posterior elements), sclerosis, edema, and cystic changes in the spinous processes. Patients present with localized back pain, worse on extension.
- Certain processes can be confused for degenerative disc disease, including:
    - Infection: discitis-osteomyelitis can cause low T1 and high T2 signal in the endplates simulating Modic type 1 changes. However, in degenerative disc disease the disc signal is often low on T2-weighted images, whereas the T2 signal of the disc is bright in infection.
    - Amyloid/spondyloarthropathy of renal failure; on radiographs, renal failure and amyloid deposition can cause irregularity of the endplates.

Central erosions with underlying OA "gullwing" pattern

Fig. 9.27 Erosive osteoarthritis of the hand with classic central erosions of the interphalangeal joints (seagull or gullwing pattern) (From Morrison W. *Problem Solving in Musculoskeletal Imaging*. Philadelphia: Elsevier; 2010.)

Table 9.12   Neuropathic Disease: Etiology and Typical Location

Leprosy: distal extremities (hands and feet)
Diabetes: feet (Lisfranc, hindfoot, MTPs)
Syrinx: upper extremities (esp. shoulders, bilateral symmetric)
Paralysis: spinal segment (esp. at junction with fixation)
Tabes dorsalis (uncommon): spine, hips, knees, ankles

Abbreviation: MTP, metatarsophalangeal.

- Less-frequent causes include multiple sclerosis, alcoholism, amyloidosis, intraarticular steroid use, congenital insensitivity to pain, and neurologic conditions such as Charcot–Marie–Tooth disease and dysautonomia (Riley–Day syndrome).
- Joints in the insensate region undergo unrecognized injury with ligament damage, osteochondral and capsular disruption, and even fracture.
- Joint injury persists and progresses due to continued stress, and arthropathy ensues.
- Loss of sympathetic control with neuropathy, or hypovascularity in the case of diabetic vasculopathy, may also play a role in disease progression.
- Neuropathic osteoarthropathy can be described in three forms: atrophic, hypertrophic, and mixed (Figs. 9.28 and 9.29).
  - The atrophic form appears as well-defined osteolysis resembling surgical resection. Proliferative response is absent, but the remaining bones are normally mineralized and the margins may be sclerotic. This pattern is classically seen in the shoulders associated with a spinal cord syrinx.
  - The hypertrophic form appears as a severe osteoarthritis with new bone production, sclerosis, fragmentation, and often subluxation.
  - The mixed form has features of bone destruction and production.

- Neuropathic disease can also be described in terms of acute, chronic, or acute-on-chronic forms (Fig. 9.30).
  - In acute neuropathic osteoarthropathy the patient presents with diffuse swelling and erythema; clinically this can simulate infection.
    - The involved joints in this early stage of disease often show little deformity or malalignment, and radiographs may just show soft tissue swelling.
    - On MRI, joint effusions are common, with prominent subchondral edema that may extend far into the medullary cavity.
    - Signal intensity changes in the bone marrow consisting of low signal intensity on T1-weighted images and high signal on T2-weighted images may be identical to those observed in septic arthritis and osteomyelitis.
    - Erosions may be seen at the margins of the joint.
    - On gadolinium-enhanced images, marrow enhancement is typically present, with predominantly subchondral distribution.
    - Periarticular soft tissue enhancement may also be seen.
    - Recent fractures related to neuropathic osteoarthropathy may create intense bone marrow edema, which lead to potential diagnostic pitfalls.
  - In chronic neuropathic osteoarthropathy, radiographic features have been summarized by words

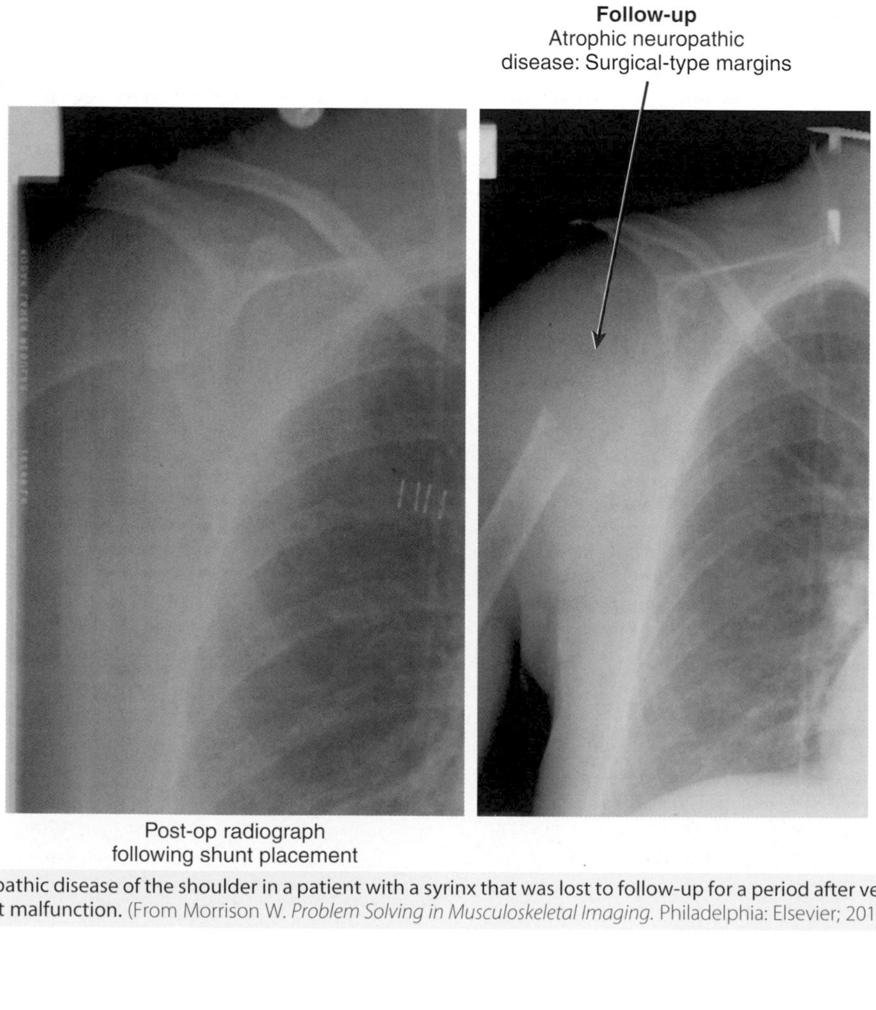

Follow-up
Atrophic neuropathic disease: Surgical-type margins

Post-op radiograph following shunt placement

Fig. 9.28 Atrophic neuropathic disease of the shoulder in a patient with a syrinx that was lost to follow-up for a period after ventriculoperitoneal shunting and subsequent shunt malfunction. (From Morrison W. *Problem Solving in Musculoskeletal Imaging.* Philadelphia: Elsevier; 2010.)

Mixed atrophic/hypertrophic
disease of THR ankle and hindfoot

Hypertrophic pattern
in the midfoot

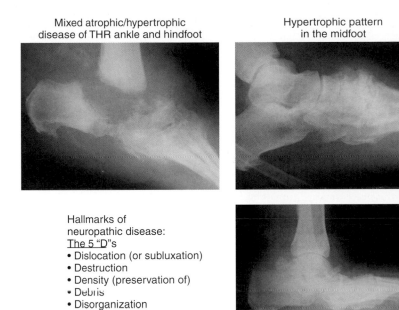

Hallmarks of
neuropathic disease:
The 5 "D"s
• Dislocation (or subluxation)
• Destruction
• Density (preservation of)
• Debris
• Disorganization

Hypertrophic pattern in the
midfoot and hindfoot

Fig. 9.29 Hypertrophic and mixed forms of neuropathic disease, common in feet of diabetic patients. (From Morrison W. *Problem Solving in Musculoskeletal Imaging.* Philadelphia: Elsevier; 2010.)

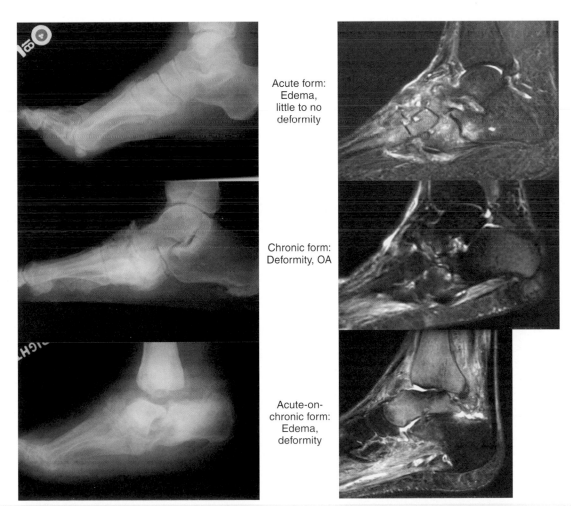

Acute form:
Edema,
little to no
deformity

Chronic form:
Deformity, OA

Acute-on-
chronic form:
Edema,
deformity

Fig. 9.30 Neuropathic disease can also be described in terms of acute, chronic, or acute-on-chronic forms. *OA,* osteoarthritis. (From Morrison W. *Problem Solving in Musculoskeletal Imaging.* Philadelphia: Elsevier; 2010.)

Table 9.13   Neuropathic Disease: the 5 'D's

Deformity
Destruction
Dislocation/subluxation
Debris
Density (preservation of)

beginning with 'D': Destruction, Debris, preserved bone Density, Disorganization, and Dislocation (or subluxation) (Table 9.13).

- The most commonly involved articulation is the Lisfranc joint (Fig. 9.31).
- Involvement here causes the metatarsal bases to migrate dorsally, and the longitudinal arch collapses, resulting in a 'rocker bottom' deformity.
- MRI features are more typical of osteoarthritis, with bone production and subchondral cystic change.

- Acute clinical presentation may be superimposed on chronic neuropathic disease, resulting in features of both on radiographs and MRI.
- In any phase of neuropathic disease, in the setting of diabetes there is often underlying diffuse soft-tissue edema or diffuse muscle atrophy, which in the absence of contrast can appear similar to diffuse cellulitis. As stated earlier, marrow changes can simulate infection.

- Additionally, osteomyelitis is frequently associated with neuropathic disease of the foot.
  - Chronic neuropathic deformity causes osseous protuberances that can produce increased friction with

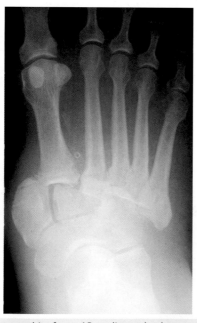

Fig. 9.31 Neuropathic foot. AP radiograph demonstrates lateral Lisfranc dislocation. Note the vascular calcification, a clue to the associated diagnosis of diabetes. There was no history of significant trauma. The tarsometatarsal joint is the most common location for a neuropathic joint in diabetic foot, but any other joint in the hindfoot, midfoot, or forefoot is at risk in the diabetic patient. (Image used with permission from BJ Manaster, MD, from the American College of Radiology Learning File.)

ill-fitting footwear and results in adjacent skin callus formation, breakdown, and ulceration; osteomyelitis ensues from contiguous spread.

- Typical locations for this to occur are the metatarsal heads, midfoot, and calcaneus. Differential features between neuropathic disease and infection are discussed in detail in Chapter 14 – Musculoskeletal Infection.

Key Concepts

Neuropathic Arthropathy

Severe, destructive
Hypertrophic or atrophic
Joint effusions
Ligamentous laxity: Subluxation, dislocation
Hypertrophic: Five Ds: bony debris, cartilage destruction, normal bone density, joint distention, joint disorganization (or dislocation or deformity)
Charcot ankle/foot: Usually diabetes mellitus
Charcot knee: Tabes dorsalis, diabetes, or congenital insensitivity/ indifference to pain
Charcot shoulder: Syringomyelia
Charcot spine: Diabetes or instrumented spinal trauma in paraplegic patients

- Neuropathic arthropathy is most common in the ankle and foot, related to diabetes. It can occur in other locations. A general rule of thumb is: if the arthritis looks so severe and complicated that it is hard to describe, think of neuropathic disease.
  - Knee: neuropathic arthropathy of the knee has historically implied tabes dorsalis as its prime cause.
    - However, it is also seen in patients with diabetes, congenital insensitivity to pain, or congenital indifference to pain.
    - The changes are usually at least partly hypertrophic.
    - Tremendous distention of the capsule with prominent debris and disorganization of the joint is the hallmark in these cases.
  - Shoulder/elbow: neuropathic arthropathy in these locations is frequently misdiagnosed.
    - A neuropathic shoulder joint most commonly develops secondary to syringomyelia (Fig. 9.32). Conversely, 20% of patients with syringomyelia develop a Charcot shoulder.
    - In advanced cases, Charcot shoulder is almost always atrophic. Thus resorption of most or all of the humeral head and neck may be seen, which may give the appearance of surgical resection of the humeral head.
    - Confirmation of syringomyelia as the cause is made with MRI of the cervical spine.
  - Spine: Historically spinal neuropathic disease was often caused by advanced syphilitic involvement (called *tabes dorsalis*); nowadays it is most frequently associated with paralysis, spinal trauma, or surgical fixation.
  - In patients with spinal cord trauma who have undergone instrumentation and fusion, the mobile segments adjacent to the fusion can undergo abnormal motion. The appearance is similar to that of other

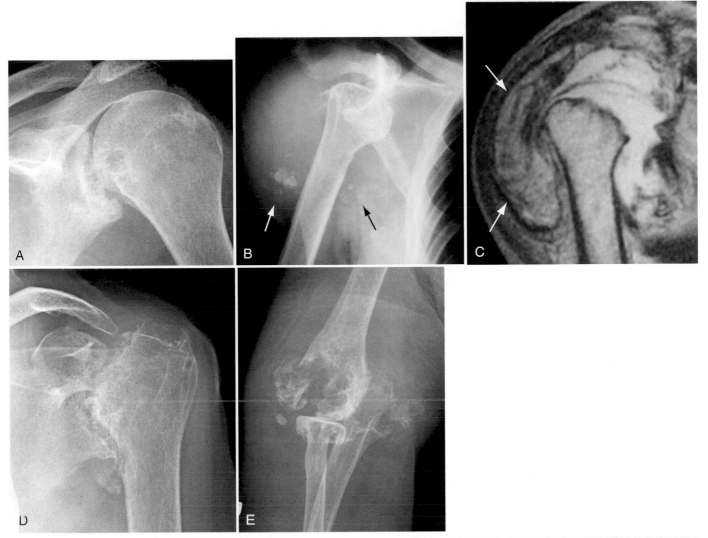

Fig. 9.32 Neuropathic shoulder and elbow. **(A)** Early findings. AP radiograph of the shoulder of a 40-year-old man with a cervical cord syrinx shows painless destruction of the glenohumeral joint. **(B** and **C)** Late findings in a different patient. The diagnosis should be based on the radiograph **(B)** in this case, which shows all the elements necessary to diagnose neuropathic shoulder. The glenohumeral joint is dislocated, there is a large effusion, and debris is seen floating in the effusion *(arrows)*. If confirmation is needed, MRI demonstrates the entire abnormality, including the debris, to be intraarticular. Coronal T2-weighted MR image **(C)** demonstrates the destroyed and dislocated humeral head surrounded by a large joint effusion, with more fluid and debris settling into the distended subdeltoid bursa *(arrows)*. With this much destruction and a confirmed articular-based process, the imaging findings are virtually pathognomonic for a neuropathic joint. Syringomyelia as the cause would be confirmed with MRI of the cervical spine. Severe shoulder **(D)** and elbow **(E)** neuropathic arthropathy in different patients.

Charcot joints, with disorganization, ligamentous instability, and bony debris (Fig. 9.33). A lesser form of this is referred to as *segmental instability*: a situation in which a combination of disc and facet disease results in abnormal, excess motion at a disc level, causing accelerated degenerative changes.

- Discitis-osteomyelitis may have identical findings.
  - The differential of neuropathic spine versus infection may be truly difficult because the two common causes of neuropathic arthropathy in the spine (diabetes and paraplegia with spinal fusion) are also associated with increased risk for development of disc space infection.
  - The presence of vacuum disc, debris, spondylolisthesis, and facet involvement can help suggest that the diagnosis is spinal neuropathic arthropathy.

- On the other hand, findings that *do not* differentiate between neuropathic and infectious arthropathy include endplate sclerosis and erosions, spurs, and decreased disc height.
- Patients undergoing long-term hemodialysis may develop a destructive process with an identical appearance, related to amyloid deposition (*dialysis-related spondyloarthropathy*).
  - Disc aspiration and biopsy may be necessary.

Inflammatory Disorders

SEPTIC ARTHRITIS

- Infection should always be considered when a monoarticular inflammatory arthropathy is seen. Imaging can

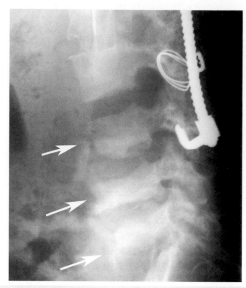

Fig. 9.33 Neuropathic spine in a paraplegic patient. This patient had a burst fracture at the level of L1 and has had an anterior partial corpectomy with strut graft placement and posterior rodding from the levels of T10-L3. Below the level of the instrumentation, note subluxation and destruction of the vertebral bodies and endplates (L3 inferior endplate, L4, and L5; *arrows*). With this much destruction in a paraplegic patient, neuropathic process must be considered.

appear identical to other inflammatory arthropathies such as rheumatoid arthritis or gout. Specific findings will be discussed in more detail in Chapter 14 – Musculoskeletal Infection.

- Unexplained effusion involving a single joint without trauma should first raise concern for septic arthritis.
- Joint infection is reviewed in Chapter 14 – Musculoskeletal Infection.

RHEUMATOID ARTHRITIS

- RA affects females more often than males at a ratio of 2–3 to 1.
- Typically, onset of adult-type RA occurs in the 20s–40s.
- Symptoms at presentation classically include joint stiffness, especially in the morning, with pain and swelling which is most commonly polyarticular and symmetric.
- Systemic manifestations include fatigue and weight loss.
- The simplified mechanism is an autoimmune attack on the synovium.
- The etiology is unknown. Genetics clearly is a factor. RA is more prevalent in cigarette smokers.
- Clinical criteria for diagnosis assesses the number of involved small and large joints, presence of rheumatoid factor (RF) or anti-citrullinated protein antibody (ACPA), inflammatory markers erythrocyte sedimentation rate (ESR) and c-reactive protein (CRP), and duration of symptoms.
  - Note that while usually present, RF is not entirely specific and is not required to make the diagnosis. Additionally, RF be falsely positive in older individuals.
- The diagnosis is frequently made and treatment started as early in the disease as possible, with the goal of preserving cartilage. Imaging may not be obtained.

- Note that the examples of later-stage disease presented here are less common today due to improved drug therapies.

Imaging Findings

- The basic pathology of RA is inflammation and proliferation of synovium (*pannus*, Figs. 9.34 and 9.35), which leads to the various radiographic appearances.
  - Periarticular swelling is due to a combination of pannus and joint effusion.
    - Fusiform soft tissue swelling is characteristic at the PIP joints of the hands, with focal soft tissue swelling at the MCP joints, at the dorsum of the wrist, and over the ulnar styloid (see Fig. 9.4).
    - In the feet, soft tissue swelling is common at the MTP joints, especially the fifth.
  - RA can affect any synovial-lined structure, including bursae and tendon sheaths.
    - Bursitis can blur soft tissue planes or create focal soft tissue prominence on radiographs; this is most evident radiographically in the retrocalcaneal bursa and olecranon bursa. Adjacent bone erosion can occur.
    - Mechanical bursitis, bursitis related to inflammatory arthritis, and septic bursitis can have an identical appearance on all modalities, including MRI; aspiration may be necessary.
    - Tenosynovitis is evident radiographically as diffuse or longitudinally oriented soft tissue swelling, commonly involving the tendons of the wrist (Fig. 9.36).
  - Inflammatory nodular soft tissue lesions may occur, called *rheumatoid nodules*.
    - Rheumatoid nodules have been reported to occur in as many as 15% of all rheumatoid patients, but appear to be uncommon today, possibly related to improved treatments.
    - Nodules appear as focal soft tissue masses, usually at sites of chronic friction, like the extensor surfaces of the forearm, as well as the hands and feet.
  - Periarticular osteopenia is a classic radiographic feature, especially in early stages of RA of the hands and feet, although a generalized pattern of osteopenia can also occur.
  - Involved joints generally demonstrate concentric, or uniform joint narrowing related to diffuse cartilage loss; however, in weight-bearing joints there may be more severe narrowing at the weight-bearing surface.
  - Axial migration can occur at the hips due to bone remodeling at the central portion of the acetabulum, with inward bowing of the iliopectineal line, called *protrusio acetabuli*.
  - Characteristic marginal erosions result from thickened, inflammatory synovial tissue (pannus) eroding the bone at the 'bare area' adjacent to the margin of the articular cartilage (Fig. 9.37).
  - Osseous proliferation is not a feature of RA; however, osteophyte formation can occur in longstanding RA, as a result of superimposed secondary osteoarthritis.

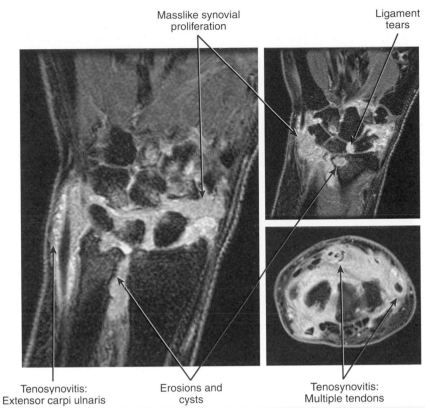

Masslike synovial proliferation

Ligament tears

Tenosynovitis: Extensor carpi ulnaris

Erosions and cysts

Tenosynovitis: Multiple tendons

Fig. 9.34 MRI is useful for evaluation of rheumatoid arthritis, to detect early erosions and track extent of synovial proliferation; MRI findings have been used to document response to treatment objectively. Intravenous contrast is helpful in that synovial pannus enhances brightly and is easily evaluated. Dynamic contrast can be used to document the degree of synovial hyperemia by plotting the time-uptake curve. MRI is also helpful in diagnosing various complications of the disease and its treatment, including ligament tears and avascular necrosis. (From Morrison W. *Problem Solving in Musculoskeletal Imaging*. Philadelphia: Elsevier; 2010.)

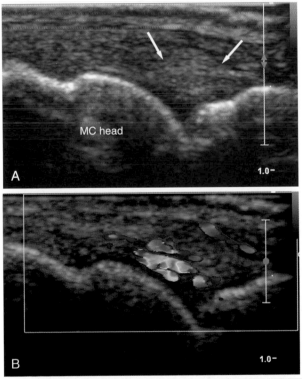

Fig. 9.35 Rheumatoid arthritis. Longitudinal images of an MCP joint with active RA. **(A)** Gray scale and **(B)** color Doppler show thickened synovium (*arrows* in A) with hyperemia.

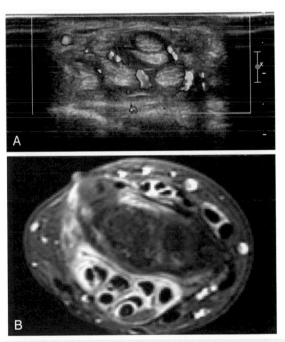

Fig. 9.36 Rheumatoid arthritis. Axial images at the wrist. **(A)** Color Doppler US. Volar is at the top of the image. Note the hyperemia within thickened, edematous synovium and hypoechoic effusions surrounding the flexor tendons. **(B)** T1-weighted, fat-suppressed image with intravenous contrast shows the same findings, with intense enhancement of thickened synovium and small effusions around the low-signal flexor and extensor tendons. Volar is at the bottom of this image.

Joint narrowing
Soft tissue swelling/effusions
Marginal rarefaction representing early erosions

Well-defined erosions
Advanced joint narrowing
Subchondral cysts

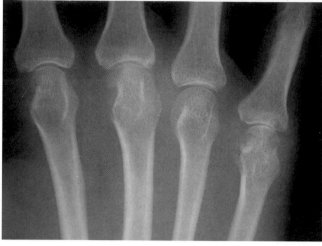

Early

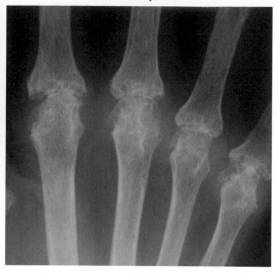

Late

Fig. 9.37 Rheumatoid arthritis—progression of disease. Involved joints generally demonstrate concentric or uniform joint narrowing related to diffuse cartilage loss. (From Morrison W. *Problem Solving in Musculoskeletal Imaging.* Philadelphia: Elsevier; 2010.)

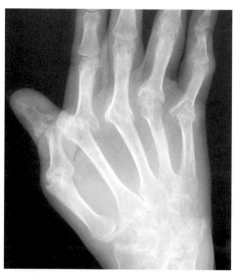

Fig. 9.38 Rheumatoid arthritis of the wrist and hand with deformity. PA radiograph demonstrates the deformity that can be seen in late rheumatoid arthritis. There is ulnar translocation of the carpus (lunate more centered over the ulna than radius) and 'Hitchhiker's thumb'. The metacarpophalangeal joints show typical volar subluxation and ulnar deviation, and the fifth finger shows a boutonnière deformity, with flexion of the proximal interphalangeal paired with extension of the distal interphalangeal. A lateral view (not shown) might show dorsal or volar flexion instability patterns of the carpus. (Image used with permission from BJ Manaster, MD, from the American College of Radiology Learning File.)

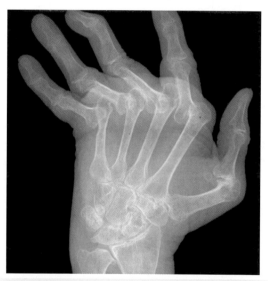

Fig. 9.39 Rheumatoid arthritis, of the hand with deformity. PA view shows metacarpophalangeal (MCP) dislocations and ulnar deviation of the second through fifth fingers, swan neck deformity of the third finger (hyperextension of the proximal interphalangeal paired with hyperflexion of the distal interphalangeal), as well as carpal and MCP erosions.

- Deformities of the hands and feet are common in RA for a variety of reasons: laxity and distension of the joint capsule; ligamentous laxity or disruption; tendinopathy or tendon tears; and altered muscle tone (Figs. 9.38 and 9.39).
  - The *swan neck deformity* is hyperextension at the PIP joint and flexion at the DIP joint. The *boutonnière* deformity is flexion at the PIP joint and hyperextension at the DIP joint. These deformities result from imbalance of the flexor and extensor tendons.
  - Subluxations at the MCP and MTP joints are also common: the digits of the hands deviate in an ulnar direction (*windswept hand* appearance); in the foot, hallux valgus is very common and may be severe, leading to overlap of the first and second toes.
  - In the wrist, carpal bone erosion may be extreme (*carpal dominant* involvement), with ligamentous disruption and laxity causing carpal instability patterns.

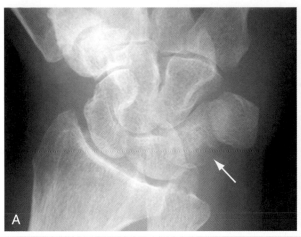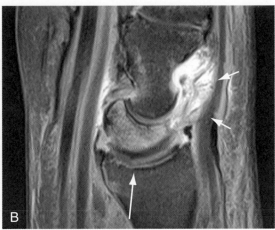

Fig. 9.40 Rheumatoid arthritis, wrist. **(A)** Norgaard (ball-catcher's) view of the wrist shows an erosion in the triquetrum *(arrow)*, which was not visible on the PA view (not shown). There were no other abnormalities on this patient's hand, but this single erosion in this typical location allows for a diagnosis of rheumatoid arthritis (RA). The pisiform, triquetrum, and ulnar styloid are classic locations for early erosions in RA. **(B)** Sagittal fat-saturated proton density–weighted MR image following direct arthrography of the radiocarpal joint shows marrow edema in the lunate *(long arrow)* and masslike pannus within the dorsal portion of the joint *(short arrows)* in a patient with early findings of RA and normal radiograph (not shown). (A, Image used with permission from BJ Manaster, MD, from the American College of Radiology Learning File.)

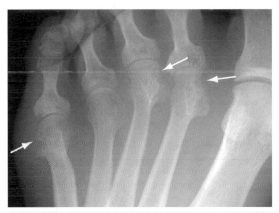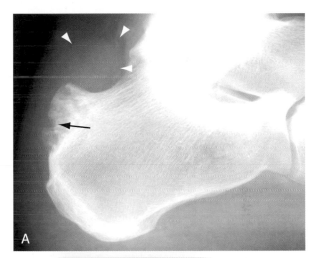

Fig. 9.41 Rheumatoid arthritis, metatarsophalangeal (MTP) joints. AP radiograph of the foot demonstrates soft tissue swelling at the MTP joints and prominent metatarsal head erosions at the second, third, and fifth metatarsals *(arrows)*. Erosions at the MTP joints are a frequent finding in rheumatoid arthritis. (Image used with permission from BJ Manaster, MD, from the American College of Radiology Learning File.)

In more severe cases this process of erosion and instability evolve to *carpal collapse* with the metacarpal bases nearly apposed to the radius.

- The entire carpus and hand may slip in an ulnar direction, referred to as *ulnar translocation.*
- Carpal collapse and dissociation, in addition to mass effect from pannus, can cause impingement on the median nerve as it passes through the carpal tunnel, resulting in carpal tunnel syndrome.

■ RA is most commonly recognized in the hands and feet (Figs. 9.40, through 9.42; see Figs. 9.4, 9.34, 9.37, 9.38, and 9.39); in fact, if there is a finding on a foot exam which is of questionable significance, it is often useful to evaluate radiographs of the hands, and vice versa.

- Distribution in the hands is characteristically more proximal than distal, commonly involving the carpus, as well as the MCP and PIP joints.

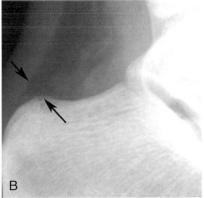

Fig. 9.42 Rheumatoid arthritis, calcaneus. **(A)** Lateral radiograph of the calcaneus demonstrates erosions at the posterior calcaneus *(arrow)*, and retrocalcaneal bursitis seen as soft tissue density in the pre-Achilles fat triangle *(arrowheads)*. These findings also can be associated with psoriasis and reactive arthritis. Most cases of retrocalcaneal bursitis are more subtle and without erosion. **(B)** Normal retrocalcaneal bursa for comparison. Note normal finding of inverted triangle of fat between the distal Achilles tendon and the superior-posterior calcaneus (between *arrows*). (A, Image used with permission from BJ Manaster, MD, from the American College of Radiology Learning File.)

- In the feet/ankles, the distribution mimics that of the hands/wrists, with the MTP joints most commonly involved (see Fig. 9.41).
  - Distribution is bilateral and symmetric; however, extent of involvement may not be the same from side to side.
- At the elbow, severe erosions can occur, resulting in a 'pencil-in-cup' appearance (Fig. 9.43), analogous to that seen in the hands with psoriatic arthritis.

- At the shoulder, erosions can occur at the margins of the humeral head; marked subacromial/subdeltoid bursitis can be seen. Inflammatory pannus may erode through the rotator cuff tendons (Figs. 9.44 and 9.45).
- The hip joints are not commonly involved; however, because of the relatively small joint capacity, involvement can result in erosions around the femoral neck. Synovitis can extend into the adjacent iliopsoas bursa (Figs. 9.46 through 9.48).

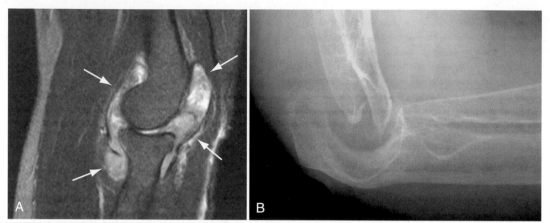

Fig. 9.43 Rheumatoid arthritis, elbow. **(A)** Sagittal T2-weighted MR image in an early case of rheumatoid arthritis shows no marrow edema or erosions, but prominent synovial pannus *(arrows)*. **(B)** Lateral radiograph of the elbow in a patient with advanced rheumatoid arthritis demonstrates the diffuse and uniform erosive change that can be seen in this disease process. There is complete resorption of the radial head, resorption of much of the distal humerus, and a large erosion of the olecranon. (A, Image used with permission from BJ Manaster, MD, from STATdx website, Amirsys, Inc.)

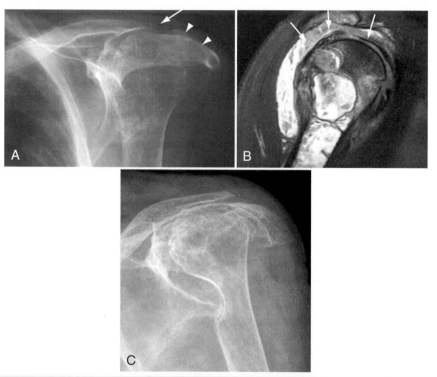

Fig. 9.44 Rheumatoid arthritis, shoulder and acromioclavicular joint. **(A)** AP radiograph of the shoulder demonstrates elevation of the humeral head caused by chronic rotator cuff tear, as well as erosions involving both the distal end of the clavicle *(arrow)* and the acromion *(arrowheads)*. **(B)** Oblique sagittal fat-saturated T2-weighted MR image shows intermediate-signal pannus filling the acromiohumeral outlet *(arrows)*. Rotator cuff is extensively torn. There are huge erosions involving the majority of the humeral head, with tremendous cyst formation extending down the shaft of the humerus. The erosions and cysts contain pannus, filling from the glenohumeral joint. **(C)** AP radiograph of the shoulder shows severe elevation of the humeral head such that it articulates with the undersurface of the clavicle and acromion, implying complete and chronic rotator cuff tear. There is a large mechanical erosion of osteoporotic bone at the medial proximal humeral metaphysis, putting the patient at risk for surgical humeral neck fracture. (B, Image used with permission from BJ Manaster, MD, from STATdx website, Amirsys, Inc.)

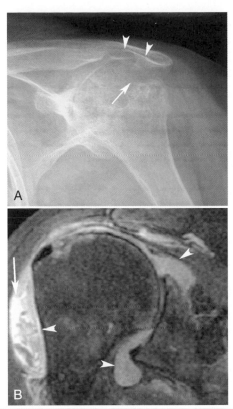

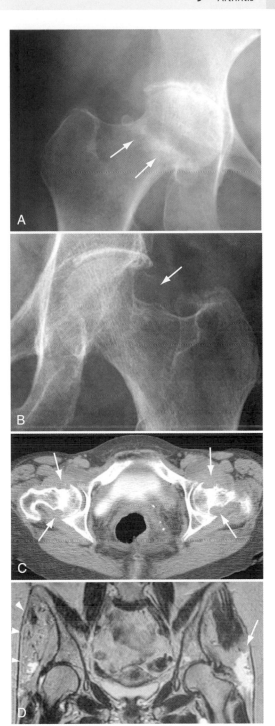

Fig. 9.45 Rheumatoid arthritis, shoulder. **(A)** AP radiograph shows osteopenia. The humeral head articulates with the undersurface of the acromion because of a chronic complete rotator cuff tear with retraction. Note the eroded undersurface of the acromion *(arrowheads)* and erosion of the humeral head and the greater tuberosity *(arrow)*. **(B)** Coronal fat-suppressed T2-weighted MR image shows intermediate-signal intensity pannus *(arrowheads)* distending the joint and subdeltoid bursa but only a small high-signal-intensity effusion extending from the glenohumeral joint into the subdeltoid bursa *(arrow)*. Also note high-riding humeral head and thin rotator cuff. There is uniform cartilage thinning. Other images (not shown) revealed cuff tears and muscle atrophy.

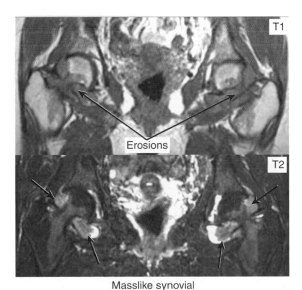

Masslike synovial
proliferation is seen in RA

Fig. 9.46 Rheumatoid arthritis (RA) of the hips with masslike pannus and symmetric involvement. (From Morrison W. *Problem Solving in Musculoskeletal Imaging.* Philadelphia: Elsevier; 2010.)

Fig. 9.47 Rheumatoid arthritis, hip. **(A)** AP radiograph shows typical rheumatoid arthritis (RA) of the hip, with uniform cartilage loss and osteopenia. There is mild axial migration and an insufficiency fracture of the femoral neck *(arrows)*. The osteopenia associated with RA and steroid therapy increases the risk for stress and insufficiency fractures. **(B)** AP radiograph shows osteoporosis and uniform cartilage loss. There is a very large superimposed erosion at the superolateral margin of the femoral head *(arrow)*. **(C)** Axial CT scan, same patient as in B, showing huge erosions of the femoral heads bilaterally *(arrows)*. Erosions of this size are unusual in RA but not unheard of; one might consider a diagnosis of superimposed amyloid deposition, but the case is proven RA. **(D)** Coronal T2-weighted MR image in a patient with long-standing RA demonstrates bilateral gluteal tendon ruptures. On the left side, note the high signal intensity at the site of the rupture *(arrow)*. The left rupture is relatively recent, because the musculature is not atrophic. On the right side, the gluteal musculature shows complete fatty atrophy, indicating a chronic tendon rupture *(arrowheads)*.

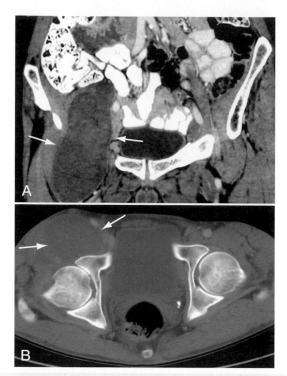

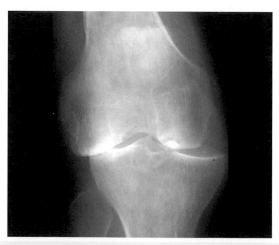

Fig. 9.48 Rheumatoid arthritis, hip, with groin mass. **(A)** Coronal CT scan shows a large low-density soft tissue mass *(arrows)* located in the right groin, extending proximally into the pelvis. **(B)** Axial CT scan shows the same low-density mass located within the iliopsoas bursa *(arrows)*, displacing the femoral neurovascular bundle anteriorly. Note that there is uniform cartilage narrowing in the right hip; compare to the normal left hip. Patients with rheumatoid arthritis of the hip may develop such a large effusion that it decompresses into the iliopsoas bursa through the relatively weak anterior hip capsule. This presents clinically as a fluctuant groin mass.

Fig. 9.49 Rheumatoid arthritis, knee. AP radiograph shows diffuse osteopenia, uniform loss of cartilage space, and medial subluxation of the tibia. Note lack of erosions due to large joint capacity. This is a typical malalignment and appearance of advanced rheumatoid arthritis involving the knee.

■ The knee joints have large capacity and may not show erosions until late in the disease (Fig. 9.49). Large joint effusion and synovitis can decompress into a Baker's cyst posteromedially (Fig. 9.50).
■ At the ankle and foot, the fifth MTP joint is most commonly involved. However, any joints can be affected. Bursitis can be present at the heel (see Fig. 9.42).

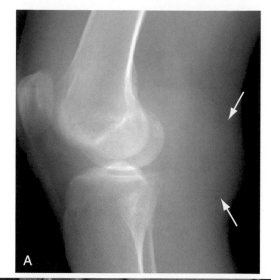

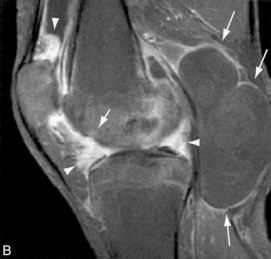

Fig. 9.50 Rheumatoid arthritis, knee. **(A)** Lateral radiograph shows osteopenia, large effusion, and mass effect posteriorly *(arrows)*. No erosions are seen. **(B)** Sagittal postintravenous contrast T1-weighted fat-saturated MR image shows much more severe disease than is apparent on the radiograph. There is bulky enhancing synovium *(arrowheads)* and bone marrow edema with subchondral cortical bone loss and erosions *(short arrow)*. The posterior mass is a large complex Baker's (popliteal) cyst, hypointense on this T1-weighted image but outlined by thin rim enhancement *(long arrows)*. **(B** Image used with permission from BJ Manaster, MD, from STATdx website, Amirsys, Inc.)

Spine Involvement

■ A major site of serious musculoskeletal complications from RA is the cervical spine (Figs. 9.51 through 9.53).
　■ The dens is surrounded by synovial tissue, both anteriorly at the junction of the dens with the anterior arch of C1, and posteriorly at the transverse ligament.
　■ Pannus at these synovial locations can cause laxity of the transverse ligament and erosion of the dens itself, leading to excessive motion and instability at C1-2.
　■ The instability may not be apparent on a neutral lateral view; lateral views in flexion and extension are generally indicated to gauge the degree of instability, although the flexion/extension motion must

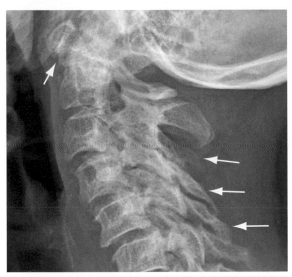

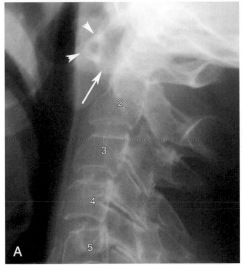

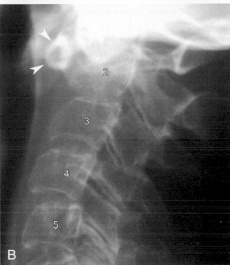

Fig. 9.51 Rheumatoid arthritis, cervical spine. Atlantoaxial subluxation is seen with widened space between the anterior arch of C1 and the anterior odontoid process *(short arrow)*. Even if it is difficult to see the odontoid process through the skull base, the disruption of the spinal laminar line at C1-C2 indicates atlantoaxial subluxation. In addition, there is atlantoaxial impaction. This is indicated by the position of the anterior arch of the atlas, located opposite the waist of the axis rather than opposite the odontoid. The other finding of rheumatoid arthritis in this patient is the lack of cortical distinctness of the facets, as well as the gracile spinous processes *(long arrows)*, acquired secondary to mechanical erosion of osteopenic bone.

be performed with great caution, always allowing the patient to flex and extend their neck voluntarily, determining their own limitation.

- This instability is very important to identify in individuals at risk, as relatively minor trauma in this setting can cause a high cervical cord injury. This is especially a concern in the preoperative setting, since prior to and during surgery the unconscious patient's neck may be extended and flexed during intubation and anesthesia.

MRI Characteristics

- On MRI, effusions are commonly seen in joints affected by RA, and synovial pannus is a characteristic finding.
  - Pannus is seen on MR images as intermediate signal on T1- and T2-weighted images with a masslike quality in the joint, distending the recesses (Tables 9.14 and 9.15).
  - Intravenous contrast typically results in intense enhancement of proliferative, hyperemic synovium (see Fig. 9.34).
  - Synovial pannus may erode through intraarticular or periarticular ligaments (e.g., causing wrist interosseous ligament tears) and tendons (e.g., causing rotator cuff tear).
  - Tenosynovitis and bursitis are common. Often multiple tendon sheaths are involved around an affected joint; if synovitis of a joint and multiple adjacent tendon sheaths is observed, a diagnosis of RA should be entertained (see Fig. 9.34).
  - In RA, synovial pannus can be observed within the tendon sheaths, with complex fluid seen on T2-

Fig. 9.52 Rheumatoid arthritis, cervical spine. **(A)** Lateral radiograph demonstrating atlantoaxial subluxation *(arrow)* and osteopenia. Note that the anterior arch of the atlas *(arrowheads)* is located at the level of the odontoid process and that at this point there is no evidence of atlantoaxial impaction. **(B)** A film of the same patient 2 years later demonstrates that severe atlantoaxial impaction has occurred, with the anterior arch of the atlas *(arrowheads)* now located opposite the inferior portion of the body of C2. Although you cannot actually see the odontoid process, it must be presumed to have impacted into the foramen magnum. Note the severe constriction of the spinal canal between the posterior aspect of the body of C2 and the anterior aspect of the spinous process of C1. Atlantoaxial impaction can be even more devastating to the patient's neurologic status than atlantoaxial subluxation. (Images used with permission from BJ Manaster, MD, from the American College of Radiology Learning File.)

weighted images, with marked distension of the sheath.

- Similarly, distension of periarticular bursae, such as the olecranon bursa or retrocalcaneal bursa, may occur, seen on MRI as complex fluid signal representing pannus within the bursal capsule (see Figs. 9.42, 9.45, and 9.48).
- In chronic RA, intraarticular bodies are occasionally observed, and may be seen as multiple fibrous ovoid structures within the joint or tendon sheath known

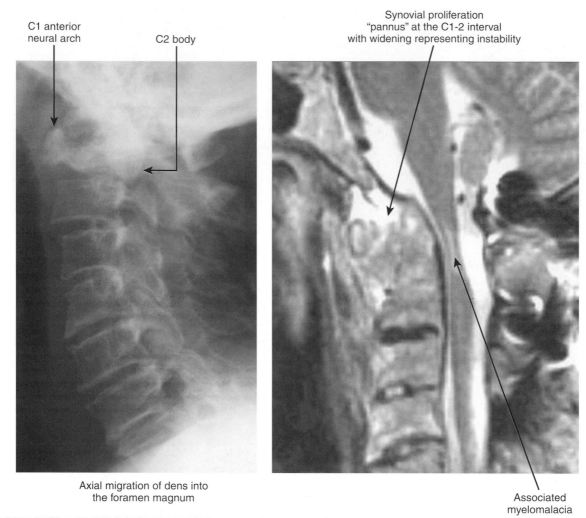

C1 anterior
neural arch

C2 body

Synovial proliferation
"pannus" at the C1-2 interval
with widening representing instability

Axial migration of dens into
the foramen magnum

Associated
myelomalacia

Fig. 9.53 Rheumatoid arthritis involving the cervical spine. There are five separate synovial compartments at C1-C2, any of which can be involved by the inflammatory pannus. Resulting erosion of the dens and ligamentous insufficiency causes atlantoaxial instability and even axial migration. (From Morrison W. *Problem Solving in Musculoskeletal Imaging.* Philadelphia: Elsevier; 2010.)

Table 9.14   Synovitis Extent and Type of Arthritis

MILD:

Osteoarthritis
Postoperative

MODERATE/MARKED:

Septic arthritis
Chronic inflammatory arthropathies

MASSLIKE

Rheumatoid arthritis
Pigmented villonodular synovitis
Synovial osteochondromatosis
Gout

Table 9.15   Soft tissue 'Masses' in Arthritis

Gouty tophi
Ganglion cysts
Rheumatoid pannus and rheumatoid nodules
Bursitis and tenosynovitis
Amyloid deposits
Sarcoid granulomas

as *rice bodies* due to their shape, number, and whitish appearance at surgery.

■ In the spine MRI is useful for determining the extent of pannus formation at C1-2, as well as the degree of compromise of the spinal canal (see Fig. 9.53).

Key Concepts

Rheumatoid Arthritis
■ Purely erosive (in the absence of superimposed osteoarthritis)
■ Fusiform soft tissue swelling
■ Periarticular osteoporosis
■ Uniform cartilage destruction
■ Bilaterally symmetric
■ Wrist: Radiocarpal joint, distal radioulnar joint; deformities
■ Hand: Proximal (MCP and PIP) deformities
■ Foot: Metatarsophalangeal (MTP) and retrocalcaneal bursa
■ Shoulder: Rotator cuff tear, erosion of distal clavicle
■ Knee: Valgus deformity
■ Hips: Uniform cartilage loss, protrusio acetabuli
■ Upper cervical spine: Facet erosions, atlantoaxial impaction, atlantoaxial subluxation

- Small volume, nondistensible joints such as the joints of the hands and feet tend to develop erosions earlier and more extensively than more distensible joints such as the knee and shoulder, which can accommodate comparatively large pannus volume before bone erosion occurs.
- It is important to note that productive bone of any type is extremely unusual in RA; specifically, periositis and enthesopathy do not occur.
- Ankylosis of a joint is extraordinarily rare in adult RA but relatively common in juvenile idiopathic arthritis. Osteophytes are not seen initially, except later in the course of disease in the setting of secondary degenerative joint disease.
- RA is remarkable for its symmetry. Although most synovial joints in the body can be affected by RA, survey radiographs for the disease should include posteroanterior (PA) and ball-catcher's (*Norgaard*) views of the hand, which is an anteroposterior (AP) oblique view with the hands internally rotated as if holding a large ball; AP and lateral views of the feet; and a lateral cervical spine radiograph, as these are the most frequent or clinically relevant sites.

ROBUST RHEUMATOID ARTHRITIS

- "*Robust*" RA (*arthritis robustus*) features large subchondral cysts and normal bone density. The distribution of abnormalities is identical to that of RA, and the abnormality seems predominantly erosive, without productive change. It is generally seen in working men with RA who maintain normal activity, thus retaining their normal bone density and forcing decompression of synovial fluid into enlarging subchondral cysts (Fig. 9.54).

STILL DISEASE

- Rare systemic autoinflammatory disease.
- Fevers, joint pain, skin rash, hepatosplenomegaly, and lymphadenopathy.
- Adult and juvenile forms are recognized. They likely are related. The juvenile form is considered a form of juvenile idiopathic arthritis, discussed in the following text.
- Destructive arthritis can be a feature (Fig. 9.55).

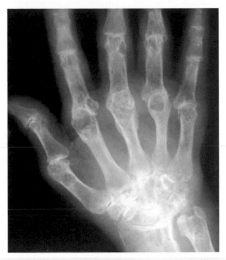

Fig. 9.54 Robust rheumatoid arthritis. PA radiograph of the hand of a 47-year-old man demonstrates extensive subchondral cyst formation, as well as erosive change in the distribution of rheumatoid arthritis. The bone density is decreased, but not as much as one might expect for the severity of disease. This is a carpenter who has continued working in his profession despite his severe rheumatoid arthritis, leading to these changes of "robust" rheumatoid arthritis. (Image used with permission from BJ Manaster, MD, from the American College of Radiology Learning File.)

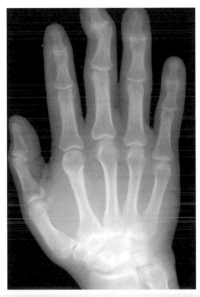

Fig. 9.55 Adult Still disease. PA radiograph demonstrates carpal and distal interphalangeal disease. The pericapitate distribution of the carpal disease is typical for adult Still disease. Note fusion of the carpal bones, more characteristic of JIA than adult-onset rheumatoid arthritis. (Image used with permission from BJ Manaster, MD, from the American College of Radiology Learning File.)

JUVENILE IDIOPATHIC ARTHRITIS

- *Juvenile idiopathic arthritis* (JIA) has replaced previously used terms such as juvenile rheumatoid arthritis (JRA, used in North America) and juvenile chronic arthritis (JCA, used in Europe).
- JIA actually includes a number of subsets of articular disease with the common characteristic that they present prior to age 16.

- These subcategories include:
  - Oligoarticular (most common, 50+%, young children, F>M).
  - Polyarticular RF-negative (next most common, about 25%), affects temporomandibular joint (TMJ) and C-spine, uveitis.
  - Polyarticular RF-positive (seropositive), basically juvenile onset of RA.
  - Systemic-onset JIA (juvenile-onset form of Still disease).
    - Extraarticular manifestations dominate, multi-focal inflammation, rash, fevers.
  - Enthesis-related arthritis, basically juvenile-onset AS.
  - Psoriatic arthritis.
  - Miscellaneous categories.
- People affected with JIA at a young age have certain manifestations on radiographic examinations related to the effects of chronic inflammation and hyperemia in growing bones.
  - Hyperemia leads to overgrowth and an enlarged appearance of the epiphyses compared to the metaphyses and diaphyses (hemophilia can result in the same pattern) (Figs. 9.56 and 9.57).
  - The hyperemic effect can also result in early fusion of the growth plate causing an abrupt transition between the epiphysis and diaphysis (i.e., short length of the metaphysis; see Fig. 9.56).
  - Early physeal fusion can cause growth disturbance, with bone shortening if the plate fuses uniformly or

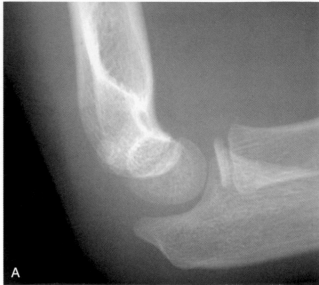

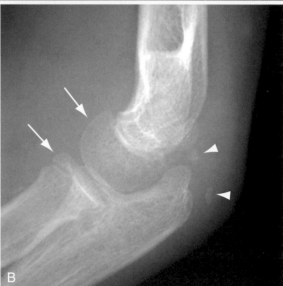

Fig. 9.57 Juvenile idiopathic arthritis (JIA), elbow. Uninvolved left **(A)** and involved right **(B)** elbow lateral radiographs in this child with JIA demonstrate relative overgrowth of the capitellum and radial head on the right side (*arrows* in B). In addition, the right elbow shows ossification of the olecranon apophysis (*arrowheads*), and an AP radiograph (not shown) demonstrated asymmetric early ossification of the lateral epicondyle on the right compared with ossification of that structure not yet occurring on the left. This acceleration of skeletal maturation is typical in a joint affected by JIA or any other cause of chronic inflammation. The adult elbow will show relative enlargement compared with the left, particularly of the radial head.

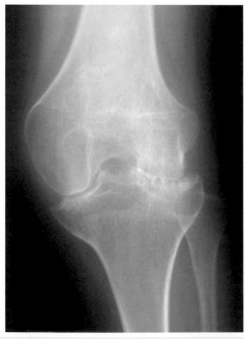

Fig. 9.56 Juvenile idiopathic arthritis, knee. AP radiograph of the knee in this 23-year-old patient demonstrates typical findings of long-standing juvenile idiopathic arthritis, with overgrown epiphyses and metaphyses, normal size of the diaphyses, wide intercondylar notch, and subchondral erosions with cartilage loss and secondary OA. The relative enlargement of the bones at the joint compared with the diaphyses is seen in juvenile idiopathic arthritis because of the chronic hyperemia occurring during skeletal growth. (Image used with permission from BJ Manaster, MD, from the American College of Radiology Learning File.)

with deformity if the fusion affects only part of the growth plate. At the ankle this can result in 'tibial tilt' (sometimes referred to as 'talar tilt') (Fig. 9.58). At the hip, chronic inflammation can lead to deformity including protrusio acetabuli (Fig. 9.59).
- The diaphyses of affected extremities may be gracile, and the combination of thin diaphyses and epiphyseal overgrowth with abrupt transition results in an 'overtubulated' pattern.
- Some radiographic findings mimic the adult form of RA and include fusiform periarticular soft tissue swelling, periarticular osteoporosis, and concentric, or uniform

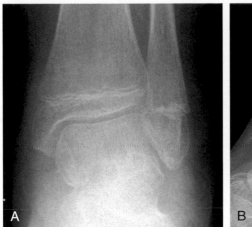
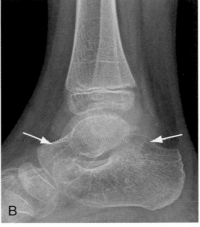

Fig. 9.58 Juvenile idiopathic arthritis (JIA), ankle. **(A)** AP radiograph shows mild valgus alignment at the distal tibia caused by growth disturbance (relative medial distal tibial overgrowth caused by hyperemia in this patient with JIA). **(B)** Lateral radiograph in a different child with JIA shows apparent large joint effusion seen as soft tissue density bulging anteriorly and posteriorly from the ankle joint *(arrows)*. The bones are osteopenic, although one must be cautious about making this assessment with radiographs in children.

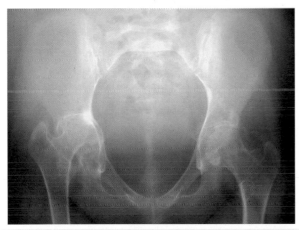

Fig. 9.59 Juvenile idiopathic arthritis (JIA), pelvis. AP radiograph of the pelvis of a 20-year-old woman with JIA demonstrates the small stature and gracile diaphyses typically seen in these patients. It also shows severe erosive change involving both hips, with protrusio acetabuli on the right side. This case does not show the valgus deformity that can occur in the femoral necks. (Image used with permission from BJ Manaster, MD, from the American College of Radiology Learning File.)

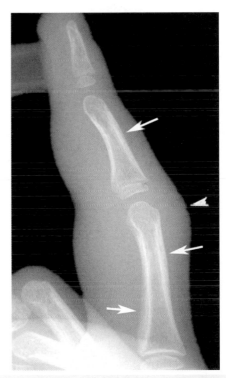

Fig. 9.60 Oligoarticular juvenile idiopathic arthritis (JIA). Lateral radiograph of the index finger in a 6-year-old girl demonstrates soft tissue swelling and dense periosteal reaction *(arrows)* and mild soft tissue swelling *(arrowhead)*. Although these changes are not pathognomonic for JIA (they could be seen in a bone infarct in a young patient with sickle cell disease, or infection), they are typical of oligoarticular JIA.

joint narrowing (although joint narrowing is typically seen only late in the disease course) (Fig. 9.60).
- However, unlike adult-onset RA, erosions are not a prominent feature.
- Additionally, in Still disease there is often periostitis adjacent to affected joints, whereas proliferation is uncommon in adult RA.
- JIA also causes joint ankylosis at a much higher frequency than in adult-onset RA (Fig. 9.61; see Fig. 9.55).
  - Any affected joint can fuse; in the cervical spine fusion of the facet joints may lead to a growth disturbance of the vertebral bodies (Fig. 9.62).
  - As vertebral bodies grow, they may become broad and flat or small and miniaturized.
  - Alternatively, hyperemia can cause the facet joints to hypertrophy resulting in tall, thin vertebrae.
  - Fusion of the carpal or tarsal bones is also common.

- In addition to early physeal closure, the ankle may show unilateral or bilateral valgus alignment due to growth disturbance, sometimes called 'tibial-talar tilt' (see Fig. 9.58).
  - Other conditions may also result in this abnormal alignment, which also may be remembered with the mnemonic "Sure Does Hurt To Jog": sickle cell anemia, skeletal dysplasias, hemophilia, and traumatic physeal injury, in addition to JIA.

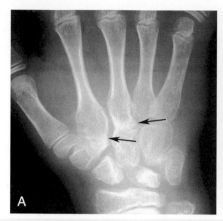
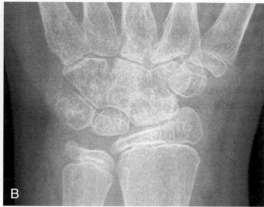

Fig. 9.61 Juvenile idiopathic arthritis (JIA), hand and wrist. **(A)** PA radiograph in this 11-year-old girl demonstrates little loss of cartilage width in the wrist or metacarpophalangeal joints but abnormal fusion between the capitate and third metacarpal, as well as between the trapezium and second metacarpal and trapezoid *(arrows)*. Early fusion in the absence of substantial erosive change or loss of cartilage is a typical finding in JIA. **(B)** PA wrist radiograph in a different child with JIA shows fusion of multiple carpal bones.

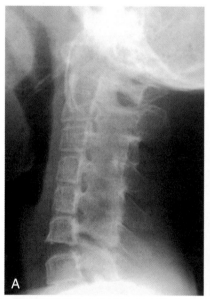
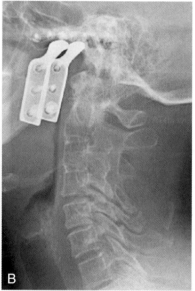

Fig. 9.62 Polyarticular rheumatoid factor (RF)-negative juvenile idiopathic arthritis (JIA), cervical spine. **(A)** Lateral radiograph of the cervical spine demonstrates complete fusion of the facets of C2 through C6. This fusion protects the endplates and disc spaces from the deterioration that is seen in advanced adult rheumatoid arthritis (RA). Fusion at an early age also results in restriction of growth of the vertebral bodies in an anteroposterior (AP) dimension (note how much smaller the bodies of C3, C4, and C5 are than C2, C6, and C7 in the AP diameter). This appearance has been termed 'waisting' of the cervical bodies. **(B)** Lateral CT localizer image in a different patient with polyarticular RF-negative JIA shows congenital fusion C2-C4 and bilateral temporomandibular joint (TMJ) arthroplasties. TMJ arthropathy occurs with both JIA and adult RA. (B, Image used with permission from BJ Manaster, MD, from the American College of Radiology Learning File.)

- The deformity and effects of cartilage damage often result in development of secondary osteoarthritis in early adulthood (see Fig. 9.56).
- As in adults, MRI of a joint affected with JIA shows a joint effusion, which may be large, as well as synovial proliferation, which is best seen after contrast administration.
  - Even without demonstration of synovial proliferation, presence of a Baker's cyst of the knee or ganglion cyst in other joints in a child should raise concern for JIA, since this finding can be associated with chronic or recurrent effusion.
  - Although synovial proliferation in a child should automatically prompt consideration of JIA, a careful history should be obtained, since infection can look similar; Lyme disease can cause a chronic synovitis and is quite common in the spring in the northeastern US.
  - Of course, internal derangement can also result in synovial proliferation, and is being seen increasingly as athletics is emphasized.
- The RF-positive polyarticular form of JIA tends to occur later, and behaves like adult RA.
- Other manifestations of JIA include a pattern resembling psoriatic arthritis, and a chronic arthropathy associated with inflammatory bowel disease.
- Imaging characteristics of these forms of JIA are similar to the corresponding adult forms.

Key Concepts

Juvenile Idiopathic Arthritis

By definition presents before age 16
Variable clinical manifestations
Most common subtype is oligoarticular, typically a 2- to 3-year-old, knee involvement common
Other forms usually appear later, with variable manifestations depending on the subtype
Knee, elbow, hip most common sites
Minority of cases are early-onset RA or AS
Periarticular osteopenia
Cartilage destruction and erosions are late manifestations
Joint contractures
Large joints: Effusions and synovitis, epiphyseal overgrowth, early growth plate closure
Hip: Valgus, protrusio acetabuli
Hand: MCP and PIP; ankylosis
Wrist: Midcarpal joint; ankylosis
Cervical spine: Atlantoaxial subluxation, odontoid erosions, ankylosis

Seronegative Spondyloarthropathies

- Seronegative spondyloarthropathy refers to a group of inflammatory conditions of the joints of the extremities and spine which are usually RF negative.

- This group includes psoriatic arthritis, reactive arthritis (previously called Reiter disease), AS, and arthropathy associated with inflammatory bowel disease (enteropathic arthropathy).
- RA and seronegative spondyloarthropathies can be thought of as existing along a spectrum:
  - RA is primarily a synovial process, rarely involving entheses; so it preferentially involves joints, tendon sheaths, and bursae.
  - AS is primarily an enthesial disease; so it preferentially involves the spine and SI joints, where ligamentous attachments are plentiful.
  - Psoriatic and reactive arthritis are in between, involving both synovial tissues and enthesial attachments.

PSORIATIC ARTHRITIS

- Approximately 5–25% of patients with skin involvement from psoriasis have *psoriatic arthritis*; conversely, most patients with articular disease have skin involvement.
- Peak age range of presentation with arthritis is 20–40 years, similar to RA.
- Psoriatic arthritis can have highly variable clinical and radiographic presentations (Figs. 9.63 and 9.64).
  - Most common distribution is oligoarticular involving the distal joints of the hands and feet.

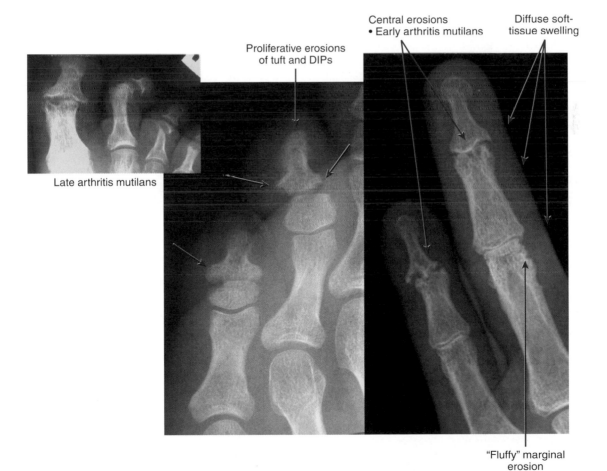

Fig. 9.63 Psoriatic arthritis. Erosions classically have a proliferative appearance, with a fluffy or whiskered quality. Central erosions can lead to joint destruction with a 'pencil-in-cup' pattern. *DIP*, distal interphalangeal joints. (From Morrison W. *Problem Solving in Musculoskeletal Imaging.* Philadelphia: Elsevier; 2010.)

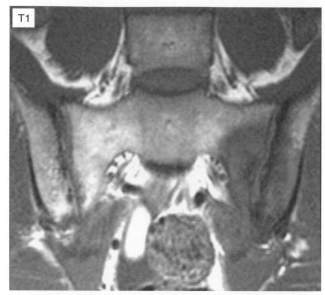

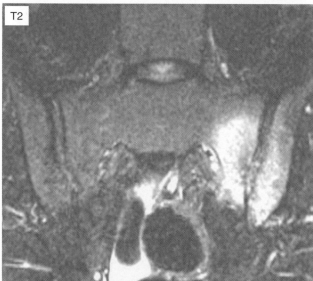

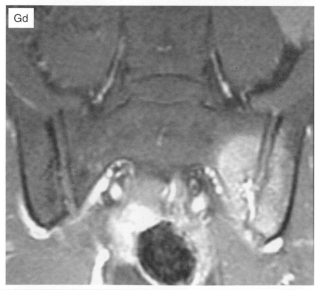

Fig. 9.64 Psoriatic arthritis involving the sacroiliac joint unilaterally. (From Morrison W. *Problem Solving in Musculoskeletal Imaging.* Philadelphia: Elsevier; 2010.)

- Polyarticular with preferential distal involvement can also be seen.
  - *Arthritis mutilans:* Severe, with destructive arthropathy and deformity. Uncommon; can also be seen in late-stage RA, JIA, multicentric reticulohistiocystosis, and systemic lupus erythematosus (SLE).
  - A large subset of cases resemble RA.
  - A small subset of cases have spondyloarthritis features that overlap with AS, with SI joint and spine involvement.
- In the distal extremities, some rays may be involved severely with sparing of other adjacent rays.
- Males and females are equally affected, but females predominate in cases of polyarticular disease and males predominate in cases with spinal disease.

Imaging Characteristics

- Radiographically, the disease is characterized by erosions with bone proliferation, similar to reactive arthritis. In fact, these two diseases are almost indistinguishable on radiographs alone.
  - One useful differentiating feature is that psoriatic arthritis commonly involves the hand, whereas reactive arthritis rarely involves the upper extremity.
  - Also, reactive arthritis is uncommon in females. Correlation with clinical history is essential.
- Diffuse joint narrowing occurs similar to other inflammatory arthropathies, related to uniform cartilage loss.
- Erosions occur at the 'bare areas' of the joint margins.
  - These erosions classically have a proliferative appearance, with a 'fluffy' or 'whiskered' quality (Fig. 9.65).
  - If the disease progresses, the erosions can become severe, with a 'sharpened pencil' appearance of the end of the bone.
    - The articular surface at the opposite side of the joint can become cupped, and there can be shortening of the digit from telescoping of one bone into the other i.e., *telescoping digits.*

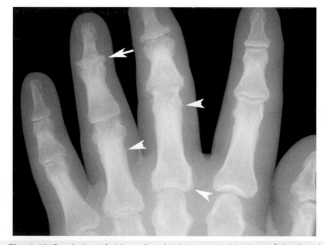

Fig. 9.65 Psoriatic arthritis, polyarthritis pattern. PA view of the hand demonstrating predominantly distal interphalangeal (DIP) joint disease, with fusion at the fourth DIP joint *(arrow).* Note also the subtle periostitis at the proximal phalanges of the third and fourth digits *(arrowheads).* Fusion and periostitis are hallmarks of psoriatic arthritis. Also note the small erosions at the third DIP joint. (Image used with permission from BJ Manaster, MD, from the American College of Radiology Learning File.)

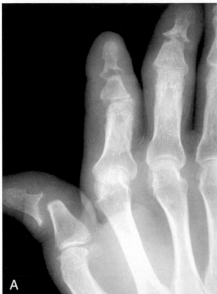

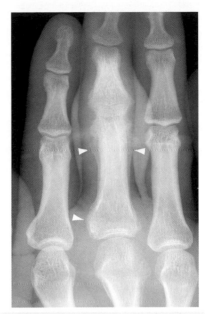

Fig. 9.67 Psoriatic arthritis, oligoarticular pattern. PA radiograph of the hand demonstrates swelling in the form of a 'sausage digit' in the third ray, with prominent periostitis along the metacarpal and proximal phalanx of the third ray *(arrowheads)*.

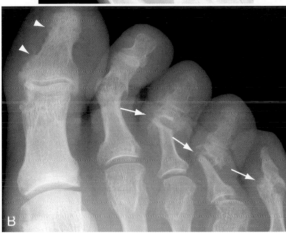

Fig. 9.66 Psoriatic arthritis, arthritis mutilans pattern. **(A)** AP radiograph of the hand shows advanced psoriatic arthritis changes, with so much destruction at the distal interphalangeal joints of digits 1, 2, and 3 that they have developed a 'pencil-in-cup' appearance. **(B)** Similar findings in a different patient, showing not only the 'pencil-in-cup' appearance of the third and fourth proximal interphalangeal joints *(arrows)* but also the new bone production (periostitis) at the distal phalanx of the great toe *(arrowheads)*. (A, Image used with permission from BJ Manaster, MD, from the American College of Radiology Learning File.)

- With severe involvement, the articular surfaces can undergo complete destruction, referred to as *arthritis mutilans* (Fig. 9.66), also termed *main-en-lorgnette* (opera hand).
- Ankylosis can occur at any involved joint, but most commonly the IP joints, the SI joints, and the facet joints of the spine.
- At the SI joints, there is early loss of the thin subchondral white line and marrow edema, which progresses to form discrete erosions, and surrounding reactive bone on both sides of the joint representing sacroiliitis (see Fig. 9.64).
  - SI involvement may be unilateral or bilateral but asymmetric.
- In addition to proliferative-type erosions, there is often periostitis adjacent to an involved joint (Fig. 9.67).

- In the spine, bulky lateral and asymmetric osseous bridging between vertebral bodies can occur (termed *parasyndesmophytes*) (Fig. 9.68).
- Erosions can also occur at the entheses.
  - Affected entheses commonly have a 'fluffy' appearance on radiographs, and on MRI demonstrate soft tissue and marrow edema, an appearance mimicking injury (e.g., plantar fasciitis).
- Distribution is characteristically distal extremities, especially the IP joints, MCP and MTP joints of the hands and feet, the spine, and SI joints; however, other joints including the wrist, ankle, elbow, knee, and shoulder can also be involved. Hip involvement is relatively uncommon.
- Unlike RA, involvement of the hand/wrist is more distal than proximal, and there can be dramatic difference in involvement of adjacent rays in psoriatic arthritis, unlike RA where involvement tends to be more uniformly distributed.
- Asymmetry of involved joints also differentiates distribution of psoriatic arthritis from the classic bilateral symmetric distribution of RA.
- Deformity in psoriatic arthritis is generally limited to the digits related to underlying bone destruction.
- Fusiform soft tissue swelling occurs around the joints of the affected digit, termed *dactylitis* or 'sausage digit' (see Fig. 9.67).
- With flexor tendon tenosynovitis, the whole digit can become swollen, also resulting in *sausage digit*.
- Focal soft tissue swelling can also be seen at entheses due to inflammatory involvement, and in periarticular tissues due to bursitis.
- Pitting of the nails may occasionally be seen on radiographs in more severe cases.
- Bone mineralization is generally preserved, although early in the disease there may be some periarticular demineralization.

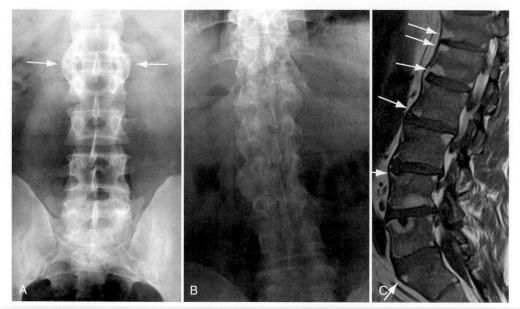

Fig. 9.68 Seronegative spondyloarthropathy of psoriasis and reactive arthritis. **(A)** AP radiograph of the lumbar spine demonstrates bilateral but somewhat asymmetric sacroiliitis, along with bulky syndesmophytes involving only the L1-L2 level *(arrows)*. This patient also had calcaneal erosive disease. Reactive arthritis and psoriatic arthritis can have an identical-appearing spondyloarthropathy, with asymmetric sacroiliitis and bulky asymmetric syndesmophytes. Contrast with the degenerative spurs in Fig. 9.23 and the fine annulus fibrosis calcification in ankylosing spondylitis (AS) in Fig. 9.77. **(B)** AP radiograph in another patient shows more extensive, but still bulky and asymmetric thoracolumbar osteophytes. **(C)** T1-weighted sagittal MR image, same patient, shows fat signal chronic corner Romanus lesions *(arrows)*. Although Romanus lesions are seen more frequently in AS, they can also be seen with other spondyloarthropathies.

Key Concepts

Psoriatic Arthritis

Varied manifestations:
- Oligoarthritis
- Polyarthritis (DIP more frequent than PIP and MCP joints)
- Symmetric type (resembles RA)
- Arthritis mutilans (deforming type, pencil-in-cup, opera hand)
- Spondyloarthropathy (bilateral, asymmetric sacroiliitis, bulky asymmetric osteophytes usually starting at the thoracolumbar junction, noncontiguous)

Most cases: Asymmetric erosive arthropathy, with superimposed bone productive changes

Bone density can be normal

Distal phalanges: Tuft resorption (acro-osteolysis) or reactive sclerosis ('ivory phalanx')

Sausage digit in the hand (due to soft tissue swelling and/or flexor tenosynovitis)

Arthropathy may precede skin changes—up to 20% of cases

REACTIVE ARTHRITIS

- *Reactive arthritis*, previously known as Reiter disease, is an oligoarticular arthritis and enthesopathy that follow an infection, usually of the genitourinary or gastrointestinal (GI) tract.
- Age of onset varies from adolescence to middle age, but peaks in the third decade.
- The clinical syndrome classically includes urethritis, conjunctivitis, and arthritis; however, frequently one of the first two is absent. A mnemonic is 'can't see, can't pee, can't bend the knee'.
- The clinical symptoms usually begin within a month of the infection, which if genitourinary is typically *Chlamydia trachomatis*, and if GI can be a number of organisms including shigella, campylobacter, or salmonella.
- The arthritis related to genitourinary disease affects males approximately five to nine times more commonly than females, whereas the syndrome following GI disease is seen in males and females equally.
- Caucasians make up approximately 80% of patients, and the HLA-B27 antigen is seen in over half of the people with the disease.
- The exact mechanism of the arthritic 'reaction' to these infections is not known but is speculated to be related to antigenic similarity between the infectious agent and an antigen in synovial joints of susceptible individuals.
- The other seronegative spondyloarthropathies, as well as RA and Behçet syndrome, also may be initiated by an unfortunate immune cross-reaction to an unknown antigen and thus also may be reactive, although such a connection is less clearly established.
- Lower extremity joints are most commonly affected; the upper extremities are rarely involved (Figs. 9.69 and 9.70).
- A knee or SI joint may be the initial site of symptoms.
- Distribution in the foot is usually distal, primarily involving the MTP and IP joints.
- Radiographic appearance is characterized by proliferative, or 'fluffy' marginal erosions and joint narrowing; as in psoriatic arthritis, severe involvement may occur, with central erosions, joint destruction, or ankylosis (Fig. 9.71).

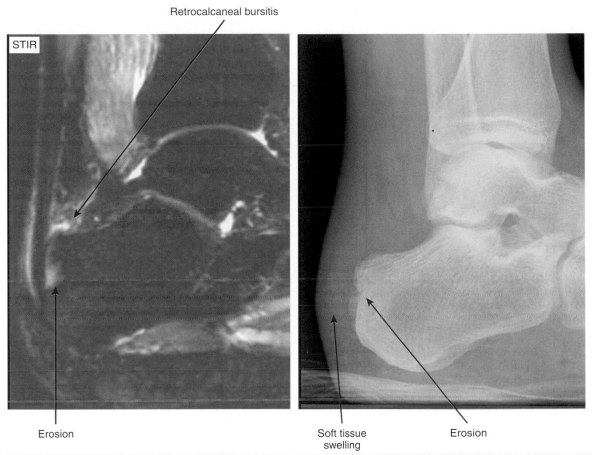

Retrocalcaneal bursitis

STIR

Erosion

Soft tissue
swelling

Erosion

Fig. 9.69 Reactive arthritis with reactive changes at the Achilles insertion. Like psoriatic arthritis, reactive arthritis often involves tendons sheaths, attachment sites of tendons/ligaments/fascia (entheses), and adjacent bursae. (From Morrison W. *Problem Solving in Musculoskeletal Imaging*. Philadelphia: Elsevier; 2010.)

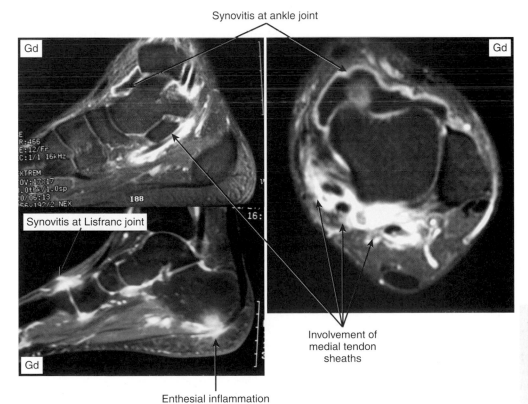

Synovitis at ankle joint

Gd

Gd

Synovitis at Lisfranc joint

Involvement of
medial tendon
sheaths

Enthesial inflammation

Fig. 9.70 Reactive arthritis involving the synovium of joints and tendon sheaths as well as the enthesis of the plantar fascia, with enhancement on post-gadolinium (Gd) MRI. (From Morrison W. *Problem Solving in Musculoskeletal Imaging*. Philadelphia: Elsevier; 2010.)

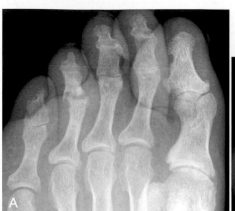
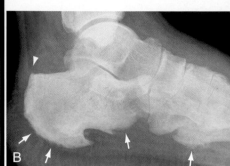
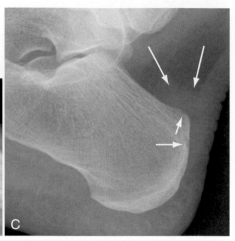

Fig. 9.71 Reactive arthritis. **(A)** PA radiograph of the toes shows erosions with new bone formation at the fourth proximal interphalangeal joint. **(B)** Lateral radiograph of the hindfoot in the same patient shows extensive new bone formation along the plantar calcaneus and fifth tarsometatarsal joint *(arrows)*, mixed erosions and new bone formation at the posterior calcaneus, and swelling of the retrocalcaneal bursa *(arrowhead)*. These findings also suggest psoriatic arthritis, which is more common, but clinical evaluation and absence of arthritis elsewhere in this patient confirmed the diagnosis of reactive arthritis. **(C)** Lateral radiograph in another patient shows much earlier changes, with inflammatory tissue at the posterior calcaneus *(long arrows)* as well as subtle erosions *(short arrows)*. Note that the bone density is normal, making psoriatic or chronic reactive arthritis more likely than rheumatoid arthritis.

- The SI joints may also be involved, usually unilateral or asymmetric similar to psoriasis.
- Diffuse soft tissue swelling can occur in one or a number of the digits, causing a 'sausage digit' but typically in the foot, not the hand.
- The appearance can be indistinguishable from psoriatic arthritis; however, most patients with psoriatic arthritis have the characteristic skin rash of psoriasis.
    - Also, psoriatic arthritis commonly involves the hand, whereas in reactive arthritis hand involvement is rare.
- Involved entheses becomes thickened, with poor definition of the adjacent fat planes (see Fig. 9.71).
- Bursae may be involved and appear distended with fluid and inflammatory synovium (see Fig. 9.71).
- On MRI, edema and enhancement can be observed at the entheses as well as the joint synovium and tendon sheaths (see Fig. 9.70).
- With more chronic disease, bursitis and enthesitis can cause erosions and bone proliferation, resulting in a classic 'fluffy' appearance.

Key Concepts

Reactive Arthritis

Formerly known as Reiter disease
Least common spondyloarthropathy
Occurs more frequently in males than in females
Radiographically identical to psoriasis but usually favors foot over hand
Calcaneal erosive disease and spur formation are prominent features

ANKYLOSING SPONDYLITIS

- AS is an inflammatory arthropathy and enthesopathy predominantly affecting the spine and pelvis; peak age is 20–40 years.
- Males are affected three to seven times more commonly than females.

- There is a strong association (90%) with the HLA-B27 antigen.
- AS typically presents as back pain and stiffness, worse in the morning, improving with exercise.
    - Patients may attempt to alleviate symptoms by avoiding bending and twisting of the spine.
- The disease can follow an intermittent course with recurrent flares.
- As ankylosis progresses the pain subsides, but stiffness often does not.
- Fractures can occur obliquely through the fused segments, and patients can suffer from a restrictive respiratory disorder caused by fusion of costovertebral joints.
- Early radiographic manifestations should be sought in any young patient with typical symptoms (Figs. 9.72 through 9.75).
- In the spine these include:
    - Squaring of the anterior vertebral bodies, usually beginning at L5 due to enthesitis and proliferation at the anterior longitudinal ligament insertion; and sclerosis at the anterosuperior endplates related to reactive bone formation at Sharpey's fiber insertions *(shiny corners)* (Fig. 9.76).
    - On MRI, edema may be seen at the anterior endplates at the sites of inflammation *(Romanus lesions)*. These are best seen on a sagittal short tau inversion recovery (STIR) sequence. Radiographs and CT show erosion initially and MRI shows edema, before healing with sclerosis (the shiny corner, low signal on MRI).
    - *Andersson lesion*, also called *inflammatory spondylodiscitis*, is an uncommon manifestation of AS, representing a fracture pseudoarthosis through a fused disc level or at a severely degenerated, unfused disc (the exact nature is debated).
    - Contrast enhancement on MRI can help detect subtle inflammation.

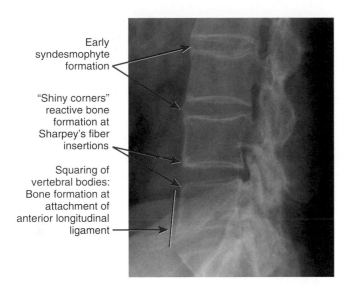

Early syndesmophyte formation

"Shiny corners" reactive bone formation at Sharpey's fiber insertions

Squaring of vertebral bodies: Bone formation at attachment of anterior longitudinal ligament

Fig. 9.72 Ankylosing spondylitis. Early radiographic manifestations should be sought in any young patient with typical symptoms. In the spine, these include squaring of the anterior vertebral bodies, usually beginning at L5 due to enthesitis and proliferation at the anterior longitudinal ligament insertion; and sclerosis at the anterosuperior endplates related to reactive bone formation at Sharpey's fiber insertions ('shiny corners'). (From Morrison W. *Problem Solving in Musculoskeletal Imaging*. Philadelphia: Elsevier; 2010.)

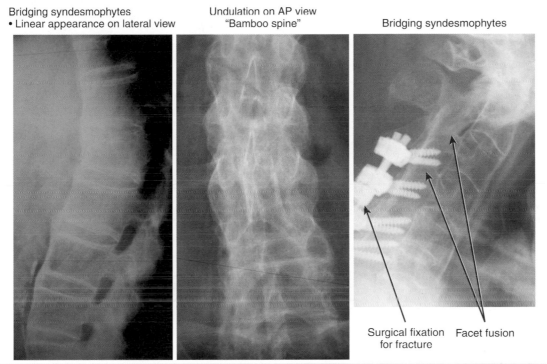

Bridging syndesmophytes
• Linear appearance on lateral view

Undulation on AP view "Bamboo spine"

Bridging syndesmophytes

Surgical fixation for fracture   Facet fusion

Fig. 9.73 Ankylosing spondylitis, late changes. Fusion with syndesmophytes; linear, close to vertebral bodies on lateral view. 'Bamboo spine' appearance on anteroposterior (AP) view. Fusion of facet and costovertebral joints may also occur. (From Morrison W. *Problem Solving in Musculoskeletal Imaging*. Philadelphia: Elsevier; 2010.)

- Eventually syndesmophytes form, bridging the discs; this is straight and closely opposed to the vertebrae on the lateral view and can be subtle; on the anteroposterior view the ossification undulates ('*bamboo spine*').
- Fusion in kyphosis often occurs.
- Cervical spine fusion can lead to laxity at C1-2 and instability.
- Facet joints and costovertebral joints often fuse as well (Fig. 9.77).
- Fractures of the fused spine in AS may involve the disc space and often run obliquely through the fused segments, termed '*chalk stick*' or '*carrot stick*' fractures (see Fig. 9.75).
- Often the first manifestations occur at the SI joints (Figs. 9.78 and 9.79); initially there is poor definition of the subchondral cortex white line and subsequently discrete erosions, which make the joint appear widened.
  - Erosions occur initially at the iliac side of the anteroinferior aspect of the joint, which is the synovial portion.
  - CT is superior to radiographs for detecting early erosions.

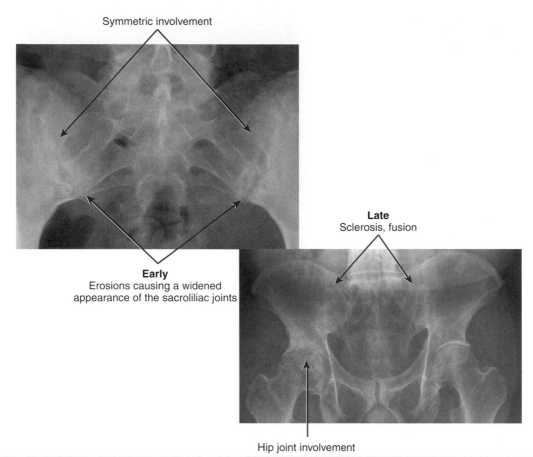

Symmetric involvement

Late
Sclerosis, fusion

Early
Erosions causing a widened
appearance of the sacroiliac joints

Hip joint involvement

Fig. 9.74 Ankylosing spondylitis, sacroiliac joint involvement. Often the first manifestations of ankylosing spondylitis occur at the sacroiliac joints. Initially, there is poor definition of the subchondral white line and subsequently discrete erosions, which make the joint look widened. Later in the course of disease, reactive sclerosis occurs around the sacroiliac joints, which ultimately may undergo fusion. Hip joint involvement may also occur. (From Morrison W. *Problem Solving in Musculoskeletal Imaging.* Philadelphia: Elsevier; 2010.)

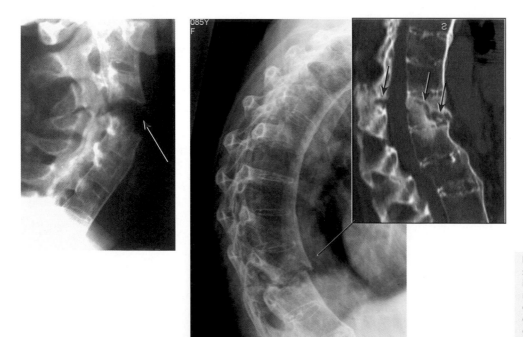

Fig. 9.75 Examples of ankylosing spondylitis with fracture. Note bridging syndesmophytes along the anterior spine; as a result, fractures often occur through the disc spaces (as seen on the left in the cervical spine) or obliquely through the vertebral elements (shown on the right in the thoracic spine). (From Morrison W. *Problem Solving in Musculoskeletal Imaging.* Philadelphia: Elsevier; 2010.)

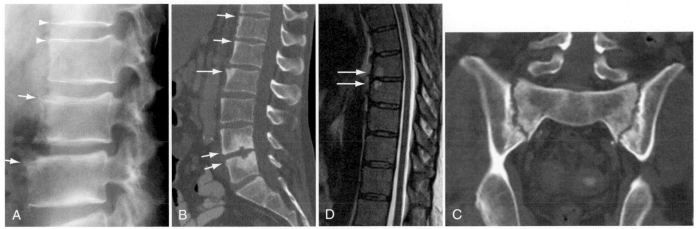

Fig. 9.76 Ankylosing spondylitis (AS), spine, early disease. **(A)** Lateral radiograph demonstrates findings in the early stages of AS. Note the squaring of some of the vertebral bodies with mild sclerosis at the corners ('shiny corners'; *arrowheads*) and the later finding of irregular new bone production at the corners of more inferior bodies *(arrows)*. A single vertical syndesmophyte is beginning to form at the inferior endplate of the lowest body seen on this image *(short arrow)*. The osteitis and resultant squaring are the first vertebral body abnormalities seen by radiograph in AS, followed by formation of the syndesmophytes. **(B)** CT in early AS shows corner osteitis and mild productive disease *(arrows)*. No syndesmophyte formation is seen at this point. **(C)** Coronal CT of the SI joints in the same patient confirms signs of AS, with joint space widening, erosions, and sclerosis. **(D)** Earliest MR changes of AS shown on sagittal STIR image as high signal at the vertebral body corners *(arrows)*; these corner abnormalities are termed *Romanus lesions*. They are typical of early AS on MR, but not pathognomonic.

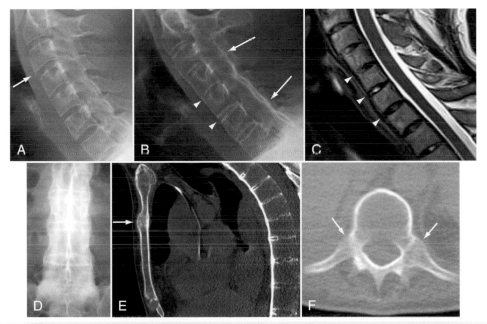

Fig. 9.77 Ankylosing spondylitis (AS), spine. **(A)** Lateral cervical spine radiograph in a young man shows minimal productive changes at the corners of the vertebral bodies, as well as a single-level syndesmophyte at C3-4 *(arrow)*. This is a common radiographic appearance in early disease. **(B)** Lateral radiograph in the same patient obtained 10 years later shows complete fusion of the spine, with thin vertical syndesmophytes at most levels *(arrowheads)* and fully fused facets *(arrows)*. **(C)** Sagittal T2-weighted MR image, same patient, shows syndesmophytes *(arrowheads)*, but they are subtle. It might be easy to miss the diagnosis if the MR image is interpreted without access to the radiograph, on which the diagnosis is obvious. **(D)** AP radiograph demonstrates advanced AS, with complete fusion of the sacroiliac joints, as well as fusion of the lumbar vertebral bodies. The thin vertical syndesmophytes seen at all levels of the lumbar spine outline the relatively dense endplates, giving the 'bamboo spine' appearance. **(E)** Sagittal CT of another end-stage AS patient, showing kyphosis and complete fusion of the thoracic spine, interspinous process fusion, and fusion of the sternomanubrial joint *(arrow)*. **(F)** Axial CT in the same patient shows costovertebral fusion *(arrows)*. Remember that axial fusion occurs not only in the spine but in the other axial joints as well.

- MRI with fluid-sensitive sequences (STIR or T2 with fat suppression) can detect marrow edema before erosions develop. Contrast enhancement can improve sensitivity.
- Later, reactive bone at the margins of the joint causes ill-defined sclerosis.
- Eventually the joint fuses and the reactive sclerosis may eventually subside.
- Both synovial and ligamentous portions of the joint eventually fuse.
- Sacroiliitis in AS (and inflammatory bowel disease) is characteristically bilateral and symmetric (MRI may show some asymmetry); sacroiliitis

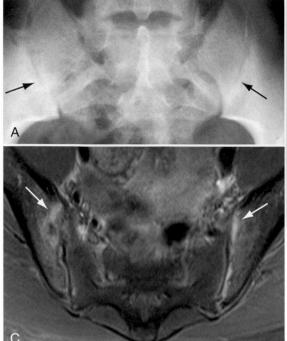

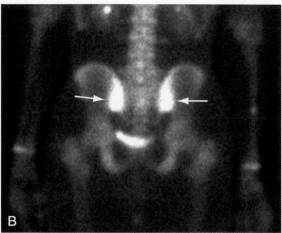

Fig. 9.78 Ankylosing spondylitis (AS), sacroiliac (SI) joints, early imaging findings. **(A)** AP radiograph of the SI joints demonstrates very early changes that can be found in the spondyloarthropathy of ankylosing spondylitis. There is loss of the normal subchondral 'white line' *(arrows)* representing erosion of the articular surfaces. **(B)** Bone scan in a child with AS shows significant and symmetric increased uptake in the SI joints *(arrows)*; note the intense radiotracer uptake relative to the anterior superior iliac spines or other apophyses/epiphyses. **(C)** Axial STIR MR image in the same child shows hyperintensity of the cortices of the SI joints bilaterally *(arrows)*, more prominent on the iliac than sacral side. No true erosions are seen at this early stage.

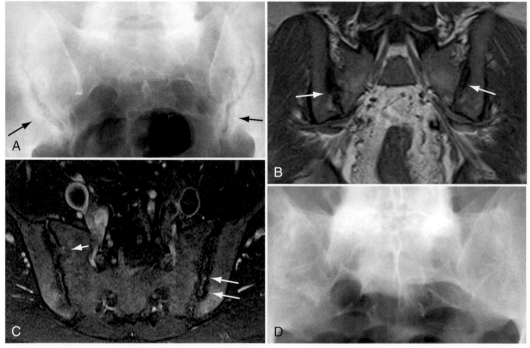

Fig. 9.79 Ankylosing spondylitis (AS), sacroiliac (SI) joints. **(A)** Intermediate phase of sacroiliitis in AS, with symmetric findings of slight widening of the SI joints, sclerosis, and erosions that are more extensive in the inferior (synovial) portion of the joints *(arrows)*. **(B)** T1-weighted coronal MR image in a 29-year-old man with AS shows bilateral hypointensity along the SI joints, with widening and erosions, more prominent on the right than the left *(arrows)*. **(C)** Fat-saturated T2-weighted axial imaging of the same patient shows marrow edema on both sides of the SI joints, as well as bilateral erosions *(arrows)*. **(D)** End-stage complete SI joint fusion. AP radiograph shows SI joints that are completely fused bilaterally.

associated with psoriatic arthritis and reactive arthritis can be unilateral, or bilateral, but is more overtly asymmetric.

■ Septic arthritis is unilateral and may also show a joint effusion and edema in adjacent soft tissues (Table 9.16).

■ In the appendicular skeleton, the hips are the most common site of involvement, typically bilateral and symmetric. Concentric bilateral joint narrowing with axial migration with minimal to no erosion is common. The peripheral large joint pattern resembles RA.

Table 9.16 Sacroiliac Joint Disease

BILATERAL SYMMETRIC

Ankylosing spondylitis
Inflammatory bowel disease
Osteitis condensans ilii (iliac side)

BILATERAL ASYMMETRIC

Psoriatic arthritis
Reactive arthritis
Rheumatoid arthritis (rare)
Osteoarthritis

UNILATERAL

Infection
Psoriatic arthritis/reactive arthritis

MIMICKERS OF SACROILIITIS

Adolescence (articular surfaces undeveloped)
Hyperparathyroidism (subchondral bone resorption)
Osteoarthritis (anterior bridging spurs)
Postop (iliac bone graft donor site)

Key Concepts

Ankylosing Spondylitis

Frequently positive for HLA-B27
Occurs more frequently in males than in females
Presents in adolescents or young adults
Bilateral sacroiliac disease hallmark; erosive early, ankylosis quickly
    follows
Bamboo spine
Affects large proximal appendicular joints more often than distal
    joints
Spine fracture at cervicothoracic and thoracolumbar junctions
    with pseudarthrosis, resulting from minimal trauma, often
    results in significant morbidity
MRI may show preradiographic findings (enthesitis, Romanus and
    Andersson spine lesions)
Romanus lesion: edema/erosion at the anterior endplates on MRI
    (subsequent sclerosis 'shiny corners' on radiographs and CT)
Andersson lesion: Fracture pseudarthrosis or severely degenerated
    disc at an unfused level
Findings can be easily overlooked in routine MRI and CT spine
    cases, even in relatively advanced disease

Key Concepts

Differential Diagnosis of Ligamentous Ossification in the Spine

Diffuse idiopathic skeletal hyperostosis (DISH; diagnosis of
    exclusion)
Ankylosing spondylitis
Severe spondylosis
Vitamin A toxicity
Fluorosis
Retinoic acid medications (classically cervical spine)

- Although AS is less common in women, the diagnosis should not be excluded on the basis of female gender. The radiographic findings tend to be neither as severe nor as typical in distribution as in male patients. The disease can present later in females and skip levels in the spine.

SPONDYLITIS OF INFLAMMATORY BOWEL DISEASE (ENTEROPATHIC ARTHROPATHY)

- The arthropathy of inflammatory bowel disease (IBD), also called *enteropathic arthropathy,* can be seen in two forms.
    - One form occurs as a result of *Salmonella, Shigella,* or *Yersinia* infections. These diseases may produce a self-limited polyarthritis, occasionally with SI joint symptoms but usually without radiographic findings.
    - A more pronounced spondyloarthropathy may occur with ulcerative colitis and less frequently with Crohn disease or Whipple disease.
        - As many as 10–15% of these patients develop chronic arthropathy.
        - Most of these patients have mild peripheral arthralgias without structural abnormalities, but one-third may develop sacroiliitis that is identical both clinically and by imaging to that of AS (Fig. 9.80).
- There is a close association of IBD spondyloarthropathy and AS because 50% of these IBD patients are positive for HLA-B27.
- In addition, 60% of AS patients have subclinical change in the large or small bowel.
- The steroids used for treatment of IBD put the patient at additional risk for osteonecrosis. Radiologic findings of osteonecrosis or bowel surgery in a study that otherwise appears classic for the diagnosis of AS should make one consider IBD spondyloarthropathy (see Fig. 9.80).

Key Concepts

Spondylitis of Inflammatory Bowel Disease

Most severe manifestations are identical to AS.
Most frequent in ulcerative colitis.

DISH and OPLL

DISH

- Diffuse idiopathic skeletal hyperostosis (DISH), previously known as Forestier disease, results in profound ossification of spinal soft tissues, including the annulus fibrosis, anterior longitudinal ligament, and paravertebral connective tissues (Fig. 9.81).
    - Ossification of the anterior longitudinal ligament results in the classic 'flowing' ossification along the anterolateral (predominantly right-sided, opposite to the aorta) aspect of the spine.
    - There is usually relative preservation of disc height of the involved segments. Degenerative disc disease, as well as facet productive change, is not as prominent as the anterior ossification.
    - Resulting fusion can cause accelerated degenerative changes at levels above and/or below fused segments.
    - Fractures can occur through areas of fusion; like AS, fractures can be atypical and obliquely oriented (the 'broken DISH') (Fig. 9.82).

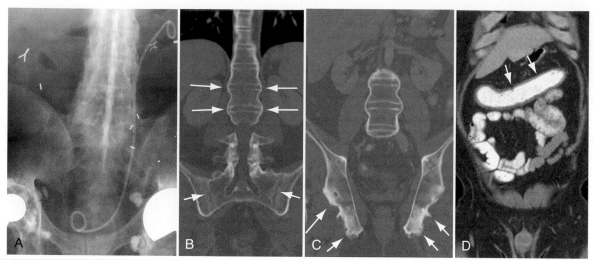

Fig. 9.80 Spondylitis of inflammatory bowel disease (IBD). **(A)** Abdominal radiograph in a patient with long-standing ankylosing spondylitis shows bilateral hip arthroplasties (likely related to avascular necrosis from steroid treatment), left ureteral stent (urolithiasis), surgical clips in the right upper quadrant (cholecystectomy for cholelithiasis), right ostomy (total colectomy for ulcerative colitis), and drain in the left abdomen (increased vulnerability to infection, in this case an abdominal abscess). Other extraarticular complications of ankylosing spondylitis include iritis, aortic valve insufficiency, and aortic root aneurysm, cardiac conduction abnormalities, and upper lung interstitial disease. **(B)** Coronal CT scan of another patient with IBD shows severe bilateral sacroiliac joint disease *(short arrows)* along with bridging vertical syndesmophytes *(long arrows)*. **(C)** Slightly more posterior coronal CT scan in the same patient again shows syndesmophytes, as well as tremendous enthesopathy along the ischii *(arrows)*. **(D)** Coronal CT scan through the abdomen, same patient, shows circumferential transverse colon wall thickening *(arrows)* in this patient with ulcerative colitis, proving IBD as the underlying cause of the spondyloarthropathy. Note that the spondyloarthropathy of IBD is identical to that of ankylosing spondylitis; hints such as bowel abnormalities may help differentiate the two.

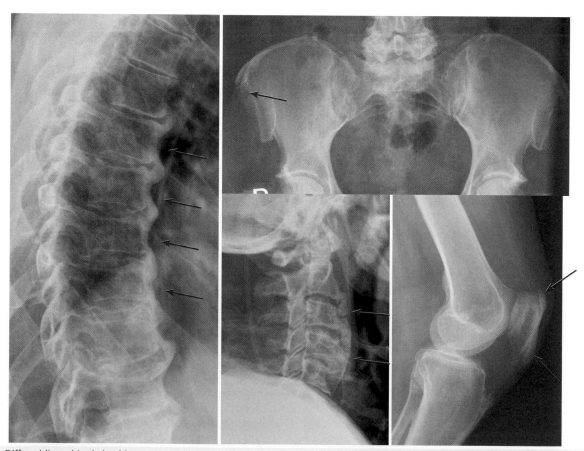

Fig. 9.81 Diffuse idiopathic skeletal hyperostosis (DISH). DISH is seen in older individuals, predominantly involving the thoracic spine with flowing anterior ossification (at least four levels); associated with enthesophytes elsewhere (especially pelvis). Patients are at increased risk for heterotopic bone formation after joint replacement. Differentiated from ankylosing spondylitis by age (older), location (C, T-spine > L-spine, no sacroiliac involvement), and morphology (loosely flowing ossification on lateral view). (From Morrison W. *Problem Solving in Musculoskeletal Imaging.* Philadelphia: Elsevier; 2010.)

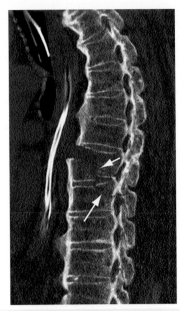

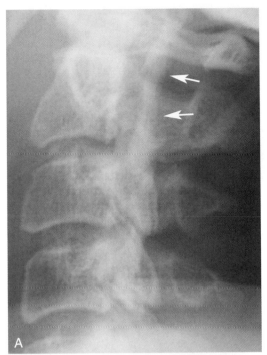

Fig. 9.82 Fracture in diffuse idiopathic skeletal hyperostosis (DISH). Sagittal CT reconstruction of the thoracic spine shows anterior flowing osteophytes along the length of the thoracic spine, effectively fusing the entire column. The bones are osteoporotic, as can occur in an older adult who has chronic DISH with extensive fusion. There is a transverse fracture extending across a disc space *(arrows)*, then into a thoracic vertebral body. This is reminiscent of the 'carrot stick' fracture that can occur with minor trauma in patients with long-column fusion and osteoporosis caused by ankylosing spondylitis. This particular patient had no evidence of ankylosing spondylitis, and there is convincing evidence of long-standing DISH; this patient's fracture occurred secondary to chest compressions during a resuscitation. (Image used with permission from BJ Manaster, MD, from STATdx website, Amirsys, Inc.)

Table 9.17   DISH Versus a Ankylosing Spondylitis

	DISH	AS
Age	Old	Young
Early distribution	T-spine	SI joints, L-spine
Lateral view	Wavy, thick	Flat, thin
Pelvic involvement	Iliac enthesophytes	Sacroiliitis
Fractures	Oblique	Oblique

Abbreviations: AS, ankylosing spondylitis; DISH, diffuse idiopathic skeletal hyperostosis; L-spine, lumbar spine; SI, sacroiliac; T-spine, thoracic spine.

- Most cases are asymptomatic.
- DISH is usually easily differentiated from AS (Table 9.17):
  - DISH is seen in an older population and is distributed mainly in the thoracic spine and cervical spine, generally sparing the lumbar spine and SI joints, whereas AS is seen in younger patients with predominant SI joint and lower spine involvement.
  - Also, while syndesmophytes in AS are thin and closely applied to the spine on the lateral view, anterior ossification in DISH is thick and undulating.
  - Patients with DISH tend to be 'bone formers'—this can manifest as enthesophytes (e.g., at the iliac crest and patella) as well as a tendency to form heterotopic ossification after surgery.

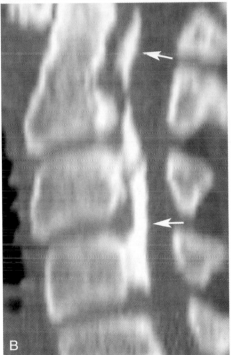

Fig. 9.83 Ossification of the posterior longitudinal ligament (OPLL). Lateral radiograph **(A)** and sagittal CT reconstruction **(B)** show OPLL *(arrows)* of the cervical spine with associated spinal stenosis.

OPLL

- Ossification of the posterior longitudinal ligament (OPLL) is another condition resulting in bone formation; this has special significance since it may result in spinal stenosis and spinal cord impingement (Fig. 9.83).
  - In OPLL, the posterior longitudinal ligament (PLL) hypertrophies and calcifies/ossifies leading to a vertically oriented 'spike' of bone extending along the

central aspect of the posterior vertebral bodies. This forms a 'heart-shaped' spinal canal and can impinge on the anterior cord.

- Calcification/ossification may extend along one or multiple levels, often with more than one site of involvement.
- OPLL occurs in the cervical spine. In most patients symptoms are insidious, with gradual onset of numbness and paresthesias in the upper extremities. Approximately 10–25% present acutely after trauma with central cord syndrome.

- DISH and OPLL may also coexist (Figs. 9.84 and 9.85), and patients with either condition also commonly exhibit prominent enthesophyte formation as well as excess heterotopic bone formation after surgery. An overlap syndrome may also exist with AS since a small proportion of patients exhibit common imaging characteristics.

- Differential considerations in DISH include:
  - *Retinoid arthropathy*, which may be a consideration in patients using retinoic acid for skin diseases and who develop skeletal hyperostoses similar to those seen in DISH.
    - In retinoid arthropathy the cervical spine is the most common site of involvement, but thoracic and lumbar involvement is seen as well (see Fig. 13.52).

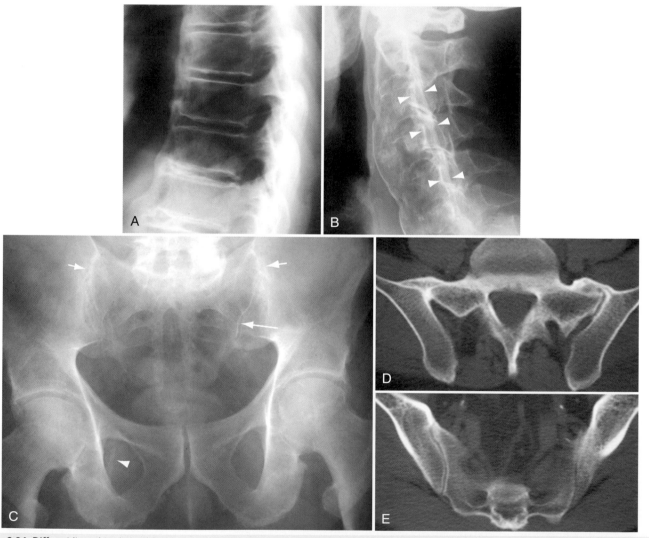

Fig. 9.84 Diffuse idiopathic skeletal hyperostosis (DISH). **(A)** Lateral thoracic spine radiograph shows dense ossification of the anterior longitudinal ligament (ALL) that is typical of DISH. **(B)** Lateral cervical spine radiograph shows mature ALL ossification, as well as ossification of the posterior longitudinal ligament (OPLL; between *arrowheads*). The two disease processes (DISH and OPLL) are frequently seen together. **(C)** AP radiograph of the pelvis shows normal inferior synovial sacroiliac (SI) joints *(long arrow)*, but fusion of the superior, nonsynovial portions of the SI joints *(short arrows)*. Also note subtle ossification of the right sacrotuberous ligament *(arrowhead)*. Both of these findings are typical of DISH. **(D** and **E)** CT in a different patient through the superior **(D)** and inferior **(E)** SI joints better demonstrates the pattern of SI disease with DISH with superior fusion and preservation of the inferior (synovial) joint.

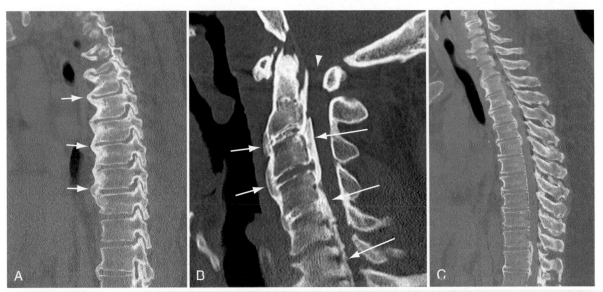

Fig. 9.85 Combined diffuse idiopathic skeletal hyperostosis (DISH) and ossification of the posterior longitudinal ligament (OPLL). **(A)** Thoracic spine sagittal CT reconstruction demonstrates typical anterior flowing osteophytes *(arrows)* on the right parasagittal side of the thoracic spine. There is no significant disc or facet disease. **(B)** Cervical spine sagittal CT reconstruction in the same patient shows mild anterior bridging osteophytes *(short arrows)* and prominent posterior longitudinal ligament ossification *(long arrows)*. Note the severe stenosis between the dens and the posterior arch of C1 *(arrowhead)*. **(C)** Left parasagittal CT reconstruction of the same thoracic spine shows ossification at several sites of the posterior longitudinal ligament. This case shows convincing presence of both DISH and OPLL, without either disease process predominating. (Images used with permission from BJ Manaster, MD, from STATdx website, Amirsys, Inc.)

- Eventually, along with the anterior osteophyte formation, anterior and PLL calcification may be seen.
- *Fluorosis* (fluoride intoxication caused by long-term ingestion) also can cause bulky paraspinous ligament calcification similar to DISH.
  - Bones affected by fluorosis may be diffusely osteopenic or sclerotic in a patchy or 'chalky' pattern.
  - Vertebral spurs are frequent, as are dental abnormalities such as mottled tooth enamel.

SAPHO Syndrome

- SAPHO syndrome (synovitis, acne, pustulosis, hyperostosis, osteitis) is an uncommon spectrum of spondyloarthropathy in which patients can have various osteoarticular manifestations, the most common being osteitis of the anterior chest wall, often with dermatologic abnormalities.
- This is seen as frequently painful hyperostosis and soft tissue ossification between the medial clavicle, anterior portion of the upper ribs, and manubrium (Fig. 9.86).
- In addition to the anterior chest wall, the axial skeleton may be involved, and rarely extraaxial tumor-simulating bone lesions are seen.
- Pustulosis, psoriatic lesions, and spondyloarthropathy may also be seen.
- More frequent in HLA-B27–positive patients.
- Shares some features with psoriatic arthritis and may be related.
- Chronic recurrent multifocal osteomyelitis (CRMO), discussed in the chapter on infection (Chapter 14 – Musculoskeletal Infection), also can share some features with SAPHO syndrome, notably clavicle sclerosis and pustulosis of the palms and soles.

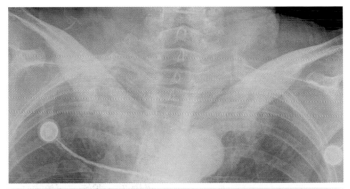

Fig. 9.86 SAPHO syndrome (synovitis, acne, pustulosis, hyperostosis, osteitis). Detail from a chest radiograph shows massive thickening of the medial clavicles and manubrium with fusion. (Courtesy of William Pommersheim, MD.)

Connective-Tissue Diseases

- The connective-tissue disorders, also known as collagen vascular diseases, are a loosely related group of multisystem diseases that have in common vasculitis, a likely autoimmune cause, a predilection for connective-tissue involvement (although not specifically collagen), and related laboratory abnormalities such as immune complexes and antinuclear antibodies (ANAs).

SYSTEMIC LUPUS ERYTHEMATOSIS

- Systemic lupus erythematosus (SLE) is an autoimmune disease occurring in a younger population (15–40 years old).
- There is a distinct gender distribution, with females more commonly affected than males (ratio ranging from 5:1 to 10:1).

- People of African descent are more commonly affected than other groups.
- Disease most commonly manifests in young adults.
- Lab markers include presence of ANAs, with certain specific subtypes frequently present. The lupus erythematosus test is no longer used due to inadequate sensitivity and specificity.
- Patients present clinically with constitutional symptoms (weakness, malaise, fever) and a rash such as the characteristic butterfly (malar) rash on the face.
- Organ system involvement includes myositis, various neurologic abnormalities, pulmonary vasculitis, pulmonary fibrosis, pleural effusions, pericarditis, cardiomyopathy, and nephritis.
- Arthropathy of SLE is common and is a nonerosive but deforming disease characterized on radiography by subluxations without erosions (Fig. 9.87).
  - The subluxations may reduce as the joints are flattened against the radiography plate and may only be seen on lateral and oblique (Nørgaard or 'ball-catchers') views.
  - *Jaccoud arthropathy* (discussed in the following section) occurs in 5% of patients with SLE.
- One of the presenting signs of musculoskeletal involvement by SLE is tenosynovitis.
  - The hands, and specifically the flexor tendons, are the most frequently involved.
  - Diagnosis is made by MRI or US.
  - Tendon disruption, and less frequently myopathy, may be seen as well.
- Another radiographic feature of SLE is the remarkably high incidence of osteonecrosis.
  - Up to one-third of patients with SLE may show osteonecrosis at MRI, although only 8% are symptomatic.

- Steroid therapy is felt to be the major etiologic factor, but the vasculitis caused by the disease process also predisposes to osteonecrosis.
- The femoral head, humeral head, and knee are common sites.
- Widespread osteonecrosis particularly if found in unusual sites (such as the talus or tibial plateau), should suggest the diagnosis of SLE.

Key Concepts

Systemic Lupus Erythematosus

Multisystem inflammation
Young adults
Occurs more frequently in females than in males
Occurs more frequently in African Americans than whites
Musculoskeletal: Polyarthritis with reversible deformities
Hand and wrist most commonly affected
Usually nonerosive (in contrast with RA)
Osteonecrosis (caused by steroid therapy and vasculitis)
Soft tissue calcification in 10% of cases, usually lower extremity

JACCOUD ARTHROPATHY

- Nonerosive reversible arthropathy with joint deformities, especially in the hand that resemble RA.
  - MCP ulnar deviation, most severe in the medial fingers, is a classic appearance.
  - Swan neck and boutonnière deformities.
  - Other joints may be involved.
  - No erosions on radiographs.
- When originally described was caused by rheumatic fever, which is now rare.
- Today occurs most frequently in SLE but can also be seen in other seronegative inflammatory arthropathies.

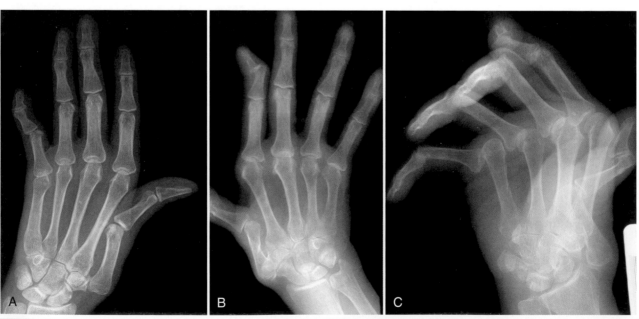

Fig. 9.87 Systemic lupus erythematosus (SLE). **(A)** PA radiograph of the hand shows multiple subluxations, including 'Hitchhiker's thumb'. **(B and C)** Reversible deformities. PA **(B)** and Norgaard **(C)** views in a patient with SLE demonstrate multiple subluxations, which appear worsened in the Norgaard view because the hand is not supported on the cassette. The bones are diffusely osteoporotic, and erosions are not seen. The findings are typical of the nonerosive but deforming arthropathy of SLE. (A, courtesy of William Pommersheim, MD.)

Approximately 5% of patients with SLE develop Jaccoud arthropathy.

SCLERODERMA (PROGRESSIVE SYSTEMIC SCLEROSIS)

- *Scleroderma* is an umbrella term for a family of autoimmune conditions that have in common hardening of the skin.
- The process may be confined to the skin or may involve several organ systems (kidneys, heart, lung, GI, and musculoskeletal), hence the term *systemic sclerosis*.
- Vascular features such as Raynaud phenomenon (episodic digital ischemia precipitated by cold or emotional stress) are common.
- The mechanism is a combination of excess collagen production, microvascular injury, and chronic inflammation.
- The etiology is unknown. Both genetic and environmental factors are involved.
- Scleroderma can be classified as diffuse or limited.
  - Skin involvement in diffuse scleroderma involves the extremities proximal to the elbows and knees, and the trunk, whereas limited scleroderma involves the distal extremities and face.
  - The *CREST syndrome* (skin calcinosis, Raynaud phenomenon, esophageal dysmotility, sclerodactyly, and telangiectasia) is a common type of limited scleroderma. CREST is an older term, and not all of the features must be present to make this diagnosis.
- Scleroderma affects females more frequently than males, in a 3:1 ratio, and is most often diagnosed in the third to fifth decades of life.
- Laboratory test results are not specific. Most patients have elevated ESR, and up to 40% are positive for RF.

- Patients with scleroderma may have coexisting SLE or polymyositis/dermatomyositis. Many features of scleroderma are also found in *overlap syndrome*, also known as *mixed connective-tissue disease*.
- Patients with scleroderma may present with Raynaud phenomenon; skin changes on the hands, feet, or face; distal joint pain and stiffness; dysphagia; and proximal myopathy.
- Esophageal atrophy and fibrosis lead to dysmotility, reflux, and reflux stricture, which may be noted as air-fluid levels within the esophagus on a chest radiograph.
- The dysmotility and 'hidebound', thickened, squared small bowel folds and pseudosacculations of the small intestine and colon are seen with GI studies.
- Soft tissue abnormalities are extremely common, seen clinically at first as edema but eventually resulting in taut, shiny, and atrophic soft tissues.
- In the hands, vasculitis and Raynaud phenomenon lead to progressive distal phalangeal tapering.
- Radiographically the acral (distal) tapering of the digits is seen both in the soft tissues and distal phalanges (Fig. 9.88), leading to an appearance like a sharpened pencil.

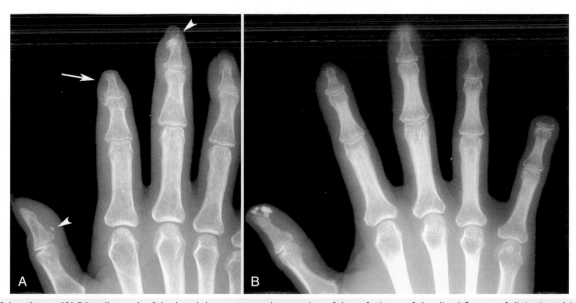

Fig. 9.88 Scleroderma. **(A)** PA radiograph of the hand demonstrates the tapering of the soft tissue of the distal fingers of digits 2 and 3, with acro-osteolysis seen at digit 2 *(arrow)*. Soft tissue calcification is seen both at the thumb and digit 3 *(arrowheads)*. This combination is typical for scleroderma. **(B)** PA radiograph of a more advanced case of scleroderma, with severe acro-osteolysis at multiple digits as well as soft tissue calcification. (A, Image used with permission from BJ Manaster, MD, from the American College of Radiology Learning File.)

Table 9.18   Acro-osteolysis Differential Diagnosis

THERMAL INJURY

- Burn (see Fig. 9.89A): May have contracture and soft tissue calcifications
- Frostbite (see Figs. 9.89B and C): Usually spares the thumb

ENVIRONMENTAL

- Polyvinylchloride (PVC)

METABOLIC

- Hyperparathyroidism: Tuft resorption, often accompanied by other signs of subperiosteal resorption, vascular calcification, or brown tumors
- Lesch–Nyhan syndrome

ARTHRITIS

- Psoriatic: There should be associated distal interphalangeal erosive disease
- Neuroarthropathy, especially diabetic

CONNECTIVE-TISSUE DISEASE

- Scleroderma: Often associated with soft tissue calcification
- Other causes of vasculitis

INFECTION

- Leprosy, associated with linear calcifications of the digital nerves (see Fig. 9.91)

- This appearance called *acro-osteolysis* may be seen in up to 80% of patients.
- Acro-osteolysis is nonspecific because it may be seen in other disorders (Fig. 9.89; Table 9.18).
- Resorption of bone, although most commonly seen in the phalangeal tufts, may also be severe at the first carpometacarpal joint, resulting in radial and proximal subluxation of the first metacarpal.

- Bone resorption can also be seen at the angle of the mandible and at the posterior ribs, particularly ribs 3–6, and diffusely about the wrist.
- In addition to distal resorption, the other distinctive radiographic feature in scleroderma is soft tissue calcification.
    - Calcification is seen in 25% of cases and may be subcutaneous, extraarticular, intraarticular, or even punctate within the terminal phalanx (Figs. 9.88 and 9.90).
    - Of those patients with calcinosis, 73–80% have hand involvement. However, soft tissue calcification in conjunction with acro-osteolysis is not specific for scleroderma (Fig. 9.91).
- Although acro-osteolysis and soft tissue calcification are the most frequent features of scleroderma, cartilage destruction and erosive changes are occasionally seen, usually late in the disease.
    - It may be difficult to attribute erosive change only to scleroderma because many patients have mixed connective-tissue disease with coexisting features of RA or other overlap syndromes that might explain the presence of erosions.
    - Overall, joint abnormalities eventually occur in nearly 50% of patients with scleroderma.
    - These joint abnormalities are usually erosive, but relatively mild, and typically lack subchondral cyst formation.
    - Mild bone productive changes and flexion contractures may be seen as well.
- Tenosynovitis is often an early finding. MRI or US may show fibrotic nodules on tendons, outlined by fluid in the tendon sheath.
- Inflammatory myopathy may be seen by MRI as well, but it is not distinguishable from other causes.

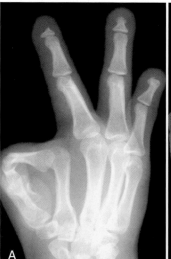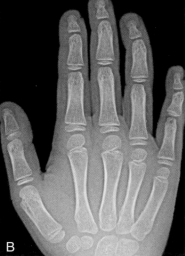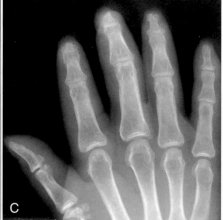

Fig. 9.89 Examples of acro-osteolysis that may mimic that seen in scleroderma. **(A)** Burn. Oblique radiograph demonstrates severe acro-osteolysis at digits 3, 4, and 5, with a contracture of digits 1 and 2. The combination is typical of burn. Soft tissue calcifications are sometimes seen as well, although not in this case. **(B)** Sequela of frostbite in a 7-year-old child. Note that the physes of the distal phalanges of digits 2–5 have closed prematurely, whereas that at the thumb is normal. The growth centers are most at risk for thermal injury, and this patient's distal phalanges will not grow further. As an adult this patient will have short distal phalanges. A thumb that is normal in size and morphologic characteristics is typical of frostbite because the thumb is protected by the cupped hand when one is cold. **(C)** Frostbite, more severe case. PA radiograph of the hand in an adult shows amputations of the distal second and third fingers and short distal phalanx of the fourth finger. Even the thumb shows some tissue loss. (A, Image used with permission from BJ Manaster, MD, from the American College of Radiology Learning File.)

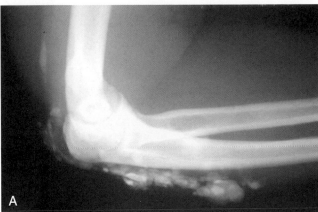

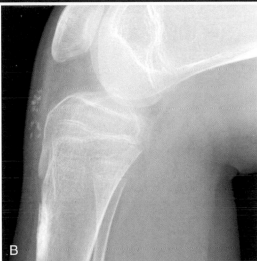

Fig. 9.90 Scleroderma. **(A)** Extensive linear and nodular soft tissue calcification at the extensor surface of the elbow and proximal forearm. **(B)** Punctate soft tissue calcification within the anterior soft tissues of the knee in a child with scleroderma. Note that the pattern or presence of soft calcifications is not specific in scleroderma.

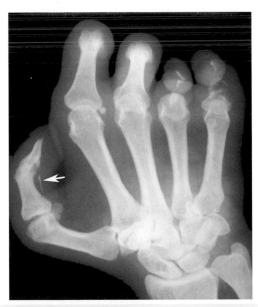

Fig. 9.91 Acro-osteolysis in leprosy shows extreme osteolysis involving all the digits, with an added feature of a calcified digital nerve *(arrow)*; digital nerve calcification is typical of leprosy.

POLYMYOSITIS AND DERMATOMYOSITIS

■ Polymyositis and dermatomyositis are autoimmune diseases that produce inflammation and muscle degeneration. In polymyositis the symptoms of proximal muscle weakness and arthralgias predominate. With dermatomyositis, a typical diffuse erythematous rash is an additional finding.

Key Concepts

Polymyositis and Dermatomyositis

Active disease: MRI shows muscle edema
Late stage: fatty infiltration/atrophy, eventual soft tissue calcifications, either subcutaneous or sheetlike in fascial planes
MRI to guide biopsy: look for sites of active inflammation
Avascular necrosis can result from corticosteroid therapy
Arthralgias, but erosions rare

■ Polymyositis and dermatomyositis usually occur in the third through fifth decades of life, and females are more frequently affected than males.
■ Dermatomyositis may also be seen in children, associated with very severe systemic symptoms. Patients with this disease show muscle weakness and tenderness with eventual contracture and atrophy.
■ The muscles involved are usually proximal limb muscles (vasti and thigh adductors particularly).
■ Early in the disease the muscles develop edema, followed later by atrophy and adjacent soft tissue calcification (Fig. 9.92).
  ▪ The early muscle disease may be identified on MRI with edema-like signal intensity in muscle, seen best with fat-saturated T2-weighted or inversion recovery sequences.
  ▪ Late-stage disease shows fatty atrophy of the muscles with increased T1 signal.
■ The calcifications that develop late in the disease are seen on radiographs.
  ▪ The most common calcification pattern is a nonspecific subcutaneous calcification. 'Sheetlike' calcifications along fascial planes are less common but are virtually pathognomonic for these diseases.
  ▪ Classically, these sheetlike calcifications are seen along the proximal large muscles.
  ▪ Occasionally, periarticular calcification may occur.
  ▪ MRI is useful in guiding a biopsy when polymyositis or dermatomyositis is suspected; an optimal biopsy should not be directed toward end-stage fatty atrophy, but rather edema related to active inflammatory cell infiltration (Fig. 9.93).
■ Although the hands, wrists, and knees are affected with arthralgias, radiographic bone or joint abnormalities are rare. However, because these patients are treated with corticosteroids, they may develop osteonecrosis and osteoporosis as a complication of therapy.

MIXED CONNECTIVE-TISSUE DISEASE AND OVERLAP SYNDROMES

■ Occasionally a connective-tissue disorder does not fall into a particular disease category, or includes features of multiple disorders.

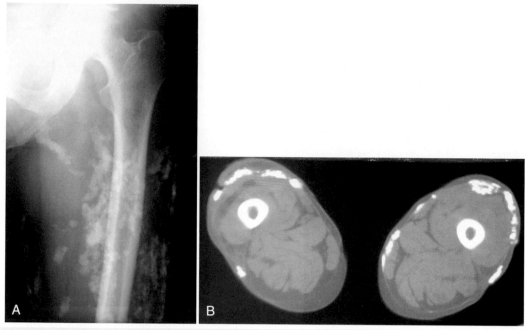

Fig. 9.92 Dermatomyositis, late-stage findings. **(A)** AP radiograph demonstrates sheetlike calcifications in the soft tissues of the thigh of this 50-year-old woman. **(B)** CT confirms the location of the calcifications to be within both the subcutaneous tissues and fascial planes. Sheetlike calcifications are typically described with late-stage dermatomyositis, but the calcifications may assume other configurations. (Images used with permission from BJ Manaster, MD, from the American College of Radiology Learning File.)

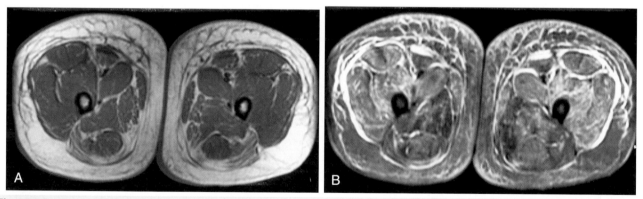

Fig. 9.93 Dermatomyositis, MRI of active disease. Axial T1-weighted **(A)** and inversion recovery **(B)** MR images of the thighs in a 35-year-old woman with new-onset dermatomyositis show extensive edema in thigh musculature, fascia, and subcutaneous tissues. Biopsy should be performed in muscles with edema but no fatty infiltration, because the latter indicates inactive, end-stage disease and may yield nonspecific biopsy results. Potential biopsy sites abound in this patient because there is little fatty infiltration.

- Conditions and terms include:
  - *Mixed connective-tissue disease* (MCTD, a combination of scleroderma, SLE, and polymyositis).
  - *Overlap syndromes* (satisfying criteria of more than one disease, such as: SLE and RA; scleroderma and RA; scleroderma and SLE; scleroderma and polymyositis) (Fig. 9.94).
  - *Undifferentiated connective-tissue syndromes* (do not satisfy criteria for any specific diagnosis).
  - Laboratory evaluation often helps establish the diagnosis in mixed connective-tissue disease. A specific autoantibody is present that also is present in scleroderma, SLE, and polymyositis.
- Imaging features reflect the disease subsets represented by the combined disease process.
  - Soft tissue swelling and coarse calcification are common.
  - The distal digits may be 'whittled' similar to scleroderma, and acro-osteolysis may be present.
  - Joint narrowing occurs as part of the inflammatory arthropathy.
  - Synovial marginal erosions develop as in RA.
  - Flexion deformities and subluxations occur.
  - Ankylosis is a late finding typically occurring at the MCP and IP joints.
  - MCTD favors small joints such as those in the hand and wrist.
- The radiologist should be aware of these overlap findings when the imaging findings do not fit neatly into a particular disease: for example, when rheumatoid-like changes are seen at the wrist while calcifications are observed in the digits.

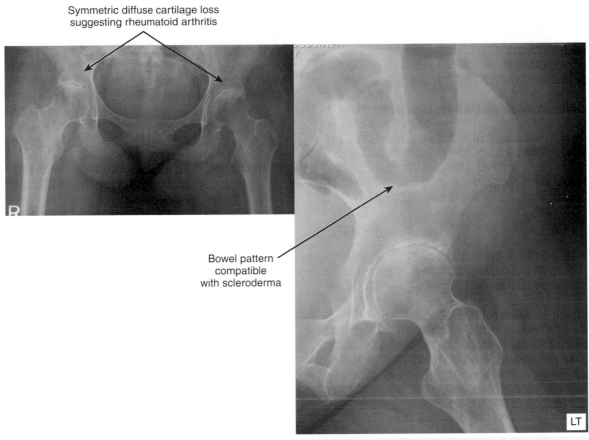

Symmetric diffuse cartilage loss
suggesting rheumatoid arthritis

Bowel pattern
compatible
with scleroderma

Fig. 9.94 Overlap syndrome. Patient exhibiting clinical, serologic, and imaging features of rheumatoid arthritis and scleroderma. (From Morrison W. *Problem Solving in Musculoskeletal Imaging.* Philadelphia: Elsevier; 2010.)

Crystalline and Deposition Diseases

GOUT

- Gout is a painful arthropathy related to monosodium urate crystal deposition in joints and periarticular soft tissues.
  - Uric acid is a normal degradation product of the metabolism of exogenous and endogenous purines, but is not further degraded because of the lack of a 'uricase' enzyme in humans.
  - Renal excretion is the main route of elimination of uric acid. Hyperuricemia may be due to overproduction, underexcretion, or most commonly a combination of the two.
  - Most patients with gout have a relatively deficient renal excretion mechanism.
    - Factors that affect renal excretion include genetic factors, drugs (diuretics, cyclosporine, salicylates), underlying chronic renal disease (most commonly hypertensive and/or diabetic nephropathy), and other conditions affecting renal function including myeloproliferative disorders.
    - Excessive alcohol consumption results in both uric acid overproduction and underexcretion.
- Gout typically occurs in middle-aged or elderly males although it may also affect females after menopause.

- There is an elevated incidence in countries with a high standard of living. The 'metabolic syndrome' of obesity, hyperlipidemia, hypertension, and insulin resistance is present in most cases. A diet high in purines likely also contributes.
- Sufficiently high urate concentration results in monosodium urate crystal formation. Urate crystals elicit an intense inflammatory reaction that generates the clinical symptoms.
- Tophi represent a focal accumulation of crystals, proteinaceous matrix, and inflammatory cells.
- Patients with gout present clinically with recurrent attacks of articular and periarticular inflammation and later with tophaceous deposits in soft tissues and joints.
- Peripheral joints (hands and feet) are most commonly involved, where lower temperatures cause urate to crystallize out of solution.

Imaging Findings

- Initially acute attacks show nonspecific radiographic findings of soft tissue swelling without articular abnormalities (Fig. 9.95). Soft tissue swelling is classically asymmetric at the joint (as opposed to 'fusiform' swelling in RA). This has been called *'lumpy-bumpy'* soft tissue swelling.
- Occasionally, periostitis occurs.

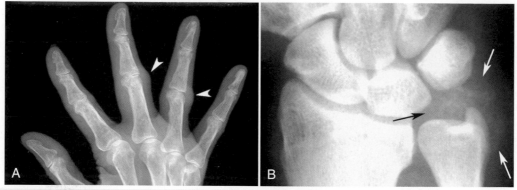

Fig. 9.95 Gout. **(A)** Oblique hand radiograph in an early case shows only eccentric juxtaarticular soft tissue swelling *(arrowheads)*. There is no cartilage narrowing, and no erosions are seen. Joint aspiration showed urate crystals. **(B)** AP radiograph of a wrist in a 44-year-old man shows a faintly calcified soft tissue mass adjacent to the ulnar styloid *(arrows)*. Bones appear normal. Differential diagnosis includes gouty tophus, but calcified neoplasm, such as synovial sarcoma or juxtacortical chondroma, is also a possibility. Aspiration proved gout.

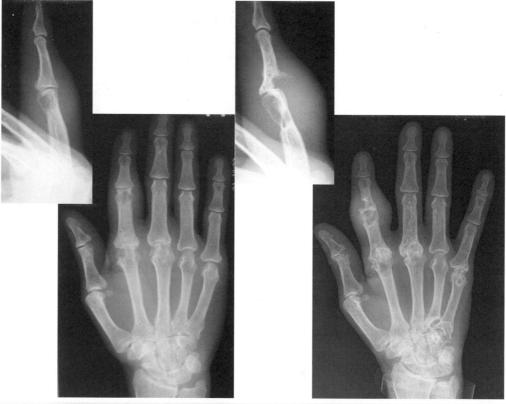

Fig. 9.96 Gout. Initial radiographs of the hand (left images) and follow-up images of the same patient (on right) show progression of tophaceous gouty erosions with a 'rat bite' pattern and overhanging edges. Note dense, asymmetric soft tissue swelling at affected joints. (From Morrison W. *Problem Solving in Musculoskeletal Imaging*. Philadelphia: Elsevier; 2010.)

- Chronic recurrent intraarticular deposition and resultant inflammation can cause marginal or central erosions and joint narrowing, eventually causing osteoarthritis in the involved joints.
- Severe involvement may cause a destructive arthropathy. Imaging can appear similar to septic arthritis (Fig. 9.96).
- Classic periarticular *'rat bite'* erosions with *'overhanging edges'* are seen in chronic tophaceous gout due to extraarticular deposits. The overhanging edge includes newly formed bone rather than simply undermined cortex and is highly specific for gout.

- The tophi are dense but usually not calcified on radiographs (Fig. 9.97). Calcification of tophi can occur in the setting of chronic tophaceous gout or severe renal disease.
- In the feet the classic joints involved are the first MTP and IP joints and the Lisfranc joint.
- In the hands there may be scattered involvement.
- The ankle, knee, and elbow are less commonly affected.
- Bursae may be involved (especially the olecranon), and unlike tophi, involvement often results in calcification of the bursa. Often there is erosion of bone at the attachment (Fig. 9.98).

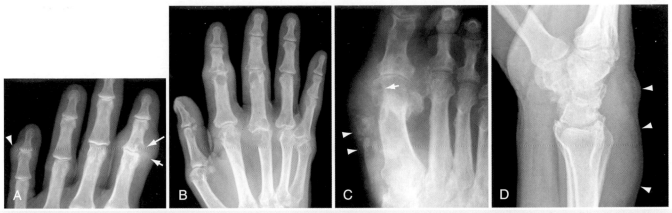

Fig. 9.97 (A) PA radiograph of the fingers demonstrates a classic appearance of gout, with dense soft tissue swelling with tophi seen at both the proximal interphalangeal (PIP) joint of the second digit *(arrows)* and the distal interphalangeal joint of the fifth digit *(arrowhead)*. In addition to the faintly calcified tophus at the second PIP joint *(short arrow)*, there is a well-defined erosion with an 'overhanging edge' at the base of the middle phalanx of the second digit *(long arrow)*. Note the normal bone density and preserved cartilage space in the second PIP joint. **(B)** Similar but more extensive gout involving metacarpophalangeal and interphalangeal joints in a different patient. **(C)** Foot radiograph in another patient with gout shows juxtaarticular erosions *(arrow)* and extensive densely calcified tophi *(arrowheads)*. **(D)** Lateral wrist radiograph in a different patient shows marked soft tissue swelling dorsal to the wrist and distal forearm *(arrowheads)* representing a large tophus without calcification or prominent erosion.

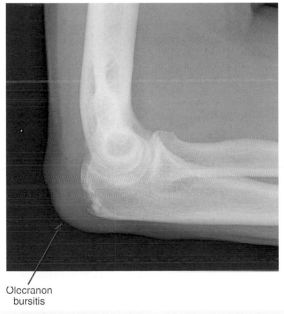

Olecranon bursitis

Fig. 9.98 Gout of the elbow with olecranon bursitis and adjacent erosion on a lateral radiograph. (From Morrison W. *Problem Solving in Musculoskeletal Imaging.* Philadelphia: Elsevier; 2010.)

- Tendon infiltration may occur and results in tendon thickening and a predisposition to tendon tear (Fig. 9.99).
- US: Tophi are often hyperechoic and poorly defined, but the appearance can vary widely, for example hyperechoic and heterogeneous. A surrounding hypoechoic 'halo' is common. Echogenic urate crystals may be seen on the surface of articular cartilage. Bone erosions and surrounding soft tissue inflammation is well detected on US.
- CT: Tophi are highly variable in attenuation, but usually much greater than soft tissue. Dual-energy CT can distinguish sodium urate from other causes of soft tissue mineralization and can be used to monitor therapy response seen as reduction in tophi size.

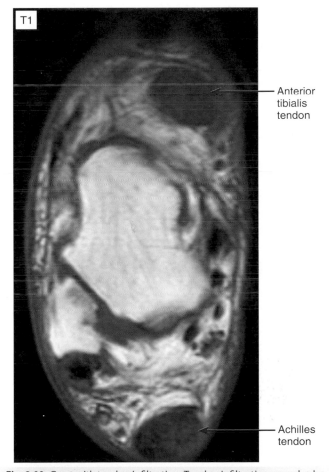

Anterior tibialis tendon

Achilles tendon

Fig. 9.99 Gout with tendon infiltration. Tendon infiltration may also be seen in amyloidosis. Tendinosis and tears are more common in these conditions, as well as with steroid and fluoroquinolone use, diabetes, and overuse. (From Morrison W. *Problem Solving in Musculoskeletal Imaging.* Philadelphia: Elsevier; 2010.)

- MRI: Tophi are generally low to intermediate signal on T1- and T2-weighted images and may enhance (Figs. 9.100 and 9.101).

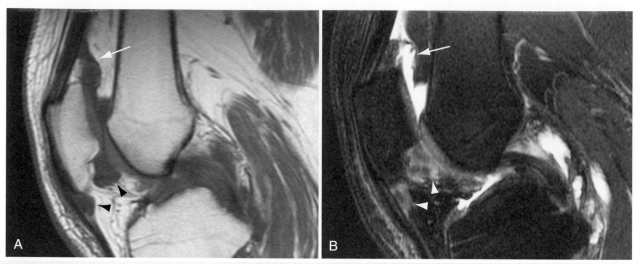

Fig. 9.100 Early gout. T1-weighted MR image **(A)** and T2-weighted fat-saturated MR image **(B)** show normal bone and cartilage and very small supra-patellar effusion *(arrow)*. However, careful observation will demonstrate two focal nodules within the anterior joint recess *(arrowheads)*. The nodules are isointense to muscle on T1-weighted MRI and mixed low and intermediate signal on T2-weighted MRI; this pattern is typical of gout, though it could be seen in nodular synovitis or pigmented villonodular synovitis as well. Aspiration proved gout.

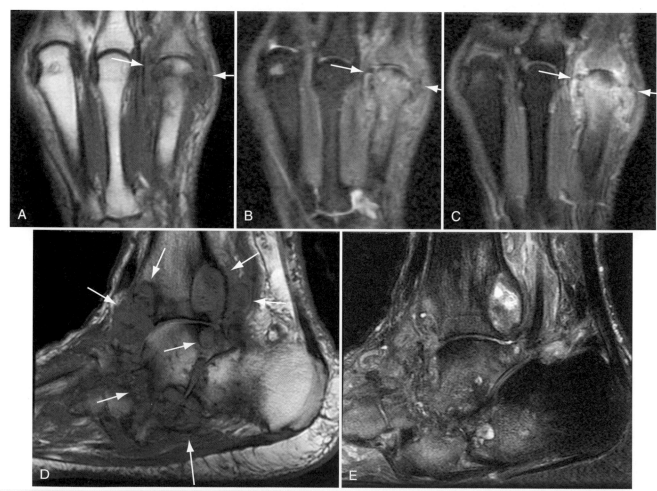

Fig. 9.101 Gout, MRI. Coronal T1-weighted **(A)**, inversion recovery **(B)**, and fat-suppressed contrast-enhanced T1-weighted **(C)** MR images in a patient with tophaceous gout of the fifth finger metacarpophalangeal joint show the tophus to have intermediate to low signal intensity in A and B *(arrows)*, and intense enhancement in C *(arrows)*, which are typical MR findings in tophaceous gout. Edema in the surrounding soft tissues reflects the inflammation and can simulate infection. (D and E) Ankle, severe tophaceous gout. T1-weighted **(D)** and fat-suppressed T2-weighted **(E)** images show large tophi in and adjacent to ankle and foot bones *(arrows in D)*. The intermediate T1-weighted and mostly low T2-weighted signal is typical for chronic tophi and could also represent pigmented villonodular synovitis or amyloid.

- Demonstration of erosions, bone marrow edema, capsular thickening and synovial inflammation, and adjacent tenosynovitis can be improved with intravenous contrast.
- This appearance, coupled with common occurrence of joint effusion and subchondral edema, can simulate infection on MR images. However, history and low-signal periarticular or intraarticular gouty aggregates should suggest the correct diagnosis. Caveat: gout and joint infection can coexist.

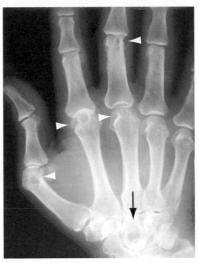

Fig. 9.102 Gout simulating rheumatoid arthritis (RA). PA radiograph of the hand in a 50-year-old man shows erosions in a proximal distribution (*arrowheads*) suggestive of RA. However, the normal bone density and the distinctness of the erosions should suggest gout as a diagnosis, even in the absence of tophus formation. Also note the carpal erosions, including a large erosion in the capitate (*black arrow*). Aspiration proved gout in this case.

Key Concepts

Gout

Monosodium urate crystal–induced arthropathy
Middle-aged to older adult men
Chronic disease processes may predispose to gout
Normal bone density
Cartilage often intact even late in the disease
Erosions: Sharply marginated and may be intraarticular or paraarticular ('nonmarginal')
Overhanging edge of a paraarticular erosion is virtually pathognomonic (the overhanging edge includes new bone formation)
First MTP, DIP, and PIP joints are the most frequently involved
Gouty tophus radiographs: May show amorphous calcification (calcium urate)
Gouty tophus MRI: Low signal intensity on T1-weighted, variably high or low signal on T2-weighted, enhances with gadolinium

---

- Gout is a relatively easy diagnosis to make when it follows all of the preceding rules, including being oligoarticular with tophi and discrete, nonmarginal erosions with overhanging edges.
- However, it may also present as a polyarticular disease, without obvious tophi but with multiple well-marginated erosions.
- This appearance in an older man should always arouse suspicion for gout but is often misdiagnosed as RA (Fig. 9.102).
- Psoriatic arthritis may produce findings suggestive of gout; serum urate level may be elevated in patients with psoriasis, serving to further confuse the issue in some cases.
- Remember that gout can have a variety of appearances and is relatively common, so it should always be kept in mind as a potential diagnosis.
- Septic arthritis in particular can have a clinical and imaging appearance that is identical to an acute gout attack.
- Definitive diagnosis is made by inspection of the synovial fluid (negatively birefringent on polarized microscopy, with long slender crystals). Both crystal analysis and microbiological evaluation may be appropriate as gout and joint infection can coexist.

CALCIUM PYROPHOSPHATE DEPOSITION DISEASE

- Calcium pyrophosphate dihydrate (CPP) crystal deposition can cause acute and chronic arthropathy, and also may create incidental findings on radiographs.
- The terminology related to clinical and radiographic features associated with CPP deposition can be confusing. The terms *chondrocalcinosis*, calcium pyrophosphate deposition disease (CPPD), pyrophosphate arthropathy, and *pseudogout* have often been used interchangeably. This ambiguity led the European League Against Rheumatism (EULAR) in 2011 to propose the following standardized terminology:
- *CPPD* is the umbrella term for all instances of CPP crystal occurrence.
- *CC*: cartilage calcification, or the equivalent term *chondrocalcinosis*.
  - Calcification in hyaline or fibrocartilage; frequently occurs in both.
  - This is a finding on imaging or histology, not a clinical condition.
  - The calcification may be CPPD or some other calcium salt.
  - CC may be an incidental finding in an otherwise normal joint, or coexist with OA.
  - CC can be associated with a variety of degenerative and metabolic processes including old age (most common), osteoarthritis, gout, renal failure, diabetes, hemochromatosis, and Wilson's disease.
- *Asymptomatic CPPD* is cartilage calcification due to CPP with or without radiographic OA findings, but clinically asymptomatic.
- *Acute CPP crystal arthritis* is an acute clinical syndrome of CPPD crystal–induced arthritis resembling gout in clinical features. *Pseudogout* is the former term for these attacks.
  - Usually monoarticular.
  - Rapid onset of joint inflammation is apparent clinically. Flares last for days or weeks.
  - Most common sites in descending order are the knee, wrist, shoulder, ankle, and elbow.

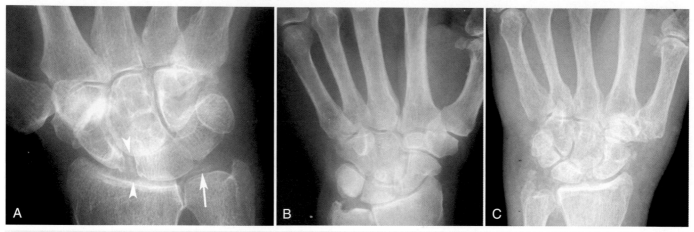

Fig. 9.103 CPPD arthropathy of the wrist. **(A)** PA radiograph of the wrist in an 81-year-old woman with pain and swelling representing acute CPP crystal arthritis. Note the chondrocalcinosis seen both in the triangular fibrocartilage *(arrow)* and between the scaphoid and lunate *(arrowheads)*. There is mild scapholunate widening. There is mild radiocarpal cartilage loss and prominent cyst formation in the scaphoid, capitate, and hamate. **(B)** Similar pattern in a different patient, with extensive chondrocalcinosis and diffuse soft tissue swelling.

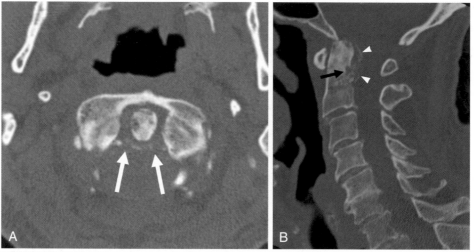

Fig. 9.104 CPPD arthropathy at the C1-2 junction. **(A)** Axial CT through the dens of the upper cervical spine shows calcification along the transverse ligament *(arrows)* posterior to the dens. **(B)** Sagittal reconstruction of the same patient reveals erosion of the posterior margin of the dens *(arrow)*. This can predispose to dens fracture in patients with CPPD involvement at C1-2. Note calcification posterior to the dens *(arrowheads)*.

- Clinically resembles acute gout.
  - Gout is more common in the feet.
- Combination of CC, joint effusion, and inflammation is suggestive of acute CPP crystal arthritis.
- Gold standard is evaluation of synovial fluid for CPP.
  - Short crystals, weakly positive birefringent.
- Remember that although uncommon, infection may coexist.
- *Chronic CPP crystal inflammatory arthritis* is a chronic inflammatory arthritis associated with CPPD.
  - Usually mono or oligoarticular.
  - Knees > wrists, shoulders, elbows, hips, midtarsal joints (Fig. 9.103).
  - CC and prominent subchondral cysts may be seen.
  - Superimposed acute attacks may occur.
  - About 10% have a symmetric polyarthritis and clinical features such as morning stiffness that resemble RA.
    - Older females.
    - MCP joints, especially the second and third.

- *OA with CPPD*: CPPD in a joint with radiographic or histologic findings of OA.
  - May or may not be symptomatic.
  - CC typically present.
  - Distribution is different than in classic OA, with less involvement of the IP joints and preferential involvement of the patellofemoral and radiocarpal articulations.
- CPPD is also common in older individuals at the atlantodens interval, with calcification and thickening of the transverse ligament and surrounding synovial tissues. This can lead to mass effect on the spinal canal, erosion of the dens, and susceptibility to dens fracture (Fig. 9.104).
- US: Echogenic CPP crystals may be seen within articular cartilage (Fig. 9.105).
- MRI: CPP deposition in menisci can have intermediate or even high signal, potentially falsely simulating a meniscal tear (Fig. 9.106).
- CT can localize sites of CPPD crystals.

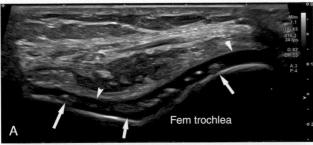

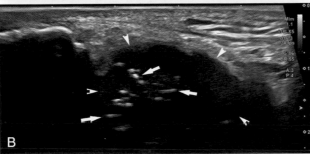

Fem trochlea

Fig. 9.105 CPPD on US. **(A)** Transverse US image of femoral trochlea articular cartilage. Anterior is at the top of the image. The cartilage is the hypoechoic band *(arrowheads)* anterior to the hyperechoic subchondral cortex. Note the echogenic foci within the cartilage, a characteristic sonographic appearance of chondrocalcinosis. **(B)** Joint effusion containing crystals. The effusion is low echogenicity surrounded by *arrowheads*. Note the small echogenic crystals (some marked with *arrows*), which swirled at real-time imaging, likened to a snowstorm.

Key Concepts

Calcium Pyrophosphate Deposition Disease (CPPD)

- Acute flares ('acute CPP crystal arthritis', formerly called 'pseudogout')
- Chronic disease shares many features with osteoarthritis (OA), but appears as 'OA with a funny distribution'
- Cartilage calcification usually (although not invariably) present, most frequent in wrist, knee, and symphysis pubis
- Large subchondral cysts, occasionally simulate a lytic neoplasm
- Knee: patellofemoral compartment predominates
- Wrist: radiocarpal, triangular fibrocartilage complex (TFCC), scapholunate ligament; can progress to scapholunate advanced collapse (SLAC) wrist
- Hand: especially second and third MCP joints

HYDROXYAPATITE DEPOSITION DISEASE (HADD)

- HADD is a crystal-mediated disease that manifests as *calcific tendinitis (tendinosis)*, *calcific bursitis*, and *calcific periarthritis*.
- Radiographically, the calcium salt deposits tend to be small, focal, dense, and somewhat cloudlike.
- It is most common at the rotator cuff (Fig. 9.107), but may be observed in virtually any tendon, ligament, or other periarticular soft tissue.

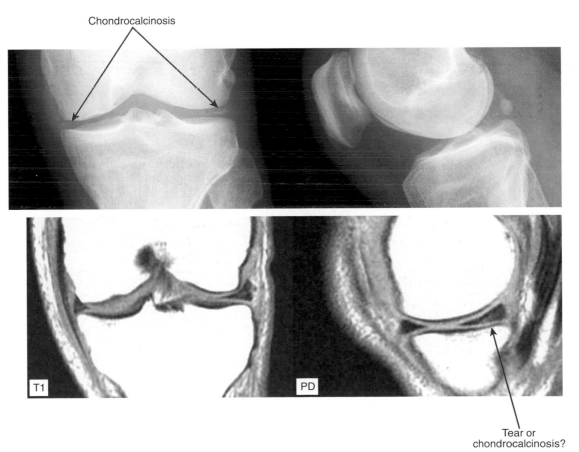

Chondrocalcinosis

Tear or chondrocalcinosis?

Fig. 9.106 Chondrocalcinosis can be hyperintense compared with normal meniscus on T1-weighted and proton density images and can potentially be misinterpreted as a meniscal tear if it appears near the superior or inferior surface. (From Morrison W. *Problem Solving in Musculoskeletal Imaging.* Philadelphia: Elsevier; 2010.)

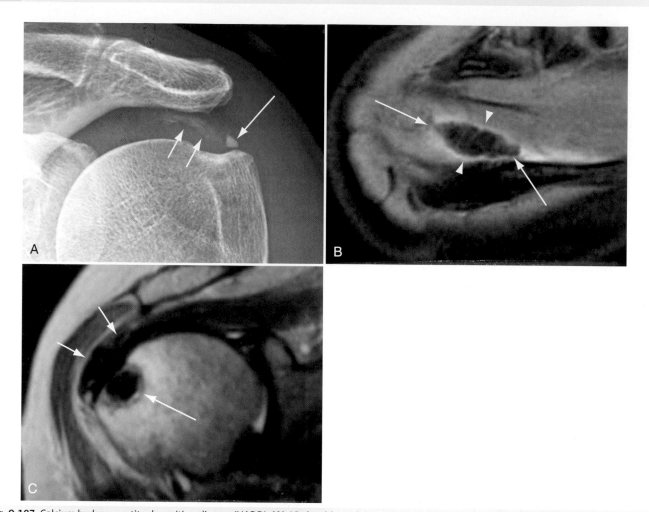

Fig. 9.107 Calcium hydroxyapatite deposition disease (HADD). **(A)** AP shoulder radiograph shows amorphous, uniform calcification above the greater tuberosity of the humerus *(long arrow)*. This is the typical appearance of HADD in a tendon (calcific tendinosis), in this case in the distal supraspinatus tendon. In addition, note the subtler calcification above the lateral humeral head *(short arrows)* representing hydroxyapatite in the subacromial/subdeltoid bursa (calcific bursitis). **(B)** Axial T1-weighted fat-saturated MR image following contrast administration, located high in the shoulder, shows a large low-signal deposit within the supraspinatus tendon *(long arrows)*. This calcific deposit is surrounded by enhancing inflamed tissue *(arrowheads)*, as can be seen in active HADD. **(C)** Coronal T2-weighted MR image shows a thickened hypointense focus within the distal supraspinatus tendon *(short arrows)* representing calcific tendinosis. Immediately adjacent, there is an erosion in the greater tuberosity that contains the same hypointense material *(long arrow)*. Although unusual, HADD deposits may erode into adjacent bone. (B and C, Images used with permission from BJ Manaster, MD, from STATdx website, Amirsys, Inc.)

- The more unusual the location, the more often it is unrecognized. Example: calcific tendinosis of the longus colli tendon anterior to the inferior margin of C1 can simulate retropharyngeal abscess on radiographs and is often overlooked on neck CT exams (Fig. 9.108).
- HA contained within a tendon is often asymptomatic until it bursts into the surrounding tissues where it incites an inflammatory reaction and acute symptoms that include pain, crepitus, erythema, swelling, and even a low-grade fever (Fig. 9.109).
- HA at the rotator cuff ruptures into the subacromial/subdeltoid bursa and then may be observed to be diffusely distributed within the bursa.
- After the rupture, hyperemia induced by the crystals results in rapid resorption of the calcification, often within a week or two.
- Intra-articular rupture of HA into the glenohumeral joint has been reported to cause a destructive arthropathy (*Milwaukee shoulder*).

- When HA causes symptoms in an atypical location such as around the hip or in the hand, it may be mistaken clinically as an infection.
- Calcific tendinitis may also cause erosion of bone at the insertion of the involved tendon, potentially simulating a tumor (see Fig. 9.107C). Regardless of location and clinical presentation, typical calcification in the region of a tendon, bursa, or in periarticular soft tissues should prompt the radiologist to suggest HADD as the diagnosis.
- Treatment involves NSAIDs and is augmented by aspiration/irrigation ('lavage' or 'barbotage') of the paste-like material through a large-gauge needle, with analgesia.
- After appropriate treatment, symptoms improve rapidly and the patient may avoid inappropriate treatment with antibiotics or more invasive surgical options (arthroscopic removal).
- Calcification associated with HADD suspected on radiographs can be confirmed on CT, but this is not usually necessary.

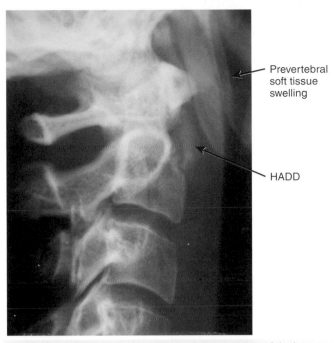

Prevertebral
soft tissue
swelling

HADD

Fig. 9.108 Hydroxyapatite deposition disease (HADD) of the longus colli tendon inferior to the C1 anterior arch. Inflammation in this location can be misinterpreted clinically and on MRI as retropharyngeal abscess. Radiographs or CT can document the correct diagnosis, facilitating prompt, appropriate treatment with nonsteroidal anti-inflammatory drugs rather than aggressive therapy. (From Morrison W. *Problem Solving in Musculoskeletal Imaging.* Philadelphia: Elsevier; 2010.)

- MRI is often ordered by referring clinicians who are not suspecting or familiar with this entity, after typical findings are missed on radiographs, or if the clinical picture simulates infection.
  - HA contained within a tendon is often found incidentally but is often overlooked on MRI because the calcification is dark like the tendon.
  - More commonly there is underlying tendinosis with intermediate signal, and the HA stands out as a focal 'lump' of low signal on all pulse sequences (see Figs. 9.107 and 9.109).
  - The calcification can be confirmed on GRE sequences; the calcium will stand out due to 'blooming' artifact.
  - When the MRI is acquired in the setting of an acute inflammatory reaction to HA, there is often bursitis (which may contain lumpy foci of low signal, a tip-off of the correct diagnosis), and surrounding edema (see Figs. 9.107 and 9.109).
  - If contrast is given, the surrounding soft tissues enhance avidly, again simulating infection.
  - Tip: look closely for a small focus or foci of low signal within an area of intense edema or enhancement.
  - If the HA has ruptured from a tendon, on MRI it will appear that there is a partial-thickness tear of the tendon, and again, the underlying cause may be overlooked.
  - Bone marrow edema is occasionally observed at the insertion of the involved tendon, and discrete erosion will be seen as a focus of fluid signal within the subcortical bone.

HADD at gluteus medius

Surrounding inflammation

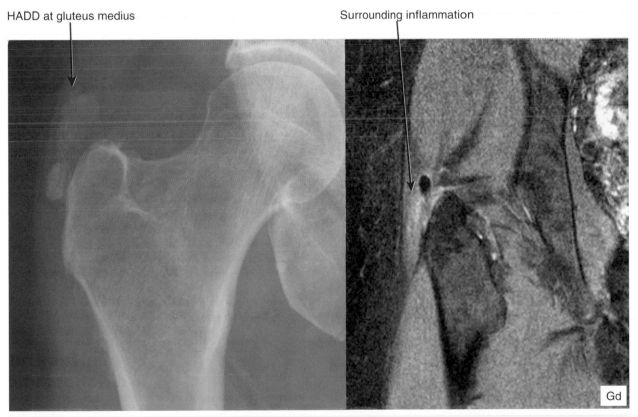

Gd

Fig. 9.109 Calcific tendinosis of the gluteus medius tendon and associated bursitis. When hydroxyapatite deposition disease (HADD) occurs in an unexpected location it can clinically simulate infection. (From Morrison W. *Problem Solving in Musculoskeletal Imaging.* Philadelphia: Elsevier; 2010.)

- CT can be helpful in some cases, as it shows the typical amorphous calcification better and with more precise localization than radiographs.
    - Upon careful inspection, one can often detect HADD in the rotator cuff and in the gluteus medius and minimus tendons on routine chest and abdomen/pelvic CT scans.
- Ultrasound is also extremely sensitive for detection, demonstrating HADD deposit as an amorphous focus of increased echogenicity with variable degrees of acoustic shadowing.

Key Concepts

Calcium Hydroxyapatite Deposition Disease (HADD)
- Amorphous, dense soft tissue calcification
- Calcific tendinitis (tendinosis), most common at the rotator cuff
- Calcific bursitis

Metabolic Conditions

AMYLOID ARTHROPATHY

- *Amyloidosis* refers to deposition of protein fibrils in organs and tissues, leading to organ enlargement and loss of function.
- A classification system based on the predisposing condition and the type of amyloid chains present has become the accepted convention. Immunostaining may allow classification into the different subtypes.
- Dozens of types have been identified, with varied sources and target organs that include the major organs, endocrine glands, and skin. Some have systemic effects, and others are more localized.
- Amyloid fibrils are amorphous under light microscopy but when stained with Congo red, a pathognomonic apple-green birefringence is observed under polarized light microscopy.
- Between 5% and 13% of patients with amyloidosis have bone or joint involvement.
- *Dialysis-related amyloid* can occur after >5 years of hemodialysis. Dialysis incompletely clears β2 microglobulin, a normal major histocompatibility antigen. Accumulated β2 microglobulin can form amyloid fibrils that are preferentially deposited in synovium and intervertebral discs, resulting in:
    - Carpal tunnel syndrome.
    - Erosive changes in joints or vertebral endplates that can mimic infection.
    - Large cyst like lesions, notably in the hip.
- Multiple myeloma and monoclonal gammopathies also can cause amyloid that may affect the musculoskeletal system.
- RA, familial Mediterranean fever, chronic infection, spondyloarthropathy, and connective-tissue disorders (e.g., SLE, scleroderma, and dermatomyositis), are other potential causes of amyloid but musculoskeletal involvement in these cases is rare.
- Imaging demonstrates similar findings regardless of the origin or type.
    - The imaging findings consist of erosions and soft-tissue masses with preservation of the articular cartilage until late in the disease process.

- Subchondral lucent lesions are common, resembling cysts but often representing solid amyloid deposits (Fig. 9.110).
- The shoulder, hip, knee, spine, and wrist are most commonly involved (Fig. 9.111).
- When an erosive arthropathy is present, this disorder should be considered if there is a history of long-term dialysis (5 years or longer). If no history is available, look for radiographic findings of chronic renal failure including vascular calcification, tuft resorption, radial side phalangeal resorption, distal clavicular or SI resorption, or *rugger jersey* spine (increased density along vertebral endplates indicating hyperparathyroidism).
- On MRI, amyloid has low to intermediate signal intensity on all pulse sequences, which helps differentiate this disease from inflammatory arthropathies and infection.
    - There are often joint effusions or soft tissue fluid collections.
    - The MRI appearance may be confusing if interpreted without history or radiographs.
    - Always consider that amyloidosis is a systemic disorder with multifocal involvement; therefore, the other exams in the patient's file may show signs of chronic renal failure and osteodystrophy.
- Involvement of the spine may cause destructive changes at the disc, which may mimic infection or neuropathic disease on all modalities, termed *erosive spondyloarthropathy* or *erosive azotemic osteoarthropathy*. (Fig. 9.112).
    - Disc narrowing is seen with endplate erosions and sclerosis that can rapidly progress to endplate destruction resulting in spondylolisthesis.
    - Vertebral collapse and paraspinal soft tissue masses also occur.
    - Multilevel involvement, which may or may not be contiguous, is typical and reflects the underlying systemic process.
- If biopsy is obtained, the pathologist should be alerted to the possibility of amyloid, so that a *Congo red* stain is used.
- Soft tissue involvement is typified by masslike deposits of amyloid in subcutaneous and periarticular tissues. Calcification is rare.
- Involvement of tendons, ligaments, and rarely muscles may also occur.
    - Tendon involvement can predispose to tendon tear; additionally, patients with renal failure are susceptible to avulsion fractures due to weakening of the underlying bone.

Key Concepts

Amyloidosis
Systemic deposition disease of abnormal protein fibrils
Classified by type of amyloid protein produced
Multiple causes, notably long-term hemodialysis, multiple myeloma and other plasma cell dyscrasias, RA, and chronic infection. Some have genetic factors
Bulky soft tissue nodules
Arthropathy: Joint space widening
Erosions and subchondral cysts: Sharply marginated
Shoulder pain and carpal tunnel syndrome are frequent presentations
Spine: May resemble discitis or neuropathic disorder

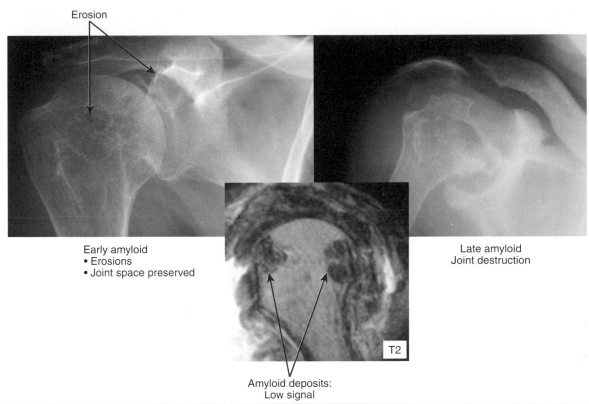

Erosion

Early amyloid
• Erosions
• Joint space preserved

T2

Late amyloid
Joint destruction

Amyloid deposits:
Low signal

Fig. 9.110 Amyloid arthropathy in the shoulder. Amyloid has low signal on T1- and T2-weighted images. Note the low-signal amyloid within large erosions and surrounding the humeral head. (From Morrison W. *Problem Solving in Musculoskeletal Imaging*. Philadelphia: Elsevier; 2010.)

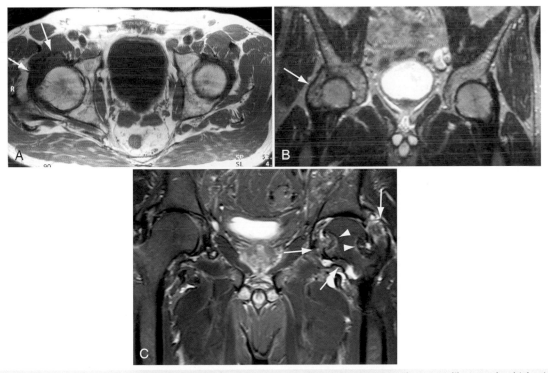

Fig. 9.111 Amyloidosis in the hips. Axial T1-weighted **(A)** and coronal inversion recovery **(B)** MR images show masslike capsular thickening of the right hip capsule *(arrows)* with intermediate to low signal intensity on both images. Biopsy showed amyloid. **(C)** Coronal fat-saturated T2-weighted MR image in a different patient shows large erosions of the left femoral head *(arrowheads)* that contain mostly hypointense material with some heterogeneous hyperintensity, with only minimal adjacent marrow edema. This material is in continuity with nodular deposits within the hip joint *(arrows)* showing the same signal characteristics. Although one might consider a diagnosis of pigmented villonodular synovitis with this appearance, amyloid deposits must also be strongly considered. This patient had been on long-term hemodialysis, and the intraarticular and osseous material proved to be amyloid.

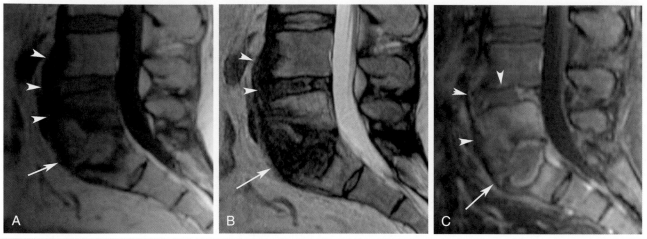

Fig. 9.112 Spinal amyloidosis (erosive spondyloarthropathy). Sagittal T1-weighted **(A)**, T2-weighted **(B)**, and contrast-enhanced fat-suppressed T1-weighted **(C)** MR images in a patient undergoing long-term dialysis show amyloid deposit in L5-S1 *(arrows)* with paravertebral extension and milder involvement of L4-L5 *(arrowheads)*. The amyloid has intermediate to low signal intensity on T1-weighted and low signal intensity on T2-weighted images, with enhancement only at the margins of the deposits.

HEMOCHROMATOSIS ARTHROPATHY

- Hemochromatosis arthropathy develops in up to 50% of patients who have hemochromatosis, thought to be caused by accumulation of iron or CPPD crystals in the joints.
- Hemochromatosis itself may be either primary, owing to increased GI absorption of iron, or secondary, owing to blood transfusions, alcoholism, or excess iron ingestion.
- Onset is usually in middle age, and men are more frequently affected than women. The clinical triad of bronze skin, cirrhosis, and diabetes may be present.
- The radiographic features of the arthropathy are essentially identical to those of CPPD arthropathy. Thus chondrocalcinosis is common in hemochromatosis.
- The disease is primarily productive, with large, "beak-like" or "hooked" osteophytes at the MCP joints (Fig. 9.113).
- However, erosions may be seen in early and active disease.
- Subchondral cysts are quite prominent, similar to those found with CPPD arthropathy.
- The joints most commonly affected are identical to those with CPPD arthropathy, including the radiocarpal joint, second and third MCP joints, and the knee (with the patellofemoral compartment predominating).

WILSON DISEASE

- Wilson disease (hepatolenticular degeneration) is an autosomal recessive (AR) genetic disorder associated with abnormal accumulation of copper in multiple organ systems.
- Degeneration of the basal ganglia, hepatic cirrhosis, and characteristic brownish-green Kayser–Fleischer rings around the cornea develop between childhood and middle age.
- Wilson disease occurs slightly more frequently in males than in females.
- The rare associated arthropathy develops later in life.
- Radiographically chondrocalcinosis may be present.

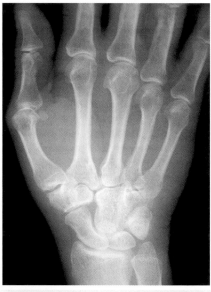

Fig. 9.113 Hemochromatosis. PA radiograph of the hand and wrist demonstrates cartilage loss and large osteophytes at the second and third metacarpophalangeal joints in a young man. This distribution is typical of hemochromatosis or CPPD arthropathy. In a younger male, as seen here, hemochromatosis is more probable.

- The bones are osteopenic.
- Cartilage destruction occurs, and the subchondral bone appears indistinct and irregular, with several small fragments or ossicles. This may give the appearance of osteochondritis dissecans.
  - The joints most frequently affected are the wrist and hand, particularly the MCPs, followed by the foot, hip, shoulder, elbow, and knee.

OCHRONOSIS (ALCAPTONURIA)

- Ochronosis results from the absence of homogentisic acid oxidase and consequent accumulation of homogentisic acid in various organs, notably connective tissues.

- Most cases are hereditary (AR), also termed *endogenous*.
- It affects males and females equally, and the arthropathy generally occurs later in life.
- The radiographic findings are of dystrophic (hydroxyapatite crystal) calcification mostly involving the discs of the spine, but calcification is also occasionally seen in cartilage, tendons, and ligaments.
- The most specific radiographic appearance is in the spine, which appears osteoporotic with dense disc calcification.
- Other joints may be involved and show changes of mild degenerative joint disease, but this is a much less specific appearance.
- Exogenous (nonhereditary) ochronosis can be caused by long-term topical use of hydroquinone in skin-whitening products.

ACROMEGALY

- Acromegaly results from an excess of growth hormone.
  - In the skeletally immature patient, excess growth hormone produces a proportional increase in the size of the bones, leading to gigantism.
  - In the skeletally mature patient, the bones cannot lengthen but respond to growth hormone by tubular bone widening and acral growth.
- In the adult, radiographic abnormalities include soft tissue thickening, especially over the phalanges and in the heel pad.
- The skull may show an enlarged sella due to the pituitary adenoma.
- The facial bones and mandible become quite prominent, as does the occipital protuberance. The paranasal sinuses may be enlarged and excessively pneumatized.
- The spine demonstrates an increased vertebral body and disc height and posterior vertebral body scalloping. There may be an exaggerated thoracic kyphosis.
- In the appendicular skeleton, hand and foot changes predominate over those in the more proximal bones. The phalanges and metacarpals may be wide, with spade-like distal phalangeal tufts (Fig. 9.114).
- Excrescences at the tendon attachments along the phalanges may be prominent. Throughout the skeleton there may be bony proliferation at the entheses.
- The hyaline cartilage increases in thickness. "Beak-like" or "hooked" osteophytes may eventually develop into secondary degenerative joint disease.

Noninflammatory Monoarticular Arthropathies

SYNOVIAL OSTEOCHONDROMATOSIS

- Synovial chondromatosis, often called synovial osteochondromatosis, involves synovial metaplasia of unknown etiology resulting in formation of cartilaginous bodies that often ossify or calcify.
- It is seen in females twice as frequently as in males and is a monoarticular disorder usually affecting large joints in the following order: knee> elbow> hip> shoulder.
- Extraarticular locations, particularly a bursa or tendon sheath, are occasionally involved.
- The disease most commonly presents in young adults.

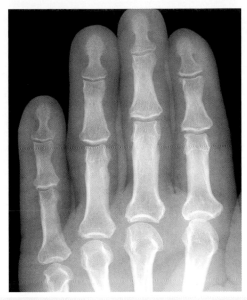

Fig. 9.114 Acromegaly. This PA radiograph demonstrates widening of the cartilage spaces, overgrowth of the soft tissues, and overgrowth of the tufts of the distal phalanges, all typical of acromegaly. (Image used with permission from BJ Manaster, MD, from the American College of Radiology Learning File.)

- Symptoms include swelling, pain, locking, and decreased range of motion.
- In long-standing disease, secondary osteoarthritis often occurs, which may cause confusion in distinguishing this process from conventional osteoarthritis with multiple bodies.
- With imaging the process is most frequently seen as an effusion with *multiple intraarticular bodies of similar size, shape, and mineralization* (Fig. 9.115).
  - The bodies are round or multifaceted and occasionally appear lamellated (calcified cartilage variant) or contain trabeculae (osseous bodies).
  - Although the individual body size may range from 1 mm to 2 cm, most are often only a few millimeters and are uniform in size (Fig. 9.116).
  - Bodies may be too small to resolve and may rather appear as amorphous periarticular density on radiographs (Fig. 9.117).
  - The bodies are usually not free-floating within the joint but rather are adherent to the synovial tissue from which they arise.
  - Occasionally bodies may form in a conglomerate focal mass.
  - In 15% of cases the bodies do not calcify, and the condition is seen on radiographs only as a soft tissue mass, which may be associated with osseous erosion. This is referred to as *synovial chondromatosis* (Fig. 9.118).
  - Osteoarthritis can form multiple bodies as well, but these typically vary in size and are few in number (this has been referred to unnecessarily as *secondary synovial osteochondromatosis*).
  - Differentiation from intra-articular bodies seen in OA is typically made by visualizing numerous intraarticular bodies of similar small size, disproportionate to the degree of OA.

Synovial osteochondromatosis
Numerous IA bodies
Similar size
Disproportionate to degree of OA

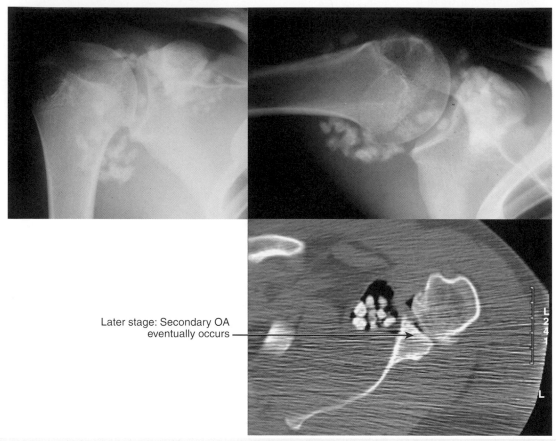

Later stage: Secondary OA
eventually occurs

Fig. 9.115 Synovial osteochondromatosis. If the bodies are calcified or ossified, radiographs show numerous bodies of similar small size, disproportionate to the degree of osteoarthritis (OA). *IA*, intraarticular. (From Morrison W. *Problem Solving in Musculoskeletal Imaging*. Philadelphia: Elsevier; 2010.)

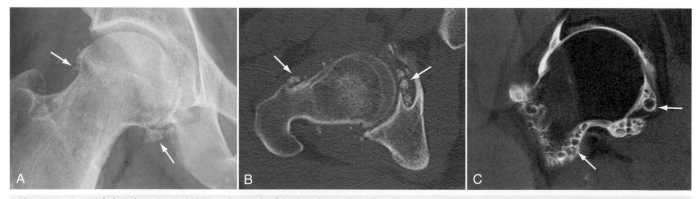

Fig. 9.116 Synovial chondromatosis. **(A)** AP radiograph of the hip shows multiple similar small, round calcified bodies *(arrows)* within the most redundant portion of the hip capsule, around the femoral neck. **(B)** Axial CT scan of the same hip shows multiple intraarticular calcified bodies *(arrows)*. The patient has developed secondary osteoarthritis. **(C)** Coronal T1-weighted fat-saturated arthrogram image shows hyperintense articular contrast surrounding multiple low-signal calcified bodies *(arrows)*.

- CT is excellent for demonstrating erosions and detecting small amounts of calcification. CT is usually not necessary to make the diagnosis, but occasionally the bodies are so small and faintly calcified that they may be missed on radiographs in large joints such as the hip.

- On MRI, the bodies are easily seen against a background of joint fluid (or intra-articular contrast in arthrography), with calcified bodies being low signal on all sequences. Chondroid tissue is bright on T2-weighted sequences and can blend with joint fluid; intravenous gadolinium contrast can be useful to

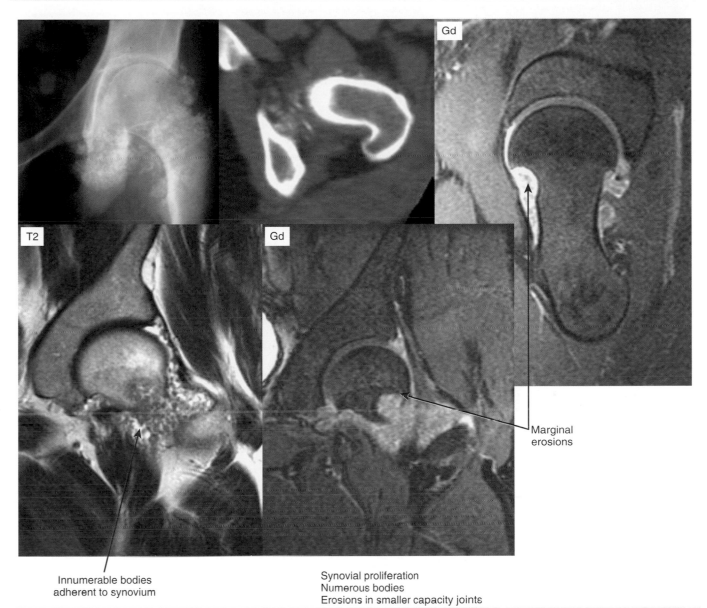

Fig. 9.117 Synovial osteochondromatosis. Erosions can occur in joints with smaller capacity such as the hip; occasionally, the bodies are so small and faintly calcified that they may be missed on radiographs. (From Morrison W. *Problem Solving in Musculoskeletal Imaging.* Philadelphia: Elsevier; 2010.)

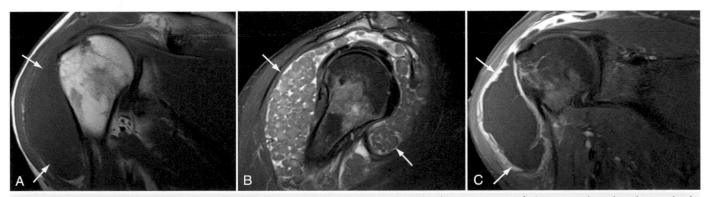

Fig. 9.118 Synovial chondromatosis, nonossified bodies. Radiograph (not shown) showed only an apparent soft tissue mass lateral to the proximal humeral metaphysis; there was no abnormal calcification. **(A)** Coronal T1-weighted image shows low-signal material distending the subdeltoid bursa *(arrows)*. There is no evidence of either low-signal calcified bodies or high-signal ossified bodies. **(B)** Sagittal T2-weighted fat-saturated MR image of the same shoulder shows the hugely distended subdeltoid bursa is packed with similar-sized round bodies *(arrows)*, surrounded by fluid. **(C)** Coronal T1-weighted fat-saturated image with intravenous gadolinium shows enhancing synovium *(arrows)* surrounding low-signal bursal 'mass'; the bodies remain isosignal to bursal fluid.

visualize areas of synovial proliferation associated with the disease process.

- The articular cartilage is preserved until late in the course of the disease and therefore the joint space is typically normal at initial presentation.
- Erosions may occur in articulations with tight capsules (e.g., the hip) or with localized involvement in smaller recesses (see Fig. 9.117).
- No periosteal reaction is associated with uncomplicated synovial osteochondromatosis.
- After synovectomy, the disease may recur in recesses or periarticular locations, with characteristic small, numerous bodies.

Key Concepts

Synovial Chondromatosis

Metaplasia of synovium into multiple small round or multifaceted cartilage intraarticular bodies
Bodies tend to be of uniform size within a joint
May undergo enchondral ossification to synovial osteochondromatosis
Usually monoarticular
Most frequent sites: knee, hip, elbow, shoulder
Secondary osteoarthritis caused by mechanical damage to joint
Radiography, computed tomography: often diagnostic if bodies are adequately mineralized; magnetic resonance imaging is diagnostic if bodies are not calcified/ossified

---

PIGMENTED VILLONODULAR SYNOVITIS (PVNS)

- Like synovial osteochondromatosis, PVNS is a benign, slowly-progressing proliferative synovial disease, probably neoplastic in etiology, occurring as a diffuse or localized form.
- PVNS and *tenosynovial giant cell tumor (TGCT)* are different terms for the same histologic lesion. The terminology in the medical literature is somewhat variable, but in both Radiology and Orthopedics, PVNS refers to the disease when located in a joint and TGCT when extraarticular, usually involving a tendon sheath or, rarely, a bursa.
- TGCT was previously called giant cell tumor of tendon sheath (GCTTS). There is no relationship to giant cell tumor of bone.
- At gross inspection, the synovium has a reddish appearance due to hemorrhage.
- Microscopically, synovial cell hyperplasia and proliferation are present. There is also subsynovial accumulation of hemosiderin-laden macrophages (related to repeated hemorrhage), multi-nucleated giant cells, and fibroblasts.
- The extraarticular form and smaller intraarticular lesions typically contain less hemosiderin than larger articular lesions.
- PVNS presents as a monoarticular arthropathy or chronic joint effusion with insidious onset, most frequently in one of the large joints of the lower extremity: knee > hip > ankle.
  - Two intraarticular forms are recognized: *localized* and *diffuse*.
  - Localized PVNS is better defined and confined to the joint, often in only part of the joint.

- Diffuse PVNS is more aggressive and may extend beyond the joint. Diffuse is much less common than localized.
- The age of presentation is typically in the 20- to 40-year-old range with no gender predilection.
- Arthrocentesis may yield serosanguineous fluid. The presence of a bloody effusion in the absence of trauma suggests PVNS.
- Tenosynovial giant cell tumor most commonly presents as an extraarticular soft tissue mass or focal swelling, typically in the hand or foot and usually related to a flexor tendon.
  - The age of presentation is older than intraarticular PVNS occurring in the fourth to sixth decades of life with a female predilection. It is the second most common soft tissue lesion of the hand after a ganglion.
  - Tenosynovial giant cell tumor is discussed further in Ch 12-Soft Tissue Tumors.
- PVNS usually does <u>not</u> calcify, which helps to separate it from synovial osteochondromatosis.
- Scalloped osseous erosions with thin, sclerotic margins may be observed, which may be large; degree of erosion is inversely proportionate to the joint capacity and is also related to extent/distribution of synovial proliferation (Fig. 9.119).
  - In a small capacity joint like the hip, erosions are often prominent.
  - In the knee, a large capacity joint, erosions may be subtle, even with extensive joint involvement.
- As with synovial osteochondromatosis, gradual cartilage loss occurs, progressing to secondary osteoarthritis. This is more likely with the diffuse form.
- CT may not be very useful except to exclude calcifications associated with synovial osteochondromatosis.
- MRI of the diffuse form is characteristic, showing synovial proliferation with low signal on T2-weighted images from hemosiderin deposition (Table 9.19). GRE sequences are especially useful to document blooming (susceptibility) artifact from the hemosiderin, to help separate it from other causes of dark synovium (Fig. 9.120). The blooming artifact may be so severe that enhancement on post-contrast imaging is obscured.
- The localized form typically appears as a noncalcified mass within the joint (Fig. 9.121).
  - On MRI the lesion has signal characteristics typical for PVNS: low T1 and T2 signal, but usually with less hemosiderin and thus less susceptibility artifact. Enhancement with gadolinium is less likely to be obscured.
  - The differential diagnosis in this case would include gout (with intraarticular tophus), synovial chondromatosis, and amyloid. Synovial biopsy may be required for diagnosis.
- First line treatment is synovectomy.
  - Recurrence rate after synovectomy is much higher in the diffuse form (30%) vs less than 10% for the localized form.
  - Supplemental therapy with intraarticular radioisotope using a beta emitter reduces recurrence. External beam radiation has been used but is falling out of favor due to potential complications.

Pigmented villonodular synovitis (PVNS)
• Monoarticular arthropathy
• Knee > hip > ankle
• Erosions
• Cysts
• Osteoarthritis

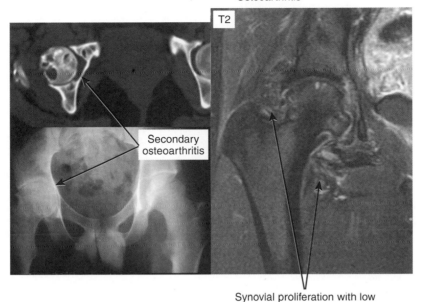

Fig. 9.119 Pigmented villonodular synovitis (PVNS). Like synovial osteochondromatosis, PVNS should be considered whenever a young adult presents with a monoarticular noninflammatory arthropathy. Similarly, the degree of erosion is inversely proportional to the joint capacity and is also related to the extent/distribution of synovial proliferation. Unlike synovial osteochondromatosis, calcification is not a characteristic of PVNS. (From Morrison W. *Problem Solving in Musculoskeletal Imaging.* Philadelphia: Elsevier; 2010.)

Table 9.19   Dark Synovium on T2-weighted MR Images

Postoperative fibrosis (usually not masslike)
Hemosiderin (blooms on GRE images):
PVNS (masslike)
Hemophilia
Gout (masslike)
RA (masslike)
Calcification (may also bloom on gradient echo (GRE) images)
Synovial osteochondromatosis (masslike with bodies)
Amyloid (masslike)

Abbreviations: GRE, gradient echo *PVNS,* pigmented villonodular synovitis; *RA,* rheumatoid arthritis.

- Newer promising medical therapies include tyrosine kinase inhibitors and monoclonal antibodies targeting tumor necrosis factor alpha (TNF-α) and colony-stimulating factor 1 (CSF1)

ADVERSE LOCAL TISSUE REACTION/SMALL PARTICLE DISEASE

- After joint replacement, release of small particles during normal use can incite an immune response, osteoclast migration, and osteolysis. In joint prostheses with a metal component this is referred to as *particle disease, aggressive granulomatous response,* or *histiocytic reaction.*

In the case of silicone plastic (*silastic*) implants used in the small joints of the hands and feet, this process is termed *silastic synovitis* or *silicone synovitis* (Fig. 9.122). There are many manifestations of this condition based on materials used and the immunologic response; the all-encompassing term is *adverse local tissue reaction* (ALTR).

- Osteolysis and loosening can occur in both large and small joint implants.
- Lucency at the prosthesis–bone (or cement–bone) interface is a hallmark of component loosening.
- Other signs of loosening include protrusio acetabuli (in the hip), fractured cement or metal, or subsidence of the prosthesis into the underlying bone.
- Areas of osteolysis are seen to be filled with tissue having inflammatory or fibrous signal characteristics, rather than fluid, and demonstrating gadolinium enhancement. Surrounding fluid collections are also common.
- Chapter 10 – Arthroplasty provides a more thorough review of these topics.

Miscellaneous Joint Disorders

LIPOMA ARBORESCANS

- *Lipoma arborescans* is a rare proliferation of lipomatous tissue within the synovium.
- May result from a chronic inflammatory synovitis with resultant hyperplasia of the fatty subsynovial tissue,

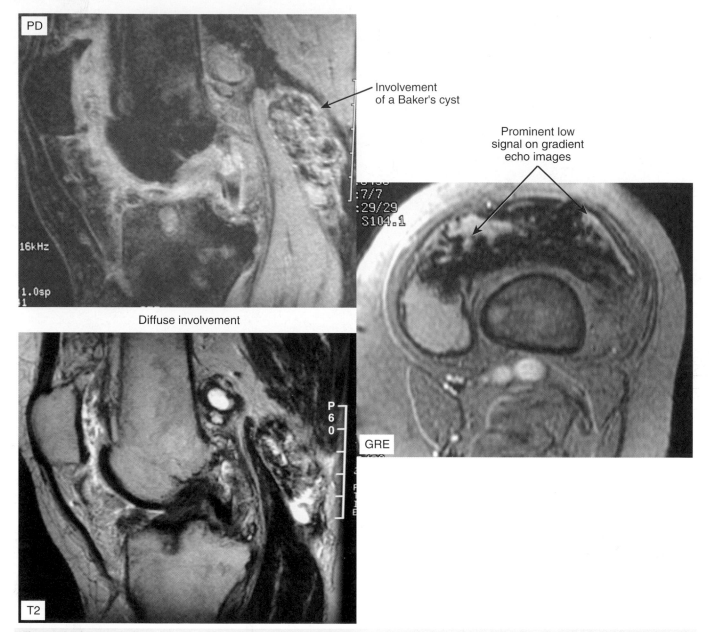

Fig. 9.120 Pigmented villonodular synovitis. In later stages with diffuse disease, extensive hemosiderin deposition is observed, which 'blooms' with low signal on gradient echo (GRE) images. (From Morrison W. *Problem Solving in Musculoskeletal Imaging.* Philadelphia: Elsevier; 2010.)

but often there is no recognized history of previous arthropathy.

- Presents as chronic masslike enlargement of the joint.
- Most common site is the knee.
- MRI shows masslike synovial proliferation with signal corresponding to fat, with numerous frondlike excrescences (Fig. 9.123).

LEAD ARTHROPATHY

- Lead-containing bullets lodged in bursae or joints can result in lead poisoning caused by dissolution of the lead by synovial fluid.
- With progressive degradation, lead particles are spread throughout the joint, lining the synovium and cartilage (see Fig. 6.69B).

- Synovial inflammation and mechanical damage to cartilage lead to productive change and secondary osteoarthritis.
- Clinical lead poisoning (*plumbism*) requires sufficient breakdown of fragments to produce a large surface area of lead and is more likely from an inflamed joint or bursa.
- Lead bullets in extraarticular soft tissues dissolve much more slowly and are not associated with lead intoxication.

HYPERTROPHIC OSTEOARTHROPATHY

- *Hypertrophic osteoarthropathy* (HOA) is periosteal new bone formation on long bones, often in association with lung cancer.

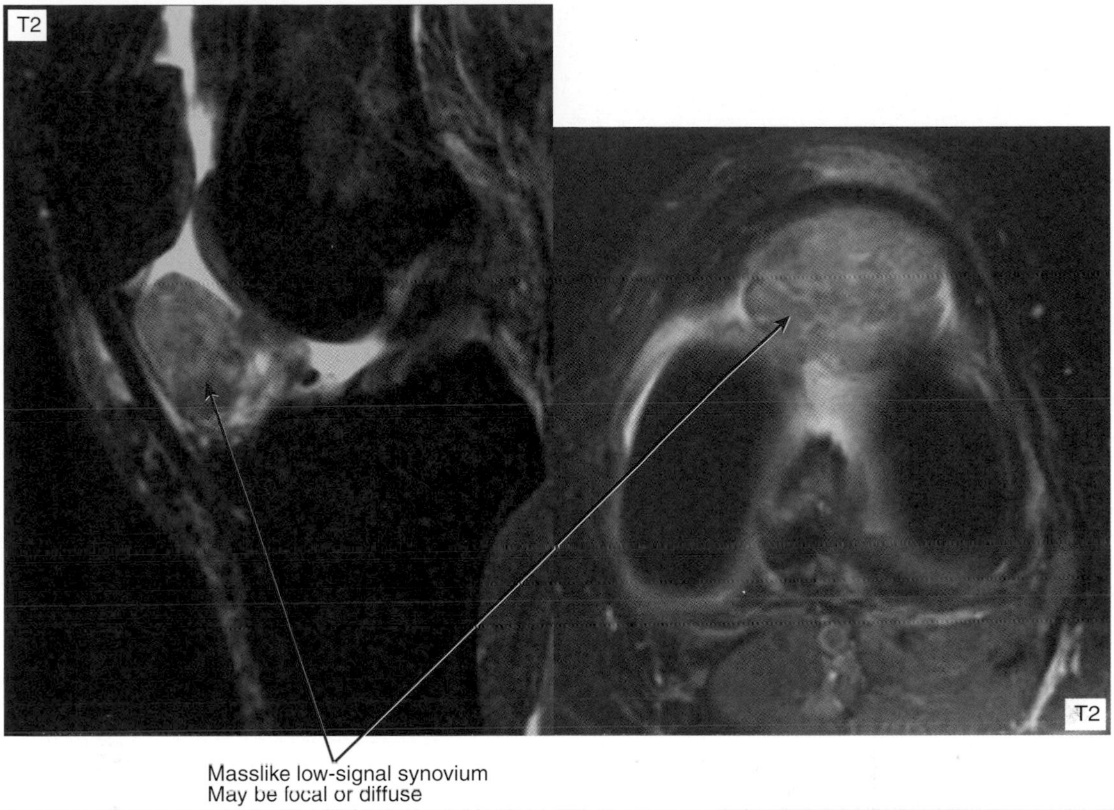

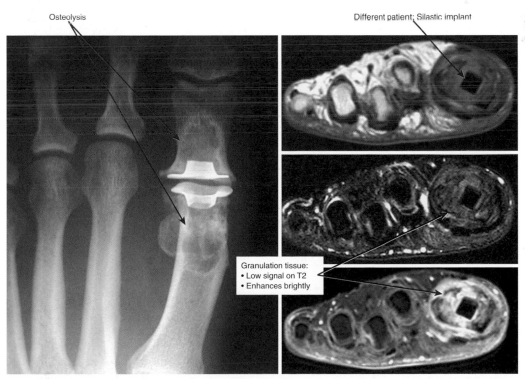

Masslike low-signal synovium
May be focal or diffuse

Fig. 9.121 Pigmented villonodular synovitis (PVNS) can be focal or diffuse; also, the amount of hemosiderin and therefore signal intensity on T2-weighted images vary. The differential for dark synovium includes PVNS, synovial osteochondromatosis, gout, hemophilia, amyloid, postoperative fibrosis, and chronic arthropathy with scarring (see also Figs. 12.44 through 12.47). (From Morrison W. *Problem Solving in Musculoskeletal Imaging.* Philadelphia: Elsevier; 2010.)

Osteolysis

Different patient: Silastic implant

Granulation tissue:
• Low signal on T2
• Enhances brightly

Fig. 9.122 Small particle disease. Radiograph (left image) shows osteolysis around a metallic prosthesis at the first MTP joint. MRI (right images) of a different patient with a silastic prosthesis shows granulation tissue surrounding the implant. (From Morrison W. *Problem Solving in Musculoskeletal Imaging.* Philadelphia: Elsevier; 2010.)

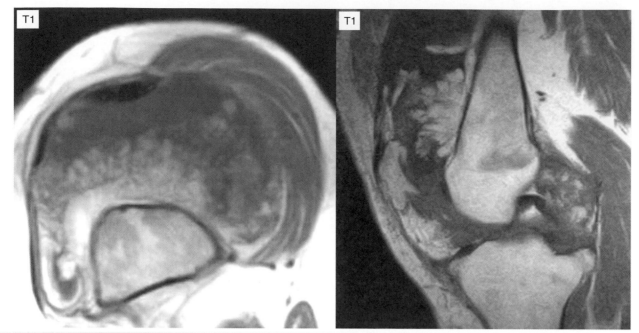

Fig. 9.123 Lipoma arborescans. MRI shows masslike synovial proliferation with signal corresponding to fat, with numerous frondlike excrescences. (From Morrison W. *Problem Solving in Musculoskeletal Imaging.* Philadelphia: Elsevier; 2010.)

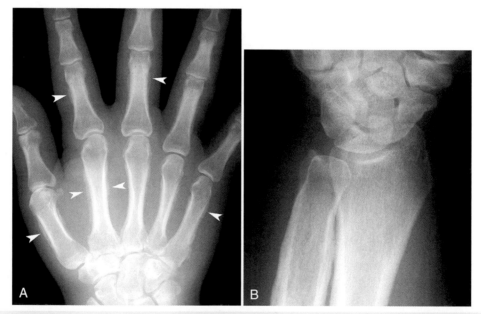

Fig. 9.124 Pachydermoperiostosis (primary hypertrophic osteoarthropathy). **(A)** PA radiograph of the hand in this 26-year-old man demonstrates thick periosteal reaction along the proximal phalanges and metacarpals *(arrowheads)*. The radiograph alone does not make the diagnosis of pachydermoperiostosis but is diagnostic when occurring in combination with the thickening of the skin over the hands and forehead seen clinically. **(B)** Distal forearm in a different patient also shows thick, solid periosteal new bone.

- Classic findings are skin thickening, long bone periostitis (periosteal new bone formation), clubbed digits, and synovial effusions.
    - Periostitis is the most consistent finding.
    - Joint effusions are not always present.
- Clinical features vary widely, and some patients are asymptomaic.
- HOA may be primary or secondary.
- *Primary HOA:*
    - Also termed *pachydermoperiostosis* and *idiopathic HOA.*

- Spectrum of diseases ranging from just periostitis to the complete process of periostitis, clubbed digits, and thickening of the skin, particularly at the forehead and dorsum of the hands (Fig. 9.124).
- Often familial and is much more common in males than in females.
- Develops during adolescence, and the process usually spontaneously arrests in young adulthood.
- Normal lifespan.
- Rare.

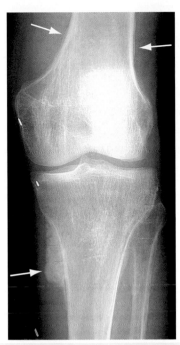

Fig. 9.125 Secondary hypertrophic osteoarthropathy. AP radiograph of the knee in a 73-year-old man with previously undiagnosed bronchogenic carcinoma who presented with knee pain. Note the solid, undulating metaphyseal and diaphyseal periosteal new bone in the distal femur and more extensively in the proximal tibia (arrows). Chest radiograph was recommended, which found the lung tumor.

- *Secondary HOA*:
  - Secondary HOA is periostitis in the extremities associated with several disease processes (Fig. 9.125).
  - Most common associations:
    - Malignancy in 90%, mainly non–small cell lung cancer.
    - Chronic infections in the chest such as tuberculosis, fungal infections, and chronic abscess, bacterial endocarditis, and infected arterial grafts.
  - There are many other, less common associations. This is a partial list:
    - Other lung maladies including chronic obstructive pulmonary disease (COPD), interstitial fibrosis, and sarcoidosis.
    - Some other malignancies in the chest or abdomen.
    - Some chronic inflammatory conditions such as IBD.
    - Chronic hypoxic conditions including cyanotic congenital heart disease, cystic fibrosis, and COPD.
    - Primary biliary cirrhosis.
- Because most cases of HOA are related to pulmonary disease, the term *hypertrophic pulmonary osteoarthropathy* (HPOA, or HPO) is also used. HOA is the preferred term.
- Patients may present with painful, swollen joints.
  - Radiographically the joints often appear normal, with possible swelling and effusions without erosive or productive changes.
  - The major abnormality of periosteal new bone formation may first be detected on the 'corner' of a joint radiograph.
  - The extent of periosteal new bone is variable, ranging from minimal to extensive, and may show onion

skinning. Longer duration of disease is associated with more extensive new bone formation.
  - Few bones or many may be involved. In general, the more extensive the periostitis, the more bones involved.
  - The bones of the leg are most commonly involved, followed by the bones of the forearm, then by the phalanges in the hand.
  - The periostitis may be painful, especially when extensive and with bronchogenic carcinoma.
  - Bone scan show increased tracer uptake in the periosteal new bone.
  - MRI may show a thin layer of intermediate or elevated T2 signal between the cortex and elevated periosteum.
- The mechanism of the periosteal new bone formation is not completely understood. Both humoral (related to growth factors) and neurologic mediators are hypothesized.
- Differential diagnosis includes other causes of symmetric periostitis such as chronic venous insufficiency, thyroid acropachy, other paraneoplastic syndromes, retinoic acid medications, vitamin A intoxication, scurvy, fluorosis, leukemia, and lymphoma.
  - The antifungal medication voriconazole used in immunocompromised transplant patients can cause periostitis resembling HOA (Fig. 9.126).
  - 'Huffing', inhalational abuse of fluorocarbons from spray cans, can produce a florid periostitis due to flouride intoxication.
  - Periosteal new bone can be seen as a physiologic finding in infants.
  - Newborn babies with congenital heart disease treated with the vasodilator prostaglandin E1 to maintain a patent ductus arteriosus develop periosteal new bone identical to HOA. The prostaglandin causes the periostitis.

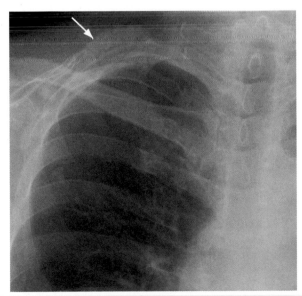

Fig. 9.126 Voriconazole-related periostitis resembling hypertrophic osteoarthropathy. AP radiograph of the shoulder demonstrates thick periosteal reaction along a rib (arrow). This developed in a patient being treated with voriconazole following liver transplantation.

■ The rare syndrome *progressive diaphyseal dysplasia* includes both periosteal and endosteal cortical thickening in long bones.

Key Concepts

Hypertrophic Osteoarthropathy

Primary or secondary, most are secondary
May present clinically as arthralgia
Radiographically normal joints
Bilaterally symmetric, solid, thick metaphyseal and diaphyseal periosteal new bone
Search for associated condition, notably lung cancer

Key Elements of a Structured Report

A structured report for a case where the primary concern is an arthropathy should include:

■ Technical note regarding body part, number of views (radiography), use of contrast (cross sectional imaging), etc.
■ Soft tissue findings (swelling, calcification).
■ Joint effusion; erosions; productive changes.
■ Alteration of joint spaces; cysts.
■ Distribution of findings; differential diagnosis with age, gender, lab data taken into account.
■ Any recommendations (additional imaging, lab tests, etc.)

Appendix: Distribution patterns in specific forms of arthritis

Key Concepts

Osteoarthritis

Productive changes: Osteophyte formation, sclerosis, and normal bone density
Most common locations: Hip, knee (medial compartment), spine, and hand (distal interphalangeal, first carpometacarpal, scapho-trapezio-trapezoidal)

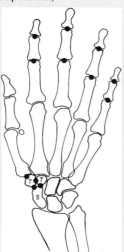

Key Concepts

Rheumatoid Arthritis

Purely erosive
Fusiform soft tissue swelling
Periarticular osteoporosis
Uniform cartilage destruction
Bilaterally symmetric
Wrist: Radiocarpal joint, distal radioulnar joint; deformities
Hand: Proximal (metacarpophalangeal and proximal interphalangeal) deformities
Foot: Metatarsophalangeal and retrocalcaneal bursa
Shoulder: Rotator cuff tear, erosion of distal clavicle
Knee: Valgus deformity
Hips: Uniform cartilage loss, protrusio acetabuli
Upper cervical spine: Facet erosions, atlantoaxial impaction, atlantoaxial subluxation

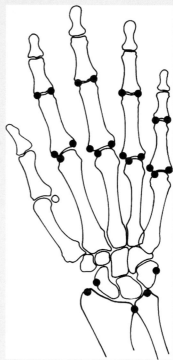

Key Concepts

Psoriatic Arthritis

Most cases: Asymmetric erosive arthropathy, with superimposed bone productive changes
Five patterns:
  Oligoarthritis (sausage digit)
  Polyarthritis (distal interphalangeal more frequent than proximal interphalangeal and metacarpophalangeal joints)
  Symmetric type (resembles rheumatoid arthritis)
  Arthritis mutilans (deforming type, pencil-in-cup)
  Spondyloarthropathy (bilateral, asymmetric sacroiliitis, bulky asymmetric osteophytes usually starting at the thoracolumbar junction, noncontiguous)
Bone density can be normal
Distal phalanges: Tuft resorption or reactive sclerosis ("ivory phalanx")
Arthropathy may precede skin changes—up to 20% of cases

Key Concepts—cont'd

Psoriatic Arthritis

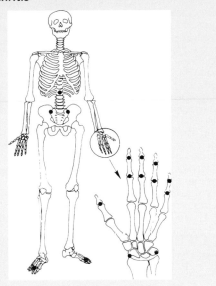

Key Concepts

Ankylosing Spondylitis

Frequently positive for HLA-B27

Occurs more frequently in males than females

Presents in adolescents or young adults

Bilateral sacroiliac disease hallmark; erosive early, ankylosis quickly follows

Bamboo spine

Affects large proximal appendicular joints more often than distal joints

Spine fracture at cervicothoracic and thoracolumbar junctions with pseudarthrosis, resulting from minimal trauma, often results in significant morbidity

Magnetic resonance imaging (MRI) may show preradiographic findings (enthesitis and Romanus spine lesions)

Findings easily overlooked in routine MRI and computed tomography spine cases, even in relatively advanced disease

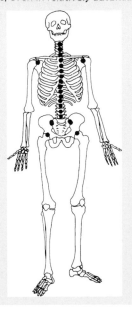

Key Concepts

Reactive Arthritis

Formerly known as Reiter syndrome

Least common spondyloarthropathy

Occurs more frequently in males than females

Radiographically identical to psoriasis but usually favors foot over hand

Calcaneal erosive disease and spur formation are prominent features

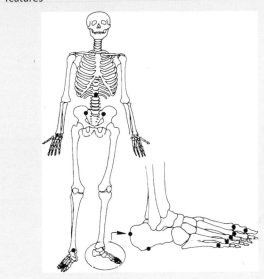

Key Concepts

CPPD Arthropathy

Shares many features with osteoarthritis (OA), but appears as "OA with a funny distribution"

Chondrocalcinosis usually (although not invariably) present, most frequent in wrist, knee, and symphysis pubis

Large subchondral cysts, occasionally simulate a lytic neoplasm

Knee: Patellofemoral compartment predominates

Wrist: Radiocarpal; can progress to scapholunate advanced collapse (SLAC) wrist

Hand: Especially second and third metacarpophalangeal joints

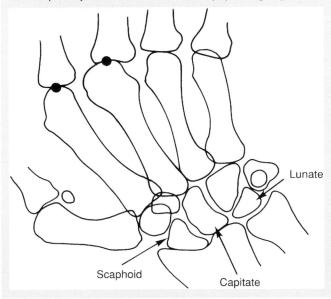

Lunate

Scaphoid   Capitate

Sources and Suggested Readings

Aringer M, Costenbader K, Daikh D, et al. 2019 European League Against Rheumatism/American College of Rheumatology Classification Criteria for Systemic Lupus Erythematosus. *Arthritis Rheumatol.* 2019; 71(9):1400–1412.

Boutry N, Lardé A, Lapègue F, et al. Magnetic resonance imaging appearance of the hands and feet in patients with early rheumatoid arthritis. *J Rheumatol.* 2003;30(4):671–679.

Campagna R, Pessis E, Feydy A, et al. Fractures of the ankylosed spine: MDCT and MRI with emphasis on individual anatomic spinal structures. *AJR Am J Roentgenol.* 2009;192(4):987–995.

Chang EY, Chen KC, Huang BK, Kavanaugh A. Adult inflammatory arthritides: what the radiologist should know. *Radiographics.* 2016;36: 1849–1870.

Choi MH, MacKenzie JD, Dalinka MK. Imaging features of crystal-indued arthropathy. *Rheum Dis Clin North Am.* 2006;32(2):427–446.

Damasio MB, Malattia C, Martini A, Tomà P. Synovial and inflammatory diseases in childhood: role of new imaging modalities in the assessment of patients with juvenile idiopathic arthritis. *Pediatr Radiol.* 2010; 40(6):985–998.

Erdem CZ, Tekin NS, Sarikaya S, et al. MR imaging features of foot involvement in patients with psoriasis. *Eur J Radiol.* 2008;67(3):521–525.

Gardner-Medwin JM, Irwin G, Johnson K. MRI in juvenile idiopathic arthritis and juvenile dermatomyositis. *Ann NY Acad Sci.* 2009;1154:52–83.

Hermann KA, Althoff CE, Schneider U, et al. Spinal changes in patients with spondyloarthritis: comparison of MR imaging and radiographic appearances. *Radiographics.* 2005;25:559–570.

Jang JH, Ward MW, Rucker AN, et al. Ankylosing spondylitis: patterns of radiographic involvement—a re-examination of accepted principles in a cohort of 769 patients. *Radiology.* 2011;258(1):192–198.

Kim NR, Choi JY, Hong SH, et al. "MR corner sign": value for predicting presence of ankylosing spondylitis. *AJR Am J Roentgenol.* 2008;191(1): 124–128.

Kiss E, Keusch G, Zanetti M, et al. Dialysis-related amyloidosis revisited. *AJR Am J Roentgenol.* 2005;185:1460–1467.

Low AH, Lax M, Johnson SR, Lee P. Magnetic resonance imaging of the hand in systemic sclerosis. *J Rheumatol.* 2009;36(5):961–964.

Maksymowych WP, Chiowchanwisawakit P, Clare T, et al. Inflammatory lesions of the spine on magnetic resonance imaging predict the development of new syndesmophytes in ankylosing spondylitis: evidence of a relationship between inflammation and new bone formation. *Arthritis Rheum.* 2009;60(1):93–102.

Matsunaga S, Nakamura K, Seichi A, et al. Radiographic predictors for the development of myelopathy in patients with ossification of the posterior longitudinal ligament: a multicenter cohort study. *Spine.* 2008; 33(24):2648–2650.

Mendenhall WM, Mendenhall CM, Reith JD, et al. Pigmented villonodular synovitis. *Am J Clin Oncol.* 2006;29(6):548–550.

Murphey MD, Vidal JA, Fanburg-Smith JC, Gajewski DA. Imaging of synovial chondromatosis with radiologic-pathologic correlation. *Radiographics.* 2007;27(5):1465–1488.

Narváez JA, Narváez J, Serrallonga M, et al. Bone marrow edema in the cervical spine of symptomatic rheumatoid arthritis patients. *Semin Arthritis Rheum.* 2009;38(4):281–288.

Narváez JA, Narváez J, Lama ED, Albert MD. MR imaging of early rheumatoid arthritis. *Radiographics.* 2010;30:143–165.

Roemer FW, Crema MD, Trattnig S, Guermazi A. Advances in imaging of osteoarthritis and cartilage. *Radiology.* 2011;260(2):332–354.

Steinbach L, Resnick D. Calcium pyrophosphate dihydrate crystal deposition disease revisited. *Radiology.* 1996;200:1–9.

Sudł-Szopińska I, Jurik AG, Eshed I, et al. Recommendations of the ESSR arthritis subcommittee for the use of magnetic resonance imaging in musculoskeletal rheumatic diseases. *Semin Musculoskelet Radiol.* 2015;19:396–411.

Takase-Minegisihi K, Horita N, Kobayashi K, et al. Diagnostic test accuracy of ultrasound for synovitis in rheumatoid arthritis: systematic review and meta-analysis. *Rheumatology.* 2018;57(1):49–58.

Taljanovic MS, Melville DM, Gimber LH, et al. High-resolution US of rheumatologic diseases. *Radiographics.* 2015;35:2026–2048.

Yap FY, Skalski MR, Patel DB, et al. Hypertrophic osteoarthropathy: clinical and imaging features. *Radiographics.* 2017;37:157–175.

Zhang W, Doherty M, Bardin T, et al. European League Against Rheumatism recommendations for calcium pyrophosphate deposition. Part I: terminology and diagnosis. *Ann Rheum Dis.* 2011;70:563–570.

10 Arthroplasty

Introduction

Joint arthroplasties are common today, especially in the hip and knee. Imaging analysis of arthroplasties includes evaluation for anatomic placement, periprosthetic fracture, prosthesis dislocation, loosening of the prosthesis, hardware failure, particle disease, mechanical wear, and infection. The following terms are used to describe arthroplasty types:

- *Total arthroplasty* refers to replacement of both sides of a joint.
- *Hemiarthroplasty* refers to replacement of only one side of a joint.
- *Unicompartmental* arthroplasties are most common in the knee and may be performed if the remaining compartments are not significantly arthritic.
- *Resurfacing arthroplasty* is a bone-sparing technique where only the articular surface and immediately subjacent bone is removed and capped with a metallic covering; this may be done for one or both sides of a joint.

This chapter will concentrate primarily on hip arthroplasties, as they are the most frequent arthroplasties encountered and the principles of evaluation are generalizable to other prostheses.

- *Hemiarthroplasty* is often performed for treatment of a hip fracture that is at risk for avascular necrosis or nonunion.
    - This is a comparatively quick and easy procedure, allowing the patient to return to weight-bearing relatively quickly compared with total arthroplasty or fracture fixation.
- *Total hip arthroplasty* (*THA*) is used most often for management of osteoarthritis, and the specific indication is refractory pain.
    - Modern hip THAs are modular, and most consist of metal alloy femoral and acetabular components lined with polyethylene plastic.

- The femoral component is composed of a stem that is inserted into the femoral shaft and a round head that is smaller than the native femoral head.
    - A separate modular neck component may also be used, which provides more operative flexibility for prosthesis positioning but increases risk for prosthesis-related complications, namely corrosion and particle disease.
- In addition to metal-on-polyethylene, ceramic-on-ceramic and ceramic-on-polyethylene prostheses are also available. Metal-on-metal prostheses are highly durable but have high complication rates and are no longer commonly used.
- Components may be *cemented* with polymethyl methacrylate (PMMA) or other cement material, or they may be *noncemented* with fixation via screws or press-fit after careful reaming of the native bone.
    - A combination of a cemented femoral component and noncemented acetabular component may be used.
- Press-fit components have a porous coating to allow ingrowth of bone for better biologic fixation; the coating may contain osteogenic substances that stimulate bony ingrowth.
    - Often the ingrowth tissue is fibrous rather than bone, which may be seen radiographically as thin lucency, but still provides good fixation.
    - For femoral stem components, the porous surface often only covers the proximal portion to help prevent proximal stress shielding and distal stress loading.

Knee arthroplasties are commonly performed for end-stage osteoarthritis.

- Similar to hip arthroplasties, these may be cemented or noncemented.
- *Total knee arthroplasties* (TKAs) may also be constrained or nonconstrained (cruciate retaining), depending on the degree of preoperative deformity and joint instability.

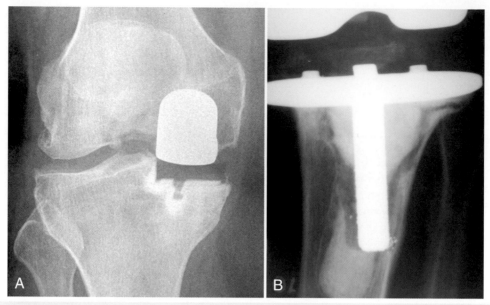

Fig. 10.1 Knee implants. **(A)** AP radiograph shows expected appearance of medial unicompartmental knee arthroplasty, with metal femoral condyle and tibial tray, with polyethylene spacer. **(B)** AP radiograph shows gross tibial component loosening, with medial tilt of the component, fractured cement, and bead shedding.

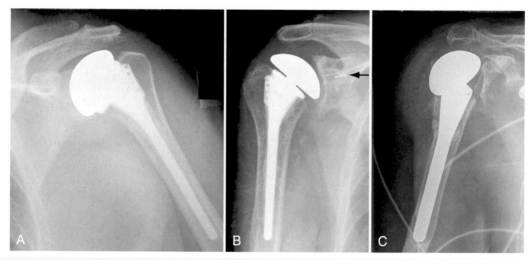

Fig. 10.2 Shoulder arthroplasty. **(A)** Hemiarthroplasty, replacing only the humeral head. **(B)** Total arthroplasty. Note the metal marker *(arrow)* in the cemented polyethylene glenoid component. **(C)** Hemiarthroplasty showing loosening, rotation, and dislocation of the humeral head component.

- *Unicompartmental knee arthroplasties* are used to treat single-compartment medial or lateral tibiofemoral osteoarthritis (Fig. 10.1A), or less commonly isolated patellofemoral compartment osteoarthritis.
  - Unicompartmental knee arthroplasties are less invasive but have higher rates of complication compared to TKAs.

Shoulder arthroplasties include hemiarthroplasties, total shoulder arthroplasties, and reverse total shoulder arthroplasties.

- *Hemiarthroplasty* (or *humeral head resurfacing*) is used to replace the humeral articular surface of the glenohumeral joint (Fig. 10.2A and C).
  - Indications for hemiarthroplasty include intraarticular humeral head fractures, humeral head avascular

necrosis, large Hill–Sachs lesions, chondrosis limited to the humeral articular surface, or congenital deformities of the humeral head.
  - Hemiarthroplasty is preferred in younger patients with pathology limited to the humeral side of the joint, primarily to preserve bone stock as many will ultimately need revision arthroplasty.
- *Total shoulder arthroplasty* is a technically more challenging surgery but has the potential to provide better function and pain relief than a hemiarthroplasty (Fig. 10.2B).
  - Total shoulder arthroplasty is most commonly performed for painful arthritis when conservative management has failed as well as for proximal humerus fractures.
  - *Anatomic total shoulder arthroplasty* is typically performed if the rotator cuff is functionally intact.

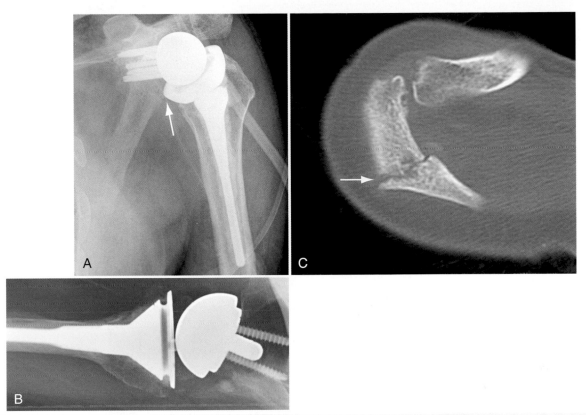

Fig. 10.3 Reverse shoulder arthroplasty. **(A)** AP radiograph shows imperfect positioning of the glenosphere (head) at the glenoid, such that there is impingement of the humeral component along the axillary border of the scapula *(arrow)*. This puts the prosthesis at risk for undercutting the gleno-sphere, followed by loosening and failure. The glenoid component should be placed more inferiorly on the glenoid. **(B)** Normal axillary lateral radio-graph of a reverse shoulder arthroplasty in a different patient, who had continued pain despite normal positioning of the components. The patient had felt a 'pop' 1 week following surgery; axial CT **(C)** shows a fracture of the acromion *(arrow)*, a relatively common site of fracture following this type of arthroplasty. (B and C, Images used with permission from BJ Manaster, MD, from STATdx website, Amirsys, Inc.)

- *Reverse total shoulder arthroplasty* is performed in patients with both irreparable massive rotator cuff tears (or otherwise functionally insufficient rotator cuff) and a functional deltoid muscle. It is another option in the management of glenohumeral joint osteoarthritis and proximal humerus fractures.
  - The convex 'head' or glenosphere is placed on the glenoid; craniocaudad placement is critical.
    - A line starting at the inferior edge of the glenosphere must continue uninterrupted along the line of the axillary border of the scapula to avoid impingement with the humeral prosthesis (Fig. 10.3).
    - In follow-up evaluation, scapular notching along the axillary border of the scapula is often a precursor to loosening and failure.
  - Reverse shoulder arthroplasty moves the center of rotation of the shoulder inferomedially, improving joint stability and mobility by enhancing action of the deltoid muscle.
    - In turn, the deltoid increases stress on the acromion; acromial stress fractures should be sought in cases of continued painful implant; they may be surprisingly difficult to identify without resorting to computed tomography (CT) (see Fig. 10.3C).

Replacement of other joints is less common because of lower frequency of disabling arthritis and difficulty in producing a functional, durable arthroplasty.

- Ankle arthroplasties often incorporate the distal fibula to use a greater surface of bone stock for implant stabilization (Fig. 10.4).
- Elbow arthroplasties are likewise less commonly performed due to the complex nature of the elbow joint.
- Small-joint arthroplasties, such as in the hands and feet, may utilize other materials besides metal alloys and polyethylene.
  - *Silastic arthroplasties* are radiolucent, flexible silicon rubber implants that were used for replacement of small joints made painful and dysfunctional by longstanding arthritis, usually rheumatoid arthritis.
    - These implants are most commonly seen at the wrist, metacarpophalangeal (MCP), and metatarsophalangeal (MTP) joints.
    - Double-stemmed silastic implants can fracture at the thinnest part, which acts as the 'hinge' at the junction of the flange and the body.
    - In addition, dislocation of the flange may occur, especially in diseases such as rheumatoid arthritis that have soft tissue imbalance or contractures.
    - Finally, repetitive motion results in silastic breakdown. Subsequent particle disease with prominent synovitis and osteolysis can develop (Fig. 10.5).
    - Uncommonly implanted presently due to these high complication rates. (Figs. 10.6 and 10.7).

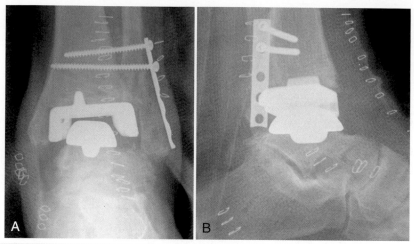

Fig. 10.4 Ankle arthroplasty. Anteroposterior **(A)** and lateral **(B)** radiographs show the dome-shaped talar component, bracket-shaped tibial component (with incorporation of the fibula), and polyethylene spacer. These arthroplasties currently have a higher failure rate than hip or knee implants.

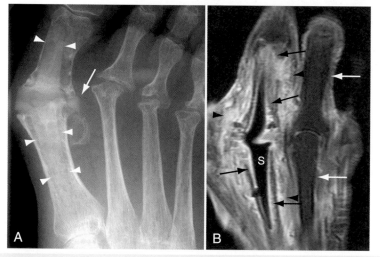

Fig. 10.5 Silastic prosthesis with particle disease. Silastic implants work best in small joints with low loads and are most often used in late-stage rheumatoid arthritis. However, there is great risk for complication. **(A)** AP radiograph of the great toe demonstrates first MTP Swanson silastic prosthesis *(arrowheads)* in a patient with late-stage rheumatoid arthritis. The prosthesis has failed, with fracture of the lateral prosthesis body *(arrow)* and osteolysis around the prosthesis. **(B)** Coronal contrast-enhanced, fat-suppressed, T1-weighted MR image shows low-signal-intensity silastic implants *(S)* in the third finger across the metacarpophalangeal joint, with intense surrounding intraosseous *(black arrows)* and extraosseous *(arrowheads)* enhancement caused by granulomatous reaction to the silastic. Contrast with the normal adjacent fourth metacarpal and proximal phalanx *(white arrows)*.

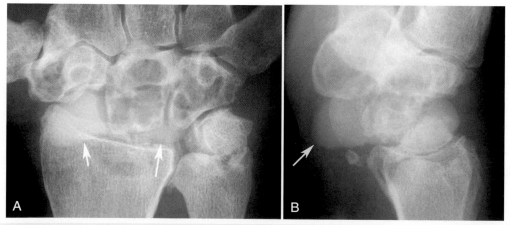

Fig. 10.6 Silastic carpal implant failure. **(A)** Posteroanterior (PA) radiograph of the wrist demonstrating resection of the scaphoid and lunate and replacement by silastic prostheses *(arrows)*. There is significant particle disease, with large cysts seen in the trapezium, capitate, and hamate. **(B)** Lateral view shows palmar dislocation of one of the carpal prostheses *(arrow)*.

■ Newer small-joint devices made with new materials and configurations are now employed, such as pyrocarbon implants and polyvinyl synthetic cartilage implants, though they have complications of their own (Fig. 10.8).

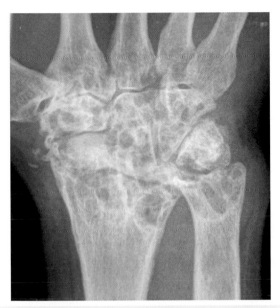

Fig. 10.7 Silastic carpal implant particle disease. PA radiograph in a different patient with a silastic carpal implant shows extensive cystlike lysis in the carpal bones. The lysis is so extensive that one might overlook the presence of the radiodense silastic scaphoid prosthesis, the source of this destructive change.

Imaging Techniques

RADIOGRAPHY

Radiography is the first-line imaging technique for evaluation of arthroplasties. Standard radiographic projections of the replaced joint are typically adequate for evaluation, though the field of view may need to be extended to include the entire extent of hardware, particularly with long-stem prostheses. Many arthroplasty complications can be diagnosed by radiographs, including improper hardware placement, periprosthetic fracture, prosthesis dislocation, hardware failure, and loosening of the prosthesis. Evidence of mechanical wear of the polyethylene liner in hip arthroplasties may be subtle but is adequately diagnosed by radiographs. Particle disease, as well as infection, may be seen as osteolysis about a prosthesis, usually prompting further evaluation with MRI or CT.

MAGNETIC RESONANCE IMAGING

Imaging the postoperative joint presents special challenges but may be necessary to detect and evaluate certain complications, particularly particle disease, infection, and other soft tissue abnormalities around the prosthesis. Interpretation of MRI following arthroplasty can be challenging due to disturbance of normal tissue planes, and artifacts from metallic prosthetic implants can be extensive. Such artifacts can be minimized by using specialized protocols employing metal artifact reduction sequences (MARS). Spin-echo and fast spin-echo sequences should be used instead of gradient

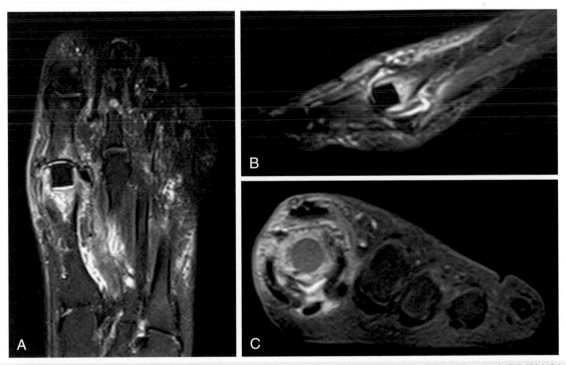

Fig. 10.8 Adverse reaction to a polyvinyl synthetic cartilage implant. Long-axis T2-weighted fat-suppressed **(A)** and sagittal STIR **(B)** MR images of the forefoot demonstrate a polyvinyl synthetic cartilage implant in the first metatarsal head, placed for first metatarsophalangeal (MTP) joint osteoarthritis. There is extensive aseptic inflammatory reaction to the implant with surrounding marrow edema, soft tissue edema, and first MTP joint effusion. **(C)** Short-axis T1-weighted fat-suppressed post-contrast MR image demonstrates associated enhancement of the surrounding bone, synovium, and periarticular soft tissues.

echo sequences. Short tau inversion recovery (STIR) or Dixon-based sequences should be used instead of frequency-selective fat-suppression techniques for fluid-sensitive imaging. Standard non–fat-suppressed T1-weighted and T2-weighted or proton density (PD) sequences are useful for evaluating the prosthesis and surrounding tissues. Other novel, proprietary MRI techniques for metal artifact suppression are offered on newer MRI scanners, which differ by manufacturer. Additional general principles to reduce metal artifact are included in Box 10.1. Keep in mind that the degree of susceptibility artifact is dependent on the metal alloy used. Titanium implants generate the least susceptibility artifact (approximately five times less than cobalt-chromium), whereas older stainless-steel implants generate enormous susceptibility artifact.

ULTRASOUND

Ultrasound (US) may be useful to evaluate for periprosthetic fluid collections, hematomas, and pseudotumors, as well as tendon tears or other soft tissue injuries about the implant. However, US may not reveal the full extent of pathology about the prosthesis, and supplemental cross-sectional imaging with MRI or CT may be required if an abnormality is detected by US. US guidance may be used for aspiration and/or biopsy in cases where infection or particle disease is suspected.

COMPUTED TOMOGRAPHY

CT is useful for evaluation of prostheses, including assessment of hardware positioning, periprosthetic fracture, loosening or osteolysis about a prosthesis, and associated fluid collections or pseudotumors. Similar to MRI, certain techniques can be employed with modern CT scanners to reduce metallic streak artifact, which is mainly caused by photon starvation and beam hardening. Several projection-based metal artifact reduction (MAR) algorithms are commercially available, which use data projection to correct artifacts primarily due to photon starvation. Dual-energy CT techniques can suppress artifact due to beam hardening by selecting virtual monochromatic images at a higher energy level. On older CT units, simply increasing the kilovolt peak (kVp) can combat photon starvation by increasing beam penetration. Doubling or tripling tube current (mAs) also improves image quality. CT arthrography following intraarticular injection of iodinated contrast may also be used for assessment of hardware loosening. Contrast extending between the bone–hardware interface suggests component loosening.

NUCLEAR MEDICINE

Nuclear medicine imaging for the evaluation of hardware complication has primarily been replaced by modern CT and MRI. A ^{99m}Technetium-methylene diphosphonate (Tc^{99}m-MDP) bone scan can be used to detect pathologic radiotracer about the prosthesis, but is not specific for infection, aseptic loosening, or other periprosthetic complication. A ^{99m}Tc-labeled white blood cell (WBC) scan is more specific for the detection of infection, but aspiration is generally quicker and ultimately necessary in such cases anyway.

Disease Processes

IMPROPER POSITIONING

Failure of a THA frequently relates to improper positioning of the components. Acetabular and femoral components should be placed in the expected anatomic sites. When evaluating a THA, the following parameters should be assessed:

- *Alignment of the acetabular component in the coronal plane.*
  - The lateral opening of the acetabulum (lateral inclination) is measured as the angle of opening relative to the transischial line (a line drawn between the two ischial tuberosities, used throughout this section as a convenient landmark for measurement).
  - The lateral opening angle of the acetabular component normally measures 40 ± 10 degrees (Fig. 10.9).

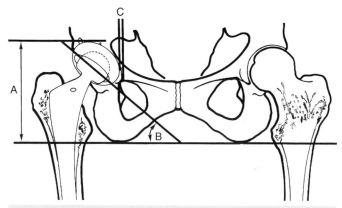

Fig. 10.9 Evaluation of total hip arthroplasty. The reference line for most of what should be evaluated in a total hip arthroplasty is the transischial line. The distance labeled *A* is used to evaluate effective limb length; another way to evaluate this would be to compare the levels of the lesser trochanters with one another. *B* indicates the opening angle (lateral inclination) of the acetabular cup. The measurements between the lines indicated by *C* are used to evaluate for either excessive or lack of medialization of the cup.

Box 10.1   Techniques for Reducing Metal Artifact on MRI

- Use fast spin-echo sequences
- For fluid-sensitive sequences, use short tau inversion recovery (STIR) or Dixon-based techniques instead of frequency-selective fat-suppression techniques
- Image on a lower field strength scanner (e.g., 1.5 Tesla instead of 3.0 Tesla)
- Use longer echo train lengths with shorter echo spacing
- Increase bandwidth
- Increase matrix
- Decrease slice thickness
- Increase number of excitations (NEX) to improve signal-to-noise ratio (SNR)
- Frequency encoding axis away from area of interest (by swapping frequency- and phase-encoding directions)

- An increased lateral opening angle puts the patient at risk for dislocation and increases risk for accelerated or asymmetric polyethylene wear of the acetabular liner.
- A decreased lateral opening angle limits abduction and may result in anterior dislocation when the hip is placed in forced abduction.
- *Angle of the acetabular component in the axial plane.*
  - As seen on a groin lateral radiograph or on an axial CT scan, the acetabulum should be anteverted (oriented anteriorly) 5 to 25 degrees.
  - Zero-degree anteversion may be acceptable if there is anteversion at the femoral neck-shaft angle, but retroversion of the acetabular component is never acceptable and predisposes to posterior dislocation.
  - It is important to note that on an anteroposterior (AP) radiograph, one can see that the acetabular component is angled, but one cannot determine whether the angulation is anteversion or retroversion without the added information from the groin lateral radiograph or axial CT scan (Fig. 10.10).

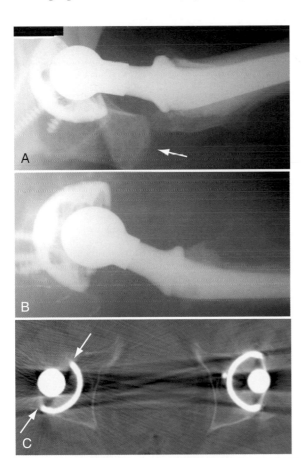

Fig. 10.10 Anteversion of the acetabular component. **(A)** Groin lateral view shows the ischium *(arrow)* that is a posterior structure and therefore showing anteversion (anterior angulation) of both the acetabular component and the femoral neck. **(B)** Groin lateral radiograph taken in a patient who chronically dislocates her hip. The reason for the dislocation is shown, with the retroverted acetabular component. **(C)** Axial CT image in a different patient shows excessive anteversion of the right acetabular component *(arrows)* and neutral alignment (inadequate anteversion) of the left acetabular component. The white disks in the center of each acetabular component are the prosthetic femoral heads.

- *Medial-lateral positioning of the acetabular component.*
  - The acetabular component should be placed such that the horizontal center of rotation of the femoral head component is similar to that of the contralateral hip (see Fig. 10.9).
  - If the acetabular component is too medial in position, there may be excessive thinning of the acetabular medial wall and risk for fracture.
  - If the acetabular component is placed too far laterally, the iliopsoas tendon will cross medial to the femoral head center of rotation, and muscle contraction will tend to force the head from the socket, increasing the risk for dislocation.
- *Limb length.*
  - Equal limb length should be maintained for both legs (within 1 cm side-to-side).
  - Limb length can be affected by placement of the acetabular component, placement of the femoral component, length and size of the femoral neck and head, and thickness of the polyethylene liner.
  - Limb length can be evaluated by choosing a femoral landmark, such as the greater or lesser trochanter, and comparing it with the opposite side relative to the transischial line (Fig. 10.11; see Fig. 10.9).
  - If the hip prosthesis (and leg) is too short, contracting muscles will be ineffective and the prosthesis is subject to dislocation.
  - If the hip prosthesis results in overlengthening of the limb, the neurovascular bundle will be stretched and the muscles likely to spasm, also subjecting the hip to dislocation.
- *Positioning of the femoral component.*
  - The femoral component should be placed in a neutral position within the femoral shaft.
  - A varus position (with the prosthesis stem resting against the lateral femoral cortex distally) predisposes the femoral component to loosening and periprosthetic fracture (Fig. 10.12).

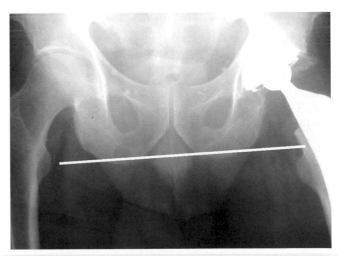

Fig. 10.11 Abnormal limb length. The transischial line is used for evaluation of effective limb length. Note that the patient's normal right hip shows the lesser trochanter to be at the level of the transischial line, whereas the total hip replacement results in extension of the lesser trochanter beyond the line. In this case the total hip replacement results in an effective overlengthening of the left leg.

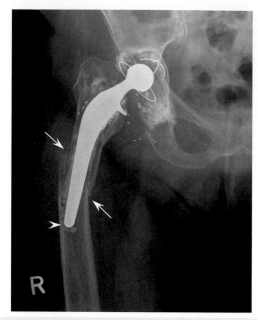

Fig. 10.12 Femoral stem varus positioning with periprosthetic fracture. AP radiograph demonstrates periprosthetic fracture about the femoral stem of a cemented right total hip arthroplasty *(arrows)*, with varus positioning of the distal femoral stem *(arrowhead)*. Osteolysis about both the femoral and acetabular cement also likely contributed to hardware failure in this case.

- *Implant size.*
  - Inappropriate sizing of implant components may result in failure of the arthroplasty hardware or component loosening.
  - Acetabular cups are sized for complete osseous coverage.
  - Uncemented stems are chosen for optimal proximal fit rather than distal canal fit, with the goal of providing maximal surface contact to promote bone ingrowth and to prevent prosthesis *subsidence* (i.e., inferior migration of the implant into the femoral shaft).
  - Inadequate reaming of the native bone or an oversized component can result in fracture intraoperatively when a press-fit prosthesis is placed.

Considerations for component positioning in TKA are as follows:

- The tibial component should be placed 90 ± 5 degrees to the long axis of the tibial shaft on the AP radiograph and ranges from 90 degrees to the long axis of the tibia to a slight posterior tilt on the lateral radiograph.
- The femoral component is placed 5 ± 5 degrees to the long axis of the femoral shaft on the lateral radiograph, with 4 to 7 degrees of valgus angulation as seen on the AP radiograph.

PERIPROSTHETIC FRACTURE

- In THAs, fracture of the host bone is uncommon but can occur in the pelvis as well as the femoral shaft (see Fig. 10.12).
  - In the femoral shaft, a fracture usually begins at the tip of the prosthetic stem and progresses longitudinally and anteriorly.

- Some periprosthetic fractures are nondisplaced and incomplete, and can be extremely subtle even with optimized CT. In some cases the only finding focal linear periosteal reaction that indicates a healing fracture.
- Fractures may occur in the setting of underlying osteolysis or hardware loosening, which weakens the native bone (Figs. 10.13 and 10.14; see Fig. 10.12).
- Patients who are osteoporotic with knee prostheses (e.g., older patients, patients with rheumatoid arthritis,

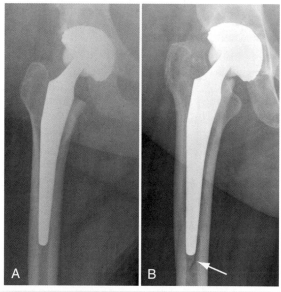

Fig. 10.13 Subsidence and fracture. **(A)** Postoperative baseline radiograph. **(B)** Several months later the patient developed acute pain. AP radiograph shows a femur fracture *(arrow)* that developed secondary to significant subsidence of the femoral component, indicating underlying hardware loosening.

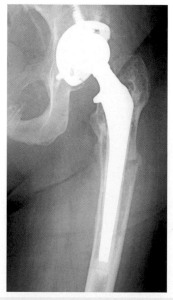

Fig. 10.14 Failed cemented femoral component. AP radiograph demonstrates a wide lucency at the cement–bone interface of the femoral component, with fracture in the proximal shaft of the femur. In addition, there is polyethylene wear, with superior migration of the femoral head within the acetabular component.

etc.) are particularly prone to developing fractures in the metaphyseal region of either the distal femur or proximal tibia.

- Fracture may be seen as a minor change in contour or a sclerotic line of fracture healing (Fig. 10.15).
- If a patient has had a previous tibial tubercle transfer, proximal tibial fracture is even more likely following placement of a TKA

DISLOCATION

- Hip arthroplasty dislocations occur most commonly in the early postoperative period (Fig. 10.16).

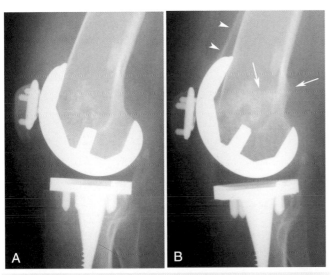

Fig. 10.15 Periprosthetic fracture. **(A)** Lateral radiograph of the knee arthroplasty at the time of placement appears normal. **(B)** The same knee several months later. The patient has developed a fracture in the distal femoral metaphysis *(arrows)*, angulation at the fracture site, and healing reaction seen at the anterior femoral cortex *(arrowheads)*.

- Prostheses using a posterior or posterolateral surgical approach are more prone to dislocation compared to those using an anterior approach.
- Dislocations are typically due to improper positioning of hardware, with specific factors including:
  - Inadequate anteversion or retroversion of the acetabular cup.
  - Increased lateral opening angle (or inclination) of the acetabular cup.
  - Lateral positioning of the acetabular cup.
- Dislocation may occur posteriorly, laterally, or anteriorly, depending on predisposing factors.
- Recurrent dislocation of a hip prosthesis is an indication for revision arthroplasty.

LOOSENING

- Mechanical (aseptic) hardware loosening is one of the most frequently encountered complications following arthroplasty and a common indication for revision arthroplasty.
- In evaluating follow-up radiographs of prostheses, it is crucial to have a comparison radiograph taken at or around the time of placement of the prosthesis.
- Loosening can be definitively diagnosed when there is migration of a component (generally superiorly and medially with an acetabular component, inferiorly with a femoral component) or a change in alignment of a component with the native bone (Box 10.2).
  - For both cemented and noncemented prostheses, the most convincing sign of loosening is progressive change in position, characterized by either subsidence or tilt (Fig. 10.17; see Fig. 10.13).
  - At follow-up, specific evaluation of limb length, lateral opening angle of the acetabulum, and positioning of the components relative to their position at the time of initial placement must be made.

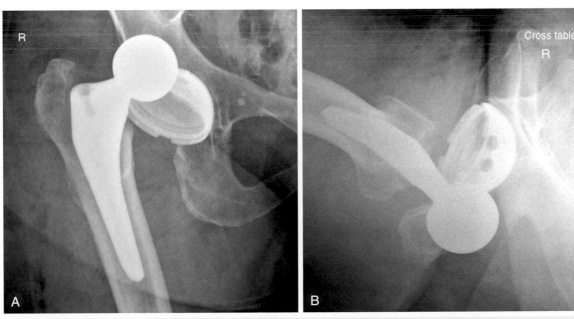

Fig. 10.16 Postoperative total hip arthroplasty dislocation. AP **(A)** and frog-leg lateral **(B)** radiographs demonstrate posterosuperior dislocation of a right total hip arthroplasty 1 day postoperatively. Note the soft tissue gas in the lateral thigh, indicating recent surgery.

Box 10.2   Radiographic Findings of Component Loosening

- Change in component alignment
- Lucency of greater than 2 mm at cement–bone or prosthesis–bone interface
- Scalloped contour of lucency around component
- Reactive change at endosteum or periosteum
- Component, bone, or cement fracture

- Comparison with initial postoperative radiographs may reveal changes in the position of a component, which may not be seen with the most recent comparison radiograph (Fig. 10.18).
- Abnormal periprosthetic lucency about a prosthesis can suggest loosening, even in the absence of positional change (Fig. 10.19).

- Periprosthetic lucency can be seen with component loosening, particle disease, and infection.
  - Loosening is generally seen as diffuse lucency about the affected component, whereas particle disease and infection tend to be more focal.
- Periprosthetic lucency >2 mm or progressively increasing lucency over sequential radiographs is consistent with component loosening.
- In both cemented and noncemented prostheses, one can expect to see a thin (1–2 mm) radiolucent zone at the cement–bone or hardware–bone interface.
  - In cemented prostheses, this radiolucent zone represents fibrous reaction to the cement and/or fibrous ingrowth.
  - In noncemented prostheses, this radiolucent zone represents fibrous ingrowth and is often outlined by a thin sclerotic line.

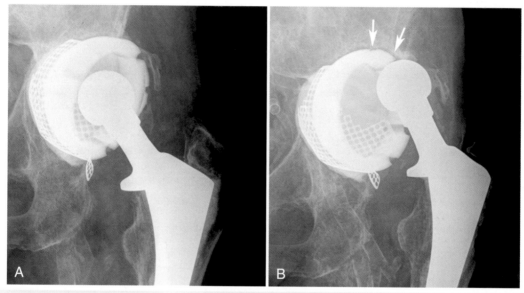

Fig. 10.17 Failed acetabular component. **(A)** Baseline AP radiograph after surgery. **(B)** One year later the acetabular component has rotated, and the femoral head is subluxed superiorly. Note the increase in lucency at the superior margin of the cup *(arrows)*.

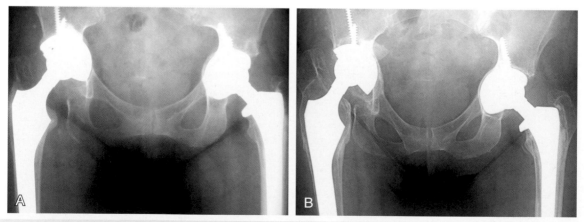

Fig. 10.18 Failed total hip arthroplasty. **(A)** Baseline examination shows noncemented right total hip arthroplasty and hybrid left total hip arthroplasty, with the components appropriately aligned and showing no evidence of loosening. **(B)** Four years later there has been a significant change, with loosening of all the components. The right acetabular component has tilted and is superiorly subsided. The right femoral component shows a lucency surrounding it at the bone–component interface with subsidence of the component by approximately 2 cm. The left acetabular component shows a 2-mm lucency surrounding it, with slight tilt, indicating loosening. The left femoral component shows a 2- to 3-mm lucency surrounding the cement–bone interface. This is loose as well. Finally, both acetabular components show superior migration of the femoral heads relative to the acetabular components, indicating polyethylene wear.

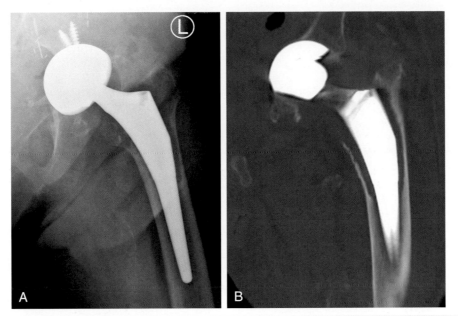

Fig. 10.19 Femoral stem component loosening. AP radiograph **(A)** and coronal CT reconstruction image **(B)** demonstrate diffuse lucency about the femoral component of a left total hip arthroplasty, indicating hardware loosening. Thinning of the medial acetabular wall with protrusio of the acetabular component is also noted.

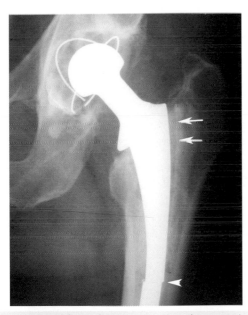

Fig. 10.20 Fractured femoral component. Note the separation of the cement from the proximal femoral component *(arrows)* and fracture across the distal prosthesis *(arrowhead)*.

- Thin lucency about a prosthesis is considered normal only when it is ≤2 mm and does not widen over time.
  - Lucency is particularly common around the superolateral portion of the acetabular component and tip of the femoral stem and is considered a normal finding unless it progresses over time.
- Additional findings of loosening of a cemented component include cement fracture (see Fig. 10.1B), separation of cement from the prosthesis, and hardware fracture (Fig. 10.20).

- Additional considerations when assessing for hardware loosening in THAs:
  - It is important to note that prominent calcar resorption is common in noncemented prostheses (recall that the calcar is the normal ridge of dense bone along the posteromedial femoral neck).
    - This resorption is caused by *stress shielding* of the proximal femur by the stiff femoral component, which transmits force from the prosthetic femoral head to the distal aspect of the stem; the bone that is not under stress is resorbed over time (see Fig. 1.2).
    - This resorption is one reason that revision THA requires a longer stem for purchase into healthy bone.
  - Femoral components may include a 'calcar shelf', which is a medial flange intended to transmit some force to the calcar to reduce bone loss caused by stress shielding.
    - Despite this and other design modifications, proximal femur bone loss caused by stress shielding remains common.
  - Cortical thickening and endosteal sclerosis are often present around the distal stem in response to locally elevated stress as normal findings, particularly in older, fully coated prostheses.
    - However, excessive cortical hypertrophy and endosteal bone bridging at the tip of the femoral stem, or excessive endosteal scalloping, probably represents component loosening, particularly if progression is shown (Fig. 10.21).
- In TKAs, the tibial component is most likely to loosen.
  - Early loosening is usually followed by tilting of the tibial component into a varus position with subsidence into the medial tibial plateau and collapse of the cancellous bone (Fig. 10.1B).

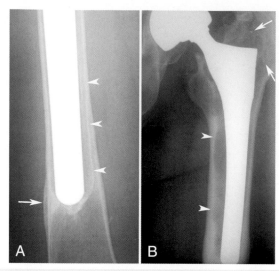

Fig. 10.21 Failed noncemented femoral component. **(A)** AP radiograph shows a wide lucency and sclerotic line surrounding the femoral component *(arrowheads)*. In addition, there is endosteal and periosteal new bone formation *(arrow)*. **(B)** AP radiograph in a different patient shows scalloping of the endosteum *(arrowheads)* as well as bead shedding *(arrows)*, indicating failure of this noncemented prosthesis. It has also subsided by approximately 1 cm.

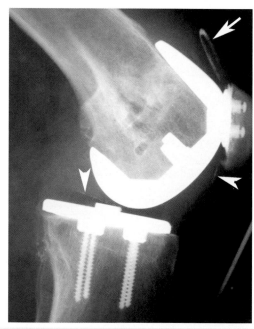

Fig. 10.22 Patellar component failure. Lateral radiograph demonstrates superior subsidence of the patellar component. It also shows dissociation of some of the metal backing, with displacement into the suprapatellar bursa *(arrow)*. Finally, the patient is developing metallosis in the joint, with metallic fragments lining the polyethylene and joint capsule *(arrowheads)*.

- Polyethylene wear, fragmentation, and dislocation may follow.
- Patellar complications occur frequently, including subsidence, polyethylene wear, polyethylene dissociation from the metal backing, disintegration of the metal backing with metallosis (metal particles lining the polyethylene and joint capsule; Fig. 10.22), and patellar avascular necrosis or fracture.

HARDWARE FAILURE

- Failure of the construct itself may constitute a complication, though is usually concomitant with other prosthetic complications.
- Fracture of the prosthesis itself is uncommon but when present tends to be of the femoral stem (Fig. 10.23; see Fig. 10.20).
- Separation of the polyethylene insert from its backing may be heralded by the presence of small wedge-shaped metallic fragments (Fig. 10.24).
- Fractures and displacement of the polyethylene can occasionally be seen.

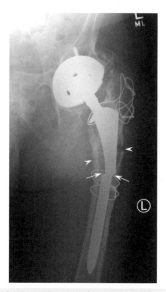

Fig. 10.23 Femoral stem component fracture with periprosthetic fracture. AP radiograph demonstrates periprosthetic fracture *(arrowheads)* about the femoral stem component of a total hip arthroplasty, as well as fracture of the femoral stem component itself *(arrows)*. Lucency is also noted about the proximal femoral stem component, predisposing to hardware failure.

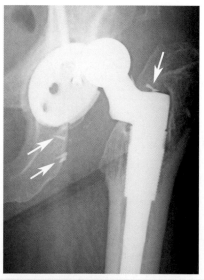

Fig. 10.24 Failed total hip arthroplasty. This patient has a dislocated total hip arthroplasty, with multiple wedge-shaped metallic densities *(arrows)*. These spikes are used to hold the polyethylene within the metallic backing of the cup. Their presence indicates failure of the cup.

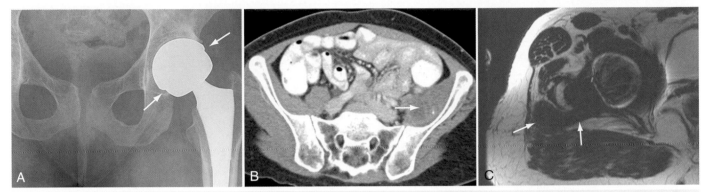

Fig. 10.25 Metal-on-metal hip arthroplasty. **(A)** AP radiograph shows a metal-on-metal prosthesis; note the absence of polyethylene liner at the interface of the head and cup *(arrows)*. The components are positioned properly, yet the patient complained of worsening pain. **(B)** Axial CT image in the same patient shows mild enhancement of an inhomogeneous iliacus mass *(arrow)*. Extensive biopsy showed debris and necrotic tissue typical of the pseudotumors that may develop in this particular type of implant. Joint fluid analysis showed abnormally high concentrations of metals. **(C)** Axial T2-weighted MRI in a different patient with metal-on-metal hip implant shows a low-signal pseudotumor located posterior to the proximal femoral shaft *(arrows)*. Either CT or MRI is essential to locate the lesions associated with complications of this type of prosthesis. (A and B, Images used with permission from BJ Manaster, MD, from Manaster BJ, Petersilge CA, Roberts CC, Hanrahan CJ. *Diagnostic Imaging: Musculoskeletal Non-Traumatic Disease*. Salt Lake City: Amirsys; 2010.)

PARTICLE DISEASE, ADVERSE LOCAL TISSUE REACTION, AND METALLOSIS

- *Particle disease* represents a group of immune-mediated disease processes resulting from small particles (including polyethylene, metal, ceramic, or cement) that are shed from a prosthesis into the joint and/or surrounding soft tissues.
- The terms *adverse local tissue reaction* (ALTR) and *adverse reaction to metal debris* (ARMD) refer to the pathologic processes that result from shedding of particles.
- ALTR is a macrophage-mediated process in which particles are engulfed by macrophages, which lyse and result in release of inflammatory cytokines, inflammatory synovitis, and stimulation of osteoclasts.
  - It is important to note that the source of the particles is not important; rather than the material, the size of the particles seems to elicit the reaction.
- ARMD, or *metallosis*, is seen in *metal-on-metal prostheses* and reflects a hapten-mediated type IV hypersensitivity reaction, characterized histopathologically by *aseptic lymphocyte-dominated vasculitis-associated lesion* (*ALVAL*).
  - ALVAL is a histopathologic diagnosis, not a radiologic one.
  - Metal-on-metal hip implants can be identified by the absence of a polyethylene cup (Fig. 10.25).
  - ARMD in chromium-cobalt arthroplasties is heralded by increased serum chromium and cobalt concentrations.
- Both ALTR and ARMD may result in periprosthetic osteolysis, fluid collections, or soft tissue masses (often called *pseudotumors*).
- Differentiating between these two processes is not critical on imaging, as both may ultimately require revision arthroplasty, though ARMD may be suggested on MRI by areas of low signal intensity or susceptibility artifact within the periprosthetic fluid collection and/or pseudotumor, reflecting the metal debris.

- Radiographs often show areas of lucency around a prosthesis, representing osteolysis (Fig. 10.26).
  - Osteolysis associated with particle disease is often localized or multifocal, compared to mechanical hardware loosening, which is more typically diffuse or circumferential.
  - Periprosthetic lucency with accompanying periostitis or rapid osteolysis about a component is concerning for infection rather than aseptic loosening or particle disease.
- Associated soft tissue damage can range from minimal to extensive, requiring evaluation by CT or MRI.
  - Imaging with CT or MRI should be optimized by using MAR techniques.
  - Images must be carefully scrutinized for periprosthetic osteolysis, fluid collections, and pseudotumors, which may be subtle (Fig. 10.27) or obvious (Figs. 10.28 through 10.30).
- Joint aspiration or aspiration of periprosthetic fluid collections may be performed to exclude underlying or superimposed infection.

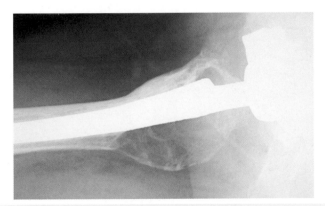

Fig. 10.26 Particle disease. Frog-leg lateral radiograph demonstrates an expanded lytic lesion in the proximal femoral metaphysis. This osteolysis most frequently is related to particle disease.

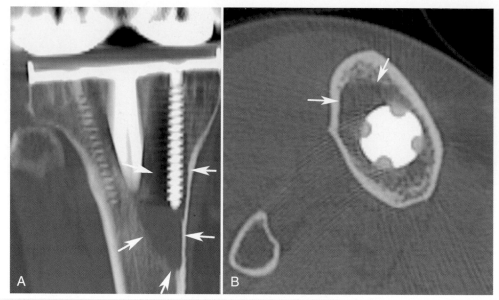

Fig. 10.27 CT of particle disease. **(A)** Coronal CT reconstruction image of the proximal tibia in a patient with a total knee arthroplasty shows well-circumscribed lysis around a tibial fixation screw *(arrows)*. **(B)** Axial CT image through the proximal leg in a different patient with a knee arthroplasty shows subtle bone lysis anterior to the cemented tibial stem component *(arrows)*.

- In cases of metallosis, aspiration may yield dark-colored fluid due to the high concentration of metal particles.
- In addition to culture and cell count analysis, fluid can be evaluated for the presence of metal ions, although concentrations may be widely variable (in contrast to serum levels for cobalt-chromium implants, which have more well-defined reference values).

POLYETHYLENE WEAR

- *Polyethylene wear* is an initially subtle radiographic diagnosis and often a trivial problem itself, though it can occasionally cause mechanical symptoms.

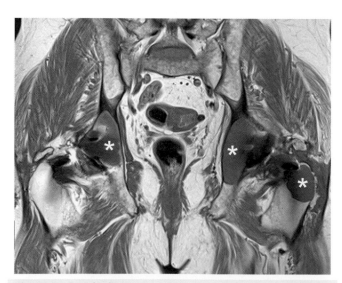

Fig. 10.28 Particle disease on MRI. Coronal T1-weighted MR image demonstrates areas of osteolysis about bilateral total hip arthroplasties *(asterisks)* indicating particle disease involving both prostheses.

- However, polyethylene wear is a major source of the small particles that can lead to component loosening and particle disease.
  - As outlined in the previous section, polyethylene particles can initiate an immune-mediated reaction that can result in osteolysis, in some cases very extensive.
- Polyethylene wear is revealed on radiographs by superolateral displacement of the femoral head within the acetabular cup, reflecting asymmetric wear of the polyethylene liner (Fig. 10.31; see Figs. 10.14 and 10.18). This is initially subtle but with greater polyethylene wear becomes more obvious.
- Acetabular component that is oriented more laterally can contribute to asymmetric polyethylene wear (lateral inclination).
- *Creep* is different from wear and reflects expected remodeling of the polyethylene liner centrally due to normal loading.
  - This occurs rather quickly and actually increases head-liner contact surface area, thereby reducing contact pressure.

INFECTION

- *Infection* is a serious complication of joint arthroplasty, requiring antibiotic therapy, hardware explantation and debridement, and often placement of an antibiotic-impregnated cement spacer until the infection has cleared and a revision arthroplasty can be safely performed.
- Radiographic findings are usually neither helpful nor specific in identifying prosthetic infections.
  - Radiographs may appear normal or demonstrate periprosthetic lucency, which may mimic loosening or particle disease.
  - Infection may ultimately result in hardware loosening and therefore have overlapping radiographic findings.

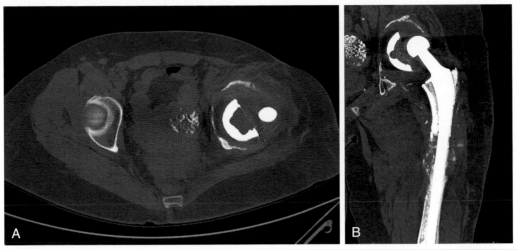

Fig. 10.29 Particle disease with extensive osteolysis. Metal artifact reduction axial **(A)** and coronal reconstruction **(B)** CT images show extensive osteolysis about both the acetabular and femoral components of a left total hip long-stem revision arthroplasty. Rotation of the acetabular component is also noted.

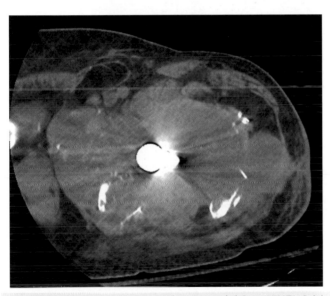

Fig. 10.30 Metallosis (adverse reaction to metal debris, ARMD). Axial CT image demonstrates extensive periprosthetic 'pseudotumor' about a metal-on-metal hip arthroplasty. Subtle hyperdensity is noted in the medial aspect of the periprosthetic soft tissue mass/fluid collection, reflecting shedding of metal debris. Fragments of the prosthesis are also noted in the surrounding soft tissues.

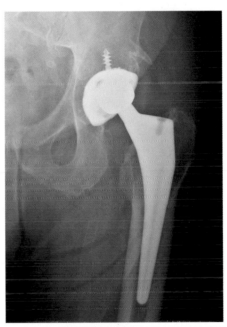

Fig. 10.31 Polyethylene liner wear. AP radiograph demonstrates superolateral positioning of the femoral head component within the acetabular component of a total hip arthroplasty, indicating asymmetric polyethylene liner wear.

- More specific findings concerning for infection include periostitis or rapidly progressive osteolysis, though these are not sensitive findings as most infections are indolent.
- CT and MRI findings may likewise overlap with other aseptic processes.
  - Osteolysis and rim-enhancing fluid collections can be seen with both infection and particle disease; identification of a draining sinus tract is more specific for infection.
  - Osteomyelitis may be seen involving the native bone around a prosthesis.
- If infection is suspected, joint aspiration under strict aseptic conditions, supplemented if necessary with nonbacteriostatic (preservative-free) saline lavage, enables detection of most prosthetic infections; additional technical considerations for performing aspiration of a THA are provided in Chapter 16—Musculoskeletal Procedures and Techniques.
  - In addition to routine Gram stain and culture, ancillary laboratory tests such as an alpha-defensin laboratory-based immunoassay may be requested to establish the diagnosis of a prosthetic joint infection.
- Nuclear medicine imaging studies for evaluation of hardware have primarily been supplanted by CT and MRI.

- In cases equivocal for infection by other imaging modalities, a ^{99m}Tc-labeled WBC scan may show increased radiotracer uptake about an infected prosthesis, but aspiration is generally quicker and easier to perform.
- For additional details regarding imaging findings of infection, see Chapter 14—Musculoskeletal Infection.

SOFT TISSUE COMPLICATIONS

In addition to complications associated with the prosthesis itself, several soft tissue complications may be encountered following arthroplasty. Careful examination of the soft tissues surrounding an otherwise normal-appearing prosthesis may reveal an alternative pain generator.

- *Hematoma* may be seen in the recent postoperative setting and can result in mass effect or compression of adjacent structures, such as nerves and vessels (Fig. 10.32).
- *Heterotopic ossification* is a common complication following arthroplasty, characterized by heterotopic bone formation in the soft tissues about the prosthesis.
  - Heterotopic ossification may be inconsequential or result in significant limitation of motion if extensive (Fig. 10.33).
- *Tendon injury*, such as tendinosis, tendon tearing, or tenosynovitis, may result from altered anatomy or mechanical wear due to placement of a prosthesis.
  - In THAs, iliopsoas tendon pathology may be encountered due to mechanical friction along the anterior margin of the acetabular cup (Fig. 10.34).
  - Gluteus medius and minimus tendon defects following THA may reflect tendon tear or surgical disruption, depending on approach.

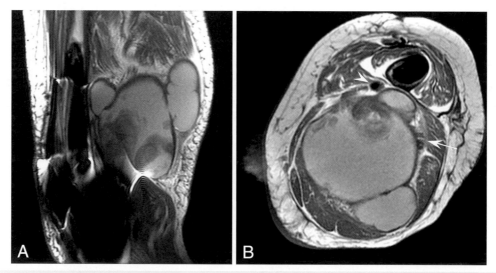

Fig. 10.32 Postoperative hematoma after total knee revision arthroplasty. Sagittal **(A)** and axial **(B)** proton density MR images demonstrate a large, complex hematoma in the posterior soft tissues following total knee revision arthroplasty. The hematoma displaces the popliteal artery (*arrowhead* in B) and tibial and common peroneal nerves (*arrow* in B).

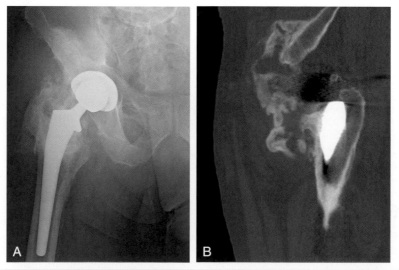

Fig. 10.33 Extensive heterotopic ossification following total hip arthroplasty. AP radiograph **(A)** and sagittal CT reconstruction image **(B)** demonstrate extensive bridging heterotopic ossification in this patient with painful restricted range of motion following total hip arthroplasty.

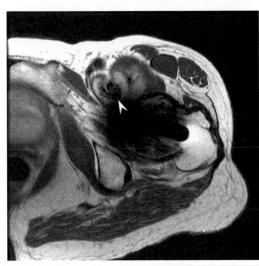

Fig. 10.34 Iliopsoas tendon injury following total hip arthroplasty. Axial proton density MR image demonstrates marked tendon thickening and interstitial tearing of the iliopsoas tendon *(arrowhead)* with surrounding iliopsoas bursitis following total hip arthroplasty.

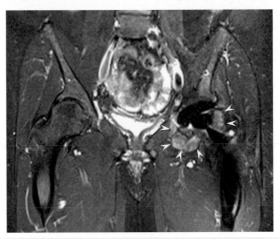

Fig. 10.36 Recurrent pigmented villonodular synovitis (PVNS) following total hip arthroplasty. Coronal STIR MR image shows masslike soft tissue *(arrows)* about a left total hip arthroplasty, which was initially placed for osteoarthritis secondary to PVNS. It was unclear on imaging whether this represented particle disease or PVNS recurrence, with image-guided percutaneous biopsy confirming the latter.

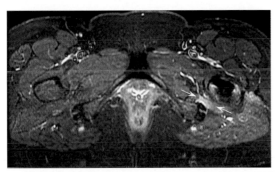

Fig. 10.35 Ischiofemoral impingement following total hip arthroplasty. Axial STIR MR image demonstrates narrowing of the left ischiofemoral space with edema in the quadratus femoris muscle *(arrows)* following total hip arthroplasty.

- *Muscle atrophy* following an arthroplasty may be due to disuse atrophy related to altered biomechanics, underlying tendon tear, or denervation.
  - Ipsilateral iliopsoas muscle atrophy is commonly seen following THA, though the exact pathophysiology and clinical significance remain unclear.
- *Nerve injury* during or after surgery may occur due to traction, compression, or ischemia.
- *Impingement syndromes* may be seen due to altered anatomy following arthroplasty, such as ischiofemoral impingement following THA due to narrowing of the ischiofemoral space (Fig. 10.35).
- *Disease recurrence* may be encountered following arthroplasty in the setting of an underlying malignancy or synovial proliferative process (Fig. 10.36).

Reporting Tips and Recommendations

- Recognize the differential diagnosis for periprosthetic lucency >2 mm, and when a specific diagnosis may be suggested.

- Make follow-up recommendations when appropriate, such as additional imaging or joint aspiration.
- Differentiate between cemented and noncemented prostheses on radiographs and be aware of their expected imaging findings.
- Communicate with the surgeon about unexpected findings on immediate postoperative radiographs, such as fracture or hardware mispositioning.
  - Keep in mind that certain findings may be suspected or known; for example, a surgeon may place cerclage wires around a proximal femoral shaft that was fractured intraoperatively, or may already be aware of a fracture caused by hardware removal.
  - Certain findings are likely not of clinical concern, such as a screw projecting beyond the cortical margin, unless extending near a major vessel, nerve, or other critical structure.
- Search for alternative causes of pain following arthroplasty, such as a hematoma causing mass effect, tendon or muscle injury, neurovascular compression, exuberant heterotopic ossification, etc.

Sources and Suggested Readings

Fritz J, Lurie B, Miller TT, et al. MR imaging of hip arthroplasty implants. *Radiographics.* 2014;34(4):E106-E132.

Fritz J, Lurie B, Miller TT. Imaging of hip arthroplasty. *Semin Musculoskelet Radiol.* 2013;17(3):316–327.

Ha AS, Petscavage JM, Chew FS. Current concepts of shoulder arthroplasty for radiologists: part 2—anatomic and reverse total shoulder replacement and nonprosthetic resurfacing. *AJR Am J Roentgenol.* 2012;199(4):768–776.

Katsura M, Sato J, Akahane M, et al. Current and novel techniques for metal artifact reduction at CT: practical guide for radiologists. *Radiographics.* 2018;38(2):450–461.

Lin DJ, Wong TT, Kazam JK. Shoulder arthroplasty, from indications to complications: what the radiologist needs to know. *Radiographics.* 2016;36(1):192–208.

Manaster B. Total hip arthroplasty: radiographic evaluation. *Radiographics.* 1996;16:645–660.

Manaster B. Total knee arthroplasty: post-operative radiographic findings. *AJR Am J Roentgenol*. 1995;165:899–904.

Mulcahy H, Chew FS. Current concepts in knee replacement: complications. *AJR Am J Roentgenol*. 2014;202(1):W76–W86.

Mulcahy H, Chew FS. Current concepts in knee replacement: features and imaging assessment. *AJR Am J Roentgenol*. 2013;201(6):W828–W842.

Mulcahy H, Chew FS. Current concepts of hip arthroplasty for radiologists: part 1, features and radiographic assessment. *AJR Am J Roentgenol*. 2012;199(3):559–569.

Mulcahy H, Chew FS. Current concepts of hip arthroplasty for radiologists: part 2, revisions and complications. *AJR Am J Roentgenol*. 2012;199(3):570–580.

Nawabi DH, Gold S, Lyman S, et al. MRI predicts ALVAL and tissue damage in metal-on-metal hip arthroplasty. *Clin Orthop Relat Res*. 2014;472(2):471–481.

Petscavage JM, Ha AS, Chew FS. Current concepts of shoulder arthroplasty for radiologists: part 1—epidemiology, history, preoperative imaging, and hemiarthroplasty. *AJR Am J Roentgenol*. 2012;199(4):757–767.

Roberts CC, Ekelund AL, Renfree KJ, et al. Radiologic assessment of reverse shoulder arthroplasty. *Radiographics*. 2007;27(1):223–235.

Roth TD, Maertz NA, Parr JA, et al. CT of the hip prosthesis: appearance of components, fixation, and complications. *Radiographics*. 2012;32(4):1089–1107.

Talbot BS, Weinberg EP. MR imaging with metal-suppression sequences for evaluation of total joint arthroplasty. *Radiographics*. 2016;36(1):209–225.

Vanrusselt J, Vansevenant M, Vanderschueren G, et al. Postoperative radiograph of the hip arthroplasty: what the radiologist should know. *Insights Imaging*. 2015;6(6):591–600.

Yanny S, Cahri JG, Barker T, et al. MRI of aseptic lymphocytic vasculitis-associated lesions in metal-on-metal hip replacements. *AJR Am J Roentgenol*. 2012;198(6):1394–1402.

11 Bone Tumors

Approach to Bone Tumors and Tumorlike Conditions

Bone tumors can be categorized as benign or malignant. Malignant tumors can be primary, secondary (i.e., because of malignant transformation of a preexisting lesion), or metastatic in origin. For many musculoskeletal neoplasms, it can be difficult both for the pathologist and the radiologist to make the distinction between benign and malignant. The pathologist often relies heavily on findings made by the radiologist and the orthopedic oncologist to make a diagnosis. In many cases the imaging features are best described in terms of the aggressiveness of the lesion rather than by specifying 'malignant' or 'benign'. The terms '*aggressive*' or '*nonaggressive*' refer to the local behavior of the tumor. While it is true that many malignant lesions have aggressive features and most benign lesions have nonaggressive features, **aggressive is not the same as malignant, and nonaggressive is not the same as benign**. Examples of benign lesions that are radiographically aggressive include Langerhans cell histiocytosis (LCH), infection, aneurysmal bone cyst (ABC), and some giant cell tumors (GCTs). Many malignant tumors do not have aggressive features on imaging studies. Multifocality raises the possibility of metastatic disease, but benign metabolic processes such as renal failure can also present with disseminated lucent or sclerotic lesions.

Evaluating bone tumors and tumorlike lesions requires a multimodality approach. Each modality has advantages and disadvantages, and a rational, tailored algorithm should be used; reflexive, simultaneous ordering of all modalities when a lesion is found or clinically suspected should be discouraged.

MODALITIES

Radiography

Radiographs remain the primary initial imaging study for detection and characterization of bone tumors. When a classically benign lesion is detected on routine radiographs, additional studies may not be required unless surgical intervention is contemplated and further anatomic information is required. In this setting either computed tomography (CT) or magnetic resonance imaging (MRI) may be most appropriate for preoperative evaluation.

CT

For bone lesions, CT is very useful for evaluation of margins, matrix mineralization, and cortical breakthrough. If an osteoid osteoma is suspected, CT is helpful to locate the lucent nidus. CT is less prone to motion artifact than MRI and thus may be preferred in evaluation of chest and anterior abdominal wall lesions.

Ultrasound

Ultrasound is valuable for evaluation of soft tissue masses but has limited utility for bone lesions. Ultrasound can be useful for biopsy of soft tissue components of a bone lesion.

MRI

When routine radiographic features of a bone lesion are indeterminate or the lesion demonstrates aggressive features or otherwise considered to be potentially malignant, MRI is useful for characterization, staging, and biopsy planning. Intravenous gadolinium-based contrast is useful for distinguishing nonenhancing cystic, myxoid, or necrotic components from solid enhancing regions. Contrast is also useful when scanned in dynamic fashion rapidly after a bolus, in order to characterize tumor vascularity: malignant tumors often enhance more rapidly than normal tissues. MRI is the modality of choice for evaluating and staging primary bone sarcomas, including compartment and neurovascular involvement. MRI is useful for determining tissue characteristics of a bone lesion, such as fat, hemorrhage, fibrous tissue, or fluid-fluid levels. However, MRI does have limitations. Although certain features on MRI can be used to narrow the differential diagnosis for bone and soft tissue masses, it is unreliable for making a specific diagnosis in most cases, and in many cases cannot reliably distinguish benign from malignant lesions. Additionally, patient size and clinical status as well as the presence of certain metallic or electrical implants may limit the utilization of MRI.

Nuclear Medicine

Tc99m methylene diphosphonate (MDP) bone scan is useful for evaluation of multiplicity of lesions. However, if the primary lesion in question (or lesion detected with another modality) shows no increased uptake on bone scan, the study is of limited value for detecting other potential sites of involvement. This is often the case with purely lytic metastases and myeloma, which are usually "cold" on bone scan. On the other end of the spectrum, diffuse involvement ('skeletal carcinomatosis'), as seen in cases of metastatic prostate or breast carcinoma, can produce such generalized uptake that the bone scan looks relatively normal except for lack of uptake by the kidneys (described as a *superscan*). Bone scan is very useful for detecting metastatic lesions of osteosarcoma, which avidly concentrate radiotracer.

Another situation in which bone scan can be useful is for the evaluation of an indeterminate sclerotic lesion. An example is distinguishing a bone island or fibrous dysplasia, which show little to no increased uptake, from a blastic metastasis, which shows high uptake.

For patients with ill-defined symptoms and normal radiographs, a radionuclide bone scan may be used to detect and localize an occult lesion. Following a positive bone scan, either MRI or CT may be selected to further characterize the lesion.

Positron emission tomography (PET)-CT scanning with bone-targeting sodium fluoride 18 produces bone scan images with superior sensitivity, specificity, and spatial resolution compared to Tc99m single-photon emission computed tomography (SPECT) images. High cost limits its use. Evaluation of prostate cancer osseous metastatic disease is a recognized application.

If a tumor is fluorodeoxyglucose (FDG)-avid, PET-CT is very useful for guiding biopsy, staging and monitoring treatment following chemotherapy, surgical resection, or ablation. Osteosarcoma, Ewing sarcoma, and multiple myeloma are examples of PET-avid malignancies. However, PET does not distinguish benign from malignant, and not all malignant tumors are FDG-avid.

Key Concepts

Summary of Modalities for Bone Tumors and Tumorlike Lesions

- Radiographs: Best exam for initial evaluation
- CT: Margins, matrix, cortical breakthrough
- US: Limited utility
- MRI: Cyst versus solid, signal characteristics, extent; can limit differential diagnosis. Biopsy planning
- Bone scan Multifocality of disease
- PET: If FDG-avid: Diagnosis, staging, follow-up of treated lesions

SPECIFIC CONSIDERATIONS

Common things are common. Primary bone malignancies are rare compared to metastatic disease and myeloma. Biopsy should be considered for equivocal cases. An important exception is when biopsy may falsely suggest an aggressive lesion, the classic example of which is a stress fracture. Some benign lesions evolve quickly and develop classically benign features or regress providing support for benignity. These lesions, if suspected, can be followed over a short term (e.g., 1 month). A second caveat regarding biopsy: If the lesion is potentially a primary tumor, percutaneous biopsy carries the risk of contamination ('seeding') of the soft tissues along the biopsy needle tract with tumor cells—consultation with the oncologic surgeon must be performed first to plan the access route. This caveat is does not apply to biopsy of metastatic lesions and myeloma.

Intraarticular Lesions

Intraarticular masslike lesions are rarely malignant; rather, they nearly always are related to an arthritis. Masslike synovial proliferation is especially common in untreated rheumatoid arthritis, but this is usually diffusely distributed. Gout can cause focal intraarticular masses, as can focal forms of pigmented villonodular synovitis (PVNS) and synovial chondromatosis.

Key Concepts

Differential Diagnosis for Synovial Masses

- PVNS
- Synovial osteochondromatosis
- Rheumatoid arthritis
- Gout
- Complex ganglion/synovial cyst
- Postoperative fibrosis (e.g., 'cyclops' lesion in the knee)
- Rare benign lesions: Lipoma arborescens, sarcoidosis and other granulomatous diseases, amyloidosis, synovial hemangioma or arteriovenous malformation, intracapsular chondroma
- Rare malignant lesions: Synovial sarcoma, synovial chondrosarcoma, synovial metastasis

---

Pathological Fracture

Pathological fracture can occur through a benign or malignant lesion (Fig. 11.1). The distinction is clinically important, but if there is no imaging prior to fracture, it can be difficult to distinguish these because hematoma, hyperemia, periosteal reaction, and bone resorption can make the lesion appear more aggressive on any imaging modality. A specific sign of benignity in a pathologic fracture is the classic radiographic sign of a *fallen fragment*, which is a fracture fragment in a dependent portion of a benign cystic bone lesion. This finding is helpful but rarely seen. If a fracture occurs in an unexpected location or due to minimal trauma, an underlying mass may be suspected. If radiographs are noncontributory, MRI with contrast shortly following the injury can visualize the underlying tumor; if delayed, hematoma at the fracture site can vascularize and simulate tumor. Whole-body imaging with bone scan, MRI, or PET-CT may be useful to search for other lesions.

'Burned-out' Lesions

Some benign lesions, as a course of their natural history or due to underlying hemorrhage, may undergo fatty involution and are eventually replaced by with fatty marrow. This can leave "ghost" of the lesion margins behind that may persist for a long period of time (Fig. 11.2). This also can be seen after fracture, orthopedic pin removal, or healing after a drilling procedure. Intraosseous lipoma and fibromyxoma

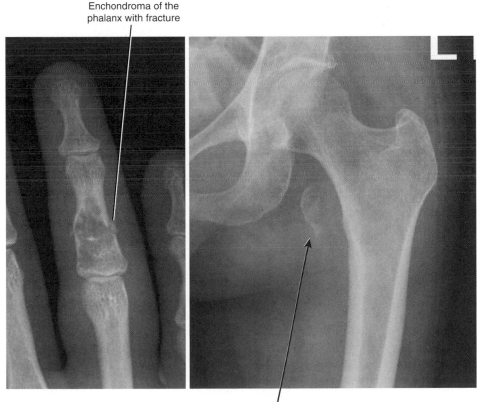

Enchondroma of the phalanx with fracture

Lung adenocarcinoma metastasis: Pathological avulsion fracture of the lesser trochanter

Fig. 11.1 Pathologic fracture can occur through benign or malignant lesions. Fracture can make the lesion appear more aggressive on all modalities. Avulsion of the lesser trochanter typically indicates underlying pathology. (From Morrison W. *Problem Solving in Musculoskeletal Imaging*. Philadelphia: Elsevier; 2010.)

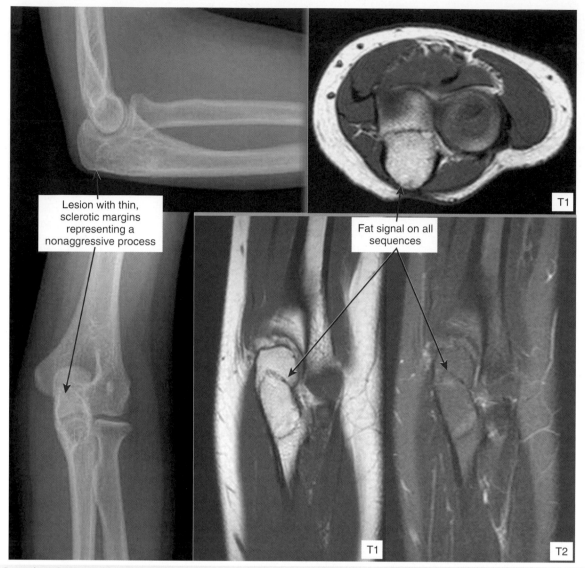

Lesion with thin,
sclerotic margins
representing a
nonaggressive process

Fat signal on all
sequences

T1

T1

T2

Fig. 11.2 Burned-out lesions—those that resemble some primary lesion on radiographs but show internal fat signal on MRI—most likely represent involuted benign lesions, although the differential includes intraosseous lipoma. Regardless, monotonous fat signal in a lesion on MRI is compatible with a benign process. Since primary bone tumors and metastatic lesions exclude, push away, or destroy marrow fat, any fat within an intraosseous lesion suggests benign etiology. (From Morrison W. *Problem Solving in Musculoskeletal Imaging*. Philadelphia: Elsevier; 2010.)

in many cases may actually reflect the sequela of a previous lesion. For example, it is likely that most calcaneal intraosseous lipomas represent regression and fatty involution of a prexisting intraosseous ganglion cyst arising from the subtalar joint.

Tumorlike Lesions on Imaging Exams

Some nonneoplastic lesions can resemble neoplams and should be considered in the differential diagnosis; alternate modalities may be needed to exclude these nonneoplastic entities. These include but are not limited to:

Infection—Occasionally infection can present with masslike features on MRI, CT, or radiography. This is especially true with 'atypical' organisms such as mycobacterial species and fungal infections like coccidioidomycosis. Appropriate history (e.g., travel) and clinical scenario (e.g., fever, immunocompromised state) should always be considered. In general, if you are considering tumor, ask yourself the question: 'Could this be infection?'

Hemophilic pseudotumor—A rare complication of hemophillia, a large hemotoma originating in a bone or adjacent muscle with erosion into bone can present as a highly aggressive-appearing lytic lesion simulating a malignant neoplasm. Clues to the correct diagnosis include the patient's age and gender (hemophilia in young males versus metastases/myeloma in an older population), MRI and CT features suggesting blood products, and arthritis associated with hemophillia. Hemophilic pseudotumor is discussed further in Chapter 13 – Bone Marrow and Metabolic Bone Disease.

Amyloid—Amyloid deposits can occur in primary or secondary forms of amyloidosis (secondary form seen in chronic renal failure) but both look the same, with soft tissue masses around joints, periarticular lytic lesions, and vertebral endplate destruction. Appropriate history is important (usually chronic kidney disease on long term dialysis), and look for other findings of chronic renal failure, such as renal osteodystrophy and imaging features of secondary hyperparathyroidism. On MRI, amyloid deposits are low signal on T1- and T2-weighted sequences.

RADIOGRAPHIC APPROACH TO BONE TUMORS

Some lesions are characteristic on radiographs, and with experience and pattern recognition the specific diagnosis can be made. In other cases the role of the radiologist is multifactorial, including:

- Determining whether the lesion is likely a neoplasm versus something else.
- Determining aggressiveness of the lesion.
- Assisting the clinician with regard to the next step in the workup.
- Ensuring that findings are reported accurately and communicated to the referring clinician with an appropriate level of urgency.

Lesion characterization:

- *Location*:
  - In long bones, diaphysis, metadiaphysis, metaphyis epiphysis; physeal involvement when present. Also location relative to the bone long axis: central, eccentric, cortical on on the bone surface.
  - When applicable, location relative to specific bone anatomy, e.g. trochanter, neck, head, tuberosity, etc.
- *Lesion density*: lytic, blastic, mixed.
- *Other features*: expansile, periosteal reaction, cotical breakthrough/soft tissue mass (these are discussed below).

- Refer to the report template at the end of this chapter.
- The following descriptors apply specifically to <u>lytic</u> lesions:
  - Matrix mineralization (if present).
  - Margin of the lesion.

Matrix Mineralization

If a lesion contains mineralization (calcification) there are a number of possibilities:

- The lesion is blastic or mixed lytic-blastic.
- The lesion is lytic and there is dystrophic calcification/residual bone.
- The lesion is forming *matrix* that is mineralizing. Matrix refers to tumor calcification in one of three specific patterns: *osteoid*, *chondroid*, or *fibrous*.

Determining the type of matrix mineralization can be very useful in narrowing the differential diagnosis. If unclear on radiographs, CT is an excellent modality for characterizing matrix.

Osteoid Matrix and Differential Diagnosis

Osteoid matrix is seen in bone-forming tumors, especially osteosarcoma, and also osteoblastoma. Osteoid matrix has a cloudlike appearance on radiographs and CT (Fig. 11.3). This should not be confused for ossification, which has a zonal phenomenon on radiographs and CT, with denser cortex peripherally and lower density trabeculae internally. In contrast, osteoid matrix has more uniform attenuation and no discernable internal architecture. Ossified lesions tend to be nonaggressive, whereas osteoid matrix can be seen in osteosarcoma.

A rare mimicker of osteoid matrix on radiographs is *tumoral calcinosis* (Fig. 11.4). Tumoral calcinosis is the

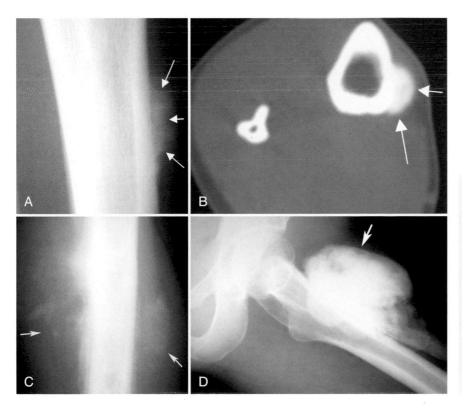

Fig. 11.3 Osteoid matrix. (A and B) AP radiograph **(A)** and axial CT image **(B)** of a surface osteosarcoma in the tibia of an 18-year-old man. The lesion arises from the surface of bone, forming amorphous osteoid matrix in the adjacent soft tissues *(arrows)*. **(C)** Subtle amorphous calcification in an osteosarcoma *(arrows)*. The matrix is less dense than bone and shows no evidence of organized bone formation. This pattern of osteoid is distinctly more aggressive than that seen in A and B, and this lesion corresponds to a conventional osteosarcoma, compared with the less-aggressive surface osteosarcoma in A and B. **(D)** Mixed pattern of dense (mature) osteoid matrix and regions of bone formation with trabeculae and cortex *(arrow)* in a 22-year-old woman. This is a parosteal osteosarcoma, much less aggressive in both appearance and behavior than conventional osteosarcoma.

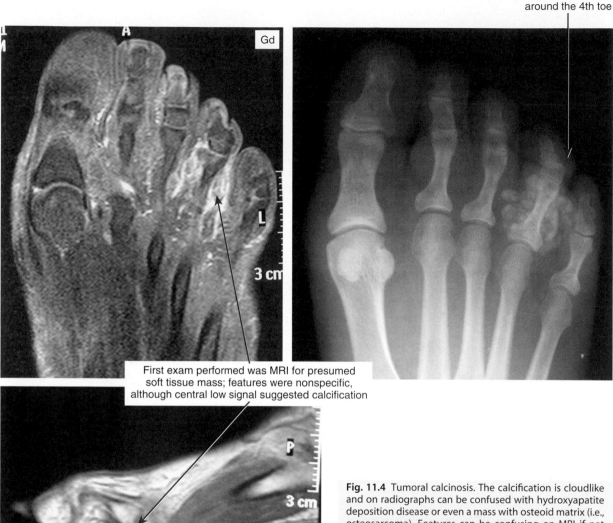

Tumoral calcinosis
around the 4th toe

First exam performed was MRI for presumed
soft tissue mass; features were nonspecific,
although central low signal suggested calcification

Fig. 11.4 Tumoral calcinosis. The calcification is cloudlike and on radiographs can be confused with hydroxyapatite deposition disease or even a mass with osteoid matrix (i.e., osteosarcoma). Features can be confusing on MRI if not correlated with radiographs. A history of metabolic disease (especially renal failure) should be sought. (From Morrison W. *Problem Solving in Musculoskeletal Imaging.* Philadelphia: Elsevier; 2010.)

deposition of calcium salts in soft tissues, usually around a joint, and is most commonly associated with chronic renal failure and secondary hyperparathyroidism, (although there is an idiopathic form seen in adolescents). CT and MRI show characteristic features of locules containing fluid and dependent sedimented calcium ("milk of calcium") adjacent to a joint. Tumoral calcinosis is discussed further in Chapter 13 – Bone Marrow and Metabolic Bone Disease.

Hydroxyapatite deposition disease (HADD, the cause of calcific tendinitis) can mimic osteoid matrix on a smaller scale. It also looks cloudlike but is limited to a small focus within a tendon or bursa. Rarely a bone erosion containing a focus of calcification can be seen with calcific tendinosis (Fig. 11.5).

Chondroid Matrix and Differential Diagnosis

Chondroid matrix is seen in cartilage forming tumors, including many (but not all) enchondromas and chondrosarcomas. Chondroid matrix is characterized by *'rings and arcs'* of calcification, arranged in circles or partial circles with a radius of 1-2 mm (Fig. 11.6). These curvilinear *'popcorn'* calcifications correspond to the lobulated architecture seen on MRI and at histology (Fig. 11.7).

A potential mimicker of chondroid matrix on radiographs is the calcification associated with bone infarction (Fig. 11.8). There are some differences that help distinguish these entities. The calcification in infarcts is sharper, better defined, serpentine, much longer, and portions may parallel the bone surface. Chondroid matrix calcification is small arcs and circles with softer margins. On MRI chondroid lesions are rounded and show lobulation with T2 hyperintensity and rim/septal enhancement, whereas infarcts may show a serpentine dark and bright line (*'double line sign'*) or just a low signal line at the lesion margin, often surrounding a central region of fat signal (so called 'mummified fat').

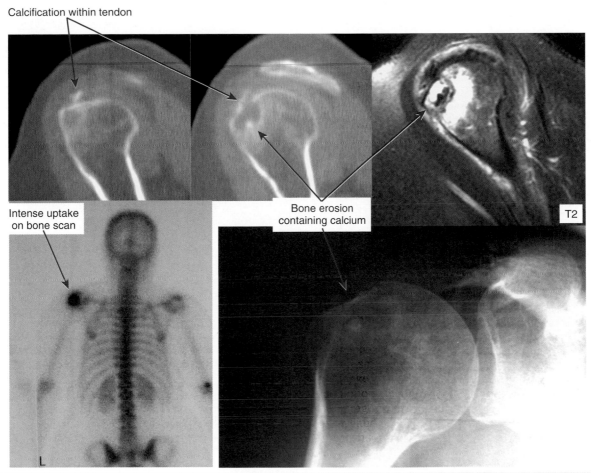

Calcification within tendon

Intense uptake on bone scan

Bone erosion containing calcium

T2

L

Fig. 11.5 Calcific tendinosis can cause erosion of bone at the tendon attachment and lead to concern for tumor. (From Morrison W. *Problem Solving in Musculoskeletal Imaging.* Philadelphia: Elsevier; 2010.)

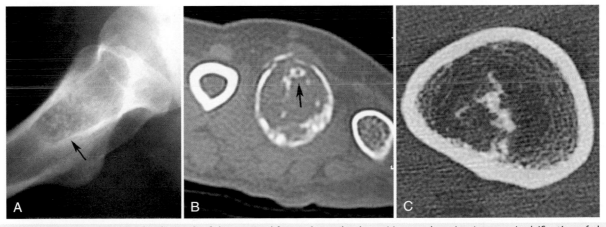

A   B   C

Fig. 11.6 Chondroid matrix. **(A)** Lateral radiograph of the proximal femur shows the dense 'rings and arcs' or 'popcorn' calcification of chondroid matrix in a grade 1 chondrosarcoma *(arrow).* **(B)** Axial CT of a metacarpal enchondroma with associated cortical expansion and fracture. Another description of chondroid matrix is 'circles or pieces of circles with a radius of 1–2 mm'. Note the centimeter markers at the right side of the image and the chondroid matrix, which includes one complete ring *(arrow).* **(C)** Axial CT of an enchondroma in the distal femoral metaphysis shows similar pattern of calcification.

Fibrous Matrix and Differential Diagnosis

Fibrous matrix is found in some fibrous lesions, especially fibrous dysplasia. Fibrous matrix has been described as a '*ground-glass*' appearance on radiographs and CT (Fig. 11.9), a description that many people have a difficult time conceptualizing. A better description is that fibrous matrix has density greater than soft tissue and has no trabeculae. Fibrous matrix is demonstrated much better with CT, which shows fairly uniform increased density, typically 60–140 HU, without trabecular architecture. On

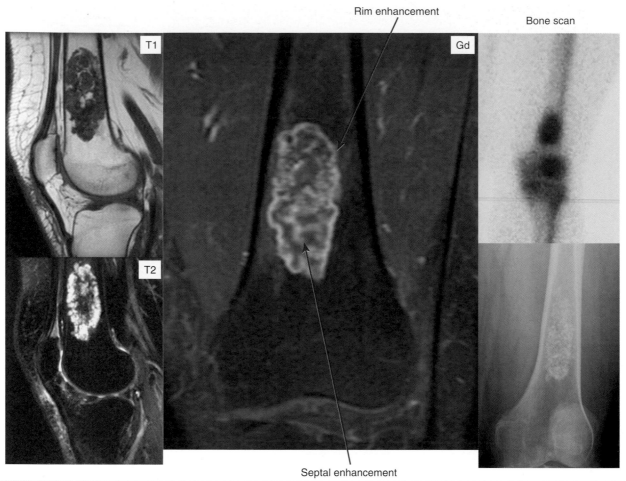

Rim enhancement

Bone scan

T1

Gd

T2

Septal enhancement

Fig. 11.7 Chondroid lesion characteristics on MRI. Note marked hyperintensity on T2-weighted images representing the prominent hydration state of the cartilage tissue. Lobulation corresponds to histologic rings of chondrocytes. Calcifications create low-signal foci. Intravenous contrast results in rim and septal enhancement around the lobules. Degree of uptake on bone scan does not correlate well with histologic aggressiveness. (From Morrison W. *Problem Solving in Musculoskeletal Imaging.* Philadelphia: Elsevier; 2010.)

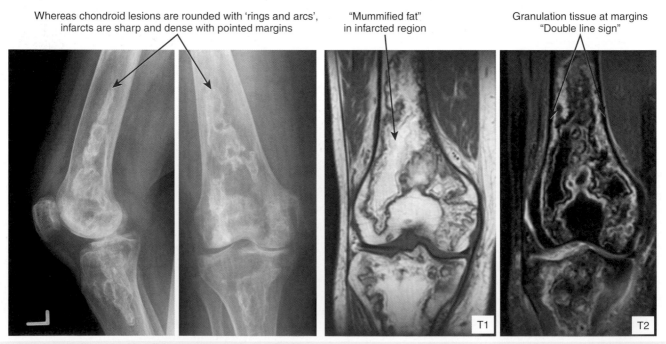

Whereas chondroid lesions are rounded with 'rings and arcs', infarcts are sharp and dense with pointed margins

"Mummified fat" in infarcted region

Granulation tissue at margins "Double line sign"

T1

T2

Fig. 11.8 Large infarcts in sickle cell disease. Well-defined sclerosis on radiographs, with geographic pattern on MRI. (From Morrison W. *Problem Solving in Musculoskeletal Imaging.* Philadelphia: Elsevier; 2010.)

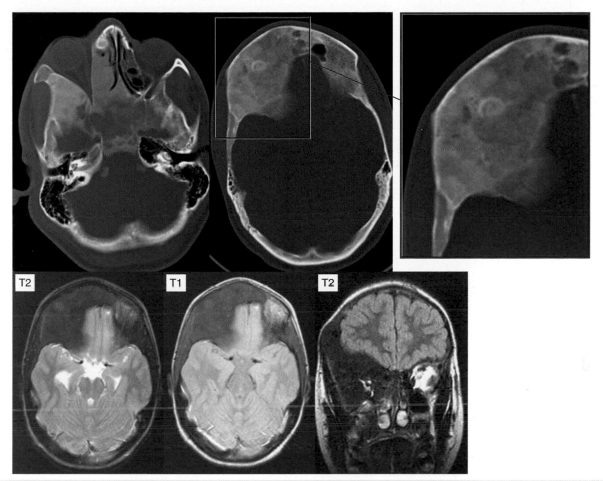

Fig. 11.9 Fibrous matrix is characterized by a ground-glass appearance (fairly uniform density greater than soft tissue, typically 60-140 HU, and without trabeculation) as seen in this case of fibrous dysplasia. (From Morrison W. *Problem Solving in Musculoskeletal Imaging.* Philadelphia: Elsevier; 2010.)

MRI the appearance is variable but is often intermediate in signal on T1- and T2-weighted sequences and homogeneously enhancing. Lesion density on CT and signal on MRI can be heterogeneous related to the presence of other elements such as cysts (in fibrous dysplasia) or chondroid tissue (in chondromyxoid fibroma).

The main differential for this appearance on radiographs is a lytic lesion surrounded by some intact native bone. The added density of the remaining normal bone may resemble uniform increased density within the lytic lesion, falsely resembling fibrous matrix. CT can clarify when needed.

Margins

Evaluation of the margins of a lytic lesion is extremely important when generating a differential diagnosis and for determining lesion aggressiveness (Figs. 11.10 through 11.13). Radiologists and orthopedic surgeons commonly classify lytic bone lesions based on the radiographic or CT appearance using the *Lodwick system*:

- Type 1 is *geographic*, i.e., has well defined margins that you could trace precisely with a pencil. Type 1 lesions are further defined based on the *zone of transition* between the lesion and host bone. 1A has a narrow zone of transition with a thin, sclerotic margin. 1B is also sharply defined, but without sclerotic borders. 1C has a

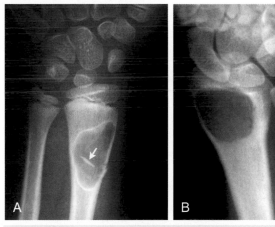

Fig. 11.10 Geographic tumor margins. **(A)** Geographic lesion (mass is easily outlined) with sharp, sclerotic (type 1A) margins. Note the 'fallen fragment sign' of a cortical fracture fragment that has fallen into this solitary bone cyst *(arrow)*. **(B)** Geographic lesion with sharp but not sclerotic (type 1B) margins in this giant cell tumor of the distal radius.

wider zone of transition with a slightly indistinct or 'fuzzy' border.
- Type 2 is 'moth-eaten' with central lucencies and irregular margins.
- Type 3 is permeative, with small lucencies; margins are hard to see.

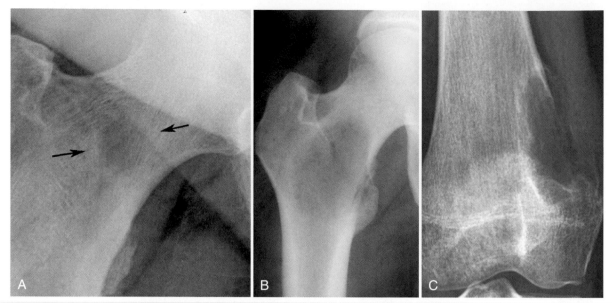

Fig. 11.11 Aggressive tumor margins: well-defined margins with broad zone of transition (type 1C margins). **(A)** Subtle femoral neck geographic lesion with 'fuzzy' margins (wide zone of transition, type 1C), a lung adenocarcinoma metastasis. **(B)** Another type 1C lesion, with a wider zone of transition and cortical breakthrough. This is a plasmacytoma. **(C)** Another lesion with a well-defined but wide zone of transition. It appears geographic in some regions but less well defined in others. This also was a lung cancer metastasis.

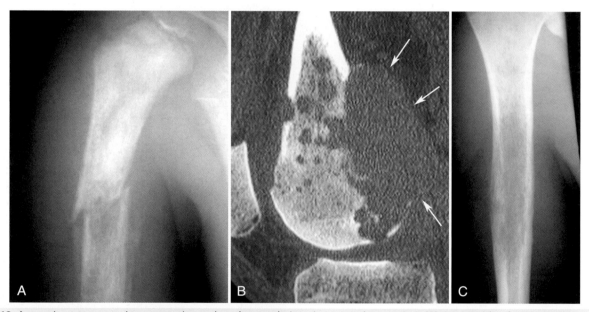

Fig. 11.12 Aggressive tumor margins: permeative and moth-eaten lesions (type 2 and 3 margins). **(A)** An example of permeative (type 3) bone destruction, with the tumor infiltrating among trabeculae, destroying some but leaving others. This metadiaphyseal lesion is an osteosarcoma arising in an 8-year-old boy. **(B)** Sagittal CT reconstruction shows a moth-eaten pattern (type 2 margin) in the distal femur due to metastatic lung cancer. Note the soft tissue mass *(arrows)*. **(C)** Lesion with permeative and moth-eaten features (type 2 and 3 margins) due to Ewing sarcoma in a 14-year-old. Note the subtle lucent areas in the proximal metaphysis. The distinction between type 2 and 3 margins is usually not significant; either indicates a highly aggressive lesion. (A, Image used with permission from BJ Manaster, MD, from the American College of Radiology Learning File.)

Type 1A lesions are nonaggressive and typically also benign. A thin, sclerotic margin is a sign that the lesion has been present for a long time without growth, allowing the bone to form a "shell" around it. This is commonly seen in cysts (simple or unicameral bone cysts, intraosseous ganglia, and subchondral cysts) and other benign lesions such as fibroxanthomas (nonossifying fibromas [NOFs] or fibrous cortical defects [FCDs]) prior to healing, and fibrous

dysplasia. A potential pitfall is a treated malignancy (e.g., a metastasis treated with chemotherapy); as growth slows, the bone reacts and may form a sclerotic rim (Fig. 11.14).

Type 1B lesions may be benign or malignant, and some benign 1B lesions may behave aggressively. As noted previously metastases and myeloma may have 1B margins. The description 'punched out lesions' is sometimes used for myeloma with multiple sharply defined lytic lesions.

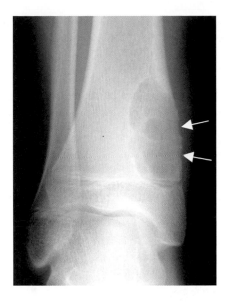

Fig. 11.13 Aggressive tumor margins: mixture of aggressive and non-aggressive margins in a 17-year-old boy. Most of the margins are sharp and sclerotic (type 1A, nonaggressive), suggesting a nonaggressive lesion. However, there is cortical breakthrough medially *(arrows)*, an aggressive finding. Despite the nonaggressive appearance of most of the lesion margin, the cortical destruction must be considered a red flag and the lesion must be worked up as an aggressive lesion. At biopsy, this was an osteosarcoma.

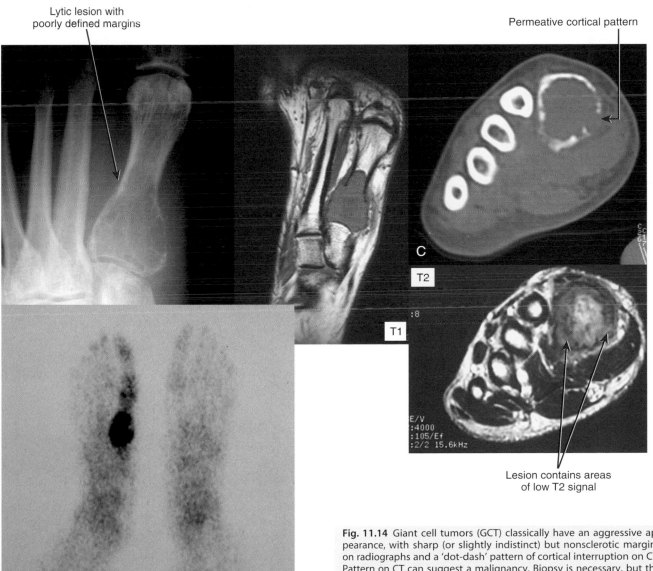

Lytic lesion with poorly defined margins

Permeative cortical pattern

T2

T1

Lesion contains areas of low T2 signal

Bone scan

Fig. 11.14 Giant cell tumors (GCT) classically have an aggressive appearance, with sharp (or slightly indistinct) but nonsclerotic margins on radiographs and a 'dot-dash' pattern of cortical interruption on CT. Pattern on CT can suggest a malignancy. Biopsy is necessary, but the diagnosis of GCT can be suggested by relatively low signal on T2-weighted MRI. (From Morrison W. *Problem Solving in Musculoskeletal Imaging.* Philadelphia: Elsevier; 2010.)

Type 1C, 2 and 3 lesions are aggressive. However, they may still be benign! The classic benign type 2 or 3 lesion is infection, which often causes ill-defined osteolysis. In this case periosteal reaction may be helpful, since infection tends to have a more mature reaction (smooth, thick) which implies a non-malignant process. LCH can also appear aggressive (ill-defined, often permeative in early phases). The type 3 permeative pattern is typically seen with small round cell lesions, with the differential including Ewing sarcoma, lymphoma/leukemia, LCH, and infection. GCT of bone may have 1B or 1C margins and is usually slow growing but can be locally highly aggressive.

Marginal patterns can be confusing if they are mixed; for example, part of the lesion has thin sclerotic margins but another area has ill-defined margins. In this case the lesion is classified by the more aggressive margin. Be aware that if a part of a benign lesion is obliquely oriented in the medullary cavity it may falsely appear ill-defined on a radiograph acquired en face. This emphasizes the importance of multiple views. If the lesion is truly partially aggressive, it may represent transformation of a benign lesion into malignancy. This may occur in chondroid lesions and rarely in other situations (e.g., sarcoma arising in a bone infarct or Paget's disease. In general, a lytic lesion should be classified by its most aggressive margin).

Key Concepts

Evaluation of Lytic Lesion Margins
- Lodwick system
- Provides information regarding lesion local aggressiveness
- Exclusively for lytic lesions, not blastic
- Radiographs or CT only
- 1A: sharp, thin sclerotic rim. Nonaggressive, and almost always benign
- 1B: sharp, non sclerotic margin. May be nonaggressive or aggressive
- 1C: well defined but fuzzy margin. Aggressive
- 2 (moth eaten) and 3 (permeative): poorly defined lesion margins. These may overlap in appearance and the distinction is not essential. Aggressive.
- If different margin types are present, judge the lesion based on the most aggressive margin.
- Aggressive does not mean malignant
  - Example: bone infection
- Nonaggressive does not mean benign
  - Example: 'punched out' lesions in multiple myeloma

Expansion/Endosteal Scalloping

'Expansion' of bone, where the cortex is deflected or remodeled outward, can be a sign of aggressiveness, but this sign is also a characteristic of many benign lesions (Fig. 11.15). Expansion is considered a type of periosteal reaction, since it occurs due to solid new bone formation by the periosteum secondary to intramedullary lesion growth. Slight focal expansion is seen in lesions such as NOF and fibrous dysplasia. Diffuse expansion of bone can be seen in Paget's disease and in marrow-packing disorders such as thalassemia and Gaucher disease. A large degree of expansion can be seen in aggressive lesions such as hemorrhagic metastases (e.g., lung, renal, thyroid

carcinoma) as well as plasmacytoma/multiple myeloma. Some benign lesions such as simple bone cyst (SBC) cause expansion and ABC and hemophilic pseudotumor can also cause significant expansion, or a so-called 'blowout lesion'. Therefore, unless there are other signs pointing to an aggressive or a nonaggressive lesion, expansion itself is not specific for malignancy.

Endosteal scalloping occurs when an intramedullary lesion grows or expands and thins the inner cortex. The classic lesion causing scalloping is a low-grade chondroid tumor, most commonly an enchondroma. However, this finding is also nonspecific and relates more to lesion rate of growth rather than histology (Fig. 11.16).

Scalloping of Outer Cortex

Scalloping of the outer cortex, in which the bone surface is concave with a sharp margin, is seen with slow-growing lesions on the bone surface or outside the bone. Because this implies slow growth, it is typically seen with benign lesions, such as tenosynovial giant cell tumor (TGCT) arising in a tendon sheath, nerve sheath tumors, and ganglia.

Periosteal Reaction

The periosteum is a layer of cells overlying the metaphysis and diaphysis of long bones. Flat bones also have a periosteum, but some bones such as the vertebrae, carpal, and tarsal bones do not have a mature periosteum so will not mount a significant periosteal reaction to similar irritation. The periosteum is responsible for appositional growth and repair of bone; that is, it lays down new bone along the cortex. When a bone undergoes stress chronically, it thickens the cortex in response. In fact, the periosteum only reacts in one way—by forming more bone. Different patterns of periosteal reaction reflect the degree of irritation of the periosteum, and how fast the periosteum is pushed away from the bone by the growth of a lesion (Figs. 11.17 and 11.18). Other synonymous terms for periosteal reaction are *periostitis* and *periosteal new bone formation*.

Types of Periosteal Reaction

Thick, undulating: implies slow growth; the periosteum has time to lay down new bone; (low aggressiveness)—for example, infection, osteoid osteoma, stress fracture.

Lamellated (onion skin): implies periodic rapid growth; periosteum periodically pushed away, lays down layer of calcium, etc.; (intermediate aggressiveness)—for example, eosinophilic granuloma (EG).

Sunburst: implies very rapid growth; periosteum forms bone as it is pushed away, creating streaks of calcium perpendicular to cortex; (very aggressive)—for example, osteosarcoma.

Codman triangle: indicates very rapid growth; at the midpoint of the mass, growth is so rapid that periosteum cannot respond. At the margins where growth is slower, the periosteum lays down bone in a triangular configuration (very aggressive)—for example, osteosarcoma, Ewing sarcoma, aggressive infections.

Cortical Breakthrough and Soft tissue Mass

Cortical breakthrough and soft tissue mass is a sign of aggressiveness. Sometimes a benign lesion such as hemophilic pseudotumor or ABC can appear to break through

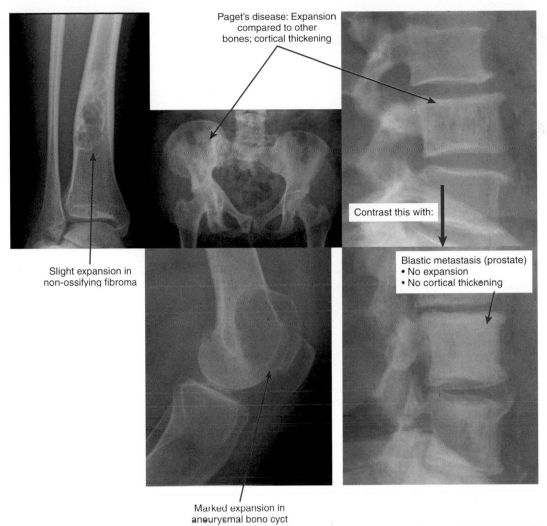

Paget's disease: Expansion compared to other bones; cortical thickening

Contrast this with:

Blastic metastasis (prostate)
• No expansion
• No cortical thickening

Slight expansion in non-ossifying fibroma

Marked expansion in aneurysmal bone cyst

Fig. 11.15 Expansion of bone can be seen in both benign and malignant conditions. Some fast-growing processes (i.e., intraosseous hemorrhage in hemophilia) can result in "blowout" lesions, as well as aneurysmal bone cyst and malignant conditions such as myeloma and metastatic disease (especially aggressive/hemorrhagic lesions such as renal, lung, and thyroid lesions). (From Morrison W. *Problem Solving in Musculoskeletal Imaging*. Philadelphia: Elsevier; 2010.)

but on CT a thin shell of cortex is seen. Soft tissue mass is seen in many bone malignancies and is especially common in Ewing sarcoma (Fig. 11.19).

GAMUTS FOR BONE TUMOR DIAGNOSIS

The imaging features described in the preceding pages are helpful for determining the aggressiveness of a bone lesion and limiting the differential diagnosis. However, the most important characteristics are the patient's age and the location of the lesion. For example, if someone calls you and says 'there is a patient with a lytic lesion in the humeral metaphysis'; you ask the age, and if they say '14' you should automatically think of a SBC; if they say '74' you should think metastasis or myeloma. Common things are common in different age groups.

Age as a Criterion for Osseous Lesions

Age   Common Lesions

1   Metastatic neuroblastoma, leukemia/lymphoma.

1–10   Ewing sarcoma; osteomyelitis, leukemia/lymphoma.

10–30   Epiphysis, skeletally immature: Chondroblastoma, LCH, osteomyelitis.
           Epiphysis, skeletally mature: GCT.
           Metaphyseal: Osteosarcoma, osteoid osteoma, fibroxanthoma (NOF or FCD), SBC, fibrous dysplasia, osteomyelitis.
           Diaphyseal, Ewing sarcoma.

30–50   Chondrosarcoma, lymphoma.

>50   Metastasis, multiple myeloma, chondrosarcoma.

Key Criteria for Categorizing a Solitary Osseous Lesion on Radiographs

- Margin/pattern of bone destruction (especially for lytic lesions).
- Matrix mineralization.
- Expansion/scalloping.
- Periosteal reaction.
- Location.
- Age of patient.

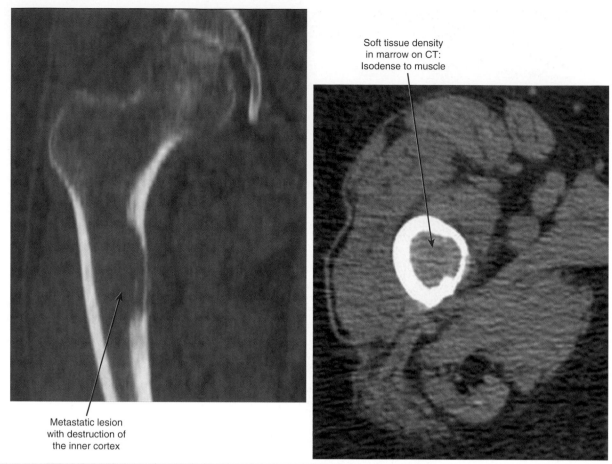

Soft tissue density
in marrow on CT:
Isodense to muscle

Metastatic lesion
with destruction of
the inner cortex

Fig. 11.16 Endosteal scalloping is seen with both slow-growing lesions such as enchondromas, as well as early involvement from malignancies—in this case a metastatic lesion from lung carcinoma. Note that here instead of expanding and remodeling the cortex, the inner cortex is being destroyed, a sign of the aggressive nature of the lesion. (From Morrison W. *Problem Solving in Musculoskeletal Imaging*. Philadelphia: Elsevier; 2010.)

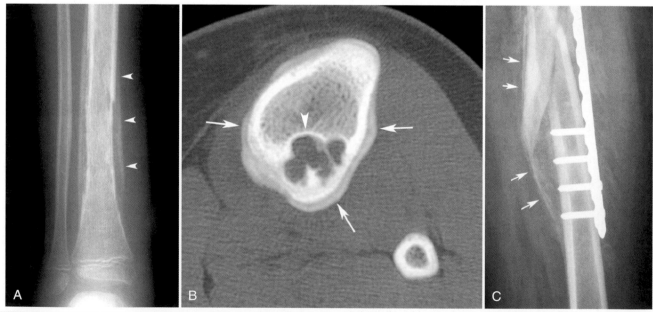

Fig. 11.17 Nonaggressive periosteal reaction. **(A)** Distal tibia radiograph in a child with osteomyelitis shows uninterrupted periosteal reaction *(arrowheads)*. Note the aggressive bone destruction. The comparatively nonaggressive solid periosteal reaction was an important clue to the correct diagnosis. **(B)** CT of a nonossifying fibroma *(arrowhead)* in the distal tibia in a child with an associated pathologic fracture (not shown). In this case the periosteal elevation *(arrows)* was not caused by the tumor but rather by healing response to a pathologic fracture through the tumor. Note the well-defined, sclerotic (type 1A) tumor margin. **(C)** Detailed view of an internally fixed femur shaft shows solid, continuous new bone *(arrows)* formed by periosteum elevated by hematoma. This will remodel into mature bone.

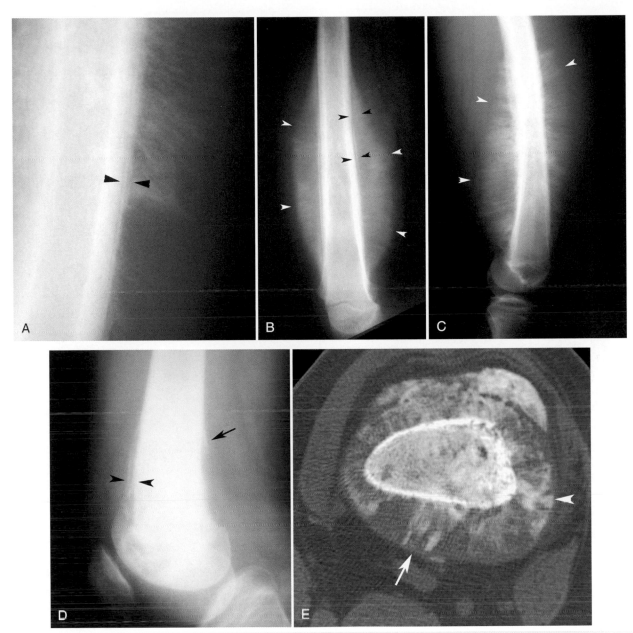

Fig. 11.18 Aggressive periosteal reaction. **(A)** Detail of a femur radiograph of a child with osteosarcoma shows subtle lamellated (between *arrowheads*) and hair-on-end periosteal reaction. **(B)** Lateral femur radiograph in a child with Ewing sarcoma shows interrupted *(black arrowheads)* and hair-on-end *(white arrowheads)* periosteal reaction. **(C)** Older child with an osteosarcoma. Note florid aggressive periosteal reaction *(white arrowheads)*. **(D)** Another older child with an osteosarcoma. Note lamellated periosteal reaction (between *black arrowheads*) and Codman triangle *(arrow)*. **(E)** Axial CT image of a teenager with distal femur osteosarcoma shows a mixture of hair-on-end periosteal reaction *(arrow)* and osteoid tumor matrix *(arrowhead)*.

Lesion Margin

Applies to lytic lesions.
Type 1 (Geographic):
  - 1A: Narrow zone of transition, thin sclerotic margin; nonaggressive.
  - 1B: Narrow zone of transition, nonsclerotic margin; may be aggressive or nonaggressive.
  - 1C: Wide zone of transition, nonsclerotic margin; aggressive.
Type 2 (moth-eaten): Multiple lytic areas; aggressive.
Type 3 (permeative): Aggressive.

Tumor Margin Differential Diagnosis

Type 1A Margin (Nonaggressive, Benign)
- Numerous benign lesions, including SBC, intraosseous ganglion cysts, NOF, enchondroma, fibrous dysplasia, chondroblastoma, LCH.

Type 1B Margin
- GCT, LCH, myeloma, metastasis.

Type 1C Margin (Aggressive)
- GCT, osteosarcoma, chondrosarcoma, osteomyelitis, brown tumor, LCH, lymphoma, metastasis.

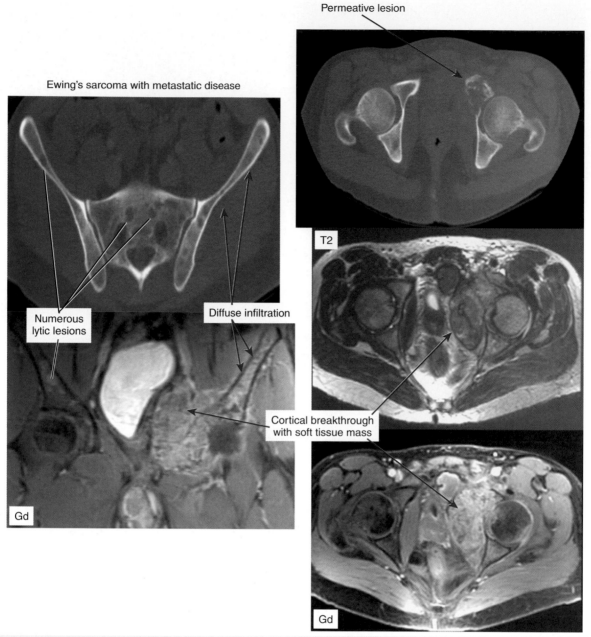

Permeative lesion

Ewing's sarcoma with metastatic disease

Numerous
lytic lesions

Diffuse infiltration

T2

Cortical breakthrough
with soft tissue mass

Gd

Gd

Fig. 11.19 Cortical breakthrough and soft tissue mass. This indicates a more aggressive process. Ewing sarcoma classically presents with a soft tissue component that is often large. Lymphoma, metastases, and other lesions can also exhibit soft tissue extension, and this finding is not specific. Some benign conditions can also show cortical breakthrough and soft tissue mass effect such as infection and fracture through a benign lesion with associated hematoma. (From Morrison W. *Problem Solving in Musculoskeletal Imaging.* Philadelphia: Elsevier; 2010.)

Type 2 (Moth-Eaten; Aggressive)
- Malignant neoplasms, primary and metastatic, osteomyelitis, LCH.

Type 3 (Permeative; Aggressive)
- Neoplastic: Round cell tumors, osteosarcoma, metastasis.
- Metabolic: Hyperparathyroidism.
- Mechanical: Fracture, aggressive osteoporosis.
- Infection: Osteomyelitis.

Tumor Matrix

Osteoid (Cloudlike, Amorphous)
- Bone-forming tumors: Osteosarcoma, osteoid osteoma, osteoblastoma.

- Also can be seen in early fracture healing.

Chondroid (Arcs and Rings)
- Cartilage-forming tumors: Enchondroma, chondrosarcoma, +/− chondroblastoma.

Fibrous (Ground Glass)
- Fibrous dysplasia.

Typical Locations for Solitary Bone Lesions

Epiphysis: Chondroblastoma, subchondral cyst, GCT (growth plate closed), clear-cell chondrosarcoma, LCH.
Metaphysis: Osteosarcoma, chondrosarcoma, enchondroma, osteochondroma, GCT (growth plate open).

Diaphysis: Round cell tumors (lymphoma, myeloma, Ewing sarcoma).

Cortical and Juxtacortical Tumors

Cortical

- Osteoid osteoma.
- Fibrous lesions: fibroxanthoma (NOF or FCD), osteofibrous dysplasia (ossifying fibroma), rare cortical fibrous dysplasia.
- Adamantinoma.

Juxtacortical (Surface Lesion)

- Osteochondroma.
- Parosteal or periosteal osteosarcoma.
- Periosteal chondroma and chondrosarcoma.
- Periosteal ganglion.
- Any soft tissue tumor near the bone.

Periosteal Reaction

- Solid: Nonaggressive process.
- Expanded shell: May be aggressive or nonaggressive.
- Lamellated ('onionskin'): Intermediate.
- Interrupted: Aggressive.
- Hair-on-end: Aggressive.
- Sunburst: Aggressive.
- Codman triangle: Aggressive.

Periosteal New Bone Formation in Children

- Infection/inflammation.
- Healing fracture; nonaccidental trauma.
- Metabolic (scurvy, hypervitaminosis A and D, Gaucher disease, others).
- Physiologic (during rapid growth).
- Solid tumors (often aggressive periosteal reaction).
- Leukemia.
- Premature birth (prostaglandin E, physiologic, metabolic disease of prematurity).
- Melorheostosis.
- Caffey disease.

MRI of Musculoskeletal Tumors: Technical Requirements

1. Surface coils must be used if possible.
2. Axial images are required for evaluation of compartments and neurovascular bundles.
3. The entire extent of the lesion must be imaged with axial sequences. One longitudinal scan that provides imaging of the entire bone is also included for evaluation of skip metastases.
4. Inclusion of an externally palpable landmark is highly desirable because it allows measurement of distance to the lesion to be accurately translated from the scan to the surgical site.
5. T1-weighted imaging must be included because it shows high tumor-to-fat contrast.
6. T2-weighted sequences, generally with fat saturation, are included, showing high tumor-to-muscle contrast.
7. Evaluation of joint involvement often requires coronal or sagittal imaging.
8. Fluid sensitive sequences such as STIR may improve lesion conspicuity.
9. Gadolinium-enhanced imaging may improve lesion conspicuity, demonstrate myxoid portions of the lesion, and assist in guiding biopsy away from necrotic portions of lesions.

Differential Diagnosis for Musculoskeletal Mass With T1 Shortening (High Signal Intensity on T1-Weighted Images)

Common

- Fat (suppresses with chemical fat suppression and inversion recovery sequences): Lipoma, liposarcoma, hemangioma, dystrophic fat.
- Methemoglobin: Hematoma, hemorrhage within a tumor.
- Gadolinium enhancement.

Uncommon

- Proteinaceous material.
- Melanin (although high signal within melanoma metastases is more likely due to methemoglobin).

Differential Diagnosis for Musculoskeletal Mass With Predominantly Low Signal Intensity on T2-Weighted Images

- Hypocellular fibrous tissue.
- Fibrous tumor (e.g., plantar fibroma, other fibromatoses).
- Scar tissue.
- Dense mineralization.
- Melanin.
- Blood products.
- Acute hematoma.
- Hemosiderin: Old hematoma, PVNS, TGCT, synovium in patients with hemophilia.
- Vascular flow void.
- Gas.
- Foreign body.
- Gouty tophus.
- Amyloidosis.
- Bone cement (i.e., methyl methacrylate).
- Highly cellular tumors such as lymphoma often have intermediate-low signal intensity.

Musculoskeletal Masses with Fluid-Fluid Levels

- GCT.
- ABC.
- Telangiectatic osteosarcoma.
- Solitary bone cyst.
- Tumor necrosis.
- Hematoma, hemorrhage within a tumor.
- Chondroblastoma.
- Hemangioma if large low-flow channels are present.
- Cystic degeneration within fibrous dysplasia.
- Tumoral calcinosis.

Lesions with Surrounding Bone Marrow Edema on MRI

- Chondroblastoma.
- Osteoblastoma.
- Osteoid osteoma.
- GCT.
- LCH.
- Osteomyelitis.
- Stress fracture.
- Pathologic fracture through a lesion.

Appearance of Lesions Recently Biopsied. Biopsy will make a lesion look more aggressive on MRI, resulting in surrounding edema and enhancement making it difficult or impossible to define the lesion's true margins. If near a neurovascular bundle, this can change a planned surgery from a limb salvage to an amputation. Thus, it is very important to obtain MRI prior to biopsy.

Appearance of Treated Lesions. The appearance of bone and soft tissue can change following treatment (Fig. 11.20). Lytic metastatic lesions can become more sclerotic (especially seen with breast metastases). Bone scan may demonstrate a paradoxical increase in activity due to bone healing (flare phenomenon).

The pattern of red marrow can change on MRI: rebound following chemotherapy, or treatment with colony-stimulating factor can result in an increase in hematopoietic marrow, which is often more cellular and thereby brighter in T2 and STIR signal than typical red marrow that may simulate new metastatic disease.

Radiation therapy results in replacement of red marrow with fatty yellow marrow. Treatment can also affect the soft tissues: radiation therapy causes soft tissue edema, especially of the underlying muscles within the port; this edema may last for years and can simulate a number of pathological conditions from trauma to infection to neurological disease; no mass effect is seen. In later follow-up, the muscles may exhibit fatty atrophy. Radiation therapy

can have other effects including osteonecrosis. Growth disturbances can occur in children. Radiation-induced sarcoma can occur as well: including osteosarcomas, chondrosarcomas, and fibrosarcomas; these are aggressive secondary malignancies that typically arise at the margins of the radiation field 10–15 years after treatment (Figs. 11.21 and 11.22).

Key Concepts

Complications of Radiation Therapy for Musculoskeletal Tumors

- Tumor recurrence
- Early growth cessation
- Growth deformities
- Radiation-induced osteochondroma
- Infection
- Radiation osteonecrosis
- Radiation-induced sarcoma

Benign Bone-Forming Tumors

OSTEOMA

- An osteoma is actually a hamartoma, an abnormal proliferation of compact bone without stromal cellular proliferation.

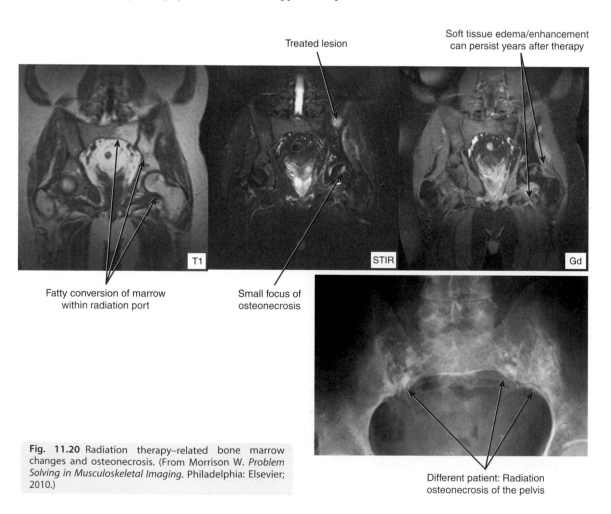

Treated lesion

Soft tissue edema/enhancement can persist years after therapy

T1   STIR   Gd

Fatty conversion of marrow within radiation port

Small focus of osteonecrosis

Different patient: Radiation osteonecrosis of the pelvis

Fig. 11.20 Radiation therapy–related bone marrow changes and osteonecrosis. (From Morrison W. *Problem Solving in Musculoskeletal Imaging*. Philadelphia: Elsevier; 2010.)

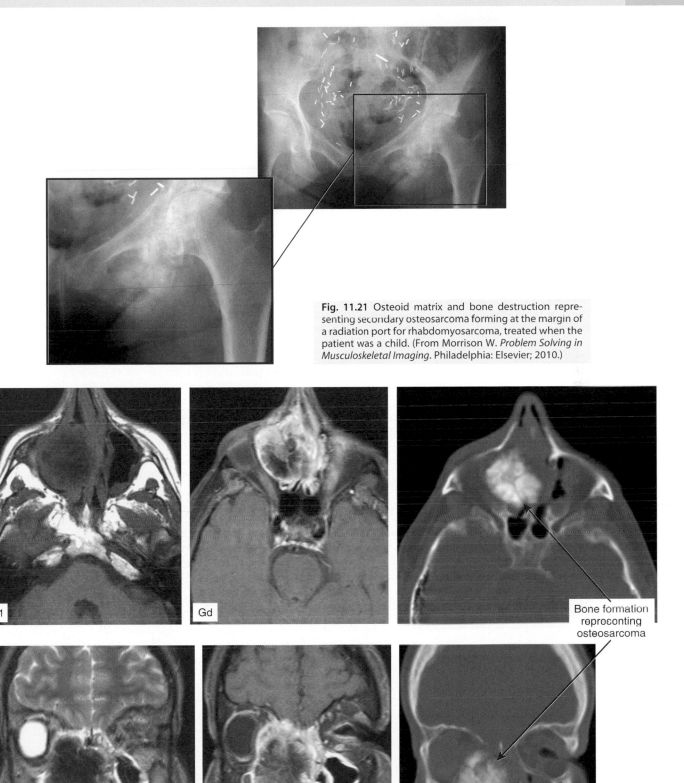

Fig. 11.21 Osteoid matrix and bone destruction representing secondary osteosarcoma forming at the margin of a radiation port for rhabdomyosarcoma, treated when the patient was a child. (From Morrison W. *Problem Solving in Musculoskeletal Imaging*. Philadelphia: Elsevier; 2010.)

Bone formation representing osteosarcoma

Fig. 11.22 A 43-year-old man with a history of enucleation and radiation therapy for retinoblastoma as a child. He now presents with secondary osteosarcoma developing at the margin of the radiation port. (From Morrison W. *Problem Solving in Musculoskeletal Imaging*. Philadelphia: Elsevier; 2010.)

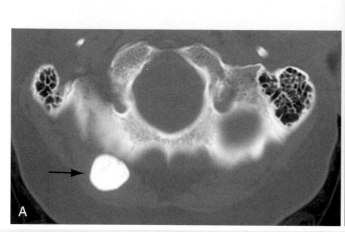
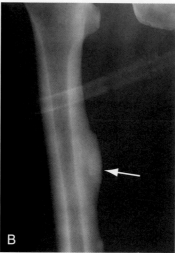

Fig. 11.23 Osteoma. **(A)** Axial CT of the head shows a very dense homogenous round suboccipital mass *(arrow)*, typical for an osteoma. **(B)** AP radiograph of the femur demonstrates dense oval surface lesions *(arrow)*. These osteomas presented in the setting of Gardner syndrome (intestinal polyposis); osteomas are rarely seen in the tubular bones unless as a part of Gardner syndrome. (B, Image used with permission from BJ Manaster, MD, from STATdx website, Amirsys, Inc.)

- Osteomas usually are found within membranous (flat) bones, either in the calvaria (usually arising from the external table) or the paranasal sinuses (Fig. 11.23A).
- Osteomas may be multifocal and rarely may develop on tubular bones, especially as part of Gardner syndrome, a disease of autosomal dominant inheritance that is associated with multiple colonic adenomatous polyps (Fig. 11.23B).
- The entire lesion is densely sclerotic with well-defined margins.
- The lesion does not behave aggressively, although it can occasionally cause expansion of adjacent bone.
- Diagnosis is made by radiographic characteristics, and no treatment is necessary.
- If an osteoma is incidentally noted on MRI, it will appear with low signal on all sequences because of its dense mineralization, though rarely there may be mild inhomogeneity.

- Differential diagnosis of an osteoma includes blastic metastasis and calvarial hyperostosis adjacent to a meningioma.

ENOSTOSIS (BONE ISLAND)

- A bone island is a region of compact bone within the medullary space, surrounded by trabecular bone.
- They may be hamartomatous proliferations, like the osteoma, or they may represent areas of failure of osteoclast activity during bone remodeling.
- The lesion is very common and is usually noted incidentally on imaging exams.
- Close inspection demonstrates spicules at the margin of the lesion that blend into the normal surrounding trabeculae (Fig. 11.24). This characteristic appearance is pathognomonic.
- CT can be helpful to evaluate margins; in addition, bone island attenuation is generally higher than most

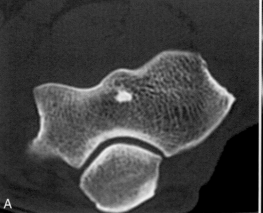
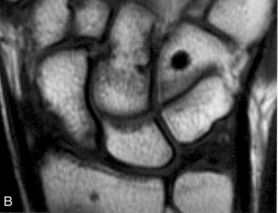

Fig. 11.24 Bone island. **(A)** Axial CT of the distal humerus, demonstrating a typical bone island in which dense bone formation is seen to be homogeneous except at its peripheral edges, where it blends into the adjacent normal trabeculae. **(B)** Coronal T1-weighted MRI shows low-signal rounded lesions within the hamate and the distal radius with the surrounding bone undisturbed. Other sequences are not shown but similarly demonstrate low signal, typical of a bone island.

untreated blastic metastases, with mean attenuation on the order of 900 HU or higher. Attenuation this high does not completely exclude a blastic metastasis.

- Bone island size varies widely, but lesions larger than 1 cm are unusual except in the pelvis, where lesions up to 2–3 cm may occur. Lesions greater than 2.0 cm in size are considered '*giant bone islands*'.
    - Large lesions or lesions increasing in size, can be evaluated with bone scan to assist in excluding blastic metastases or osteosarcoma (Fig. 11.25).
    - A normal bone scan excludes the possibility of osteosarcoma. Note that a large bone island may show mild tracer uptake, which can make a positive bone scan unreliable in excluding the diagnosis. However, blastic malignancies are typically much 'hotter' and the distinction is readily made.
    - Correlation with prostate-specific antigen also can be helpful in men because it is usually although not always elevated when metastatic prostate cancer to bone is present.
    - If a bone island is noted on MRI, it will have low signal intensity on all sequences, identical to normal cortical bone.
- *Osteopoikilosis* is a condition characterized by multiple bone islands clustered in the epiphyses around joints.

Key Concepts

Bone Island

- Small round or oval focus of dense bone within medullary space
- Blends into surrounding trabeculae
- Occasionally enlarge slowly or present with large size; may therefore need to be differentiated from slow-growing low-grade osteosarcoma. Negative bone scan excludes osteosarcoma

OSTEOID OSTEOMA

- Osteoid osteoma is a small lytic lesion (the nidus) surrounded by dense reactive bone formation.
- Almost all present between the ages of 10 and 25 years.
- The male-to-female ratio is 3:1.

- Osteoid osteomas have a typical clinical presentation of aching pain lasting weeks, months, or years.
    - The pain is often worse at night and is relieved with nonsteroidal anti-inflammatory drugs. This presentation is not unique but suggests the diagnosis.
    - These symptoms are dramatically relieved by complete excision or ablation of the lesion.
    - Although painful, osteoid osteoma is a benign lesion and may spontaneously involute after about 3 years. However, the symptoms are usually so severe that most lesions are treated.
- In children, lesions can result in growth disturbances and can also be a cause of "painful scoliosis" when located in the spine.
- Histologically, osteoid osteoma is similar to osteoblastoma, with the latter usually >2 cm in size and more often affecting the axial skeleton.
- The most common location of osteoid osteoma is the cortex of tubular bones (65–70%).
    - The femoral and tibial cortices represent 60% of all osteoid osteomas.
- Imaging appearance is fairly characteristic: focal cortical sclerosis with a lucent center (nidus).
    - The nidus is composed of highly vascular fibrous tissue, osteoid, and immature bone.
    - The nidus is the central lucent area on radiography or CT, although it may mineralize partially or nearly completely, potentially obscuring the lesion.
    - The local sclerotic reaction of a cortical osteoid osteoma may be so dense that the nidus may be masked on radiographs (Fig. 11.26).
    - If the nidus is not seen, these lesions could be confused with prominent healing bone formation about a stress fracture or other etiologies.
    - CT shows the nidus and reactive bone exquisitely (Figs. 11.27 and 11.28) and can be confirmatory when diagnosis is obscure by MRI (Figs. 11.29 and 11.30).
    - MRI shows hypointense nidus and adjacent low signal on T1-weighted images; fluid-sensitive images may show either hypointensity or hyperintensity of the nidus; the high signal of the surrounding edema

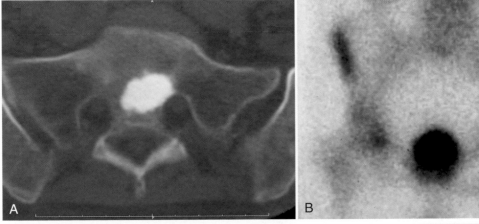

Fig. 11.25 Bone scanning as problem solver for giant bone island. **(A)** Detail from abdominal CT image in a patient with breast cancer shows a large sclerotic lesion in the sacrum. **(B)** Diphosphonate bone scanning shows minimal tracer uptake by the lesion, excluding an active blastic metastasis or osteosarcoma. Larger bone islands can show mild uptake on bone scan.

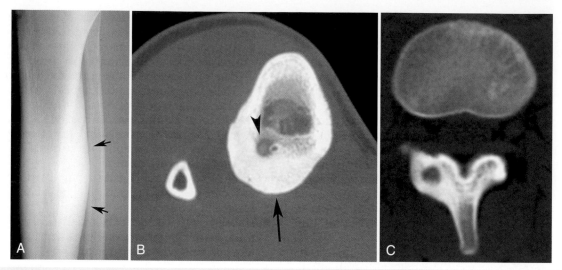

Fig. 11.26 Osteoid osteoma. (A and B) Typical, cortically-based osteoid osteoma. Lateral radiograph **(A)** shows focal cortical thickening of the posterior diaphysis of the tibia in this 14-year-old boy *(arrows)*. The cortical thickening is so dense that the nidus of the osteoid osteoma is not seen. It is, however, easily seen on CT; *(arrowhead in B)*. Note again the dense cortical thickening adjacent to the osteoid osteoma nidus *(arrow)*. **(C)** Osteoid osteoma in the vertebral posterior elements of L1. CT shows findings similar to those in B, with small, round lucent lesion with dense surrounding sclerosis. Osteoid osteoma occurs in the posterior elements of the spine; the pain may result in splinting, with the patient developing a nonrotational scoliosis, concave on the side of the lesion.

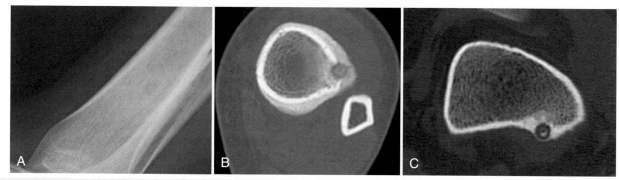

Fig. 11.27 Comparison of reactive change at cortical osteoid osteoma. **(A)** Radiograph of the leg shows a small but distinct lytic lesion within the tibia, with dense surrounding sclerosis. **(B)** Axial CT of the same lesion shows the lytic nidus and the full extent of the reactive change, which involves periosteum, endosteum, and marrow. This reactive change is typical of osteoid osteoma but need not be this severe. **(C)** Axial CT of another lesion, in the cortex of the distal femur, showing a round lytic lesion with dense central nidus, surrounded by much less impressive sclerotic reaction. This may represent a subperiosteal osteoid osteoma, which typically raises the periosteum and excavates the underlying cortex but does not arise within the cortex and does not elicit much bone reaction. These cases illustrate the varying amount of osseous reactive change one can expect in osteoid osteoma.

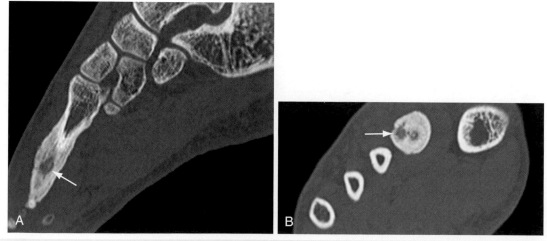

Fig. 11.28 Osteoid osteoma mimicking stress fracture. Sagittal CT **(A)** and coronal CT **(B)** show severe endosteal and periosteal thickening along the length of a single metatarsal. This appearance suggests healing and reactive change typical of stress fracture. However, both views show a focal lytic lesion located within the cortex *(arrows)* of the bone, proving osteoid osteoma as the instigator of the reactive change.

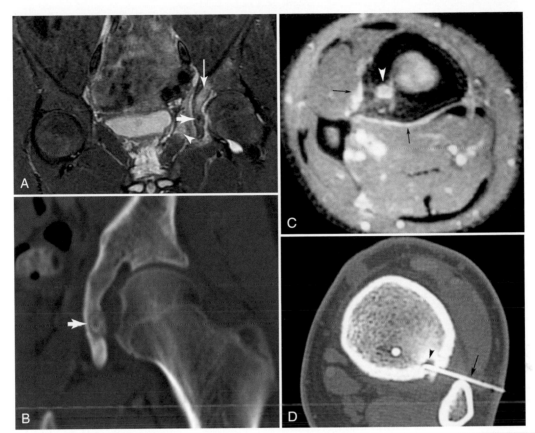

Fig. 11.29 Osteoid osteoma on MRI. **(A)** Coronal T2-weighted, fat-saturated image demonstrates a left hip effusion. There is high signal within the medial acetabular wall *(thin arrow)* and the adjacent soft tissues *(arrowhead)*. Hidden within all this hyperintense signal is a focal round low signal *(wide arrow)* that represents the osteoid osteoma nidus. This nidus is easily overlooked on MRI and could even lead to an unrewarding biopsy of the edematous muscle or acetabular wall. **(B)** Coronal CT of the same lesion clearly shows the focal nidus *(arrow)*, showing this is the true lesion, with all the surrounding abnormality seen on MRI representing only reactive change. **(C)** Axial fat-suppressed T1-weighted image with intravenous gadolinium in a different patient shows intensely enhancing nidus *(arrowhead)* in the posterolateral tibial cortex and intense periosteal enhancement *(small arrows)* overlying the thickened cortex adjacent to the nidus. As in this case, osteoid osteoma virtually always shows intense enhancement of at least part of the nidus, as well as less intense enhancement of the reactive tissue. **(D)** Axial CT of a different tibial osteoid osteoma *(arrowhead)* shows electrode placed *(arrow)* for percutaneous radiofrequency ablation; this is the typical and very effective treatment for osteoid osteoma.

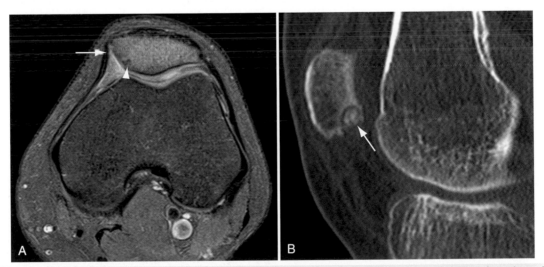

Fig. 11.30 Comparison of MRI and CT of osteoid osteoma. **(A)** Axial PD, fat-saturated MRI of the knee shows edematous hyperintensity of the entire patella *(arrow)*. It would be easy to overlook the tiny round low-signal lesion along the medial facet of the bone *(arrowhead)*. **(B)** Sagittal CT of the same lesion shows the nidus *(arrow)* much more clearly, with a lytic round lesion containing central calcification. The CT makes the diagnosis much more easily than MRI; in fact, in this case it was performed following the suggestion of a very astute radiologist who raised the question of osteoid osteoma rather than simply relegating the case to 'patellofemoral syndrome'. Contrast enhanced MR images, appropriately not obtained with routine knee imaging, would have made the osteoid osteoma more conspicuous. When osteoid osteoma is suspected, contrast enhanced images can be helpful.

may obscure the nidus itself (see Figs. 11.29 and 11.30). Gadolinium-based contrast is helpful as the nidus of osteoid osteoma enhances avidly.

■ Bone scan shows very intense tracer uptake in the nidus surrounded by less intense uptake. Note that CT or MRI are preferred for lesion identification and localization.

Key Concepts

Osteoid Osteoma

■ Small round or ovoid lytic lesion (the nidus), less than 1.5 cm. Nidus may contain sclerotic focus

■ Painful, worse at night, relieved with nonsteroidal anti-inflammatory drugs (NSAIDs)

■ Intense reactive sclerosis in long bone diaphyseal lesions. This may obscure nidus on radiographs. Computed tomography or magnetic resonance imaging may be needed

■ Reactive bone formation may occur at some distance from nidus if lesion is intracapsular

■ Most common locations: Femoral diaphysis, tibial diaphysis, femoral neck, posterior elements of spine

■ Treatment: NSAIDs; image-guided percutaneous ablation (usually CT-guided radiofrequency ablation [RFA] or cryoablation); surgical excision in refractory cases or locations that are unsafe for ablation; MRI-guided focused US surgery (MRgFUS) is a promising new noninvasive technique

■ Osteoid osteoma also may occur within a joint capsule, especially along the femoral neck.

■ These lesions can be difficult to diagnose. Unlike the extraarticular cortical osteoid osteomas, intracapsular lesions elicit little marginal sclerosis or periosteal bone formation because there is no periosteum inside the joint.

■ However, new bone formation is often found at a distance from the nidus, more distally along the cortex, much like the remote periosteal reaction found in chondroblastoma (Figs. 11.31 and 11.32).

■ In addition, host reaction in the form of chronic synovitis can be intense with joint effusion and, over a long period, cartilage loss and osteoarthritis (see Fig. 11.31).

■ If chronic synovitis and lateral subluxation of the femoral head occur in a child with an intracapsular osteoid osteoma, irreversible limb-length discrepancy and a valgus configuration of the femoral neck can result (see Fig. 11.32).

■ Because the sclerotic bone reaction is found at some distance from the nidus and the articular reaction can be extreme, the actual culprit in this variety of osteoid osteoma, the nidus, can be easily missed.

■ MRI is the best 'problem solver' test when an intraarticular osteoid osteoma is suspected. Surrounding bone marrow edema helps to locate the lesion. Intravenous contrast also can help localize the nidus.

■ The least common variety of osteoid osteoma is found in a subperiosteal location.

■ These are manifest as a round, soft tissue mass located immediately adjacent to bone with underlying scalloping, irregular bone resorption, and little reactive change (see Fig. 11.27C).

■ The talus is the most common site of this rare variety of osteoid osteoma.

■ Osteoid osteomas also occur in the spine, especially the posterior elements (see Fig. 11.26C).

■ The patient can develop painful scoliosis, with the lesion located at the concave margin of the apex of the curve, with no rotatory component.

■ Because of the sclerotic reaction to the underlying nidus, an osteoid osteoma in the posterior elements of the spine can be mistaken for a blastic metastasis or sclerosis related to abnormal stress, particularly in a patient with contralateral spondylolysis.

■ By definition, the nidus of an osteoid osteoma is less than 2 cm in size, and most are only a few millimeters in size

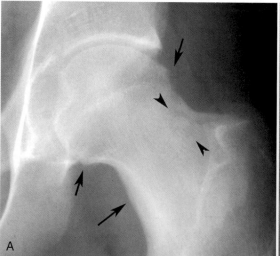
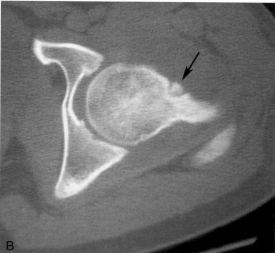

Fig. 11.31 Intracapsular osteoid osteoma. (A and B) Seventeen-year-old boy. AP hip radiograph **(A)** shows reactive change in the form of femoral head osteophytes and calcar buttressing (thickening of the medial femoral neck cortex; *short arrows*). The nidus of the osteoid osteoma is in the anterior femoral neck cortex *(arrowheads)*, better seen with CT *(arrow in* **B).** Note that the reaction from an intracapsular osteoid osteoma manifests as an arthritis.

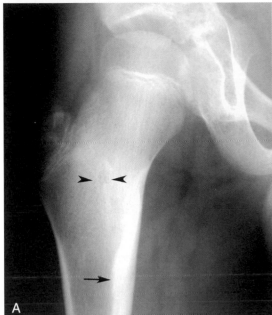

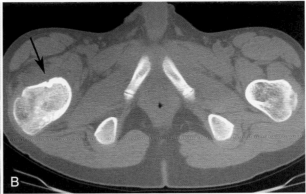

Fig. 11.32 Osteoid osteoma with resulting growth deformities in a 10-year-old boy. **(A)** AP radiograph of the hip shows dense and remote cortical reactive bone formation *(arrow)*, a wide and valgus femoral neck, and the faintly seen lucent nidus of the osteoid osteoma *(arrowheads)*. **(B)** The intracapsular nidus is localized with CT *(arrow)*. Growth disturbance can also occur with extracapsular lesions but is less frequent and tends to be less severe. (Images used with permission from BJ Manaster, MD, from the American College of Radiology Learning File.)

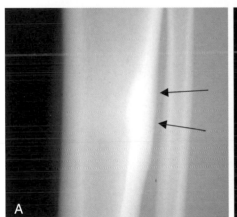

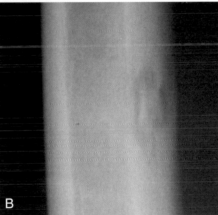

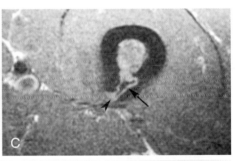

Fig. 11.33 Osteoid osteoma mimics. **(A)** Stress fracture. Lateral radiograph of the leg in a 16-year-old girl, which demonstrates thickening of the cortex of the tibia in the posterior medial position in its proximal third *(arrows)*, identical to the radiographic appearance of osteoid osteoma in Fig. 11.26A. This is a typical location for a stress fracture, which it proved to be. However, the radiographic appearance is not always distinguishable from an osteoid osteoma with the nidus obscured. **(B and C)** Intracortical abscess with sequestrum. Lateral radiograph **(B)** of the middiaphysis of the femur in a 15-year-old boy demonstrates thickening of the cortex, this time with an irregularly shaped lytic lesion and central density. Although this could represent an osteoid osteoma with central calcified nidus, the fat-suppressed, contrast-enhanced, T1-weighted MR image **(C)** demonstrates an irregularly shaped, low-signal-intensity sequestrum *(arrow)* with surrounding enhancement, and interruption of the cortex *(arrowhead)*.

(larger lesions are considered osteoblastomas). Osteoid osteoma may not be truly neoplastic because it has limited growth potential and does not metastasize.

- Bone scan in extraarticular osteoid osteoma shows intense tracer uptake in the nidus, as well as in the reactive bone. Classically the nidus uptake is greater, resulting in the *'double-density sign'* of punctate intense activity at the nidus surrounded by a larger region of less intensely increased activity.
- The differential diagnosis of a cortical osteoid osteoma includes osteoblastoma, chronic osteomyelitis, and stress fracture (Fig. 11.33).
    - Chronic infection may have a percutaneous draining sinus. CT may show a small channel between the nidus of infection and the adjacent soft tissues

termed a 'cloaca' (sewer) that is not present in osteoid osteoma.
    - The temporal pattern of pain associated with a stress fracture is different from that associated with an osteoid osteoma because pain with the former improves at night and with rest.
- The differential diagnosis of an intraarticular osteoid osteoma includes any cause of monoarticular synovitis such as infection and inflammatory arthritis. In children, early Legg–Calvé–Perthes disease may have similar clinical features.
- The radiologist often plays a key role in the treatment of these lesions. CT-guided resection with a drill, or radiofrequency ablation, cryoablation or thermoablation, is effective and generally causes less morbidity than

surgical resection (see Fig. 11.29D). MRI-guided focused US surgery (MRgFUS) is a promising new noninvasive technique.

OSTEOBLASTOMA

- Osteoblastoma is a rare benign bone-forming tumor that may be difficult to differentiate from osteoid osteoma histologically.
- Osteoblastoma may be characterized by its common location in the posterior elements of the spine (40–55% occur in the spine or flat bones and, of those arising in the spine, 94% are found in the posterior elements). The remainder occur mostly in long bones.
- Osteoblastomas are usually type 1A geographic lesions with a narrow zone of transition and sclerotic margin, with expansion of the underlying bone. Lesions appear nonaggressive, with only occasional cortical breakthrough. However, there is occasional aggressive behavior.
- Although these are bone-forming tumors, they have a wide range of density on radiography and CT, from lucent to a mixed pattern to a completely blastic appearance (Figs. 11.34 and 11.35).
- Because of this range of mineralization, signal intensity on T1- and T2-weighted MRI can vary widely.
- MRI may demonstrate prominent adjacent marrow and soft tissue edema (see Fig. 11.35).
- Treatment is with curettage or marginal excision, and recurrence is rare.
- Differential diagnosis includes osteoid osteoma, osteomyelitis, and ABC in the spine; in addition, because of the occasional finding of osteoid matrix and the flare phenomenon on MRI mimicking soft tissue mass, these lesions can be mistaken for osteosarcoma.

- Secondary ABC may arise in greater than 10% of lesions.
- Unlike osteoid osteomas, they may rarely undergo malignant transformation ("aggressive osteoblastoma").

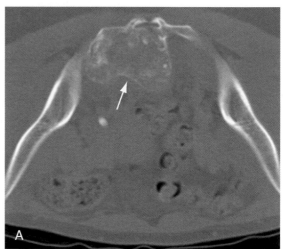

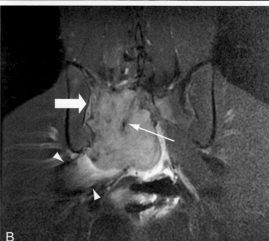

Fig. 11.35 Osteoblastoma with flare phenomenon. **(A)** Axial CT in the prone position shows an expanded, predominantly lytic lesion *(arrow)* within the sacrum. There is some calcification within the lesion. The lesion statistically is most likely a chordoma, but osteoblastoma must be considered. **(B)** Coronal T1-weighted, fat-saturated postgadolinium image of the same lesion shows enhancement of the entire lesion *(large arrow)* with hypointensity of the calcifications *(thin arrow)*. This is not a specific appearance. However, there is also very intense signal seen within adjacent soft tissues *(arrowheads)*. This represents the 'flare phenomenon' that may be seen in bone and soft tissues adjacent to osteoblastoma. (Images used with permission from BJ Manaster, MD, from STATdx website, Amirsys, Inc.)

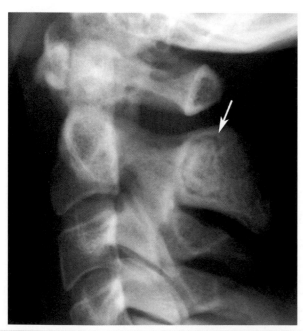

Fig. 11.34 Osteoblastoma. Lateral radiograph shows mixed lytic and blastic lesions expanding the spinous process of C2 *(arrow)*; this is a typical location bone appearance of osteoblastoma in this 36-year-old woman.

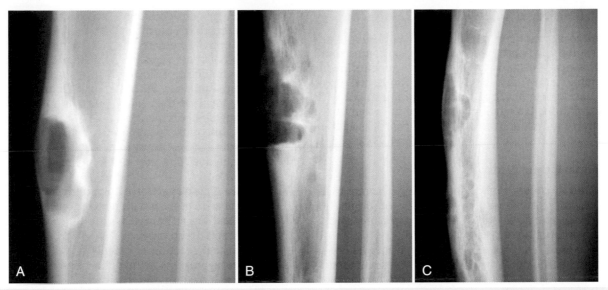

Fig. 11.36 Similarity of imaging appearance of osteofibrous dysplasia, cortical fibrous dysplasia, and adamantinoma. **(A)** AP radiograph of a cortically-based lytic lesion in the proximal tibia of a 12-year-old girl. This is typical of osteofibrous dysplasia (also known as ossifying fibroma). However, it is not always radiographically distinguishable from a cortically-based fibrous dysplasia or adamantinoma. **(B)** Cortically-based lytic lesion in the anterior tibia of a 12-year-old girl. This lesion has adjacent daughter lesions and at biopsy was found to be fibrous dysplasia. **(C)** Cortically-based lytic lesions in the anterior tibia, this time in a 10-year-old boy, which proved to be adamantinoma.

OSTEOFIBROUS DYSPLASIA (OSSIFYING FIBROMA)

- Osteofibrous dysplasia (formerly termed 'ossifying fibroma') is an extremely rare, benign fibro-osseous dysplasia found almost exclusively in the anterior proximal tibia.
- It most often appears in the first through second decades of life and appears as a cortically-based geographic, oval lesion.
- It is associated with anterior cortical bowing and generally causes local expansion of bone.
- The lesion has a sclerotic rim and may be entirely lucent or may contain osteoid matrix (appearance is described as 'ground glass').
- This lesion can be histologically and radiographically similar to cortically-based fibrous dysplasia and adamantinoma. These three lesions are believed by some authors to represent a spectrum of disease, although there are subtle histologic differentiating characteristics.
- The radiologist should consider osteofibrous dysplasia with classic features described earlier, with adamantinoma in the differential diagnosis if there is a more aggressive appearance (Fig. 11.36).
- MRI of osteofibrous dysplasia confirms cortical origin of the lesion and can evaluate for soft tissue/medullary invasion associated with the more aggressive adamantinoma (Fig. 11.37).

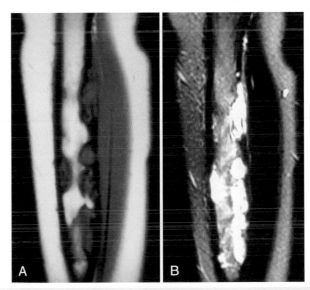

Fig. 11.37 MRI of osteofibrous dysplasia. Oblique sagittal T1-weighted **(A)** and T2-weighted **(B)** MR images of the tibia in a patient with osteofibrous dysplasia show cortically-based lesions to have intermediate T1-weighted and high T2-weighted signal. The radiograph in this patient (not shown) resembles findings in Fig. 11.36, with well-defined lytic lesions corresponding to the MRI abnormalities. The MRI findings, like the radiographic findings, are not specific for osteofibrous dysplasia versus adamantinoma or cortically-based fibrous dysplasia.

Malignant Bone-Forming Tumors (Osteosarcomas)

In general, primary bone malignancies are rare; osteosarcoma is the most common primary malignant bone tumor in adolescents. Among all ages it is second only to myeloma in frequency of primary bone malignancy (15–20%). Several types of osteosarcoma are described, and, because of their varying prognosis, treatment, and imaging features, we consider them individually. The World Health Organization (WHO) classifies osteosarcoma into central (intramedullary) and surface lesions, with subtypes and histologic variants in each group. Osteosarcoma classification is also divided into primary and secondary lesions.

CENTRAL (INTRAMEDULLARY) OSTEOSARCOMA

Central osteosarcoma types include conventional, telangiectatic, small cell, and low-grade osteosarcoma. Small cell and low-grade osteosarcoma are rare, accounting for approximately 2% of all osteosarcomas. Small cell osteosarcoma can appear similar to Ewing sarcoma, but with osteoid formation. Low-grade osteosarcoma occurs later in the third to fourth decade and can appear less aggressive, confused for benign lesions such as fibrous dysplasia.

Conventional Osteosarcoma

- As with all sarcomas, pathologists classify a tumor as an osteosarcoma not according to its site of origin but rather by histologic features, in this case bone, specifically the production of osteoid.
- Osteosarcomas can be histologically quite heterogeneous, and pathologists further classify these tumors on the basis of predominant features: 50% produce enough osteoid to be termed 'osteoblastic', whereas 25% produce predominantly cartilage (chondroblastic) and 25% produce predominantly spindle cells (fibroblastic).
- Conventional osteosarcoma makes up 85% of all osteosarcomas (Figs. 11.38 through 11.42).
  - Most (75%) arise in children and young adults between 10 and 25 years of age.
- Arise from the medullary cavity.
- Most (91%) are metaphyseal in origin, but they can be diaphyseal. Despite a metaphyseal origin, the tumor frequently crosses the physis to involve the epiphysis; the physis is not an effective barrier to this tumor (see Fig. 11.40).
  - Such epiphyseal involvement is found in 75% of cases and, although infrequently detected by radiography, can be easily seen on MRI.
  - Epiphyseal spread of tumor must be sought because there are significant therapeutic implications in the skeletally immature patient (the preferred allograft often cannot be used because of both growth and articular considerations; rather, osteoarticular graft or a prosthesis must be placed).
- Conventional osteosarcoma occurs most frequently at the sites of most rapid growth: the distal femur is the most common site, followed by the proximal tibia and the proximal humerus. Although flat bones are less frequently involved than long bones, osteosarcoma of the iliac wing deserves mention.
- Though one must be prepared to make the diagnosis on early, subtle cases, conventional osteosarcomas have a very rapid doubling rate and frequently are large when first noticed.
- They are highly aggressive in imaging appearance:
  - Permeative pattern with a wide zone of transition.
  - Cortical breakthrough is usually seen, often with a large soft tissue mass.
  - Periosteal reaction is usually present and often appears aggressive, with a hair-on-end, sunburst, or Codman triangle pattern.
  - Tumor osteoid matrix is visible on radiograph or CT in 90% of the cases and pathognomonic when present in the soft tissue mass.
    - The matrix characteristically has amorphous density, without an organized trabecular pattern.
    - The amount of matrix and the degree of matrix calcification vary widely, so the radiographic appearance may range from densely blastic to nearly completely lytic (see Fig. 11.41). Lytic lesions have aggressive (1C or higher) margins.

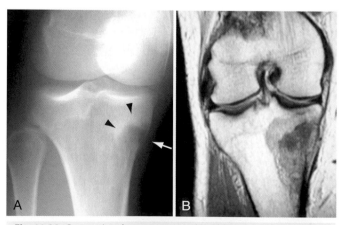

Fig. 11.38 Conventional osteosarcoma. **(A)** Oblique radiograph shows an aggressive, predominantly lytic lesion in the proximal tibia metaphysis. Note cortical breakthrough *(arrow)* and wide zone of transition. A very small region of sclerosis within the bone *(arrowheads)* could represent either tumor matrix or reactive bone formation. **(B)** Coronal proton density–weighted MRI shows that the lesion is larger than suggested by radiography and confirms cortical breakthrough medially.

Key Concepts

Conventional Osteosarcoma

- Most common primary bone sarcoma in the adolescent age group
- Frequently located about the knee, originating centrally in the metaphysis and often extending across the physis to the epiphysis
- Highly aggressive, rapid growth
- Permeative margins, cortical breakthrough, and soft tissue mass
- Most show osteoid matrix (varies from extremely subtle to significantly dense), but occasionally presents as a purely lytic lesion
- Aggressive periosteal reaction: Hair-on-end, sunburst, or Codman triangle; may be absent
- Spread: Direct invasion, local lymphatic; hematogenous metastasis to bone, lung

- The radiographic appearance often (but not always) corresponds to these histologic findings, with the matrix calcification in the cartilage and spindle cell variety being subtler relative to that of the osteoblastic variety.
- Radiographs are pathognomonic if the lesion is typical in location and shows osteoid matrix in an aggressive osseous lesion with osteoid within the soft tissue mass.
- The differential diagnosis for osteosarcoma can include Ewing sarcoma. Although Ewing sarcoma tends to be diaphyseal in location, it can be metadiaphyseal. Furthermore, Ewing sarcoma can elicit an extensive reactive bone formation that can mimic osteoid matrix. However,

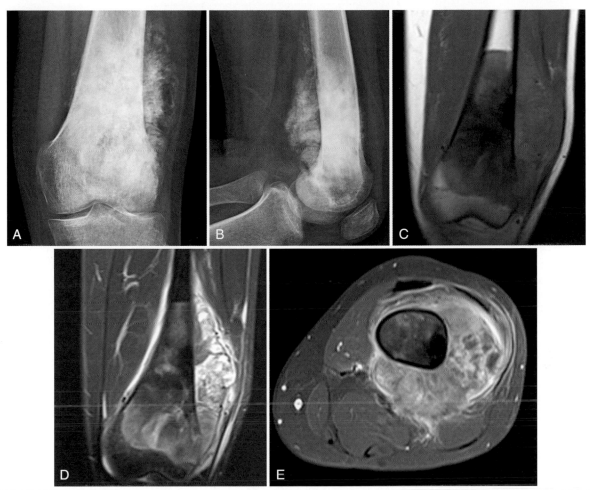

Fig. 11.39 Conventional osteosarcoma in a 20-year-old woman. AP **(A)** and lateral **(B)** radiographs demonstrate a classic appearance of osteosarcoma. The lesion originated eccentrically in the distal femoral metaphysis and has produced aggressive-appearing immature tumor osteoid in both the bone and soft tissue mass. There is aggressive periosteal reaction and a wide zone of transition. There is no possible diagnosis other than conventional osteosarcoma. Note the difference in sclerosis in this lesion compared with that shown in Fig. 11.38; both lesions are osteosarcoma and have similar prognoses. **(C)** Coronal T1-weighted MRI of the lesion shows the signal to be lower than that of skeletal muscle, as expected for this heavily ossified tumor. **(D)** Coronal STIR MR image shows mixed low and high signal in both the bone and soft tissue mass. **(E)** Axial T1-weighted, fat-saturated, post-contrast image shows significant heterogeneous enhancement, with a few regions of low-signal necrosis in the soft tissues. Note that axial imaging is far preferable to longitudinal imaging in determining muscle/anatomic compartment and neurovascular involvement.

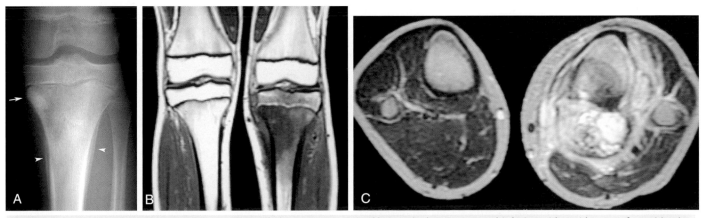

Fig. 11.40 Conventional osteosarcoma. **(A)** AP radiograph demonstrates a mixed lytic and sclerotic geographic lesion with a wide zone of transition in the metadiaphysis of the tibia in this 14-year-old boy. The lesion is highly aggressive, with abundant periosteal reaction *(arrowheads)* that is interrupted medially and lamellated laterally. Tumor matrix *(arrow)* causes the increased density in the medial metaphysis. By radiographic criteria this is the classic appearance of osteosarcoma. Also, by radiographic criteria the epiphysis appears spared. However, MRI better demonstrates the true tumor size. The T1-weighted coronal MR image **(B)** shows abnormal signal in the epiphysis and more extensively in the metaphysis and diaphysis because of tumor extension. The axial T2-weighted MR image **(C)** demonstrates the large soft tissue mass involving both the anterior and posterior compartments, as well as the popliteal neurovascular bundle.

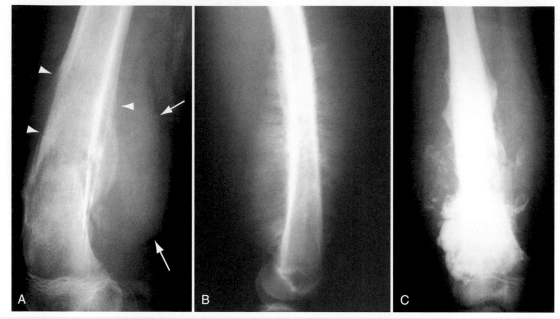

Fig. 11.41 Conventional osteosarcomas, demonstrating the variety of appearance of tumor osteoid matrix. **(A)** Lateral radiograph of a highly aggressive lesion involving the distal metaphysis of the femur in a 12-year-old girl. Note interrupted periosteal reaction *(arrowheads)*. A large soft tissue mass extends well beyond the periosteal reaction *(arrows)*, containing very subtle amorphous tumor matrix; amorphous matrix is seen within the osseous portion as well. It is important to recognize this subtle matrix as osteoid. **(B)** Lateral radiograph of an osteosarcoma in a different patient shows much more obvious tumor osteoid matrix emanating in a hair-on-end pattern throughout the large soft tissue mass. The intraosseous portion of the lesion extends proximal to the end of the radiograph. **(C)** AP radiograph of another osteosarcoma in a different patient that shows even greater density in the osteoid matrix, with regions that are much less amorphous, yet not forming organized trabeculae. This illustrates that the range of density of osteoid can be wide, and periosteal reaction also contributes to tumor density on radiographs.

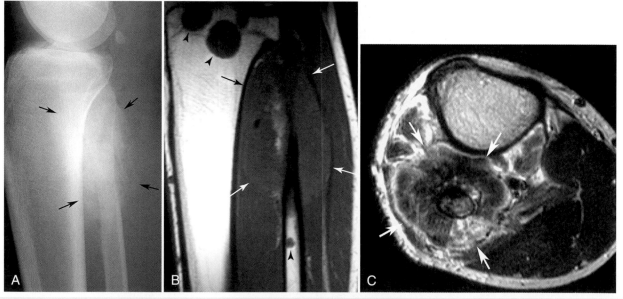

Fig. 11.42 Conventional osteosarcoma with skip lesions. **(A)** Lateral radiograph in a 17-year-old boy shows cloudlike osteoid matrix surrounding the proximal fibula. Sagittal T1-weighted **(B)** and axial T2-weighted **(C)** MR images show the tumor mass *(arrows)* and also show marrow 'skip' metastases in the proximal tibia and fibular shaft *(arrowheads in B)*.

the reactive bone formation is restricted to the involved bone and does not extend into the soft tissue mass in an Ewing sarcoma. This usually helps differentiate the two.

■ MRI signal intensity is variable depending on composition.

  ■ Hyperintensity can be seen on T1-weighted images if there is hemorrhage contained within the lesion. This

can also be seen after initial chemotherapy treatment if there has been favorable response with necrosis.

■ T2-weighted signal intensity varies. Densely calcified tumors can have low signal intensity in much of the lesion on all sequences, but there are invariably regions of hyperintensity on fluid-sensitive sequences.

- Contrast enhancement is intense and differentiates solid active tumor from sclerotic bone formation and necrotic regions of the lesion.
- Because so many of these lesions occur around the knee, coronal or sagittal imaging is useful to evaluate for joint involvement.
- In addition, careful attention must be paid to imaging the remainder of the involved or adjacent bone to detect 'skip' lesions (i.e., metastatic lesions to the same or immediately adjacent bone), which occur in 1–10% of cases (see Fig. 11.42).
- PET-CT can guide biopsy and assist with staging, and is very useful in assessing tumor response to therapy and follow-up surveillance.
- Any lesion that produces immature bone can be confused with osteosarcoma on histopathology, including healing fractures, early myositis ossificans, the avulsive cortical irregularity (or tug lesion) of the posteromedial distal femur, and some metastases.
  - It is important to recognize these lesions to avoid or help interpret biopsy, because tissue obtained during the active repair phase of these lesions may be difficult to distinguish histologically from osteosarcoma. Careful evaluation, including patient history and radiographic analysis, may mitigate a potentially confusing biopsy report.

Osteosarcoma: What the Clinician Wants to Know

- Tumor margins: MRI often better for showing medullary and soft tissue/joint involvement than other modalities.
- Epiphyseal spread.
- Muscle/compartment involvement.
- Joint involvement.
- Neurovascular bundle involvement.
- *Skip lesions*: synchronous lesions within the same or an immediately adjacent bone.
- Metastases: Lung (CT), bones (PET or bone scan), local lymph nodes.

- The metastatic potential of conventional osteosarcoma is high, with hematogenous spread to lungs and bones and lymphatic spread locally.
  - Metastases at any of these sites may produce tumor osteoid.

- Metastases are found in 5–10% of patients at clinical presentation.
- As with most sarcomas, pulmonary metastases tend to be small, so chest CT is required for staging.
- Eighty percent of tumor relapses occur in the lung, and 20% occur in bone. Both local recurrence and systemic disease usually occur within 2 years after initial diagnosis.
- Current 5-year survival is about 75% in patients without metastasis, lower in patients who present with metastatic disease.
- Regardless of the success of chemotherapy (or radiation, if that is chosen), wide surgical excision is required to prevent local recurrence. Limb salvage is preferred if possible because it improves the quality of life without significantly affecting longevity. The patient concludes therapy with adjuvant multidrug chemotherapy.
- As with most sarcomas, follow-up imaging is performed more frequently during the first 2–5 years after treatment because most recurrences occur during this time.

Telangiectatic Osteosarcoma

- Telangiectatic osteosarcoma is a rare osteosarcoma variant that occurs in the same age range and location as conventional osteosarcoma.
- Telangiectatic osteosarcoma is expansile (75% show aneurysmal expansion) and mostly lytic (subtle matrix may be seen as small foci in the periphery of the lesion in 58%) with cortical breakthrough (Fig. 11.43).
- A geographic pattern can mislead the unwary into underdiagnosis; it is essential to identify any region with a broad zone of transition, which may raise a 'red flag' that it represents an aggressive lesion.
- On MRI fluid fluid levels are common (90%). Telangiectatic osteosarcoma is highly vascular and contains necrotic tissue and large pools of blood, with tumor usually located only at the periphery and along septations.
  - T1-weighted sequences may show high signal due to hemorrhage.
  - The peripheral tumor can be seen to appear nodular in some areas and irregular in others.
  - Contrast enhancement is seen in the periphery, as well as in any nodular masses.

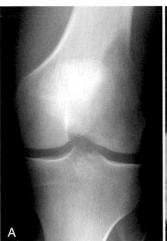
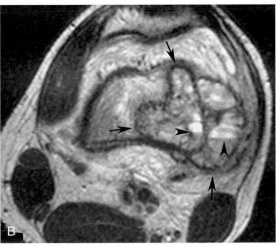

Fig. 11.43 Telangiectatic osteosarcoma. (A) AP radiograph demonstrates a geographic lytic lesion with a wide zone of transition (type 1C margin) in the distal femoral metaphysis extending to the subchondral region. This aggressive pattern of bone destruction is sometimes erroneously interpreted as nonaggressive, particularly when compared with the highly aggressive osteosarcomas seen in Figs. 11.38 to 11.42. (B) Axial T2-weighted MR image demonstrates the large extraosseous soft tissue mass *(arrows)* that contains fluid-fluid levels *(arrowheads)*. This is the classic MR appearance of telangiectatic osteosarcoma, but this appearance may be seen in other lesions, notably aneurysmal bone cysts and giant cell tumors. Combined with the aggressive radiographic appearance, telangiectatic osteosarcoma is a likely preoperative diagnosis.

- Careful observation is required to avoid misdiagnosing telangiectatic osteosarcoma as the less aggressive ABC or even GCT, both lesions that can contain fluid-fluid levels. ABCs usually do not have tumor nodules along the periphery. In these lesions the zone of transition on radiographs is narrower than for an osteosarcoma.
- The metastatic potential, workup, prognosis, and therapy are identical to those for conventional osteosarcoma.

Osteosarcomatosis

- Osteosarcomatosis is an older term coined to describe the apparent synchronous appearance of osteosarcoma at multiple sites, often bilaterally symmetric.
- Now understood to be widely metastatic disease at presentation.
- The lesions are high grade and prognosis is poor.

SURFACE OSTEOSARCOMA

Surface osteosarcoma subtypes include parosteal, periosteal, and high-grade surface osteosarcoma.

Parosteal Osteosarcoma

- Parosteal osteosarcoma (Figs. 11.44 through 11.47) is a surface lesion that represents the second most common variety of osteosarcoma (4–5% of all osteosarcomas) and the most common surface osteosarcoma (65% of these lesions).
- Arises from the outer (fibrous) layer of the periosteum.
- Although there is a wide age range, including adolescence, more than 80% of cases occur between the ages of 20 and 50 years. Thus the median age is older than is found with conventional osteosarcoma.
- The lesion also tends to be of low grade and is better differentiated than conventional and telangiectatic osteosarcoma.
- This surface osteosarcoma is found most frequently at the posterior distal femoral metaphysis (65%); other common locations are the proximal tibia and proximal humerus.

- It is metaphyseal in 90% of cases.
- Most of the tumor is located in the adjacent soft tissues, usually with lobulated margins.
  - As the lesion enlarges, it tends to 'wrap' around the bone; parts of the lesion may be adjacent to the underlying cortex without being adherent to it, resulting in a cleavage plane or 'cleft' between much of the lesion and the underlying bone.
- There is marrow involvement in nearly all cases; this is usually not seen on radiography but is confirmed on MRI. Although marrow involvement per se does not change the prognosis, it is crucial to describe the extent of involvement so that initial surgical resection is complete, thus preventing recurrence and possible worsening of the grade of the lesion.
- The tumor matrix is usually densely sclerotic centrally, whereas peripherally the matrix may be less mature or even nonossified.
  - CT can demonstrate this zonal phenomenon, as may MRI
  - The MRI appearance varies depending on the degree of matrix ossification. If it is hypocellular, there will be low signal on all sequences. However, more cellularity is usually present, in addition to soft tissue components, which results in an inhomogeneous appearance.
  - The lesion enhances with contrast, in both the marrow and soft tissue portions. The extent of marrow involvement should be carefully assessed, along with regions that are more cellular; these might suggest a focus of higher grade or dedifferentiation.
- Parosteal osteosarcomas tend to be slow growing and low grade and generally have an excellent result with adequate treatment (90–95% survival at 5 years); they can be ideal for limb salvage techniques with wide resection.
- Because of the low-grade nature of the lesion, chemotherapy is generally not necessary. However, with inadequate excision, the lesion may recur locally in a more aggressive form.

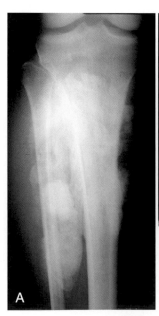

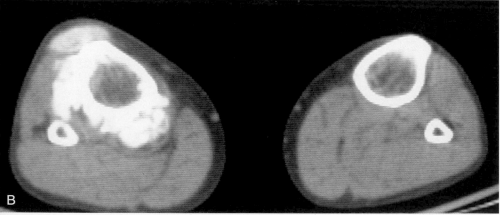

Fig. 11.44 Parosteal osteosarcoma. (A and B) Extensive lesion with dense matrix. **(A)** AP radiograph shows a dense, well-defined osteoid matrix forming this tumor, which appears to 'wrap around' the proximal tibial metadiaphysis in this 41-year-old man. **(B)** The appearance of the tumor as a surface lesion wrapping around the underlying bone is confirmed on CT. This is a large parosteal osteosarcoma in a typical location with characteristic dense osteoid formation.

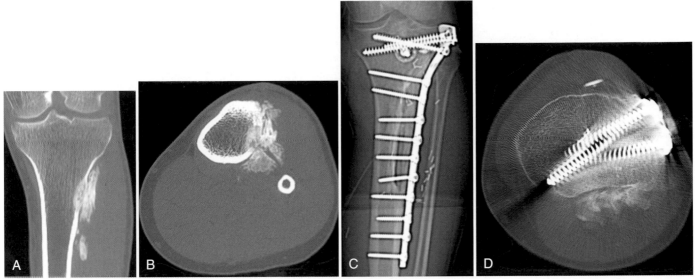

Fig. 11.45 Parosteal osteosarcoma. Smaller lesion than that shown in Fig. 11.44, also with dense matrix. **(A)** Coronal CT reconstruction shows a surface lesion producing dense, fairly mature osteoid along the lateral tibial cortex. There is some involvement of the adjacent marrow. **(B)** Axial CT better demonstrates the character of the tumor bone formation, as well as the marrow involvement. However, be aware that the extent of marrow involvement is better evaluated on MRI than on CT. The lesion is beginning to wrap around the tibia. The appearance is typical of parosteal osteosarcoma. **(C and D)** CT 2 years later. CT scout image **(C)** shows the lesion management with limb salvage surgery. The tumor was resected en bloc, and the resulting defect in the tibia was partially filled in with a vascularized fibular graft and additionally supported with a plate and screws. This surgery, if tumor resection was complete, preserves limb function with prognosis identical to amputation. However, the resection specimen margins were not completely clear of tumor when reviewed by pathologic examination after the surgery. Axial CT image **(D)** shows tumor recurrence with new soft tissue calcification posterior to the tibia.

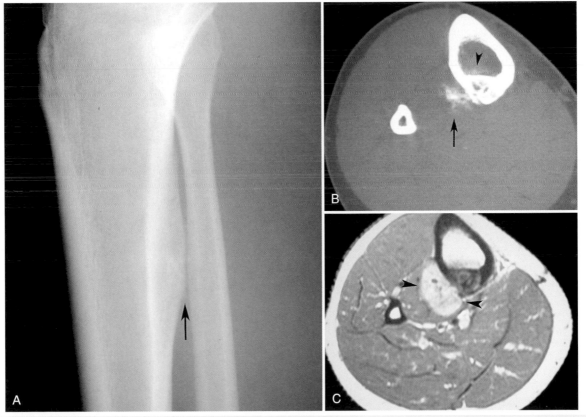

Fig. 11.46 Parosteal osteosarcoma, with only minimal visible tumor calcification. **(A)** Lateral radiograph shows prominent focal cortical bone formation in the posterior tibial metadiaphysis, a location that is typical for a stress fracture in this active 28-year-old man. There is extremely subtle osteoid matrix posterior to the thickened cortex *(arrow)*. **(B)** CT demonstrates the matrix in the soft tissues *(arrow)* and subtle new bone formation within the medullary canal *(arrowhead)*. The dense cortical new bone formation is also demonstrated. CT confirms the diagnosis of an early parosteal osteosarcoma. **(C)** Axial T2-weighted MR image shows the soft tissue mass *(arrowheads)*. Because this sequence was performed without fat suppression, the marrow extension is difficult to distinguish from normal marrow fat.

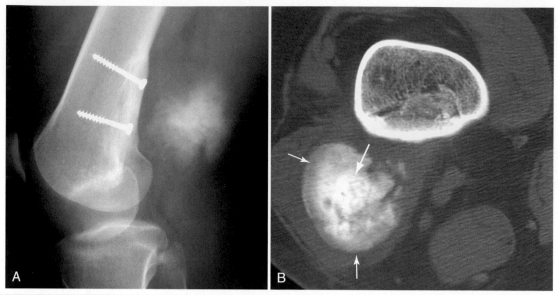

Fig. 11.47 Recurrent parosteal osteosarcoma. **(A)** Lateral radiograph demonstrating a previously resected parosteal osteosarcoma with bone graft secured with screws at the posterior cortex, now incorporated. The recurrent tumor is in the soft tissues and demonstrates the zoning phenomenon typical of parosteal osteosarcoma; the more mature bone formation is located centrally in the mass, and the periphery shows less mature osteoid formation. **(B)** The zoning phenomenon is emphasized on CT, where the dense center *(long arrow)* is surrounded by less mature peripheral osteoid formation *(short arrows)*.

- With multiple recurrences, may dedifferentiate into a high-grade sarcoma.
- In addition, parosteal osteosarcomas may even initially contain foci that are of higher grade or are dedifferentiated to conventional osteosarcoma.
- Metastases to the lung in uncomplicated parosteal osteosarcoma occur both later and with considerably lower frequency compared with metastases in conventional osteosarcoma.
- Parosteal osteosarcoma is generally not a difficult diagnosis to make radiographically. In its earliest stages it could be mistaken for myositis ossificans or heterotopic ossification. These conditions demonstrate a zonal phenomenon denser at the periphery, whereas osteosarcoma is denser centrally.
- Parosteal osteosarcoma is easily distinguished from an osteochondroma because the latter should show cortical and marrow continuity with the underlying bone.

Periosteal Osteosarcoma

- Periosteal osteosarcoma is a rare surface osteosarcoma (<2% of all osteosarcomas, 25% of surface osteosarcomas).
- Arises from the inner (bone forming) layer of the periosteum.
- Periosteal osteosarcomas generally arise in the second or third decade of life, slightly later than conventional osteosarcomas.
- They frequently show some chondroid differentiation at histologic analysis and are usually of intermediate grade.
- Periosteal osteosarcomas are usually located in a more diaphyseal position than either conventional or parosteal osteosarcomas.
- The femur and the tibia are the most common locations for periosteal osteosarcoma, followed by the humerus.

- It has a distinct radiographic appearance compared with parosteal or conventional osteosarcomas.
  - Because it is a surface lesion, it usually causes scalloping of the underlying cortex, although occasionally cortical thickening is seen at the proximal or distal ends of the lesion (Fig. 11.48).
  - The lesion tends to wrap around the circumference of the bone, though less extensively than a mature parosteal osteosarcoma.

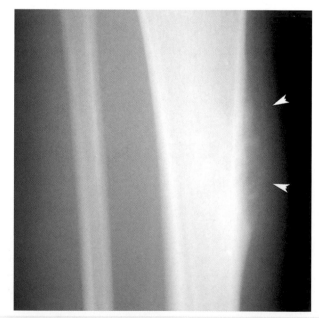

Fig. 11.48 Periosteal osteosarcoma. AP radiograph demonstrates the surface periosteal osteosarcoma in a 12-year-old girl, with the typical tumor osteoid arising from the surface of the lesion and a faint thickening of the cortex at the edge of the lesion but scalloping of the cortex centrally in the lesion *(arrowheads)*. Compare with Fig. 11.3.

- At the knee, periosteal osteosarcoma may be suggested rather than parosteal osteosarcoma by medial rather than posterior location.
- The soft tissue mass extends from the surface of the lesion, usually with spicules of bone emanating in a sunburst pattern.
- Aggressive periosteal reaction is common, often in the form of a Codman triangle.

Key Concepts

Osteosarcoma Subtypes by Location

Intramedullary types:
- *High-grade intramedullary* (conventional, central) (85%)
- *Telangiectatic*: Expansile with fluid-fluid levels; high grade
- *Low-grade*: Rare, older patient population (3rd and 4th decades), less aggressive, can be confused for fibrous dysplasia
- *Small cell*: Rare, can appear similar to Ewing sarcoma but with osteoid formation.
- *Secondary*: Poor prognosis; Common causes: Paget's disease, radiation, dedifferentiated chondrosarcoma; Rare causes: Fibrous dysplasia, preexisting bone infarct

Surface types:
- Parosteal > periosteal > high-grade surface
- *Parosteal*:
  - Low grade unless recurrent
  - Posterior distal femur > proximal tibia > humerus or proximal femur
  - Surface mass
  - Usually calcifies densely (especially centrally)
- *Periosteal*:
  - Intermediate grade
  - Medial distal femur, tends to wrap around the bone
  - Cortical scalloping, bone spicules radiating from cortex
  - Intraosseous involvement rare
- Parosteal and periosteal: Older mean age and better prognosis than conventional osteosarcoma

Extraosseous: Rare; soft tissue mass, may calcify; high grade; poor prognosis

- MRI demonstrates the extent of the soft tissue mass and usually shows no intramedullary extension of the lesion, although the rare intramedullary extension of lesion should be sought because this will affect limb salvage plans.
  - The MRI signal is nonspecific: low intensity on T1-weighted images and high intensity on T2-weighted images.
  - The sunburst type bone formation may be seen as low-signal linear rays on all sequences.
- Treatment is by wide excision. Their prognosis is better than that of conventional osteosarcomas, although not as good as that of parosteal osteosarcomas.
- The major differential diagnosis is periosteal chondroma, another surface lesion that can have a very similar appearance (Fig. 11.49). The rare high-grade surface osteosarcoma can be difficult to differentiate as well.

High-Grade Surface Osteosarcoma

- High-grade surface osteosarcoma is rare (<1% of all osteosarcomas, 10% of all surface osteosarcomas).
- Arises from the outer cortex.

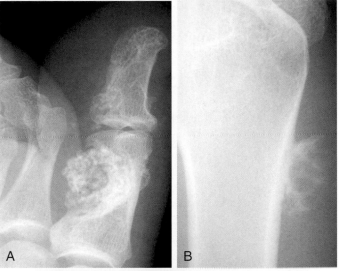

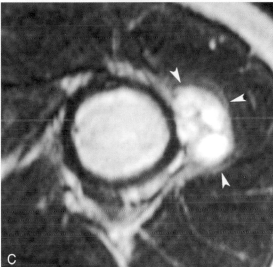

Fig. 11.49 Periosteal chondromas. **(A)** Lateral radiograph of the great toe in a 50-year-old woman. Note the lesions in both the proximal and distal phalanx, with each showing scalloping of the underlying bone and a densely calcified chondroid matrix. These findings are of a surface lesion, and each is a typical example of a periosteal chondroma. It is unusual to see two adjacent lesions. **(B)** Another example, with a somewhat different appearance, is seen in an AP radiograph of the proximal humerus in an 18-year-old woman. Again, a surface lesion is demonstrated, this time without scalloping and with prominent matrix extending into the soft tissues. **(C)** Axial T2-weighted MR image shows a juxtacortical mass with high-signal-intensity lobules *(arrowheads)*, which is suggestive of cartilage but is not specific. Although this proved at biopsy to be a periosteal chondroma, an imaging diagnosis of parosteal osteosarcoma, periosteal osteosarcoma, or periosteal chondrosarcoma might be reasonable on the basis of the imaging characteristics.

- Like periosteal osteosarcomas, these lesions tend to involve the diaphysis of long bones, most frequently the femur and humerus (Fig. 11.50).
- The majority contain osteoid matrix, and there may be partial destruction of the underlying cortex.
- Periosteal reaction, often aggressive, is common.
- They are similar in appearance to early parosteal or more mature periosteal osteosarcomas, although intramedullary involvement is more frequent in the high-grade surface lesions.

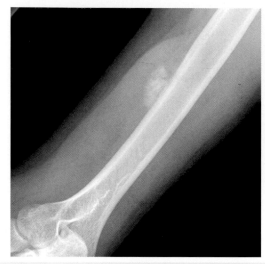

Fig. 11.50 High-grade surface osteosarcoma. AP radiograph demonstrates tumor osteoid formed at the surface of the humerus. The MR image (not shown) demonstrated a soft tissue mass extending beyond the tumor matrix. Although the appearance is suggestive of the more common parosteal osteosarcoma, the location of the lesion at the humeral diaphysis rather than metaphysis might raise questions about this diagnosis. Pathologic examination proved it to be a high-grade surface osteosarcoma. (Image used with permission from BJ Manaster, MD, from Manaster BJ, Petersilge CA, Roberts CC, Hanrahan CJ. *Diagnostic Imaging: Musculoskeletal Non-Traumatic Disease.* Salt Lake City: Amirsys; 2010.)

- High-grade surface osteosarcomas have the same prognosis as conventional osteosarcoma and are managed similarly.

EXTRASKELETAL OSTEOSARCOMA

- Extraosseous osteosarcoma is a rare form of osteosarcoma occurring in the soft tissues (1–2% of soft tissue tumors, 2–4% of osteosarcomas).
- The lesion is found most frequently in the thigh, with less frequent occurrence in the upper extremity and retroperitoneum.
- The soft tissue mass has variable amounts of mineralized osteoid (seen in 50% of the cases; see Fig. 11.51).
- MRI appearance is nonspecific. Treatment is with wide resection and adjuvant chemotherapy or radiation therapy; tumors are high-grade and prognosis is poor, worse than that for conventional osteosarcoma.

OSTEOSARCOMA IN THE OLDER AGE GROUP

- Osteosarcomas arising in patients older than age 60 years often do not have the classic appearance of conventional osteosarcoma.
- Their location tends to be different (one-fourth in the axial skeleton, often in the cranial/facial bones, and with greater frequency in the soft tissues).
- Eighty percent of the bone lesions present as purely lytic with aggressive margins.
- Although some are primary osteosarcomas, about half arise in preexisting lesions (termed *secondary osteosarcoma*).
  - Common preexisting lesions for secondary osteosarcoma include Paget's disease (67–97% of secondary

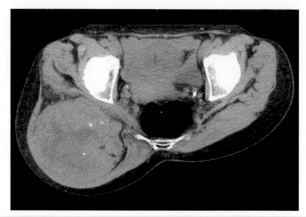

Fig. 11.51 Extraskeletal osteosarcoma. Axial CT demonstrates a large soft tissue mass within the gluteus maximus of an older male patient. The mass contains calcified matrix that is nonspecific in appearance. Biopsy demonstrated a rare extraskeletal osteosarcoma. (Image used with permission from BJ Manaster, MD, from STATdx website, Amirsys, Inc.)

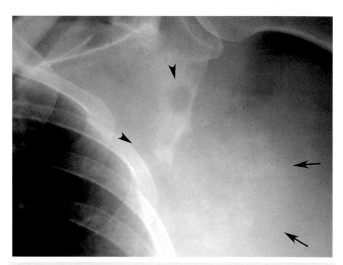

Fig. 11.52 Secondary osteosarcoma. AP radiograph of the shoulder demonstrates destruction of the scapula (*arrowheads*), along with a large soft tissue mass in the axilla containing subtle osteoid matrix (*arrows*). This 66-year-old woman had axillary radiation for breast carcinoma and 12 years later developed a radiation-induced osteosarcoma.

osteosarcoma), previously irradiated bone (6–22% of secondary osteosarcoma), and dedifferentiated chondrosarcoma.
- Secondary osteosarcomas tend to be high-grade and aggressive.
- It is likely that no more than 1% of patients with Paget's disease are at risk for developing osteosarcoma, and when osteosarcoma does occur in these patients, there is generally long-standing and severe Paget's disease.
- Postradiation osteosarcomas (Fig. 11.52) have locations that parallel those of commonly irradiated areas (shoulder girdle for breast carcinoma, pelvis for genitourinary tumors).
- Osteosarcoma is the most frequent malignancy to arise from radiated bone, with the interval between radiation and diagnosis ranging from 3 to 40 years (average, 14 years).

Other sarcomas that occur in radiated bone include undifferentiated pleomorphic sarcoma and chondrosarcoma.
- Up to 10% of well-differentiated chondrosarcomas can dedifferentiate into osteosarcoma or other high-grade sarcoma.
  - Imaging studies often show a sharp transition between the well-differentiated chondrosarcoma and the highly aggressive dedifferentiated tumor. This tumor may contain elements of fibrosarcoma, pleomorphic sarcoma, and high-grade chondrosarcoma, as well as osteosarcoma.
  - Osteosarcoma may also rarely arise from benign conditions, including osteochondroma, osteoblastoma, bone infarct, and fibrous dysplasia.
- Treatment of osteosarcoma in the older patient is with radical excision and chemotherapy. However, the tumors are usually high-grade and survival is poor, averaging less than 40% at 5 years in older patients with primary osteosarcoma and 7.5% in patients with osteosarcoma arising in a preexisting lesion.

Cartilage-Forming Tumors

- Cartilage-forming tumors are very common and most are benign.
- Many have chondroid matrix (see Fig. 11.6) or other features discussed later that allow easy diagnosis.
- However, the distinction between benign cartilage-forming tumor and chondrosarcoma can be extremely difficult in some situations.
- Chondrosarcoma is the third most common primary malignant bone tumor following multiple myeloma and osteosarcoma; it is frequently misdiagnosed, often as a benign lesion.

ENCHONDROMA

- Enchondromas are common benign cartilaginous neoplasms originating in medullary bone; they are the second most common benign bone tumor and constitute 10–25% of all benign bone tumors.
- Enchondromas are most frequently discovered incidentally on radiographs because they are usually asymptomatic in the absence of pathologic fracture or malignant transformation.
- They are thought to arise in the medullary canal owing to continued growth of residual benign cartilaginous rests that are displaced from the growth plate.
- Location:
  - Enchondromas are especially common in the tubular bones of the hands or feet, and up to 50% of all enchondromas occur in one of those locations (Fig. 11.53).
  - They are also commonly distributed among metaphyseal (uncommonly diaphyseal) regions of the long tubular bones, especially the proximal humerus, proximal or distal femur, and proximal tibia, but occur only rarely in the axial skeleton.
  - Enchondromas are so rarely located in the epiphysis that should one be diagnosed as such by pathologic examination, one should suggest that the pathologist reevaluate the cells for evidence of chondroblastoma or chondrosarcoma.
  - Similarly, enchondromas are extremely rare in the axial skeleton; a lesion with cartilage matrix in the pelvis or ribs should be considered suspicious for chondrosarcoma.
- Enchondromas are usually monostotic. They may, however, be multiple when found in the hands or feet (see Fig. 11.53). Patients with multiple enchondromatosis (Ollier disease; see later discussion) have more than one enchondroma in locations other than the hands or feet.

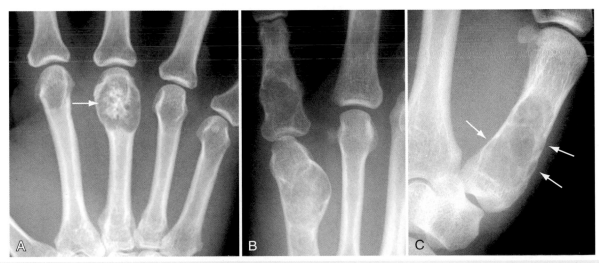

Fig. 11.53 Enchondroma in the hand. Fifty percent of enchondromas arise in the hands or feet. Note the wide variety of appearance of cartilaginous matrix in these cases (see also Fig. 11-6B). **(A)** AP radiograph of the middle phalanx of a finger in a 35-year-old man. In this case there is a geographic lesion with a narrow zone of transition with dense punctate calcifications *(arrow)*. This is a pathognomonic appearance of an enchondroma. **(B)** AP radiograph of the fourth and fifth fingers in a different patient, a 23-year-old man. In this case the matrix is much less dense, and the lesions are expanded. These also are typical for enchondroma. A patient can have more than one enchondroma in the hands or feet without a suggestion of multiple enchondromatosis. **(C)** AP radiograph of the thumb in a third patient shows a lytic central lesion, without matrix, with endosteal scalloping and minimal expansion *(arrows)*. Because there is no matrix, a complete differential diagnosis for this lesion includes solitary bone cyst, giant cell tumor, aneurysmal bone cyst, or fibrous dysplasia, but the location in the hand makes enchondroma by far the most likely diagnosis.

Key Concepts

Enchondroma

- Common, usually incidental benign cartilage-forming neoplasm
- Central, metaphyseal location
- Chondroid matrix, but may be entirely lytic (especially in the hand or foot)
- Geographic, although often without a sclerotic margin
- MRI shows lobulated bright signal on T2-weighted images, with low-signal-intensity calcifications.
- Fifty percent of cases occur in tubular bones of hands and feet, which may exhibit bone expansion with cortical thinning, often with pathologic fracture.
- Small risk for malignant transformation, more common in multiple enchondromatosis (Maffucci syndrome > Ollier disease)

- Imaging appearance:
  - The most common appearance of an enchondroma is that of a discrete geographic lesion, often with lobulated margins (Figs. 11.54 and 11.55; see Figs. 11.6 and 11.53), though the margin is usually not sclerotic on radiograph.
  - The lesion in long tubular bones may mildly expand bony margins, with cortical thinning, but significant expansion is not expected in the long bones.
  - Sclerotic margins are more common in the hands and feet, and lesions in the small tubular bone may expand significantly and present with a pathologic fracture.
  - Enchondromas usually contain cartilaginous matrix, which may appear as stippled (punctate), curvilinear ('rings and arcs'), or flocculent ('popcorn') calcification, generally appearing denser than normal bone (see Fig. 11.54).
  - However, enchondromas can also appear lytic and be discovered only incidentally by MRI or inferred radiographically by cortical thinning or endosteal erosion (see Fig. 11.53C).

- Enchondromas show no cortical breakthrough, soft tissue mass, or host response in the absence of pathologic fracture; these findings suggest chondrosarcoma.
  - Endosteal scalloping can be seen with both enchondroma and chondrosarcoma. More extensive scalloping is suggestive of chondrosarcoma.
  - Growth or other change over time—especially development of lytic areas—also suggests aggressiveness.
  - Pain in the region of a chondroid lesion, especially pain at night, and without other potential sources of pain should be considered suspicious for chondrosarcoma.
- Bone scan does not help differentiate enchondroma from chondrosarcoma because, unless the lesion is very small, 30% of enchondromas show increased uptake on bone scan.
- PET-CT generally shows higher standard uptake value (SUV) in higher-grade (2 or 3) chondrosarcoma than low-grade chondrosarcoma or enchondroma, but the difference is small.
- On MRI an enchondroma appears as a mass with lobules of intermediate (isointense to muscle) signal intensity on T1-weighted images and very high signal intensity on T2-weighted images (Figs. 11.55 and 11.56).
  - The very high T2-weighted signal intensity is caused by the high water content of the mucopolysaccharide extracellular matrix of the tumor cartilage.
  - The periphery as well as stroma between the chondroid nodules may enhance with gadolinium, but the nodules themselves do not enhance.
  - Occasional internal septations, and punctate signal voids representing matrix calcifications, are also seen. However, this appearance is not specific for enchondroma, because a low-grade chondrosarcoma can be indistinguishable from enchondroma on all imaging studies.
- The differential diagnosis of an enchondroma in the hands or feet is different from that of an enchondroma in the more proximal tubular bones.

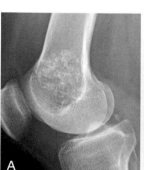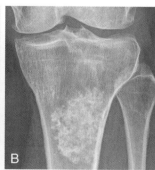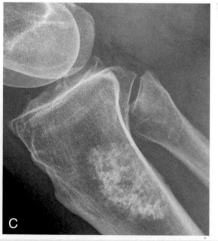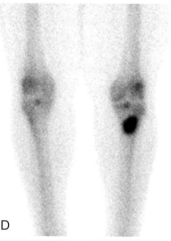

Fig. 11.54 Enchondroma. (A) Lateral radiograph demonstrates a central metaphyseal lesion containing punctate chondroid matrix. Note that the matrix is slightly denser than bone and that the lesion appears geographic, though there is no sclerotic margin. AP **(B)** and lateral **(C)** radiographs of another enchondroma in a middle-aged individual. The punctate chondroid matrix appears almost conglomerate. The lesion is slightly eccentric, and there is a slight amount of scalloping of the posterior cortex seen on the lateral view. The apparent 'halo' of lucency surrounding the chondroid matrix holds no prognostic meaning. **(D)** Bone scan of same lesion shows significant uptake; this has no diagnostic value in distinguishing enchondroma versus chondrosarcoma.

- If the lesion shows no matrix calcification, one might also consider a diagnosis of GCT, epidermoid inclusion cyst, ABC, solitary bone cyst, and fibrous dysplasia.
- Statistically GCT is the second most common neoplasm in the small tubular bones.
- Enchondroma may appear quite aggressive in the digits, but chondrosarcoma is extremely rare in the hands or feet, regardless of the radiographic appearance.

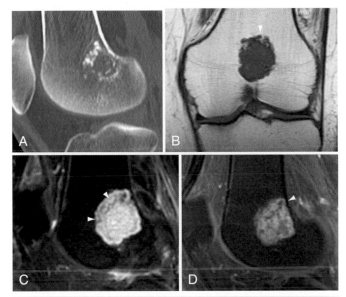

Fig. 11.55 Enchondroma, MRI appearance. **(A)** Sagittal CT reconstruction shows a lytic lesion located eccentrically in the distal femoral metaphysis. The lesion contains scattered punctate chondroid matrix and is typical of enchondroma. **(B)** Coronal T1-weighted MRI of the same lesion shows a hypointense lesion. There are small nodular regions along the periphery (arrowhead); these can be seen in enlarging enchondromas and do not necessarily suggest degeneration to chondrosarcoma. **(C)** Sagittal T2-weighted, fat-saturated image shows the lesion to have hyperintense nodular regions scattered throughout (arrowheads). These are small typical benign cartilage nodules. **(D)** Sagittal postcontrast T1-weighted, fat-saturated image shows enhancement of the periphery of the lesion (arrowhead), as well as of the internal stroma. The cartilage nodules themselves do not enhance. This is a typical enhancement pattern of enchondroma.

- Symptomatic enchondromas of the hands and feet are generally treated with curettage and bone grafting. Lesions that present with pathologic fracture are usually allowed to heal before curettage.
- In sites other than the hands or feet, enchondroma may occasionally be confused on radiograph with bone infarct, although the sharp, serpentine pattern of calcification found in a mature bone infarct usually allows clear differentiation, as does the MRI (see Fig. 11.8).
- Solitary enchondroma of the pelvis, ribs, or sternum is exceedingly rare. A solitary lesion with chondroid matrix in any of these locations should be considered a chondrosarcoma until proven otherwise.

Key Concepts

Enchondroma Versus Chondrosarcoma

Strongly favors enchondroma:
- Location in hands or feet

Favors enchondroma:
- Small lesion, stable over time
- No endosteal cortical scalloping
- Asymptomatic

Favors chondrosarcoma:
- Proximal location
- Large size
- Enlarging
- Pain without mechanical cause
- Destruction of previously present matrix
- Endosteal cortical scalloping greater than two thirds of cortical thickness
- Cortical breakthrough
- Pelvic, sternum, or rib location

- Differentiating enchondroma from low-grade chondrosarcoma is difficult.
  - As noted earlier, radiologic studies may fail to identify specific findings for differentiating benign from low-grade malignant lesions.
  - Radiographically, besides the obvious (cortical breakthrough, soft tissue mass, periostitis), signs that suggest aggressive nature include large size (>5 cm

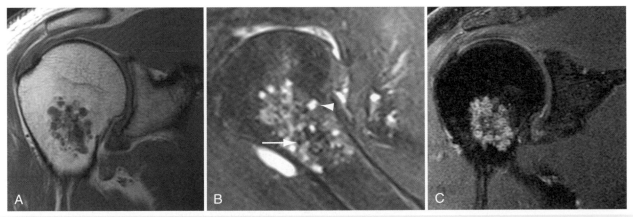

Fig. 11.56 Enchondroma, MRI appearance. **(A)** Coronal T1-weighted MRI shows a hypointense nodular pattern of a nonencapsulated lesion in the proximal humeral metaphysis. **(B)** Sagittal T2-weighted, fat-saturated image of the same lesion shows hypointense calcified matrix (arrow), as well as the punctate hyperintense cartilage nodules (arrowhead). Note that the cartilage nodules do not appear as numerous as those in Fig. 11.55; there is more stroma present. **(C)** Coronal postcontrast T1-weighted, fat-saturated image shows typical enhancement surrounding the lesion as well as the nodules; there is no additional confluent enhancement as might be found if this were a chondrosarcoma rather than enchondroma.

should raise concern), and significant endosteal scalloping (e.g., greater than 2/3 of cortical thickness). Of course, any change over time is suspicious, including increase in size and/or scalloping, or change in internal mineralization pattern. Pain arising from the lesion also raises suspicion.

- Although histology is the gold standard, the pathologist may also have difficulty; sampling bias of a percutaneously acquired specimen, along with histologic criteria (number of mitoses per high power field), reflecting the ill-defined spectrum of benign to malignant, often causing the pathologist to seek out the radiologist to make the final call.

- If the lesion is indeterminate by imaging and there is pain unexplained by adjacent pathology, tissue sampling is generally advised.
  - Because of potential sampling bias (percutaneous biopsy can only sample a small region of the tumor), these lesions typically proceed to open biopsy; however, high-risk location may prompt an initial effort at imaging-guided percutaneous needle sampling.
  - As with any primary tumor if percutaneous needle biopsy is requested, the approach should be discussed with the bone tumor surgeon to ensure that no potential flaps are compromised and that the tract is along the potential incision line.
  - Surgical resection can yield a definitive diagnosis, but may cause significant morbidity depending on the location.

- If a lesion has imaging features of a benign enchondroma but the patient has pain that cannot be easily attributed to other musculoskeletal pathology (e.g., adjacent joint pathology), follow-up is prudent.
  - Follow-up is also recommended a large but otherwise nonaggressive-appearing lesion without pain.
  - If prior radiographs are available for comparison, diagnosis may be facilitated; any change over time after skeletal maturity should be cause for concern.

- Follow-up is not needed for asymptomatic lesions with no concerning imaging features or for lesions in the hands or feet.

- Unfortunately there is no good data on time interval for follow-up imaging of an indeterminate chondroid lesion, and when it is safe to stop.
  - The interval can also be based on level of concern.
  - Since low-grade lesions are slow growing, it is probably reasonable to re-image annually.
  - In some cases radiographs are adequate, but if the imaging finding that generated the concern is visualized best on CT or MR, then that modality is preferred as a follow-up exam.

MULTIPLE ENCHONDROMATOSIS (OLLIER DISEASE AND MAFFUCCI SYNDROME)

Ollier Disease

- Multiple enchondromatosis (Ollier disease) is a rare developmental abnormality characterized by the presence of enchondromas in the metaphyses and diaphyses of multiple bones.

- The disease appears in early childhood and is neither hereditary nor familial and is considered to be a dysplasia.

- Most cases are unilateral and localized to one extremity. They may look like typical enchondromas or may be much larger and may appear grotesque, especially in the fingers.

- Lesions in the metaphyses of the long bones frequently do not have a typical appearance of enchondroma but rather appear striated, with vertical lucencies and densities. Most have some chondroid matrix (Fig. 11.57).

- The involved limb usually is short and frequently deformed.

- The risk for malignant transformation (usually chondrosarcoma) approaches 35% by age 40, so surveillance is recommended.

- The disease probably results from the ectopic deposition of cartilage rests from the physis, which continue to grow, causing the bony deformities. Loss of physeal cartilage accounts for the limb shortening.

Maffucci Syndrome

- Rare syndrome which falls in the spectrum of multiple enchondromatosis, in which enchondromatosis is found in combination with soft tissue and visceral hemangiomas.

- Phleboliths may be present, which, in addition to the features of enchondromatosis, make the radiographic diagnosis (Fig. 11.58).

- Maffucci syndrome is believed to have a much higher malignant potential than enchondromatosis alone; in addition to the enchondromas, the hemangiomas may degenerate to sarcoma. Surveillance is required.

OSTEOCHONDRAL EXOSTOSIS (OSTEOCHONDROMA)

- *Exostosis* is a general term for an excrescence from the bone surface; this can be from a traumatic origin (e.g., malunion of fracture), developmental (i.e., avian spur at the elbow), or tumor (osteochondroma).

- Osteochondromas are one of the most common benign tumors, seen in approximately 3% of the population.

- Osteochondromas are the result of displaced physeal cartilage, which causes lateral bone growth from the metaphyseal region.
  - The displaced physeal cartilage produces new bone, creating an excrescence from the underlying metaphyseal bone.
  - This results in the essential feature of an osteochondroma: continuity of the normal marrow, cortex, and periosteum between the osteochondroma and the host bone (Fig. 11.59).
  - The osteochondroma is covered by a cartilaginous cap, which is its source of growth.
  - Growth may continue up until skeletal maturation, but no lesional growth should occur after that time.
  - Chondroid matrix may be seen within the cartilaginous cap, but otherwise the appearance is that of deformed but otherwise normal bone.
  - The size may range from small to very large, and soft tissues are displaced by the bony mass.

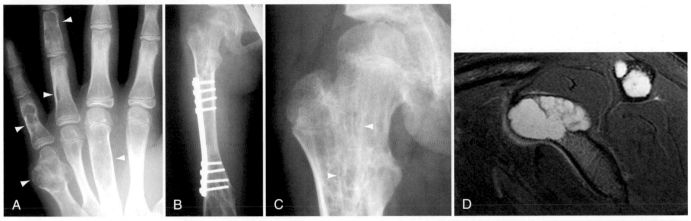

Fig. 11.57 Multiple enchondromatosis (Ollier disease). **(A)** AP radiograph of the hand in a 13-year-old boy shows several enchondromas *(arrowheads)*. Several of these show chondroid matrix typical of enchondromas. Bone expansion by enchondromas in Ollier disease can be much greater than in this example, to the point of being grotesque. **(B)** AP radiograph of the femur in a 9-year-old patient with Ollier disease. Note that the dysplasia involves the metaphyses and epiphyses but not the diaphyses. In this case the patient has undergone limb lengthening, which is the reason for the lateral plating. **(C)** Detail of the proximal femur from B. The vertical striations that can be seen in multiple enchondromatosis are shown *(arrowheads)*. Notice that the appearance of the dysplasia in multiple enchondromatosis can be very different from that of a routine enchondroma (e.g., Fig. 11.54). Chondroid matrix need not be seen in multiple enchondromatosis. **(D)** Sagittal T2-weighted, fat-saturated image through the scapula demonstrates two distinct lobulated, expanded hyperintense lesions within the coracoid process and acromion. The appearance is typical of benign cartilage; this is a case of multiple enchondromatosis (Ollier disease). (B and C, Images used with permission from BJ Manaster, MD, from the American College of Radiology Learning File.)

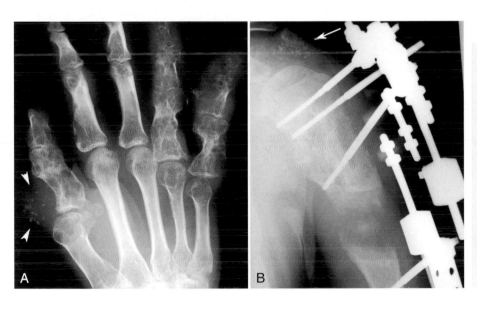

Fig. 11.58 Maffucci syndrome. **(A)** AP radiograph of the hand in a 31-year-old patient with Maffucci syndrome. Note the multiple, fairly typical-appearing enchondromas. There also are soft tissue hemangiomas, the most prominent seen at the proximal phalanx of the thumb, where phleboliths are seen in the soft tissue mass *(arrowheads)*. **(B)** AP radiograph of the proximal humerus in an 11-year-old girl with Maffucci syndrome. Note the dysplastic appearance of the proximal humerus, which would be typical of either Ollier disease or Maffucci syndrome. However, the soft tissue hemangioma in the shoulder (note the phleboliths, *arrow*) leads to the diagnosis of Maffucci syndrome. The external fixation hardware is related to limb lengthening to compensate for severely shortened limbs in Maffucci syndrome, which are caused by diversion of growth plate cartilage to the enchondromas.

Key Concepts

Osteochondroma

- Metaphyseal: Osteochondroma usually points away from adjacent joint
- Around knee most common location, but can occur anywhere
- Ninety-five percent of cases found in extremities; most are solitary
- Distinct appearance, with normal marrow, cortex, and periosteum extending from the underlying bone into the osteochondroma, and a cartilage cap, which may or may not show chondroid matrix
- Growth ceases at skeletal maturity
- Mechanical complications are common
- Pain or continued growth after skeletal maturity warrants exclusion of sarcomatous transformation

- An osteochondroma can be *pedunculated* (cauliflower-like; Figs. 11.59 and 11.60) or *sessile* (broad-based; Fig. 11.61).
  - Pedunculated osteochondromas usually grow away from the adjacent joint.
  - Sessile osteochondroma may be mistaken for metaphyseal dysplasia because they result in apparent broadening (undertubulation) of the bone.
- Ninety-five percent of cases occur in the extremities, and 40% are found around the knee. Ninety percent are solitary.
  - The most common locations of osteochondromas are the distal femur (30%), proximal humerus (10–20%), tibia (20%), and fibula, all regions of rapid growth, though they are seen involving many other bones, including the pelvis, scapula, spine, and small tubular bones.

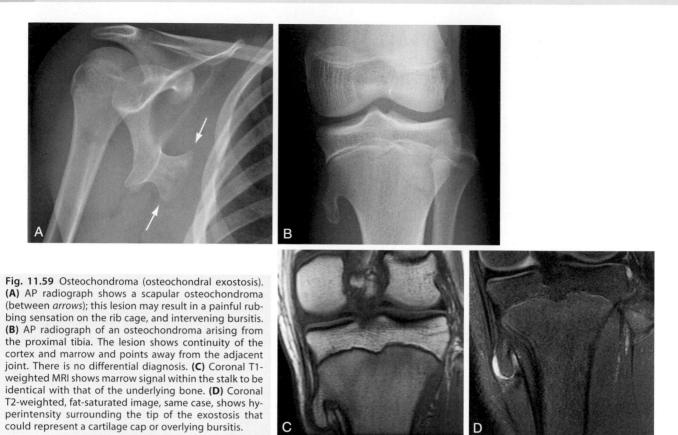

Fig. 11.59 Osteochondroma (osteochondral exostosis). **(A)** AP radiograph shows a scapular osteochondroma (between *arrows*); this lesion may result in a painful rubbing sensation on the rib cage, and intervening bursitis. **(B)** AP radiograph of an osteochondroma arising from the proximal tibia. The lesion shows continuity of the cortex and marrow and points away from the adjacent joint. There is no differential diagnosis. **(C)** Coronal T1-weighted MRI shows marrow signal within the stalk to be identical with that of the underlying bone. **(D)** Coronal T2-weighted, fat-saturated image, same case, shows hyperintensity surrounding the tip of the exostosis that could represent a cartilage cap or overlying bursitis.

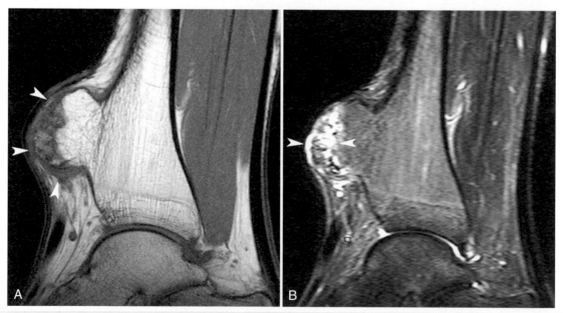

Fig. 11.60 Pedunculated osteochondroma. Sagittal T1-weighted MRI **(A)** and sagittal T2-weighted, fat-saturated MRI **(B)** show a pedunculated anterior tibial osteochondroma with overlying cartilage cap. The cap is isointense to muscle on T1-weighted image but hyperintense on T2-weighted image *(arrowheads)*. The cap is thicker than that seen on the osteochondroma pictured in Fig. 11.59, but the cap remains less than 1 cm in thickness. Some low-signal material is seen within the cap, representing calcified chondroid matrix.

- The imaging appearance of an osteochondroma usually is pathognomonic.
  - The pedunculated or cauliflower variety can be differentiated from a parosteal osteosarcoma by the type of matrix and the lack of continuity of the cortex and marrow with host bone seen in the osteosarcoma.

- Occasionally myositis ossificans that is adjacent to the cortex may be confused with an osteochondroma, but careful examination demonstrates no cortical or marrow continuity with myositis ossificans.
- CT may be helpful when differentiation is difficult. The broad-based sessile type of osteochondroma may

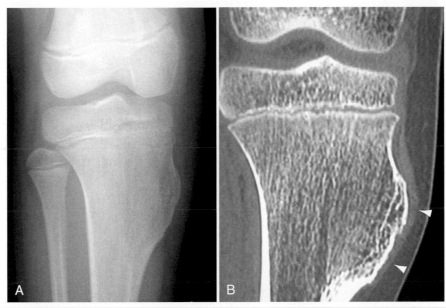

Fig. 11.61 Sessile osteochondroma. AP radiograph **(A)** and coronal CT reformat **(B)** show typical bulgelike sessile osteochondroma at the medial proximal tibial metaphysis. Note thin, presumed cartilage cap *(arrowheads* in B).

be confused with old postfracture deformity, a metaphyseal dysplasia, or the occasional cortically-based fibrous dysplasia.

- The MRI appearance of an osteochondroma is characteristic, with continuity of normal-appearing host bone marrow and cortex extending into the lesion.
  - The overlying hyaline cartilage cap is high signal on T2-weighted MR images, typical of cartilage, and is uniform or gently undulating in thickness, generally less than 1 cm thick in adults (see Figs. 11.59 through 11.61), though it may be up to 3 cm thick in children.
  - The cap is covered by a thin perichondrium that is hypointense on T1- and T2-weighted sequences.
  - Contrast enhancement is seen only in the thin tissue covering the cap and in septae within the cap.
- Complications of a solitary osteochondroma (Fig. 11.62) include:
  - Formation of an overlying adventitial bursa that may become inflamed. Bursa formation can be painful and cause an apparent palpable lesion enlargement.
  - Mechanical complications such as limitation of motion and compression of adjacent nerves, muscles, or blood vessels.
    - Nerve impingement and pseudoaneurysm formation can occasionally occur, especially around the knee in the popliteal fossa.
    - Scapular blade lesions that protrude anteriorly can cause pain and palpable friction with motion as they slide over the ribs.
  - Fracture of the neck of a pedunculated lesion.
  - Very rarely, malignant transformation of the cartilage cap.
    - Few (probably far fewer than 1%) solitary osteochondromas undergo malignant transformation of the cartilage cap to chondrosarcoma (accounting for 8% of all chondrosarcomas).
    - Specific findings include destruction of exostosis bone, destruction of previously present matrix in

the cartilage cap, a thick (>1 cm) or irregular cartilage cap, or growth of the cartilage cap after skeletal maturity.
  - However, osteochondromas at the pelvis have a higher likelihood for malignant transformation, and these are usually treated aggressively with resection.
  - More frequently there is no early radiographic change, but the patient reports pain or growth of the osteochondroma after skeletal maturity.
  - In the absence of mechanical reasons for pain or the formation of a bursa simulating the growth of the osteochondroma, such clinical symptoms indicate malignant transformation until proved otherwise.
  - If malignant degeneration is suspected, a chondrosarcoma workup is done, which includes MRI.
- Symptomatic osteochondromas are treated with resection. The entire cartilage cap must be removed to prevent recurrence.

MULTIPLE HEREDITARY OSTEOCHONDROMAS

- Multiple hereditary osteochondromas, also called multiple hereditary exostosis (MHE), is an uncommon autosomal dominant disorder resulting in multiple osteochondromas, usually numerous.
- Patients present with multiple osteochondromas and short stature, the latter caused by diversion of physeal cartilage to the osteochondromas with consequent diminished longitudinal bone growth.
- The lesions first appear in childhood as lumps adjacent to joints. Long bones are affected most frequently, but the spine is also involved in up to 27%.
- Although some of the osteochondromas are cauliflower-like, most are broad-based sessile lesions. These sessile osteochondromas result in a greater circumference of the metaphyses (Fig. 11.63); the deformity may simulate

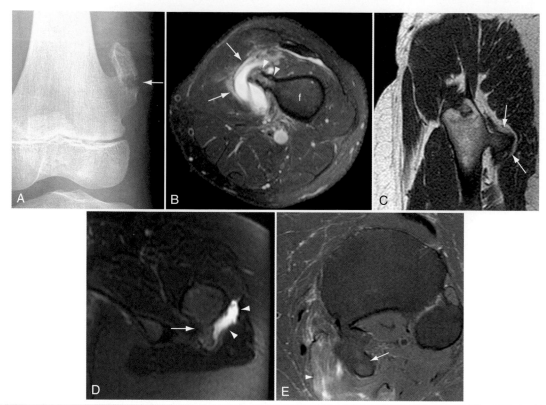

Fig. 11.62 Osteochondroma: benign complications. **(A)** Fracture through the base of a pedunculate osteochondroma *(arrow)*. **(B)** Bursitis. Axial fat-suppressed T2-weighted MR image shows fluid-distended bursa *(arrows)* that has formed over a pedunculated medial distal femoral **(f)** osteochondroma *(arrowheads)*. **(C)** Sagittal T1-weighted MR image shows a posterior proximal femoral osteochondroma *(arrows)*; this was a symptomatic lesion that the patient felt was enlarging. **(D)** Axial T2-weighted, fat-saturated image of the same lesion as in C shows the posterior osteochondroma *(arrow)* with adjacent fluid-filled bursa *(arrowheads)*. It is the distension of this bursa that mimicked growth of the exostosis. **(E)** Axial T2-weighted, fat-saturated image of a different osteochondroma *(arrow)*. The adjacent gastrocnemius muscle is edematous *(arrowhead)*; this is denervation edema, related to interference of the nerve by the osteochondroma.

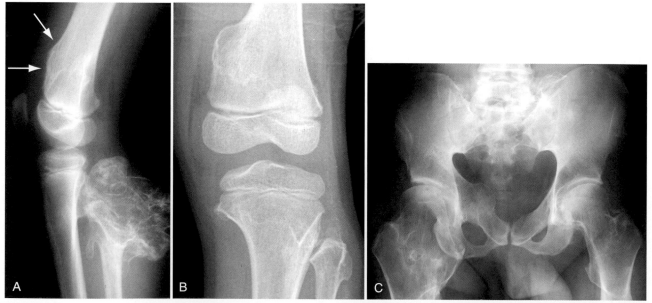

Fig. 11.63 Multiple osteochondromas. **(A)** Lateral radiograph of the knee in a 7-year-old girl demonstrates the large cauliflower-like osteochondroma of the proximal fibula and a sessile lesion of the distal femur *(arrows)*. These sessile osteochondromas occasionally are mistaken for a metaphyseal dysplasia, leading to a missed diagnosis of multiple hereditary osteochondromas. **(B)** AP radiograph of a different child, showing sessile osteochondroma at the distal femur and more pedunculated osteochondromas arising from the tibia and fibula. **(C)** AP radiograph of the pelvis shows an older child with multiple osteochondromas, including lesions arising from the pubic rami. The right pubic ramus lesion is obvious, whereas the left appears only as broadening of the bone. Similarly, the right femoral neck has an obvious large, somewhat sessile lesion, whereas the left may simply give the appearance of calcar buttressing, though it is in fact a more subtle sessile lesion. If the right hemipelvis in this case matched the appearance of the left, the abnormalities might be either overlooked or called an undertubulation dysplasia.

a bone dysplasia, particularly because the lesions are usually bilateral.

- Coxa valga and Madelung deformity may also be seen.
- The elbow and wrist joints are often dislocated and/or deformed.

■ Due to the multiplicity of osteochondromas, patients with multiple hereditary osteochondromas are at higher risk for development of chondrosarcoma. Current estimate is a less than 1% lifetime risk, which is lower than previously thought.

- The imaging findings suggesting degeneration are identical to those of a solitary osteochondroma, including underlying bone destruction, scattering of previously noted cartilage matrix (termed 'snow-storm' appearance), and enlargement of the cartilage cap over time.

■ Treatment of multiple exostoses depends on circumstances, with local resection as necessary for mechanical problems. The patients are observed for sarcomatous transformation because prophylactic resection of all lesions is not a realistic option.

DYSPLASIA EPIPHYSEALIS HEMIMELICA (TREVOR DISEASE)

■ Dysplasia epiphysealis hemimelica (DEH), also known as Trevor disease or Trevor–Fairbank disease, has been described as an intraarticular epiphyseal osteochondroma leading to articular deformity (Fig. 11.64). A more precise description is epiphyseal cartilage overgrowth, sometimes with multiple ossification centers and metaphyseal involvement.

■ Rare (1:1,000,000), M>F.

- The lesions may occur in single joint or multiple joints in a single extremity. The knee and ankle are the most common sites of occurrence.
- Histologically, the lesions are identical to osteochondromas. Radiographically, they have the appearance of a lobulated mass arising from the epiphysis, which is usually well mineralized.
- MRI can help define the extent of the lesion and its relationship to the joint surfaces. Not surprisingly, Trevor disease causes joint deformity, pain, and limited range of motion.
- Management is surgical, with resection of the bony excrescences.

PERIOSTEAL (JUXTACORTICAL) CHONDROMA

■ Periosteal chondroma is a benign cartilaginous lesion originating from the inner layer of the periosteum (see Fig. 11.49).

■ The lesion produces a soft tissue mass and cortical pressure erosion that can be difficult to differentiate from that seen in periosteal osteosarcoma.

■ Calcification is produced in the soft tissue mass in about 50% of periosteal chondromas, also potentially resembling a periosteal osteosarcoma.

■ Periosteal chondromas occur in a wide age range and are seen in both large and small tubular bones (70% occur in the humerus or femur, 25% in digits).

■ Periosteal reaction can be striking, falsely leading one to believe the lesion to be aggressive.

■ Buttressing of the cortex may be found at the ends of the lesion.

■ The MRI appearance may be useful, showing cartilage nodules on fluid-sensitive sequences; however, the soft

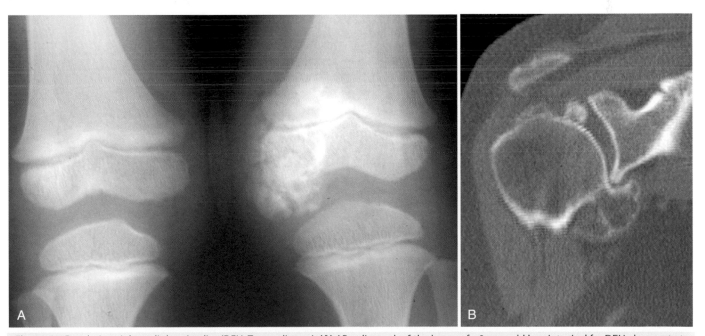

Fig. 11.64 Dysplasia epiphysealis hemimelica (DEH, Trevor disease). **(A)** AP radiograph of the knees of a 9-year-old boy is typical for DEH, demonstrating an osteochondroma-like lesion arising from the epiphysis. This intraarticular process is usually solitary. **(B)** Coronal CT reconstruction of the proximal right humerus in a different patient shows similar findings, with multiple osteochondroma-like lesions arising from the humeral head. (A, Image used with permission from BJ Manaster, MD, from the American College of Radiology Learning File.)

tissue mass adjacent to the bone destruction may make the lesion appear more aggressive by MRI than by radiograph.

- Heterogeneous contrast enhancement is seen, particularly at the periphery of the lesion, and there is marrow involvement in 20% of cases. The clinical behavior, however, is benign.
- The lesion is treated with wide excision, whenever possible, to preclude recurrence.
- The major differential diagnosis, as noted previously, is periosteal osteosarcoma. Periosteal chondrosarcoma is extremely rare, and the two cannot be reliably differentiated by imaging; this serves as another reason to treat with wide excision. TGCT can cause cortical 'saucerization' (i.e., scalloping of the external bone surface), with a soft tissue mass that occasionally appears to be a surface lesion, but MRI should serve to differentiate this tendon-based lesion.

CHONDROBLASTOMA

- Chondroblastoma (Codman tumor) is a rare benign cartilaginous tumor found almost exclusively in the epiphysis in skeletally immature patients and young adults.
- This is one of the few neoplasms characteristically found in the epiphysis.
- Chondroblastoma tends to be eccentrically located within the epiphysis. If there is partial physeal closure, the lesion may extend into the metaphysis.
- The most common site of involvement is the proximal humerus, followed by the proximal tibia, and proximal and distal femur. The patella or bones of the hindfoot may also be involved.
- The lesion typically has geographic and sclerotic margins. Margins are often lobulated, best appreciated with MRI or CT, typical of cartilaginous lesions.

- The tumor is predominantly lytic, although 25–50% show some amount of chondroid matrix. This may be very subtle, seen only by CT. Even though the lesion is nonaggressive in appearance, most chondroblastomas elicit a thick periosteal reaction along the metaphysis, a location remote from the lesion (Fig. 11.65).
  - The cause for this finding is uncertain, but the reaction may be mediated by hormone-like factors released by the tumor.

Key Concepts

Chondroblastoma

- Epiphyseal location, skeletally immature patients and young adults
- Proximal humerus most common location
- Chondroid matrix present in up to 50% of cases
- May contain fluid-fluid levels, usually related to secondary ABC
- May elicit prominent periosteal reaction in the metaphysis
- Differential diagnosis: LCH and infection (epiphyseal osteomyelitis) in children; GCT or articular-based process (e.g., PVNS) in adolescents and young adults

- MRI shows signal intensity isointense with muscle on T1-weighted images and high cartilage-type signal intensity on T2-weighted images, often in a lobulated pattern characteristic of a chondroid lesion.
  - 30% contain secondary ABC with fluid-fluid levels.
  - A joint effusion and adjacent bone marrow, periosteal, and soft tissue edema and enhancement are often present.
  - Because of the adjacent bone marrow and soft-tissue reaction, MRI often suggests a more aggressive lesion than is demonstrated by radiography; in general radiographic features are more reliable than MR in assessing the aggressiveness of a tumor.

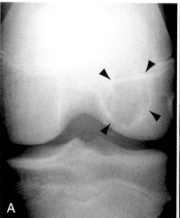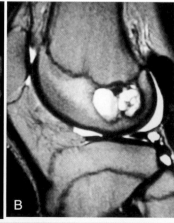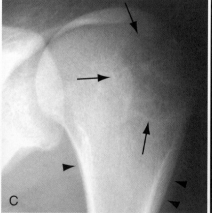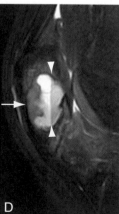

Fig. 11.65 Chondroblastoma. **(A)** AP radiograph of the knee in a 14-year-old boy shows a geographic lytic lesion in the epiphysis with a narrow zone of transition and sclerotic (type 1A) margin *(arrowheads)*, a typical appearance of chondroblastoma with the open physis. **(B)** T2-weighted sagittal MR image demonstrates the epiphyseal location, as well as the largely homogeneous high-signal appearance that can be typical of cartilage lesions. Also note surrounding high-signal bone marrow edema and joint effusion. **(C)** AP radiograph of a chondroblastoma in a different patient, an 18-year-old man. In this case the lytic lesion is again located predominantly in the epiphysis and has a partially nonsclerotic margin *(arrows)*. Note the very dense, mature periosteal reaction in the metaphysis *(arrowheads)*, remote from the tumor. Both the location of the lesion in the proximal humerus epiphysis and the dense periosteal reaction away from the tumor are typical of chondroblastoma. **(D)** Sagittal T2-weighted, fat-saturated MR image shows a lesion within the patella that has a solid component anteriorly *(arrow)*, with fluid-fluid levels posteriorly *(arrowheads)*. This represents an aneurysmal bone cyst arising in a solid chondroblastoma. Chondroblastoma is one of the more common original lesions in which an aneurysmal bone cyst may arise. (D, Image used with permission from BJ Manaster, MD, from STATdx website, Amirsys, Inc.)

- Diagnosis is made by radiography, and CT can be helpful in confirming matrix calcification.
- MRI may also demonstrate other features of chondroblastoma, such as a superimposed ABC (see Fig. 11.65D).
- Patients with chondroblastoma present with localized pain.
- Treatment is by curettage and bone graft. Recurrence rate is as high as 15%, but this can be reduced with presurgical injection of phenol, alcohol, or similar adjuvant. Polymethylmethacrylate (PMMA) can be used in larger lesions. Metastatic potential is negligible, with only isolated case reports of metastatic spread.
- The major differential diagnoses in the adolescent or young adult include GCT crossing into the epiphysis, articular lesions with large cysts (e.g., PVNS), and clear-cell chondrosarcoma. In children the differential diagnosis includes LCH and epiphyseal osteomyelitis.

CHONDROMYXOID FIBROMA

- Chondromyxoid fibroma is a very rare benign cartilaginous lesion that also contains fibrous and myxoid tissue.
- This lesion is so rare that it should very infrequently be offered as a likely differential diagnostic possibility.
- Although the age range is wide, it is most frequently seen in the second and third decades.
- Fifty percent of the lesions are found about the knee, with the majority in the proximal tibia and the others distributed in the proximal femur, flat bones, tarsal bones, and other small bones of the hand or foot.
- Lesion margins are geographic and sclerotic, often lobulated. The tumor usually occurs eccentrically in the metaphysis.
- Chondromyxoid fibroma usually has a thick sclerotic margin and may cause mild cortical expansion (Fig. 11.66B).
- Although this is a cartilaginous lesion, it is rare to find calcified tumor matrix within it.
- The MRI appearance is nonspecific, with low signal intensity on T1-weighted images and high signal intensity on T2-weighted images, which is often inhomogeneous.
- Patients present with local pain and swelling.
- The lesion follows a benign course and undergoes malignant transformation only rarely.
- Treatment is with curettage and bone grafting. The recurrence rate is high (approximately 25%) following curettage, perhaps because of incomplete removal of this lobulated lesion.

CHONDROSARCOMA

- Chondrosarcoma (also called *central chondrosarcoma* or *conventional chondrosarcoma*) is the third most common primary malignant bone tumor.
- The peak incidence is 50–70 years of age, but the range is wide; because of the frequent occurrence of this tumor, age should not be used to dismiss this diagnosis in a teenager or young adult.
- Chondrosarcoma may be either primary or secondary (i.e., arising de novo or from malignant degeneration from a preexisting benign cartilaginous lesion, most often an enchondroma) (Figs. 11.67 through 11.70).

- These lesions are usually metaphyseal in location and are particularly common in the proximal long bones as well as the pelvis and the shoulder girdle.
- Although enchondroma is common in the hands and feet, it is extremely rare for these lesions to undergo malignant transformation; chondrosarcoma is rare in the peripheral extremities.
- Matrix mineralization is present in 78% of chondrosarcomas, but the amount of chondroid tumor matrix varies, ranging from completely lytic lesions to lytic lesions with only a few flecks of calcification, to dense aggregates of chondroid matrix (see Figs. 11.67 and 11.68).
- Ninety percent of chondrosarcomas are low grade.
  - Although even low-grade chondrosarcomas are generally large (>5 cm) at presentation, they tend to be well defined.
  - Like enchondromas, low-grade chondrosarcomas may show only mild endosteal scalloping. However, endosteal scalloping that removes more than two-thirds of the cortical thickness favors a chondrosarcoma over an enchondroma. (Please see further discussion of distinguishing enchondroma from chondrosarcoma in the section on 'Enchondroma').
  - Low-grade chondrosarcomas can have a narrow zone of transition, without sclerotic margins.
  - Low-grade chondrosarcoma usually shows no cortical breakthrough or soft tissue mass; however these characteristics can be seen in 50% of higher-grade lesions.
  - In general, low-grade tumors contain more myxoid tissue and therefore tend to have less chondroid matrix.
- Adjacent cortical thickening by combined periosteal and endosteal new bone formation may occur (see Fig. 11.68). Endosteal thickening is seen in only a few other aggressive lesions in patients of this age group, including primary lymphoma of bone, Ewing sarcoma in a younger age group, and osteomyelitis.
- It is very important to be aware that chondrosarcomas are common malignant tumors of bone, and most are not aggressive in radiographic appearance. Therefore if a central lesion in the correct age group appears slightly to moderately aggressive, with a questionable widened zone of transition or endosteal scalloping, the diagnosis of chondrosarcoma should be offered, whether or not definite chondroid matrix is found.
- This lesion is commonly underdiagnosed because it so often appears nonaggressive. Underdiagnosis results in delayed treatment, which puts the patient at risk for recurrence or metastatic disease.

Key Concepts

Chondrosarcoma

- Third most primary malignant bone tumor
- Usually demonstrates chondroid tumor matrix
- Usually low grade and radiographically nonaggressive
- Central, metaphyseal, with endosteal thickening
- Increasing pain or lesion growth in an adult exostosis or centrally located enchondroma should suggest diagnosis

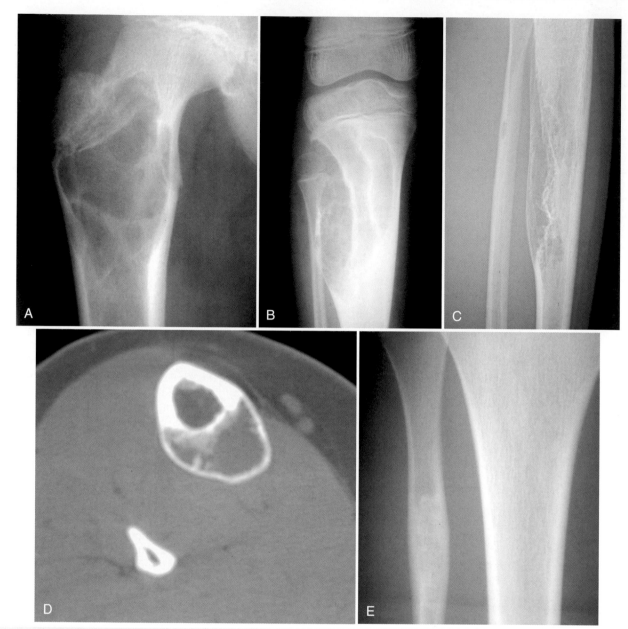

Fig. 11.66 Transverse locations of tumors in long bones. **(A)** AP radiograph showing a central lesion in the proximal femur, a solitary bone cyst in an 11-year-old boy. **(B)** AP radiograph demonstrating an eccentric location of a metaphyseal lesion, in this case a chondromyxoid fibroma in an 18-year-old woman. **(C)** A cortically-based lesion in the midshaft of the tibia in a 14-year-old girl. Although from the radiograph alone one may not be able to determine that the lesion is completely cortically-based, CT in D confirms this. **(D)** In this case, the lesion is an unusual manifestation of fibrous dysplasia, which can occasionally be cortically-based. **(E)** AP radiograph demonstrating a nonossifying fibroma that is healing with sclerosis. Nonossifying fibroma is usually a cortically-based lesion; however, when it occurs in very small bones such as the fibula, it fills the entire marrow space and gives the appearance of being a central lesion. For an example of a juxtacortical (surface) lesion, see Fig. 11.3A and B.

- On MRI well-differentiated chondrosarcoma usually shows the lobulated T2-bright features of hyaline cartilage typical of benign cartilage lesions (seen in 72% of chondrosarcomas).
  - The fibrous stroma between the chondroid nodules often enhances intensely, as does the periphery of the lesion, but this is nonspecific because benign enchondromas have a similar pattern of enhancement.
  - Some authors believe that 'puddling' or confluent enhancement may help to differentiate some low-grade chondrosarcomas from enchondroma (see Figs. 11.69 and 11.70). Higher-grade lesions will

appear nonspecific and have inhomogeneous high signal intensity on T2-weighted imaging; the lesion appears more disorganized, and lobulation may not be detectable. Mineralized matrix will be seen as low signal intensity on all sequences. Enhancement in higher-grade lesions is more generalized, surrounding regions of low-signal necrosis.
- The major differential diagnosis of chondrosarcoma is enchondroma. Distinguishing features were discussed previously.
  - The lesion can also be confused with a bone infarct if the bone infarct matrix does not have its typical

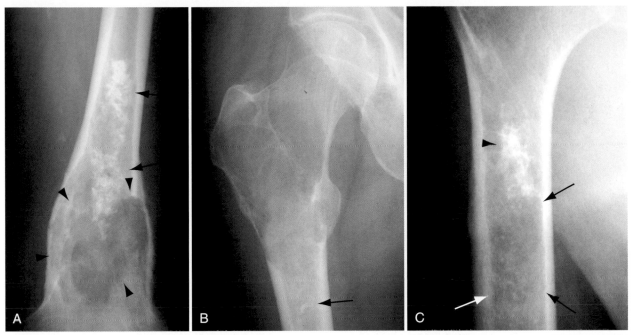

Fig. 11.67 Intramedullary chondrosarcoma arising in enchondroma, with obvious degeneration. **(A)** AP radiograph of the distal femur in a 79-year-old man. This demonstrates the typical matrix of an enchondroma in its proximal portion *(arrows)*, extending into a highly destructive lesion more distally *(arrowheads)*. This is a chondrosarcoma arising in an enchondroma (see also Fig. 11.56). **(B)** AP radiograph of a geographic lytic lesion with a mildly widened zone of transition (type 1C) margin in the proximal femur of a 52-year-old man. There is subtle chondroid matrix in the proximal femoral shaft *(arrow)*. With the aggressive lesion margins, chondroid matrix, proximal location, and patient's age, the diagnosis can only be chondrosarcoma. **(C)** AP radiograph of the proximal humerus in a 58-year-old man. Note the chondroid matrix in the proximal portion of the lesion *(arrowhead)*, which represents a benign enchondroma. However, lytic change distal to the matrix *(arrows)* represents destruction of bone and the distal portion of the parent enchondroma by chondrosarcoma. This more distal portion of the enchondroma has transformed to a chondrosarcoma. Note the spectrum of chondroid matrix one might expect to see in chondrosarcoma, comparing these three lesions as well as those shown in Fig. 11.68.

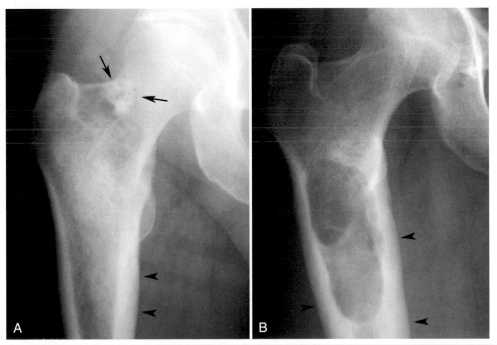

Fig. 11.68 Intramedullary chondrosarcoma arising in enchondroma, with subtle signs of sarcomatous degeneration. **(A)** AP radiograph of the proximal femur in a 38-year-old man. There is chondroid matrix in the proximal portion of the lesion *(arrows)*, and the lesion shows a destructive pattern with a somewhat wide zone of transition. These features alone make it a chondrosarcoma. In addition, there is prominent thickening of the cortex *(arrowheads)*, also a finding that may be seen in intramedullary chondrosarcoma, although it is not specific. **(B)** AP radiograph of the hip in a 51-year-old woman, also an intramedullary chondrosarcoma. In this case there is no visible chondroid matrix. The zone of transition is narrow but not sclerotic (type 1B margin), and there is cortical thickening with mild expansion related to slow tumor growth *(arrowheads)*. The location, age of the patient, and endosteal and periosteal thickening suggest the diagnosis of chondrosarcoma despite the absence of chondroid matrix or aggressive features. This is the type of lesion that is often misdiagnosed as a benign lesion.

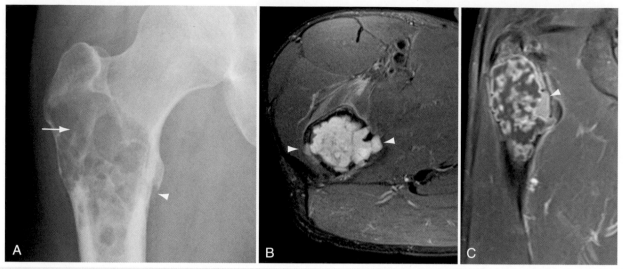

Fig. 11.69 Central chondrosarcoma, MRI appearance. **(A)** AP radiograph shows a lytic lesion arising in the proximal femoral metadiaphysis. There is no matrix. The lesion has expanded the bone slightly, and there is a tiny region of cortical breakthrough *(arrowhead)*. Distally there is cortical thickening, whereas proximally there is significant endosteal thinning *(arrow)*. Despite the absence of chondroid matrix, one must presume chondrosarcoma. **(B)** Axial T2-weighted, fat-saturated image through the subtrochanteric portion of the lesion shows hyperintense lobulations typical of benign cartilage. However, there is also significant cortical thinning and even cortical breakthrough *(arrowheads)*; this is concerning for degeneration to chondrosarcoma. **(C)** Coronal postcontrast T1-weighted, fat-saturated image of the lesion shows enhancement surrounding the nodules and the periphery as expected for enchondroma. However, there is also a region of confluent enhancement at the periphery of the lesion *(arrowhead)*, as well as proximally and distally; this, along with the cortical breakthrough, makes the diagnosis of chondrosarcoma. Pathologic evaluation showed low-grade chondrosarcoma arising in enchondroma.

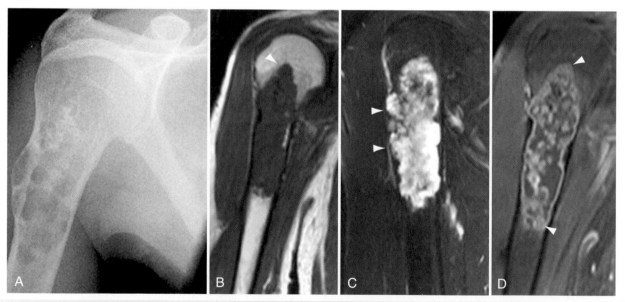

Fig. 11.70 Chondrosarcoma, low grade. **(A)** AP radiograph shows a predominantly lytic central lesion of the proximal humeral metadiaphysis. There is punctate chondroid matrix within the proximal portion of the lesion. There is expansion and an extensive area of endosteal scalloping. **(B)** Coronal T1-weighted MR image shows homogeneous hypointensity *(arrowhead)*. **(C)** Coronal T2-weighted, fat-saturated image shows typical hyperintense cartilage nodularity. There is diffuse endosteal scalloping and focal cortical breakthrough *(arrowheads)*. **(D)** Coronal postcontrast T1-weighted, fat-saturated MR image shows perilobular and peripheral enhancement, typical of enchondroma. However, there are small confluent regions of contrast enhancement *(arrowheads)* superimposed on this pattern. This is suspicious for chondrosarcoma. Pathologic evaluation showed enchondroma with small areas of degeneration to low-grade chondrosarcoma.

sharp, serpentine pattern, but MRI or CT will differentiate the two.

■ If no chondroid matrix is present, the differential diagnosis includes metastasis, plasmacytoma, pleomorphic sarcoma, fibrosarcoma, and lymphoma. If the lesion is less aggressive in appearance and without matrix, aggressive GCT might be considered.

■ Peripheral (exostotic) chondrosarcomas either may be primary or may secondarily arise as malignant transformation of an osteochondroma.

■ They are seen most frequently in the third, fourth, and fifth decades of life.

■ They are large extraosseous lesions, arising from the metaphyses of long bones, as well as the pelvis,

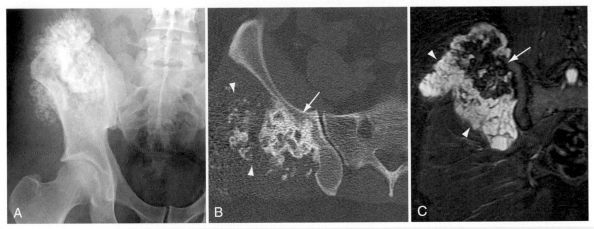

Fig. 11.71 Peripheral (exostotic) chondrosarcoma. **(A)** AP radiograph shows a large exostosis arising from the right iliac wing. Based on the radiograph, one is unlikely to be able to differentiate between osteochondroma and chondrosarcoma. **(B)** Axial CT of the same lesion shows that there is a well-defined osteochondroma *(arrow)*, but that peripherally there is a 'snowstorm' effect of less-organized chondroid matrix *(arrowheads)*. This is diagnostic of degeneration of the osteochondroma to chondrosarcoma, but MRI is required to fully evaluate the soft tissue mass. **(C)** Coronal T2-weighted, fat-saturated image of the same lesion shows the osteochondroma *(arrow)* arising from the iliac wing, with a very thick and irregular hyperintense cartilage cap and soft tissue mass *(arrowheads)* extending from the underlying lesion, confirming the diagnosis of chondrosarcoma. Axial imaging is required to fully evaluate muscle and neurovascular involvement.

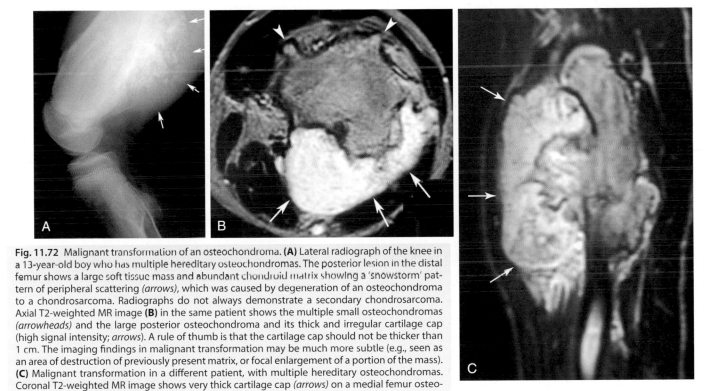

Fig. 11.72 Malignant transformation of an osteochondroma. **(A)** Lateral radiograph of the knee in a 13-year-old boy who has multiple hereditary osteochondromas. The posterior lesion in the distal femur shows a large soft tissue mass and abundant chondroid matrix showing a 'snowstorm' pattern of peripheral scattering *(arrows)*, which was caused by degeneration of an osteochondroma to a chondrosarcoma. Radiographs do not always demonstrate a secondary chondrosarcoma. Axial T2-weighted MR image **(B)** in the same patient shows the multiple small osteochondromas *(arrowheads)* and the large posterior osteochondroma and its thick and irregular cartilage cap (high signal intensity; *arrows*). A rule of thumb is that the cartilage cap should not be thicker than 1 cm. The imaging findings in malignant transformation may be much more subtle (e.g., seen as an area of destruction of previously present matrix, or focal enlargement of a portion of the mass). **(C)** Malignant transformation in a different patient, with multiple hereditary osteochondromas. Coronal T2-weighted MR image shows very thick cartilage cap *(arrows)* on a medial femur osteochondroma in the patient.

shoulder girdle, sternum, and ribs (Figs. 11.71 and 11.72).

- They most frequently show normal-appearing underlying host bone extending into an exostosis but with a thick cartilaginous cap.
- The thickness of the cartilaginous cap has attracted much commentary. One series showed that cartilaginous caps less than 1.5 cm in thickness correlate with benign lesions, whereas those greater than 2.5 cm are more likely to be malignant.

- Changes over time in the appearance of chondroid calcification in an osteochondroma may help to diagnose transformation to a chondrosarcoma, but MRI may frequently be necessary to evaluate the cartilaginous cap thickness.
- Higher-grade lesions may show destruction of the stalk as well as soft tissue mass beyond that of the cartilaginous cap (see Fig. 11.72).
- As described with osteochondromas, transformation to chondrosarcoma may produce no distinct

radiographic signs. Therefore clinical signs of new-onset nonmechanical pain and increased size after growth plate closure should be considered of primary importance in suggesting the diagnosis of peripheral chondrosarcoma.

- Ninety percent of chondrosarcomas, either central or peripheral, are low-grade lesions. Therefore local recurrence is more common than is metastatic disease.
- If the tumor recurs, it may appear as a higher-grade tumor.
- Prognosis is worse for proximal and axial lesions than distal lesions.
- Five-year survival is approximately 75% (89% for grade 1 lesions), and this can be improved by a more prompt radiologic diagnosis and meticulous surgical technique.
- Chondrosarcoma can be readily implanted in soft tissues because it does not need a blood supply to survive. Therefore recurrences may be due to tumor spill at the time of biopsy or resection.
- Wide excision is the therapy of choice. Radiation and chemotherapy do not improve survival or decrease local recurrence rates of low-grade lesions; they are reserved for high-grade lesions, cases with inadequate surgical margins, or recurrences.

CLEAR-CELL CHONDROSARCOMA

- Clear-cell chondrosarcoma is a very rare lesion that is most often mistaken for a chondroblastoma because it can be identical in imaging appearance and location in the epiphyses, especially of the proximal femur and humerus.
- Clear-cell chondrosarcoma occurs in patients who are older than those with chondroblastoma, peaking in the third decade.
- Presents clinically with slow onset of pain.

- Long-bone epiphysis (proximal femur most common), in contrast with other long-bone chondrosarcomas, which are mostly metaphyseal.
- It is usually geographic in appearance, with a narrow zone of transition and sclerotic margin. Periosteal reaction and cortical breakthrough are rare. Chondroid matrix may be present but is usually absent.
- MRI shows high T2 signal.
- Main differential diagnosis is chondroblastoma (chondroblastoma patients typically are younger).
- If left untreated, clear-cell chondrosarcoma may become much more aggressive. Treatment is wide excision; curettage alone can result in an aggressive recurrence.

DEDIFFERENTIATED CHONDROSARCOMA

- A portion of a low-grade chondrosarcoma may dedifferentiate into a high-grade, highly aggressive lesion. This dedifferentiation results in a neoplasm that may have several elements, including fibrosarcoma, pleomorphic sarcoma, high-grade chondrosarcoma, and osteosarcoma, superimposed on a well-differentiated cartilage tumor. As many as 10% of chondrosarcomas dedifferentiate.
- The radiographic appearance of dedifferentiated chondrosarcoma follows the pathologic findings.
- Fifty-three percent show areas with features of low-grade chondrosarcoma, with other areas with highly aggressive features such as bone lysis (Fig. 11.73).
- It is important to choose a biopsy site that includes the more aggressive portion of the lesion.
- Prognosis of dedifferentiated chondrosarcoma is poor, with a 5-year survival rate of only 24%. Metastases to the lung are common. Treatment is with radical excision and chemotherapy.

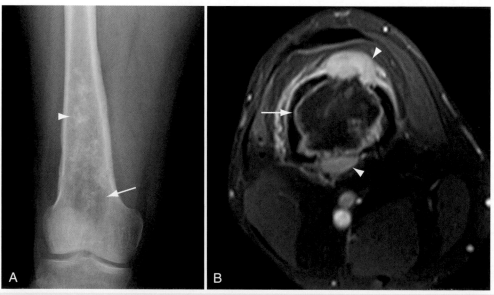

Fig. 11.73 Dedifferentiated chondrosarcoma. **(A)** AP radiograph shows typical chondroid matrix within a large lytic lesion *(arrowhead)*. There is thickened cortex, typical of low-grade chondrosarcoma. Superimposed on this is a lytic lesion, having a distinctly different appearance *(arrow)*. **(B)** Axial postcontrast T1-weighted, fat-saturated image through the lytic region shows peripheral and some central enhancement of the underlying chondrosarcoma *(arrow)*. However, there is also an intensely enhancing soft tissue mass breaking through the cortex anteriorly and posteriorly *(arrowheads)*. This changing character should alert the reader to dedifferentiation of the lesion. At biopsy the underlying lesion was low-grade chondrosarcoma; the more aggressive mass proved to be a high-grade spindle cell sarcoma. This fits the definition of dedifferentiated chondrosarcoma.

Fibrous Tumors and Tumorlike Conditions

FIBROUS DYSPLASIA

- Fibrous dysplasia is not a neoplasm but rather a hamartomatous fibro-osseous metaplasia or dysplasia consisting of a fibrous stroma with islands of osteoid and woven bone.
- The lesion is relatively common. Although there is a wide age range of occurrence, it most often is detected in the second and third decades of life.
- Fifteen to twenty percent of cases of fibrous dysplasia are polyostotic.
  - Polyostotic fibrous dysplasia has a more aggressive clinical and radiographic appearance and usually becomes symptomatic before the age of 10 years.
  - In 90% of polyostotic cases the lesions are monomelic (i.e., involve a single limb).
- Fibrous dysplasia can be found in any bone but is uncommon in the spine.
  - The most common areas of involvement include the tubular bones (in which the lesions are usually central and metadiaphyseal), ribs, pelvis, skull (particularly the base of skull), and facial bones.
- The lesions range from being completely lucent, to 'ground-glass density' (discussed previously), to densely sclerotic.
  - The density depends on the amount of woven bone present in the fibrous stroma.
- Fibrous dysplasia has a range of radiographic appearances, depending on whether it is found in the skull, pelvis, or tubular bones.
  - Lesion density tends to depend on location. In general, lesions in the base of the skull tend to be sclerotic (Fig. 11.74).

- Calvarial lesions range from lytic to dense and show a nonaggressive expansion of bone.
- Fibrous dysplasia in the ribs and tubular bones tends to have ground-glass density (Figs. 11.75 and 11.76).
- Pelvic and scapular lesions may be bubbly and expansile (Fig. 11.77).
- Bones involved with fibrous dysplasia are frequently expanded, often with cortical thinning (see Fig. 11.76).
  - The thin expanded bones are 'soft', and long bones may develop bowing and angulation deformities with weight-bearing, often resulting in limb-length discrepancy. This may result in a *shepherd's crook deformity*, with severe varus of the femoral neck (see Fig. 11.76C), though this can also be seen in Paget's disease and osteogenesis imperfecta.
  - Polyostotic disease with deformed bones, often with a ground-glass density and lacking trabecular definition, makes for a distinct radiographic appearance.
  - Although the lesions in the long bones are usually central, fibrous dysplasia can also be cortically-based. When this occurs in the tibia, it can appear identical to osteofibrous dysplasia (ossifying fibroma) and adamantinoma (see Fig. 11.36).

Key Concepts

Fibrous Dysplasia

- Long bones: Expansile, cortical thinning, mildly opaque (ground glass), bowing. 'Long lesion in a long bone'
- Skull: May be densely sclerotic, decreases size of orbit and sinuses. CT shows expansion, ground glass
- Pelvis: Lytic and bubbly, often large, or mildly expansile
- Fifteen to twenty percent polyostotic, usually unilateral
- Treatment is for symptoms only
- McCune–Albright syndrome: Fibrous dysplasia + hormonal disorder + 'coast of Maine' café-au-lait spots

---

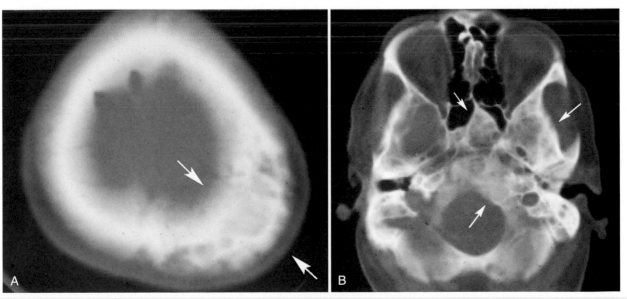

Fig. 11.74 Fibrous dysplasia, skull. **(A)** Axial CT through the skull reveals widening of the diploic space and mixed density *(arrows)*. **(B)** CT of the skull base shows mild enlargement and sclerosis of the left skull base compared with the right *(arrows)*, with ground-glass density. The enlargement and sclerosis are typical of fibrous dysplasia in the skull.

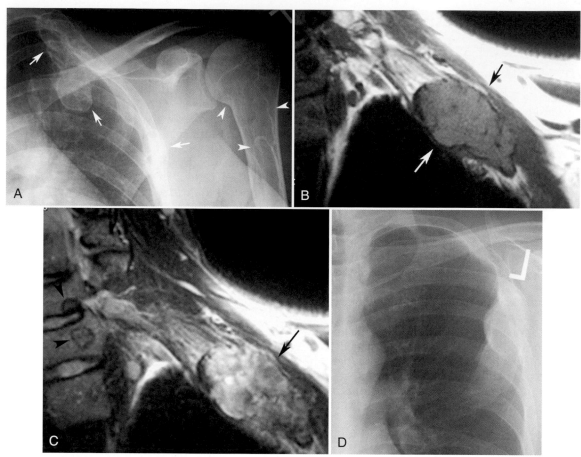

Fig. 11.75 Fibrous dysplasia, rib. Ribs are a common location for fibrous dysplasia. This 24-year-old woman had a brachial plexopathy. **(A)** AP radiograph demonstrates expanded ribs *(arrows)*, as well as typical lesions in the proximal humerus *(arrowheads)*. Coronal T1-weighted **(B)** and T2-weighted **(C)** MR images in the same patient show masslike enlargement of the first rib *(arrows)*, which is isointense with muscle on T1-weighted images and has heterogeneous signal intensity on T2-weighted images. This mass compresses the brachial plexus. Note additional lesions in the adjacent vertebrae *(arrowheads)*. **(D)** AP radiograph in a different patient with fibrous dysplasia shows a significantly expanded and sclerotic third rib. This appearance is so typical of fibrous dysplasia that it needs no further workup.

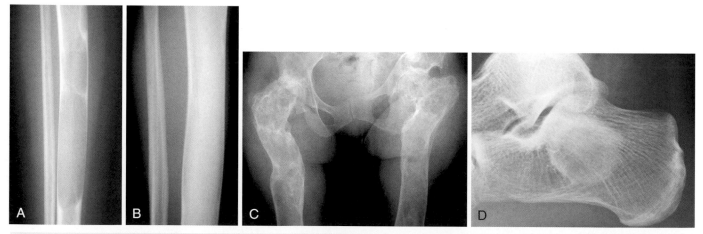

Fig. 11.76 Fibrous dysplasia, tubular bones. **(A)** AP radiograph of the tibia in a 10-year-old girl demonstrates mild expansion with uniform ground-glass density. This is a typical appearance of fibrous dysplasia in the long bones. **(B)** AP radiograph in another patient with fibrous dysplasia shows even greater ground-glass density, again with mild expansion of the tibia. The juxtaposition of these two cases demonstrates the spectrum of ground-glass density of fibrous dysplasia. Both lesions are relatively long compared with the degree of bone expansion. The zone of transition is narrow, and there is no cortical interruption. Remember that although most cases of fibrous dysplasia are central medullary lesions, fibrous dysplasia can occasionally be cortically-based. These cortically-based lesions can be significantly different in appearance. For examples please see Fig. 11.66C and D and Fig. 11.48. **(C)** AP radiograph in another patient with fibrous dysplasia shows intermediate density, with unusually marked expansion of the diaphyses. Note the bilateral femoral neck varus configuration, which has been termed a 'shepherd's crook' deformity and is typical of fibrous dysplasia. Femoral neck varus is also seen with other bone-softening conditions, such as osteomalacia and Paget's disease. **(D)** Lateral radiograph of the calcaneus shows a sclerotic focus adjacent to the physiologic central calcaneal lucency. This lesion is small enough that no expansion has occurred.

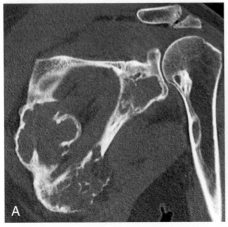
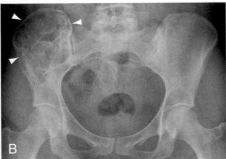
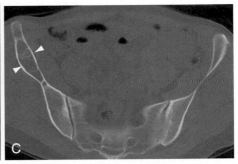

Fig. 11.77 Fibrous dysplasia, flat bones. **(A)** Coronal CT reconstruction shows a bubbly lytic expanded lesion in the scapula and smaller more sclerotic lesions in the humerus. Fibrous dysplasia of the scapula or pelvis most frequently appears as a bubbly and expanded lesion. **(B)** AP pelvis shows mild expansion of the right iliac wing *(arrowheads)* compared with the left. The lesion is ill-defined but appears to be lytic. **(C)** Axial CT confirms the mild expansion of the entire right iliac wing *(arrowheads)*. Although this does not show the degree of expansion that can sometimes occur, the expanded nonaggressive lesion is typical of fibrous dysplasia.

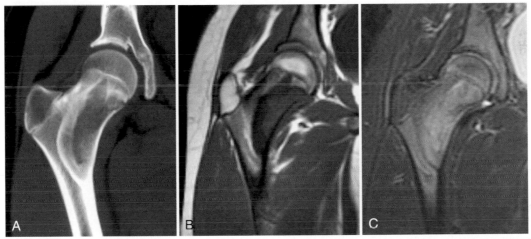

Fig. 11.78 Fibrous dysplasia of the proximal femur in a 12-year-old girl. Coronal CT reformat **(A)**, coronal T1-weighted **(B)**, and inversion recovery MR **(C)** images show the typical broad sclerotic margin. This lesion has fairly dense mineralization peripherally, with associated low signal intensity on the MR images. The less densely mineralized central region has MR signal intensity that is commonly seen in fibrous dysplasia and other fibrous lesions, which is intermediate on T1-weighted images and only mildly increased on fat-suppressed T2-weighted images or inversion recovery.

- Craniofacial involvement can occur, especially in patients with polyostotic fibrous dysplasia, with predilection for the sphenoid bones. The bone expansion may cause facial deformity, cranial nerve compression, and exophthalmos. In extreme cases facial involvement is known as leontiasis ossea, or leonine facies ('lion face'). The radiographic appearance may suggest Paget's disease, but the cortex is not as thickened, and ground-glass density rather than trabecular thickening is frequently present.
- Bone scans of fibrous dysplasia generally show mildly increased tracer uptake when lesions are active.
- MRI is nonspecific, with low to intermediate signal on T1-weighted and variable signal on T2-weighted sequences (Fig. 11.78; see Fig. 11.75).
  - Contrast enhancement is variable and may be heterogeneous.
  - Cystic degeneration occurs occasionally, including superimposed ABC, which can result in a fluid-fluid level.
- Fibrous dysplasia is usually easily diagnosed with radiography. Visualization of skull lesions may benefit from CT.
- Differential diagnosis may include Paget's disease, neurofibromatosis type 1 (NF1), and, for localized disease, other fibrous lesions.
- Most lesions remain quiescent throughout life, neither improving nor resolving.
- Only 5% continue to enlarge after skeletal maturity.
- Malignant transformation, usually to fibrosarcoma or osteosarcoma, is rare.
- Treatment is generally reserved for symptomatic lesions such as fractures or deformities.
- Limb-length discrepancy, angular deformity, and pseudarthrosis seen in the tibia of young children with fibrous dysplasia may require osteotomy, bone grafting, and immobilization. Resection or curettage of an asymptomatic site of fibrous dysplasia is usually both futile and unnecessary.

- Fibrous dysplasia (usually the polyostotic form) may be associated with a variety of endocrine disorders, including hyperthyroidism, hyperparathyroidism, acromegaly, diabetes, and Cushing syndrome.
  - *McCune–Albright syndrome* is polyostotic fibrous dysplasia, endocrine disorder (most often precocious puberty or hyperthyroidism), and café-au-lait spots with irregular 'coast of Maine' margins (as compared with the 'coast of California' margins of NF1).
  - *Cherubism* is a rare, familial, congenital fibrous dysplasia–like enlargement of the mandible with associated abnormal dentition. The jaw usually assumes more normal morphologic characteristics by adolescence.
  - The rare *Mazabraud syndrome* is fibrous dysplasia associated with intramuscular myxomas.
    - The myxomas usually occur near the abnormal bones.
    - A myxoma is a rare benign mass in the extremities, typically found within skeletal muscle, composed predominantly of myxoid tissue, which has very high T2 signal intensity (see Fig. 12.35).

NONOSSIFYING FIBROMA/FIBROUS CORTICAL DEFECT (FIBROXANTHOMA)

- Non-ossifying fibroma (NOF) and fibrous cortical defect (FCD) are histologically identical, nonneoplastic cortically-based lesions that are thought to arise secondary to physeal defects that migrate away from the physis with growth.
- Both are referred to as fibroxanthomas. The distinction between NOF and FCD is based on size; NOF is the larger version, > 2cm.
- Very common, occurring in 30–40% of children older than age 2 years.
- The cause may be related to trauma at muscle attachment sites in the growing skeleton that results in self-limited fibrous proliferation.
  - A manifestation of this is seen at the posterior femoral metaphysis at the knee, corresponding to the gastrocnemius attachment near the physeal plate; this

had been previously referred to as cortical desmoid, now called *avulsive cortical irregularity*.

- The large majority are asymptomatic and incidental, although larger lesions may present with pathologic fracture.

Key Concepts

Fibroxanthoma (Nonossifying Fibroma, Fibrous Cortical Defect)

- Very common, often found incidentally in pediatric radiographs, especially around the knee and ankle. Does not require further workup
- Bubbly lytic lesion with sclerotic margins
- Cortical metadiaphyseal lesion
- Larger lesions may present with pathologic fracture
- Most common natural evolution is to be replaced by bone ('heal') over a few years with mild residual sclerosis

- Eighty percent occur in the metaphysis or metadiaphysis of the long bones of the lower extremity.
- Eccentric, cortically-based lesions. Although they may arise in the cortex, they can enlarge to involve the intramedullary region and even appear central when found in thin bones such as the fibula or ulna (see Fig. 11.66E).
- Geographic, 'bubbly' lytic lesions with a sclerotic margin and no matrix calcification (Fig. 11.79).
- Expansile lesions can be associated with reactive cortical thickening. Otherwise, there is no periosteal reaction unless pathologic fracture has occurred.
- The lesions involute spontaneously, with dense bone replacing the fibrous tissue. The resulting 'healed' NOF/FCD may demonstrate homogeneous sclerosis (Fig. 11.80; see Fig. 11.66E).
- MRI shows low signal intensity on T1-weighted images and variable signal intensity on T2-weighted images, depending on the extent of hypercellular fibrous tissue and healing bone that is present (see Fig. 11.80B). Eighty percent of NOFs/FCDs show hypointensity in at least part of the lesion on fluid-sensitive sequences.

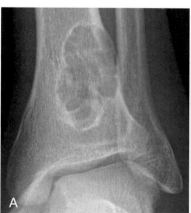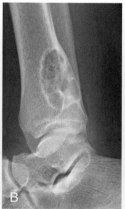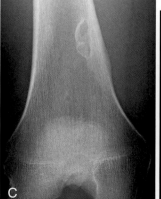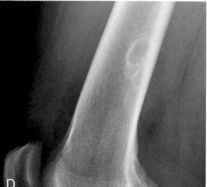

Fig. 11.79 Nonossifying fibroma (NOF). AP **(A)** and lateral **(B)** radiographs show a cortically-based geographic metaphyseal lesion that has a well-defined sclerotic rim. This mildly expanded lesion is a typical nonossifying fibroma. AP **(C)** and lateral **(D)** radiographs show a lytic cortically-based metadiaphyseal lesion with sclerotic rim. Note that the lesion is filling in with normal bone peripherally and particularly inferiorly. This represents the natural history of NOF.

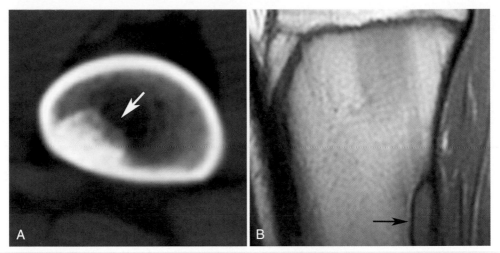

Fig. 11.80 **(A)** Axial CT through the distal femoral metaphysis in a 21-year-old man shows eccentric uniform sclerosis *(arrow)*. This is a healed nonossifying fibroma (NOF); the bone will eventually remodel to a normal appearance. **(B)** Sagittal T1-weighted MR image shows a small, cortically-based intermediate-signal-intensity mass *(arrow)* at the posterior proximal tibial metadiaphysis. The tumor had intermediate signal intensity on T2-weighted images as well (not shown); this is the typical MR appearance of NOF.

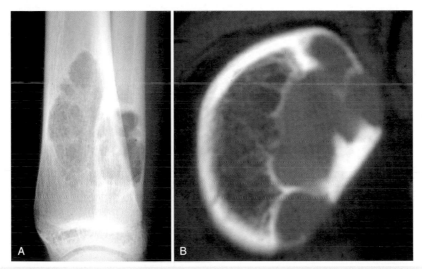

Fig. 11.81 Multiple nonossifying fibromas (NOFs). Lateral ankle radiograph **(A)** and axial CT **(B)** through one lesion show multiple NOFs. Note the typical well circumscribed 'bubbly' lytic appearance of NOF. NOFs are usually solitary or few in number; numerous lesions should prompt an evaluation for neurofibromatosis type 1.

- Many children have more than one lesion. However, a finding of multiple fibroxanthoma-like bone lesions (Fig. 11.81) should cause consideration for associated conditions, such as NF1 and Jaffe–Campanacci syndrome.
  - Jaffe–Campanacci syndrome is characterized by multiple NOFs/FCDs with café-au-lait-spots but without neurofibromatosis.
  - Other associations reported with Jaffe–Campanacci syndrome include mental retardation, precocious puberty, hypogonadism, and cardiovascular and ocular abnormalities.

LIPOSCLEROSING MYXOFIBROUS TUMOR (POLYMORPHIC FIBRO-OSSEOUS LESION OF BONE)

- Liposclerosing myxofibrous tumor (LSMFT) is a benign fibro-osseous bone lesion that usually occurs in the fourth through sixth decades of life and is most specifically characterized by its location.
  - More than 90% of these lesions occur in the central portion of the proximal (intertrochanteric) femur.
- The lesion consists of a mixture of tissues, any of which may predominate on imaging.
- Histologically, LSMFT is composed of a complex mixture of immature bone and fibrous tissue. Xanthomatous and myxoid elements are frequently present. Ischemic ossification may be found within altered fat.
- LSMFT may be related to fibrous dysplasia or represent an endstage degeneration of an intraosseous fibrous lesion.
- The lesion usually appears as a lytic or ground-glass (though there may be a dense sclerotic portion) geographic lesion with a type 1A margin, often with a thick sclerotic border (Fig. 11.82).
- Amorphous mineralization is present in most (72%) lesions.

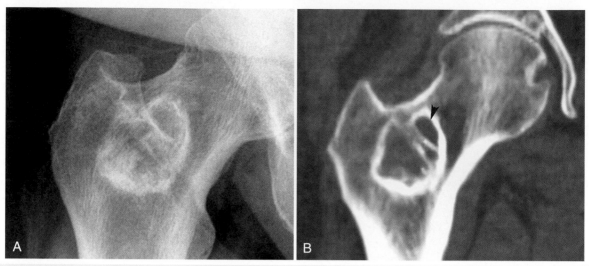

Fig. 11.82 Liposclerosing myxofibrous tumor (LSMFT). AP radiograph **(A)** and coronal CT reconstruction **(B)** show a geographic mixed-density lesion with a fairly broad sclerotic margin in the proximal femur. This is the classic appearance and location of LSMFT. Note that a portion of the lesion has fat attenuation (*arrowhead* in B). A geographic lesion containing both sclerosis and fat in this location is the typical appearance of LSMFT.

- The matrix appears globular and irregular. There may also be cystic regions, as well as areas containing fat density.
- The MRI appearance is nonspecific, with heterogeneous T2-weighted imaging signal. T1-weighted images are more homogeneous, and isointense to muscle. The condition occurs over a wide age range, but most cases are found in adults.
- An important feature of this lesion is its small potential for malignant transformation, despite the initial nonaggressive radiographic appearance.
- The lesion may present with pain or may be incidental. Because malignant potential has been reported, clinical and imaging follow-up has been recommended.

Fibroblastic Tumors

DESMOPLASTIC FIBROMA

- Desmoplastic fibroma is the rare form of fibromatosis in bone.
- Most of these lesions present in the second decade of life and have a geographic pattern with cortical expansion and endosteal erosion.
- The lesions are located centrally in the metaphysis, most frequently in the long bones but also in the pelvis and mandible.
- There is no tumor matrix and generally no significant host response. Because these can be radiographically aggressive, they can be difficult to distinguish radiographically as well as histologically from a well-differentiated fibrosarcoma.
- Their behavior is not malignant, but recurrence is very common.
- The large soft tissue mass is best evaluated by MRI. There are often large blood vessels and hypervascularity; focal regions of hemorrhage or necrosis are common.
- Although the imaging and histologic character is of a highly aggressive lesion, the patient's age should suggest

the correct diagnosis and associated relatively good prognosis.
- Treatment ranges from observation to curettage with grafting to complete resection.

FIBROSARCOMA

- Fibrosarcoma is a malignant spindle cell tumor that may arise in either bone or soft tissue.
- Osseous fibrosarcoma involves the long tubular bones in 70% of cases and the pelvis in 9%.
- Radiographically, it is a lytic permeative lesion with a wide zone of transition, located either centrally or eccentrically in the metaphysis.
- The lesion may contain sequestered bone fragments and may or may not elicit periosteal reaction. Cortical breakthrough and soft tissue mass are common.
- MRI characteristics are nonspecific, with T1-weighted signal isointense to muscle, hyperintense inhomogeneous fluid-sensitive appearance, and enhancement. It may contain myxoid, cystic, or necrotic regions. Contrast enhancement is usually avid (Fig. 11.83).

Fibrohistiocytic Tumors

BENIGN FIBROUS HISTIOCYTOMA

- Benign fibrous histiocytoma is a rare geographic osseous lesion that has a histologic appearance very similar to that of fibroxanthoma, but demonstrates different features:
  - It arises centrally in the metaphyseal region of long bones.
  - Both CT and MRI features are nonspecific.
  - Unlike NOF, benign fibrous histiocytoma has a tendency to recur after curettage and may be symptomatic.
  - Benign fibrous histiocytoma may also originate in soft tissue, where it may be located either subcutaneously, within deep soft tissues, or within organs.
  - Treatment is surgical excision, but recurrence risk is high.

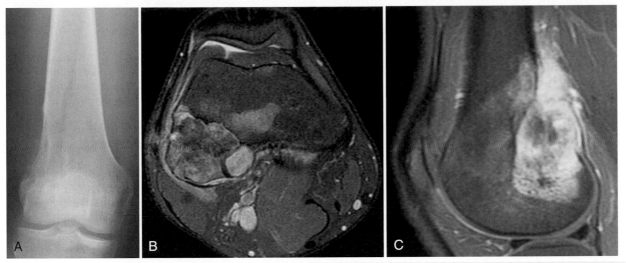

Fig. 11.83 Osseous fibrosarcoma. **(A)** AP radiograph shows an eccentric metaphyseal lytic lesion in a 22-year-old man. There is a wide zone of transition and cortical breakthrough. **(B)** Axial intermediate–weighted, fat-saturated MR image shows the lesion to be highly heterogeneous, with both low- and high-signal regions. There is posteromedial cortical breakthrough. **(C)** Sagittal T1-weighted, fat-saturated postgadolinium MR shows intense enhancement in the mass, along with edema in the adjacent bone. There is cortical breakthrough with a large posterior soft tissue mass; central necrosis is seen.

PLEOMORPHIC SARCOMA

- Undifferentiated pleomorphic sarcoma, or simply pleomorphic sarcoma is an aggressive sarcoma that contains both fibroblastic and histiocytic elements in varying proportions. Pleomorphic refers to the heterogeneous appearance of the tumor cell nuclei. This lesion is much more common in soft tissues. It was formerly termed malignant fibrous histiocytoma (MFH), although this term has fallen out of favor after reclassification by the WHO.
- Pleomorphic sarcoma of bone is relatively rare, making up 2–5% of all primary malignant bone tumors.
- Osseous pleomorphic sarcoma may arise either primarily or secondarily.
- The age range is wide, but the peak prevalence is in 30- to 60-year-old patients.
- Most osseous pleomorphic sarcoma lesions occur in the long tubular bones (75%; femur most frequent), usually centrally in the metaphysis or diaphysis.
- Imaging appearance (Fig. 11.84A):
  - They generally appear geographic, with a wide zone of transition seen in at least part of the lesion.
  - The lesion is lytic, although dystrophic calcification may be seen in as many as 15% of cases.
  - MRI is nonspecific, with low signal intensity on T1-weighted and heterogeneous high signal intensity on T2-weighted images, with occasional low-signal-intensity regions relating to dystrophic calcification.
- Although most osseous pleomorphic sarcoma arises as a primary lesion, up to 28% arise as secondary lesions.
  - Underlying lesions include Paget's disease, previously radiated bone, dedifferentiated chondrosarcoma, fibroxanthoma (NOF/FCD), fibrous dysplasia, enchondroma, chronic osteomyelitis, and bone infarct (osteonecrosis).
  - With these secondary forms of pleomorphic sarcoma, an aggressive lesion will be found in contiguity with

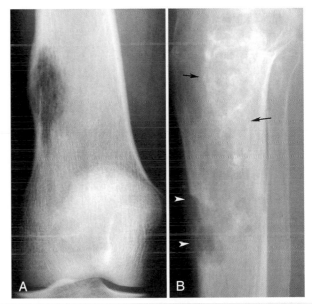

Fig. 11.84 Osseous pleomorphic sarcoma, primary and secondary. **(A)** AP radiograph of a moderately aggressive-appearing lesion (note the somewhat wide zone of transition without sclerotic margin) in the distal metadiaphysis of the femur in a 22-year-old man. There is no matrix. This is a nonspecific appearance, but an aggressive lytic lesion in an adult should include primary osseous pleomorphic sarcoma as a diagnostic consideration. **(B)** Lateral radiograph of the proximal tibia in a 66-year-old woman demonstrates dystrophic calcific matrix in a serpiginous pattern typical of bone infarct *(arrows)*. However, a more destructive lesion is found in contiguity but slightly distal to the bone infarct *(arrowheads)*. This aggressive lesion arising from a bone infarct represents a secondary osseous pleomorphic sarcoma (Images used with permission from BJ Manaster, MD, from the American College of Radiology Learning File.)

the benign lesion from which it arises. For example, pleomorphic sarcoma arising in bone infarct may demonstrate the nonaggressive serpiginous pattern of calcification commonly seen in bone infarct, immediately contiguous with a highly destructive pattern (Fig. 11.84B).

- Most pleomorphic sarcomas are high-grade tumors, with a 5-year survival rate of 34–50%.
- Metastases involve lung, bone, lymph nodes, and liver.
- Local recurrence after resection is common.
- Treatment consists of aggressive surgical excision and chemotherapy, often supplemented by radiation therapy.

Fatty Tumors

INTRAOSSEOUS LIPOMA

- Intraosseous lipoma is a benign bone lesion consisting of adipocytes, and in some cases may represent fatty involution of a 'burned-out' benign lesion that previously occupied the same site.
- The majority of lesions (71%) arise in the lower extremity, most frequently the femur, followed by the tibia and calcaneus.

- Within the calcaneus the lesion arises centrally, below the subtalar joint, in an area that normally shows physiologic lucency.
- Intraosseous lipoma initially is a lytic lesion, showing fat density on radiograph or CT and fat signal on all MRI sequences, isointense to subcutaneous fat.
- Lesions are geographic, usually with a thin sclerotic margin (Fig. 11.85).
- The lesions may undergo changes as they involute, developing regions of fat necrosis and central calcification (Fig. 11.86).
- On MRI, lesions show fat signal in the majority of the lesion with low signal in any regions of calcification; regions of fat necrosis are hypointense on T1-weighted and hyperintense on T2-weighted imaging.

PAROSTEAL LIPOMA

- Parosteal lipoma is a fatty lesion arising from the bone surface, strongly adherent to the underlying periosteum.

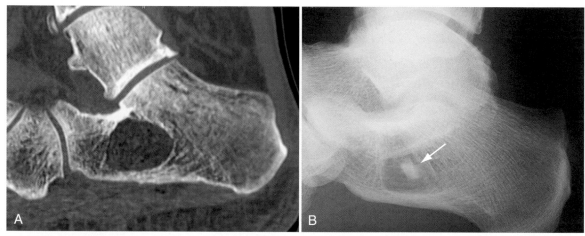

Fig. 11.85 Intraosseous calcaneal lipoma. **(A)** Sagittal CT reconstruction shows sharply marginated fat attenuation mass in the central calcaneus. Cysts and numerous other tumors can occur in this location, but the fat attenuation in this case is pathognomonic. **(B)** Lateral radiograph of another case shows dystrophic calcification centrally *(arrow)* within a lesion containing fat density, a classic feature of calcaneal intraosseous lipoma during involution.

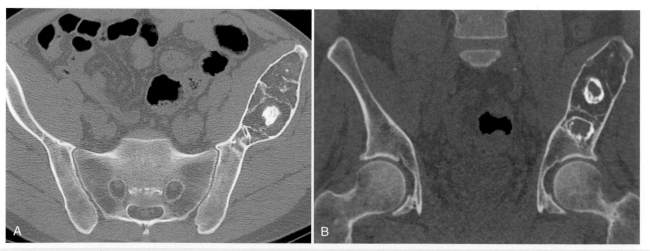

Fig. 11.86 Intraosseous lipoma, in an involutional stage. Axial **(A)** and coronal **(B)** CT reformat shows an expanded left anterior iliac lesion with fat attenuation and no evidence of aggressive behavior. There are several foci of calcification, some solid and some with circumferential calcification; these represent regions of fat necrosis within the lesion.

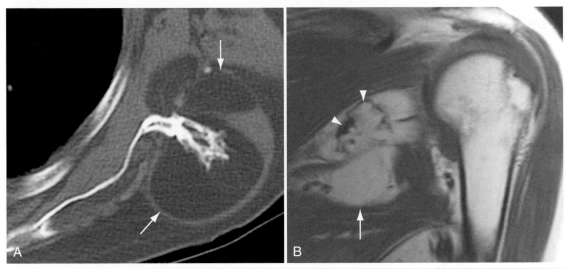

Fig. 11.87 Parosteal lipoma. **(A)** Axial CT shows a branching osseous excrescence arising from the scapula, surrounded by a lobulated fat-density lesion *(arrows)*. **(B)** Coronal T1-weighted MR image of the same shoulder shows the high-signal fat density of the lesion *(arrow)* and the low signal of the bony reaction *(arrowheads)*.

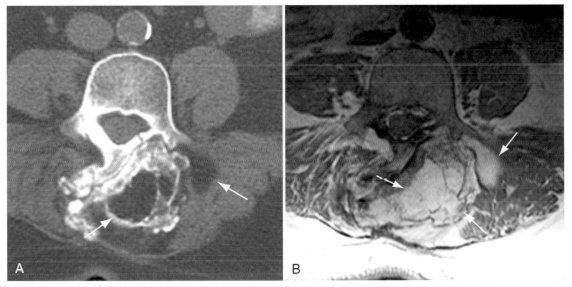

Fig. 11.88 Parosteal lipoma. **(A)** Axial CT shows prominent osseous reaction arising from the posterior elements with surrounding areas of fat attenuation *(arrows)*. **(B)** Axial T1-weighted MR image shows the hyperintense fat within the posterior spinous muscles *(arrows)*; all findings are typical of parosteal lipoma.

- The fat-density soft tissue mass is typical of lipoma on all types of imaging.
- The characteristic feature of this lesion (seen in 67–100% of cases) is an osseous excrescence that arises from the adjacent cortex (Figs. 11.87 and 11.88).
- This excrescence may be solid or spiculated. The lesion is benign but may cause mass effect on adjacent tissues including nerves.

Vascular Tumors

HEMANGIOMA (VASCULAR MALFORMATION)

- Vascular malformations in general are benign proliferations of large (cavernous) or small (capillary) endothelium-lined spaces filled with blood.

- Although *hemangioma* is engrained in the literature, it is contained by the umbrella term *vascular malformation*.
- Vascular malformations are divided into high-flow and low-flow malformations, which incorporate the older terms capillary hemangioma, cavernous hemangioma, arteriovenous malformation, and venous angioma or malformation.
- Vascular malformations may arise anywhere and may be either osseous or soft tissue in origin.
- Although the osseous lesions are detected most frequently in the fourth and fifth decades of life, the age range is wide; the vast majority are incidentally found, especially in the spine.
- Soft tissue vascular malformations are described in Chapter 12 – Soft Tissue Tumors.

- The vast majority of osseous vascular malformations are cavernous hemangiomas and are found in the vertebral bodies, skull, and facial bones.
- In the vertebral bodies the number of trabeculae are reduced, leaving only prominent vertical trabeculae that are reduced in number but are thickened.
  - This gives a vertical striated appearance referred to as 'corduroy sign' or 'jail-bar sign' on radiographs and coronal and sagittal CT imaging.

- These prominent trabeculae on a lucent background also cause a 'polka dot' or 'starry sky' appearance on axial CT
- In the skull there is classically a 'spokewheel' pattern of trabeculae, extending from the center to the periphery.
- On MRI, macroscopic fat signal is seen on T1-weighted images. T2 signal is variable and depends on the quantity of vascular tissue. The classic hemangioma is hyperintense on T1- and T2-weighted images (Fig. 11.89).
- These appearances are pathognomonic for benign hemangioma.
- Some lesions do not contain obvious fat signal on MRI or do not have characteristic morphologic features described earlier, so-called *atypical hemangiomas* due to their atypical imaging appearance (Fig. 11.90).
  - Lesions often enhance on postcontrast MRI, therefore Gadolinium-based contrast administration is not useful for diagnosis in indeterminate cases.
  - Opposed-phase MRI (chemical shift imaging or 'in-and out-of-phase' imaging) can be used to detect very small quantities of intralesional fat, which can help

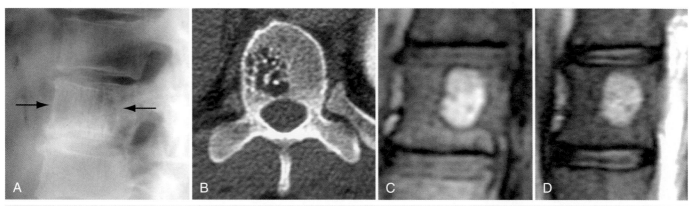

Fig. 11.89 Vertebral body hemangioma. **(A)** Lateral radiograph of a lower thoracic vertebral body hemangioma *(arrows)* showing the vertical striations that are typical of hemangioma. **(B)** Axial CT image shows typical CT appearance, a well-circumscribed lesion with fatty or water density tissue between trabeculae that are thick but few in number. Sagittal T1-weighted **(C)** and T2-weighted **(D)** MR images show high signal on both sequences, reflecting the fat and free water within these lesions. (A, Image used with permission from BJ Manaster, MD, from the American College of Radiology Learning File.)

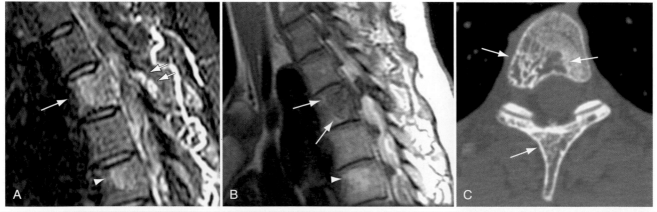

Fig. 11.90 Atypical spinal hemangiomas. **(A)** Fat-suppressed T2-weighted MR image shows high signal intensity in hemangiomas in T3 *(arrows)* and T5 *(arrowhead)* owing to free water and slowly flowing blood within the tumors. This appearance is nonspecific, because a metastasis could have identical appearance. Note that the T3 lesion involves the vertebral body *(long arrow)* and posterior elements *(short arrows)*. **(B)** Sagittal T1-weighted MR image shows the usual finding of high signal intensity throughout the T5 lesion *(arrowhead)* because of fat within the tumor stroma. However, the T3 lesion has only a thin peripheral rim of high signal intensity *(arrows)*. This is enough to make the diagnosis of hemangioma. Some spinal hemangiomas contain no high T1-weighted signal and can be difficult to diagnose. **(C)** CT through T3 lesion shows the typical thickened vertical trabeculae, with extension through the posterior elements *(arrows)*.

confirm the diagnosis; a Dixon fat–water separation sequence is used to acquire 'fat plus water' (in-phase) and 'fat minus water' (out-of-phase) images. Region of interest (ROI) measurements of the lesion are acquired. If the signal drops more than 20% on out-of-phase images compared to in-phase images, this is a sign that there is significant fat within the lesion.

- Rarely hemangiomas can exhibit locally aggressive characteristics with expansion and occasionally a soft tissue mass, which may lead to neurologic symptoms. These are referred to as *aggressive hemangiomas*. They may require surgical removal and spinal stabilization; however, if a lesion occurs in a location difficult to remove, they may be followed to ensure stability.
- *Klippel–Trénaunay–Weber* syndrome is the classic triad of bone and soft tissue hypertrophy, cutaneous hemangioma, and congenital varicose veins. Imaging findings include hemihypertrophy or macrodactyly, phleboliths, subcutaneous fat hypertrophy, abnormal superficial-to-deep vein connections, and lack of venous valves (Fig. 11.91).
- The rare intraarticular *synovial hemangioma* may cause repetitive bleeding into the joint and an appearance

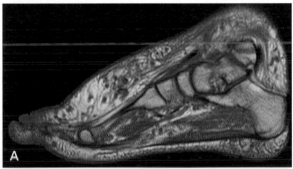
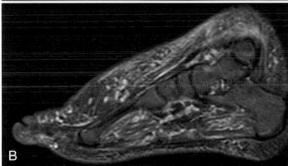
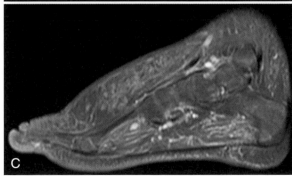

Fig. 11.91 Klippel–Trénaunay–Weber syndrome. Sagittal T1-weighted **(A)**, STIR **(B)**, and postcontrast T1-weighted fat-saturated **(C)** images of the foot show fatty overgrowth and prominent low-flow vessels.

similar to hemophilia. The knee and elbow are favored sites for synovial hemangioma; this site preference also makes it difficult to differentiate from the appearance of hemophilia.

- Other benign osseous vascular tumors of the extremities are rare, including osseous lymphangioma; *cystic angiomatosis* is a rare benign multicentric manifestation of hemangiomatosis or lymphangiomatosis, often with severe visceral involvement.
  - The multiple lytic lesions of bone are nonspecific in appearance unless calcified phleboliths are present in the soft tissues.
  - Another variant is *Gorham disease*, or massive osteolysis. This is a disease of multicentric angiomatosis with regional dissolution of bone, which is rapid and severely destructive, spreading contiguously across joints.

HEMANGIOPERICYTOMA AND HEMANGIOENDOTHELIOMA

- Hemangiopericytoma and hemangioendothelioma fit within the category of vascular lesions with aggressive features.
- *Hemangiopericytoma* is a malignant vascular tumor that most often originates from the meninges, sinuses, or elsewhere in the head and neck. Peak incidence is in the fourth and fifth decades.
  - Primary hemangiopericytoma of bone is very rare and may have a variety of radiographic appearances that range from nonaggressive to aggressive.
  - The axial and proximal appendicular skeletons are the most frequent sites.
  - Discovery of a skeletal hemangiopericytoma should prompt a search for a meningeal or head and neck primary tumor.
- *Hemangioendothelioma* is also a low-grade malignant lesion, which can be difficult to differentiate histologically from angiosarcoma.
  - Patients are typically younger (third and fourth decades).
  - As with hemangiopericytoma, the soft tissue portions of the mass usually are not mineralized.
  - Radiographs of an osseous lesion show osteolysis—sometimes multifocal, sometimes expansile—with variably aggressive tumor margins.
- The MRI appearance of these tumors is variable and nonspecific, although vascular channels are occasionally seen. There is no underlying fatty stroma, as there is in hemangioma.
- These vascular tumors may be multicentric and can metastasize. When they are multicentric, they tend to involve several bones of a single extremity, often the feet. Interestingly, the lesions that are multicentric tend to have a better prognosis than the solitary lesions.

ANGIOSARCOMA

- Angiosarcoma is a rare malignant vascular tumor that usually occurs in elderly patients in soft tissues, but can occur in bone, and can occur in much younger patients.

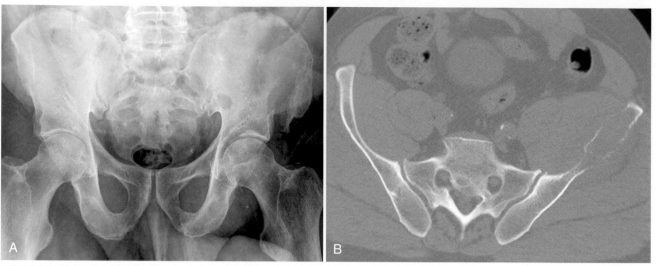

Fig. 11.92 Angiosarcoma. **(A)** AP radiograph shows a large lytic lesion of the left iliac wing. There is a pathologic fracture, and the zone of transition is wide, suggesting that the lesion is aggressive. **(B)** Axial CT of the same lesion shows the lesion to be permeative, with cortical breakthrough. The appearance is of an aggressive lesion but is otherwise nonspecific.

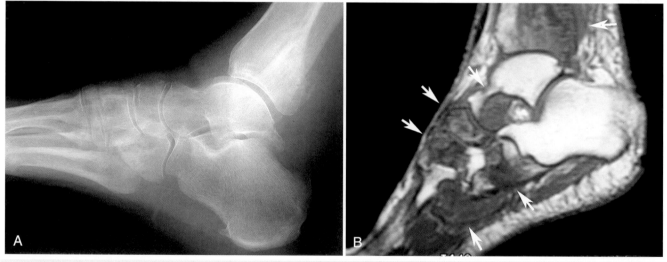

Fig. 11.93 Angiosarcoma. **(A)** Lateral radiograph of the foot in a 67-year-old man shows an ill-defined destructive lesion involving the posterior aspect of the distal tibia. One might consider that the lucencies seen throughout the bones of the hindfoot and midfoot represent disuse osteopenia. **(B)** T1-weighted MR image demonstrates low-signal-intensity lesions involving the multiple bones of the foot and ankle *(arrows)*. Multiple lesions involving the lower extremities frequently prove to be vascular tumors. In this case the diagnosis is multifocal angiosarcoma.

- Angiosarcoma may be difficult to differentiate histologically from the less aggressive hemangioendothelioma.
- Osseous angiosarcomas are extremely rare, permeative, aggressive-appearing lesions without matrix. The most common location is metaphyseal, in the femur, tibia, humerus, and pelvis (Figs. 11.92 and 11.93).
- Thirty-eight percent of angiosarcomas are multifocal; it is unclear whether this represents synchronous or metastatic disease. When multifocal, the lesions tend to be regional in distribution. Furthermore, the prognosis is somewhat improved if the lesions are multifocal.
- Five-year survival is poor for patients who have solitary lesions, with metastases spreading to the lungs or skeleton. Treatment consists of wide resection.

Marrow Tumors

EWING SARCOMA

- Ewing sarcoma is a highly malignant neoplasm found primarily in children and adolescents.
- Ewing sarcoma is the most common primary malignant bone tumor found in children in the first decade of life. In the second decade it is second only to osteosarcoma.
- Ninety-five percent occur between the ages of 4 and 25 years, with the most frequent occurrence between 5 and 14 years.
- Along with lymphoma, leukemia, primitive neuroectodermal tumor (with which Ewing sarcoma shares a specific

chromosome 11;22 translocation and is histologically highly similar but not identical), and metastatic neuroblastoma, Ewing sarcoma is sometimes termed a 'small round cell tumor' in reference to a similar histologic appearance.

- These malignancies, along with osteomyelitis and LCH, also have a similar radiographic appearance (*small round cell* pattern, Lodwick type 3).

- Ewing sarcoma occupies the central medullary compartment, most commonly within the diaphysis or metadiaphysis when in long bones.
- Seventy-five percent of cases involve the pelvis or long tubular bones.
    - Other sites of involvement include the shoulder girdle, rib, and vertebral body.
    - Location is related to the age at presentation; Ewing sarcoma tends to involve the tubular bones in children younger than age 10 and the axial skeleton, pelvis, and shoulder girdle in patients older than age 10.
    - Rarely, Ewing sarcoma arises in soft tissues.
- The tumor is classically permeative, with a large soft tissue mass (Fig. 11.94). In fact, this presentation is fairly

characteristic of Ewing sarcoma in the appropriate age group.
- No calcified tumor matrix is produced.
- Most Ewing sarcomas are completely lytic, but one-fourth have minimal reactive bone, and about 15% have marked sclerotic reactive bone (Fig. 11.95).
    - The presence of this sclerotic reactive bone might falsely suggest osteosarcoma as the diagnosis.
    - However, the reactive bone in Ewing sarcoma is found only within the intraosseous portion of the tumor and is not produced within the soft tissue components.
        - This feature helps to differentiate a sclerotic Ewing sarcoma from an osteosarcoma, which most frequently shows tumor matrix formation in both the permeative osseous lesion and the extraosseous soft tissue mass.
- Aggressive periosteal reaction is a prominent feature of Ewing sarcoma.
- Systemic reaction may be prominent as well, because one-third of the patients present with fever, leukocytosis, and elevated erythrocyte sedimentation rate. This clinical presentation simulates infection.

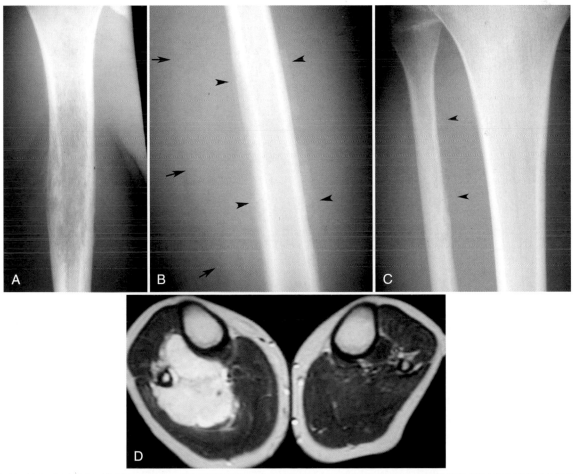

Fig. 11.94 Ewing sarcoma. **(A)** Classic appearance of Ewing sarcoma is a highly permeative lesion in a long bone, as seen in this humerus tumor in a 14-year-old girl. **(B)** Sagittal radiograph of the middiaphysis of the femur in a 10-year-old girl. The permeative change in the bone is almost impossible to see, but there is aggressive, interrupted periosteal reaction *(arrowheads)* as well as a large soft tissue mass *(arrows)*. This is also a common radiographic appearance of Ewing sarcoma. An even more subtle case of Ewing sarcoma is seen in an AP radiograph **(C)** of the proximal fibula in a 23-year-old woman. There is subtle permeative change in the medial cortex with equally subtle periosteal reaction *(arrowheads)*. Axial T2-weighted MR image **(D)** shows the true tumor size, which is larger than that suggested by the radiograph.

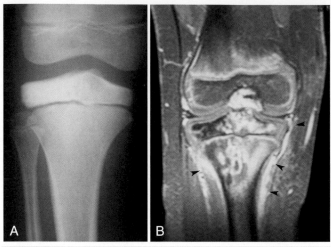

Fig. 11.95 Sclerotic Ewing sarcoma. **(A)** AP radiograph of the knee in a 9-year-old boy. The proximal epiphysis of the tibia is sclerotic, but no definite destructive change is seen. Ewing sarcoma can elicit such dense reactive bone formation that the permeative change can be obscured. **(B)** Coronal fat-suppressed, contrast-enhanced, T1-weighted MR image shows that the lesion not only involves the proximal tibial epiphysis but also extends far into the metaphysis. There is an enhancing soft tissue mass *(arrowheads)*, although it is not as large as was seen in Fig. 11.94D.

Key Concepts

Ewing Sarcoma

- Most common primary malignant bone neoplasm in the first decade of life
- Highly aggressive: Permeative pattern, large soft tissue mass, aggressive periosteal reaction. Occasional host bone sclerosis and sunburst periosteal reaction may resemble osteosarcoma
- Tubular bones more frequently involved in the younger age group; flat bones and axial skeleton more frequently involved in adolescents and young adults
- Central and diaphyseal or metadiaphyseal
- Systemic symptoms are frequent and may be confused clinically with osteomyelitis
- Bone and lung metastases are common

- The MRI appearance of Ewing sarcoma is nonspecific, with low signal intensity on T1-weighted images and high signal intensity on T2-weighted images. The soft tissue component of the mass is typically large and may contain central necrosis.
  - However, as mentioned earlier, an aggressive bone lesion with a large soft tissue mass in the appropriate age group should elicit the diagnosis.
- The differential diagnosis primarily consists of the other 'small round cell' lesions (neuroblastoma metastases, lymphoma, primitive neuroectodermal tumor, and leukemia), osteomyelitis, and LCH.
  - Although benign and highly malignant lesions are included in this same differential diagnosis, each of these lesions mentioned previously can have a highly aggressive permeative appearance and require biopsy for diagnosis.
  - The duration of symptoms may be helpful in differentiating among these round cell lesions. LCH may be

one of the most locally aggressive, with the shortest time course of osseous destruction (1–2 weeks). Osteomyelitis also has a relatively short course of osseous destruction (2–4 weeks). Ewing sarcoma, although highly aggressive, has a somewhat slower course, with destructive changes seen at 6–12 weeks. Occasionally Ewing sarcoma has a slower course early in the disease.
- Ewing sarcoma is initially monostotic, but metastases to bone are common so that the lesion may present initially as a polyostotic disease. This can contribute to difficulty in diagnosis.
  - Fifteen to thirty percent have identifiable metastases at the time of diagnosis; the actual number likely is higher due to metastases too small to detect with imaging. This likely accounts for the poor response to local therapy only.
  - Metastases affect lung and bone with equal frequency. Of all the primary bone sarcomas, Ewing sarcoma most frequently metastasizes to other bones.
- Treatment includes aggressive chemotherapy with surgery and/or radiation therapy. Ewing sarcoma is highly responsive to radiation therapy, but recurs without adjuvant chemotherapy. Amputation and limb salvage surgery with wide resection are secondary options.
- Ewing sarcoma has the highest SUV on PET– CT of all malignant primary bone tumors, so PET is used to restage and assess response.
- The 5-year survival of patients with Ewing sarcoma has improved to 70%. Central and larger lesions, lesions with more aggressive histologic features, and tumors expressing certain cellular receptors are associated with a worse prognosis.

PRIMARY LYMPHOMA OF BONE

- Primary lymphoma of bone is an uncommon presentation of lymphoma and must be distinguished from secondary osseous involvement by extraosseous primary disease, because the latter requires more aggressive therapy and is associated with a worse prognosis.
- Extraosseus lymphoma metastatic to bone is far more common than primary lymphoma of bone.
- Most cases present between age 30 and 60 years.
- Initial presentation can be monostotic or polyostotic.
- Polyostotic initial presentation is more common in children.
- Patients present with bone pain, and a mass may be apparent on physical examination.
- The lesion tends to arise in appendicular central diaphyseal or metadiaphyseal sites, particularly the femur, tibia, and humerus, but also can occur in the pelvis, scapula, and spine.
- The classic appearance of primary lymphoma of bone is lytic, most frequently moth-eaten or permeative (Fig. 11.96), but it can appear to be of mixed density because of reactive bone formation and prominent endosteal thickening.
- Other patterns can be seen that are suggestive of the diagnosis:
  - One pattern is a large mass surrounding a bone with comparatively little bone changes except for a subtle

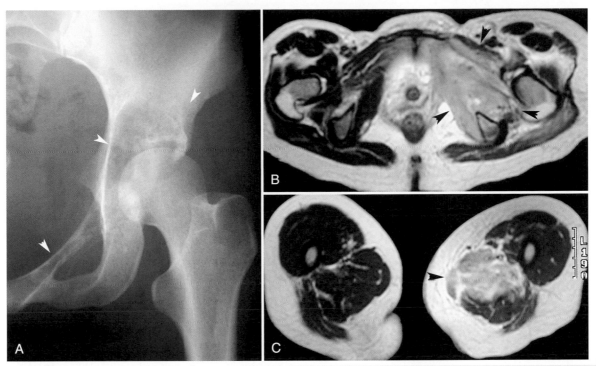

Fig. 11.96 Primary lymphoma of bone. **(A)** AP radiograph of the left hip shows a highly permeative lesion involving the acetabulum and extending into the superior pubic ramus in a 31-year-old woman *(arrowheads)*. Axial T2-weighted MR images obtained through the low pelvis **(B)** and thighs **(C)** demonstrate an unusually extensive soft tissue mass *(arrowheads)* associated with this lesion. In its proximal portion the soft tissue mass involves both the obturator internus and externus, and the mass extends well down into the proximal half of the thigh, involving the adductor musculature. Such a large, infiltrative soft tissue mass is typical of primary lymphoma.

permeative pattern or cortical thickening. CT or MRI may show tumor extension through small cortical channels without overt cortical destruction (only 28% show cortical destruction), with an associated circumferential soft tissue mass.

- Another pattern, seen on MRI, resembles diffuse marrow infiltration. The MRI appearance generally is not specific for diagnosis, but MRI is needed for staging because radiographs do not show the true size and extent of the lesion. Lymphoma lesions show increased tracer uptake on bone scanning, sometimes before radiographs show any changes.

- The major differential diagnosis relates to other aggressive lesions occurring in this age range: in adults, metastases, myeloma, and high-grade sarcomas; in younger patients, osteomyelitis, osteosarcoma, LCH, and Ewing sarcoma.

- Primary lymphoma of bone can metastasize to lymph nodes and bone. Lung metastases are uncommon but when present may increase in size and number quickly.

- Treatment is chemotherapy, potentially including rituximab (antilymphoma monoclonal antibodies), often supplemented with radiation therapy. Surgical stabilization of associated pathologic fractures is often needed.
  - Lesions often become sclerotic when successfully treated.
  - Five-year survival rates are among the best for all primary bone tumors.

- Metastatic non-Hodgkin lymphoma to bone indicates an aggressive tumor with poorer prognosis (Fig. 11.97).

Key Concepts

Primary Lymphoma of Bone

- Permeative. Enormous soft tissue mass with relative preservation of cortex
- Long bones: Usually diaphyseal
- Large tubular bones, pelvis, and scapula
- Sequestra of normal bone surrounded by tumor
- Most common age range: 30–60 years

HODGKIN DISEASE

- Hodgkin disease in bone is almost always metastatic in etiology.
- Twenty percent of patients with Hodgkin disease have radiographic evidence of bone involvement, but it is extremely rare as a primary bone tumor.
- Metastatic Hodgkin disease can involve bone either by hematogenous dissemination or by contiguous spread from adjacent nodes.
- The sternum is a common site of contiguous tumor involvement.
- Hodgkin disease of bone is seen most frequently in the second through fourth decades of life.
- Lesions are most frequently found in the axial skeleton, especially vertebral bodies.
  - They may be lytic but most frequently are either blastic or mixed lytic and blastic.
  - The '*ivory vertebra*' (Fig. 11.98) is a classic manifestation of Hodgkin disease, although it is also seen in blastic metastatic disease and Paget's disease.

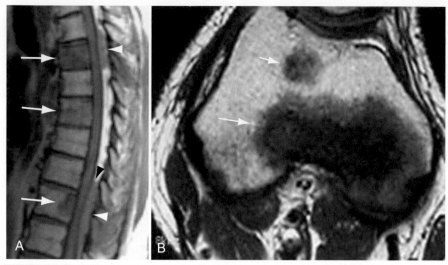

Fig. 11.97 Metastatic non-Hodgkin lymphoma. **(A)** Spine. Sagittal T1-weighted MR image in the thoracic spine of a 50-year-old man shows low signal in vertebral bodies *(arrows)* and epidural tumor *(arrowheads)* with cord compression. Epidural extension is common in lymphoma but is not specific because many tumors may grow within the epidural space. **(B)** Distal femur. Axial T1-weighted MR image shows low-signal lesions *(arrows)* with some preservation of trabeculae, reflecting the infiltrative behavior of lymphoma.

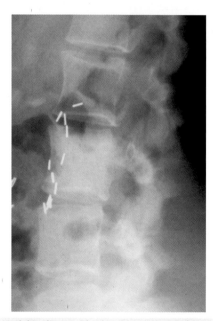

Fig. 11.98 Hodgkin disease. This lateral radiograph of the spine demonstrates an ivory vertebra at L3. Although ivory vertebra can be seen in other disease processes, the periaortic lymph node dissection suggested by the position of the clips helps to make the diagnosis of Hodgkin disease in this case. (Image used with permission from BJ Manaster, MD, from the American College of Radiology Learning File.)

- Two thirds of cases are polyostotic.
- The lesions may be moderately aggressive in appearance and may show a soft tissue mass.

MULTIPLE MYELOMA

- Multiple myeloma represents neoplastic proliferation of plasma cells and is the most common primary bone tumor.
- The solitary form is called *plasmacytoma*; the multiple form is much more frequent.
- Ninety-five percent of patients are older than 40 years of age.

Key Concepts

Multiple Myeloma

- Most common appearance: Multiple punched-out lytic lesions
- May present as diffuse osteopenia, without focal lytic lesion
- Occasionally presents as a focal lytic expansile lesion (plasmacytoma)
- Radiographic skeletal series less sensitive than whole-body MRI

- Plasmacytomas are lytic expansile geographic lesions (Fig. 11.99).
- They have a relatively narrow zone of transition without sclerotic margins (Lodwick 1B or 1C).
- No matrix calcification is present.
- The most common sites of occurrence for plasmacytoma reflect the distribution of red (hematopoietic) marrow in the skeleton: the vertebral bodies, pelvis, femur, and humerus.
- The differential diagnosis of plasmacytoma depends on its radiographic appearance. Other lesions that fit this description include metastasis, high-grade chondrosarcoma, GCT, and brown tumor of hyperparathyroidism.
- 70% of patients with plasma cell neoplasia have multiple myeloma, which most often presents with numerous focal, punched-out lytic lesions with a narrow zone of transition.
  - These lesions are generally less than 5 cm in size, often less than 1 cm (Fig. 11.100).
  - Occasionally lesions present as large, expansile 'blowout' lesions.
  - Less commonly, multiple myeloma presents as generalized osteopenia (Fig. 11.101), with no visible focal lesions. Finding unexplained generalized osteopenia, perhaps with a compression fracture in a patient who is not expected to have osteoporosis (i.e., a middle-aged man), should suggest the diagnosis of multiple myeloma.

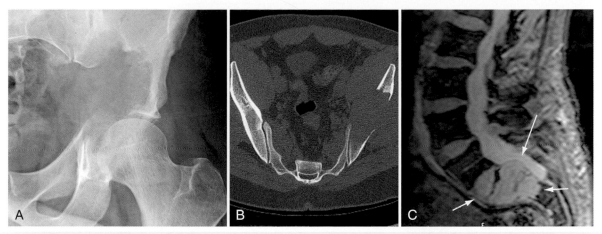

Fig. 11.99 Plasmacytoma. (A and B) Solitary large lytic lesion of the iliac wing. Radiograph **(A)** and CT scan **(B)** show a large, sharply marginated, purely lytic lesion with cortical breakthrough ('blowout lesion'). **(C)** Sagittal T2-weighted MR image of sacral plasmacytoma *(arrows)* in a different patient. This lobulated, 'mini-brain' appearance is typical for plasmacytoma.

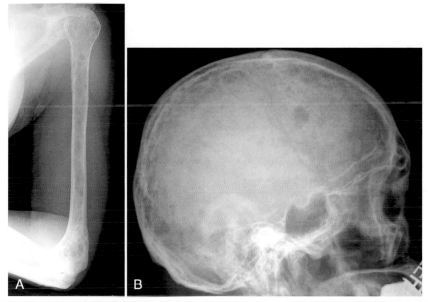

Fig. 11.100 Multiple myeloma. The humerus **(A)** and lateral skull **(B)** show multiple 'punched-out' round lytic lesions with a very narrow zone of transition typical of myeloma.

- A *variegated* (or "salt and pepper") pattern on MRI refers to diffuse marrow infiltration with numerous tiny T1-hypointense, T2-hyperintense lesions.
- Whether it presents as focal punched-out lesions, blowout lesions, or as generalized osteopenia, multiple myeloma originates in the red marrow but then progresses to the cortex and other areas.
- The major differential diagnosis for multiple myeloma is metastatic disease and the less-frequent multiple brown tumors of hyperparathyroidism.
- Some manifestations of multiple myeloma are unusual.
  - Ten to fifteen percent of cases of multiple myeloma are associated with symptomatic amyloidosis. When amyloid is deposited in the synovium, the radiographic picture may simulate rheumatoid arthritis. (Amyloidosis is further discussed in Chapter 9 – Arthritis and Chapter 13 – Bone Marrow and Metabolic Bone Disease).

  - Rarely, multiple myeloma may have a sclerotic pattern, with either a sclerotic margin around lytic lesions or entirely sclerotic round lesions. Such 'sclerosing myeloma' (Fig. 11.102) is associated with the POEMS syndrome. This acronym stands for the syndrome of polyneuropathy, organomegaly, endocrinopathy, M protein, and skin changes.
- The role of imaging in myeloma detection, staging, and restaging is evolving.
  - Radiographic skeletal survey is still advocated as the gold standard by one important clinical oncology organization, in part because of universal availability, with MRI having a more limited role.
  - However, total body MRI survey with STIR and T1-weighted sequences clearly is more sensitive in detection of small lesions and more reliably assesses overall tumor burden than radiographs or CT and thus is now the standard procedure at many centers.

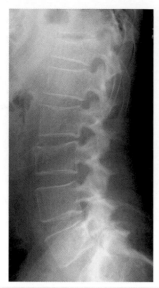

Fig. 11.101 Myeloma. A subtle example, where one sees only diffuse osteopenia and compression fractures of the superior endplates of T12 and L3. However, this radiograph is of a 32-year-old man who has no known metabolic disease or steroid use. When severe generalized osteopenia is seen in a patient whose age and gender do not suggest senile osteoporosis, multiple myeloma should be strongly considered.

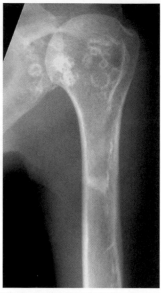

Fig. 11.102 Sclerosing myeloma. Multiple myeloma very rarely has lesions that are entirely sclerotic or show a sclerotic rim. Sclerosing myeloma is rare and is part of the POEMS syndrome, discussed in the text. This appearance can also be seen following successful treatment and healing of the lesions.

- MRI also demonstrates complications of therapy, including steroid complications (osteonecrosis), bisphosphonate complications such as mandible osteonecrosis and impending proximal femur shaft fractures, and epidural spread of disease, which can be an oncologic emergency.
  - A potential weakness of MRI is false-positives: myeloma lesions are generally bright on T2-weighted images and intermediate on T1-weighted images, a nonspecific appearance shared by many lesions, including atypical hematopoietic bone marrow. Specificity is improved with chemical shift (in- and out-of-phase) imaging for indeterminate lesions.
  - Adding FDG PET-CT further improves the specificity of MRI survey, and in combination they offer extremely high accuracy.
  - FDG PET-CT is the most accurate test for assessing disease response and posttreatment surveillance.
- Most cases of plasmacytoma progress to multifocal or generalized disease within a few years, although a few remain localized.
- Whole-body MRI at the time of diagnosis will upstage many plasmacytoma patients to multiple myeloma, which may offer these patients a better chance at survival. Going forward, this technique will likely become the standard of care in the workup.
- Multiple myeloma 5-year survival rates are improving, now >50% in the US.
  - Poor prognostic features include more than one bone lesion, high tumor burden, elevated serum tumor markers, renal failure, and more aggressive tumor genetics.
- Treatment depends on stage and disease activity.
  - Focal lesions and spinal cord compression are treated with radiation therapy, with occasional ablative surgery for plasmacytomas.

- Active disease is managed with aggressive chemotherapy with stem cell transplantation.
- Newer drugs including immune modulators, monoclonal antibodies, and others may avoid the need for stem cell transplants in some patients.
- Milder disease (smoldering myeloma) is treated less aggressively or observed.
- Bisphosphonates to preserve bone mineral density.
- Surgical stabilization of pathologic fractures or weakened bones with risk of fracture (i.e., large lesions or those involving greater than 50% of cortical width).
  - Prophylactic placement of an intramedullary nail may be used to prevent an impending long-bone fracture.
  - CT can better quantify the degree of cortical destruction in an individual lesion.
- Vertebroplasty or kyphoplasty can stabilize painful spine fractures.

METASTATIC DISEASE OF BONE

- Osseous metastasis occurs in 20–35% of malignancies.
- Metastases to bone are significantly more common (in a ratio of 25:1) than primary bone tumors.
- Over age 50, an aggressive bone lesion has a high likelihood of representing a metastasis or multiple myeloma.
- About 80% of bone metastases arise from primary tumors of the lung, breast, prostate, and kidney. Other common primary lesions metastasizing to bone include gastrointestinal, thyroid, and small round cell malignancies.
- Bone scan is highly sensitive for detection of blastic metastases and can be useful in differentiating blastic metastases (i.e., prostate) from benign sclerotic foci such as a giant bone island. Sensitivity of bone scan is lower

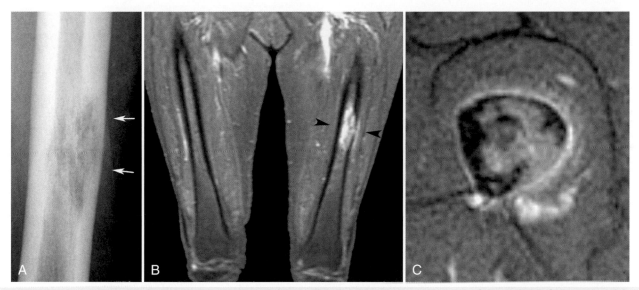

Fig. 11.103 Lytic metastasis. Lung adenocarcinoma metastasis to femur midshaft. **(A)** Permeative lytic lesion in femoral midshaft. Note cortical destruction *(arrows)*. The lesion was painful, and the patient was at risk for pathologic fracture. **(B)** Coronal inversion recovery MR image shows the lesion in the left femoral midshaft (between *arrowheads*). Note cortical lateral breakthrough. **(C)** Axial fat-suppressed, postcontrast T1-weighted MR image shows the enhancing tumor permeating through the normally low-signal cortex. This lesion was managed with radiation and prophylactic femoral nail placement.

for lytic metastases such as lung. Overall specificity of bone scan in screening for metastases is poor.

- PET-CT (in FDG-avid malignancies) and whole-body MRI screening examinations are alternatives to bone scan but are less widely used. PET-CT is very useful for detection of recurrent disease in FDG-avid tumors after treatment.
- Most commonly, radiographs, CT, and MRI are used in a complementary fashion with clinical findings and bone scans in an effort to improve accuracy.
- MRI is highly sensitive and moderately specific for evaluation of metastases.
- A lytic metastasis with bone pain warrants special attention because of risk for pathologic fracture.
  - Radiographic signs of impending fracture include lesions that occupy the majority of the medullary space and those showing 50% or greater cortical thickness destruction, especially in a weight-bearing region.
  - CT and MRI can be very useful in assessing the degree of cortical destruction and true tumor extent.
- It is important to remember that metastasis to bone can resemble a variety of primary bone tumors, both lytic and blastic.
- Most bone metastases have a moth-eaten or geographic pattern with an ill-defined or wide zone of transition, no sclerotic margin, and often little periosteal reaction or soft tissue mass (Fig. 11.103).
- Occasionally a metastasis may present as a geographic, bubbly, expansile mass (Fig. 11.104).
- Expansile solitary metastases are often caused by highly vascular lesions such as renal cell or thyroid carcinoma. Presurgical embolization can reduce the risk of hemorrhage with these metastases.
- The density of metastases varies.
  - Purely lytic metastases are most frequently of lung origin but are also seen with kidney, breast, thyroid, gastrointestinal, and neuroblastoma.

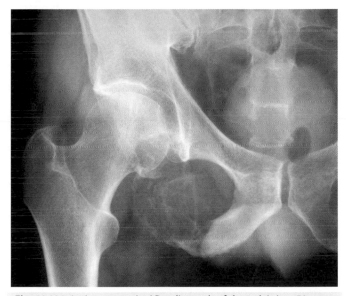

Fig. 11.104 Lytic metastasis. AP radiograph of the pelvis in a 50-year-old man demonstrates an expansile lytic renal cell carcinoma metastasis in the right ischium. Renal cell and thyroid metastases are often highly vascular and may bleed significantly after biopsy. When presented with a lytic lesion and a request for percutaneous biopsy, many experts advise a search for a primary tumor with physical examination, chest radiography, and abdomen CT before biopsy. Because this patient had a renal mass at CT (not shown), a smaller biopsy needle would be used to reduce the risk for hemorrhage.

  - Blastic metastases (Fig. 11.105) include prostate, breast, bladder, gastrointestinal (adenocarcinoma and carcinoid), lung (usually small cell), and medulloblastoma.
  - Mixed lytic and blastic metastases can be seen in breast (Fig. 11.106), lung, prostate, bladder, and neuroblastoma metastases.
  - With therapy or radiation necrosis, one may see changing patterns of density.

Fig. 11.105 Blastic metastases. **(A)** Multiple prostate metastases in the spine. **(B)** Subtle prostate metastases in a 45-year-old man. Note the small blastic lesion in the right femoral neck *(arrow)* and subtle sclerotic areas in the ischium *(arrowheads)*. These lesions are not clearly bone islands because they do not blend into surrounding trabeculae. Bone scan (not shown) showed high tracer uptake in these lesions, excluding bone islands. The prostate-specific antigen (PSA) level was elevated, and biopsy of a bone lesion showed prostate cancer. The PSA level is frequently, but not necessarily, elevated with metastatic prostate cancer. **(C)** Unusual bladder transitional cell carcinoma metastasis to the proximal ulna resembles a primary osteosarcoma with hair-on-end appearance.

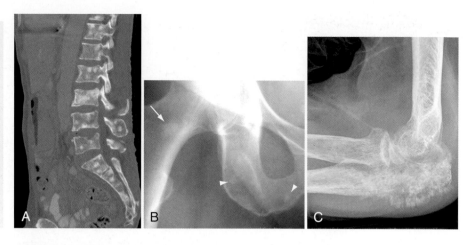

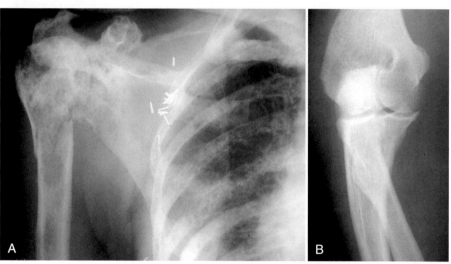

Fig. 11.106 Mixed-density metastases and distribution of metastatic disease. **(A)** Lytic and blastic destructive lesions involving the ribs and shoulder girdle bones in this 45-year-old woman with widespread metastatic breast carcinoma. Note the pathologic fracture of the proximal humeral shaft. **(B)** In contrast, the elbow and adjacent bones in the same extremity obtained at the same time are normal. This case typifies the distribution of metastases to sites of hematopoietic marrow, which in an adult are the axial and proximal appendicular skeleton.

Key Concepts

Metastases

- Purely lytic: Lung most frequent, followed by kidney, breast, thyroid, gastrointestinal (GI), neuroblastoma.
- Blastic: Prostate, breast, bladder, GI (adenocarcinoma and carcinoid), lung (usually small cell), medulloblastoma.
- Mixed lytic and blastic: Breast, lung, prostate, bladder, and neuroblastoma.
- Therapy or radiation necrosis can change the lesion density (e.g., lytic metastases heal to more normal density).
- Most metastases occur where red bone marrow is found, therefore 80% of metastases are located in the axial skeleton (ribs, pelvis, vertebrae, and skull) (Fig. 11.107; see Fig. 11.106), and proximal humerus and femur (see Figs. 11.94 and 11.106). Epiphyses are rarely involved.
- Lesions distal to the elbows or knees are usually caused by primary lung cancers that have accessed the pulmonary venous system.
- Although most metastases are central medullary lesions, occasionally a cortically-based metastasis can occur, most often of lung or breast origin (Fig. 11.108).
- Metastases are frequently found in the spine, where they may appear as nonspecific compression fractures caused by vertebral body destruction.
- Bone or PET-CT scan and MRI are the preferred modalities for detection of vertebral metastases. MRI also provides assessment of spinal cord compression.

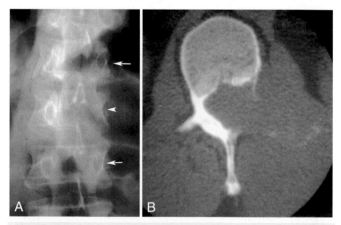

Fig. 11.107 Spinal metastasis with absent pedicle. **(A)** AP radiograph shows absent left L1 pedicle *(arrowhead)*. Contrast with the normal ovoid densities of the T12 and L2 pedicles *(arrows)*. **(B)** Axial CT image shows the destroyed left L1 pedicle and associated soft tissue mass. Most metastases to the spine occur in the vertebral body and are very difficult to detect on radiographs until bone loss is extensive.

- Some specific sites are worthy of mention with respect to metastatic disease.
    - First, a lesser trochanter avulsion fracture in an adult should be considered pathologic until proven otherwise (Fig. 11.109).

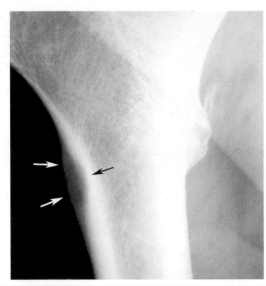

Fig. 11.108 Unusual site of metastasis. AP radiograph of the proximal femur in this 65-year-old man demonstrates a cortically-based lytic lesion *(arrows)*. Cortical metastases are uncommon, but when they occur, they are most likely caused by pulmonary or breast primary lesions.

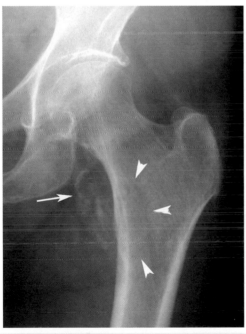

Fig. 11.109 Lesser trochanter avulsion *(arrow)*, in this case a result of metastatic lung cancer. Note the subtle adjacent lytic lesion *(arrowheads)*. This is a classic presentation for lung cancer, but myeloma, renal carcinoma, or aggressive tumors could also present this way. See also Fig. 5.29.

- Second, in patients with known breast cancer, a solitary sternal lesion is rare but, if present, has an 80% probability of being caused by metastatic disease.
- Finally, the presence of a transverse fracture in a long bone, especially without significant prior trauma, should alert the radiologist to the possibility of a pathologic fracture.

Miscellaneous Tumors and Tumorlike Lesions

GIANT CELL TUMOR OF BONE

- Giant cell tumor (GCT) is a relatively common, usually benign but frequently locally aggressive neoplasm constituting 5% of primary bone tumors.
- It consists of connective tissue, multinucleated osteoclastic giant cells resembling osteoclasts, and a fibrous stroma. The neoplastic cell is not the giant cell but rather a spindle cell in the stroma, which helps to distinguish GCT from the many other lesions that may contain reactive giant cells.
- GCTs nearly always occur after physeal fusion; 80% occur between 20 and 50 years of age.
- GCT is one of the few musculoskeletal tumors that is slightly more common in women (female-to-male ratio, 1.1 to 1.5:1).
- The tumors are eccentric and arise in the metaphysis (Fig. 11.110), then enlarge.
  - In the skeletally mature, extension into the epiphysis is a hallmark feature, with tumor typically extending to subchondral bone.
  - In skeletally immature patients, GCT may be confined to the metaphysis.
- Most (50–65%) occur about the knee, with most of the remainder at distal radius and ulna or proximal humerus.
- The vast majority of GCTs are solitary. Multiple lesions can occur, especially in skull and facial bones affected by Paget's disease.
  - Note that in a bone with Paget's disease, an aggressive lytic lesion should be considered sarcomatous transformation until proven otherwise, though differential diagnosis includes secondary GCT.
- GCTs also occur in the spine (7% of all GCTs), where they most often involve the sacrum or body of a vertebra (Fig. 11.111).
  - Ninety percent of spinal GCTs arise in the sacrum.
  - GCT is the second most common primary bone tumor of the sacrum (after chordoma) and is the most common benign primary sacral tumor (71% are GCT).
  - Within the sacrum, GCT tends to involve the upper elements (S1 or S2); it may involve adjacent vertebral bodies and/or cross the sacroiliac joint.

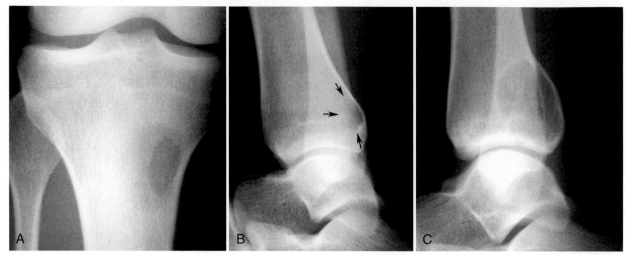

Fig. 11.110 Metaphyseal giant cell tumor (GCT). **(A)** AP radiograph of the proximal tibia in a 22-year-old woman demonstrates a lytic lesion arising eccentrically in the metaphysis having a narrow zone of transition but no sclerotic margin. Some might have a difficult time arriving at the diagnosis because the lesion does not extend all the way to the subchondral bone. It should be remembered that GCTs arise in the metaphysis and may only reach the subchondral bone when they are moderately large. (B and C) Different case showing moderate growth of GCT. Lateral radiograph **(B)** in an 18-year-old man shows a very subtle, small lytic lesion, with a narrow zone of transition lacking a sclerotic margin centered in the posterior distal tibial metaphysis extending toward the epiphysis *(arrows)*. Eighteen months later, lateral radiograph of the same ankle **(C)** shows the lesion has enlarged and now extends to the distal articular surface. This rate of growth is expected and does not imply aggressive or malignant GCT. (A, Image used with permission from BJ Manaster, MD, from the American College of Radiology Learning File.)

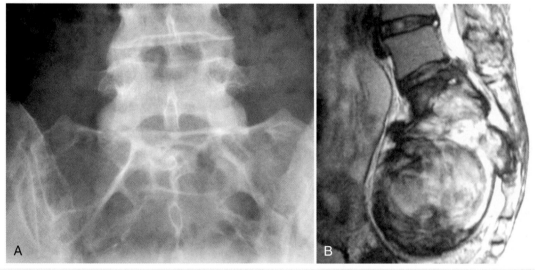

Fig. 11.111 Giant cell tumor (GCT) in the spine. **(A)** AP radiograph of the lumbar spine demonstrates an expanded lytic lesion occupying the superior sacrum. The extent of the lesion is seen better with MRI. **(B)** Sagittal T2-weighted MR image demonstrates a very large mass with heterogeneous signal intensity extending anteriorly from the sacrum. Note the densely whorled hypointense regions within the lesion; this is a typical appearance of GCT on fluid-sensitive sequences, likely caused by dense hemosiderin or collagen within the lesion. The spine and particularly the sacrum are favorite locations for GCT in the axial skeleton.

- GCT generally is a slowly growing tumor, but rapid growth has been reported during pregnancy.
- The typical radiographic appearance of GCT is a lytic geographic lesion with a narrow zone of transition and no marginal sclerosis (type 1B margin) at the end of a long bone, often with mild bone expansion (Figs. 11.112 and 11.113; see Figs. 11.110 and 11.111).
- A broader zone of transition (type 1C margin) can be seen, and areas of margin sclerosis are occasionally seen. (Remember to evaluate the aggressiveness of a lytic bone lesion by the most aggressive portion of its margin.)

- The lesion can also appear even more aggressive, with cortical breakthrough; however, extraosseous extension with a soft tissue mass is uncommon (Fig. 11.114).
- On CT a classic 'dot-dash' appearance of the cortex reflecting cortical bone loss is observed, leading to a permeative appearance of the cortex but without associated soft tissue mass.
- Though microscopic foci of calcification can be present, there is no calcified matrix seen on imaging.

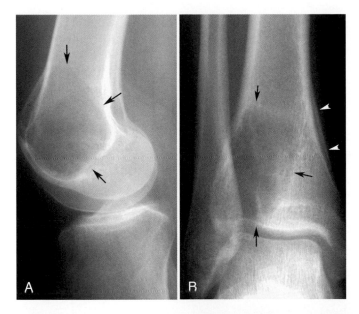

Fig. 11.112 Giant cell tumor (GCT). (A) Lateral knee radiograph shows a large lytic lesion in the distal femoral metaphysis *(arrows)*, extending to the subchondral bone at the anterior portion of the femoral condyle and the roof of the intercondylar notch. There is no matrix, and the zone of transition is narrow and lacks a sclerotic margin (type 1B margin). This is a typical appearance of GCT, seen in a 31-year-old woman. (B) GCT in the distal tibia of a 16-year-old boy *(arrows)*, with similar features. Note the mature periosteal new bone formation *(arrowheads)*, which is a normal stress response to structural weakening of the distal tibia rather than a direct response to the tumor.

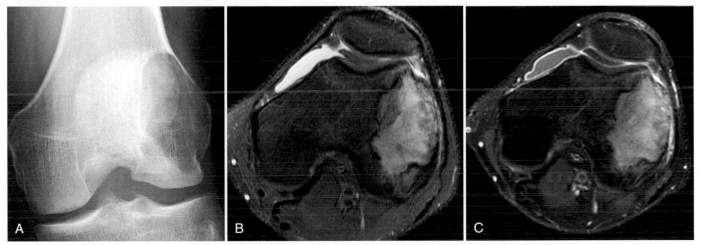

Fig. 11.113 Typical giant cell tumor (GCT). (A) AP radiograph demonstrates an eccentrically located lytic lesion arising within the distal femoral metaphysis and extending to the subchondral bone plate. The zone of transition is narrow, but the margin is not particularly sclerotic. There is no host reaction. Appearance is typical of GCT. (B) Axial T2-weighted fat-saturated MR image of the same lesion shows a heterogeneously hyperintense lesion with mild osseous expansion. There are nodular regions of low signal within about one fourth of the lesion, a finding characteristic of GCT. (C) Axial postcontrast T1-weighted fat-saturated image at the same level shows inhomogeneous enhancement of the lesion.

Key Concepts

Giant Cell Tumor (GCT)

- Typical lesion lytic geographic at the end of a long bone, without margin sclerosis. In the skeletally mature the lesion extends to the subchondral bone
- MRI: mostly intermediate on T1- and T2-weighted images, with areas of low T2 signal. Solid portions enhance intensely. Secondary ABCs in can show fluid-fluid levels
- Most common sites: About the knee, distal radius or ulna, vertebral body, or sacrum
- Originates in the metaphysis
- Rare before physeal fusion, most commonly between 20 and 40 years of age
- Most are benign, but may metastasize to lung
- Approximately 25–50% local recurrence rate; higher with less-aggressive surgery. Recurrent tumors may behave more aggressively

- MRI appearance:
  - The typical MRI appearance is uniform, intermediate-low signal intensity on T1-weighted images. High cellularity, hemosiderin, and collagen deposition result in relatively low T2-weighted signal (in 63–90%) within the lesion.
  - Areas of relatively low T2-weighted signal intensity are seen in at least 20% of lesions. This feature can help to distinguish GCT from other common subchondral lesions such as subchondral cyst or a Brodie abscess, which are usually uniformly bright on T2-weighted images.
  - Fluid-fluid levels also may be seen in GCTs due to secondary ABCs, which occur in approximately 14%.
  - Enhancement is seen in all cases following contrast administration and is usually heterogeneous.
  - Intense bone marrow edema and enhancement around the radiographically apparent margins of the

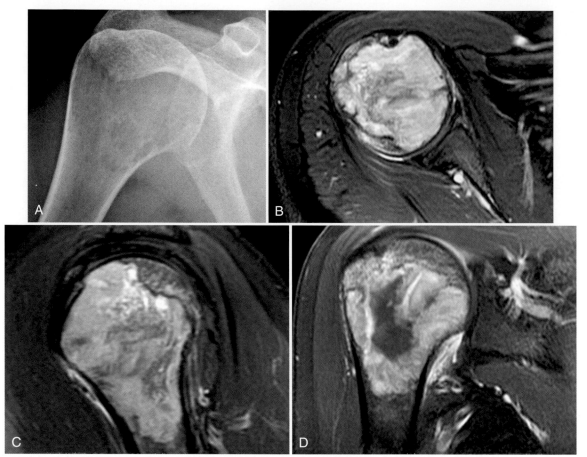

Fig. 11.114 Aggressive giant cell tumor. **(A)** AP radiograph shows a faintly seen lytic lesion within the proximal humerus of a 27-year-old woman. The lesion has a rather indistinct zone of transition, giving it an aggressive appearance. **(B)** Axial T2-weighted fat-saturated MR image of the same lesion shows a heterogeneously hyperintense lesion containing whorled low-signal foci. There is a small region of cortical breakthrough posteriorly. **(C)** Sagittal T2-weighted fat-saturated image shows the regions of hypointensity even more distinctly. **(D)** Coronal postcontrast T1-weighted fat-saturated image shows strong enhancement of the lesion, as well as a portion that has broken through the cortex. The central portion is partially necrotic.

lesion. This does not indicate marrow infiltration but rather represents reactive edema.

- The diagnosis is often made with imaging. In the long bones, differential diagnosis includes ABC, especially when fluid-fluid levels are present. As noted above, GCT and ABC may coexist.
  - A subchondral cyst or Brodie abscess might be considered but should have a more prominent sclerotic margin and should not show bone expansion.
  - Chondroblastoma also is a subchondral tumor and also may contain fluid-fluid levels, but chondroblastoma is generally found in skeletally immature patients and arises in the epiphysis (remember that GCT originates in the metaphysis, though it usually extends across the epiphysis to the subchondral bone after physeal closure). Chondroblastoma also typically has sclerotic margins and often contains chondroid matrix calcification.
  - Brown tumor of hyperparathyroidism may have a radiographic appearance similar to that of GCT. However, these patients have appropriate clinical history and will manifest typical radiographic features of hyperparathyroidism.
  - Other lytic lesions, such as plasmacytoma, metastasis, or a sarcoma without matrix, may resemble GCT.

- Nonossifying fibroma is an eccentric metaphyseal lesion. Its slightly different location, as well as its sclerotic border, should easily differentiate this lesion from GCT.
- In the spine and sacrum, GCT could be confused most frequently with chordoma or chondrosarcoma because the location in the body of the sacrum or vertebra is similar.
- Spinal ABC and osteoblastoma usually occur in the posterior elements rather than the body, which is the typical site of GCT.
- Almost all GCTs are benign with low histologic grade, but despite this approximately 2% are malignant.
- These are notoriously unpredictable tumors. Lesion local aggressiveness is not well-predicted by histology or imaging appearance.
- Five percent metastasize to the lung, including from benign lesions (*benign metastasizing giant cell tumor*). The lung metastases are very slow growing and have benign histology identical to the primary tumor. An hypothesized mechanism for this bizarre situation is venous embolization. Among patients with histologically benign lesions that metastasize, the prognosis is excellent with surgical resection of the lung metastases.

- The mainstay of management of the primary tumor has long been resection and curettage, but local recurrence rates were as high as 40% and recurrent tumor often was more aggressive than the original tumor.
  - Adding bisphosphonates stabilizes bone adjacent to the tumor and reduces recurrence rates.
  - The next advance was to supplement currettage with ablative therapy (thermal, phenol, hydrogen peroxide, PMMA, burring), reducing local recurrence rates to 10% or less.
    - If PMMA is used, it supports the thin residual overlying articular bone, and it cures at high temperature, enhancing tumor kill at the surgical margins.
    - Follow-up radiographs will show a thin radiolucent halo around the PMMA as a normal finding.
- *Denosumab* is an immunotherapy monoclonal antibody medication that inhibits production of multinucleated osteoclasts, and is remarkably effective treating GCT. It is possible that a large proportion of cases will be treated medically in the near future.
- Evaluation of GCT local recurrence: New, enlarging, asymmetric lytic regions in the tumor bed or surgical margins indicate recurrence (Fig. 11.115).
  - MRI: recurrent tumors are enhancing, intermediate-signal-intensity lesions that can be obscured by the surrounding post surgical change. However, if the tumor was treated methyl methacrylate, the recurrant tumor is easily seen adjacent to the dark cement.
  - Treatment options for recurrent tumor include aggressive surgical therapy with wide resection and replacement of the resected bone with an osteoarticular graft or a long-stem custom prosthesis, but in a young patient, such prosthesis might require multiple revisions throughout life, causing considerable morbidity.
  - Moreover, tumors can recur despite such wide resection. Because of the difficulty of resection, spine GCT may be treated with radiation.

- Radiation therapy carries a risk of tumor malignant transformation.
- *Giant cell reparative granuloma* is a nonneoplastic reactive lytic lesion that occurs primarily in the jaw, maxilla, hands, and feet.
  - The radiographic features may be similar to those of GCT, but the lesion is otherwise unrelated to GCT (except of course that both contain giant cells at histologic evaluation).
  - The similarity in tumor names is a potential source of confusion.

SIMPLE BONE CYST (UNICAMERAL OR SOLITARY BONE CYST)

- Simple bone cyst (SBC), also termed 'solitary or unicameral bone cyst', is a very common nonneoplastic lesion of childhood, most frequently discovered in the first and second decades of life (85%).
- It is a benign fluid-filled (serous or serosanguineous) cystic osseous lesion that is often found incidentally or may present with a pathologic fracture.
- In children 90% occur in the long bones, with the most common sites being the proximal humerus (50%), followed by the proximal femur (20%).
- SBC is a geographic lytic lesion with sharp margins that typically are sclerotic (type 1A) but occasionally nonsclerotic (type 1B).
- It may be mildly expansile with thinning of the endosteal cortex and has no tumor matrix.
- In the absence of pathologic fracture, there is no periosteal reaction.
- The lesion does not cross the growth plate.
- SBC is a central lesion that initially is metaphyseal in location, abutting the growth plate.
- With advancing skeletal maturation, an SBC 'migrates' into the diaphysis (Fig. 11.116).
  - This 'migration' actually represents growth of normal bone away from the cyst.

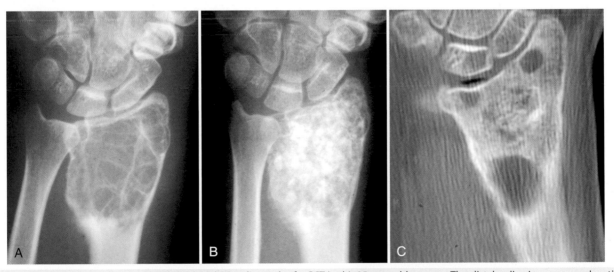

Fig. 11.115 Recurrent giant cell tumor (GCT). **(A)** Initial AP radiograph of a GCT in this 25-year-old woman. The distal radius is a common location for GCT, and this case is atypical only in the degree of pseudotrabeculation seen. **(B)** The lesion was treated with curettage and grafting, as shown in the radiograph. **(C)** One year later, direct coronal CT demonstrates that, although much of the bone graft has incorporated and matured, three separate sites of lucency are tumor recurrence within the distal radius.

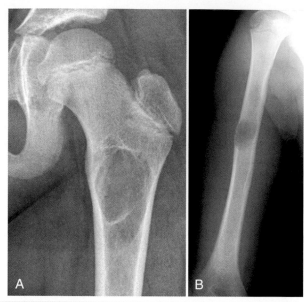

Fig. 11.116 Simple bone cyst (SBC). **(A)** AP radiograph of the proximal femur in a child demonstrates a central mildly expansile lytic lesion, located in the metadiaphysis. Note the thinned cortex, lack of matrix, and narrow zone of transition. **(B)** AP radiograph of the humerus in a different child demonstrates an SBC that has 'migrated away' from the metaphysis, with a pathologic fracture through the lesion.

- As the name implies, the lesions are fluid-filled.
- Lesions may contain internal bone septations or pseudo-trabeculations (Fig. 11.117), but the lesion usually consists of a single communicating space, hence the terms 'simple' and 'unicameral'.
- Lesions presenting with pathologic fracture may have the *fallen fragment sign*, which represents a fracture fragment that settles inferiorly in the dependent portion of the fluid-filled cyst (see Figs. 11.10A and 11.117). In a young patient with a well-circumscribed

lytic lesion in a typical location, this finding is pathognomonic for SBC.
- SBC rarely can be found in adults, often in locations that are unusual for this lesion in children, such as the iliac wing, calcaneus, or talus (Fig. 11.118).
- MRI is rarely required for diagnosis of SBC. However, the MRI appearance is typical of a cyst with low-signal T1 and fluid-like T2 signal with occasional fluid-fluid levels representing internal hemorrhage if the cyst has been previously traumatized (Fig. 11.119). Fibrous septations may be seen.
  - Only a very fine rim of peripheral enhancement may be seen on postcontrast MRI.
- It is important to note that fewer than 50% of proven SBC cases meet all the criteria of 'simple' cysts.
  - On T1-weighted imaging, 40% show heterogeneity and may contain small regions of high signal, presumably related to blood products related to pathologic fracture. Signal on fluid-sensitive sequences may be inhomogeneous.
  - Lesions may contain septa that enhance with contrast. The septa may be incomplete and fluid may communicate through the entire lesion, though 75% may have loculated regions.
  - Thus many SBCs do not fully meet the criteria of a simple fluid-filled cyst on MRI.
  - Such complex MRI features should not deter consideration of SBC as the diagnosis if this is the most reasonable diagnosis by characteristic radiographic features in the appropriate age group.
- The major radiographic differential diagnosis includes fibrous dysplasia (if there is no matrix present to give the typical ground-glass appearance of fibrous dysplasia) and LCH.
  - ABC is usually not part of this differential diagnosis because it is eccentrically located rather than the centrally located SBC.

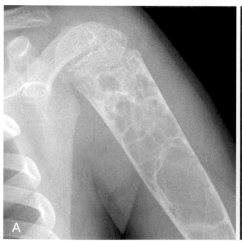
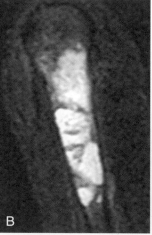
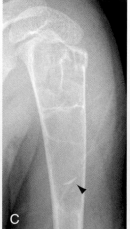
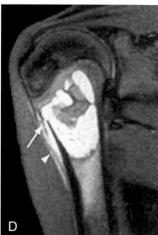

Fig. 11.117 Simple bone cyst (SBC). **(A)** AP radiograph of the humerus shows a lytic central metadiaphyseal lesion causing mild expansion of the bone. There is a narrow zone of transition and sclerotic margin. There are regions of loculation and pseudotrabeculation, making the lesion appear more complex than a 'simple' bone cyst, but often seen in this lesion. **(B)** Sagittal T2-weighted fat-saturated image of the same lesion shows high signal within the lesion that appears to have septa and loculated regions. **(C)** AP radiograph of another patient with SBC. The lesion is again typical, showing a lytic geographic appearance expanding the bone concentrically. In addition, there is a small fragment of bone floating within the cyst *(arrowhead)*. This is a 'floating fragment'; the fragment is a small fractured piece and is thought to be pathognomonic for SBC. See also Fig. 11.10A for an example of the fallen fragment sign. **(D)** Coronal T2-weighted fat-saturated image of SBC in another patient shows pathologic fracture *(arrow)* along with subperiosteal fluid *(arrowhead)*. The contents of this SBC are not as 'simple' as the name implies.

- SBC occurring in the adult calcaneus may resemble an intraosseous lipoma or a pseudocyst. (A pseudocyst is an area of relative lucency seen on a radiograph between areas of primary bone trabeculae).
- SBCs are treated with corticosteroid injections. Multiple injections may be required over several months. In most cases the lesions shrink and disappear.
- Surgical curettage and bone grafting are reserved for lesions that do not respond to injections or are at risk of pathologic fracture. Surgery is avoided if possible for SBCs adjacent to a physis to avoid physeal injury and growth disturbance.

- The recurrence rate following curettage is high (35–50%). The likelihood of recurrence relates predominantly to patient age, with younger patients (those younger than age 10) having a much higher likelihood of recurrence. SBC with pathologic fracture in the proximal humerus is treated with immobilization. Fracture healing can also induce 'healing' of the SBC.

Key Concepts

Simple Bone Cyst

- First and second decades of life
- Central metaphyseal or metadiaphyseal proximal humeral location most common
- Expansile, geographic, nonaggressive
- 'Fallen fragment' sign if fracture
- Often does not have the appearance of a 'simple' cyst
- Treated with serial steroid injections, or curettage if needed
- High recurrence rate following curettage

ANEURYSMAL BONE CYST

- An aneurysmal bone cyst (ABC) is a benign, expansile (often extremely, hence the term 'aneurysmal'), eccentric bone lesion consisting of blood-filled cystic cavities separated by connective tissue septa.
- ABC is found most frequently in the first through third decades of life, with 70% of cases occurring between 5 and 20 years of age.
- ABC may be primary or secondary.
  - At least a subset of ABCs are related to genetic translocation, suggesting that these represent primary neoplasms.

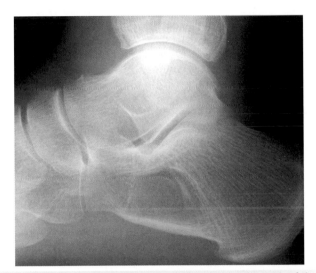

Fig. 11.118 Adult simple bone cyst (SBC). Lateral radiograph of the calcaneus in a 43-year-old man, demonstrating a lytic lesion in the anterior portion of the calcaneus. This is a typical location for either SBC or intraosseous lipoma. Biopsy in this case demonstrated SBC.

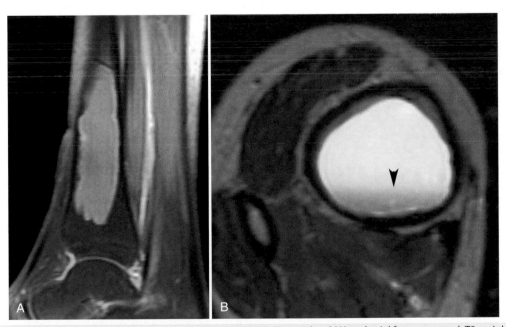

Fig. 11.119 Adult simple bone cyst (SBC). Sagittal fat-suppressed, postcontrast, T1-weighted **(A)** and axial fat-suppressed, T2-weighted **(B)** MR images show the typical features of a cyst, with uniform high T2 signal and fluid-fluid level in B *(arrowhead)*, and intermediate-low T1 signal and enhancement only of the rim of the tumor in A. Absence of surrounding marrow or periosteal edema or enhancement suggests that despite the bone loss caused by the lesion, there is no stress reaction in the surrounding bone.

- Secondary ABC arises within a preexisting tumor, most frequently GCT, chondroblastoma, fibrous dysplasia, osteoblastoma, or nonossifying fibroma.
- These associations may be found in up to 30% of cases.
- These observations underlie the need for careful radiologic evaluation of ABCs so that the presence of an associated tumor is not missed during biopsy. Excisional biopsy is often preferred because it avoids this pitfall.

Key Concepts

Aneurysmal Bone Cyst (ABC)

- Expansile (often extremely), lytic, narrow zone of transition, eccentric, metaphyseal in long bones. Thin, intact shell of expanded overlying bone
- Also found in posterior elements in the spine
- Generally younger than 30 years of age
- CT and MRI demonstrate fluid-fluid levels in most cases
- Occasionally it is rapidly progressive, simulating a more aggressive lesion
- May be posttraumatic (often cortically-based) or secondary within a preexisting tumor—look for a solid enhancing component that might represent the primary tumor

---

- The lesion is usually located in the metaphysis of a long bone (70–80%). Femur, tibia, and humerus are the most common locations.
  - They are rarely found in the flat bones; 50% of these are in the pelvis.
  - Ten to fifteen percent are located in the hands or feet (Fig. 11.120).
  - Fifteen percent arise in the spine, where they originate in the posterior elements but may extend to involve the body.

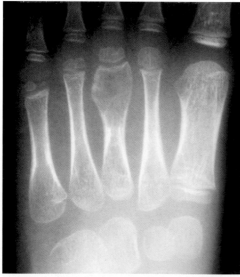

Fig. 11.120 Aneurysmal bone cyst (ABC). Foot radiograph in a child shows an expansile lesion in the distal third metatarsal metadiaphysis. There is no matrix or cortical breakthrough. A solitary bone cyst (SBC) could be considered as well, although there is more bone expansion than usually seen with SBC. Completely lytic enchondroma is another possibility, but ABC was proven in this case.

- ABC is usually a geographic lesion with a narrow zone of transition, often large with extreme ('aneurysmal') bone expansion, a narrow zone of transition, and a fine sclerotic rim (type 1A margin) (Fig. 11.121).
  - This sclerotic rim may not be seen on radiographs (see Fig. 11.121) but is more completely seen with CT; nonetheless, the margin appears complete in only 63%
- There is no tumor matrix.
- Both CT and MRI usually show fluid-fluid levels (Figs. 11.122 through 11.125), but it should be noted that such levels are not specific for ABCs; they also have been described in SBC, GCT, telangiectatic osteosarcoma, osteoblastoma, chondroblastoma, and rarely in other lesions.
  - These are also some of the tumors associated with ABC, and thus a fluid-fluid level seen in these tumors may be within a secondary ABC
  - The presence of an associated tumor may be suggested by a thick rind, thick septations, or a peripheral nodule or mass (see Figs. 11.123D and 11.125).
- A solid variety of ABC (5%) does not show fluid-fluid levels; these lesions have aggressive imaging features.
- The major differential diagnosis of ABC includes nonossifying fibroma, fibrous dysplasia, and SBC in the long bones; osteoblastoma in the spine; and lesions that may contain fluid-fluid levels as noted previously (see Box 29.13).
  - It is particularly important to avoid underdiagnosing a telangiectatic osteosarcoma as ABC, because the treatment is radically different.
- As with GCT, ABC management is advancing. Historically, the main management therapy was curettage, with or without bone grafting depending on size and location of the lesion. However, recurrence is common, as high as 59%.
- Adjuvant therapies have been developed that reduce recurrence:
  - High speed burr: after curettage, burring can cause mechanical disruption of the interior of the lesion.
  - Argon beam coagulation: induces desiccation and coagulation within the cavity after curettage.
  - Phenol injection: 'sterilizes' the interior of the lesion, destroying residual neoplastic cells.
  - Cryosurgery: freezing provides a cytotoxic effect.
  - PMMA: undergoes an exothermic reaction which can also provide a cytotoxic effect.
  - Sclerotherapy: agents including polidocanol and Ethibloc cause thrombosis and coagulation.
  - Selective arterial embolization of the lesion reduces intraoperative bleeding and may instead be combined with percutaneous sclerosant injection.
  - Bisphosphonates and Denosumab also may assist with management.
  - Radiotherapy has also been proposed for unresectable lesions.

LANGERHANS CELL HISTIOCYTOSIS

- Langerhans cell histiocystosis (LCH), formerly known as histiocytosis X or eosinophilic granuloma (EG), is one of a variety of rare disorders that occur predominantly in

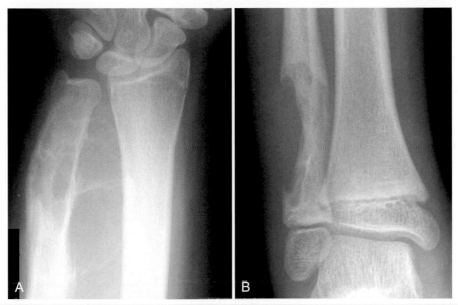

Fig. 11.121 Aneurysmal bone cyst (ABC). **(A)** AP radiograph of the distal forearm in a 16-year-old boy demonstrates an eccentrically located metaphyseal expansile lesion. This is a large but nonaggressive lesion, typical for ABC. Outer expanded 'rim' is only incompletely seen. **(B)** AP radiograph of the ankle in an adolescent shows an eccentric lytic metaphyseal fibular lesion. The lateral cortical rim is so thin that it is not visible on the radiograph, giving the lesion an aggressive appearance.

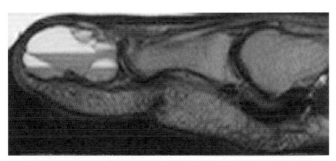

Fig. 11.122 Aneurysmal bone cyst (ABC) of the great toe. Sagittal inversion recovery MR image shows an expansile lesion of the great toe distal phalanx with multiple fluid-fluid levels.

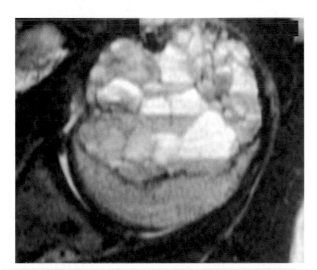

Fig. 11.123 Aneurysmal bone cyst (ABC) of the proximal humerus. Axial T2-weighted MR image of the left shoulder shows an ABC in the proximal humerus of a 35-year-old woman, with the typical bone expansion and multiple fluid-fluid levels.

children, characterized by histiocytic infiltration of various organ systems.

- The defining infiltrating cell is the Langerhans cell, which is a specific type of immunologic cell. Neutrophils, eosinophils, and macrophages also are found in the infiltrates.
- The cause of LCH is poorly understood, and it is not agreed whether the condition is reactive or neoplastic.
- Overall, LCH is more common in males, and, although it can affect patients of any age, it usually presents in patients younger than 15 years.
- The most common manifestation of LCH is a localized, often solitary, lytic bone lesion.
- More aggressive, clinical variations of LCH with multi-organ system involvement include *Letterer–Siwe* and *Hand–Schüller–Christian* disease. Other forms of LCH have been described, and many patients do not fit clearly into any category.
  - *Letterer–Siwe disease.*
    - The most severe and least common (10%) clinical form of LCH is Letterer–Siwe disease, which is aggressive multisystem involvement in infants and toddlers younger than 2 years. Letterer–Siwe is more common in boys.
    - Radiographic bone findings consisting of small lytic lesions primarily in the skull are present in only about half of children with Letterer–Siwe disease, although marrow infiltration is frequent.
    - Clinical findings include hepatosplenomegaly, lymphadenopathy, pancytopenia (caused by histiocytic infiltration of the marrow space), and skin infiltration.
    - Mortality exceeds 50%.

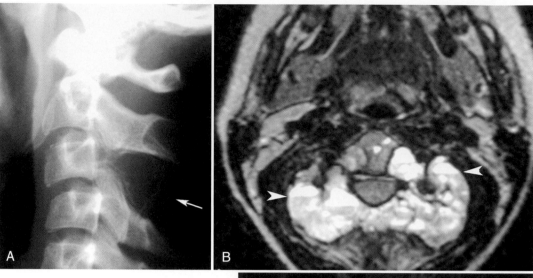

Fig. 11.124 Aneurysmal bone cyst (ABC) of the spine. **(A)** Lateral radiograph of the cervical spine in an adolescent demonstrates expansion and near-complete destruction of the posterior elements of C3 *(arrow)*. **(B)** Axial T2-weighted MR image shows the large lesion size. Note the numerous fluid-fluid levels throughout *(arrowheads)*. The age of the patient, along with the location of the lesion in the posterior elements of the spine and the presence of multiple fluid-fluid levels, makes the diagnosis of ABC. **(C)** Sacral ABC in a different patient *(arrowheads)*. Axial T2-weighted MR image shows fluid-fluid levels throughout the lesion.

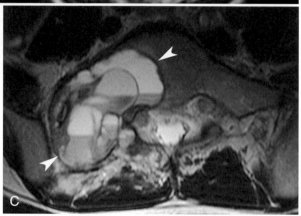

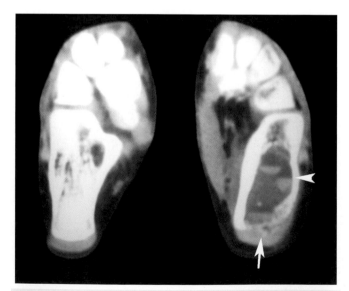

Fig. 11.125 Secondary aneurysmal bone cyst (ABC). Axial CT shows a mass in the left calcaneus that contains areas with fluid-fluid levels *(arrowhead)*. Also note the posterior cortical destruction *(arrow)*. The appearance suggests telangiectatic osteosarcoma, but this was a giant cell tumor with a large secondary ABC that occupied most of the lesion.

Key Concepts

Langerhans Cell Histiocytosis (LCH)

- Rare spectrum of disorders in children related to histiocytic infiltration of various organ systems. Not all patients match the classic subtypes
- Letterer–Siwe disease: Aggressive multiorgan system disease, age 0–2 years, high mortality rate
- Hand–Schüller–Christian disease: Intermediate, chronic multiorgan system disease
- LCH of bone: Single organ system involvement in bone
- Bone lesions may have a variety of appearances. One classic pattern of long-bone lesions begins with a highly aggressive appearance, with a permeative pattern and soft tissue mass, but often heal spontaneously over 6–24 months
- Ten to twenty percent are polyostotic
- Spine: Vertebra plana
- Skull: Beveled-edge sharply defined lytic lesion
- Differential diagnosis depends on lesion appearance. Often includes Ewing sarcoma, osteomyelitis, and metastatic neuroblastoma

- *Hand–Schüller–Christian disease.*
  - Hand–Schüller–Christian disease is a clinically less-aggressive, more common (20%) form of LCH, with chronic multiorgan system involvement.

- Clinical onset is usually age 2–10 years.
- Classical clinical features include proptosis, diabetes insipidus, and lytic bone lesions. Thymus, liver, and lung involvement may occur.
- Spontaneous pneumothorax and eventual pulmonary fibrosis can occur.
- Mortality is low in the absence of pulmonary involvement.
- The most common expression of LCH is isolated bone involvement.
- The discrete bone lesion has long been termed EG of bone, but LCH of bone is now the preferred term. 'EG' is so embedded in the terminology that it maintains clinical relevance and is likely to persist, but the remainder of this discussion uses the term LCH of bone.
- Most occur at age 5–15 years, but the disorder can present late into the 20s or in younger children.
- Younger age at presentation is associated with greater chance of progression to polyostotic disease.
- Clinically, the lesions are painful, and there may be a palpable lump.
- Most cases of bone involvement present with a single lesion, but 25–34% develop polyostotic disease within 6 months of developing the first lesion.
- The skull and flat bones are the most common site (65–70%), followed by the long bones (25–30%, femur most common); spine is involved in 9%.
- The radiographic appearance of LCH of bone varies; thus it appears in the differential diagnosis of many types of lesions.
  - Long-bone lesions usually begin with a highly aggressive moth-eaten or permeative pattern. These lesions are usually central and metadiaphyseal, but any part of the bone may be involved. (Recall that LCH of bone is included in the short differential diagnosis of a lytic epiphyseal lesion in a child, along with infection and chondroblastoma.) There may be a soft tissue mass.

- When LCH is confined to bone, the lesions may heal spontaneously over months to 2 years. The margin becomes well defined, and periosteal reaction, which can be highly aggressive in appearance at presentation, becomes solid (Figs. 11.126 and 11.127).
- Thus, depending on when a lesion is studied, the appearance can vary from aggressive to nonaggressive.
- Discordant findings of solid (nonaggressive) periosteal reaction around a permeative (highly aggressive) lesion in a long-bone diaphysis in a child is a classic appearance in a spontaneously healing LCH (see Fig. 11.126).
- Skull lesions have a narrow zone of transition with nonuniform involvement of the inner and outer skull tables, giving a beveled-edge appearance when viewed on edge, or concentric lytic disks when viewed en face.
- The lesions tend not to have a sclerotic margin. There is no tumor matrix, but rarely a fragment of bone may be left centrally, resembling a sequestrum. Periosteal reaction is common, and a soft tissue mass may be seen.
- LCH can also involve the vertebral body (Figs. 11.128 and 11.129).
  - The vertebral body involvement can have a classic radiographic appearance of a compressed vertebral body (*vertebra plana*), with intact posterior elements and disks and lack of an associated soft tissue mass (see Fig. 11.128).
  - However, if the collapse is recent, paraspinous hematoma may mimic soft tissue mass.

Key Concepts

Vertebra Plana

- LCH (no associated soft tissue mass on cross-sectional imaging unless acute collapse with hematoma)
- Tumor (metastases, myeloma, leukemia, hemangioma)
- Fracture (osteoporosis, osteogenesis imperfecta)
- Infection

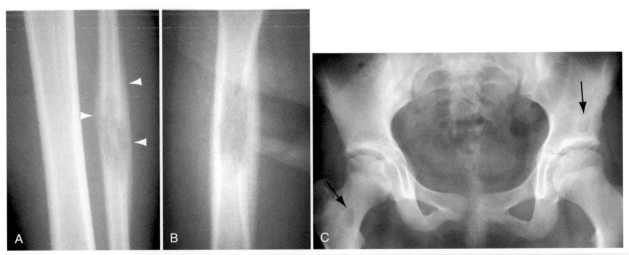

Fig. 11.126 Langerhans cell histiocytosis (LCH) of bone. This condition can have a wide variety of appearances, ranging from highly aggressive to completely nonaggressive. **(A)** AP radiograph showing a highly aggressive permeative lesion in the fibular middiaphysis of a 3-year-old girl, suggesting Ewing sarcoma. However, there is a discordant finding of nonaggressive solid periosteal reaction *(arrowheads)*. This unusual juxtaposition indicates a healing lesion, in this case a spontaneously healing Langerhans cell histiocytoma. **(B)** Similar pattern in the femur in of a 2-year-old, showing an aggressive lytic diaphyseal lesion that could easily be either LCH or Ewing sarcoma. LCH was proven at biopsy. **(C)** Another pattern of LCH in a different patient, a 12-year-old girl. In this case the disease is polyostotic and the lesions have a narrow zone of transition but lack sclerotic margins *(arrows)*.

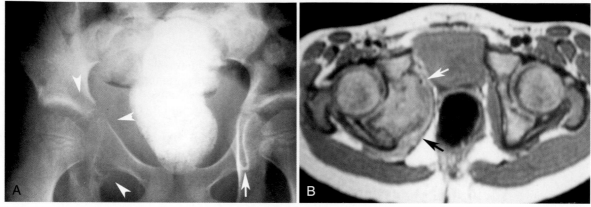

Fig. 11.127 Langerhans cell histiocytosis (LCH). **(A)** AP radiograph of the pelvis in a 6-year-old boy demonstrates a geographic lytic lesion with broad zone of transition involving the right acetabulum *(arrowheads)*. Note that the radiographic teardrop in the right hip has been destroyed, compared with the left side *(arrow)*. **(B)** Axial proton density–weighted MR image demonstrates a large soft tissue mass *(arrows)*. With this aggressive pattern of osseous destruction and soft tissue mass in a patient of this age, Ewing sarcoma should be most strongly considered, but it should be remembered that LCH can also have an aggressive appearance. This was proven to be LCH at biopsy. (Images used with permission from BJ Manaster, MD, from the American College of Radiology Learning File.)

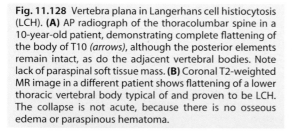

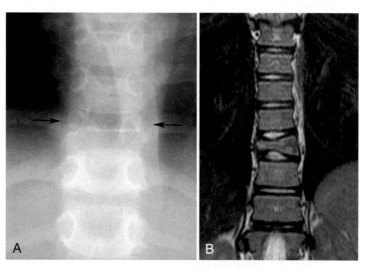

Fig. 11.128 Vertebra plana in Langerhans cell histiocytosis (LCH). **(A)** AP radiograph of the thoracolumbar spine in a 10-year-old patient, demonstrating complete flattening of the body of T10 *(arrows)*, although the posterior elements remain intact, as do the adjacent vertebral bodies. Note lack of paraspinal soft tissue mass. **(B)** Coronal T2-weighted MR image in a different patient shows flattening of a lower thoracic vertebral body typical of and proven to be LCH. The collapse is not acute, because there is no osseous edema or paraspinous hematoma.

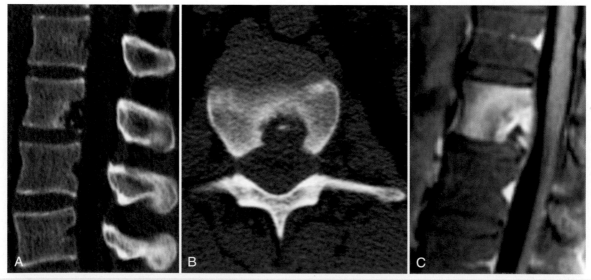

Fig. 11.129 Langerhans cell histiocytoma (LCH), spine. Sagittal **(A)** and axial **(B)** CT scans show a lytic lesion within the posterior inferior body of L2. There is a small bony sequestrum within the lytic portion of the lesion; the sequestrum and location of the lesion are strongly suggestive of LCH. **(C)** Sagittal postcontrast T1-weighted fat-saturated image shows significant peripheral enhancement of the lesion and a small epidural soft tissue mass. There is edema seen throughout the vertebral body.

- Because LCH of bone can be highly aggressive in its radiographic appearance as well as its rapid evolution, the differential diagnosis includes Ewing sarcoma, lymphoma, osteomyelitis, and aggressive bone metastases.
- Although LCH of bone can have a soft tissue mass and an aggressive appearance, it is a benign lesion. Radiography may suggest the diagnosis, particularly when the lesion is polyostotic or has radiographic features noted previously, but biopsy may be required for definitive diagnosis.
- Predictors of clinical outcome in children with LCH include the number of organ systems involved and the child's age.
  - Children with multiorgan system disease, especially with pulmonary disease, and those younger than 2 years of age fare more poorly.
  - Many therapeutic regimens have been used, and therapy for LCH is not standardized.
  - For a single organ system bone disease with a single LCH, curettage, wide excision, and intralesional steroid injection all have been effective.
  - However, because solitary osseous LCH often heals spontaneously, there is some debate as to whether any treatment is needed if the patient has no painful lesion or widespread bone disease.
  - Optimal treatment for aggressive multisystem disease may include chemotherapy.
  - Radiation may be used for vertebral disease with cord compression.
- *Erdheim–Chester disease* is a rare, non-Langerhans histiocytosis that presents with painful sclerosis of the long bones sparing the epiphyses.
  - Multiorgan system infiltration with lipid-laden macrophages, multinucleated giant cells, lymphocytes, and histiocytes bears some resemblance to LCH at histologic examination.
  - However, Erdheim–Chester is a disease of adults rather than children.
  - This condition is fatal, causing organ failure such as cardiac or renal failure or pulmonary fibrosis.

BROWN TUMOR OF HYPERPARATHYROIDISM

- Brown tumors are localized accumulations of osteoclasts that produce expanded lytic lesions in patients with hyperparathyroidism or renal osteodystrophy.
- Radiographically and pathologically, a brown tumor may be difficult to differentiate from a GCT.
- The untreated lesion is lytic, geographic, and nonspecific on MRI. However, other manifestations of hyperparathyroidism are usually present as well, making the diagnosis possible (Fig. 11.130; see also Fig. 13.36).
- Brown tumors are thought to occur with greater frequency in primary hyperparathyroidism, but because secondary hyperparathyroidism is so much more common, most brown tumors occur in secondary hyperparathyroidism.
- Following treatment of hyperparathyroidism, a brown tumor may ossify, sometimes densely.

CHORDOMA

- Chordoma is a low-grade malignant neoplasm that arises from notochord remnants, most often in adults (fourth through seventh decades of life).
- Chordoma is the most common primary malignant bone tumor in the spine (20–34%).
- It is more frequent in men (male-to-female ratio, 2:1).
- Because of the cell of origin, it is specifically restricted in location to the clivus, spine, and sacrum.
  - The greatest number (50%) arise in the sacrum and coccyx; indeed, chordomas represent 40% of all sacrococcygeal tumors. It tends to involve the lower sacral elements.
  - Chordomas are next most frequently found in the clivus (35%), and 15% occur in the spine, most frequently the lumbar region.
  - Spine chordomas begin in the midline in the vertebral body but may extend into the posterior elements.
- Chordomas cause extensive local bone destruction, often with a large soft tissue mass, extending into either the spinal canal or the paraspinal soft tissues (Fig. 11.131).
- The tumor infiltrates surrounding soft tissues and may present with neurologic symptoms or, in the sacrum, rectal bleeding or bowel or bladder symptoms.
- Extension to adjacent bodies is common, as is extension across the sacroiliac joint.
- Skull base chordomas are usually small when detected.
- Metastasis is uncommon (to the lung when it occurs), but chordoma can have a high morbidity because of local neurologic involvement.

Key Concepts

Chordoma

- Arises from notochord remnants; sacrococcygeal, skull base/clivus, vertebral bodies, especially C2
- Large lytic lesion with soft tissue mass; usually contains fine calcifications (nonspecific pattern)
- May metastasize, but local morbidity of greater concern; difficult to resect completely; frequent local recurrence

Intratumoral calcifications are common; they are seen in 50–70% of cases by radiograph and 90% by CT.

- CT or preferably MRI with contrast is needed to define the extent of bone and soft tissue involvement.
- On MRI internal hemorrhage and cyst formation may be seen.
  - MRI shows low to intermediate T1 signal, but there may be areas of high signal intensity because of hemorrhage and high protein content.
  - T2 hyperintensity is seen but may be altered by calcification and hemosiderin; generalized low signal intensity is not characteristic (Fig. 11.132).
  - There is moderate, heterogeneous enhancement.
- Chordomas may show little or no activity on bone scan.
- Chordomas grow slowly and may have a narrow zone of transition with a sclerotic margin, but the tumor size, predominant osteolysis, and location are clues to the diagnosis.
  - In the vertebral body metastatic disease, multiple myeloma, GCT, and lymphoma belong in the differential diagnosis.
  - Sacrococcygeal chordomas are often large at presentation; frequently calcify in an amorphous pattern

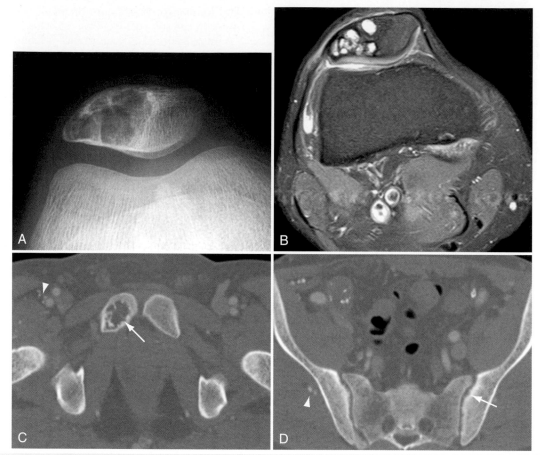

Fig. 11.130 Brown tumors. **(A)** Axial view of the knee shows multiple lytic lesions within the patella of a 30-year-old. The lesions are well marginated and do not elicit osseous reaction. **(B)** Axial intermediate–weighted fat-saturated image of the same knee shows the lesions to be hyperintense, a nonspecific pattern. **(C)** Axial CT scan in the same patient shows a nonaggressive lytic lesion within the right pubic bone *(arrow)*. There are also scattered soft tissue calcifications *(arrowhead)*, not expected in a patient of this age. **(D)** Axial CT scan located higher in the pelvis shows subchondral resorption and collapse of the sacroiliac joints *(arrow)*, mimicking erosions. There is soft tissue calcification *(arrowhead)*; note that the bone density is decreased and trabeculae indistinct relative to that expected in a 30-year-old. The findings are of renal osteodystrophy; the lytic lesions are brown tumors (see also Fig. 13.36).

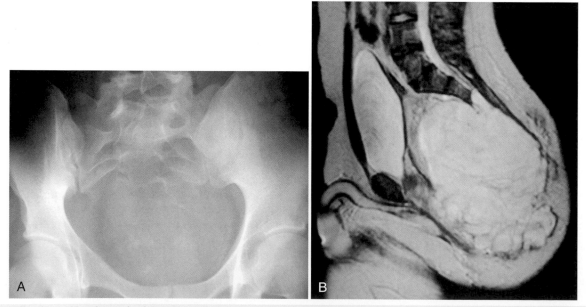

Fig. 11.131 Chordoma. AP radiograph of the pelvis **(A)** and sagittal T2-weighted MRI **(B)** demonstrate how large and locally aggressive a chordoma can be. Note the extensive destruction of the distal sacrum and a large soft tissue mass. The radiograph shows subtle calcification in the mass that is difficult to reproduce in a textbook.

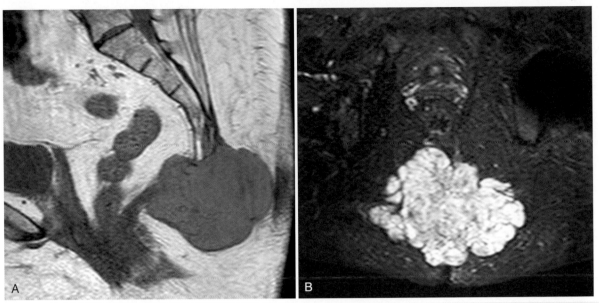

Fig. 11.132 Chordoma. **(A)** Sagittal T1-weighted MR image shows a large mass originating at the sacrococcygeal junction, involving the entire coccyx, with large circumferential mass. T1 hypointensity is relatively homogeneous in this case. **(B)** Axial STIR MR image of the same lesion shows it to be large and heterogeneous; location and appearance are typical of sacral chordoma.

(not chondroid or osteoid matrix); and may resemble chondrosarcoma, GCT, or plasmacytoma. However, assessment of matrix may be difficult in the pelvis because of overlying structures, and a chondrosarcoma might be considered in some cases.

- Chondrosarcomas in the pelvis tend to occur off the midline, whereas chordomas arise from the midline.
- An incidentally-detected small T2 hyperintense lesion in the clivus, vertebrae, or sacrum/coccyx on MRI may present a diagnostic dilemma. These lesions often represent *benign notochordal cell tumors* (previously called *giant vertebral notochordal rests*), though differentiation from a small chordoma may be impossible.
  - Benign notochordal cell tumors do not demonstrate aggressive features and are less likely to enhance on postcontrast MRI than small chordomas.
  - Benign notochordal cell tumors may rarely transform into or coexist with chordomas, and thus routine interval follow-up MRI is often recommended.
- Treatment is early wide resection, if possible, or surgical debulking, with radiation often used for recurrence.
  - Five-year survival is 74%, but higher for the chondroid variant.
  - Chordomas recur frequently in the surgical bed, and tumor seeding along biopsy tracts and surgical incisions also occurs. This can result in multicentric local recurrences.

ADAMANTINOMA

- Adamantinoma is a rare epithelioid lesion of unknown pathogenesis, containing elements of squamous, alveolar, and vascular tissue (Fig. 11.133).
- Adamantinoma is a low-grade and sometimes multicentric malignant neoplasm.

- Twenty percent metastasize to the lung, lymph nodes, or skeleton.
- However, it is generally locally nonaggressive, and the lesion may be present for several years before developing metastatic lesions.
- The most frequent location of adamantinoma is in the mid or proximal anterior tibial diaphysis (80–90%), usually eccentric or cortically-based. This may be the most distinctive feature of adamantinoma. It may also be quite large at presentation.
- The early pattern of bone destruction is geographic but may appear more aggressive with more advanced or recurrent disease.
- There is generally a sclerotic margin, and the lesion often has a bubbly lytic appearance.
- A soft tissue mass may occur as the lesion becomes larger.
- Although the lesion is monostotic, it may have satellite foci adjacent to the initial lesion in the tibia or even in the adjacent fibula.
- The major differential diagnosis of adamantinoma is fibrous dysplasia and ossifying fibroma (osteofibrous dysplasia). In fact, many investigators believe there is a spectrum of all three of these diseases.
  - All may be cortically-based and located in the tibia and appear somewhat aggressive (Figs. 11.133 and 11.134).
  - These lesions are also similar but not identical histologically, because the epithelial tumor cell will always be found with adamantinoma (see Fig. 11.36).
- Recurrence is common after surgery. The ideal treatment is wide excision; however, because the lesion is often mistaken as nonaggressive, the initial treatment is often an inadequate curettage.
- Lesions in older patients tend to be more aggressive. Overall 5-year survival is 60%.

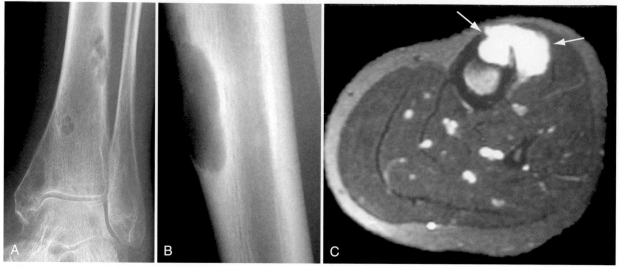

Fig. 11.133 Adamantinoma. **(A)** AP radiograph demonstrates a cortically-based lytic lesion in the tibia in a 17-year-old girl. The lesion appears to have adjacent sister lesions. Although it is typical of adamantinoma, it cannot be radiographically distinguished from osteofibrous dysplasia or cortically-based fibrous dysplasia (see Fig. 11.36). **(B)** Lateral radiograph in another case of adamantinoma shows a cortically-based lytic lesion in the tibia. **(C)** Axial T2-weighted MR image of the same lesion as in B confirms the cortical location of the lesion, as well as cortical breakthrough with a soft tissue mass *(arrows)*; this indicates an aggressive lesion and is typical of adamantinoma.

Fig. 11.134 Adamantinoma. **(A)** AP radiograph of the tibia in an adolescent shows multiple cortically-based lytic lesions with a pathologic fracture *(arrow)*. **(B)** Axial T1-weighted MR image of the lesion demonstrates that this is indeed a cortically-based lesion that wraps around the cortex *(arrows)*. As with the other cases shown, although this lesion is typical of adamantinoma, it cannot be radiographically distinguished from osteofibrous dysplasia or cortically-based fibrous dysplasia.

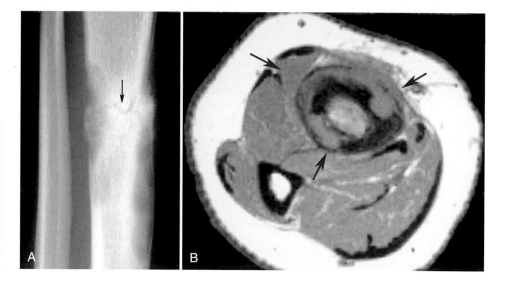

- *Ameloblastoma* is a histologically benign, locally aggressive lytic lesion of the mandible that was formerly termed 'adamantinoma of the mandible'.
  - This condition is unrelated to adamantinoma and is mentioned here only because the overlapping terminology may lead to confusion.

INTRAOSSEOUS GANGLION CYST

- Lobulated intraosseous cystic lesions are commonly found around the wrist, knee, ankle, and other joints with a narrow neck that connects the lesion to the joint or an adjacent ligament or tendon attachment site, referred to as intraosseous ganglion cysts—analogous to soft tissue ganglion cysts arising from joint capsules and tendon sheaths.
- A common location is at the tibial spines related to mucoid degeneration of the anterior cruciate ligament

(ACL), and at the posterior tibia related to the posterior cruciate ligament (PCL) insertion. Another common location is the body of the calcaneus, arising from the subtalar joint.
- Fluid-sensitive MRI sequences typically show very bright, well-circumscribed, unilocular or multilocular masses. Intravenous contrast shows enhancement only of the thin ganglion wall. Communication with the adjacent joint is sometimes demonstrated at arthrography.
- May communicate with soft tissue (extraosseous) ganglia.

Template

The following is a sample template of a radiographic description of a solitary bone tumor:

There is a —— cm (central, eccentric, surface, exophytic) (lytic, blastic, mixed-density) lesion in the (specific bone and location within the bone: diaphysis, etc.). The lesion begins ____ cm (distal, proximal) to the (identify a clinically palpable osseous landmark, such as a joint line or apophysis). The tumor margin/pattern of bone destruction (if lytic) is (1A, 1B, 1C, 2, or 3/'geographic with a sclerotic margin', etc.). The tumor contains (chondroid, osteoid, no) tumor matrix. There is (no, solid, interrupted, lamellated, hair-on-end, etc.) periosteal reaction. There is/is no (bone expansion, cortical breakthrough, extraosseous soft tissue mass). Overall, the lesion has (nonaggressive, aggressive, highly aggressive) radiographic features.

A complete report will also include diagnostic possibilities and recommendations for additional imaging, biopsy, and laboratory and clinical evaluation, if appropriate. For example, some lesions are 'don't touch' lesions (i.e., benign with malignant features at histology, such as MO and healing fracture).

Sources and Suggested Readings

Alípio GOF, Carneiro BC, Pastore D, et al. Whole-body imaging of multiple myeloma: diagnostic criteria. *Radiographics.* 2019;39:1077–1097.

Axoux EM, Saigal G, Rodriquez MM, Podda A. Langerhans cell histiocytosis: pathology, imaging and treatment of skeletal involvement. *Pediatr Radiol.* 2005;35:103–115.

Costelloe CM, Macapinlac HA, Madewell JE, et al. 18F-FDG PET/CT as an indicator of progression-free and overall survival in osteosarcoma. *J Nucl Med.* 2009;50(3):340–347.

Costelloe CM, Chuang HH, Madewell JE. FDG PET/CT of primary bone tumors. *AJR Am J Roentgenol.* 2014;202:W521–W531.

D'Anastasi M, Notohamiprodjo M, Schmidt GP, et al. Tumor load in patients with multiple myeloma: β2-microglobulin levels versus whole-body MRI. *AJR Am J Roentgenol.* 2014;203:854–862.

Degnan AJ, Ho-Fung VM. More than epiphyseal osteochondromas: updated understanding of imaging findings in dysplasia epiphysealis hemimelica (Trevor disease). *AJR Am J Roentgenol.* 2018;211:910–919.

Espinosa LA, Jamadar DA, Jacobson JA, et al. CT-guided biopsy of bone: a radiologist's perspective. *AJR Am J Roentgenol.* 2008;190(5):W283–W289.

Fayad LM, Jacobs MA, Wang X, et al. Musculoskeletal tumors: how to use anatomic, functional, and metabolic MR techniques. *Radiology.* 2012;26(2):340–356.

Ganeshan D, Menias CO, Lubner MG, et al. Sarcoidosis from head to toe: what the radiologist needs to know. *Radiographics.* 2018;38:1180–1200.

Gupta P, Potti TA, Wuertzer SD, et al. Spectrum of fat-containing soft tissue masses at MR imaging: the common, the uncommon, the characteristic, and the sometimes confusing. *Radiographics.* 2016;36:753–766. Hanrahan CJ, Christensen CR, Crim JR. Current concepts in the evaluation of multiple myeloma with MR imaging and FDG PET/CT. *Radiographics.* 2010;30(1):127–142.

Jelinek J, Murphey M, Kransdorf M, et al. Parosteal osteosarcoma: value of MR imaging and CT in the prediction of histologic grade. *Radiology.* 1996;201:837–842.

Jesus-Garcia R, Osawa A, Filippi RZ, et al. Is PET–CT an accurate method for the differential diagnosis between chondroma and chondrosarcoma? *SpringerPlus.* 2016;5:236. DOI 10.1186/s40064-016-1782-8

Liu PT, Valadez SD, Chivers FS, et al. Anatomically based guidelines for core needle biopsy of bone tumors: implications for limb-sparing surgery. *Radiographics.* 2007;27(1):189–205:discussion 206.

Manaster BJ, Petersilge CA, Roberts CC, Hanrahan CJ. *Diagnostic Imaging: Musculoskeletal Non-Traumatic Disease.* Salt Lake City: Amirsys; 2010.

Manaster BJ, Dalinka M, Alazraki N, et al. Follow-up examinations for bone tumors, soft tissue tumors, and suspected metastasis post therapy. American College of Radiology ACR Appropriateness Criteria. *Radiology.* 2000;215(suppl):379–387.

Methta M, White L, Knapp T, et al. MR imaging of symptomatic osteochondromas with pathological correlation. *Skeletal Radiol.* 1998;27:427–433.

Matsuo M, Ehara S, Tomakawa Y, et al. Muscular sarcoidosis. *Skeletal Radiol.* 1995;24:535–537.

Moore SL, Teirstein AE. Musculoskeletal sarcoidosis: spectrum of appearances at MR imaging. *Radiographics.* 2003;23:1389–1399.

Moore SL, Kransdorf MJ, Schweitzer MJ, et al. Can sarcoidosis and metastatic bone lesions be reliably differentiated on routine MRI? 2012. *AJR Am J Roentgenol.* 2012;198(6):1387–1393.

Mulligan M, McRae G, Murphey M. Imaging features of primary lymphoma of bone. *AJR Am J Roentgenol.* 1993;173:1691–1697.

Murphey M, Flemming D, Boyea S, et al. Enchondroma vs chondrosarcoma in the appendicular skeleton: differentiating features. *Radiographics.* 1998;18:1213–1237.

Murphey MD, Jelinek JS, Temple HT, et al. Imaging of periosteal osteosarcoma: radiologic-pathologic comparison. *Radiology.* 2004;233:129–138.

Patel NB, Stacy GS. Musculoskeletal manifestations of neurofibromatosis type 1. *AJR Am J Roentgenol.* 2012;199(1):W99–W106.

Ryu K, Jaovisidha S, Schweitzer M, et al. MR imaging of lipoma arborescens of the knee joint. *AJR Am J Roentgenol.* 1996;167:1229–1232.

Shah JN, Cohen HL, Choudhri AF, et al. Pediatric benign bone tumors: what does the radiologist need to know? *Radiographics.* 2017;37:1001–1002.

Springfield D, Rosenberg A, Mankin H. Relationship between osteofibrous dysplasia and adamantinoma. *Clin Orthop.* 1994;309:234–244.

Stacy GS, Mahal RS, Peabody TD. Staging of bone tumors with illustrative examples. *AJR Am J Roentgenol.* 2006;186(4):967–976.

Tannenbaum MF, Noda S, Cohen S et al. Imaging musculoskeletal manifestations of pediatric hematologic malignancies. *AJR Am J Roentgenol.* 2020;214:455–464.

Tavare AN, Robinson P, Altoos R, et al. Postoperative imaging of sarcomas. *AJR Am J Roentgenol.* 2018;211:506–518.

Ulano A, Bredella MA, Burke P, et al. Distinguishing untreated osteoblastic metastases from enostoses using CT attenuation measurements. *AJR Am J Roentgenol.* 2016;207:362–368.

Wu JS, Hochman MG. Soft tissue tumors and tumorlike lesions: a systematic imaging approach. *Radiology.* 2009;253(2):297–316.

12 *Soft Tissue Tumors*

Introduction

This chapter provides an introduction of how to approach soft tissue masses encountered on imaging, various imaging techniques, and an overview of many commonly encountered soft tissue masses. The goal of this chapter is to equip the radiologist with an adequate fund of knowledge and lexicon necessary to narrow the differential diagnosis and provide guidance to the referring clinician for patient management. Finally, the topics of soft tissue tumor staging, tumor biopsy, and assessment of tumor response to therapy are discussed.

There are a large variety of benign and malignant soft tissue tumors, only some of which have characteristics that are specific enough to make an imaging diagnosis. Fortunately, there are few entities that make up the majority of the commonly encountered soft tissue tumors, many of which are benign. Malignant soft tissue tumors can be primary, secondary (due to malignant transformation of a preexisting lesion), or metastatic in origin. Of the numerous primary soft tissue malignancies that may be encountered, many are exceedingly rare, often with a nonspecific imaging appearance, and are thus beyond the scope of this text. Lastly, keep in mind that there are a variety of nontumor lesions that may present as soft tissue masses. Such tumor mimics (i.e., musculoskeletal mass lesions that are not true neoplasms) can be considered as another category.

The first step in the evaluation of a soft tissue mass is to determine whether the lesion is a tumor or a "pseudotumor", i.e., a non-neoplastic space occupying lesion that

resembles a neoplasm. If truly a tumor, the next question is whether the lesion is unquestionably benign. Many pseudotumors and benign tumors will require no further workup by imaging or biopsy. If not, the function of the radiologist adjusts from analytical to descriptive, detailing the anatomic location, compartments involved, margins, proximity to neurovascular structures, and vascularity. Accompanying findings, such as mass effect, soft tissue edema, and invasion of adjacent structures should be reported. A specific diagnosis by imaging is not essential, as several soft tissue tumors have no specific features and histopathologic analysis is often required for definitive diagnosis. However, providing a concise description of such imaging features is invaluable for narrowing the differential diagnosis considerations, biopsy planning, and definitive treatment by the orthopedic oncologist. Lastly, if the lesion is indeterminate, the radiologist may recommend alternative imaging modalities, short-term follow-up imaging, or biopsy, depending on the level of clinical and imaging suspicion.

Magnetic resonance imaging (MRI) is the modality of choice for evaluation of soft tissue masses. However, MRI is not reliable for differentiation of benign from malignant lesions, unless it displays imaging characteristics specific for particular benign processes. Malignant soft tissue tumors are not always infiltrative; in fact, most appear well defined. Certain MRI characteristics may be useful in narrowing the differential diagnosis for soft tissue masses. A summary of T1-hyperintense lesions is provided in Box 12.1, T2-hypointense lesions in Box 12.2, and T2-hyperintense lesions in Box 12.3.

Box 12.1 Soft tissue Lesions With Hyperintensity on T1-Weighted Imaging

Common

- Fat (suppresses with chemical fat suppression or inversion recovery)
  - Fatty tumors
    - Lipoma
    - Liposarcoma
  - Fatty mature marrow
    - Myositis ossificans
    - Heterotopic ossification
  - Hemangioma/vascular malformation
- Methemoglobin
  - Hematoma
  - Hemorrhage within a tumor
- Gadolinium enhancement (with IV contrast administration)

Uncommon

- Proteinaceous material
- Melanin (high signal within melanoma metastases is more likely due to methemoglobin)

Box 12.2 Soft tissue Lesions With Hypointensity on T2-Weighted Imaging

- Hypocellular fibrous tissue
  - Fibroma other fibromatoses
  - Scar tissue
- Dense mineralization
- Melanin
- Blood
  - Acute hematoma
  - Hemosiderin
  - Old hematoma
  - Pigmented villonodular synovitis (PVNS) and tenosynovial giant cell tumor (TGCT)
  - Hemosiderotic synovitis in patients with hemophilia
- Vascular flow void
- Gas
- Foreign body
- Gouty tophus
- Amyloidosis
- Methacrylate

Box 12.3 Soft tissue Lesions With Hyperintensity on T2-Weighted Imaging

Benign

- Cysts
  - Ganglion cyst
  - Parameniscal cyst
  - Paralabral cyst
- Fluid collections
  - Bursitis
  - Seroma
  - Lymphocele
  - Hematoma
  - Abscess
  - Morel-Lavallée lesion (closed degloving injury)

- Vascular and lymphatic malformations
- Myxoma (typically intramuscular)
- Peripheral nerve sheath tumors (PNST), most commonly schwannoma and neurofibroma
- Glomus tumor (typically in the digits)

Malignant

- Synovial sarcoma
- Myxoid sarcoma
- Undifferentiated pleomorphic sarcoma
- Cystic or necrotic components of any malignant tumor

Imaging Techniques

RADIOGRAPHY

While radiographs are essential in the diagnostic workup of bone tumors, they are generally less helpful in evaluating soft tissue tumors. In certain cases, radiographs may show calcification or fat density associated with a soft tissue lesion or involvement of adjacent bones.

MAGNETIC RESONANCE IMAGING

Due to its superb soft tissue contrast and multiplanar capability, MRI is the best imaging modality for evaluation of a soft tissue mass, and for local staging in cases of malignancy. A high-quality examination including the entire lesion is necessary. The relationship of the tumor to critical adjacent structures such as muscle compartments, neurovascular structures, and joints must be discernable. Imaging in three planes with T1-weighted and T2-weighted fat-suppressed sequences is necessary for a complete examination. Postcontrast imaging following the intravenous administration of gadolinium-based contrast solution may be required to distinguish a solid from cystic lesion and to characterize viable (enhancing) versus necrotic or hemorrhagic (nonenhancing) tumor. Dynamic contrast-enhanced MRI has been advocated by some investigators to assist in differentiating malignant tumor from reactive tissue, or benign from malignant masses, as malignant tumors tend to enhance more rapidly due to neovascularity. Additionally, incorporating the use of diffusion-weighted imaging (DWI) into routine MRI protocols for tumor imaging has been steadily gaining popularity. DWI can be useful as a functional imaging technique without the use of contrast, as highly cellular tumors tend to restrict diffusion and have lower apparent diffusion coefficient (ADC) values.

MRI may exaggerate or underestimate tumor size because peritumoral edema signal cannot reliably be differentiated from adjacent tumor. Also, tumor microinvasion into adjacent tissues may not be demonstrated by MRI. MRI is not absolutely reliable for diagnosis or for predicting tumor grade. However, MRI may provide clues to the diagnosis (see Boxes 12.1 to 12.3). For example, uniformly monotonous fat signal intensity in a soft tissue mass, confirmed with chemical fat suppression, indicates a lipoma. MRI may reveal flow voids within a lesion, such as with arteriovenous malformations. Highly cellular lesions such as lymphoma tend to have relatively low signal intensity on T2-weighted imaging compared with other (noncalcified) malignancies.

Hemorrhage, hematoma, and inflammatory change may produce abnormal signal intensity patterns that can be confused with tumor. Infection can involve several compartments, appear highly invasive, and incite prominent tissue reaction, mimicking tumor. Infections may have nonspecific signal intensity on MRI unless there is an encapsulated abscess (which is best demonstrated with postcontrast imaging). Similarly, hematoma, especially in a chronic stage, may be misdiagnosed as a neoplasm by MRI. Chronic hematomas often incite tremendous adjacent tissue reaction and may appear to involve many compartments with a highly inhomogeneous mass. However, it is also important to remember that tumors may bleed, and thus hemorrhage can mask an underlying tumor. In situations where the clinical history or imaging features raise any concerns as to whether a lesion is truly a hematoma, biopsy or close follow-up with MRI until complete resolution is recommended.

ULTRASONOGRAPHY

Ultrasonography (US) can depict, localize, and characterize relatively superficial soft tissue masses. Smaller lesions and clearly cystic lesions may be adequately characterized on US alone. However, larger or deeper lesions may be only partially evaluated and may require further evaluation with MRI. Tumor vascularity can be assessed with Doppler interrogation on US. US is often used for image-guided biopsy of accessible soft tissue masses.

COMPUTED TOMOGRAPHY

Generally, MRI is preferred to computed tomography (CT) for evaluation soft tissue tumors. CT is not very useful for characterization of soft tissue lesions due to poor soft tissue contrast, though it may be useful for demonstrating macroscopic fat within a lesion (such as a lipoma) or associated soft tissue calcification. Noncontrast CT may be useful to detect hematoma (hyperdense blood products) in the posttraumatic setting, though spontaneous hematoma should be investigated to evaluate for underlying soft tissue mass.

NUCLEAR MEDICINE

Positron emission tomography (PET) integrated with CT (PET-CT) using ^{18}F-fluorodeoxyglucose (^{18}F-FDG) is a functional imaging technique used to evaluate tumor metabolic activity based on glucose uptake and retention. PET-CT is used in many types of cancers, including lung, colorectal, breast, and head and neck cancers, as well as melanoma and lymphoma. PET-CT is also useful for the evaluation of some soft tissue sarcomas. Applications include initial tumor metabolic characterization, staging, and assessment of treatment response.

Soft Tissue Masses

GANGLION CYST

- Cysts are commonly found around the wrist, knee, and many other joints, and they are often described with the umbrella term *ganglion*.
- Represent loculated accumulation of viscous fluid around a joint, tendon, ligament, or other collagenous structure.
  - Despite the name, these masses are unrelated to neural elements.
  - Most periarticular ganglia originate from small capsular or tendon sheath defects that act as a one-way valve, allowing fluid and debris to leave the joint but not return.
  - Degenerated ligaments such as the anterior cruciate ligament and posterior cruciate ligament of the knee may have associated adjacent or intrasubstance ganglion cysts. These ganglia can be large.
  - Rarely, a ganglion can arise within the substance of a tendon and remain completely within the tendon sheath.
- Vary in size from a few millimeters to several centimeters and may be unilocular or multilocular; in the latter the locules typically communicate.
- Ganglion cyst is the most common mass around the hand and wrist.
- Similar lesions occur in association with glenoid or acetabular labral or meniscal tears, termed *paralabral cysts* or *meniscal cysts*, respectively.
  - Meniscal cysts may be *parameniscal* (adjacent to the meniscus) or occasionally *intrameniscal* (contained within the meniscal substance).
- MRI features are characteristic (Fig. 12.1):
  - Fluid-sensitive MRI sequences show a very bright, well-circumscribed, unilocular or multilocular mass.
  - Usually hypointense on T1-weighted imaging, though may be intermediate or hyperintense due to proteinaceous debris or hemorrhage.
  - Intravenous contrast shows enhancement only of the thin ganglion wall.
- US demonstrates an anechoic or hypoechoic thin-walled lesion with acoustic enhancement, sometimes with internal septations.
- Sometimes a thin 'neck' connecting the ganglion to an adjacent joint or tendon sheath may be evident on MRI, which should be sought, as successful resection of the ganglion requires resection of the neck to avoid recurrence of the lesion.
  - This can also be useful to reliably diagnose a ganglion cyst when trying to differentiate between other soft tissue masses.
  - MR arthrography may demonstrate communication with the injected joint, or no communication if the cyst has become loculated.
- Occasionally, it may be difficult to distinguish between a ganglion cyst and normal joint recess filled with joint fluid.
  - Presence of internal septations, thin neck, or mass effect on adjacent structures are imaging characteristics that suggest a ganglion cyst rather than a joint recess.

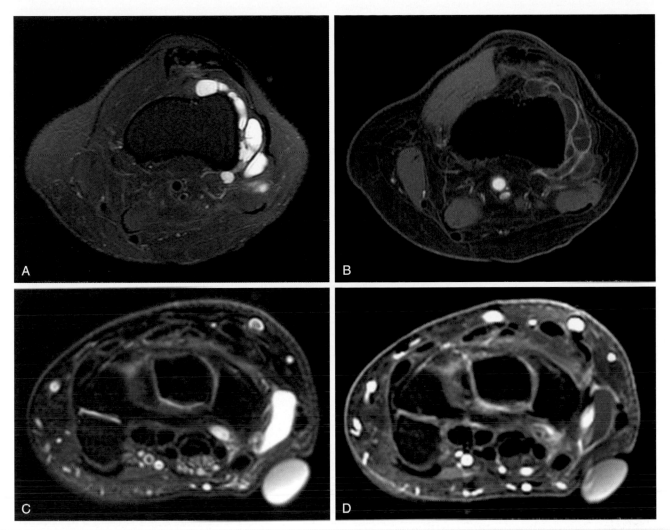

Fig. 12.1 Ganglion cyst. Axial T2-weighted fat-suppressed **(A)** and T1-weighted fat-suppressed postcontrast **(B)** MR images of the knee demonstrate a multilocular fluid-bright ganglion cyst insinuating along the lateral aspect of the distal femur, with thin peripheral and septal enhancement. Axial T2-weighted fat-suppressed **(C)** and T1-weighted fat-suppressed postcontrast **(D)** MR images of the wrist in another patient demonstrate a ganglion cyst at the radial aspect of the wrist, again fluid-bright with thin peripheral enhancement. Note that contrast is not generally required to make the diagnosis.

- Complete description of the location is important for presurgical planning, especially the relationship with adjacent neurovascular structures.
- Complex ganglion cysts can occasionally be difficult to differentiate from soft tissue tumors.
  - May be complex and heterogeneous, containing synovial debris or chronic blood products.
  - Ganglion cysts are very common, whereas malignant tumors arising from joints or tendon sheaths are very rare.
  - If the cystic lesion is not clearly connected to a synovial compartment, contrast-enhanced MRI or biopsy may be necessary.

TUMOR MIMICS AND PSEUDOMASSES

Accessory Muscles

- An accessory muscle or hypertrophied muscle can sometimes simulate a soft tissue mass.
- US and MRI show expected muscle architecture and typical echotexture/signal characteristics.

Fascial Defects

- Fascial defects may be caused by trauma or surgery, leaving a rent in the fascia that allows the muscle to herniate through, termed a *myofascial hernia* (Fig. 12.2).
- MRI may show muscle tissue protruding through the fascial defect with associated intramuscular or perifascial edema.
- US offers the added flexibility for dynamic evaluation if the herniation is intermittent and only evident with certain activities.

Lymph Nodes

- Normal and enlarged lymph nodes may be mistaken clinically for soft tissue masses if palpable.
- Commonly encountered lymph nodes around joints include popliteal fossa lymph nodes behind the knee and epitrochlear lymph nodes at the medial elbow.
- Normal and inflammatory lymph nodes typically demonstrate a characteristic reniform configuration with a normal fatty hilum; loss of these features can be seen with neoplasm.

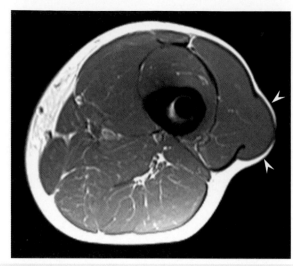

Fig. 12.2 Myofascial hernia. Axial T1-weighted MR image demonstrates a vastus lateralis muscle hernia *(arrowheads)* following intramedullary rod placement for a femur fracture.

- Lymph nodes may become enlarged as a reactive inflammatory process, such as infection distally in the extremity.
- Classic infections associated with epitrochlear lymphadenopathy include cat-scratch disease (*Bartonella henselae*) and rose gardener's disease (*Sporothrix schenkii*), though any infection of the distal extremity can result in this finding.
- Noninfectious causes of peripheral lymphadenopathy are broad and include lymphoma, metastatic disease, autoimmune diseases, amyloidosis, sarcoidosis, and other miscellaneous conditions.

Inflammatory Pseudotumors and Deposition Diseases

- Inflammatory arthropathies, including rheumatoid arthritis, gout, and Lyme arthritis, can present with soft tissue masses around tendons, bursae, and joints.

- Noninflammatory arthropathies, such as pigmented villonodular synovitis (PVNS) and amyloidosis, can also present as periarticular soft tissue masses.
- Masses may be due to masslike synovial proliferation (termed *pannus* in rheumatoid arthritis), tophi in tophaceous gout, and amyloid deposits in amyloidosis.

Hematomas

- Hematomas may be encountered in the musculoskeletal system both spontaneously and due to trauma.
- Acute hematoma on noncontrast CT is hyperdense compared to background muscle.
- On MRI, hyperintensity on T1-weighted imaging not due to presence of fat is characteristic of acute or subacute blood products, which can be confirmed with a noncontrast T1-weighted fat-suppressed sequence (Fig. 12.3).
  - Unlike in the central nervous system, blood products in the musculoskeletal system do not follow a predictable time course, and acute and chronic blood products commonly coexist.
  - In chronic stages, blood eventually transforms to low signal on both T2-weighted and T1-weighted sequences.
  - Blood products can persist for days to weeks (or even months) and areas of hyper- and hypointensity are often mixed.
  - When a hematoma begins to 'organize', it becomes vascularized and may enhance heterogeneously, which often simulates a soft tissue tumor.
    - If bland organizing hematoma is suspected, follow-up may still be required to document resolution and exclude an underlying hemorrhagic mass, unless the clinical presentation is unequivocal.
    - Keep in mind that soft tissue sarcomas can present following minor trauma, which can bring them to the patient's attention or cause intralesional hemorrhage.
- Although there is little in the literature regarding workup of suspected but not definitive hematoma encountered

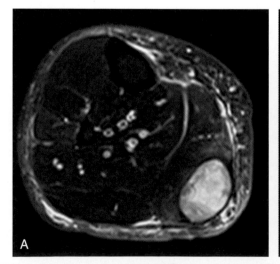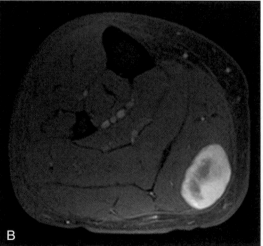

Fig. 12.3 Intramuscular hematoma. Axial STIR **(A)** MR image in a runner with a calf injury demonstrates a heterogeneously T2-hyperintense collection with a thin rim of hypointensity centered within the medial head gastrocnemius muscle. Axial T1-weighted fat-suppressed **(B)** MR image obtained without contrast demonstrates intrinsic T1 hyperintensity, confirming the diagnosis of an intramuscular hematoma.

in the musculoskeletal system, diagnostic options include short-term interval follow-up MRI (in 1–2 months), pre- and postcontrast MRI, PET-CT, or aspiration and/or biopsy depending on the degree of clinical suspicion.

Myositis Ossificans and Heterotopic Ossification

- Myositis ossificans and the similar process of heterotopic ossification represent heterotopic formation of nonneoplastic bone and cartilage in soft tissue due to metaplasia of connective tissue.
- *Myositis ossificans* refers specifically to ossification within muscle, whereas *heterotopic ossification* is a more general term for any soft tissue ossification.

- The cause is usually blunt trauma, sometimes only minor, most commonly in areas prone to such injury, such as the thigh and around the elbow.
- Myositis ossificans also can be associated with burns and neurologic disorders, with greater than one-third of paraplegic patients showing extensive, nontraumatic myositis ossificans.
- The histologic evolution of myositis ossificans parallels the radiographic evolution (Figs. 12.4 – 12.6; see also Fig. 1.57).
  - During the first 4 weeks of evolution, myositis ossificans has a pseudosarcomatous appearance in its central zone, which may suggest malignant neoplasm.

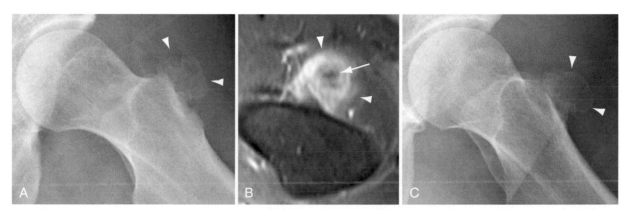

Fig. 12.4 Myositis ossificans. **(A)** Frog-leg radiograph of the hip shows an amorphous ossific density adjacent to the posterior greater trochanter *(arrowheads)*. This patient had trauma 9 weeks earlier; organizing bone within myositis ossificans has this somewhat amorphous appearance within this time frame. **(B)** Axial intermediate-weighted fat-saturated image obtained at the same time shows central hypointensity *(arrow)* with peripheral hyperintensity *(arrowheads)*. This is the MRI appearance of myositis ossificans as it evolves its ossification, before showing the organized peripheral bone formation of the mature process. **(C)** Frog-leg radiograph of the same lesion obtained 20 weeks following the traumatic episode shows mature peripheral ossification of the lesion *(arrowheads)*. This pattern of zoning is pathognomonic for myositis ossificans and signals that the lesion is mature.

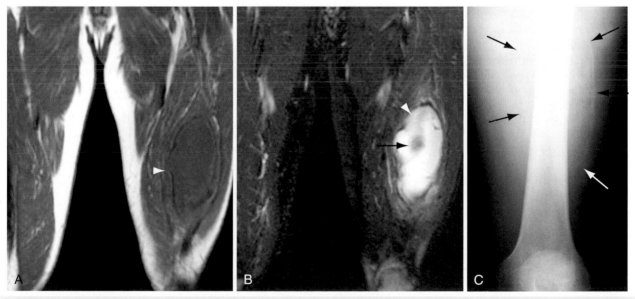

Fig. 12.5 Myositis ossificans. Coronal T1-weighted **(A)** and fat-suppressed T2-weighted **(B)** MR images in an athlete who sustained a deep bruise to the anterior thigh 2 weeks earlier show a thigh mass that is hypointense to skeletal muscle *(arrowhead in A)*. On T2-weighted image, the majority of the lesion is hyperintense *(arrowhead in B)*, with a central region of hypointensity *(arrow)*. Radiographs at this time were normal. The timing is such that one would expect to see the earliest hints of osteoid formation on MR images, but one does not expect to see ossification by radiograph until 3 to 4 weeks post injury. **(C)** Radiograph obtained 2 months later shows classic peripheral, mature ossification of myositis ossificans *(arrows)*. (Reproduced with permission from May DA, Disler DG, Jones EA, et al. Abnormal signal intensity in skeletal muscle at MR imaging: patterns, pearls, and pitfalls. *Radiographics.* 2000;20 Spec No:S295–S315.)

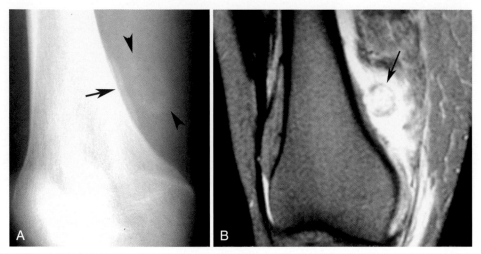

Fig. 12.6 Myositis ossificans. **(A)** Oblique radiograph of the distal thigh in a 15-year-old girl with a painful mass demonstrates faintly seen osteoid within a mass *(arrowheads)*, as well as periosteal reaction along the adjacent femur *(arrow)*. This is a nonspecific appearance and could represent either myositis ossificans or an early surface osteosarcoma. **(B)** MRI is extremely helpful, with the T2-weighted coronal image showing a ring of low signal *(arrow)* surrounding and surrounded by extensive soft tissue edema. The ring of low signal intensity represents maturing osteoid and is the zoning phenomenon of myositis ossificans.

- During the first 2 weeks, only a soft tissue mass is present, which clinically may be painful, warm, and doughy.
- Weeks 3–4 begin to show amorphous density within the mass, often with periosteal reaction of adjacent bone, which may be mistaken for an early surface osteosarcoma.
- During weeks 4–8, histologic examination shows a centrifugal pattern of maturation, where the periphery of the lesion is demarcated by immature osteoid formation that with time gradually organizes into mature bone.
  - Amorphous osteoid matures into compact bone peripherally that surrounds a lacy pattern of less mature bone.
  - Maturation proceeds centrifugally, as is seen both radiologically and histologically.
  - *Zonal phenomenon* seen on radiographs as a radiodense mass with rim-like calcification that appears denser at the periphery than the center.
  - Over ensuing months, the osseous mass reaches full maturity, often with reduction in size and migration toward the periosteum of nearby bone.
  - History and timeframe are crucial in supporting the early diagnosis of myositis ossificans and avoiding a potentially disastrous misdiagnosis of osteosarcoma.
- The MRI appearance of myositis ossificans relates to the age of the lesion and is similar to the radiographic appearance (see Figs. 12.4 –12.6).
  - Early lesions show a mass that is isointense to muscle on T1-weighted imaging and high signal or heterogeneous on T2-weighted imaging.
  - Surrounding soft tissue edema is prominent.
  - Periosteal reaction and bone marrow edema may be seen if the myositis is located near bone.
  - More mature lesions (over 8 weeks) are better defined; the center remains heterogeneous, but there may be either central hypointensity or the central lesion may demonstrate a rimmed halo of decreased signal on all sequences (MRI equivalent of zonal phenomenon).
- Differential diagnosis considerations of myositis ossificans include surface osteosarcoma (parosteal or periosteal osteosarcoma), juxtacortical chondroma, osteochondroma, and tumoral calcinosis.
  - *Parosteal osteosarcoma* typically shows the reverse of the zonal phenomenon seen with myositis ossificans, with denser calcification in the center than in the periphery.
  - *Periosteal osteosarcoma* usually appears more aggressive, often scalloping the underlying cortex.
  - *Juxtacortical chondroma* also often presents with scalloped underlying cortex and juxtacortical calcific densities; early myositis ossificans could possibly mimic this appearance.
  - *Osteochondroma* is easily distinguished from myositis ossificans because an osteochondroma arises from the underlying bone, with continuation of cortical and medullary bone into the lesion.
  - *Tumoral calcinosis* presents as periarticular calcified soft tissue masses, usually around the hip, shoulder, and elbows, typically found in patients with renal failure.
    - Calcifications in tumoral calcinosis are amorphous and often show fluid-fluid levels on cross-sectional imaging.
- *Fibrodysplasia ossificans progressiva*, formerly known as *myositis ossificans progressive*, is a hereditary mesodermal disorder characterized by progressive ossification of striated muscles, tendons, and ligaments.
  - Typically appears as a spontaneous mutation, though may be inherited in an autosomal dominant mode with a wide range of expression.
  - Characterized by heterotopic ossification of muscles, tendons, fascia, and ligaments.
  - Most frequent presenting symptom and location is acute torticollis, with a painful mass seen in the

sternocleidomastoid muscle, with subsequent progression to the shoulder girdle, rib cage, upper arms, spine, and pelvis.

- Heterotopic bone often bridges between adjacent bones of the skeleton and causes severe restriction of motion, disability, and eventually death.

EXTRASKELETAL SOFT TISSUE TUMORS OF OSSEOUS OR CARTILAGINOUS ORIGIN

Very rarely, typically osseous-based tumors may arise in the soft tissues, such as extraskeletal osteosarcoma, Ewing's sarcoma, or chondrosarcoma. Similarly, there can be extramedullary involvement of multiple myeloma or even a solitary extramedullary plasmacytoma. Benign extraskeletal soft tissue tumors, such as soft tissue osteoma or soft tissue chondroma, are also exceedingly rare. Extraskeletal tumors of osseous or cartilaginous origin often have imaging characteristics and internal matrix similar to their skeletal counterparts.

- *Extraskeletal osteosarcoma.*
  - Rare (1–2% of soft tissue tumors, 2–4% of osteosarcomas), generally occurring later in life (40+ years).
  - Found most frequently in the thigh, with less frequent occurrence in the upper extremity and retroperitoneum.
  - Soft tissue mass has variable amounts of mineralized osteoid (seen in 50% of the cases) and MRI appearance is often nonspecific (Fig. 12.7).
  - Treatment is with wide resection and adjuvant chemotherapy or radiation therapy; prognosis is poor, worse than that for conventional osteosarcoma.

VASCULAR MALFORMATIONS

- The terminology of vascular malformations has been historically varied, most recently updated by the International Society for the Study of Vascular Anomalies (ISSVA) in 2018.
- As per the current classification scheme, vascular malformations (which are classified separately from vascular tumors) are subdivided into simple vascular malformations, combined vascular malformations,

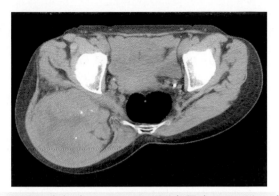

Fig. 12.7 Extraskeletal osteosarcoma. Axial CT demonstrates a large soft tissue mass within the gluteus maximus of an older male patient. The mass contains calcified matrix that is nonspecific in appearance. Biopsy demonstrated a rare extraskeletal osteosarcoma. (Image used with permission from BJ Manaster, MD, from STATdx website, Amirsys, Inc.)

vascular malformations of major named vessels, and vascular malformation syndromes associated with other anomalies.

- Simple vascular malformations include capillary malformations, venous malformations, lymphatic malformations, primary lymphedema, arteriovenous malformations (AVMs), and arteriovenous fistulas (AVFs).
- Combined vascular malformations include two or more distinct malformation types within a single lesion.
- Differentiation between various types of vascular malformations may not be possible by imaging.
  - Many soft tissue vascular malformations present as a mass, which may contain fatty stroma, feeding or draining vessels, and phleboliths.
    - Intralesional fat is characterized by high signal intensity on both T1- and T2-weighted imaging, with corresponding hypointensity on fat-suppression sequences.
  - Many soft tissue vascular malformations include numerous tortuous vessels, packed closely together, resulting in a characteristic 'can of worms' appearance on CT or MRI (Figs. 12.8 and 12.9).
    - On MRI the tortuous vessels are seen either as high signal or flow void, depending on the rate of flow.

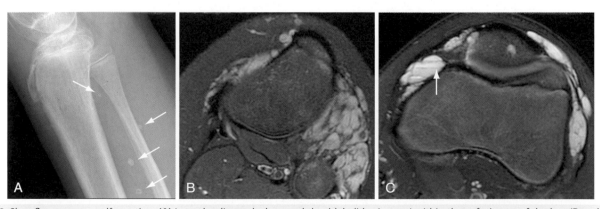

Fig. 12.8 Slow-flow venous malformation. (**A**) Lateral radiograph shows subtle phleboliths *(arrows)* within the soft tissues of the leg. (**B** and **C**) Axial intermediate-weighted fat-saturated images through the knee in the same patient demonstrate multiple tortuous vessels coursing through the anterior portion of the limb, seeming to wrap around the knee. The flow in this huge malformation is so slow that fluid-fluid levels are seen (*arrow* in **C**).

- Dynamic contrast-enhanced MRI can help differentiate between high-flow and slow-flow vascular malformations.
- If a vascular malformation occurs in a skeletally immature patient, it may cause focal bone overgrowth due to chronic hyperemia.
- *Arteriovenous malformation.*
  - High-flow vascular lesion arising in childhood or early adulthood, ranging in size and extent, often

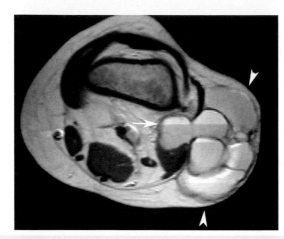

Fig. 12.9 Slow-flow venous malformation. Low-flow vascular malformation in the distal medial thigh *(arrowheads)*. Axial T2-weighted image shows dilated vascular channels. The channels are enhanced after intravenous contrast administration, excluding a lymphangioma. The flow is so slow that the cellular components are layering, producing fluid-fluid levels *(arrow)*.

with poorly defined margins and infiltration of soft tissues.
  - When located in the deep soft tissues, these lesions can be associated with limb overgrowth (because of increased blood flow through the arteriovenous malformation), with large feeding and draining vessels.
  - Computed tomography angiography (CTA) or magnetic resonance angiography (MRA) may be requested for delineation of vascular supply prior to embolization (Fig. 12.10).
- *Venous malformation.*
  - Colloquially known as soft tissue hemangiomas, though this term is reserved for true hemangioma tumors by the ISSVA.
  - Soft, compressible, nonpulsatile mass arising in childhood or early adulthood.
  - Slow-flow vascular lesion with slow, gradual enhancement; may contain pheboliths and fluid-fluid levels (see Figs. 12.8 and 12.9).
  - Intramuscular lesions may be associated with regional muscle atrophy.
- *Lymphatic malformation.*
  - Benign developmental lesions composed of dilated lymphatic channels.
  - 75% occur in the head, neck, or axilla.
  - Majority of the mass follows fluid signal (Fig. 12.11).
- *Klippel–Trénaunay–Weber syndrome* is the triad of localized gigantism (bone and soft tissue hypertrophy), cutaneous hemangioma ('port wine stain'), and congenital varicose veins or venous malformations.

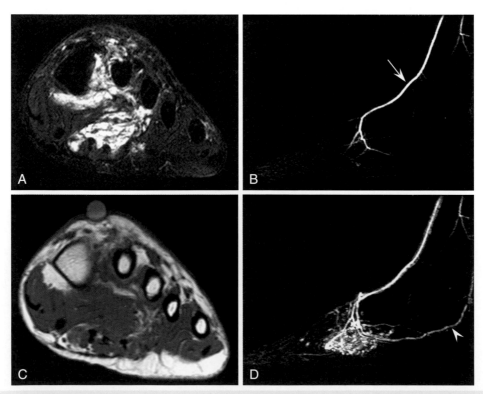

Fig. 12.10 Arteriovenous malformation. Short-axis T2-weighted fat-suppressed **(A)** and T1-weighted **(B)** MR images of the foot demonstrate a large T2-hyperintense mass insinuating throughout the midfoot with interspersed T1-hyperintense intralesional fat. Dynamic MRA using time-resolved imaging of contrast kinetics (TRICKS) following intravenous contrast administration shows the feeding arterial supply from the anterior tibial artery **(C, arrow)** and venous drainage into the greater saphenous vein (D, arrowhead).

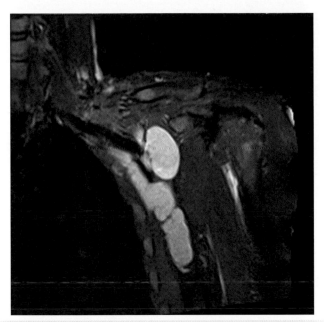

Fig. 12.11 Lymphatic malformation. Coronal STIR image of the chest obtained for pectoralis major tear demonstrates a large, lobulated T2-hyperintense lymphatic malformation tracking along the brachiocephalic and axillary neurovascular bundle, which was an incidental finding.

- Imaging findings include hemihypertrophy or macrodactyly, phleboliths, subcutaneous fat hypertrophy, abnormal superficial to deep vein connections, and lack of venous valves (Fig. 12.12).
- The knee and elbow are favored sites for synovial hemangioma; this site preference also makes it difficult to differentiate from the appearance of hemophilia.

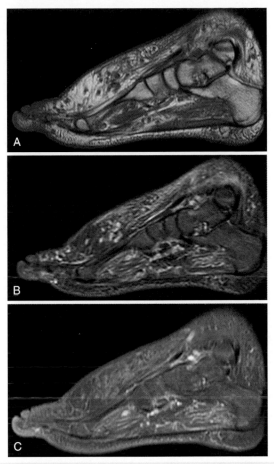

Fig. 12.12 Klippel–Trénaunay–Weber syndrome. Sagittal T1-weighted (**A**), short-tau inversion recovery (**B**), and postcontrast T1-weighted fat-saturated (**C**) images of the foot show fatty overgrowth and prominent low-flow vessels.

GLOMUS TUMOR

- *Glomus tumor* (*glomangioma* or *neuromyoarterial glomus*) is a benign perivascular lesion consisting of neural, muscle, and arterial components similar to glomus body cells.
  - Should not be confused with *paragangliomas*, which are neuroendocrine tumors that are sometimes also referred to as glomus tumors.
- Although they have been reported throughout the body, there is a strong propensity for the subungual region of the fingers (Fig. 12.13).
  - Most commonly occur in patients between 30 and 60 years of age.
  - Present as a tender red-blue nailbed nodule with paroxysms of excruciating pain, often exacerbated by changes in temperature.
- May cause a well-marginated scalloped defect on the dorsal aspect of the terminal phalanx.
- MRI demonstrates a small mass (typically <1 cm) in the subungual region with intense T2 bright signal and robust contrast enhancement following the administration of intravenous contrast.
- Treated by local excision; MRI used to detect and accurately localize the lesion and for follow-up postsurgical imaging to ensure complete resection and/or evaluate for local recurrence.

LIPOMATOUS TUMORS

Soft tissue Lipoma

- Lipomas are common tumors (representing 50% of all soft tissue tumors) consisting of fatty tissue.
- 80% of lipomas are found in the subcutaneous tissues; most others are intermuscular or intramuscular.
  - If inter- or intramuscular, may infiltrate fascial planes and muscle compartments.
- Lipomas typically present as a painless, soft, compressible, mobile mass (Figs. 12.14 and 12.15).
- Imaging features are characteristic:
  - If they are large enough to be seen on radiographs, they may appear as radiolucent (fat tissue density) masses.
  - Show fat attenuation on CT (between −120 and −90 Hounsfield units).
  - MRI shows a sharply bordered lesion with high-signal-intensity matching that of subcutaneous fat on both T1- and T2-weighted imaging, which suppresses with fat saturation.
  - Ultrasound likewise shows a defined lesion with echogenicity and echotexture similar to subcutaneous fat.
- Some subcutaneous lesions can be difficult to differentiate from surrounding fat.

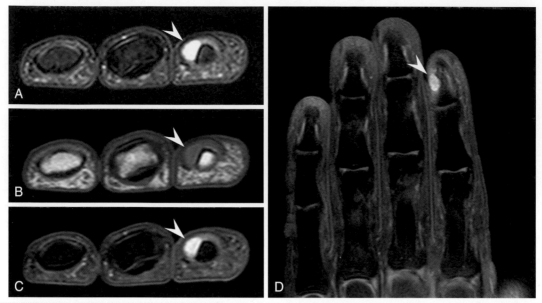

Fig. 12.13 Glomus tumor. Axial T2-weighted fat-suppressed **(A)**, axial T1-weighted **(B)**, and axial and coronal postcontrast T1-weighted fat-suppressed **(C** and **D)** MR images show a T2-hyperintense, T1-hypointense, avidly enhancing lesion in the subungual region of the index finger *(arrowheads)*, consistent with a glomus tumor. The diagnosis is most suggested by the location at the nail bed.

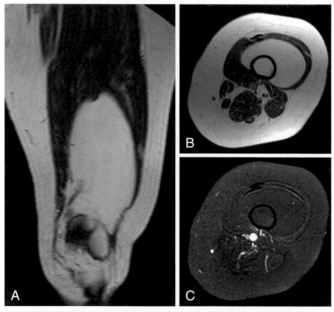

Fig. 12.14 Lipoma. Coronal **(A)** and axial **(B)** T1-weighted MR images demonstrate a large mass with uniform high signal and a few thin internal septations centered within the distal vastus lateralis muscle. The signal matches that of the subcutaneous fat. Axial T2-weighted fat-suppressed MR image **(C)** of the same lesion shows complete suppression, matching that of the subcutaneous fat. This is a classic lipoma.

- Imaging with a marker over a palpable lesion and enlarging the field of view to include both sides to compare symmetry can be helpful for evaluating a small lesion.
- Lipomas may contain calcification and ossification, usually representing dystrophic calcification caused by prior trauma and hemorrhage.
  - Such calcification is usually very dense and often is block-like or in the form of small lines and angles.

- Traumatized subcutaneous fat may show a similar pattern of calcification.
- *Chondroid lipoma* is an extremely rare, benign soft tissue tumor containing variable amounts of fat and chondroid tissue, which may demonstrate internal chondroid matrix calcification.
- The most important role of the radiologist in evaluating lipomatous lesions in the musculoskeletal system on imaging is detecting the rare atypical lipomatous tumor or low-grade, well-differentiated liposarcoma.
  - MR images should be carefully scrutinized to detect any site within a lipoma where typical fat signal is not shown, such as nodules, thickened septa, or areas of irregular or nodular enhancement that may raise concern for low-grade liposarcoma (Box 12.4).
  - Lipomas may contain thin enhancing septa (<2 mm thick) but otherwise do not enhance.
  - Intramuscular lipomas may entrap muscle fibers (Fig. 12.16); it is important to avoid misdiagnosing traversing muscle tissue as thickened septa or nodules.
- The term *nonencapsulated lipoma* is often used informally to descibe asymmetric distribution of fat in obesity, though true nonencapsulated lipomas do exist.
  - Imaging findings include a region of fat with fewer septations than the surrounding subcutaneous fat, as well as deflection of fascial planes reflecting mass effect.

Lipomatosis

- *Lipomatosis* is a condition characterized by excessive fat distributed either randomly or symmetrically over the body.
- *Macrodystrophia lipomatosa* is a localized form of gigantism with overgrowth of fat and vascular elements; associated increased blood flow results in overgrowth of the soft tissues and bone, usually in the hand or foot (Fig. 12.17).

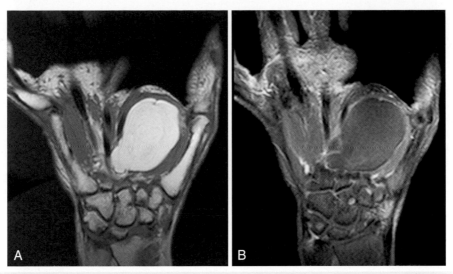

Fig. 12.15 Lipoma. Coronal T1-weighted **(A)** and postcontrast fat suppressed T1 weighted **(B)** images show a lipoma in the palm of the hand. Note that the signal of the tumor is identical to that of the subcutaneous fat. This holds true on all sequences, including sequences with chemical fat suppression. Also note lack of enhancing nodule or thick septation within the masses, findings that may indicate a liposarcoma.

Box 12.4   Lipoma Versus Atypical Lipomatous Tumor (Well-Differentiated Liposarcoma)

Lipoma

- Fat density and signal intensity
- May contain thin septations (<2 mm in thickness)
- No nodularity
- No enhancement

Atypical lipomatous tumor (well-differentiated liposarcoma)

- Majority of tissue is adipose, following fat density and signal intensity
- Thick (>2 mm), irregular enhancing septations
- Nodules that enhance

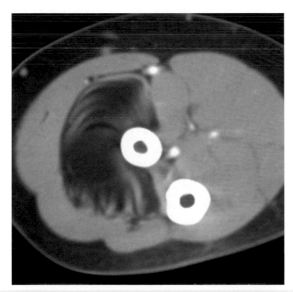

Fig. 12.16 Intramuscular lipoma. Axial CT shows a low-attenuation mass in the forearm. Note that the lesion arises within rather than adjacent to the muscle. There are several muscle fibers entrapped within the lesion. It is important to recognize these as muscle fibers rather than misdiagnose them as thickened septa within the lipoma.

- Lipomatosis of the nerve (*fibrolipomatous hamartoma*) is usually associated, classically involving the median nerve in the hand, discussed later.
- Bony proliferation generally ceases after skeletal maturation, but soft tissue overgrowth continues into adulthood.

Atypical Lipomatous Tumor

- Atypical lipomatous tumor (ALT) is a low-grade malignancy composed predominantly of fat, also termed *well-differentiated liposarcoma*.
- ALT is the most common type of liposarcoma (40–50%).
- Usually painless and most frequently is located in the deep tissues of the extremities; the thigh is most common (Fig. 12.18).
- Composed of >75% fat, with variably thickened septa and nodularity (see Box 12.4).
  - Septa and nodules have increased signal intensity on fluid-sensitive imaging and usually show enhancement.
- Treatment is with wide excision; recurrence rates are related to location, relatively low in the extremities (23–43%) and surprisingly high in the retroperitoneum (90–100%).

Liposarcoma

- Soft tissue liposarcomas are common and are the second most common malignant soft tissue tumor in adults after undifferentiated pleomorphic sarcoma.
- Soft tissue liposarcoma may range from a well-differentiated (i.e., ALT) to a high-grade lesion.
- Various subtypes, the most common after ALT being myxoid liposarcoma (33% of liposarcomas, 10% of all adult soft tissue sarcomas).
- Most common age range is 30–60 years, and most cases arise in the lower extremity (75%), most frequently the thigh; retroperitoneal location is less frequent.
- Liposarcoma may have a widely variable appearance on imaging studies, depending on the grade and histologic features of the lesion.

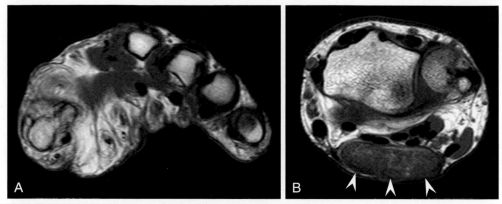

Fig. 12.17 Macrodystrophia lipomatosa. Axial T1-weighted MR image of the hand **(A)** demonstrates overgrowth (localized gigantism) of the radial-sided structures. Axial T1-weighted MR image of the wrist **(B)** demonstrates a fibrolipomatous hamartoma of the median nerve *(arrowheads)* with marked nerve enlargement, predominantly with low-signal fibrous components and interdigitating T1-hyperintense fat.

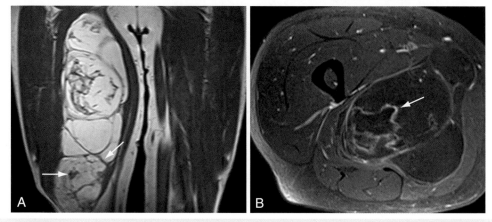

Fig. 12.18 Atypical lipomatous tumor. **(A)** Coronal T1-weighted image shows a very large adipose lesion located within the thigh. The lesion has prominent nodularity and thick septa *(arrows)*, which must alert one to the diagnosis of atypical lipomatous tumor. **(B)** Axial T1-weighted fat-saturated postcontrast image through the same lesion shows enhancement of the septa *(arrow)*. Septa within a simple lipoma should not be thick and should not enhance in this manner. (Images used with permission from BJ Manaster, MD, from STATdx website, Amirsys, Inc.)

- Low-grade, well-differentiated lesion may show fat density at radiography and CT, and fat signal intensity on MRI; such well-differentiated liposarcomas fall into the spectrum of ALT.
- Higher-grade liposarcomas typically contain less than 25% fat and may contain far less than that.
  - One might have to search hard-to-find regions of fat signal (Fig. 12.19), and in some cases none is found (Fig. 12.20).
  - Thus, a high-grade liposarcoma may be completely nonspecific at MRI, having low signal intensity at T1-weighted imaging and high inhomogeneous signal intensity at T2-weighted imaging.
- Myxoid liposarcoma may contain large foci of myxoid tissue that mimic fluid on T2-weighted sequences; postcontrast imaging is crucial to demonstrate that these regions are in fact myxoid rather than cystic.
  - There are often round cell components that have variable MRI appearance.
  - Degree of enhancement varies with cellular composition.
- The uncommon pleomorphic liposarcoma is highly undifferentiated and may contain little or no visible fat on imaging studies.

- Liposarcoma can metastasize to other soft tissues, including the lung, liver, and other solid organs, and can also metastasize to bone.
- May locally invade adjacent structures.
- High-grade liposarcomas are aggressive and require wide excision and chemotherapy, often combined with radiation therapy.
  - Prognosis is relatively poor and worsens with greater round cell components at histology.

FIBROUS TUMORS AND TUMORLIKE CONDITIONS

Benign fibrous soft tissue tumors consist of fibromatoses and fibroblastic proliferations. There are variants that are rare and others that depend on histologic rather than imaging differentiation. The most commonly encountered and recognizable of these lesions are discussed in the following text. Keep in mind that benign fibrous tumors are often hypocellular with dense collagenous components, and thus generally have lower signal on T2-weighted imaging than other, more cellular soft tissue tumors. Malignant fibrous tumors, such as dermatofibrosarcoma protuberans and fibrosarcoma, are also discussed.

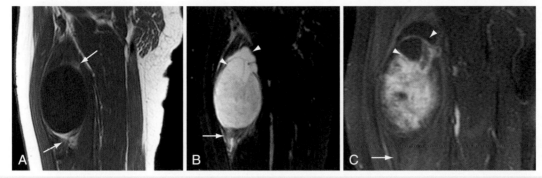

Fig. 12.19 Liposarcoma showing minimal amount of fat. **(A)** Sagittal T1-weighted MR image shows large lesion within the anterior thigh that is predominantly hypointense to skeletal muscle. However, there are two subtle regions of fat density *(arrows)*; this amount of fat within the lesion makes the diagnosis of liposarcoma. **(B)** Sagittal short-tau inversion recovery MR image through the same level shows the mildly heterogeneous hyperintense lesion. The region that showed fat density on the T1-weighted image now saturates out *(arrow)*, confirming that it indeed represents a small amount of fat. There are regions that appear particularly fluidlike *(arrowheads)* adjacent to the mass itself; these are the myxoid foci. **(C)** Sagittal T1-weighted fat-saturated postcontrast image again shows complete saturation of the fatty region *(arrow)*. There is relatively little enhancement of the myxoid regions *(arrowheads)*, but the remainder of the lesion shows intense though heterogeneous enhancement. The findings are typical of myxoid liposarcoma.

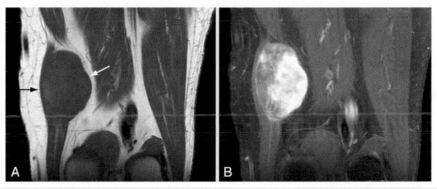

Fig. 12.20 Liposarcoma with no discernible fat. **(A)** Coronal T1-weighted MR image shows a large hypointense soft tissue mass *(arrows)*; there is no fat density. **(B)** Coronal T1-weighted fat-saturated postcontrast image shows heterogeneous intense enhancement of the lesion. The appearance is nonspecific; it could easily represent either undifferentiated pleomorphic sarcoma or liposarcoma, the two most common soft tissue sarcomas. Biopsy proved high-grade liposarcoma.

Superficial Fibromatoses

- These are locally infiltrative benign fibroblastic lesions, most commonly found arising from the palmar or plantar fascia/aponeuroses.
- *Palmar fibromatosis*, also known as *Dupuytren's contracture*, is fibromatosis of the palmar hand.
  - Fibrotic bands affecting the palmar aponeurosis tether the hand flexor tendons, causing flexion contractures, most frequently the fourth and fifth digits (Fig. 12.21).
  - Most common type of superficial fibromatosis, typically seen in older adults, and in particular those of northern European descent.
- *Plantar fibromatosis*, also known as *Ledderhose disease*, can be seen in both children and adults.
  - Characterized by benign but potentially locally aggressive lobular tumorlike growth of the plantar fascia.
  - May be seen as a solitary plantar fibroma or multiple plantar fibromas.
- Growths in superficial fibromatoses typically have low signal intensity on T1-weighted imaging and generally low (but more variable) signal on fluid-sensitive sequences; postcontrast enhancement is variable and relates to lesion maturity (Fig. 12.22).

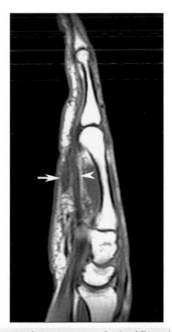

Fig. 12.21 Dupuytren's contracture. Sagittal T1-weighted MR image in the hand shows a low-signal-intensity fibrous band *(arrow)* palmar to the flexor tendons *(arrowhead)* typical of fibromatosis.

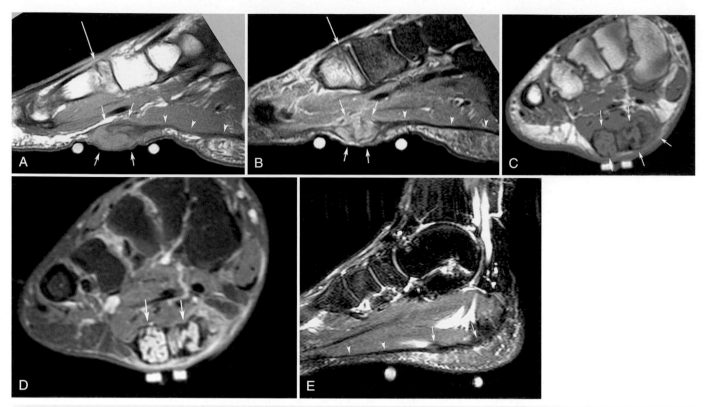

Fig. 12.22 Plantar fibromatosis. Sagittal T1-weighted **(A)** and fat-suppressed, T2-weighted **(B)** images show multilobulated mass *(arrows)* with heterogeneous relatively low signal intensity arising from the plantar fascia *(arrowheads)*. Also note the stress fracture in the proximal first metatarsal *(long arrows)*. **(C)** Short-axis T1-weighted image in another patient shows a heterogeneous hypointense plantar mass *(arrows)*. **(D)** Contrast-enhanced, fat-suppressed, T1-weighted MR image of the same lesion shows heterogeneous intense enhancement *(arrows)*. **(E)** Sagittal fat-suppressed T2-weighted MR image in a different patient shows predominantly low signal in the plantar fibroma *(arrows)* and normal plantar fascia more distally *(arrowheads)*. This mass had low signal intensity on T1-weighted images and did not enhance (not shown). Either pattern may be seen with plantar fibromatosis.

- Significant enhancement and higher signal on T2-weighted imaging suggest lesion immaturity and increased risk for recurrence following excision.
- Superficial fibromatoses are also visible with ultrasonography (Fig. 12.23).
  - Soft tissue nodules or thickened cords identified along the affected fascia.
- Diagnosis is usually easy, but this condition can be difficult to treat because of a tendency for local invasion and recurrence.
- Palmar and plantar fibromatoses may coexist in the same patient.

Deep (or Desmoid-Type) Fibromatoses

- *Deep (or desmoid-type) fibromatoses*, also known as *desmoid tumor* and *aggressive fibromatosis*, are benign fibroblastic tumors that are locally aggressive and infiltrative but do not metastasize.
  - Characterized by a fibrotic band-like or tendon-like composition; histologically composed of sheets of fibroblasts with a herringbone pattern, without significant numbers of mitoses.
  - As a group, soft tissue fibromatoses tend to be large, locally infiltrative, and occasionally multicentric.
  - Tumor often infiltrates through compartmental barriers and has no visible capsule either at surgery or with imaging.

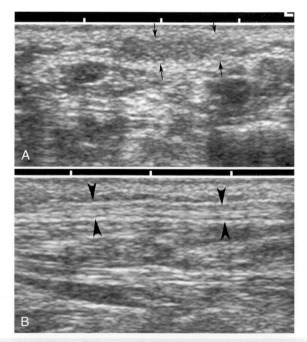

Fig. 12.23 Plantar fibroma on ultrasound. Longitudinal US images are displayed as they were obtained, with plantar surface of foot at top of the image. Note irregularly thickened hypoechoic plantar fascia (**A**, *arrows*). Contrast with normal thin, uniform, echogenic plantar fascia (**B**, *arrowheads*) at a different site in the same patient.

- Desmoid tumor typically presents as a painless, infiltrative soft tissue mass, which can originate anywhere but is subdivided by location: intraabdominal, abdominal wall, and extraabdominal.
  - *Intraabdominal* lesions most frequently involve the small bowel mesentery and may result in bowel obstruction.
  - *Abdominal* lesions typically occur in young women within the abdominal wall muscles and fascia, usually during or following pregnancy, or related to oral contraceptive use.
  - *Extraabdominal* lesions most frequently involve the extremities (70%), usually in an inter- or intramuscular location.
- Extraabdominal desmoid tumors are commonly referred to in the musculoskeletal literature as *aggressive fibromatosis* (Figs. 12.24 and 12.25).
  - Aggressive appearance may lead to a misdiagnosis of a malignant lesion; however, MRI signal characteristics can be helpful in making the correct diagnosis.
    - In up to 80% of cases, signal intensity is low on both T1-weighted and T2-weighted imaging due to tumor hypocellularity.
    - In the remaining 20% of cases, nonspecific low or intermediate signal intensity on T1-weighted sequences and high signal intensity on T2-weighted sequences make the diagnosis more difficult (see Fig. 12.24).
    - Enhancement is variable but often intense.
    - Lesions tend to grow along fascial planes, which can be a clue to the diagnosis.
  - Regardless of location, lesions may be large by the time they are detected and show aggressive local infiltration of adjacent muscle, vessels, nerves, and tendons.
    - Direct extension of tumor may affect adjacent bone, either via bony remodeling (pressure erosion) or by stimulating a 'frondlike' periosteal reaction.
    - Although lesions do not metastasize, they are locally highly aggressive, with a postresection recurrence rate of 19–88%.
- Because these tumors are infiltrative and unencapsulated, margins can be difficult to assess with imaging studies or by direct palpation at surgery, necessitating wide surgical margins.
- Adjuvant therapies include nonsteroidal antiinflammatory drugs (NSAIDs), hormone therapy (antiestrogens and prostaglandin inhibitors), chemotherapy agents, and newer kinase inhibitors.
- For those cases recurring in locations likely to result in significant morbidity, external beam radiation or thermal ablation may be considered.

Nodular Fasciitis

- Benign, highly cellular, nonneoplastic fibrous lesions arising in the subcutaneous tissues along the superficial fascia, which may simulate a rapidly growing sarcomatous neoplasm, both clinically and histopathologically.
- Most commonly encountered in the upper extremities and trunk, less frequently in the head and neck region and lower extremities.
- Seen in children and adults up to approximately 40 years of age; may have a history of trauma to the affected area.
- Condition is usually self-limited with spontaneous regression following the period of rapid growth, though

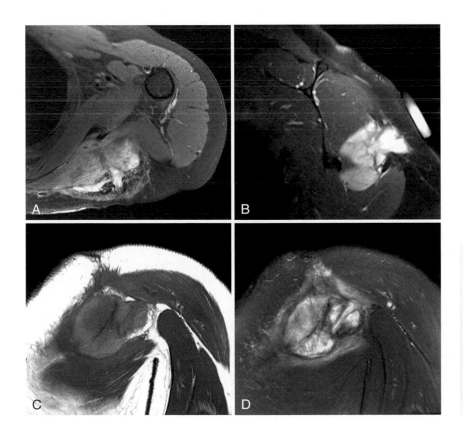

Fig. 12.24 Aggressive fibromatosis (desmoid tumor) arising at a site of prior lipoma excision. Axial proton density fat-suppressed **(A)**, sagittal T1-weighted fat-suppressed postcontrast **(B)**, coronal T1 **(C)**, and coronal T2 fat-suppressed **(D)** MR images of the left shoulder demonstrate a heterogeneously T2-hyperintense aggressive-appearing mass centered in the infraspinatus and teres minor muscles. The mass is intermediate signal on T1-weighted imaging **(C)**, with internal bands of low T1 and T2 signal (C and D). Tissue sampling obtained via image-guided core needle biopsy revealed a low-grade spindle cell lesion, consistent with desmoid-type fibromatosis, also termed *desmoid tumor* or *aggressive fibromatosis*.

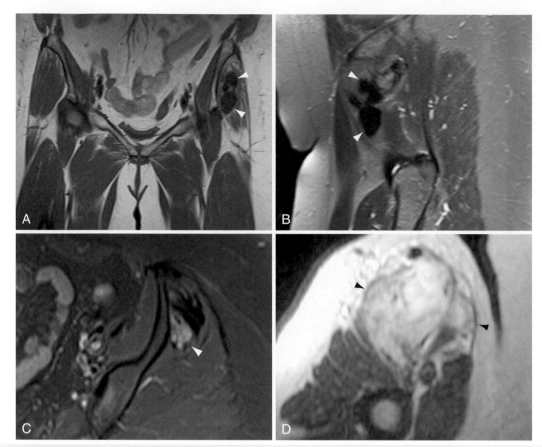

Fig. 12.25 Aggressive fibromatosis (desmoid tumors). **(A)** Coronal T1-weighted MR image shows three adjacent round masses *(arrowheads)*, hypointense to skeletal muscle. **(B)** Sagittal T2-weighted, fat-saturated image shows the multiple lesions to be contiguous and to remain hypointense in signal *(arrowheads)*. **(C)** Axial T1-weighted, fat-saturated postcontrast image shows parts of the lesion remaining hypointense while other portions enhance avidly *(arrowhead)*. This case shows typical signal characteristics of desmoid tumors. **(D)** Axial T2-weighted MR image in a different patient shows an invasive high-signal-intensity mass *(arrowheads)* in the proximal arm of a 42-year-old man. At biopsy this proved to also be aggressive fibromatosis. This case demonstrates that aggressive fibromatosis (desmoid tumors) can have a variety of signal characteristics on both fluid-sensitive and postcontrast imaging.

may require fine-needle aspiration or percutaneous biopsy to confirm the diagnosis.
- If performed, surgical resection is usually curative with low rate of recurrence.
- Intralesional injection of corticosteroid may result in involution.
- MRI or US imaging demonstrate a small (<4 cm) subcutaneous mass along the superficial fascia (Fig. 12.26).
- MRI features are variable, depending on histologic subtype:
  - Myxoid and cellular subtypes demonstrate T2-hyperintensity and signal on T1-weighted imaging isointense to muscle.
  - Fibrous subtype is generally hypointense to muscle on both T2- and T1-weighted sequences.
  - Contrast enhancement is usually diffuse but may be peripheral if there are central cystic or myxoid components.

Elastofibroma Dorsi

- Benign fibrous pseudotumor that results from chronic mechanical friction between the scapula and posterior chest wall.
- Presents characteristically on imaging as an ill-defined triangular or ovoid-shaped soft tissue mass deep to the

serratus anterior and latissimus dorsi muscles, interspersed with fat.
- Most frequently encountered in middle to older-aged females and may be bilateral in up to 25–30% of cases.
- CT and MRI demonstrate a well-defined, heterogeneous soft tissue mass inferomedial to the scapula, with fibrous components similar in appearance to skeletal muscle and interspersed fatty streaking (Fig. 12.27).
- Treated with excision if symptomatic.

Fibroma of Tendon Sheath

- Benign, slow-growing mass arising along a tendon in the extremities, particularly the hand.
- May be clinically and radiologically indistinguishable from a giant cell tumor of tendon sheath, which has overlapping imaging features (discussed later in this chapter).
- MRI demonstrates a soft tissue mass with attachment to a tendon or tendon sheath, which is iso- or hypointense to muscle on T1- and T2-weighted sequences.
- Treated with excision, which confirms the diagnosis on histopathology; may recur if incompletely excised.

Dermatofibrosarcoma Protuberans

- Low-grade spindle cell malignant sarcoma that involves the dermis and subcutaneous tissues.

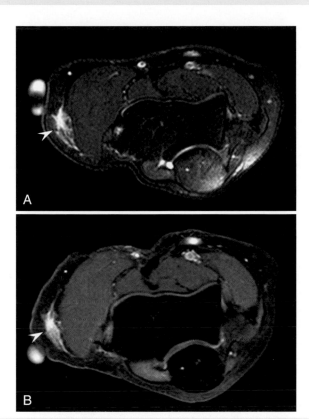

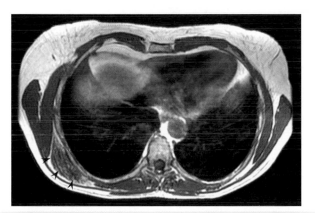

Fig. 12.26 Nodular fasciitis. Axial T2-weighted fat-suppressed **(A)** and T1-weighted fat-suppressed postcontrast **(B)** MR images of the elbow demonstrate an irregularly marginated, T2-hyperintense enhancing mass along the superficial fascia of the brachioradialis muscle *(arrowheads)*.

Fig. 12.27 Elastofibroma dorsi. Axial T1-weighted MR image of the chest demonstrates an ovoid-shaped, intermediate-signal soft tissue mass *(arrowheads)* deep to the right serratus anterior and latissimus dorsi muscles with interspersed T1-hyperintense fat.

- 50% arise in the chest, back, and abdominal wall; 35–40% involve the upper extremity; head/neck/scalp involvement is also common.
- Mass is usually exophytic, but otherwise imaging appearance is nonspecific.
  - Does not contain calcification.
  - Hypointense on T1-weighted imaging and moderately hyperintense on fluid-sensitive sequences (Fig. 12.28); most show moderate enhancement.
  - Larger lesions tend to be more heterogeneous.

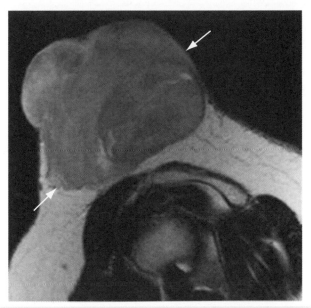

Fig. 12.28 Dermatofibrosarcoma protuberans. Sagittal T2-weighted MR image of the shoulder demonstrates a large exophytic mass arising in the superficial soft tissues *(arrows)*. The signal is moderately hyperintense to muscle and mildly heterogeneous. This is typical of dermatofibrosarcoma protuberans. (Image used with permission from BJ Manaster, MD, from Manaster BJ, Petersilge CA, Roberts CC, Hanrahan CJ. *Diagnostic Imaging: Musculoskeletal Non-Traumatic Disease.* Salt Lake City: Amirsys; 2010.)

- Diagnosis is most suggested by the location and exophytic nature of the lesion.
- Though the lesions grow slowly, they may develop ulceration and satellite lesions in advanced cases.
- Wide excision is required to prevent recurrence; rarely the lesions may transform to fibrosarcoma.

Fibrosarcoma

- Malignant spindle cell tumor that may arise in either bone or soft tissue.
- Fibrosarcoma originating in the soft tissues is relatively uncommon and tends to be located in the deep regions of the extremities.
- MRI characteristics are entirely nonspecific:
  - T1-weighted signal isointense to muscle, hyperintense inhomogeneous fluid-sensitive appearance, and enhancement.
  - May contain myxoid, cystic, or necrotic regions.

UNDIFFERENTIATED PLEOMORPHIC SARCOMA

- *Undifferentiated pleomorphic sarcoma*, or simply *pleomorphic sarcoma*, was formerly known as malignant fibrous histiocytoma (MFH) and is the most frequent soft tissue sarcoma in adults, representing about 25–40% of all adult soft tissue tumors.
- Occurs over a wide age range (10–90 years of age), with most patients between 30 and 60 years of age.
- Most common site is the extremities, and 50% of all cases are found in the lower extremity; 90% are deep lesions.
- Highly aggressive tumor; usually painless and may be large by the time of presentation.

- Radiographic appearance is nonspecific, with distorted fat planes around the mass.
  - Up to 15% of pleomorphic sarcomas may contain dystrophic calcification, mimicking either myositis ossificans or synovial sarcoma.
  - When adjacent to a long bone, tumor may cause a smooth cortical pressure erosion.
- MRI appearance is generally nonspecific:
  - T1-weighted images appear isointense to muscle and T2-weighted images show inhomogeneous high signal intensity (Fig. 12.29).
  - Contrast enhancement is intense, but there are often large areas of necrosis (Fig. 12.30).
  - Hemorrhage may be identified as T1-weighted hyperintensity; there may be fluid-fluid levels in regions of hemorrhage.
    - It is crucial not to misdiagnose the lesion as a hematoma.
  - Lesions may appear to have a reactive pseudocapsule but must be considered aggressive, with tumor cells invariably infiltrating locally at the margins.
- Lesions are treated with wide surgical excision and adjuvant chemotherapy; there is a high recurrence rate (19–31%), and 5-year survival ranges between 50% and 70%.

SYNOVIAL SARCOMA

- *Synovial sarcoma* represents 2.5–10% of all malignant soft tissue sarcomas, and it is one of the most common soft tissue sarcomas in younger adult patients (15–35 years of age).
- Although the name of the lesion suggests an articular process, 90% of synovial cell sarcomas do not originate from a joint but are often found in the soft tissues near a joint.
  - Tumor is named by the predominant histologic differentiation, in this case tumor cells that resemble synovioblastic cells.
- Most occur in the lower extremity, especially at or distal to the knee, but can occur in any extremity or rarely at other sites.
- Synovial cell sarcomas have a higher prevalence of dystrophic calcification than do the other soft tissue sarcomas.
- Age (young adult), location (lower extremity, juxtaarticular), and calcification, if present, can suggest this tumor (Figs. 12.31 to 12.33).

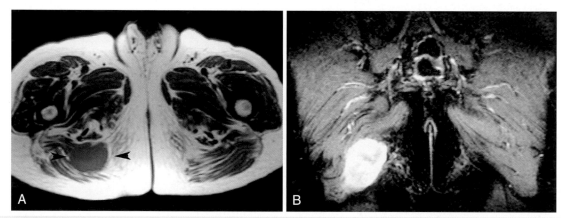

Fig. 12.29 Undifferentiated pleomorphic sarcoma. **(A)** Axial T1-weighted MR image showing an intramuscular soft tissue mass in the right gluteus maximus that is isointense with muscle *(arrowhead)*. **(B)** Coronal T2-weighted MR image shows slightly heterogeneous but mostly high signal intensity. This is a nonspecific appearance, but a sarcoma must be considered.

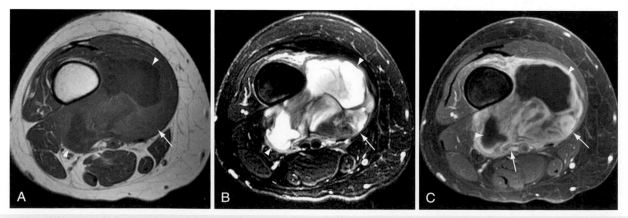

Fig. 12.30 Undifferentiated pleomorphic sarcoma in a 76-year-old woman. **(A)** Axial T1-weighted MR image shows a large posterior thigh mass with regions of density isointense to muscle *(arrow)* and other regions hypointense to muscle *(arrowheads)*. **(B)** Axial intermediate-weighted, fat-saturated image at the same level shows heterogeneous hyperintensity in the mass *(arrow)* and intense fluidlike signal in the regions that were of particularly low signal on the T1-weighted image *(arrowheads)*. **(C)** Axial T1-weighted, fat-saturated postcontrast image proves that the enhancing mass *(arrows)* surrounds two large regions of necrosis *(arrowheads)*.

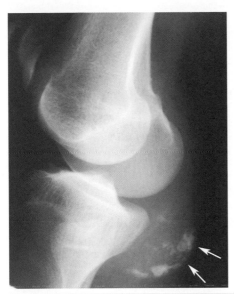

Fig. 12.31 Synovial sarcoma with dystrophic calcification. Oblique radiograph of the knee in an 18-year-old man, demonstrating a soft tissue mass containing dystrophic calcification *(arrows)*. Synovial sarcoma calcifies more frequently than other soft tissue sarcomas. The location, calcification, and age of the patient should yield a strong suspicion of synovial sarcoma. (Image used with permission from BJ Manaster, MD, from the American College of Radiology Learning File.)

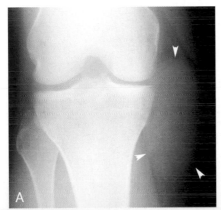

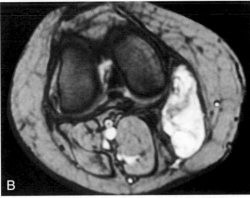

Fig. 12.32 Synovial sarcoma without calcification. (A) AP radiograph of the knee in a 17-year-old girl demonstrates a soft tissue mass adjacent to but not within the knee joint *(arrowheads)*. **(B)** Axial gradient-echo image of the lesion, demonstrated here to be juxtaarticular. There is a large cystic component. Despite the lack of calcification and the encapsulated appearance of this lesion, the age of the patient, location, and prevalence of the lesion lead one to suspect that the diagnosis is synovial sarcoma, which was proved at biopsy.

- Radiographs may be unrevealing or show only a subtle soft tissue mass, though soft tissue calcification is present in up to 30% of cases.
    - If present, calcification is dystrophic and tends to occur in the periphery or eccentrically in the mass.
    - Adjacent bone may exhibit periosteal reaction or a pressure erosion; osseous invasion is seen in 5%.
- MRI features include:
    - T1-weighted signal isointense to muscle.
    - Hyperintensity on T2-weighted images, which may be markedly heterogeneous.
        - Heterogeneity of the high T2 signal intensity is marked, often with areas of internal hemorrhage, internal cystic regions, and occasional fluid-fluid levels (see Fig. 12.33).
    - *Triple sign* has been attributed to this lesion, with three varieties of T2 signal intensity caused by hemorrhage/necrosis, solid tissue, and calcification.
    - *Bowl of grapes* refers to a multiloculated appearance of the mass with internal septa on T2-weighted imaging.
        - The cystic component may be dominant, showing very bright signal intensity on T2-weighted images, which may falsely suggest a ganglion cyst (see Fig. 12.32).
        - Contrast enhancement is helpful in distinguishing a solid mass from a ganglion cyst, because the latter enhances only faintly at the lesion margins.
- Synovial cell sarcomas are treated with wide excision, often with adjuvant chemotherapy and occasional radiation therapy.
- Calcified tumors tend to have a better prognosis, but outcome is generally poor, with pulmonary metastasis encountered frequently, including late metastases, and local recurrence in about 25% of patients despite aggressive local therapy.

LYMPHOMA

- Musculoskeletal involvement of lymphoma may be secondary or present as the primary site of disease (extranodal lymphoma).
- Primary lymphoma of bone always involves the osseous structures but may have large associated soft tissue components.
    - CT or MRI may show tumor extension through small cortical channels without overt cortical destruction (only 28% show cortical destruction), with an associated circumferential soft tissue mass.
    - Systemic lymphoma with bone involvement is usually treated with chemotherapy.
- Muscular lymphoma may occur in the setting of disseminated lymphoma, local extension from osseous or nodal disease, or, rarely, as primary muscular lymphoma.
    - Predilection for the extremities (particularly the thigh) and trunk.
    - MRI is the best imaging modality for assessment of muscle involvement (Fig. 12.34).
        - May show a focal intramuscular mass or diffuse muscle infiltration and enlargement.
        - Due to hypercellularity, tumor is often iso- or slightly hyperintense to muscle on T1-weighted

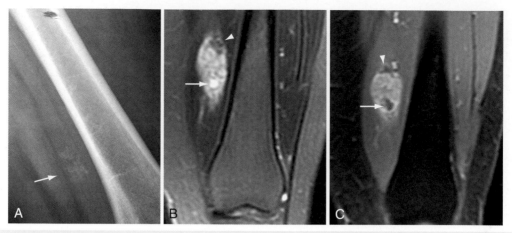

Fig. 12.33 Synovial sarcoma in a young adult woman. (A) Lateral radiograph shows nonspecific dystrophic calcification *(arrow)* located posterior to the distal femoral metadiaphysis. No other abnormality is seen. **(B)** Coronal T2-weighted fat-saturated image of the same location shows a highly heterogeneous lesion located deep in the soft tissues of the thigh. There is a small focus of very high signal *(arrow)* and another hypointense focus related to the calcification *(arrowhead)*. **(C)** Coronal postcontrast T1-weighted fat-saturated image shows the lesion to have heterogeneous intense enhancement, with the low-signal calcification *(arrowhead)* and a round low-signal focus confirming cystic component *(arrow)*. This heterogeneity has been termed the *triple sign*. These MRI characteristics, along with the combination of patient age (young adult), location (lower extremity, adjacent to but not involving the knee joint), and dystrophic calcification, all point to the proven diagnosis of synovial sarcoma.

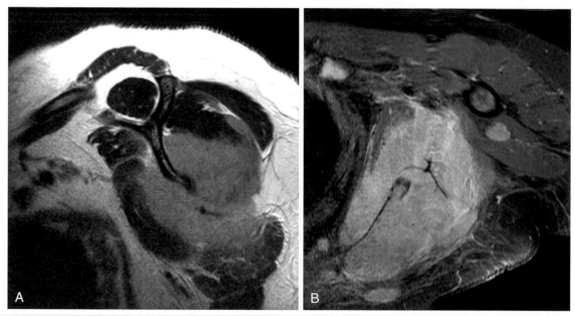

Fig. 12.34 Diffuse large B-cell lymphoma in a 51-year-old woman. Sagittal T2-weighted **(A)** and axial T1-weighted fat-suppressed postcontrast **(B)** MR images of the shoulder demonstrate a T2-intermediate, enhancing mass centered about the scapula with osseous destruction and a large soft tissue component with extensive involvement of the rotator cuff musculature.

imaging and intermediate signal (hyperintense to muscle) on T2-weighted imaging.

- Postcontrast imaging may demonstrate diffuse or thick peripheral/septal enhancement.

INTRAMUSCULAR MYXOMA

- Generally painless, benign soft tissue neoplasm that has a predilection for large muscles, being most frequently seen in the thigh, buttocks, and shoulder.
- Occurs most frequently in women (2:1 female-to-male ratio) within the age range of 40–70 years.
- No risk for malignant degeneration.

- On CT, attenuation of the mass falls between that of fluid and muscle.
- MRI is most frequently used for diagnosis and characterization.
  - Appearance on T1-weighted imaging is usually homogeneous with a low to intermediate signal intensity.
  - Very hyperintense on T2-weighted imaging (may be mistaken for a cystic lesion).
    - One of the most helpful characteristics on fluid-sensitive imaging is high signal extending beyond the lesion itself, caused by leakage of myxomatous tissue (Fig. 12.35).

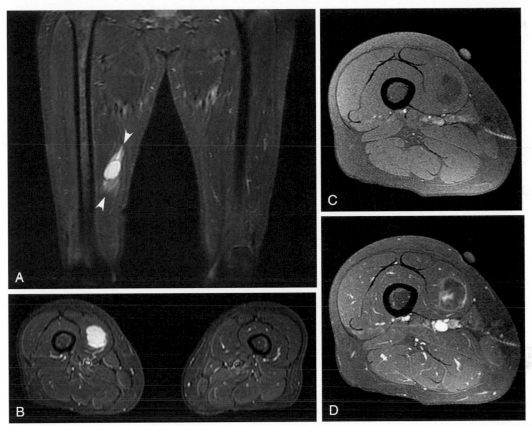

Fig. 12.35 Intramuscular myxoma. Coronal **(A)** and axial **(B)** STIR MR images demonstrate a homogeneously hyperintense mass within the vastus medialis muscle. Most characteristic of the myxoma is the 'tail' of hyperintensity extending from the lesion (A, *arrowheads*), indicating leakage of myxomatous material into the surrounding soft tissues. Axial precontrast **(C)** and postcontrast **(D)** T1 weighted fat-suppressed images show mild, heterogeneous enhancement of the lesion, typical of myxoma.

- Frequently has a high-signal rim of fat, especially around the superior and inferior margins of the lesion.
- Enhancement is mild-to-moderate; there may be septa and purely cystic foci within the lesion.
- *Mazabraud syndrome* is characterized by multiple intramuscular myxomas and fibrous dysplasia (usually polyostotic).

NEUROGENIC TUMORS

- Peripheral nerve sheath tumors (PNSTs), whether benign or malignant, are most classically distinguished by their fusiform shape.
  - Mass tapers at one or both ends to accommodate the nerve entering and exiting the tumor; the nerve is often seen as a 'tail' extending from the tumor proximally and/or distally (*tail sign*).
- Benign PNSTs include *neurofibromas* and *schwannomas*.
  - Together, these represent about 10% of all benign soft tissue tumors, with neurofibroma being slightly more common than schwannoma.
  - Both types of benign PNSTs most frequently affect patients 20–30 years of age.
  - Both show initial slow growth and usually are relatively small when detected.
  - Tumors can be exquisitely painful, particularly when biopsied.

- There are three MRI signs that are typical of, though not pathognomonic for, PNSTs.
  - *Fascicular sign*: Enlarged nerve fibers are seen in cross section as multiple small ringlike structures, like fibers in a cable (Fig. 12.36A and B).
  - *Target sign*: Low signal seen centrally on a fluid-sensitive sequence that appears as a target (Fig. 12.36C).
  - *Split-fat sign*: Lesion surrounded in part by a thin peripheral rim of fat, separating it from adjacent muscles, best seen at a tapering margin of the tumor.
- Keep in mind that these signs do not help distinguish these tumors from one another, either histologically or benign from malignant, and some PNSTs may not exhibit any of these signs (Fig. 12.36D).

Neurofibroma

- *Neurofibromas* are composed of Schwann cells, fibroblasts, and collagen that surround and engulf the fibers of the associated nerve (Fig. 12.37; see Fig. 12.36).
- Neurofibromas may be localized, diffuse, or plexiform.
- *Localized neurofibroma*.
  - 90% of all neurofibromas are localized and solitary, most often arising in the superficial cutaneous nerves, and are not associated with neurofibromatosis type 1 (NF1).
  - Patients with NF1 may have hundreds of localized neurofibromas, in addition to diffuse and plexiform neurofibromas (Fig. 12.38).

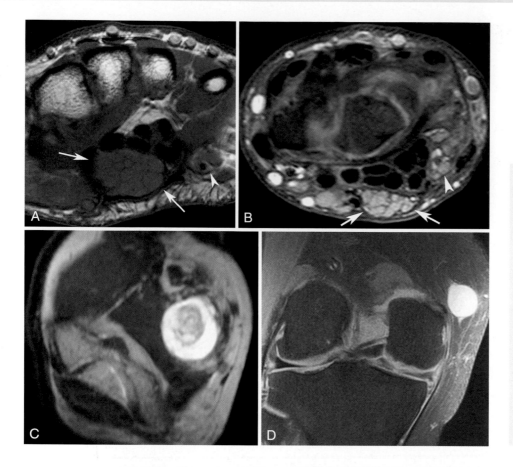

Fig. 12.36 Signs of peripheral nerve sheath tumors (PNSTs). Axial T1-weighted **(A)** and fat-suppressed T2-weighted **(B)** MR images of the wrist in a patient with neurofibromatosis 1 show multiple small fascicle-like structures ('fascicular sign') within neurofibromas of the median *(arrows)* and ulnar *(arrowhead)* nerves. **(C)** Peripheral neurofibroma with 'target sign'. Axial T2-weighted MR image shows a mass in the antecubital soft tissues in a 52-year-old man. Note the high signal intensity peripherally with central low signal, resembling a target. The target sign is frequently seen in neurofibroma but can also be seen in other PNSTs. **(D)** Coronal T2-weighted fat-saturated image shows a schwannoma with tail-like nerve exiting the tumor both proximally and distally ('tail sign'); this particular lesion shows neither a target nor fascicular sign, but the fusiform shape with nerve exiting the lesion is typical of PNST.

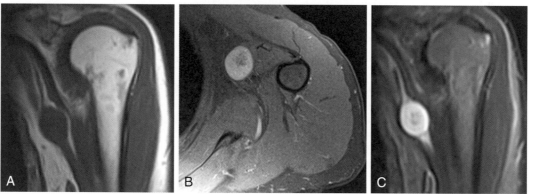

Fig. 12.37 Localized solitary neurofibroma in an older adult man who complained of tingling down his arm. **(A)** Coronal T1-weighted MR image shows a fusiform mass, hypointense to skeletal muscle, in the distribution of the median nerve, with nerve seen entering and exiting the lesion. **(B)** Axial intermediate-weighted, fat-saturated lesion shows the lesion to be hyperintense, with central low signal, a typical target sign. **(C)** Coronal postcontrast T1-weighted fat-saturated image shows enhancement of the lesion, with target features; the nerve entering and exiting the lesion is also enlarged and enhances, making it easy to discern. The lesion is typical in appearance for peripheral nerve sheath tumor; biopsy proved neurofibroma.

- Neurofibromas invade the nerve fascicles, which become separated and intimately involved with tumor.
- CT typically shows a near-water density mass.
- MRI shows low signal intensity on T1-weighted images and heterogeneously increased signal intensity on T2-weighted images.
- Nerve fascicles may be visible within the tumor, seen on MRI as multiple small ringlike structures, known as the *fascicular sign* (see Fig. 12.36).
- *Split-fat sign* is the finding of fat separating the tumor from adjacent muscles, best seen at a tapering margin of the tumor.

- *Tail sign* is the finding of tapered proximal and distal margins.
- *Fascicular sign*, *split-fat sign*, and *tail sign* are characteristic of PNSTs, but not specific for neurofibromas as other PNSTs have these findings as well.
- More frequently seen *target sign* is characterized by low signal intensity centrally with a ring of higher signal intensity peripherally on T2-weighted MR images (see Fig. 12.36).
  - This pattern reflects the histologic features of the tumor, with peripheral myxomatous tissue (with high T2 signal) surrounding a fibrocollagenous core.

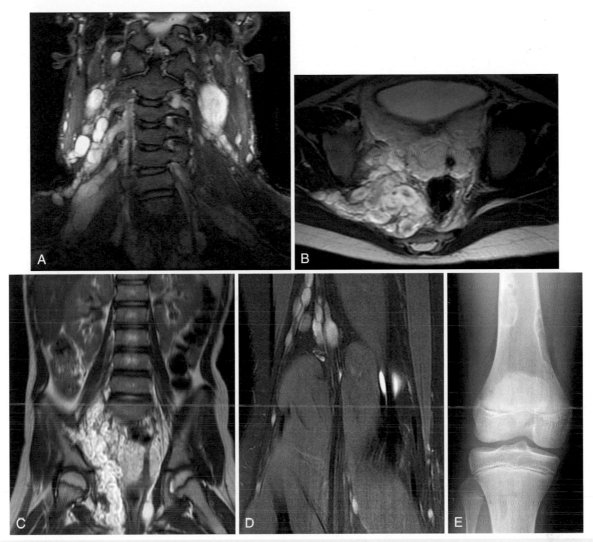

Fig. 12.38 **Neurofibromatosis type 1. (A)** Coronal inversion recovery MR image in the cervical spine shows innumerable bilateral high-signal-intensity neurofibromas. Note the enlarged neural foramina on the left side. Axial T2-weighted **(B)** and coronal T2-weighted **(C)** images in a child with neurofibromatosis 1 show similar findings along the sciatic nerve roots. The individual enlarged nerves can be distinguished on the axial image, assuring the diagnosis. **(D)** Coronal intermediate-weighted fat-saturated image shows innumerable neurofibromas in the popliteal fossa along the paths of the tibial and peroneal nerve distributions, as well as in subcutaneous positions. The appearance is typical of neurofibromatosis. **(E)** AP radiograph shows multiple nonossifying fibromas in typical metadiaphyseal position, arising from the cortex. Nonossifying fibroma is usually a solitary lesion; when it is multiple, neurofibromatosis should be considered, as proved to be the case here.

- This pattern is more specific for neurofibromas, though may occasionally be encountered with schwannomas and malignant PNSTs.
- Enhancement may be heterogeneous or follow a similar or reverse pattern to the *target sign* on T2-weighted imaging.
- Cutaneous neurofibromas are less likely to demonstrate typical signs than are deeper lesions.
- *Diffuse neurofibroma.*
  - Presents as plaque-like skin elevation.
  - Much more likely to arise sporadically than in association with NF1 (similar to localized neurofibromas).
  - On MRI, diffuse neurofibroma is nonspecific, infiltrating or expanding the subcutaneous tissues.
- *Plexiform neurofibroma.*
  - Unlike localized and diffuse types, plexiform neurofibromas are highly associated with NF1.

- Presents as long segments of diffusely and irregularly enlarged nerves and nerve branches and clinically may result in limb disfigurement and dysesthesia.
- High risk for malignant transformation (8–12%).

Schwannoma

- *Schwannoma*, also known as neurilemoma, neurinoma, perineural fibroblastoma, and peripheral glioma, is the other common benign PNST.
- Histologically schwannomas are composed of Schwann cells and variable amounts of myxoid material and collagen and are positive for S-100 protein.
- In contrast with neurofibromas, schwannomas do not engulf the associated nerve and therefore often can be 'peeled off' the associated nerve at surgery.
  - As schwannomas cannot be reliably distinguished from neurofibromas at imaging, biopsy is often required prior to operative management.

- Schwannomas are most commonly found in spinal and sympathetic nerve roots, and in the extremities they usually affect nerves in the flexor surfaces of the upper and lower extremities, particularly the ulnar and peroneal nerves (Fig. 12.39).
- Schwannomas, like neurofibromas, are usually solitary.
- If there are multiple schwannomas, they generally occur in a cutaneous distribution, with a very small proportion of these associated with NF1 (note that intracranial schwannoma is associated with NF2).
- *Schwannomatosis* is a rare syndrome of multiple peripheral schwannomas.
- As with neurofibromas, fusiform shape, association with a nerve, and the *target sign*, *split-fat sign*, and *tail sign* are variably seen at MRI.
- Schwannomas are typically heterogeneously T2 hyperintense, though some have fairly uniform intermediate-low signal on T2-weighted images.
- *Ancient schwannomas* are slow-growing schwannomas of long duration often with cystic degeneration and calcification.

Malignant Peripheral Nerve Sheath Tumors

- *Malignant PNSTs* (MPNSTs; also called *neurofibrosarcomas* or *malignant schwannomas*) make up 5–10% of all soft tissue sarcomas.
- Generally seen in patients 20–50 years of age and are slightly more common in women, though MPNST in NF1 patients shows a marked male predominance.
- MPNST associated with NF1 may approach 50% of the cases; these present earlier and with a wider age range than MPNST not associated with NF1.
- Although some of these lesions arise from a preexisting neurofibroma, it should be emphasized that the malignant potential of a neurofibroma is very low.

- Malignant PNSTs are usually deep lesions, involving the major nerve trunks such as the sciatic nerve, brachial plexus, and sacral plexus (Fig. 12.40).
  - Large size, irregular margins, and heterogeneous signal intensity of many malignant PNSTs may suggest a malignant lesion, although these findings are nonspecific.
  - *Target sign* is occasionally present.
  - Rapid growth in a previously stable neurofibroma and invasion or destruction of adjacent tissues may be present and are more specific signs.
- Malignant PNSTs are aggressive lesions, requiring wide surgical excision, chemotherapy, and often radiation therapy.
- Local recurrence and distant metastases to lung, bone, and lymph nodes are common; 5-year survival rate is 23–44%.

Morton Neuroma

- *Morton neuroma* (or *intermetatarsal neuroma*) is not a neoplasm but rather perineural fibrosis and plantar digital nerve degeneration occurring in the interdigital space of the foot between the metatarsal heads.
- Cause is thought to be repetitive trauma, with the digital nerve abraded by the intermetatarsal ligament that connects adjacent metatarsal heads.
- Association of Morton neuroma with high-heeled shoes may account for the gender frequency (18:1 female-to-male ratio).
- Lesions are most frequently found between the second and third or third and fourth metatarsal heads (second and third intermetatarsal spaces, respectively).
- Diagnosis can be made clinically but may be mimicked by other lesions such as stress fractures, intermetatarsal bursitis, metatarsophalangeal arthrosis, and tendinitis.

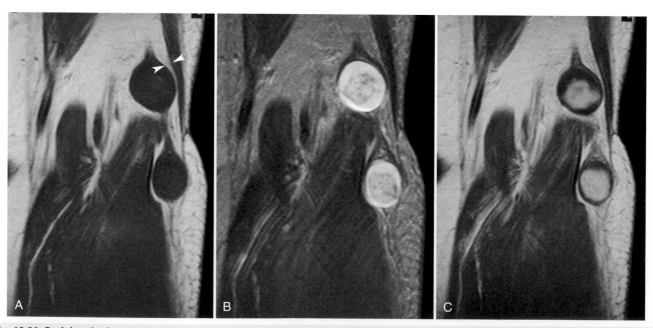

Fig. 12.39 Peripheral schwannomas. Coronal T1-weighted **(A)**, T2-weighted **(B)**, and contrast-enhanced T1-weighted **(C)** MR images through the posterior knee region show two schwannomas in the peroneal nerve. Note the fusiform shape with tapering proximal and distal tumor margins, target appearance, and 'split fat' between the tumors and adjacent muscles (*arrowheads* in A). Although these could easily be neurofibromas, biopsy proved schwannomas; schwannomas are multiple in 2% of cases. The peroneal nerve is a particularly common site for schwannoma.

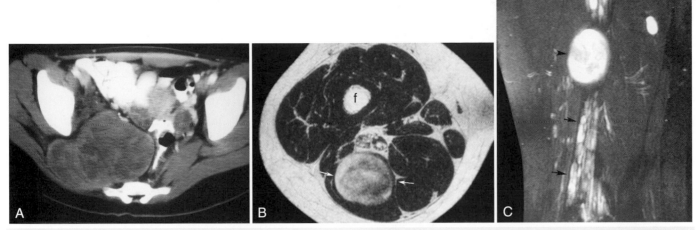

Fig. 12.40 Malignant peripheral nerve sheath tumors (MPNSTs). **(A)** CT image shows a large mass in the right sciatic notch that on biopsy was shown to be a neurofibrosarcoma arising from the sciatic nerve. Management of this lesion is difficult because wide excision is required, and the sciatic nerve is sacrificed. (B and C) Neurofibromatosis with MPNST. Axial T2-weighted MR image **(B)** shows mass *(arrows)* with heterogeneously high signal intensity and a target sign. Coronal fat-suppressed T2-weighted MR image **(C)** demonstrates the mass *(arrowhead)*, which at biopsy was a MPNST, and also demonstrates multiple smaller neurofibromas arising from the tibial and common peroneal nerves of the thigh *(arrows)*. f, femur.

- MRI is helpful in differentiating these possibilities.
  - MRI shows a small dumbbell-shaped mass between the metatarsal heads on short-axis imaging, hypointense to fat and clearly demarcated on T1-weighted images, usually with hypointense or intermediate signal on T2-weighted images (Fig. 12.41).
  - Lesions enhance variably, though contrast is often unnecessary to make the diagnosis.
- Morton neuromas are easily detected as hypoechoic, noncompressible masses on US imaging using a high-frequency transducer (Fig. 12.42).
- Larger lesions are more likely to be symptomatic; smaller lesions may be detected incidentally.

Fibrolipomatous Hamartoma (Neural Fibrolipoma)

- *Fibrolipomatous hamartoma*, or *neural fibrolipoma*, is a tumorlike hamartomatous overgrowth of mesodermal and epidermal elements resulting in nerve enlargement, with fatty tissue interposed between thickened nerve bundles.
- Usually seen in children or young adults, and there is a marked predilection for the median nerve.
- MRI appearance is pathognomonic, with high T1- and T2-signal lipomatous tissue surrounding longitudinally oriented low-signal thickened nerve bundles (Fig. 12.43).

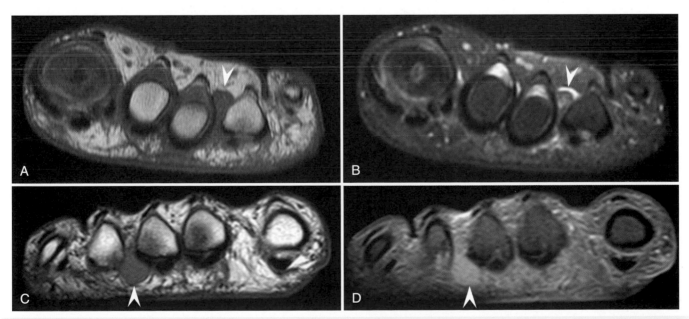

Fig. 12.41 Morton neuroma. Short-axis T1-weighted **(A)** and T2-weighted fat-suppressed **(B)** MR images show a Morton neuroma *(arrowheads)* in the third intermetatarsal space, between the third and fourth metatarsal heads. The neuroma is most conspicuous on the T1-weighted image, as it is outlined by fat. Short-axis T1-weighted **(C)** and T1-weighted fat-suppressed postcontrast **(D)** MR images in another patient show a Morton neuroma in the third intermetatarsal space *(arrowheads)*, demonstrating mild postcontrast enhancement.

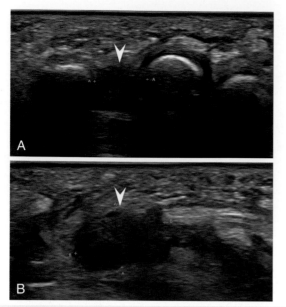

Fig. 12.42 Morton neuroma on ultrasound. Transverse **(A)** and longitudinal **(B)** US images demonstrate a hypoechoic intermetatarsal mass *(arrowheads)*. Neuromas are noncompressible on US, differentiating them from intermetatarsal bursitis.

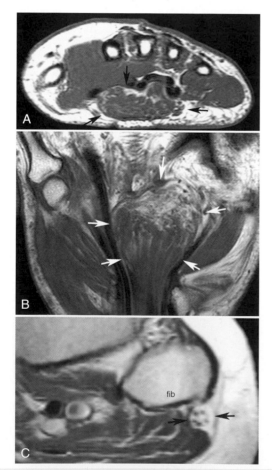

Fig. 12.43 Fibrolipomatous hamartoma (neural fibrolipoma). Axial **(A)** and coronal **(B)** T1-weighted MR images of the wrist and proximal hand demonstrate massively enlarged median nerve with multiple nerve fascicles surrounded by bright lipomatous signal *(arrows)*. **(C)** Axial T1-weighted MR image in the proximal left leg shows a similar lesion in the peroneal nerve *(arrows)*. *fib*, fibular head.

- May be associated with macrodactyly and *macrodystrophia lipomatosa* (see Fig. 12.17).

TENOSYNOVIAL GIANT CELL TUMOR

- *PVNS* is a monoarticular benign tumorlike proliferation of synovium that occurs in joints, bursae, and tendon sheaths.
- The condition is termed *tenosynovial giant cell tumor* (TGCT; previously called *giant cell tumor of tendon sheath*) when it is extraarticular within a tendon sheath.
- Thought to be a nonmalignant neoplastic process; it is histologically identical to PVNS (Fig. 12.44) and some pathologists use the term TGCT for both.
- TGCT is a common lesion, representing 5% of all soft tissue tumors, presenting as a painless, slow-growing synovial proliferation within a tendon sheath, usually of the finger (85%).
- Radiographs show a noncalcified soft tissue mass; about 10–20% have associated bony pressure erosion (Figs. 12.45 and 12.46).
- MRI shows a low-signal lobulated mass on T1-weighted image with variably low to high signal intensity on fluid-sensitive sequences; contrast enhancement is usually intense (Fig. 12.47; see Figs. 12.44 and 12.46).
- TGCT usually hemorrhages much less than does intraarticular PVNS, and therefore tends to have less specific findings on MRI.
- The tendon itself is uninvolved and moves freely from the tumor on dynamic US evaluation.
- Diagnosis is usually made by clinical and imaging features, particularly when the mass is seen to extend along a tendon sheath.
- Treatment is with surgical excision, though local recurrence may be seen in up to 20% of cases.
- Malignant TGCT (occurring de novo or due to malignant transformation of TGCT) is a rare but extremely aggressive sarcoma that is locally destructive and frequently metastatic.

SOFT TISSUE METASTASES

- Metastases to the extranodal soft tissues are uncommon but can be seen with certain entities such as melanoma (metastases may have hyperintensity on T1-weighted images, either due to the paramagnetic properties of melanin or intralesional hemorrhage), lymphoma (diffuse soft tissue infiltration mimicking cellulitis), and rarely other various aggressive malignancies.
- Multiplicity of soft tissue lesions should raise concern for soft tissue metastatic disease.

DERMAL AND SUBCUTANEOUS LESIONS

- Dermal and subcutaneous lesions are typically small and notoriously difficult to differentiate by imaging.
- Diagnoses range from benign (epidermal inclusion cyst, foreign body granuloma, traumatic fat necrosis) to malignant (melanoma, invasive skin cancer, dermatofibrosarcoma protuberans).
- Generally, direct inspection and correlation with clinical course is required; biopsy may be required for indeterminate lesions.

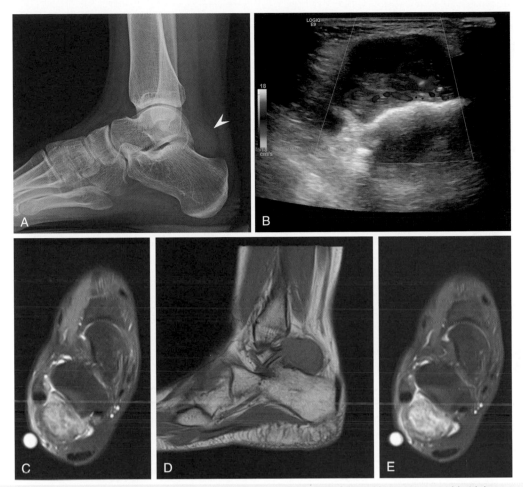

Fig. 12.44 Pigmented villonodular synovitis (PVNS), localized form. **(A)** Lateral radiograph of the ankle in a 15-year-old girl demonstrates a soft tissue mass as the posterior aspect of the ankle *(arrowhead)*. **(B)** Color flow Doppler US image of the mass demonstrates internal vascularity. Axial T2-weighted fat-suppressed **(C)**, sagittal T1-weighted **(D)**, and axial T1-weighted fat suppressed postcontrast **(E)** MR images of the ankle demonstrate a heterogeneously T2-hyperintense, T1-isointense, enhancing mass at the posterolateral aspect of the subtalar joint. Biopsy showed PVNS, localized form, histologically identical to tenosynovial giant cell tumor.

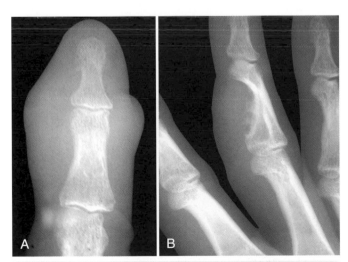

Fig. 12.45 Tenosynovial giant cell tumor (TGCT). **(A)** AP radiograph of the finger in a 52-year-old woman demonstrates a nodular soft tissue mass with normal underlying bone. This is the most typical appearance for TGCT. However, these lesions occasionally cause scalloping of adjacent bone, resulting in an appearance such as that seen in a finger in a 20-year-old man **(B)**.

- Imaging (ultrasound or MRI) may occasionally suggest a specific diagnosis and can be useful to evaluate deep extension for surgical management of malignant processes.

Tumor Staging, Biopsy, and Follow-Up

TUMOR STAGING

The American Joint Committee on Cancer (AJCC) has produced the system most frequently used to stage primary malignant soft tissue musculoskeletal tumors. The Eighth Edition of the *AJCC Cancer Staging Manual* was initially published in October 2016, with staging relevant to primary malignant musculoskeletal soft tissue tumors summarized in Boxes 12.5 and 12.6.

- Staging is based on histologic grade (G), lymph node involvement (N), and presence of metastases (M).
- Four tumor locations for soft tissue sarcomas were introduced into the Eighth Edition: (1) trunk and extremity,

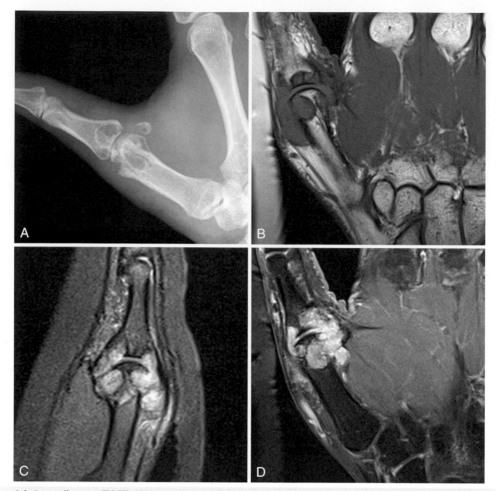

Fig. 12.46 Tenosynovial giant cell tumor (TGCT). **(A)** Lateral image of the thumb shows large, well-defined 'erosions' of the head of the metacarpal and base of the proximal phalanx. These might initially make one consider an arthritic process such as gout. Note that the cartilage width is maintained, as is the bone density. **(B)** Coronal T1-weighted MR image of the hand in the same patient shows the large 'erosions' with hypointense adjacent soft tissue mass. **(C)** Sagittal T2-weighted fat-saturated image of the thumb shows the large hyperintense 'erosions' and elevation of the extensor tendon by a high-signal mass. **(D)** Oblique postcontrast T1-weighted fat-saturated image of the thumb again shows the hyperintense erosions and soft tissue mass. Even though the mass does not extend far down the flexor tendon sheath, one must consider TGCT in this young patient. The 'erosions' are mechanical scalloping of the underlying bone in this case that is not a true arthritis.

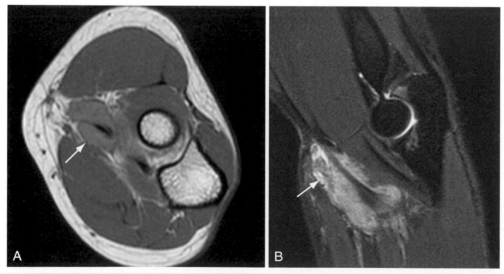

Fig. 12.47 Tenosynovial giant cell tumor. **(A)** Axial intermediate-weighted MR image shows fluid signal slightly hyperintense to skeletal muscle surrounding the biceps tendon *(arrow)*. **(B)** Sagittal T2-weighted fat-saturated image in the same patient shows the hypointense nodular-appearing proliferation *(arrow)* with surrounding hyperintense fluid extending along the biceps tendon, typical of giant cell tumor of tendon sheath.

Box 12.5   AJCC Staging of Primary Malignant Musculoskeletal Soft Tissue Tumors in the Trunk and Extremity: T, N, M, and G Definitions

T (primary tumor) is based on the tumor's longest dimension
   T1: ≤5cm
   T2: >5-10 cm
   T3: >10-15 cm
   T4: >15 cm
   Additional terms: TX = primary tumor cannot be assessed;
      T0 = no evidence of primary tumor
N (nodal spread)
   N0: no nodal spread
   N1: nodal spread present.
   If nodal status is not known, N0 is used
M (distant metastasis)
   M0: no distant metastasis
   M1: distant metastasis present
G (histologic grade) is based on the grading system reviewed in Box 12.7
   G1: total score 2-3
   G2: total score 4-5
   G3: total score 6-8
   Additional term: GX = grade cannot be assessed

Data from AJCC Cancer Staging Forms, Eight Edition

Box 12.6   AJCC System for Staging of Trunk and Extremity Sarcomas

Based on tumor size, histology, and lymph node or distant metastasis
Stage IA: Small tumor (<5cm), low-grade histology
Stage IB: Any size tumor, low-grade histology
Stage II: Small tumor, intermediate or high-grade histology
Stage IIIA: Intermediate tumor size (5-10cm), intermediate or high-grade histology
Stage IIIB: Larger tumor (>10cm), intermediate or high-grade histology
Stage IV: Presence of any nodal or distant metastasis.

Box 12.7   FNCLCC Histologic Grading System

Tumor differentiation	
Score 1	Sarcoma closely resembling normal adult mesenchymal tissues
Score 2	Sarcomas for which histologic typing is certain
Score 3	Embryonal and undifferentiated sarcomas, synovial sarcoma, and sarcomas of uncertain type
Mitotic count	
Score 1	0–9/10 HPF
Score 2	10–19/10 HPF
Score 3	≥20/10 HPF
Tumor necrosis	
Score 0	No necrosis
Score 1	<50% tumor necrosis
Score 2	≥50% tumor necrosis

FNCLCC, Fédération Nationale des Centers de Lutte Contre Cancer; *HPF*, high-power field

The largest difference between this and the AJCC system is in the primary tumor (T) definition. Rather than tumor size, this system emphasizes tumor encapsulation and whether it extends beyond its compartment of origin. Note that the concept of *extremity compartments* as used in sarcoma staging is different than for compartment syndrome. In the latter, extremity compartments are defined by indistensible fascia, as discussed in Chapter 1 – Introduction to Musculoskeletal Imaging. In tumor staging, the term is used differently, as it refers to a portion of an extremity with shared blood and lymphatic drainage that is relevant for surgical management (e.g., the anterior compartment of the thigh includes the vastus medialis, lateralis, and intermedius muscles, which incidently are not vulnerable to compartment syndrome). As used in sarcoma staging, understanding and accurately reporting the tumor location in terms of a compartment is critical, because an aggressive sarcoma can potentially contaminate an entire compartment. In addition to compartment involvement, the MSTS system evaluates tumor proximity or involvement with neurovascular bundles. These are critical factors when considering limb salvage surgery. Cross-sectional imaging, usually MRI, is used for this site evaluation, with axial plane imaging being most useful. Regardless of whether one prefers to use the AJCC or the MSTS system, neurovascular bundle and specific muscle/compartment involvement must be included in the imaging report, as these elements reflect patient prognosis and are used to develop a surgical plan.

The algorithm for soft tissue musculoskeletal lesion workup is shown in Fig. 12.48. This is a much simpler algorithm compared to that for osseous lesions. It also starts with a radiograph, with the recognition that this modality will usually not add much information (one looks for fat density, soft tissue calcification, character of fat plane distortion, and secondary involvement of adjacent osseous structures). US may be obtained if the lesion is superficial and likely benign. The workup then proceeds to MRI, followed by biopsy if the lesion is not definitively benign. Once

(2) retroperitoneum, (3) head and neck, and (4) visceral sites.

- For trunk and extremity sites, tumor (T) is rated by size, now divided into four categories: (a) ≤5 cm, (b) >5 cm and ≤10 cm, (c) >10 cm and ≤15 cm, and (d) >15 cm.
- Depth relative to the superficial fascia has been eliminated from the Eighth Edition.
- For trunk and extremity tumors, lymph node metastases are now classified as stage IV regardless of histologic grade or tumor size (i.e., anyTN1M0anyG = stage IV).
- Histologic grade is based on the Fédération Nationale des Centers de Lutte Contre Cancer (FNCLCC) system, which takes into account tumor differentiation, mitotic count, and tumor necrosis (Box 12.7).

The Musculoskeletal Tumor Society (MSTS) surgical tumor staging system (also know as the Enneking staging system) may be preferred by some orthopedic oncologists.

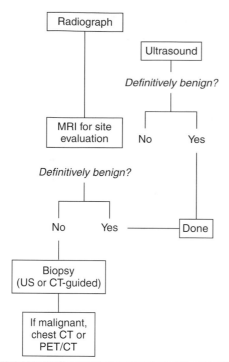

Fig. 12.48 Suggested algorithm for soft tissue musculoskeletal lesion workup.

malignancy is established, the workup for metastatic disease is performed, which typically includes chest CT, although whole-body ^{18}F-FDG PET-CT may be appropriate with certain malignancies.

TUMOR BIOPSY

Both tumor staging and treatment decisions require confidence that representative tissue is obtained in the biopsy. Soft tissue tumors are often biopsied under US if accessible, though CT-guidance may be preferable for deeper lesions. Whether the biopsy is performed percutaneously by the radiologist or by surgical incision, imaging contributes significantly to the biopsy planning process. Targeting viable enhancing, nonnecrotic, nonhemorrhagic regions of tumor provides optimal tissue sampling for accurate histologic diagnosis. It is worth noting that some investigators have recently suggested that avoiding areas of necrosis could theoretically downgrade tumor stage, as the FNCLCC histologic grading system includes tumor necrosis as a factor for overall score (see Box 12.7). Thus, in addition to targeting viable tumor components, it may be worthwhile to sample multiple areas of the tumor, particularly in those that are substantially heterogeneous on imaging.

Consideration of needle approach is crucial for suspected primary bone and soft tissue sarcomas to avoid compartment contamination and potential tumor seeding. One must work with the surgeon to determine the needle approach that will avoid contaminating more than one compartment or any of the soft tissues that the surgeon may require for reconstruction. The soft tissue compartments, as well as specific structures to be avoided during biopsy, are outlined in the article by Liu et al. listed in Sources and Suggested Readings. Careful review of the pre-procedure MRI

and consultation with the surgical oncologist performing the definitive treatment is essential for optimizing patient outcomes.

See Chapter 16 – Musculoskeletal Procedures and Techniques for additional principles, site-specific recommendations, and technical considerations related to biopsy of musculoskeletal lesions.

RESTAGING AND ASSESSING TUMOR RESPONSE

Although surgical resection is the definitive treatment for most malignant musculoskeletal soft tissue tumors, many are initially treated with chemotherapy to obtain systemic control and radiation therapy for tumor debulking, which in many tumors is believed to help achieve local control. These lesions must be restaged before surgical resection, evaluating both the site for surgical planning and the response to treatment. Restaging generally includes chest CT to evaluate for pulmonary metastases and MRI of the primary site (with and without contrast, in all three planes). Primary site reevaluation includes imaging the entire area of involvement on pretreatment scans, as well as a direct comparison of key components with the initial MRI to determine any change in lesion size and degree of tumor response to therapy.

Imaging interpretation is difficult during the initial treatment phase of tumors treated with chemotherapy to determine response. The most important indicator of response is a high percentage of tumor necrosis, though this is difficult to reliably quantify by imaging. Some imaging findings are associated with a good response to chemotherapy. Decrease in tumor size, indicated by a 50% decrease in the product of the two largest perpendicular diameters, is consistent with a favorable treatment response. Dynamic contrast-enhanced MRI, which evaluates the rate of enhancement after an intravenous gadolinium-based contrast bolus, has been advocated to assess tumor response to chemotherapy because malignant tumors tend to enhance more rapidly than other tissues. PET-CT can also offer critical information regarding treatment response by providing an objective, semiquantitative measurement of ^{18}F-FDG uptake if the tumor is FDG-avid.

SURGICAL TREATMENT CONSIDERATIONS

Although chemotherapy and radiation are frequently used as adjuvant therapy, resection of the primary lesion is considered for almost all musculoskeletal sarcomas. There are three surgical treatment options for soft tissue masses:

1. *Marginal excision*
   - Plane of dissection passes through the reactive tissue or pseudocapsule of the lesion.
   - Satellites of residual tumor may be left behind.
   - Inadequate treatment for malignant tumors or lesions with a high recurrence rate but may occasionally be chosen for reasons of functionality if combined with radiation or chemotherapy.
2. *Wide excision*
   - Entire lesion is removed, including a surrounded cuff of intact normal tissue.

- Plane of dissection is well beyond the reactive tissue surrounding the lesion as depicted on imaging studies, but the entire muscle or bone is not removed.
- Considered adequate for recurrent tumors, aggressive benign tumors, as well as most sarcomas.

3. *Radical resection.*
   - Lesion is removed along with the entire muscle, bone, or other tissues in the affected compartment(s).
   - Radical resection is not commonly required for treatment of musculoskeletal tumors.

Although wide excision is required for optimal treatment of aggressive tumors, compromises may be made to retain limb functionality by achieving only a marginal excision but supplementing it with radiation or chemotherapy. Please note that the term *limb salvage* is not a specific treatment option. Rather, limb salvage procedures are simply those that offer tumor control without sacrifice of the limb. Most fall into the category of wide excisions, but marginal excisions are also limb salvage procedures. Consideration of limb salvage is based on the staging of the lesion, anatomic location, age and expected growth of the patient, extent of local disease, and expected function after the procedure.

TUMOR FOLLOW-UP

Timing and type of imaging used for follow-up examination is a crucial issue and ideally should be individualized for each tumor type and indeed each patient. Follow-up imaging should relate to the hazard rate (i.e., the likelihood of timing of recurrence) of tumor recurrence in that individual. The individual hazard rate is related to tumor type, grade, size, and location; patient age and sex; tumor stage; type of treatment; and surgical margins.

The goal of a follow-up imaging protocol is to concentrate testing when the recurrence is most likely to occur. However, models relating to the hazard rate and utility/risk analysis do not exist for most individual extremity tumor types, and the best the literature offers is to consider the sarcomas as a group. Most reports agree that approximately 80% of sarcomas that recur locally or systemically will do so within 2 years of primary treatment. This suggests that the most frequent follow-up should occur in the first 2 years, with tapering of imaging frequency after that time. Certain tumor types have notoriously high rates of late recurrence and metastasis, thus requiring routine long-term surveillance. For example, mean time of recurrence and metastasis for synovial sarcoma is 3.6 years and 5.7 years, respectively.

For local recurrence of malignant or aggressive musculoskeletal soft tissue tumors, the most recent American College of Radiology (ACR) Appropriateness Criteria recommends MRI without and with contrast be performed 3–6 months after initial surgery or treatment as a baseline study. Continued MRI surveillance is recommended every 3–6 months for 10 years. After the first 5 years, MRI surveillance may decrease in frequency to yearly examinations, or earlier if the patient becomes symptomatic. Note that the presence of orthopedic hardware may limit the usefulness of MRI, in which case using metal suppression techniques or the addition of radiography, CT, and/or ultrasonography may be necessary. Whole-body ^{18}F-FDG PET-CT may be appropriate for evaluation of local recurrence of FDG-avid tumors if MRI is suboptimal due to metal artifact or imaging findings are otherwise equivocal.

For both low-risk and high-risk patients, ACR Appropriateness Criteria guidelines recommend a baseline noncontrast chest CT performed within 3–6 months after initial surgery or treatment for evaluation of pulmonary metastasis. Subsequent follow-up noncontrast chest CT should be performed every 3–6 months for the first 10 years, although reduction in frequency to 6–12 months may be considered after 5 years depending on individual circumstances. For higher-risk patients, ^{18}F-FDG PET-CT may be used as a problem-solving tool for evaluation of pulmonary metastasis. Routine imaging surveillance for evaluation of osseous metastatic disease is not recommended in asymptomatic patients, with the caveat being patients with myxoid liposarcoma due to high rates of soft tissue and osseous metastasis. In such patients, screening with whole-body MRI is preferred, as PET-CT has a high false-negative rate for this particular tumor type.

When MRI is used to follow treated tumors, it is important to recognize that high signal intensity on T2-weighted sequences is not specific for tumor recurrence and can be seen with several nonneoplastic post-treatment effects. Examples include postoperative seroma, hematoma, changes related to radiation therapy, fat necrosis, packing material, scar tissue, or herniation of other tissue into the tumor bed. Enhancement alone is not necessarily a sign of recurrence, particularly if it is not masslike, as postsurgical scarring and postradiation effects may enhance. Narrowing the search to enhancing nodules improves specificity for recurrent tumor. Dynamic contrast-enhanced MRI has been advocated, because recurrent tumor in general tends to enhance more rapidly than benign lesions. Reference to the initial MRI examination prior to treatment is paramount, as recurrent tumor often has similar imaging characteristics to the original tumor. Review of the pretreatment MRI for initial tumor extent and margins may point to sites of potential recurrence. PET-CT is also a useful technique for detection of recurrent tumor and is advocated as a problem-solving tool in cases that are equivocal by other imaging methods. Biopsy of suspicious postoperative lesions may be necessary to rule out tumor recurrence in some cases.

Follow-up examination of a limb salvage with allograft is an art form, both in terms of obtaining high-quality images and interpreting these images. MRI artifact caused by metal implants can be mitigated with the strategies discussed in Chapter 1 – Introduction to Musculoskeletal Imaging and Chapter 10 – Arthroplasty. MRI usually provides useful information even when limited by metal artifact. CT with contrast or ultrasonography may be useful in specific cases.

Reporting Tips and Recommendations

- Characterize lesions as benign or not definitively benign on imaging.
  - If not definitively benign after imaging options have been exhausted, biopsy should be recommended for histopathologic diagnosis.

- Describe lesion characteristics, including location, size and extent, margins, compartments involved, and relationship to or involvement of major neurovascular bundles.
  - T1-weighted images are essential for evaluation of fat planes potentially separating the mass from other compartments and neurovascular bundles.
- For cases requiring percutaneous biopsy, consult with the orthopedic oncologist providing definite treatment prior to biopsy to plan the needle biopsy approach.
  - The biopsy procedure can contaminate tissues along the needle track and thus any compartment the needle passes through, potentially affecting surgical planning and tissue reconstruction options if the lesion is a primary sarcoma.
  - Surgeon may request the biopsy tract be positioned along the line of the intended surgical incision so the needle track can be resected at surgery, or through a compartment that is already involved.
- Provide an accurate differential diagnosis when possible or acknowledge when a differential is broad.
  - Many soft tissue sarcomas look similar on MRI; in some cases, an educated guess regarding histology can be made based on patient age, tumor location, and imaging features.

Sources and Suggested Readings

Amin MB, Edge, SB, Greene FL, et al (eds). *AJCC Cancer Staging Manual.* 8th ed. New York, NY: Springer Publishing; 2017.

Anderson MW, Temple HT, Dussault RG, et al. Compartmental anatomy: relevance to staging and biopsy of musculoskeletal tumors. *AJR Am J Roentgenol.* 1999;173(6):1663–1671.

Baheti AD, O'Malley RB, Kim S, et al. Soft tissue sarcomas: an update for radiologists based on the Revised 2013 World Health Organization Classification. *AJR Am J Roentgenol.* 2016;206(5):924–932.

Bakril A, Shinagare AB, Krajewski KM, et al. Synovial sarcoma: imaging features of common and uncommon primary sites, metastatic patterns, and treatment response. *AJR Am J Roentgenol.* 2012;199(2):W208–W215.

Beaman FD, Kransdorf MJ, Andrews TR, et al. Superficial soft tissue masses: analysis, diagnosis, and differential considerations. *Radiographics.* 2007;27(2):509–523.

Bermejo A, De Bustamante TD, Martinez A, et al. MR imaging in the evaluation of cystic-appearing soft tissue masses of the extremities. *Radiographics.* 2013;33(3):833–855.

Blacksin MF, Ha DH, Hameed M, et al. Superficial soft tissue masses of the extremities. *Radiographics.* 2006;26(5):1289–1304.

Chhabra A, Soldatos T. Soft tissue lesions: when can we exclude sarcoma? *AJR Am J Roentgenol.* 2012;199(6):1345–1357.

Del Grande F, Subhawong T, Weber K, et al. Detection of soft tissue sarcoma recurrence: added value of functional MR imaging techniques at 3.0 T. *Radiology.* 2014;271(2):499–511.

Dinauer PA, Brixey CJ, Moncur JT, et al. Pathologic and MR imaging features of benign fibrous soft tissue tumors in adults. *Radiographics.* 2007;27(1):173–187.

Eary JF, Hawkins DS, Rodler ET, Conrad EU 3rd. (18)F-FDG PET in sarcoma treatment response imaging. *Am J Nucl Med Mol Imaging.* 2011;1(1):47–53.

Fayad LM, Jacobs MA, Wang X, et al. Musculoskeletal tumors: how to use anatomic, functional, and metabolic MR techniques. *Radiology.* 2012;26(2):340–356.

Flors L, Leiva-Salinas C, Maged IM, et al. MR imaging of soft tissue vascular malformations: diagnosis, classification, and therapy follow-up. *Radiographics.* 2011;31(5):1321–1340; discussion 1340–1341.

Garner HW, Bestic JM. Benign synovial tumors and proliferative processes. *Semin Musculoskelet Radiol.* 2013;17(2):177–178.

Garner HW, Kransdorf MJ, Bancroft LW, et al. Benign and malignant soft tissue tumors: posttreatment MR imaging. *Radiographics.* 2009;29(1):119–134.

Gaskin CM, Helms CA. Lipomas, lipoma variants, and well-differentiated liposarcomas (atypical lipomas): results of MRI evaluations of 126 consecutive fatty masses. *AJR Am J Roentgenol.* 2004;182(3): 733–739.

International Society for the Study of Vascular Anomalies (ISSVA) Classification of Vascular Anomalies. Approved at the 20th ISSVA Workshop, Melbourne, April 2014, last revision May 2018. Available at https://www.issva.org/UserFiles/file/ISSVA-Classification-2018.pdf. Accessed 2020 Mar 20.

Kransdorf M. Benign soft tissue tumors in a large referral population: distribution of specific diagnosis by age, sex, and location. *AJR Am J Roentgenol.* 1995;164:395–402.

Kransdorf M. Malignant soft tissue tumors in a large referral population: distribution of specific diagnosis by age, sex, and location. *AJR Am J Roentgenol.* 1995;164:129–134.

Kransdorf M, Meis J, Jelinek J. Myositis ossificans: MR appearance with radiologic pathologic correlation. *AJR Am J Roentgenol.* 1991;157:1243–1248.

Kransdorf MJ, Bancroft LW, Peterson JJ, et al. Imaging of fatty tumors: distinction of lipoma and well-differentiated liposarcoma. *Radiology.* 2002;224(1):99–104.

Kransdorf MJ, Murphey MD. Imaging of soft tissue musculoskeletal masses: fundamental concepts. *Radiographics.* 2016;36(6):1931–1948.

Krieg AH, Hefti F, Speth BM, et al. Synovial sarcomas usually metastasize after >5 years: a multicenter retrospective analysis with minimum follow-up of 10 years for survivors. *Ann Oncol.* 2011;22(2):458–467.

Lee JC, Thomas JM, Phillips S, et al. Aggressive fibromatosis: MRI features with pathologic correlation. *AJR Am J Roentgenol.* 2006;186(1): 247–254.

Lim CY, Ong KO. Imaging of musculoskeletal lymphoma. *Cancer Imaging.* 2013;13(4):448–457.

Lim HJ, Johnny Ong CA, Tan JW, et al. Utility of positron emission tomography/computed tomography (PET/CT) imaging in the evaluation of sarcomas: a systematic review. *Crit Rev Oncol Hematol.* 2019;143:1–13.

Liu PT, Valadez SD, Chivers FS, et al. Anatomically based guidelines for core needle biopsy of bone tumors: implications for limb-sparing surgery. *Radiographics.* 2007;27(1):189–205; discussion 206.

Macpherson RE, Pratap S, Tyrrell H, et al. Retrospective audit of 957 consecutive (18)F-FDG PET-CT scans compared to CT and MRI in 493 patients with different histological subtypes of bone and soft tissue sarcoma. *Clin Sarcoma Res.* 2018;8:9.

Manaster BJ. Soft tissue masses: optimal imaging protocol and reporting. *AJR Am J Roentgenol.* 2013;201(3):505–514.

May DA, Disler DG, Jones EA, et al. Abnormal signal intensity in skeletal muscle at MR imaging: patterns, pearls, and pitfalls. *Radiographics.* 2000;20 Spec No:S295–S315.

Middleton WD, Patel V, Teefey SA, et al. Giant cell tumors of the tendon sheath: analysis of sonographic findings. *AJR Am J Roentgenol.* 2004;183(2):337–339.

Moulton J, Blebea J, Dunco D, et al. MR imaging of soft tissue masses: diagnostic efficacy and value of distinguishing between benign and malignant lesions. *AJR Am J Roentgenol.* 1995;164:1191–1199.

Mulligan ME, McRae GA, Murphey MD. Imaging features of primary lymphoma of bone. *AJR Am J Roentgenol.* 1999;173(6):1691–1697.

Murphey M, Gross T, Rosenthal H. Musculoskeletal malignant fibrous histiocytoma: radiologic pathologic correlation. *Radiographics.* 1994;14:807–826.

Murphey M, Smith W, Smith S, et al. Imaging of musculoskeletal neurogenic tumors: radiologic pathologic correlation. *Radiographics.* 1999;19:1253–1280.

Murphey MD, Arcara LK, Fanburg-Smith J. From the archives of the AFIP: imaging of musculoskeletal liposarcoma with radiologic-pathologic correlation. *Radiographics.* 2005;25(5):1371–1395.

Murphey MD, Gibson MS, Jennings BT, et al. From the archives of the AFIP: imaging of synovial sarcoma with radiologic-pathologic correlation. *Radiographics.* 2006;26(5):1543–1565.

Murphey MD, Rhee JH, Lewis RB, et al. Pigmented villonodular synovitis: radiologic-pathologic correlation. *Radiographics.* 2008;28(5):1493–1518.

Nieweg O, Pruins J, Von Ginkel R, et al. FDG-PET imaging of soft tissue sarcoma. *J Nucl Med.* 1996;37:257–261.

Patel NB, Stacy GS. Musculoskeletal manifestations of neurofibromatosis type 1. *AJR Am J Roentgenol.* 2012;199(1):W99–W106.

Petscavage-Thomas JM, Walker EA, Logie CI, et al. Soft tissue myxomatous lesions: review of salient imaging features with pathologic comparison. *Radiographics.* 2014;34(4):964–980.

Roberts CC, Kransdorf MJ, Beaman FD, et al. ACR Appropriateness Criteria® Follow-up of Malignant or Aggressive Musculoskeletal Tumors.

Available at https://acsearch.acr.org/docs/69428/Narrative/. American College of Radiology. Accessed 2020 Mar.

Shapeero L, Vanel D, Couanet D, et al. Extra skeletal mesenchymal chondrosarcoma. *Radiology.* 1993;186:819–826.

Sookur PA, Naraghi AM, Bleakney RR, et al. Accessory muscles: anatomy, symptoms, and radiologic evaluation. *Radiographics.* 2008;28(2):481–499.

Steiner JE, Drolet BA. Classification of vascular anomalies: an update. *Semin Intervent Radiol.* 2017;34(3):225–232.

Subhawong TK, Jacobs MA, Fayad LM. Diffusion-weighted MR imaging for characterizing musculoskeletal lesions. *Radiographics.* 2014;34(5):1163–1177.

Tanaka K, Ozaki T. New TNM classification (AJCC eighth edition) of bone and soft tissue sarcomas: JCOG Bone and Soft Tissue Tumor Study Group. *Jpn J Clin Oncol.* 2019;49(2):103–107.

Tavare AN, Robinson P, Altoos R, et al. Postoperative imaging of sarcomas. *AJR Am J Roentgenol.* 2018;211(3):506–518.

Wu JS, Hochman MG. Soft tissue tumors and tumorlike lesions: a systematic imaging approach. *Radiology.* 2009;253(2):297–316.

Zhao F, Ahlawat S, Farahani SJ, et al. Can MR imaging be used to predict tumor grade in soft tissue sarcoma? *Radiology.* 2014;272(1):192–201.

13 Bone Marrow and Metabolic Bone Disease

Bone Marrow Imaging

Key Concepts

Bone Marrow

Components: Red marrow (cellular, hematopoietic), yellow marrow (fatty), trabecular bone
Symmetric left and right
Newborns: Widely distributed red marrow
Infants: Epiphyses and epiphyseal equivalents (apophyses) undergo fatty conversion during first few months
Children: Progressive replacement of red marrow by fatty marrow, distal to proximal and diaphyseal to metaphyseal

Adults: Red marrow is normally found in the axial skeleton and the proximal portions of the appendicular skeleton; red marrow is more widely distributed in women, smokers, endurance athletes, patients with chronic anemia, obese patients, and persons living at high altitudes
Marrow reconversion (yellow to red): Acquired anemia, medication, hypoxia

Basic components of the marrow cavity from an imaging standpoint:

- *Yellow (fatty)* marrow.
- *Red (hematopoietic)* marrow.
- Trabecular bone.
- In certain disease states: tumor, pus, fibrosis, or deposition of products of abnormal metabolism.

Yellow marrow:

- Approximately 80% fat.
- Magnetic resonance imaging (MRI) signal intensity is similar to fat on all sequences.

Red marrow:

- Contains cellular elements and fat (40%) and is vascular.
- MRI signal:
  - T1-weighted and T2-weighted: intermediate.
  - Higher in signal than yellow marrow on fluid-sensitive sequences such as fat-suppressed T2-weighted and short-tau inversion recovery (STIR) (Fig. 13.1).
  - Chemical shift imaging (in- and out-of-phase) shows signal dropout on out-of-phase images due to mixture of fat and water elements within each voxel.
- Red marrow may fill the entire marrow cavity, or may have a 'wispy', ill-defined configuration, or may occasionally be rounded and well circumscribed, simulating a metastasis (termed *focal nodular marrow hyperplasia*).

Trabecular bone:

- Can be directly visualized, especially on high-resolution images.
- Also contributes to marrow signal intensity by causing susceptibility artifact.
  - This is most evident on gradient-echo sequences, which show signal loss in regions of extensive trabecular bone.

MARROW CONVERSION

- Bone marrow is a highly dynamic part of the musculo-skeletal system that changes during growth and in response to local and systemic conditions.
- Local change from red to yellow or vice versa is *marrow conversion.*

Age-Related Marrow Conversion

- Red to yellow.
- Follows a predictable pattern during growth (Fig. 13.2).
- At birth: Red marrow is widely distributed.
- Infants and toddlers: The earliest conversion to fatty marrow occurs in the epiphyses and apophyses within the first few months after these centers begin to ossify.
  - Useful rule of thumb: Epiphyses and apophyses should contain only yellow marrow within 6 months after ossification begins. (Notable exception: proximal humerus, which can contain red marrow well into adulthood).
  - The terminal phalanges convert next.
- During childhood and adolescence: Conversion in the long bones begins in the diaphyses and progresses toward the metaphyses, and also progresses from distal to proximal (Figs. 13.2 and 13.3).
  - Red marrow may become distributed in patterns that are potentially confusing.
    - Small islands of preserved red marrow may have a variety of configurations that might be confused with metastases.
    - Bands of red marrow can extend from the physis into the metaphysis. These have been compared to flames ('*marrow flames*').
- Conversion of marrow in the flat bones lags behind that of the long bones.

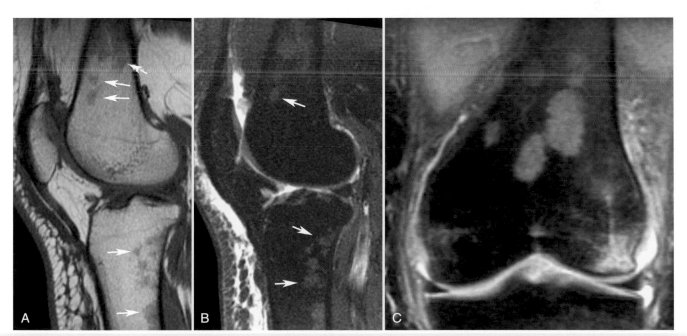

Fig. 13.1 MRI of bone marrow. **(A** and **B)** Sagittal T1-weighted **(A)** and fat-suppressed T2-weighted **(B)** MR images of the knee in an obese 39-year-old woman with heavy menses because of fibroids. The hematopoietic (red) marrow has intermediate T1 and T2 signal intensity, in this case in a nodule-like configuration *(arrows)*. The fatty (yellow) marrow has typical fat signal intensity. This is a normal pattern. **(C)** Another example of normal marrow simulating metastatic deposits, in this case also in the distal femur.

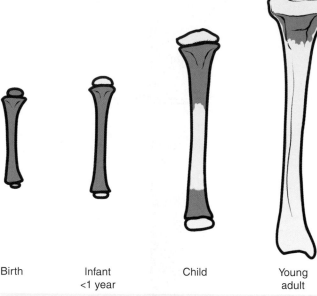

Birth   Infant   Child   Young
             <1 year   adult

Fig. 13.2 Normal sequence of marrow conversion during growth. The images show typical distribution of red (shaded) and yellow (unshaded) marrow at birth, in an infant less than 1 year, a child, and in a young adult (left to right).

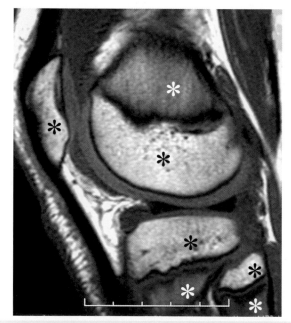

Fig. 13.3 Normal hematopoietic marrow distribution in an older child. Sagittal T1-weighted MR image of the lateral aspect of the knee in a 12-year-old boy shows uniform high signal intensity of fatty marrow in the epiphyses and the patella *(black asterisks)*, and uniform intermediate signal intensity of hematopoietic marrow in the metaphyses *(white asterisks)*.

- Adult pattern:
  - Conversion to fatty marrow is mostly complete by age 25, with red marrow concentrated in the axial skeleton and the proximal humeral and femoral metaphyses. Red marrow may also be found in the metaphyses around the knees and in the humeral heads, especially in pre-menopausal women and obese patients.

- In later adulthood:
  - Slow continuation of the fatty conversion process.
  - By the eighth decade of life, even the pedicles and posterior elements of the vertebrae contain fatty marrow.
- This normal progression may be delayed or arrested in women or in persons who are chronically anemic, obese, cigarette smokers, or who have other causes of hypoxia.

MARROW RECONVERSION (YELLOW TO RED)

- Fatty marrow is quite labile and easily reconverts to hematopoietic marrow when stressed (Fig. 13.4).
- Reconversion to hematopoietic marrow usually follows an orderly pattern that is the reverse of the original conversion, beginning in the spine and flat bones and extending toward the appendicular skeleton.
  - Reconversion may be spotty or complete, especially in the femurs and humeri. Conditions associated with extensive marrow reconversion include acquired anemias (hemolytic, related to chronic disease, or related to chronic blood loss), heavy cigarette smoking, hypoventilation hypoxia, poorly compensated heart disease, acquired immunodeficiency syndrome (AIDS), and 'sports anemia' (physiologic response in endurance athletes such as marathon runners).
  - Marrow-stimulating medications such as erythropoietin or granulocyte colony-stimulating factor can cause extensive marrow reconversion.
  - Reconverted marrow can have a nodular configuration, simulating metastatic disease. *Focal nodular marrow hyperplasia* is a descriptive term for normal red marrow distributed in a nodular pattern. MRI with in- and out-of-phase imaging shows lipid within the red marrow, excluding malignancy.

MARROW INFILTRATION

- Replacement of normal marrow elements with abnormal cells or abnormal metabolites.
- Examples: myeloma, polycythemia vera, lymphoma, leukemia, hemochromatosis, amyloidosis, Gaucher disease, myelofibrosis, and metastases.
  - Note that metastases are usually found in red marrow.
- Infection also can cause focal marrow infiltration.
- Pathologic marrow infiltration can mimic marrow reconversion on MRI.
  - Marrow-packing disorders such as Gaucher disease may be intermediate on both T1-weighted and T2-weighted images.
  - In contrast, with infection or neoplastic infiltration, T1-weighted images usually show low signal and fluid-sensitive images usually show high signal.
- *Serous atrophy*, also termed *gelatinous transformation*, can resemble diffuse marrow infiltration with diffuse low T1 and high T2 signal that may be heterogeneous.
  - Caused by severe malnutrition, eating disorders.
  - Marrow fat is metabolized and replaced by gelatinous material.

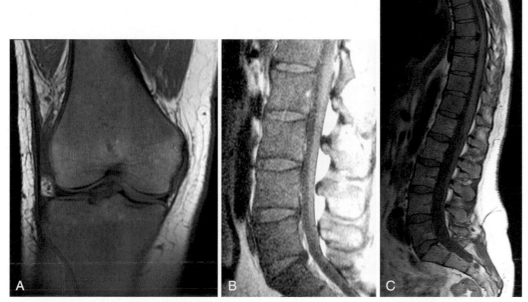

Fig. 13.4 Abnormal marrow signal due to cellular infiltration. **(A)** Severe chronic anemia. Coronal T1-weighted MR image of the knee in a young adult with a rare hemoglobinopathy demonstrates low marrow signal because of massively increased marrow cellularity, in this case hematopoietic marrow. This is most clearly abnormal in the epiphyses, which should contain only fat and trabeculae in an adult. **(B)** Marrow replacement because of acute myeloid leukemia (AML). Sagittal T1-weighted MR image in a 30-year-old man who had severe low back pain but normal radiographs show diffuse uniform low signal intensity in the lumbar vertebrae. A rule of thumb is that on a T1 image the vertebral body should have higher signal than the disc. The patient was not known to have a chronic anemia so a peripheral blood smear was recommended, which showed AML. **(C)** Sagittal T1-weighted image of a 45-year-old man shows less uniform marrow infiltration because of widespread non-Hodgkin lymphoma. The extensive areas of low marrow signal are abnormal.

TOOLS FOR DISTINGUISHING NORMAL MARROW FROM PATHOLOGIC CONDITIONS

- Distribution: Normal distribution changes with age (see previous text).
- Anything other than yellow marrow in an epiphysis or apophysis 6 months after it begins to ossify is suspicious for pathology (exception: humeral head).
- Rule of thumb: Normal red marrow has T1-signal intensity higher than skeletal muscle or normal intervertebral disc.
  - Exceptions include repetition time (TR) greater than 700 ms (not a true T1), the spine in infants, and conditions associated with extensive marrow reconversion (e.g., severe anemia, bone marrow transplant).
- Unusually high or low signal intensity on fluid-sensitive sequences suggests a pathologic marrow process.
- Evidence of bone destruction or extraosseous mass is never normal.
- *Chemical shift imaging* (in- and out-of-phase) MRI.
  - *Dixon imaging* uses similar physics to produce in- and out-of-phase images, as well as fat-only and water-only images.
  - Excellent problem solver for indeterminate marrow (red marrow vs. tumor).
  - Short acquisition time, less than 1 minute.
  - Normal red marrow contains a mixture of fat and cellular elements.
  - The fat and water elements within each voxel cause signal loss on the opposed phase of in- and out-of-phase MRI (Fig 13.5).

- Tumors contain no fat and do not show signal drop-off.
- At least 20% signal drop-off from in-phase to out-of-phase indicates a benign process with high accuracy (Fig. 13.5).
- Experience has shown that a smaller or no signal drop-off is not predictive either way. In other words, drop-off of less than 20% is indeterminate for benign versus malignant.
- *Diffusion-weighted images* (DWI) can show abnormal diffusion restriction (bright signal) in malignant vertebral compression fractures, whereas benign osteoporotic compressions usually do not. Spatial resolution is low.
- 18F-fluorodeoxyglucose (18F-FDG) positron emission tomography-computed tomography (PET-CT) may also help to distinguish benign from malignant vertebral compressions.
- Dual-energy CT can distinguish fat-containing marrow from denser metastases, but is less sensitive than MRI.
- Technetium-99m (Tc-99m) sulfur colloid is taken up by the red marrow and therefore can be used to distinguish marrow infiltration from reconversion. However, this is not commonly performed.

MYELOID DEPLETION

- Marrow space devoid of hematopoietic elements.
- Seen in patients with aplastic anemia, in regions treated with radiation therapy, and with some chemotherapy regimens.
- Marrow signal is that of fat on all sequences (Fig. 13.6).

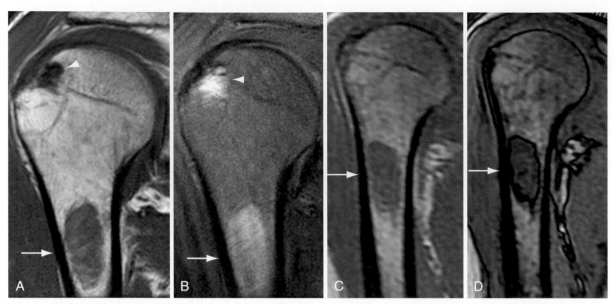

Fig. 13.5 Chemical shift MRI. This technique takes advantage of the different precession frequencies of fat and water. (A and B) Oblique coronal T1-weighted **(A)** and fat-suppressed T2-weighted **(B)** images from routine shoulder MRI show marrow edema in the greater tuberosity related to rotator cuff impingement *(arrowhead)*. Also note the unexpected ovoid lesion in the proximal humeral metaphysis with bright T2- and intermediate T1-signal intensity that raises concern for an aggressive lesion such as a metastasis *(arrow)*. Radiographs were normal. The patient had no history of malignancy and the lesion was not considered to be the cause of his shoulder pain. (C and D) Chemical shift images. In-phase image **(C)** and out-of-phase image **(D)** again show the lesion *(arrow)*. In-phase image C is obtained with the lipid and water elements in phase, so the signal of each voxel is the sum of both elements. Out-of-phase image D is obtained with lipid and water 180 degrees out of phase, so a voxel containing both lipid and water (e.g., marrow fat and cells) loses signal because the lipid signal nulls the water signal. Note the significant signal drop-off throughout the lesion between C and D, which essentially excludes metastases because they generally do not contain significant lipid. The lesion was stable on follow-up MRI 6 months later. Because an unnecessary biopsy was avoided, a definite diagnosis is not available. The MRI findings are compatible with atypical hematopoietic marrow.

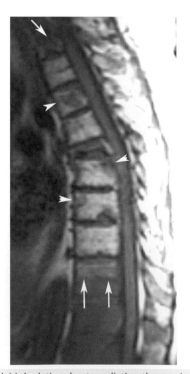

Fig. 13.6 Myeloid depletion due to radiation therapy in a 50-year-old woman with a history of breast cancer. The patient had previously received radiation treatment of metastatic disease in the midthoracic spine. Sagittal T1-weighted MR image shows fatty replacement in the radiation field (between *arrows*). The areas of low signal intensity within the treated vertebrae *(arrowheads)* could represent treated, healed blastic metastases or active metastases. In this case, the lesions were recurrent metastatic disease.

MARROW EDEMA

- Used as a generic term for increased marrow signal on fluid-sensitive sequences in a localized or regional pattern.
- Common causes include trauma (fracture or osseous contusion), mechanical osseous stress response, infection, inflammation, and reactive to adjacent bone or soft tissue pathology.
- Strictly speaking, not all such signal change reflects true extracellular edema, and additionally the term *bone marrow edema* has a specific narrow definition in pathology; therefore some authors prefer to use the term *edema-like signal*.

HEMOSIDERIN DEPOSITION

- Chronic hemolytic anemias or multiple transfusions can cause marrow hemosiderin deposition with decreased marrow signal intensity on all sequences (Fig. 13.7).
- Other reticuloendothelial sites (i.e., the liver and spleen) will show similar changes.

MYELOFIBROSIS

- A myeloproliferative disorder that results in fibrosis in areas of the skeleton that normally are involved in hematopoiesis.
- This forces hematopoiesis farther peripherally (e.g., marrow reconversion in the femoral and humeral diaphyses) and extramedullary hematopoiesis.
- The reconverted marrow sites, in turn, may become fibrotic.

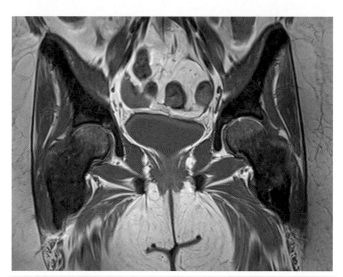

Fig. 13.7 Hemosiderosis caused by multiple transfusions. Note the signal void throughout all visualized marrow space. This is a T1-weighted sequence, but the findings were similar on all sequences.

- The appearance varies according to the severity and stage of the disease. Extramedullary hematopoiesis causes hepatosplenomegaly and paraspinous masses.

BONE AND MARROW CHANGES FOLLOWING RADIATION THERAPY

- Directly toxic to rapidly dividing myeloid elements.
- Also toxic to intraosseous blood vessels.
- Toxicity is dose dependent and changes over time.
- Days:
  - Marrow edema and hemorrhage, or no change.
- Weeks to months:
  - Higher doses: permanent conversion to yellow marrow (myeloid depletion).
  - Lower doses: conversion to yellow marrow but with eventual reconversion to red marrow after months or many years.
    - Elimination of myeloid elements from the radiation field may lead to marrow reconversion elsewhere that might simulate disease.
- A few months to 2+ years:
  - *Radiation osteonecrosis* (radiation osteitis):
    - Osteopenia, mottled bone density, conversion from fatty to heterogeneous MRI signal on T1 and T2.
    - Periosteal new bone formation.
    - Increased risk of osteomyelitis.
    - Findings may resemble osteomyelitis and/or recurrent tumor.
  - Insufficiency fracture.
    - Pelvis and sacrum are classic sites (Fig. 13.9).
  - Growth disturbances in children (physeal injury).
- Many years:
  - Insufficiency fractures.
  - Secondary tumors:
    - Adults: rarely sarcomas, usually high-grade.
    - Young children: osteochondromas.

- Imaging findings:
  - Radiographs: symmetric sclerotic trabeculae (either diffusely or patchy local increased density with cortical thickening) in the hematopoietic bones (vertebrae, pelvis, ribs, and the long tubular bones), without bone expansion (Fig. 13.8).
  - MRI: low signal on both T1- and T2-weighted images due to marrow fibrosis in the hematopoietic bones, with reconversion of fatty marrow to red marrow in the shafts and more distal portions of the large tubular bones.

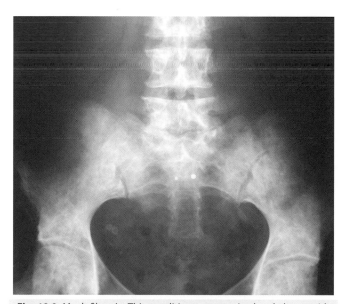

Fig. 13.8 Myelofibrosis. This condition presents in the skeleton with fibrosis in the regions normally involved in hematopoiesis (axial skeleton), with subsequent compensatory hematopoiesis in the fatty marrow of the large tubular bones. The latter sites may in turn become fibrotic. The involved bones show mixed sclerosis and lucency, as do all the bones on this AP radiograph.

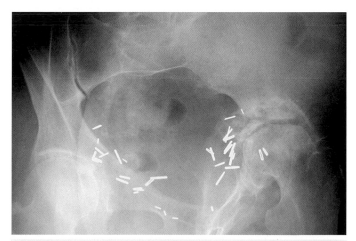

Fig. 13.9 Osteonecrosis, radiation injury. The left femoral head and acetabulum show the mixed sclerosis and lucency of radiation osteonecrosis, with collapse of the femoral head and fragmentation of the acetabular roof in this 64-year-old man who underwent radiation for prostate cancer. The pelvic clips indicate a lymph node dissection.

Osteonecrosis (Avascular Necrosis)

Key Concepts

Osteonecrosis

Radiographs: Sclerosis, followed by subchondral lucency, fracture, articular surface collapse, and secondary osteoarthritis
Magnetic resonance imaging: Double-line sign
CT: Slender serpentine sclerotic line
Cartilage remains normal until secondary degenerative disease
Causes are numerous. Mnemonic ASEPTIC: sickle cell anemia, steroids, ethanol abuse, pancreatitis, trauma, idiopathic or infection, and caisson disease (*dysbaric avascular necrosis*). Also remember Gaucher disease and radiation. Most common causes are trauma, steroids, alcoholism, sickle cell disease; many cases idiopathic
Most common sites are femoral head, lunate, proximal pole of the scaphoid, humeral head, vertebral body

Osteonecrosis (*avascular necrosis [AVN], ischemic necrosis, aseptic necrosis,* or *bone infarct*) is an incompletely understood phenomenon that may be related to traumatic or compressive interruption of arterial inflow, increased marrow pressure with impeded venous drainage, or intraluminal vascular obstruction. The outcome is necrosis of the cellular elements of bone.

Dead bone is as strong as live bone, but only temporarily. Normal wear and tear, especially in weight-bearing bones, results in microfractures that weaken the bone over time. Perhaps more importantly, the repair process following osteonecrosis can weaken the bone substantially before creating new bone. This creates a window of vulnerability to fracture and collapse that is the feared consequence of osteonecrosis.

Associations:

- Mnemonic 'ASEPTIC' for sickle cell **a**nemia, corticosteroids, **e**thanol abuse, **p**ancreatitis, **t**rauma (dislocation, nearby fracture), **i**diopathic or **i**nfection, and **c**aisson disease (decompression sickness where nitrogen bubbles occlude small vessels; see note in the following text).
- Gaucher disease, hypercoagulable states, and radiation therapy can be added to this list.
- Osteonecrosis is more common in patients with renal transplants, perhaps only because of steroid use.
- Most common causes are trauma, steroids, alcoholism, sickle cell disease, and many cases are idiopathic.
- Occurs in parts of bones extensively covered by articular cartilage:
  - Limited vascular supply, as blood vessels do not cross articular surfaces.
  - Femoral head.
  - Lunate.
  - In trauma: scaphoid proximal pole, talar dome, humeral anatomic head.
- Epiphyses with convex contours experience increased intramedullary pressure with weight-bearing.
  - This elevated hydraulic pressure contributes to bone strength but may increase vulnerability to vascular occlusion and osteonecrosis.
  - Femoral head, talar dome, and lunate.

- Osteonecrosis is not limited to these small bones and epiphyses. May occur anywhere, notably:
  - Vertebral bodies.
  - Metaphyses of long bones of the lower extremity.
    - These infarcts are clinically less important, as they are much less associated with fracture.
    - *Bone infarct* is a commonly used term for osteonecrosis in a metaphysis or diaphysis. *AVN* is commonly used for osteonecrosis in an epiphysis.

Historical note: *Caisson disease* is nitrogen embolization following rapid decompression after breathing pressurized air. Rapid decompression causes nitrogen dissolved in the blood to form microbubbles that occlude small vessels. This condition was common during construction of New York City's Brooklyn Bridge. The footings for the bridge were dug out by hand under waterproof caissons that contained pressurized air. The workers were decompressed rapidly at the end of each shift. Today it is divers who most frequently have this condition. Before the epidemic of caisson disease in New York, most cases of hip osteonecrosis were caused by infection, especially tuberculosis, hence the alternate term *aseptic necrosis* for today's most frequent causes.

The histologic finding in osteonecrosis is that the lacunae within lamellar bone that are normally occupied by osteocytes are empty (*empty lacunae*).

OSTEONECROSIS HEALING

- Osteonecrosis heals by slow replacement of dead bone by new immature bone in a process termed *creeping substitution*.
- After bone necrosis, revascularization and granulation ingrowth occur along a reactive interface, advancing into the bone infarct, initially replacing dead bone with weaker reparative tissue, then walling off the necrotic bone with a shell of sclerosis.
- Healing usually is limited, and the sclerotic line remains fixed in position on follow-up studies. Complete healing of some small infarcts has been reported but is rare.
- The healing process temporarily weakens the bone. Additionally, necrotic bone also becomes weaker than living bone over time, as microfractures are not repaired.
- Subchondral fractures may occur, with progressive subchondral fragmentation, flattening, and deformity.
- Initially the articular cartilage is unaffected by osteonecrosis because it is nourished by synovial fluid. Secondary osteoarthritis (OA) may occur later if the articular surface becomes deformed by a subchondral fracture.

IMAGING OF ADULT FEMORAL HEAD OSTEONECROSIS

Osteonecrosis of the hip is discussed here as the prototypical example of the imaging features of osteonecrosis.

Radiography

- The first radiographic sign in the hip osteonecrosis is sclerosis, generally in the center of the femoral head (see Fig. 13.10).
  - Occurs weeks or months after the bone infarction.

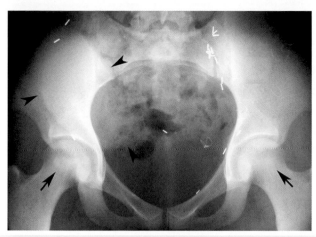

Fig. 13.10 Osteonecrosis, renal transplant. AP radiograph of the pelvis in this 27-year-old woman demonstrates central sclerotic areas within both femoral heads *(arrows)*, the earliest radiographic finding of osteonecrosis. The cause of osteonecrosis is apparent, with the soft tissue mass of the renal transplant seen in the right iliac fossa *(arrowheads)*.

- Initially, the sclerosis is relative in nature as the vascularized bone surrounding the necrotic bone becomes osteopenic because of local hyperemia.
- Later in the process the reactive interface develops, with bone formation and repair causing a zone of increased density. The new bone is relatively sclerotic.
- *Crescent sign.*
  - Thin band of subchondral lucency.
  - Fracture of subchondral trabecular bone.
  - Thought to be initiated by subchondral bone resorption by the repair process.
  - Most often anterolateral femoral head, best seen on a frog-leg lateral radiograph but is often visible on an anteroposterior view as well (Figs. 13.11 and 13.12).
  - High likelihood of progression to collapse.
- More advanced osteonecrosis:
  - Progressive subchondral fragmentation, flattening, and deformity.
  - Secondary OA.

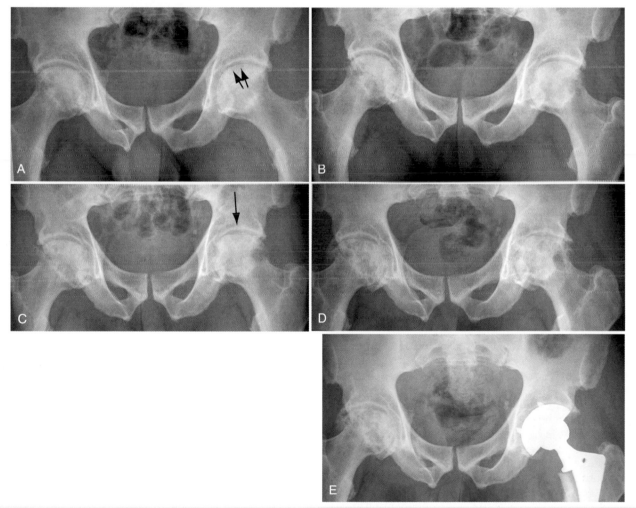

Fig. 13.11 Hip osteonecrosis. Radiographic progression over time in a 45-year-old man with bilateral AVN. **(A)** Initial radiograph shows sclerosis in both femoral heads and a left femoral head subchondral crescent with early collapse *(arrows)*. **(B)** Three months later the left crescent is no longer visible because of further collapse. Note the flattening of the right femoral head. **(C)** One year after the image in B, bilateral femoral head collapse is progressing, more evident on the left *(arrow)*, and secondary osteoarthritis (OA) is developing, with subchondral sclerosis and osteophyte formation. **(D)** Twenty months after the image in C, collapse and secondary OA are more prominent. **(E)** Five months later a left total arthroplasty has been placed. The right will be replaced soon.

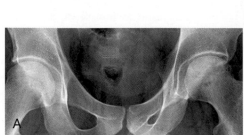
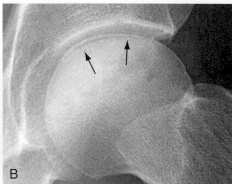

Fig. 13.12 Osteonecrosis radiographic evaluation, value of frog-leg lateral view. **(A)** AP radiograph of the left hip in a 29-year-old man with bilateral osteonecrosis. Note the characteristic but very subtle mottled density of the bilateral femoral heads. **(B)** Left hip frog-leg lateral radiograph shows a subchondral crescent lucency *(arrows)*, making the diagnosis of osteonecrosis easy. The right hip lateral was identical.

MRI

- Highly sensitive and specific for osteonecrosis (Figs. 13.13 and 13.14).
- The most common finding is a well-defined area of normal-appearing fatty marrow surrounded by a thin rim with low signal on T1- and T2-weighted images.
  - The low signal line is the shell of sclerosis that walls off the necrotic bone.
  - *Double-line sign*: A rim of increased signal intensity on T2-weighted sequences is usually present along the inner side of the serpentine line.
    - Represents granulation tissue along the interface.
    - Seen in most but not all cases of osteonecrosis.
    - Virtually pathognomic for osteonecrosis.
  - The line contour may be wavy and ring-like, wedge-shaped, and/or serpentine. The line often connects with subchondral bone in epiphyseal osteonecrosis. The line in metaphyseal osteonecrosis is usually highly serpentine.
  - The infarct may be extensive or localized to a small segment of the femoral head (often superior).
  - Marrow inside the infarct zone maintains normal fat signal initially, but later may become edematous, and in late stages fibrotic, with low T1 and T2 signal intensity.
- Marrow edema may also be present, especially later in the process, and correlates with pain.
  - When subchondral collapse is present, extremely intense marrow edema may be present throughout the femoral head and neck and extend into the intertrochanteric femur.
- MRI has 98% specificity in differentiating normal from abnormal bone but only 85% specificity in differentiating osteonecrosis from nonosteonecrosis disease unless the double-line sign is present, in which case specificity is nearly 100%.
- The superb sensitivity of MRI in detection of AVN has led to an interesting observation that osteonecrosis can be clinically occult. Therefore the value of screening at-risk but asymptomatic patients has not been established.

Computed Tomography

- The line is seen as a thin, serpentine sclerotic line (Fig. 13.15).

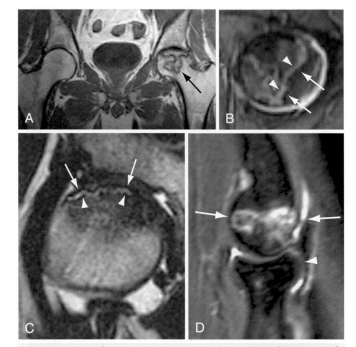

Fig. 13.13 MRI of osteonecrosis. **(A)** Coronal T1-weighted MR image of the hips shows classic serpentine lines *(arrow)* in the left femoral head. Also note mild flattening of the superior aspect of the left femoral head. **(B)** Sagittal T2-weighted MR image in a different patient shows the double-line sign of serpentine low *(arrows)* and high *(arrowheads)* signal intensity. **(C)** Axial fat-suppressed T2-weighted MR image in the same left hip as shown in A also shows the bright *(arrowheads)* and dark *(arrows)* lines, although the latter are less conspicuous with fat suppression. **(D)** Humeral capitellum osteonecrosis after trauma. Sagittal fat-suppressed T2-weighted MR image in a patient with ongoing pain after successful reduction of a radial head dislocation several months previously shows osteonecrosis of the capitellum *(arrows)*. The normal radial head is marked by an *arrowhead*.

- The crescent sign and subchondral collapse when present are easily seen.

Radionuclide Bone Scanning

- May detect osteonecrosis before it is visible on radiographs.
- Seen initially as a photopenic region.
- Later increased activity with revascularization and repair and secondary OA.

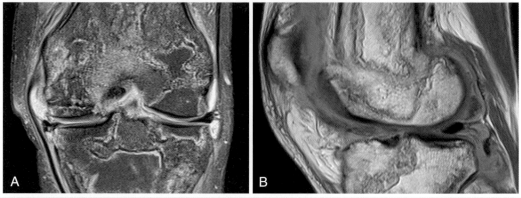

Fig. 13.14 MRI of osteonecrosis: knee. Coronal fat-suppressed T2-weighted MR image **(A)** and sagittal proton density–weighted image **(B)** show the classic serpentine double-line sign of bone infarct.

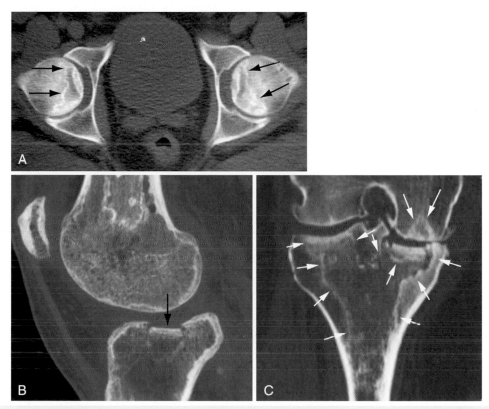

Fig. 13.15 CT of osteonecrosis. (A) Bilateral hip osteonecrosis. The serpentine lines of osteonecrosis on MRI are seen on CT as thin sclerotic lines *(arrows)*. **(B)** Knee. Patient with sickle cell anemia shows similar findings. Also note the lateral tibial plateau fracture *(arrow)* that occurred after only moderate trauma. **(C)** Medial tibial plateau fracture in a patient on long-term steroid therapy. Note the relationship of the infarct *(short arrows)* with the depressed fracture. Also note the small focus of subchondral osteonecrosis in the knee *(long arrow)*.

The serpentine line of osteonecrosis can occasionally overlap in appearance with a subchondral fracture.

- The distinction is important because subchondral fractures, if managed with non–weight-bearing, can heal without collapse.
- Subchondral fractures are usually straight, gently uniformly curved, or zigzag, and may be discontinuous and not serpentine.
- Subchondral fractures may be convex relative to adjacent subchondral cortex, whereas osteonecrosis lines may be concave to the overlying cortex.

- Marrow edema frequently precedes a subchondral fracture, whereas marrow edema appears after the serpentine line in osteonecrosis.

Femoral Head Osteonecrosis Staging

- Before MRI, staging was radiographic (Ficat).
- Current staging combines radiographic and MRI findings.
  - The widely used Steinberg system is in Box 13.1.
- The Ficat and Arlet system and the Association Research Circulation Osseous (ARCO) system additionally incorporate clinical findings.

Box 13.1 Steinburg System for Staging of Femoral Head Osteonecrosis

Stage 0: Radiographs, MRI, and bone scan are normal
Stage I: Radiographs normal, abnormal bone scan and/or MRI
Stage II: Radiographs: femoral head sclerosis and/or lucencies (but not a subchondral crescent)
    Modifiers for stages I and II:
    A: mild: <15% head involvement as seen on radiograph or MRI
    B: moderate: 15–30%
    C: severe: >30%
Stage III: Subchondral crescent sign (present or impending subchondral collapse)
    A: mild: collapse/crescent beneath <15% of articular surface
    B: moderate: 15–30%
    C: severe: >30%
Stage IV: Flattening of femoral head, with depression graded into
    A: mild: <15% of surface has collapsed and depression is <2 mm
    B: moderate: 15–30% collapsed or 2–4 mm depression
    C: severe: > 30% collapsed or > 4 mm depression
Stage V: Secondary osteoarthritis with joint space narrowing and femoral head flattening
Modifiers: Average the extent of femoral head involvement (same as stage IV) and acetabular abnormality to derive A (mild), B (moderate), or C (severe)
Stage VI: Severe secondary osteoarthritis

Source: Steinberg DR, et al. A quantitative system for staging avascular necrosis. *The Bone and Joint Journal.* 1995;77:34-41.

Useful information in an Imaging Report

- The extent of osteonecrosis roughly corresponds to the amount of femoral head at risk for collapse.
    - Report the extent of disease in coronal and sagittal planes (clock-face analogy).
    - This helps the surgeon to determine whether the patient can be best treated by core decompression (Fig. 13.16), osteotomy with realignment to a non-collapsed weight-bearing portion, or prosthesis placement.
- Femoral head flattening/collapse and its extent.
- Any progression over time.
- Development of secondary OA.
- Contralateral side involvement (may be clinically silent).

OSTEONECROSIS AT SITES OTHER THAN THE HIP

- Lunate: 'lunate malacia', *Kienböck disease.*
    - Caused by a combination of trauma, anatomy that increases mechanics stress on the lunate, notably ulna minus variance, and anatomic variations in lunate blood supply (Fig. 13.17).
- Bones that are extensively covered with articular cartilage are especially vulnerable to AVN after trauma. These include the femoral head, proximal pole of the scaphoid, humeral anatomic head, and talar body and dome (see Fig. 1.28).
- *Freiberg disease* (also called *Freiberg infraction*) is subchondral collapse of metatarsal heads, most often the second. The role of osteonecrosis is debated, but likely is a component, especially in younger patients. The process is initiated by trauma, women wearing high-heeled shoes most commonly. Microfractures interrupt local blood vessels.
- Sickle cell disease and systemic lupus erythematosis (SLE) are common causes of osteonecrosis of the humeral head and talus.
- *Kümmell disease* is posttraumatic osteonecrosis in the spine.
    - The classic finding is transversely oriented gas within a partially collapsed lower thoracic or upper lumbar vertebral body.
    - Thought to be caused by a vacuum phenomenon, similar to gas in a joint.
    - The gas-containing space is dark on all MRI sequences but may be filled with fluid or granulation (Fig. 13.18).
    - Gas in a vertebral body fracture usually indicates benign rather than malignant etiology of the fracture.
- Sickle cell disease and Gaucher disease produce an 'H-shaped' vertebra in which the midportion of the superior and inferior end plates of osteonecrotic vertebrae are impacted.

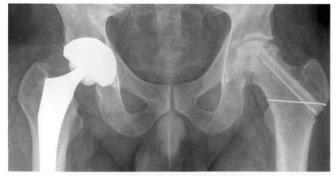

Fig. 13.16 Vascularized fibular graft within left hip core decompression was placed several years previously. Note the subtle left femoral head collapse. The right hip arthroplasty was for avascular necrosis.

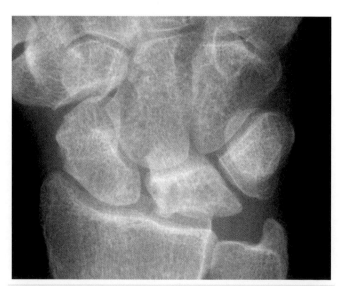

Fig. 13.17 Kienböck disease (lunate osteonecrosis). PA radiograph of the wrist shows a dense lunate with proximal collapse, representing osteonecrosis.

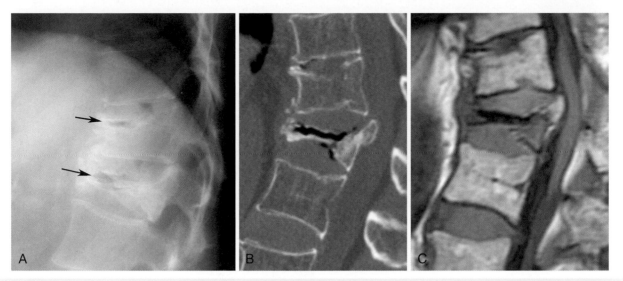

Fig. 13.18 Osteonecrosis: spine. **(A)** Lateral radiograph of the spine in a man taking steroids for an organ transplant demonstrates gas in the collapsed T12 and L1 bodies *(arrows)*. The presence of gas in a collapsed vertebral body is known as Kümmell disease and is considered pathognomonic for benign collapse rather than neoplasm. Sagittal CT reformat **(B)** and T1-weighted MR image **(C)** in a different patient with collapse of T12 show similar findings. Note the signal void of the gas in C. Another possible cause of a fairly linear signal void in a vertebral body is methyl methacrylate from a vertebroplasty.

ADULT OSTEONECROSIS MIMICS

- A stress-related insufficiency fracture of the subchondral femoral head may simulate osteonecrosis clinically and on imaging studies. The overlying fragment may impact, simulating osteonecrosis with collapse.
  - With or without collapse, a subchondral insufficiency fracture line usually has a relatively uniform or zigzag contour, as opposed to the serpentine, undulating line or lines seen with osteonecrosis.
- A subchondral fracture in the anterior weight-bearing medial femoral condyle was initially thought to represent osteonecrosis and therefore misnamed 'spontaneous osteonecrosis of the knee' (SONK). This condition is now understood to be initiated by trauma.
- Transient osteoporosis of the hip may resemble hip osteonecrosis at presentation, discussed later.

TREATMENT OF ADULT OSTEONECROSIS

- Femoral head:
  - Physical therapy.
  - Bisphosphonates. Evidence of efficacy is limited.
  - Core decompression.
    - To decrease intramedullary pressure.
    - Some living bone and an electrical stimulator may be inserted.
    - Can be combined with drilling small holes from the core into the infarct zone to stimulate neovascularization.
    - Seen radiographically as a cylindrical lucency extending from the intertrochanteric femur through the neck into the head.
    - Somewhat controversial regarding effectiveness.
  - A vascularized fibular graft may be placed into the decompression core to stimulate healing and revascularization (see Fig. 13.16).
  - Rotational osteotomy.

- Small lesions only.
  - Femoral head is rotated relative to the neck to move the dead bone away from a weight-bearing site.
  - Arthroplasty.
- Scaphoid:
  - Splinting.
  - Revascularization.
- Lunate:
  - Osteotomies to reduce mechanical load on the lunate such as correction of ulna minus ulna lengthening or radius shortening.
  - Revascularization.

LEGG–CALVÉ–PERTHES DISEASE (LCP, PERTHES)

- Osteonecrosis of the pediatric hip (Fig. 13.19 through 13.21).
- Typically presents during age 4–8 years, when the vascular supply to the femoral head is most at risk.
- M>F 5:1.
- May be bilateral in 10+% of cases, although the presentation in such cases is usually asymmetric.
- The first radiographic sign may be effusion, and the clinical presentation may mimic infection.
- Later the involved capital femoral epiphysis ossification center may appear smaller than the contralateral normal side. The joint space appears wider medially.
- Later still, mechanical forces combined with weakening of the capital femoral epiphysis by the necrosis and healing process result in fragmentation and flattening of the femoral head. The lateral femoral head is often less affected.
- Metaphyseal irregularity and lucent metaphyseal 'cysts' adjacent to the physis (see Fig. 13.19B) are manifestations of growth abnormality that results in a short, wide femoral neck. The latter was emphasized in an old term for LCP, *coxa magna*.

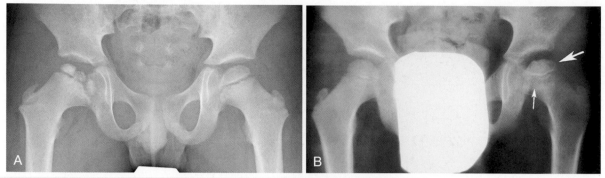

Fig. 13.19 Legg–Calvé–Perthes (LCP) disease. **(A)** AP radiograph of the hip in a 7-year-old girl shows fragmented, flattened, and widened right capital femoral epiphysis. **(B)** This case is earlier in the disease process. Note the left capital femoral epiphysis is smaller and denser and has irregular margins *(large arrow)*. Also note the small lucent 'metaphyseal cyst' *(small arrow)* adjacent to the physis, a frequent finding in LCP.

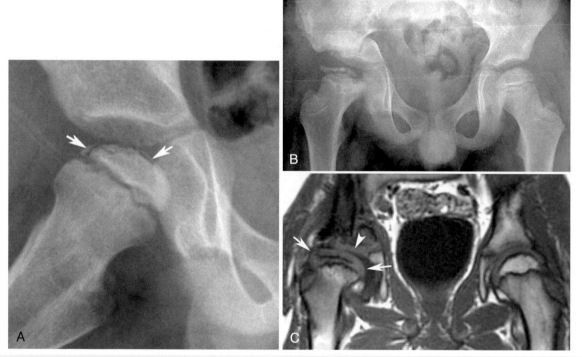

Fig. 13.20 Legg–Calvé–Perthes disease, progression over time. **(A)** Frog-leg lateral radiograph shows subchondral lucencies *(arrows)* in the right capital femoral epiphysis. **(B)** AP radiograph over 1 year later shows typical progression, with broad, fragmented capital femoral epiphysis, wide femoral neck, and irregular acetabulum. **(C)** Coronal T1-weighted MR image shows similar findings. Note the greater thickness of the intermediate-signal-intensity cartilage of the right femoral head *(arrows)* and acetabulum *(arrowhead)* compared with the normal left.

- Femoral head deformity induces secondary deformity in the acetabulum, with flattening and irregularity.
- Intraarticular bodies may occur.
- The outcome varies. Some cases have a normal or near-normal outcome. However, most children have some lasting decrease in range of motion, and early OA is common.
- Prognostic factors in LCP:
  - Older children at the time of diagnosis and girls (who are generally more skeletally mature than boys of the same age) have a poorer prognosis because they have less remaining growth, and thus less time for the hip to remodel back to a more normal configuration.
  - Involvement of greater than 50% of the femoral head also indicates a worse prognosis. Incomplete coverage

of the femoral head ossification center by the acetabular roof also indicates a greater risk for early OA.
- MRI can be used to assess the extent of femoral head osteonecrosis, femoral head coverage by the acetabulum, and secondary changes in the acetabulum (Fig. 13.20). Despite these benefits, MRI is not frequently used in managing LCP because most management is conservative, with salvage procedures such as femoral or acetabular osteotomy performed only after a clinical problem has developed.

LCP Mimics in Children

- *Meyer dysplasia* is delayed and irregular ossification of the capital femoral epiphysis ossification centers that can simulate LCP. Radiographic findings are usually seen

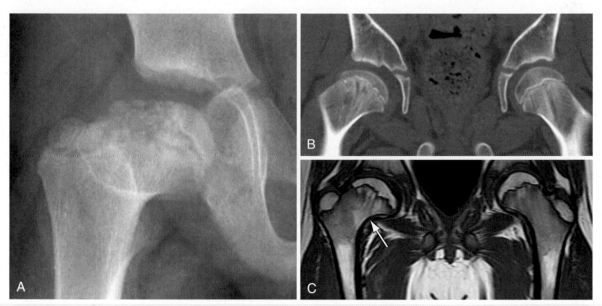

Fig. 13.21 Legg–Calvé–Perthes (LCP) disease, progression over time. **(A)** A 6-year-old with LCP of the right hip, with extensive fragmentation of the superior head. The left hip was normal. Six years later, coronal CT scan **(B)** and T1-weighted MR image **(C)** of healed LCP. The right femoral neck is wider than the left (*arrow* in C). The right capital femoral epiphysis is wider and shorter longitudinally than the left but has smooth contour and normal density in B and normal signal in C. Note the compensatory change in the right acetabulum. The deformed right hip is vulnerable to labral tear and early osteoarthritis.

in a younger age group (2–4 years). The radiographic findings in this benign condition resolve spontaneously during childhood.

- Hypothyroidism, sickle cell disease, Gaucher disease, and epiphyseal dysplasias can cause fragmentation of the capital femoral epiphyses in children. In contrast with LCP, the fragmentation is usually bilateral in these conditions.

OSTEONECROSIS AND OSTEONECROSIS MIMICS AT OTHER SITES IN THE GROWING SKELETON

- Fragmentation and/or sclerosis in epiphyses and in epiphyseal equivalents (apophyses and small bones of the hands and feet) can be seen at numerous sites in the growing skeleton as a normal and as a pathologic finding.
  - Sever's disease (calcaneus apophysis).
  - Blount disease (proximal medial tibia).
  - Femoral condyles.
  - Panner disease (capitellum).
  - Sinding–Larsen–Johansson (patellar lower pole).
  - Osgood–Schlatter (at the proximal and distal ends of the patellar tendon.
  - Scheuermann disease (vertebral endplates).
  - Elbow medial epicondyle.
  - Köhler bone disease (tarsal navicular).
  - Frieberg (metatarsal heads).
- Fragmentation at the tibial tubercle, calcaneal apophysis, tarsal navicular, and within the ossifying femoral condyles may occur as normal variants during during development.
  - MRI can assist in distinguishing normal variation from pathologic cases. Normal variant cases tend to have no associated edema, whereas edema, often intense, is associated with true pathology.

- Legg–Calvé–Perthes, Köhler, and Panner are currently understood to be initiated by osteonecrosis, whereas the others are initiated by trauma. Frieberg in children has features of both but in adults may be purely traumatic.
- It was originally hypothesized that these were all manifestations of osteonecrosis and associated growth disturbance and repair. The term *osteochondroses* was applied.
  - Current understanding is that these conditions are quite varied in etiology, natural history, and clinical significance, and the grouping is of questionable utility. The authors do not prefer this term. However, the term appears in the American Board of Radiology (ABR) study guide and therefore is included here.

Osteoporosis

Key Concepts

Generalized Osteoporosis

Major worldwide health problem
Major complication is fracture: Spine, hip, forearm most frequent
Diagnosis: Dual x-ray absorptiometry (DEXA)
T-score: Relative to normal young adults
World Health Organization criteria: −1 to −2.5 indicates osteopenia; lower than −2.5 indicates osteoporosis
Z-score: Relative to age-matched reference group; less useful
Diagnosis: Other quantitative tests: quantitative computed tomography; ultrasonography for calcaneus and radius
Radiography is insensitive
Radiographic findings
Semiquantitative: Cortical tunnels, cortical thinning
Qualitative: Decreased bone density, accentuated trabecular bone contrast, and increased contrast between cortical and medullary bone

Osteoporosis is a disease of diminished bone quantity, with increased risk of fracture.

- Bone is living tissue that is constantly turning over via removal by osteoclasts and new bone formation by osteoblasts.
- Overall bone mass increases during growth and reaches a maximum at about age 30 years in both men and women.
- Later, for reasons that are not fully understood, bone turnover becomes unbalanced, with bone loss exceeding bone production.
- Bone loss typically begins in the fourth decade in women and in the fifth or sixth decades in men. 30–50% of women older than 60 years show evidence of significant bone loss.
- The metabolically active portion of bone is the bone surface, as osteoblasts and osteoclasts are located mainly on the bone surface. Trabecular bone has much more surface area than cortical bone, and thus is most vulnerable to bone loss in imbalanced bone turnover.
- In contrast with osteomalacia, the ratio of osteoid matrix to hydroxyapatite mineral in osteoporosis is normal. Histologically, there is less of both, with cortical thinning and diminished quantity and thickness of trabecular bone.
  - Consequently, the bone is weaker, mainly simply due to less bone, and to a lesser degree loss of trabecular integrity and microelasticity.
- The major complication of osteoporosis is *fragility fracture*.
- The most common locations of osteoporotic fragility fractures are at sites of high trabecular bone content: spine, hip, proximal humerus, distal forearm.
- It is this fracture risk that makes osteoporosis a major health issue throughout the world because of its high prevalence in the elderly, especially women, and its enormous impact on morbidity, mortality, and societal cost.

OSTEOPOROSIS ASSOCIATIONS

- Advancing age ('senile osteoporosis').
- Postmenopausal osteoporosis: associated with the diminished estrogen levels in postmenopausal women.
- For women, any cause of decreased estrogen, such as bilateral oophorectomy, prolonged amenorrhea in young female endurance athletes; hypogonadal syndromes such as Turner syndrome.
- Low testosterone in men.
- Low body weight.
- Low levels of weight-bearing exercise, immobilization.
- Family history of osteoporosis.
- Greater incidence among white and Asian women than Black women.
- Endocrine: hyper- and hypothyroidism, Cushing disease, hyperparathyroidism.
- Malnutrition, low-calcium diet, eating disorders, malabsorption due to celiac disease, inflammatory bowel disease, biliary disease, surgical bowel shortening or bypass.
- Inborn errors of metabolism: for example, hemochromatosis, hypophosphatasia, homocystinuria.

- Drugs (partial list):
  - Corticosteroids (or Cushing disease).
  - Antiseizure: phenobarbital, phenytoin.
  - Anticoagulants: heparin and warfarin.
  - Proton pump inhibitors.
- Alcoholism.
- Smoking.
- Osteogenesis imperfecta.
- Amyloidosis.
- Mastocytosis.
- Multiple myeloma can cause extensive bone loss.
- Rare idiopathic juvenile forms of osteoporosis.

TERMINOLOGY

- *Osteopenia* is often used as subjective term for diminished bone density as perceived on radiographs due to *decreased bone mineral density* (BMD).
- *Osteoporosis* is a more specific term for decreased bone mass with deteriorated bone architecture and associated increased prevalence of fragility fractures.
- Both terms are also used in a somewhat different and very specific way in interpreting dual-energy x-ray absorptiometry (DEXA) bone density scans (discussed in the following text).
- Osteoporosis is the most common cause of decreased BMD, but one must keep in mind that there are other causes, such as osteomalacia.

OSTEOPOROSIS TREATMENT

- Bisphosphonate drugs inhibit osteoclast activity.
  - Some osteoclast activity is necessary for normal bone turnover and maintenance of bone strength, so currently used for no longer than 3–4 years.
  - Rare potential complications of long-term use: otherwise unusual stress fractures of the lateral proximal femoral shaft (Fig. 5.34D) and osteonecrosis of the mandible.
- Dietary supplementation with calcium and/or vitamin D is helpful if deficient, but has not been clearly shown to be helpful if not deficient.

FRACTURE RISK ASSESSMENT TOOL (FRAX®)

- **F**racture **R**isk **A**ssessment Tool.
- Combines a patient's BMD T-score and clinical information to provide a risk estimate of hip fracture and other osteoporotic fractures in the following 10 years.
- Based on actuarial data.
- Available free online and with apps.
- Used to assist decision-making regarding whether or not to start a patient on bisphosphonates.
- Mainly used if the patient is not already taking bisphosphonates.

QUANTITATIVE MEASUREMENT OF BONE MINERAL DENSITY

Dual-Energy X-ray Absorptiometry (DEXA)

Current scanners use two different tube voltages with effective voltages ranging from about 40 to 100 keV depending on the system. Comparing the total beam attenuation for each energy allows the lean and adipose soft tissue contribution to be subtracted with reasonable (although not perfect) precision. Patient ionizing radiation exposure is minimal, measured in μSv.

- Patient positioning:
  - Supine, with care to avoid obliquity.
  - Proximal femur: leg abducted 15 degrees and internally rotated 25 degrees.
    - Goal is to have the femoral neck parallel to the table, perpendicular to the beam.
    - Frequently used measurement sites include the femoral neck, Ward's area (inferior femoral neck), greater trochanter, and intertrochanteric femur.
  - Spine: hips and knees flexed, to minimize lumbar lordosis.
- DEXA measures bone density in g/cm² (area), so strictly speaking not actual BMD.
- World Health Organization guidelines for diagnosis of osteoporosis using DEXA:
  - Well-validated predicator for fracture risk.
  - Measure bone density at several sites, including proximal femur and spine (Fig. 13.22A,B).
  - Compare with normal young adults (the standard deviation is the *T-score*).
  - Compare with age- and sex-matched reference populations (the standard deviation is the *Z-score*).
  - *Osteopenia*: T-scores between −1 and −2.5 (i.e., bone density between 1 and 2.5 standard deviations below the average of normal young adults of the same sex).
  - *Osteoporosis*: T-scores below −2.5.
- Be aware that these definitions of osteopenia and osteoporosis are specific to reporting on DEXA scans.

DEXA pitfalls:

- DEXA measures bone density in area. Consequently, DEXA overestimates BMD in patients with larger bones and underestimates BMD in patients with smaller bones.
- Falsely elevated BMD measurements:
  - Spine osteophytes (Fig. 13.22C).
  - Vertebral compression fractures.
  - Soft tissue calcifications such as abdominal aorta.
  - Diffuse idiopathic skeletal hyperostosis (DISH).
  - Bone islands.
- Falsely lowered BMD measurements:
  - Prior laminectomies.
  - Small patients.
- Measurements at each site of risk are more predictive of fracture risk at that site than is a measurement from a remote site. For example, the risk for hip fracture is best determined from a BMD measurement of the hip.
- Limited validation in children.
- Older units used radionuclides, which caused higher patient exposure.

Quantitative CT (QCT)

- Measures true BMD (mg/cm³).
- BMD alone does not completely describe bone strength. Trabecular architecture also is an important factor in overall bone strength (or perhaps more precisely, bone fragility, in osteoporosis). Quantitative CT (QCT) densitometry allows evaluation limited to trabecular bone where generalized osteoporosis is most greatly manifested.
- Patient is scanned with a reference calibration phantom.
- T-score derived from an established QCT database.
- Also reports absolute BMD:
  - Normal >120 mg/cm³; osteopenia 80–120; osteoporosis <80 as per American College of Radiology (ACR) guidelines.
- Avoids the DEXA pitfall of overestimating bone density in the presence of DISH, aortic calcification, spine fracture, and degenerative osteophyte formation.
- DEXA is more widely used because it is less expensive and uses less radiation (DEXA: 0.001 mSv hip and spine vs. 0.2 mSv or greater for QCT spine only).

Semiquantitative Measurement of BMD in Routine CT of the Abdomen and Pelvis

- Uses routine body CT scans.
- Opportunistic: no additional radiation.
- Simple and fast: Draw region of interest around trabecular bone in lumbar vertebral bodies or femur (exclude cortex). Measured Hounsfield units (HU) can be used as a rough screening test for osteoporosis.
- Less precise than QCT or DEXA.
- Specific values for osteoporosis and osteopenia vary based on which vertebral body was measured, and also vary between studies.
- Trabecular bone density measurements vary with kV.
- At 120 kV, a suggested threshold value for osteoporosis and significantly increased fracture risk is 90–100 HU in L1.

Ultrasound

- Specialized US equipment can evaluate BMD.
- Can also provide information about trabecular structure and bone microelasticity, which also contribute to fracture risk.
- Limited to superficial sites: calcaneus, tibia, distal radius, and phalanges.
- Advantages:
  - Inexpensive.
  - Portable.

MRI

- High-resolution MRI can evaluate trabecular architecture.
- Specialized sequences are required and are technically challenging.
- For quantitative assessment, MRI is primarily a research tool.
- Some commercially available sequences can rival CT for semi-quantitative and qualitative evaluation of bone morphology and trabecular density, with potential to replace CT for some common indications such as glenoid bone stock assessment prior to shoulder arthroplasty.

NONQUANTITATIVE FINDINGS IN OSTEOPOROSIS

Long Bones

- Fragility fracture (fracture from trauma that would not break a normal bone).

Birth Date		64.5 years	**Referring Physician:**	
Height / Weight	66.0 in.	180.0 lbs.	**Measured:**	(13.60)
Sex / Ethnic:	Female	White	**Analyzed:**	(13.60)

DualFemur Bone Density Trend

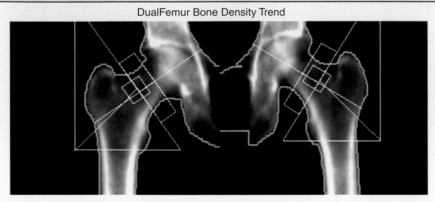

Image not for diagnosis

Densitometry Ref: Neck (BMD)   Trend: Neck Mean (BMD)
BMD (g/cm²)   YA T-score   %Change vs Baseline

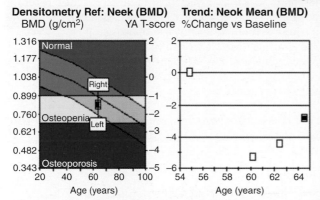

Hip Axis Length Comparison (mm)

Left = −3.6   Right = −1.5

−30 −20 −10 Mean 10 20 30

(Right = 106.4 mm) (Mean = 107.9 mm) (Left = 104.3 mm)

COMMENTS:

Region	BMD[1] (g/cm²)	Young-Adult[2,7] T-score	Age-Matched[3] Z-score
Neck			
Left	0.823	−1.5	−0.5
Right	0.830	−1.5	−0.4
Mean	0.826	−1.5	−0.4
Difference	0.007	0.0	0.0
Total			
Left	0.893	−0.9	−0.1
Right	0.906	−0.8	0.0
Mean	0.900	−0.9	−0.1
Difference	0.013	0.1	0.1

Trend: Neck Mean

Measured Date	Age (years)	BMD[1] (g/cm²)	Change vs Previous (g/cm²)	Previous (%)
	64.5	0.826	0.014	1.7
	62.5	0.812	0.007	0.9
	60.2	0.805	−0.045*	−5.3*
	54.8	0.850	−	−

∗. Indicates significant change based on 95% confidence interval.
1. Statistically 68% of repeat scans fall within ISD (± 0.012 g/cm² for DualFemur Neck)
2. USA (Combined NHANES (ages 20–30) / Lunar (ages 20–40)) Femur Reference Population (v112)
3. Matched for Age, Weight (females 25–100 kg), Ethnic
7. DualFemur Total T-score difference is 0.1. Asymmetry is None.
11. World Health Organization - Definition of Osteoporosis and Osteopenia for Caucasian Women: Normal = T-score at or above −1.0 SD; Osteopenia = T-score between −1.0 and −2.5 SD; Osteoporosis = T-score at or below −2.5 SD; (WHO definitions only apply when a young healthy Caucasian Women reference database is used to determine T-scores.)

Printed;   (13.60); Filename: 4xsy2q6gya.dfx; Right Femur; 18.5:%Fat=31.9%; Neck Angle (deg)=55; Scan Mode: Standard 37.0 μGy; Left Femur; 19.0:%Fat=33.2%; Neck Angle (deg)=59; Scan Mode: Standard   37.0 μGy

A

Fig. 13.22 (A and **B)** Sample automatically generated DEXA report. The patient is taking bisphosphonates.

Birth Date:	64.5 years	**Referring Physician:**	
Height / Weight:	66.0 in. 180.0 lbs.	**Measured:**	(13.60)
Sex / Ethnic:	Female White	**Analyzed:**	(13.60)

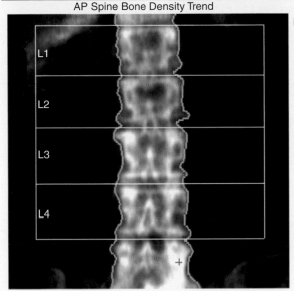

AP Spine Bone Density Trend

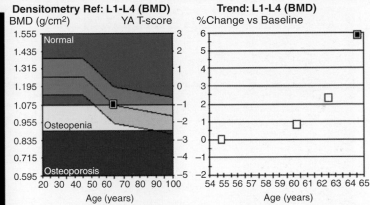

Densitometry Ref: L1-L4 (BMD)

BMD (g/cm²)   YA T-score

Trend: L1-L4 (BMD)

%Change vs Baseline

Region	BMD[1] (g/cm²)	Young-Adult[2] T-score	Age-Matched[3] Z-score
L1	1.002	−1.1	−0.1
L2	0.927	−2.3	−1.3
L3	1.179	−0.3	0.7
L4	1.147	−0.6	0.4
L1-L4	1.071	−1.0	0.0

COMMENTS:

		Trend: L1-L4	**Change vs**	
Measured Date	Age (years)	BMD[1] (g/cm²)	Previous (g/cm²)	Previous (%)
	64.5	1.071	0.036*	3.5*
	62.5	1.035	0.015	1.5
	60.2	1.020	0.008	0.8
	54.8	1.012	−	−

Image not for diagnosis

(13.60)76:3.00:50.03:12.0 0.00:11.10

0.60x1.05 23.5:%Fat=46.7%
0.00:0.00 0.00:0.00
Filename: 4xsy2q6gya.dfx
Scan Mode: Standard;OneScan   37.0 µGy

*. Indicates significant change based on 95% confidence interval.
1. Statistically 68% of repeat scans fall within ISD (± 0.010 g/cm² for AP Spine L1-L4)
2. USA (Combined NHANES (ages 20–30) / Lunar (ages 20–40)) AP Spine Reference Population (v112)
3. Matched for Age, Weight (females 25–100 kg), Ethnic
11. World Health Organization - Definition of Osteoporosis and Osteopenia for Caucasian Women: Normal = T-score at or above −1.0 SD; Osteopenia = T-score between −1.0 and −2.5 SD; Osteoporosis = T-score at or below −2.5 SD; (WHO definitions only apply when a young healthy Caucasian Women reference database is used to determine T-scores.)

B

Fig. 13.22, cont'd

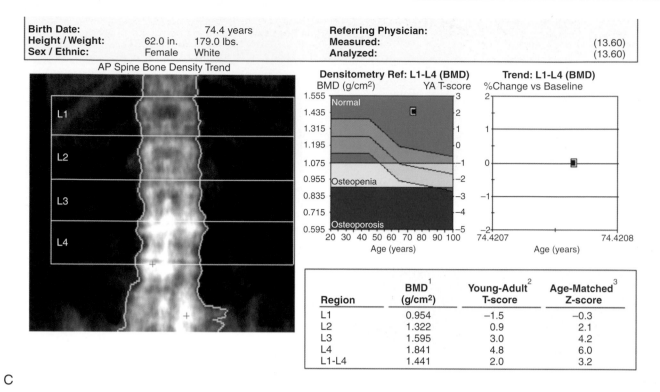

Birth Date:		74.4 years	Referring Physician:	
Height / Weight:	62.0 in.	179.0 lbs.	Measured:	(13.60)
Sex / Ethnic:	Female	White	Analyzed:	(13.60)

Region	BMD[1] (g/cm²)	Young-Adult[2] T-score	Age-Matched[3] Z-score
L1	0.954	−1.5	−0.3
L2	1.322	0.9	2.1
L3	1.595	3.0	4.2
L4	1.841	4.8	6.0
L1-L4	1.441	2.0	3.2

C

Fig. 13.22, cont'd (C) False elevation of measured lumbar spine bone mineral density caused by hypertrophic degenerative change. Note the wide range of T-scores from L1 to L4. L1 is the only level that might be accurate.

- Fairly specific for osteoporosis in an appropriate setting.
  - Nondisplaced fragility fractures can be occult on radiographs and occasionally on CT.
  - MRI is highly sensitive: fracture line is low signal on T1-weighted, with surrounding marrow edema on fluid-sensitive sequences.
  - Fragility fractures in osteoporosis may be incomplete.
- Cortical thinning in the second and third metacarpal shafts.
  - Normal mid-diaphyseal cortical thickness should account for at least 50% of transverse bone width in individuals with normal bone density (Fig. 13.23).
  - Less is suggestive of osteoporosis.
- *Cortical tunnels and cavities.*
  - Also termed *intracortical lucencies.*
  - Cortical tunnels are subtle linear lucencies in cortical bone, parallel to the bone long axis, several millimeters in length, and often less than 0.5 mm in diameter (Fig. 13.24). They are part of the normal bone turnover process, as aggregates of osteoclasts create these cylindrical defects in lamellar bone that normally are promptly filled in with new bone by osteoblasts.
  - *Cortical cavities* are like cortical tunnels but larger and less uniform.
  - Radiographically visible cortical tunnels and cavities reflect the delayed and diminished osteoblastic activity in osteoporosis.
  - Can also be seen in high bone turnover and/or relatively rapid bone loss associated with hyperparathyroidism, hyperthyroidism, regional hyperemia, and complex regional pain syndrome (formerly called

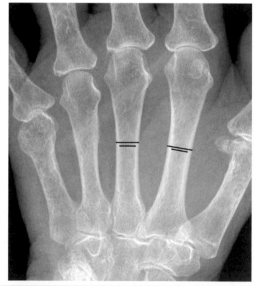

Fig. 13.23 Cortical thickness in the metacarpals and metatarsals can serve as a rough guide to the presence or absence of generalized osteoporosis in adults. In this elderly woman with osteoporosis, the transverse width of the medullary spaces (illustrated by *short lines* across the second and third metacarpals) exceeds one-half the transverse width of the shafts *(long lines)* because of cortical bone loss. This generalization does not apply to children.

reflex sympathetic dystrophy). Small, discrete areas of endosteal or subperiosteal cortical bone loss also may be seen in these conditions.
- Progressive loss of trabeculae in the proximal femur (Fig. 13.25).

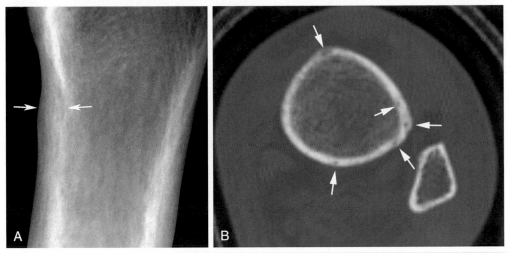

Fig. 13.24 Intracortical lucencies (cortical tunnels) in osteoporosis. **(A)** Detail view of the femur in a 65-year-old man immobilized for a fracture shows subtle radiolucent lines parallel to the cortex (between *arrows*). **(B)** CT of the distal tibia in a 95-year-old woman shows tunnels in the cross section *(arrows)*.

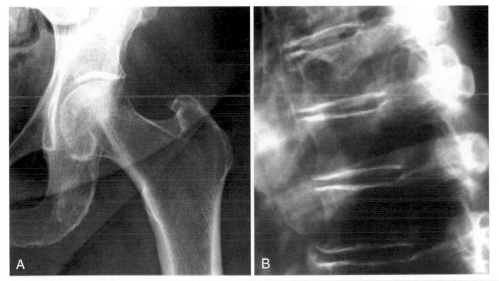

Fig. 13.25 Osteoporosis. **(A)** AP view of the hip shows an exaggerated trabecular pattern in the primary compressive lines of force. The tensile lines of force are largely absent, indicating advanced osteoporosis. **(B)** Lateral radiograph of the spine shows exaggerated contrast between the end plates and the medullary bone.

- Accentuation of stress- or load-bearing trabeculae that are the last to be resorbed.
- Transverse trabeculae in the diaphysis or metaphysis, termed *bone bars* or *reinforcement lines*.

Spine

- Vertebral endplates may appear thinned, with exaggerated contrast between the vertebral body end plate and the central density (Fig. 13.25).
- Compression fractures can take the shape of anterior wedging, biconcavity of endplates, or generalized loss of height.
- Increased conspicuity of vertically oriented trabecular bone in the spine due to generalized loss of horizontally oriented trabeculae.
- Vertebral body marrow often has a mottled appearance on T1-weighted MR images in patients with osteoporosis, but this appearance is neither sensitive nor specific.

VERTEBRAL BODY COMPRESSION FRACTURE IMAGING

- Radiography and CT:
  - Fracture detection. Comparison with prior studies is one marker of fracture acuity.
- MRI:
  - Fracture detection.
  - Marrow edema on fluid-sensitive sequences is a useful marker of a recent, active (acute or subacute), or potential impending compression fracture.
  - Can be helpful in management: recent fractures respond best to vertebroplasty.
- Bone scan:
  - Becomes positive a few days after a fracture.
  - Bone scans in patients with primary osteoporosis usually are normal.
  - MRI is preferred for fracture dating.

DECREASED BONE MINERAL DENSITY IN CHILDREN

- Easily overestimated on radiographs.
- Quantitative evaluation is limited.
- Causes:
  - Drugs (same list as adults, in children most likely to be corticosteroids, antiseizure, and immune suppression medications).
  - Rickets.
  - Neuromuscular conditions (disuse).
  - Osteogenesis imperfecta.
  - Diabetes.
  - Juvenile idiopathic arthritis (JIA).
  - Malnutrition (specifically deficient dietary calcium and vitamin D) as can be seen in malabsorption conditions and anorexia nervosa.
  - Renal disease.
- *Idiopathic juvenile osteoporosis* is a diagnosis of exclusion.
  - Pain, fractures, long bone, and spine deformities.
  - Bone density eventually recovers, but deformities may persist.

REGIONAL OSTEOPOROSIS

- Decreased BMD confined to a portion of the skeleton.

Causes:

- Disuse.
  - Wolff's Law (use it or lose it) applies locally.
- Increased local blood flow.
  - Hyperemia induces osteoclast activation and thus bone resorption.
  - Examples: inflammatory arthropathy, hypervascular tumors, complex regional pain syndrome, and healing fractures with immobilization (Fig. 13.26).
  - Bone loss can develop rapidly, producing an 'aggressive osteoporosis' pattern.
    - Radiography and CT: prominent small foci of obvious demineralization resembling the permeative pattern of an aggressive bone tumor.
    - MRI may show patchy edema signal.

- At least initially, this aggressive osteoporosis pattern (Fig. 13.27) is due to loss of bone mineral, but with preservation of the osteoid matrix. This allows for relatively rapid remineralization if the stimulus is removed.

Key Concepts

Regional Osteoporosis

Local osteopenia, often symptomatic, may appear radiographically aggressive

Regional migratory osteoporosis

Transient osteoporosis of the hip

Complex regional pain syndrome

Local hyperemia: Healing fracture, hypervascular tumor, infection, synovitis

Diminished loading, disuse

TRANSIENT OSTEOPOROSIS OF THE HIP (TOH, IDIOPATHIC TRANSIENT OSTEOPOROSIS OF THE HIP, ITOH)

- Patients present with sudden onset of severe unilateral hip pain.
- Occurs most commonly in middle aged men and pregnant women in the third trimester.
- Radiographs:
  - Asymmetric diminished bone density.
  - Subchondral bone resorption.
  - Preserved cartilage space.
- Bone scan: intense tracer uptake (in contrast with osteonecrosis, which initially has diminished tracer uptake).
- MRI:
  - Intense marrow edema in the femoral head and neck with diminished signal on T1-weighted images (Figs. 13.28 and 13.29).
  - Gadolinium contrast enhancement throughout the femoral head and neck.
  - Joint effusion frequently present.
- Bone marrow edema may be extensive and extend below the femoral neck.
- Femoral neck fractures occur rarely, most commonly in pregnant women.

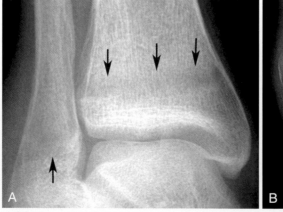
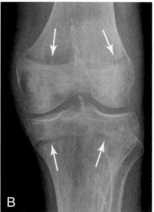

Fig. 13.26 Osteoporosis related to disuse and local hyperemia. **(A)** Disproportionate focal demineralization of the metaphysis after casting. This radiograph was obtained during a cast change for a fifth metatarsal fracture. Note the transverse bands of demineralization *(arrows)* in the distal tibia and fibula metaphyses, reflecting the rich vascular supply of this portion of a bone. **(B)** Similar finding around the knee of an older adult *(arrows)*.

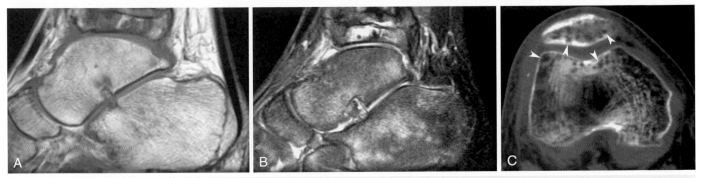

Fig. 13.27 'Aggressive' osteoporosis related to disuse and local hyperemia. (A and B) Marrow changes on MRI in a 14-year-old boy after casting and internal fixation of a distal tibial fracture. Sagittal T1-weighted **(A)** and inversion recovery **(B)** MR images of the hindfoot show a 'mottled' pattern of decreased T1-weighted **(A)** and increased T2-weighted **(B)** marrow MR signal intensity that might suggest an aggressive infiltrative process or infection. Radiographs (not shown) depicted a corresponding subtle permeative pattern of bone demineralization. These changes were reversed when weight-bearing was resumed. **(C)** Axial CT image in an adult with a recently operated, healing tibial plateau fracture shows multiple tiny lytic areas *(arrowheads)* that can falsely suggest a highly aggressive infiltrating tumor or infection.

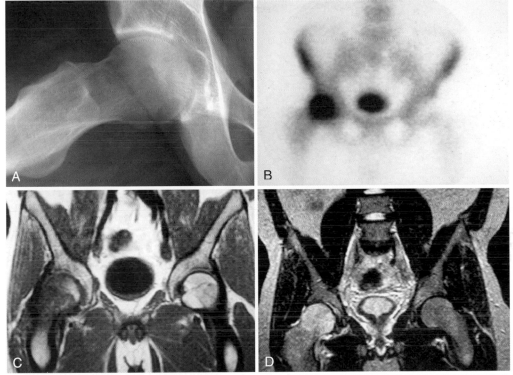

Fig. 13.28 Transient osteoporosis of the hip. **(A)** AP radiograph of the right hip in a 45-year-old man shows subtle demineralization. **(B)** Radionuclide bone scan shows intense uptake in the right femoral head (see also Fig. 13.29).

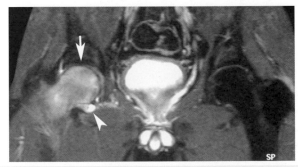

Fig. 13.29 Transient osteoporosis of the hip. Coronal inversion recovery MR image shows intense edema in the femoral head *(arrow)* and neck, and an effusion *(arrowhead)*.

- A recent observation is that high resolution MRI often demonstrates a small subchondral trabecular fracture early in the course of this condition in many patients. This observation may change our understanding of TOH, as it suggests a femoral head subchondral fracture maybe a cause rather than an effect in TOH.
- Adding to the confusion is that some cases of TOH progress to radiographic findings of osteonecrosis with subchondral collapse, but most do not.
- Self-limited, usually reversing after several months. Treated with non-weight bearing, pain management, and bisphosphonates.

Transient regional osteoporosis (TRO, Transient regional migratory osteoporosis, TRMO)

- Lower extremity joint pain with bone marrow edema similar to TOH.
- Multiple episodes at different sites.
- Clinical course in each joint is similar to TOH.

Complex regional pain syndrome (CRPS), previously known as *reflex sympathetic dystrophy* (RSD) and Sudeck's atrophy.

- Swelling, extreme pain, and hyperesthesia, often in a 'glove' or 'stocking' distribution that extends to the distal aspect of the involved extremity.
- Local osteoporosis.
- Most cases follow an injury. Hemiplegia also can precede CRPS.
- Pathophysiology is complex and incompletely understood, with alterations in the central, somatic, and autonomic nervous systems.
  - Sympathetic and parasympathic imbalance is thought to contribute to the local osteoporosis.
- Imaging (Fig. 13.30):
  - Radiographs: rapid-onset local osteopenia.
    - *Aggressive osteoporosis* pattern that resembles an aggressive permeative process.
    - May appear within 2 weeks of onset.
  - Bone Scan: abnormal earlier than radiographs. All three phases are hot.
  - MRI: patchy marrow edema–like signal.

Disorders of Calcium Homeostasis

Bone is mostly mineral (*calcium hydroxyapatite*) deposited on a matrix composed primarily of collagen (*osteoid*). Both the mineral and collagenous components must be normal and present in normal amounts for normal bone strength.

Metabolic, hormonal, or genetic conditions can alter the composition or quantity of the matrix or the calcium hydroxyapatite, resulting in bones that are weak, deformed, or demineralized, often in a characteristic pattern.

NORMAL CALCIUM AND PHOSPHATE HOMEOSTASIS

Calcium–phosphate balance and sodium–phosphate balance are critical in cellular electrolyte equilibrium and maintenance of numerous energy-dependent cellular transactions, including adenosine triphosphate production and muscle action.

Not only is bone important structurally; it also provides a large reserve for calcium and phosphate. Most bone calcium is bound up in calcium hydroxyapatite, which is deposited or released relatively slowly. However, a small portion of bone mineral is in the form of soluble bone salts, available in minutes as needed to maintain serum calcium levels.

- Calcium and phosphate are found in serum in both bound and free (unbound) forms.
- Free calcium and phosphate levels are constant.
- Normal levels are maintained by gut absorption of electrolytes, use of mobile bone reserves, and kidney tubular action.
- The hormones responsible for interacting with these targets are *parathyroid hormone* (PTH, parathormone), *vitamin D*, and *calcitonin*.

Key Concepts

Calcium Homeostasis

Parathyroid hormone and vitamin D are the two main regulators of calcium and phosphate homeostasis

Parathyroid hormone acts on bone and kidney to increase serum calcium while mildly decreasing phosphate levels

Vitamin D acts on bone and gut to calibrate serum calcium and phosphate levels for phosphate balance

Vitamin D is dependent on dietary intake and normal function in small bowel, liver, and kidney

Parathyroid Hormone (PTH)

- Produced by the four parathyroid glands.

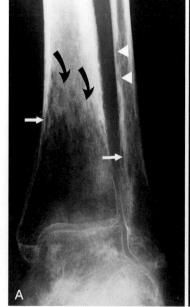
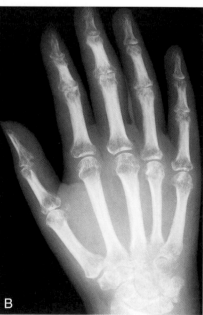

Fig. 13.30 Complex regional pain syndrome (formerly reflex sympathetic dystrophy). **(A)** AP view of the ankle shows pronounced bone demineralization in the distal leg and hindfoot with aggressive features, including intracortical lucency *(straight arrows)*, endosteal resorption of bone *(arrowheads)*, and a broad zone of transition *(curved arrows)* to more normal-appearing proximal tibial and fibular diaphyses. **(B)** PA radiograph of the hand of another patient shows pronounced periarticular osteopenia and diffuse soft tissue swelling in the wrist and hand.

- Low serum levels of calcium induce the glands to produce the hormone.
- PTH acts on several sites to increase calcium levels in the serum.
  - Renal: PTH acts on the proximal tubules to enhance phosphate excretion and calcium reabsorption through calcium–phosphate pumps. PTH also acts as a cofactor to enhance the synthesis of the fully active form of vitamin D, 1,25-hydroxyvitamin D (*1,25 vitamin D₃*), thus indirectly increasing calcium levels through vitamin D action.
  - Bone: PTH stimulates osteoclast-mediated bone resorption, which results in hydroxyapatite dissolution and thus increases calcium and phosphate levels in the blood.
- *Bottom line*: <u>PTH acts to increase calcium and mildly decrease phosphate levels in the blood.</u>

Vitamin D

- The endogenous form (*cholecalciferol, vitamin D₃*) is derived from cholesterol and is synthesized in the skin after exposure to ultraviolet light.
- Most vitamin D, however, comes from dietary supplementation.
- Exogenous forms of vitamin D are absorbed through the gut and converted in the liver to 25-hydroxyvitamin D.
- The active form of the vitamin is subsequently produced in the kidney, where it is 1-hydroxylated.
- The 1,25-hydroxylated form is the active form of the hormone (*1,25 vitamin D₃*).
  - Acts on bone, gut, kidney, parathyroid glands, and other tissues, including the skin.
  - In bone the vitamin binds with intranuclear receptors and causes transcription of osteocalcin, osteopontin, and alkaline phosphatase. This action results in mobilization of calcium and phosphorus and also promotes maturation and mineralization of osteoid matrix. For this activity, vitamin D requires the presence of PTH as a cofactor.
    - *Osteocalcin* is a hormone produced by osteoblasts. In addition to contributing to bone formation, osteocalcin has multiple other effects including reducing insulin resistance and enabling the acute stress response ('fight or flight').
    - *Osteopontin* is a linking protein produced by a variety of cells including osteoblasts and osteocytes. In addition to contributing to bone formation, osteopontin has other effects including promoting inflammatory cell activation in rheumatoid arthritis and inflammatory bowel disease.
  - In the gut *1,25 vitamin D₃* causes the production of calcium-binding protein and thus increased intestinal calcium transport, with passive absorption of phosphate. This action of vitamin D requires PTH as a cofactor.
  - Acts to increase phosphate resorption in the proximal renal tubules, also requiring the presence of PTH.
  - Inhibits the release of PTH from the parathyroid glands and is a cofactor of action of PTH in bone.
- *Bottom line:* <u>Vitamin D acts to increase calcium and phosphate levels in the blood.</u>

Calcitonin

- Less important than PTH and vitamin D.
- Produced primarily by the parafollicular cells of the thyroid gland.
- Antagonist to PTH.
  - Action: inhibit osteoclast-mediated bone resorption and to stimulate renal calcium clearance.
- Increased blood levels of calcium result in increased levels of calcitonin.
- *Bottom line:* <u>Calcitonin acts to decrease calcium levels in the blood.</u>

HYPERPARATHYROIDISM

Key Concepts

Hyperparathyroidism

Normal proportion of mineralized bone to osteoid (vs. osteomalacia)
Primary hyperparathyroidism: Usually due to hyperfunctioning adenoma; associated with multiple endocrine neoplasia
Secondary hyperparathyroidism: Usually by renal disease that causes physiologic activation of the hormone
Tertiary hyperparathyroidism: Autonomous overproduction after correction of the initial stimulus. Typical presentation is four-gland overproduction in a renal transplant patient
Radiographs:
Demineralization at multiple sites, most classically subperiosteal demineralization of radial aspects of second and third middle phalanges
Clues to primary versus secondary:
Calcium pyrophosphate deposition, brown tumors more frequent in primary
Bone sclerosis, periostitis, soft tissue calcification more frequent in secondary
There are three forms: primary, secondary, and tertiary.

Primary Hyperparathyroidism

- Parathyroid gland adenoma (60–90% of cases).
- Remainder: parathyroid gland hyperplasia or, rarely, glandular adenocarcinoma.
- In about 10% of cases, adenomas can be multiple.
- Occurs in 95% of patients with multiple endocrine neoplasia (MEN) type 1 and about 25% of patients with MEN type 2A.
- *Labs:* Serum levels of calcium are elevated whereas serum levels of phosphate are decreased.
- Clinical: Patients usually present clinically with generalized weakness, urolithiasis, peptic ulcer disease, pancreatitis, and bone and joint pain and tenderness ('bones, stones, and groans').
- Sestamibi nuclear medicine scans may localize a primary adenoma. Treatment is surgical to remove the adenoma.

Secondary Hyperparathyroidism

- Gland stimulation in reaction to low calcium levels.
- By far the most common cause of secondary hyperparathyroidism is renal failure.
  - Mechanism: tubular dysfunction and diminished capacity to excrete phosphate. Elevated serum phosphate levels result in calcium–phosphate binding and

sometimes nonmeasurable diminished serum calcium levels, which in turn promote PTH synthesis.

- Treatment can be medical or surgical (renal transplant).
- *Labs:* low to normal serum calcium levels; elevated phosphate levels.

Tertiary Hyperparathyroidism

- Occurs in long-standing secondary hyperparathyroidism.
- Continued overproduction of hormone despite correction of the cause of secondary hyperparathyroidism (e.g., renal transplant).
- The parathyroid glands function autonomously, producing hormone despite a lack of calcium imbalance to induce hormone synthesis.
- Four-gland hyperplasia in a renal transplant patient is the classic presentation.
- Treatment is surgical gland removal.
- *Labs:* serum calcium level is normal or high, phosphate decreased.

Hyperparathyroidism Imaging Findings

- Generalized bone demineralization (Fig. 13.31).
- Bone loss is most apparent at sites of greatest surface area because osteoclasts are located on the bone surface. Therefore bone loss is most apparent at subperiosteal, intracortical, endosteal, trabecular, subchondral, and subligamentous locations (Fig. 13.32 see Fig. 13.31).

- Subperiosteal:
  - *Bone resorption that is specific for hyperparathyroidism:* subperiosteal along the radial aspects of the second and third middle phalanges.
  - Distal phalanx tuft bone resorption (*acro-osteolysis,* see Fig. 13.31).
  - Other sites of subperiosteal bone resorption include the medial aspect of the humerus, femur, and tibia; the superior and inferior aspects of the ribs; and the lamina dura of the teeth.
- Subchondral:
  - Can mimic inflammatory arthropathy and is especially seen in the sacroiliac, acromioclavicular, sternoclavicular, and temporomandibular joints, and at the pubic symphysis (see Fig. 13.32).
- Subligamentous:
  - Most common at the trochanters, ischial tuberosities, inferior surfaces of the calcaneus and distal clavicle, and elbow.
- Intracortical and subperiosteal resorption can mimic highly aggressive neoplasia, and endosteal bone resorption can mimic endosteal erosion that is seen in marrow dyscrasias, such as multiple myeloma (Fig. 13.33).
- Additional classic findings:
  - Skull: 'salt-and-pepper' appearance (Fig. 13.31B).
  - Soft tissue calcification (due to elevated calcium–phosphate product).

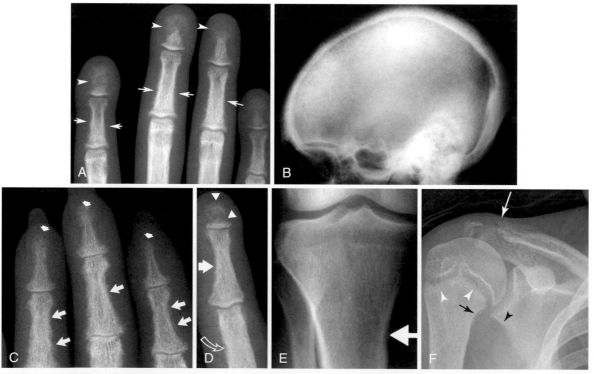

Fig. 13.31 Radiographic features of hyperparathyroidism. **(A)** PA radiograph of fingers reveals diffuse bone demineralization. The trabeculae are fuzzy because of diffuse resorption. Note the presence of localized resorption of bone at the distal phalangeal tufts *(arrowheads)* and along the middle phalanges *(arrows).* **(B)** Lateral skull radiograph shows salt-and-pepper appearance. **(C)** PA radiograph of fingers demonstrating subperiosteal bone resorption in phalanges *(arrows)* and subcortical tuft resorption *(arrowheads).* **(D)** PA radiograph of finger demonstrates subperiosteal bone resorption *(closed arrow)* that is greater on the radial side (left side of the image). Also note intracortical *(open arrow)* and tuftal *(arrowheads)* bone resorption. **(E)** AP radiograph of proximal tibia demonstrates subperiosteal bone resorption at the medial aspect of the proximal tibial metaphysis *(arrow).* **(F)** AP shoulder radiograph in a child shows resorption of the lateral clavicle *(white arrow),* subperiosteal resorption of the medial proximal metaphysis *(black arrow),* and medial inferior glenoid neck *(black arrowhead),* all with fuzzy margins. Also note the widened proximal humeral physis with fuzzy margin of the proximal metaphysis *(white arrowheads).*

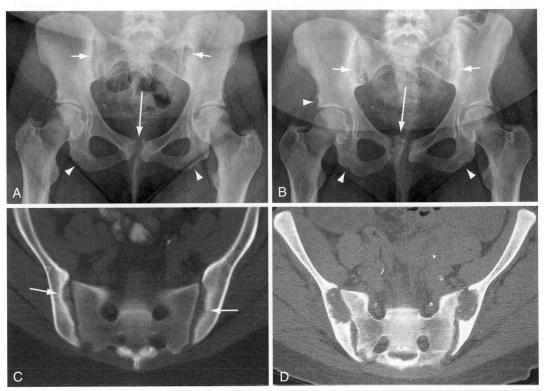

Fig. 13.32 Radiographic features of hyperparathyroidism, pelvis. AP radiographs in a patient with primary hyperparathyroidism at the time of diagnosis **(A)** and 6 months later **(B)**. The patient initially declined treatment. Note the progression of bone resorption at the pubic symphysis *(long arrow)*, iliac bones at the sacroiliac (SI) joints *(short arrows)*, and ischial tuberosities at the hamstring tendon origins *(arrowheads)*. (C and D) CT images in different patients show bilateral subchondral bone resorption *(arrows* in C). In these cases the resorption involves the fibrous portions of the SI joints, in contrast with inflammatory arthropathy.

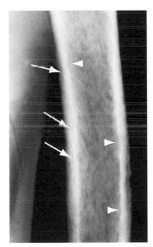

Fig. 13.33 AP radiographic view of the humerus in patient with secondary hyperparathyroidism shows numerous intracortical lucencies *(arrows)* and endosteal bone resorption *(arrowheads)* mimicking aggressive neoplasia.

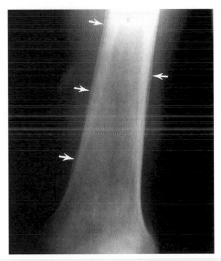

Fig. 13.34 AP radiograph of distal femur in patient with secondary hyperparathyroidism shows solid periosteal new bone formation *(arrows)*.

- Periostitis (Fig. 13.34).
- Calcium pyrophosphate dihydrate deposition and bone sclerosis (Fig. 13.35). Soft tissue calcification, periostitis, and osteosclerosis are more frequently seen in secondary hyperparathyroidism related to elevated calcium–phosphate product.
- Insufficiency fractures can occur in bones weakened by hyperparathyroidism.

- *Brown tumors* (Fig. 13.36).
  - Accumulations of osteoclasts and fibrous tissue with variable cystic change.
  - May contain blood products, hence the name.
  - Imaging: eccentric, lytic, occasionally intracortical, and often expansile lesions that can be confused radiographically with giant cell tumor or fibrous dysplasia. Can be multiple and tend to heal after treatment of the underlying disorder.

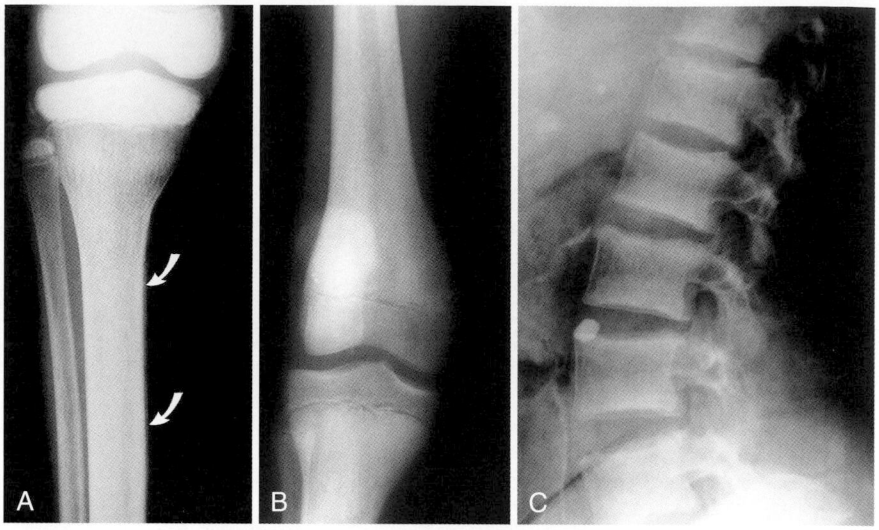

Fig. 13.35 Secondary hyperparathyroidism and bone sclerosis. **(A)** AP radiograph of proximal tibia shows epiphyseal bone sclerosis and tibial diaphyseal solid periosteal new bone *(arrows)*. **(B)** AP radiograph of knee shows generalized increased bone density. Note increased thickness of cortical bone. **(C)** Lateral radiograph of lumbar spine shows typical features of rugger jersey spine with alternating bands of density and lucency. The denser bone is located adjacent to the end plates.

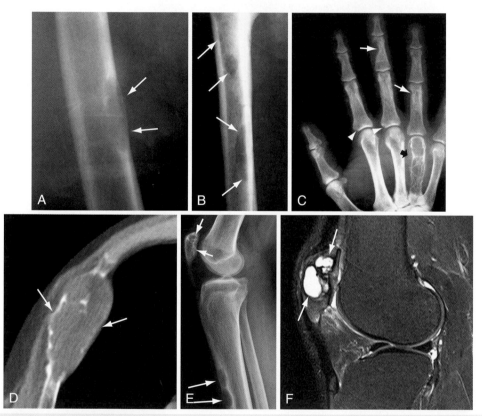

Fig. 13.36 Brown tumors of hyperparathyroidism. **(A)** AP view of femur shows mildly expansile intracortical lytic mass *(arrows)*. **(B)** AP view of femur shows multiple brown tumors *(arrows)*. **(C)** PA view of hand shows brown tumors in fourth metacarpal bone *(black arrow)*. Typical features of hyperparathyroidism are also shown with diffuse bone demineralization, subperiosteal bone resorption, and marginal subchondral bone resorption *(arrowheads)*. Two additional brown tumors are shown in the third middle phalanx and the fourth proximal phalanx *(small arrows)*. **(D)** Axial CT scan of a right rib shows typical brown tumor as expansile lytic mass *(arrows)*. **(E)** Radiograph shows sharply marginated lucent lesions in the patella *(short arrows)* and anterior tibial cortex *(long arrows)* in a patient with hyperparathyroidism compatible with brown tumors. **(F)** Sagittal fat-suppressed T2-weighted MR image in the same patient as in E shows bright T2-weighted signal in the brown tumors *(arrows)*. The MR appearance of brown tumors varies with relative amounts of hemorrhage, cystic change, and fibrous tissue in the tumor. Note that no soft tissue mass is present.

- Prevalence is highest in primary hyperparathyroidism (up to 40%) but also occur in secondary hyperparathyroidism. Because secondary hyperparathyroidism is much more prevalent than primary hyperparathyroidism, most Brown tumors occur in secondary hyperparathyroidism.

- *Osteiits fibrosa cystica* is a combination of osteopenia, bone deformity, and Brown tumors and is a classic manifestation of chronic hyperparathyroidism (Fig. 13.37). Rarely seen nowadays due to earlier intervention.
- Tendon and ligament laxity and rupture (Fig. 13.38).

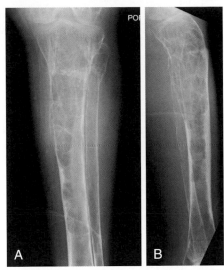

Fig. 13.37 Osteiits fibrosa cystica. AP and lateral radiographs of the leg show severe bone loss and multiple lucent brown tumors.

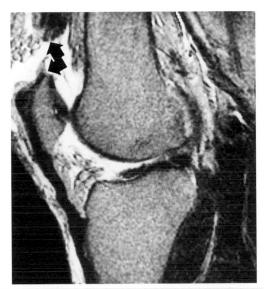

Fig. 13.38 Tendon rupture in hyperparathyroidism. Sagittal T2-weighted MR image of knee in a patient with primary hyperparathyroidism shows acute rupture of quadriceps tendon at patellar insertion *(arrows)*.

OSTEOMALACIA AND RICKETS

Vitamin D deficiency produces *osteomalacia* in adults and *rickets* in children.

Key Concepts

Osteomalacia

Vitamin D deficiency
Multiple causes that interfere with synthesis of the active form of vitamin D
Decreased mineral relative to osteoid matrix
Diminished bone density and pseudofractures (Looser zones)

Osteomalacia ('Soft Bones')

- Diminished bone mineral, with preserved osteoid.
- Generalized bone demineralization is a major feature.

- Contrast with hyperparathyroidism and osteoporosis: all cause diffuse loss of bone mineral that is visible on radiographs. Hyperparathyroidism and osteoporosis reduce bone mineral *and* bone osteoid matrix. Osteomalacia reduces mineral but with (relatively) preserved osteoid. This occurs in osteomalacia because of the loss of osteoblastic capacity to deposit hydroxyapatite crystals on the cartilaginous matrix. Thus, osteomalacia is a pathologically distinct disease.
- Causes: Any of these conditions in a mother may result in rickets in a newborn or infant:
  - Lack of dietary intake.
  - Lack of sunlight exposure: dark skin, cultural (body covered), seasonal.
  - Diminished gut absorption of vitamin D or of calcium, in malabsorption syndromes such as Crohn's disease, Celiac disease, or small bowel resection. Biliary disease also can reduce gut absorption.
  - Hepatocellular disease: interferes with 25 hydroxyl ation of vitamin D.
  - Renal disease: interferes with 1-hydroxylation of 25-vitamin D.
  - *X-linked hypophosphatemia.*
    - A form of *vitamin D–resistant rickets.*
    - Reduced production of 1,25-hydroxyvitamin D and phosphate reabsorption by the kidneys due to a genetic defect.
    - Results in decreased phosphate available for bone mineralization.
    - There is also an intrinsic defect in osteoblast function that further impairs bone production.
  - Receptor resistance to vitamin D action (rare).
  - Drugs such as phenytoin (Dilantin) and phenobarbital can interfere with vitamin D hydroxylation.
  - *Oncogenic osteomalacia* is caused by hormone production by a usually benign tumor that interferes with tubular reabsorption of phosphate (e.g., fibroblast factor 23).
    - Most of these tumors are small, benign, and asymptomatic.
    - Examples: hemangioma, nonossifying fibroma, giant cell tumor of bone, hemangiopericytoma, and phosphaturic mesenchymal tumor. The osteomalacia is cured by resection of the lesion.
    - Imaging diagnosis can be challenging. Octreotide scanning with PET or single-photon emission computed tomography (SPECT) finds some tumors. Whole body MRI is also used.
  - Oncogenic osteomalacia is rare.

Radiographic Features of Osteomalacia:

- *Generalized bone demineralization.*
- Radiographs: Osteomalacic bone appears lucent, coarsened, and smudgy (Fig. 13.39), which is probably caused by a mixture of decreased bone density and possibly radiographic density contributed by nonmineralized osteoid.
- *Looser zones*, or *pseudofractures*:
  - Highly specific for osteomalacia.
  - Linear foci of undermineralized osteoid at sites of mechanical loading (Fig. 13.40). Often bilateral and symmetric.

- Linear lucencies perpendicularly oriented to the cortex of the bone, with incomplete penetration of the full bone width.
- Usually occur along the concave (compressive) margins of the curvature of the bone.
  - In contrast with many stress fractures or pseudofractures of Paget's disease.

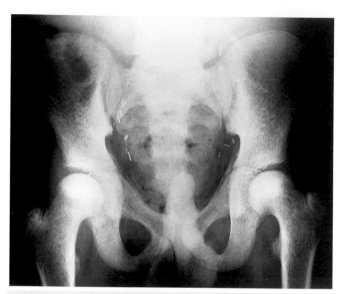

Fig. 13.39 AP radiograph shows diffuse bone demineralization and coarsened appearance of bone typical for osteomalacia.

- Characteristic locations of Looser zones include the medial aspects of the proximal femurs, the pubic bones, the dorsal aspect of the proximal ulnae, the distal parts of the scapulae, and the ribs.

Rickets

- Rickets is osteomalacia in the growing skeleton.
- Vitamin D deficiency in rickets reduces mineralization in the zone of provisional calcification at the physis. The disease is especially well demonstrated at sites of rapid bone growth, such as the proximal and distal femur, the proximal tibia, the proximal humerus, and the distal radius.

Radiographic Findings in Rickets

- Diminished mineralization and physeal cartilage overgrowth (wide physis) often with flaring of the metaphysis are classic findings (Fig. 13.41A).
- Rib ends: Flared rib bends create the *rachitic rosary* appearance (Fig. 13.40B).
- Generalized 'bone softening': femoral bowing, sometimes bizarre deformities after the onset of weight-bearing, which result from repeated insufficiency fractures (Fig. 13.41C). Severe cases may have short, squat bones that suggest a skeletal dysplasia.
- Salter–Harris I fractures (slipped capital femoral epiphyses), occur most commonly bilaterally at the hips.
- Correcting the metabolic deficiency will reverse the findings at the growth plates, although bone deformities frequently persist to some degree (Fig. 13.42).

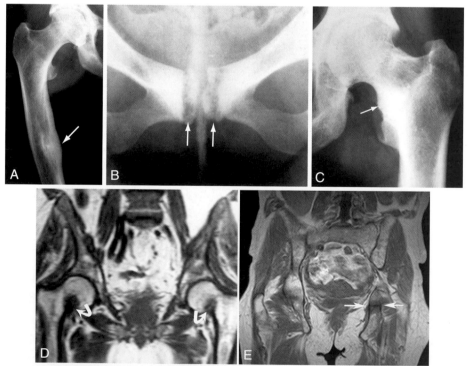

Fig. 13.40 Pseudofractures (Looser zones). **(A)** AP radiograph of femur shows typical appearance of pseudofracture as incomplete linear transverse lucency along the concave, or weight-bearing, aspect of the femur *(arrow)*. **(B)** AP radiograph of pelvis shows bilateral symmetric linear lucencies in the medial pubic bones *(arrows)* consistent with pseudofractures. **(C)** AP radiograph of the left femur shows ill-defined linear lucency at weight-bearing, medial margin of the basicervical femoral neck with surrounding sclerosis *(arrow)*. **(D)** Coronal T1-weighted MR image of hips in the same patient as in C shows bilateral, symmetric pseudofractures in the femoral necks. The broad zones of diminished signal *(arrows)* correlate with sclerosis on the radiographs. **(E)** Coronal T1-weighted MR image of the pelvis in a different patient shows Looser zone in the left ischium (between *arrows*).

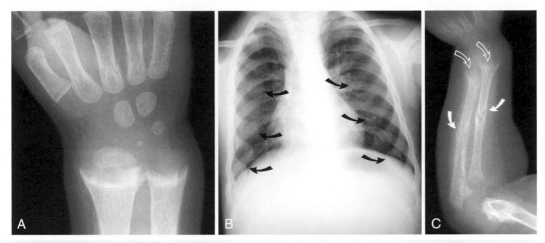

Fig. 13.41 Radiographic features of rickets. **(A)** PA radiograph of wrist shows widened physes, irregular zones of provisional calcification, and flaring of the metaphyses in distal radius and ulna. Note diffuse osteopenia and coarsened appearance of trabecular bone. **(B)** AP radiograph of chest shows rachitic rosary with diffuse bilateral costochondral enlargement *(arrows)*. **(C)** AP radiograph of the forearm shows radial and ulnar insufficiency fractures *(closed arrows)* associated with typical features of rickets. Note diffuse bone demineralization, coarsened trabeculae, flared metaphyses, and irregular margin of zones of provisional calcification *(open arrows)*.

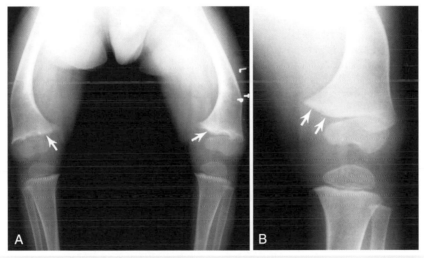

Fig. 13.42 Rickets before and after treatment. **(A)** AP radiograph of knees shows irregular contour of femoral metaphyseal zones of provisional calcification *(arrows)*, metaphyseal flaring, and varus deformity of distal femurs. **(B)** After treatment, AP radiograph of left knee shows narrowing of physes, restored smooth contour of distal femoral metaphyseal zones of provisional calcification *(arrows)*, and diminished metaphyseal flaring. Femoral varus deformity persists.

Key Concepts

Rickets

Rickets = osteomalacia in children
Wide physes (unmineralized zone of provisional calcification)
Metaphyseal irregularity, fraying; metaphyses may become dense with treatment
Leg bone bowing (other causes: congenital, Blount disease, neurofibromatosis type 1, osteogenesis imperfecta, achondroplasia)
Large rib ends (rachitic rosary)
Salter–Harris I fractures, slipped capital femoral epiphysis

Differential Diagnosis in Rickets

- *Schmid-type metaphyseal chondrodysplasia,* which looks similar to rickets, with growth plate widening, but this disease is caused by an inborn error in enchondral ossification. Laboratory values and bone mineralization are normal.

- *Hypophosphatasia,* in which bone is severely osteopenic, growth plates are wide, and multiple fractures are seen. However, in this disease serum alkaline phosphatase level is low, unlike other causes of rickets in which the enzyme level is elevated. This condition is rare.

RENAL OSTEODYSTROPHY

Key Concepts

Renal Osteodystrophy

Long-standing renal failure
Combined features of hyperparathyroidism and osteomalacia; one or the other may dominate
Increased bone density
Soft tissue calcification: vascular, tumoral calcinosis
Amyloidosis

Chronic renal failure results in complex hormonal and electrolyte imbalances and alterations in calcium homeostasis. The current conceptualization is *chronic kidney disease–mineral and bone disorder (CKD-MBD)*, which unifies the hormonal and serum calcium and phosphate alterations, osseous abnormalities, and soft tissue calcifications.

- Renal osteodystrophy is an essential part of this syndrome.
- The imaging findings in renal osteodystrophy variably include features of hyperparathyroidism, osteomalacia, and bone sclerosis (Figs. 13.43 and 13.44).

Renal osteodystrophy pathophysiology, simplified:

- Renal failure results in hyperphosphatemia and thus increased synthesis of PTH and decreased 1,25-hydroxyvitamin D production in the kidney.
- Diminished vitamin D production activates PTH synthesis.
- Thus, renal failure patients will experience both elevated PTH and diminished active vitamin D.
- The interaction of these various hormonal and metabolic imbalances (and other factors omitted in this simplified discussion) manifests differently in different patients, so the clinical and imaging findings are varied.
    - Some patients have a variation of renal osteodystrophy characterized by *high bone turnover*. In these patients, imaging findings of hyperparathyroidism are most evident. PTH, phosphate, and alkaline phosphate (a marker of bone turnover) are increased. Serum calcium is decreased.
    - Other patients have *low bone turnover* and normal parathyroid levels. Osteomalacia findings are dominant in these patients. PTH can be normal.
    - Many patients will have a combination of hyperparathyroid and osteomalacia findings on imaging studies.
- Also, elevated calcium–phosphate product results in calcium deposition in bone and soft tissues (curiously termed *metastatic calcification*), leading to increased bone density, extensive vascular calcification, and varied additional soft tissue calcification in many patients.
- Management is determined in part by the degree of bone turnover, mineralization, and osteoid percentage

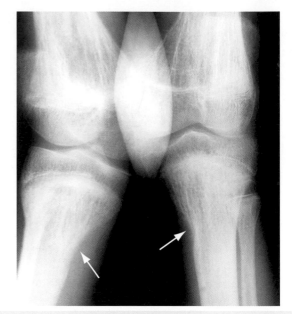

Fig. 13.43 AP radiograph of both knees in a boy with renal osteodystrophy shows combined features of osteomalacia and hyperparathyroidism. Note coarsened trabecular appearance typical of osteomalacia, and subperiosteal bone resorption in the concave cortex of the proximal tibias (*arrows*) typical of hyperparathyroidism. Genu valgum, as shown in this case, is often found in children with hyperparathyroidism.

of bone volume. As noted earlier, imaging findings can provide evidence of high or low bone turnover, but bone biopsy may be required for accurate evaluation of current status.

Historical note: Aluminum from hemodialysis and oral phosphate binders was another contributing factor to renal osteodystrophy in the past, but is no longer used.

Additional Morbidities

- *Dialysis-related amyloidosis* (DRA) can be seen in patients undergoing long-term dialysis. Beta-2 microglobulin is a normal cell surface antigen that is incompletely cleared by dialysis. Long-term dialysis leads to accumulation of beta-2-microglobulin that forms into amyloid fibrils. The amyloid is deposited in and around

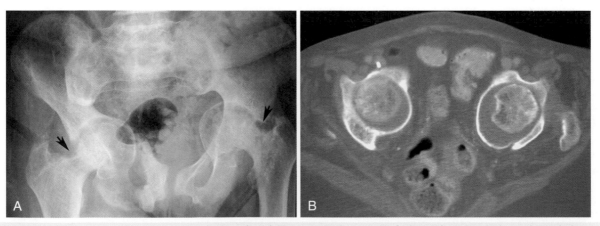

Fig. 13.44 Renal osteodystrophy. AP pelvis radiograph **(A)** and axial CT image **(B)** show severe findings of renal osteodystrophy, including protrusio acetabuli, sacroiliac and pubic symphysis subchondral bone resorption, bilateral femoral neck subperiosteal bone resorption (*arrows* in A), rugger jersey spine, right pubic insufficiency fractures, diffuse coarsening of trabeculae, and mixed pattern of increased and decreased bone density.

joints and intervertebral discs leading to imaging findings that can simulate infection (Fig. 13.45, see also Figs. 9.110, 9.111, and 9.112).

- ▪ Amyloid is discussed further in Chapter 9 – Arthritis.
- ■ Increased risk for osteomyelitis and septic arthritis because of chronic immune suppression.
- ■ Increased risk for AVN if on long-term steroid therapy.
- ■ Pathologic fractures and subchondral bone collapse in osteopenic bone.
- ■ *Calciphylaxis (calcific uremic arteriolopathy, CUA).*
  - ▪ Metastatic calcification in small arteries that supply the skin, followed by thrombosis for unknown reasons, with resulting skin necrosis. (recall that metastatic calcification = calcification due to high calcium–phosphate product, not malignancy).
  - ▪ Numerous associated risk factors include medications, diabetes, obesity, female sex, protein S or C deficiency, and others.
  - ▪ Despite the name, is not immune-mediated.

Renal Osteodystrophy Imaging Findings

Usually includes features of hyperparathyroidsim and osteomalacia, plus variable bone sclerosis:

- ■ Mixed bone density with areas of decreased bone density and osteosclerosis. Overall density often increased (see Box 13.2).

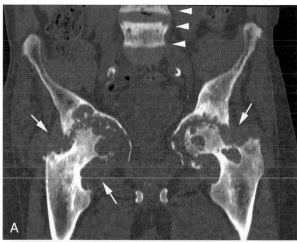

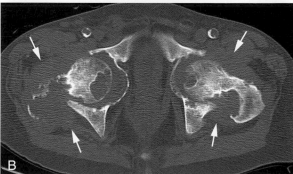

Fig. 13.45 Coronal **(A)** and axial **(B)** CT images in a patient with renal osteodystrophy show masslike amyloid deposition in both hip joints *(arrows)*. Note the large erosions in the femoral heads and left femoral neck due to the amyloid. Also note the rugger jersey spine *(arrowheads in A)*, protrusio acetabuli, and the enthesial bone resorption on the superior greater trochanters.

Box 13.2   Differential Diagnosis of Diffuse Increased Bone Density (Mnemonic: 3MsPROF)

Myelofibrosis
Mastocytosis
Metastatic disease, rarely myeloma
Sickle cell anemia
Paget's disease, pyknodysostosis
Renal osteodystrophy
Osteopetrosis
Fluorosis

- ■ Vertebral body endplate sclerosis: *rugger jersey spine.* ('Rugger' is British slang for rugby. The traditional rugby jersey has broad horizontal stripes.)
- ■ Extensive soft tissue calcifications:
  - ▪ Vascular calcifications, especially arterial.
  - ▪ Paraarticular accumulations of calcium–phosphate precipitates, which can occasionally take on a liquid form as *milk of calcium*; when massive and multicystic, these are referred to as *tumoral calcinosis* (Fig. 13.46).
- ■ Looser zones and other insufficiency fractures and can be found in addition to the classic features of hyperparathyroidism.

HYPOPARATHYROIDISM

- ■ Incapacity of the parathyroid glands to produce sufficient hormone for calcium homeostasis.
- ■ Occurs most commonly after parathyroid gland resection for hyperparathyroidism.
- ■ *Labs*: hypocalcemia and hyperphosphatemia.
- ■ Clinical manifestations: irritability, seizures, and tetany.
- ■ Imaging findings:
  - ▪ 'Metastatic' deposition of calcium phosphate salts, often in subcutaneous locations or the basal ganglia of the brain.
  - ▪ Osteosclerosis can be localized or generalized. Osteoporosis is rarely seen.

Pseudohypoparathyroidism

- ■ Target cell resistance to PTH.
  - ▪ Clinical features resemble hypoparathyroidism.
- ■ *Labs*: high serum levels of PTH.
- ■ These patients have a characteristic body type: they are short and obese, with short metacarpals and metatarsals, especially in the first, fourth, and fifth metatarsals (Fig. 13.47).
- ■ Short stature and short metacarpals are caused by early physeal closure.
- ■ Thick calvaria and intracranial and soft tissue calcifications can be seen. Also seen are unusual small osteochondromas, projecting at right angles to the shafts of the bones (see Fig. 13.47D).
- ■ Radiographic features are otherwise similar to those seen with hypoparathyroidism.

Pseudopseudohypoparathyroidism

- ■ Clinically and radiologically the same as pseudohypoparathyroidism.
- ■ *Labs*: serum hormone levels of PTH and calcium are normal.

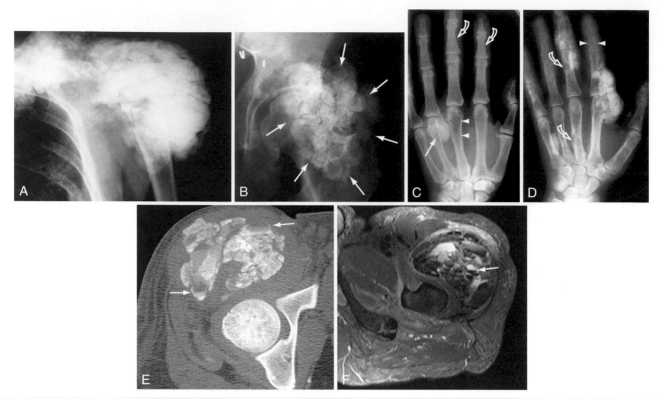

Fig. 13.46 Examples of tumoral calcinosis. **(A)** AP radiograph of the left shoulder demonstrates massive paraarticular soft tissue calcification caused by tumoral calcinosis. Note the diffuse demineralization of bone and multiple left rib fractures. **(B)** AP radiograph of the left hip shows multiple paraarticular calcifications *(arrows)* caused by tumoral calcinosis. **(C)** PA radiograph of the right hand shows soft tissue deposit of tumoral calcinosis *(closed arrow)* and features of hyperparathyroidism with diffuse demineralization of bone, subperiosteal bone resorption *(open arrows)*, and third metacarpal brown tumor *(arrowheads)*. **(D)** PA radiograph of the right hand shows multiple deposits of tumoral calcinosis, diffuse bone demineralization, third metacarpal and phalangeal brown tumors *(open arrows)*, and Looser zone in second middle phalanx *(arrowheads)*. **(E)** CT image of patient undergoing long-term dialysis who has tumoral calcinosis anterior to the right hip. Note the subtle layering within some of the calcium-filled cysts *(arrows)*. **(F)** Fat-suppressed T2-weighted MR image also shows fluid levels within loculations *(arrow)*. The dependent calcium has low signal on all sequences.

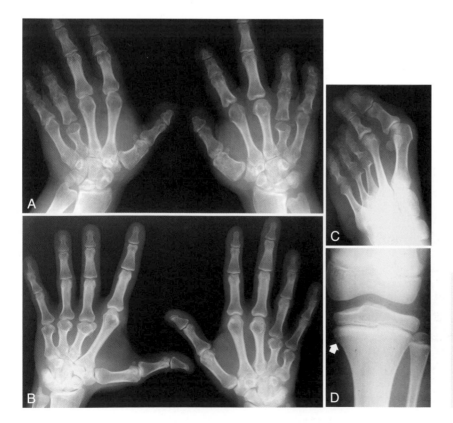

Fig. 13.47 Characteristic features of pseudohypo-parathyroidism. **(A)** PA radiograph of hands shows characteristic shortening and mild widening of multiple small tubular bones, particularly the first and fourth metacarpals in this patient. **(B)** PA radiograph of hands in another patient shows pronounced shortening of the right third through fifth and the left fourth and fifth metacarpal bones. **(C)** Frontal radiograph of foot shows third through fifth metatarsal shortening. **(D)** AP radiograph of knee shows tiny osteochondroma *(arrow)*.

Thyroid-Related Conditions

HYPOTHYROIDISM

- Adults: mild osteoporosis, soft tissue edema, and myopathy.
- Children: severe delay in skeletal maturity (Fig. 13.48A).
- Dental development is also severely delayed.
- Wormian bones (intrasutural ossicles).
- A *bullet-shaped vertebra* at the thoracolumbar junction (Fig. 13.48B).
- Epiphyseal fragmentation (which in the proximal femur can mimic Legg–Calvé–Perthes disease).

HYPERTHYROIDISM

- Increased bone turnover, decreased BMD.

THYROID ACROPACHY

- Rare sequela of treatment for thyrotoxicosis.
- Can manifest as prominent, fluffy, solid periosteal new bone deposition, particularly in the metacarpals/tarsals and phalanges in the hands and feet (Fig. 13.49).
- Also: clubbing and soft tissue swelling such as in the orbits (exophthalmos) and lower extremities (myxedema).

Additional Metabolic Conditions

SKELETAL FLUOROSIS

- Fluoride or compounds containing fluorine are ingested from ground water or other sources or inhaled. High

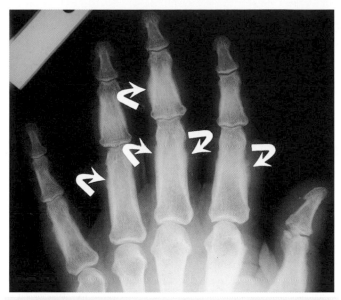

Fig. 13.49 PA radiograph of hand in woman with thyroid acropachy shows exuberant fluffy periosteal new bone formation *(curved arrows)* in the proximal and middle phalanges and generalized swelling of the fingers.

levels in ground water are common in many parts of the world.
- Fluoride is incorporated into bone. The resulting fluoride-containing salt is relatively insoluble and hard to remove, which interferes with normal bone turnover and normal calcium metabolism.
- Long-term toxic exposure can result in bones that are radiographically denser but are weaker (Fig. 13.50). Fracture risk is increased.

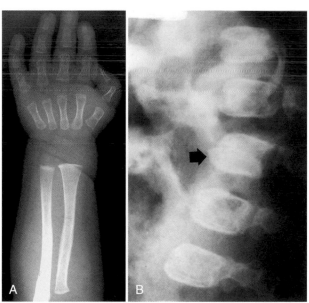

Fig. 13.48 Eleven-month-old girl with congenital hypothyroidism. **(A)** PA radiograph of hand and forearm shows severe delay in skeletal maturity, with complete absence of ossification of the carpal bones and epiphyses. **(B)** Lateral radiograph of thoracolumbar junction shows bullet-shaped vertebra *(arrow)* arising at a right angle from medial aspect of proximal tibial metaphysis.

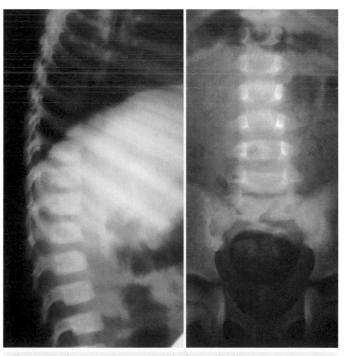

Fig. 13.50 Fluorosis. This 4-year-old African child lives in an area with elevated fluoride in drinking water. Note the diffusely increased bone density, best appreciated on the lateral radiographic view.

■ Soft tissue calcification, notably in connective tissues and along periosteum.

■ Impaired calcium metabolism can result in secondary hyperthyroidism.

■ *Dental fluorosis* is caused by milder exposure during early childhood. The teeth are mottled in appearance and highly resistant to caries.

HYPERVITAMINOSIS A

■ Cause: overingestion.

■ Children are especially vulnerable to vitamin A toxicity.

■ Increased bone turnover.

■ Elevated serum calcium, soft tissue calcification.

■ Periosteal new bone formation can be very prominent in (Fig. 13.51).

■ Findings may mimic Caffey disease (infantile cortical hyperostosis). However, the mandible is usually spared in hypervitaminosis A, whereas mandible periosteal new bone formation is a classic finding in Caffey.

■ In the spine, can mimic DISH and seronegative spondyloarthropathy.

■ Hepatosplenomegaly and jaundice due to liver toxicity.

■ Hydrocephalus in acute toxicity.

RETINOIDS

■ Retinoic acid derivatives are related to vitamin A and are used for treating acne and as a chemotherapeutic agent in neuroblastoma.

■ In children, bone growth and maturation are accelerated.

■ As with hypervitaminosis A, florid new bone formation in the spine may resemble DISH. With retinoids, this occurs most commonly in the cervical spine (Fig. 13.52).

■ Ligament and tendon calcification or ossification has been observed.

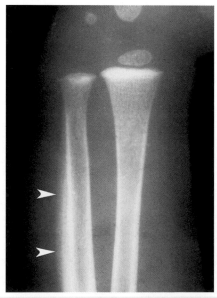

Fig. 13.51 Hypervitaminosis A. Note the solid periosteal new bone formation on the distal ulna *(arrowheads)*, which is a nonspecific finding. This child had been given excessive oral vitamin A.

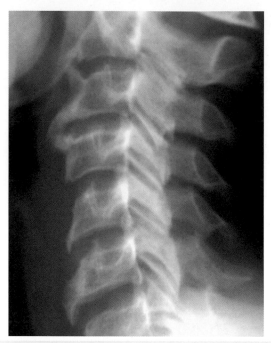

Fig. 13.52 Retinoid arthropathy. The lateral cervical spine in this 22-year-old man demonstrates prominent anterior osteophyte formation in the cervical spine, an incongruent finding in a patient of this age. He was using retinoids, which are vitamin A analogues, for a skin condition. (Image used with permission from BJ Manaster, MD, from the American College of Radiology Learning File.)

HYPERVITAMINOSIS D

■ *Labs*: hypercalcemia, hypercalciuria, and phosphaturia.

■ Causes:
  ■ Overingestion.
  ■ Occasionally granulomatous diseases such as sarcoid and, rarely, lymphoma are capable of extrarenal activation of vitamin D.

■ Imaging findings mostly are related to the hypercalcemia: soft tissue metastatic calcification, nephrolithiasis, and pancreatitis.

■ Generalized osteopenia may occur.

■ In children, the zone of provisional calcification widens, creating a dense transverse metaphyseal band.

HEAVY METAL POISONING

■ Several heavy metals, most notably lead, are osteoclast poisons that result in increased bone density and undertubulation in the metaphyses because of lack of normal remodeling.

■ *Dense metaphyseal bands* (Box 13.3) can also be seen physiologically in growing children, although their presence in non–weight-bearing long bones such as proximal fibula and distal ulna strongly suggests lead poisoning (Fig. 13.53).

■ Healing rickets can also cause dense metaphyseal bands. The clinical history, as well as other findings of rickets (e.g., metaphyseal widening), may help to make the correct diagnosis.

■ Rarer causes of dense metaphyseal bands include hypervitaminosis D, treated hypothyroidism, and, very rarely, scurvy.

Box 13.3 Dense Metaphyseal Bands (Partial Listing)

Heavy metal poisoning (e.g., lead)
Healing rickets or hyperparathyroidism
Treated leukemia
Trauma
Chemotherapy
Growth recovery lines (slender and sharply defined)
Normal variant in weight-bearing bones
Chronic anemia
Hypervitaminosis D
Osteopetrosis
Bisphosphonate therapy, e.g., for osteogenesis imperfecta

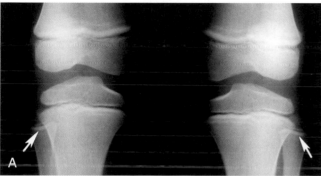

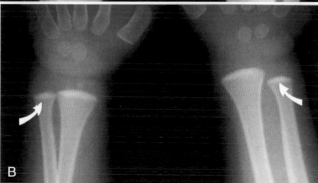

Fig. 13.53 Two patients with lead poisoning. **(A)** AP radiograph of knees shows multiple dense metaphyseal bands bilaterally in the femur, tibia, and fibula *(arrows)*. The presence of the increased density in the fibular metaphyses strongly suggests heavy metal poisoning. Note mild metaphyseal undertubulation. **(B)** AP radiograph of wrists shows dense metaphyseal bands in distal radius and ulna *(arrows)* bilaterally. The presence of the increased density in the distal ulnar metaphyses is highly suggestive of lead poisoning.

SCURVY

- Cause: low dietary intake of vitamin C.
- Vitamin C is required for collagen synthesis and therefore is needed for bone matrix (osteoid), cartilage, tendon, and ligament synthesis. Without the vitamin, production of collagen and thus bone production is diminished.
- Imaging: diffuse bone demineralization.
- Increased tendency toward insufficiency fracture.
- Children:
    - Extensive pronounced subperiosteal hemorrhage and subsequent periosteal ossification.
    - Decreased trabeculae cause the thin cortex of long bones to appear unusually well defined on radiographs.

- *Wimberger ring sign*, which is a sclerotic epiphyseal rim related to disorganized bone production at the epiphyseal ossification center. (Not to be confused with the *Wimberger sign* of multifocal metaphyseal destruction in congenital syphilis).
- *Frankel line*, which is a dense metaphyseal line adjacent to the physis.
- *Trummerfeld zone*, which is lucency proximal to the Frankel line.
- *Pelkan spur*, which extends distally from the metaphysis.
- The differential diagnosis includes congenital syphilis and neuroblastoma.

Hematologic Disorders

HEMOPHILIA

- A group of related bleeding disorders that result from clotting factor deficiencies.
- The two most common types of hemophilia, *hemophilia A* (factor VIII deficiency) and *hemophilia B* (factor IX deficiency, 'Christmas disease') are inherited X-linked recessive inheritance and therefore occur only in males.
- Musculoskeletal manifestations include hemarthroses, growth deformities, arthropathy, and tumorlike hematomas.

Key Concepts

Hemophilia

A group of related bleeding disorders that result from clotting factor deficiencies.
The two most common types of hemophilia, *hemophilia A* (factor VIII deficiency) and *hemophilia B* (factor IX deficiency, 'Christmas disease'), are inherited through an X-linked recessive pattern and therefore are only found in males.
Musculoskeletal manifestations include hemarthroses, growth deformity, arthropathy, and tumorlike hematomas.

Hemophilic Arthropathy

- May occur in several joints.
- Often asymmetric.
- Can be caused by trivial trauma.
- Most commonly involved joints: knee, elbow, and ankle.
- Less common: hip and shoulder.
- Multiple episodes of hemarthrosis result in hypertrophied synovium, which often contains hemosiderin deposits.
- Radiographs: increased density in joint soft tissues (see Fig. 13.54).
- MRI: hemarthrosis can have elevated T1 signal due to methemoglobin. Hemosiderin-laden synovium has low T1 signal, intermediate to low T2 signal intensity, and characteristic 'blooming' effect on gradient-echo imaging of very low signal intensity (see Fig. 13.56), similar to pigmented villonodular synovitis.
- Hemarthroses cause synovial inflammation, which in turn causes local hyperemia.

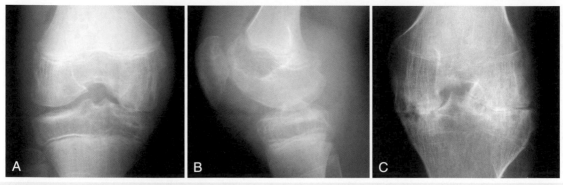

Fig. 13.54 Hemophilia. **(A** and **B)** AP and lateral radiographs of a knee in a 13-year-old boy with hemophilia show typical findings. Note the large dense effusion, enlarged and 'squared' epiphyses, large metaphyses, widened intercondylar notch, and subchondral erosions. Also note the relatively narrow physes, which are closing prematurely. **(C)** Typical progression of findings is seen in this 16-year-old boy. These findings are radiographically indistinguishable from juvenile idiopathic arthritis (JIA), but in these cases were bilateral (not shown), which is unusual for JIA.

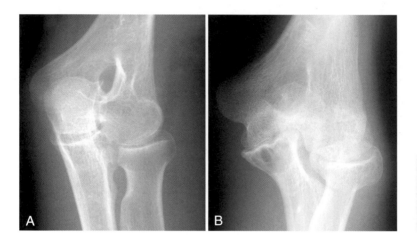

Fig. 13.55 Hemophilia: elbow. **(A)** Oblique radiograph of the elbow in an 18-year-old man demonstrates classic but mild changes of hemophilia, with a wide intercondylar notch, radial head overgrowth, and mild cartilage loss. **(B)** Similar but more severe changes in a 34-year-old man. Note the enlarged radial head and much more advanced erosive change.

- Findings related to hyperemia:
  - Local osteopenia.
  - Epiphyseal overgrowth. Flared metaphyses and enlarged ('balooned') epiphyses, with comparatively gracile (slender) diaphysis. Classic findings include enlarged radial head in the elbow, wide intercondylar notch in the knee (see Fig. 13.55; see also Fig. 13.54).
  - Accelerated growth.
  - Early physeal fusion (growth plate closure).
  - Articular cartilage destruction, with erosions and subarticular cysts caused by synovial inflammation (see Fig. 13.56).
  - Secondary degenerative arthritis.

JIA may have an identical pattern of overgrowth and destructive change, which is not surprising as both are caused by inflammatory synovitis in a growing skeleton. The two processes may not be distinguishable radiographically. Clinically, however, the two diseases are distinct.

Pseudotumor of Hemophilia

- Hematoma (interosseous, subperiosteal, or soft tissues), with bizarre MRI signal due to blood products.
- Can erode the surface of adjacent bone, may resemble an aggressive neoplasm.
- Femur, pelvis, tibia, and calcaneus most common locations.
- Caused by repeated bleeding in the same area.

- Radiographic patterns:
  - Extrinsic or intrinsic scalloping and pressure erosion at the cortical margin of an adjacent bone.
  - Bone destruction and expansile periosteal reaction that may be extensive, but margins are generally sharply circumscribed and become sclerotic during healing.
  - MRI appearance may be quite bizarre because of the presence of blood products of varying ages (Fig. 13.57). MRI may show a hypointense rim because of a fibrous capsule and hemosiderin deposits, whereas the central signal will vary according to the age of the hematoma and the presence of clot contained therein. Usually many different combinations of signal intensities are seen, reflecting the process of remote and recurrent bleeding as well as clot organization.

THALASSEMIA

- A group of inherited hemoglobinopathies that occur most commonly in individuals of Mediterranean heritage, but which also occur in persons of African descent.
- Most severe form is *thalassemia major* (*Cooley anemia*, β-thalassemia).
  - Autosomal recessive.
  - Clinically manifested early in life; death often occurs during childhood.

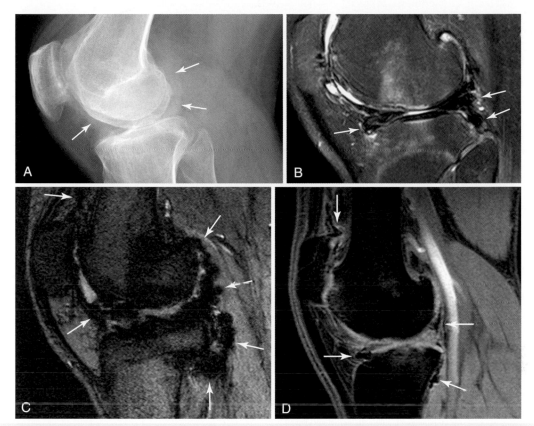

Fig. 13.56 Hemophilic arthropathy, chronic findings. **(A)** Lateral knee radiograph in a young adult with hemophilia demonstrates cartilage loss, irregular subchondral bone, and subtle high-density synovium *(arrows)*. **(B)** Sagittal fat-suppressed T2-weighted MR image in the same patient demonstrates similar findings. Note the very low signal synovium *(arrows)*. The findings resemble pigmented villonodular synovitis. **(C)** Gradient-echo sequence in the same patient shows the classic 'blooming' signal void caused by hemosiderin-laden macrophages in the synovium. **(D)** Sagittal fat-suppressed spoiled gradient-echo (SPGR) image in a different young adult with milder hemophilia. This patient had less hemosiderin in the synovium. The fast spin-echo sequences (not shown) did not show the synovial signal void seen in B, but it is seen on this image *(arrows)*. The vulnerability of gradient-echo sequences to susceptibility artifact caused by hemosiderin can be useful when searching for evidence of old or chronic hemorrhage.

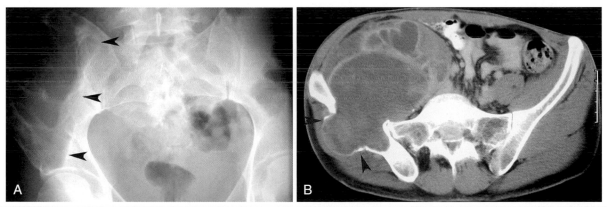

Fig. 13.57 Pseudotumor of hemophilia. **(A)** AP radiograph of the pelvis in a 35-year-old man demonstrates a well-defined lytic lesion in the right iliac wing *(arrowheads)*. There is pseudotrabeculation within the lesion and no matrix. **(B)** CT demonstrates the large soft tissue mass with heterogeneous attenuation, enhancing margin, and well-defined lytic margins. The CT scan shows no trabeculae within the mass. The radiograph appearance is because of the shell of expanded bone at the posterior margin of the pseudotumor *(arrowheads)*.

- Marrow hyperplasia with an expanded marrow space is the major radiographic feature and may be spectacular (Fig. 13.58).
- Skull: cranial diploic space is widened and may show dense striations with a hair-on-end appearance. Marrow expansion obliterates the paranasal sinuses, alters dentition, and causes hypertelorism.

- Appendicular skeleton: osteopenia and enlarged marrow cavities. The distal femurs may show an *Erlenmeyer flask deformity*, as with other marrow-packing disorders. Multiple transfusions lead to hemochromatosis, potentially with associated calcium pyrophosphate dihydrate arthropathy and marrow hemosiderosis (Box 13.4).

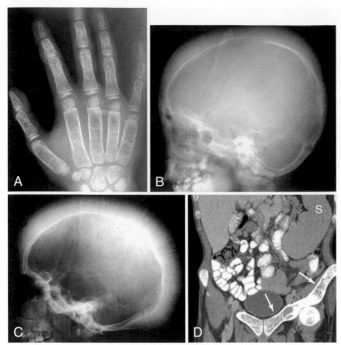

Fig. 13.58 Thalassemia major: marrow space expansion. **(A)** PA radiograph of a hand demonstrates diffuse osteopenia and widening and squaring of the metacarpals and phalanges. These features are seen in diseases where there is severe marrow hyperplasia with enlargement of the marrow space. **(B)** Skull shows widened diploic space and obliteration of the maxillary sinuses. **(C)** Similar findings in a different patient. Marrow expansion this profound is most often associated with thalassemia major. **(D)** Coronal CT reconstruction shows enlarged pubic bones *(arrows)* and spleen *(S)* related to increased hematopoiesis. (C, Image used with permission from BJ Manaster, MD, from the American College of Radiology Learning File.)

Box 13.4   Erlenmeyer Flask Deformity of the Distal Femurs

Expansion of the distal metaphysis with straight rather than
    concave contour
Storage diseases
    Gaucher disease
    Niemann–Pick disease
Some severe anemias such as sickle cell and thalassemia
A variety of skeletal dysplasias
    Notably Pyle disease, metaphyseal dysplasia that results in
        expanded metaphyses of the tubular bones, especially
        about the knee, with normal diaphyses.
Osteopetrosis
Achondroplasia
Osteoclast poisons, notably heavy metals such as lead, can cause
    failure of tubulation during skeletal growth, leaving a wide
    metaphysis.

- Milder forms of thalassemia have milder or absent radiologic manifestations.

SICKLE CELL ANEMIA

- Autosomal recessive inherited hemoglobinopathy found in 0.2% of African-American newborns and slightly less than 0.1% of Hispanic-American newborns.

- Hemoglobin can polymerize, deforming the red blood cell (RBC) and occluding microvasculature.
- Heterozygous protects against malaria.
- Hallmarks:
  - Anemia.
  - Bone and soft tissue infarcts.
- Increased risk of osteomyelitis (salmonella > staph, enteric Gram negatives).
- Imaging findings:
  - Related to chronic hemolytic anemia.
  - Increased bone marrow cellularity on MRI.
  - Hemosiderosis from multiple transfusions.
  - Related to microvascular occlusion created by sickled cells when exposed to low oxygen tension:
    - Bone infarcts (Figs. 13.59 and 13.60).
    - H-shaped endplate central vertebral endplate collapse (due to osteonecrosis, Fig. 13.61).

Dactylitis, also termed *hand-foot syndrome,* occurs in 10%–20% of young children with sickle cell disease, as early as the first year of life.

- Radiographs: periosteal reaction and soft tissue swelling (Fig. 13.62).
- Osteomyelitis, bone infarcts, and dactylitis can have overlapping clinical and radiographic features. MRI can be helpful, but sometimes radionuclide scanning with tagged leukocytes and/or biopsy are necessary.
- Diphosphonate bone scans often show diffusely increased tracer uptake, with focal 'hot spots' in healing infarcts or at regions of infection.
- Nonmusculoskeletal radiographic findings in sickle cell disease include renal papillary necrosis, cholelithiasis (red cell lysis leads to calcium bilirubinate caculi), splenic autoinfarction, cardiomegaly, stroke, and pulmonary infarction.

Sickle cell trait (one sickle cell gene and one normal gene) causes few musculoskeletal findings. Bone infarcts are occasionally seen.

Sickle Cell Hemoglobin C

- Heterozygous for both sickle cell disease and hemoglobin C.
- Marrow hyperplasia of the skull.
- Subchondral osteonecrosis. Metadiaphyseal bone infarcts are less common.
- Splenomegaly.

MASTOCYTOSIS

- Rare proliferative disorder of mast cells.
- Clinical manifestations may be limited to the skin (skin rash *urticaria pigmentosa*), usually without radiologic manifestation, or may be systemic. Systemic disease may result from a hyperplastic response to an unknown stimulus or may be an exceedingly rare variant of leukemia.
- Clinical findings related to histamine release include flushing, nausea, and vomiting.
- Marrow infiltration and histamine release by mast cells in the systemic form may result in generalized or localized osteoporosis, nonspecific lytic lesions, or focal or generalized sclerosis (Figs. 13.63 and 13.64).

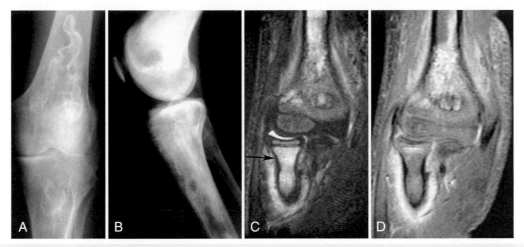

Fig. 13.59 Sickle cell disease: long-bone infarct. Bone infarcts can be seen either as a serpentine calcification **(A)** or as a generalized but patchy increase in bone density **(B)**. The latter is the more common appearance of bone infarct in patients with sickle cell anemia. **(C and D)** Coronal inversion recovery **(C)** and fat-suppressed postcontrast T1-weighted **(D)** MR images show acute bone infarcts in a child with sickle cell disease. Note the uniform marrow edema in the proximal radius *(arrow* in C), yet only minimal enhancement in D. Also note the intense periosteal edema and enhancement around the infarct. There are similar findings in the distal humeral metaphysis and diaphysis. These findings could represent infection, but in this case were acute infarcts. The classic serpentine double-line sign of avascular necrosis is not seen early in the process.

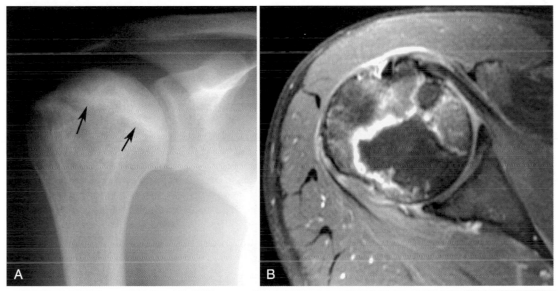

Fig. 13.60 Sickle cell disease: osteonecrosis. Avascular necrosis, particularly of the humeral head and femoral head, is a typical finding of sickle cell disease. **(A)** AP shoulder radiograph shows patchy sclerosis *(arrows)*. There is no collapse. **(B)** Axial T2-weighted MR image in a different patient shows the classic serpentine double-line sign of avascular necrosis.

- Treatment is guided by the clinical aggressiveness of the disease and includes histamine blockers. More aggressive forms are also treated with steroids and chemotherapy.

LEUKEMIA

- Heterogeneous group of neoplastic proliferation of leukocytes.
- The most common malignancy of childhood.
- Clinical presentation may include bone or joint pain (hip most often), which can be confused with juvenile rheumatoid arthritis.
- Imaging:
  - Hepatosplenomegaly.

- Marrow infiltration.
- Hemorrhage (because of low platelet counts).
- Opportunistic infections.
- Generalized osteoporosis is usually present.
- Cranial sutures may be widened.
- Metaphyseal lucencies.
- *Leukemic lines* are lucent transverse metaphyseal bands adjacent to the physis (Fig. 13.65). These usually occur in older children and are thought to represent disturbed endochondral ossification with diminished mineralization of new bone rather than erosion of bone by leukemic infiltration.
- Growth recovery lines related to remissions and chemotherapy cycles are often pronounced.

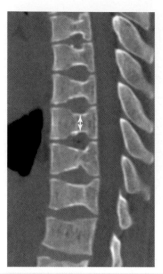

Fig. 13.61 Sickle cell: spine. Sagittal CT reformat demonstrates the classic central endplate collapse termed an *H-shaped vertebra (arrows)* at multiple levels. The sickled cells may sludge in the looping arcades at the end plates of the vertebral bodies, causing them to collapse in their central portion.

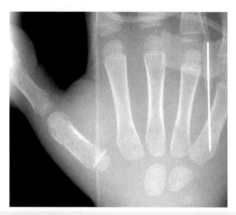

Fig. 13.62 Sickle cell dactylitis. Radiograph of the thumb in a 3-year-old girl with sickle cell disease and acute pain and swelling demonstrates subtle heterogeneous density and periosteal reaction in the first metacarpal. These findings could represent infection, but in this case represent the early changes of the bone infarct in this child with the clinical findings of hand-foot syndrome. (Image used with permission from BJ Manaster, MD, from the American College of Radiology Learning File.)

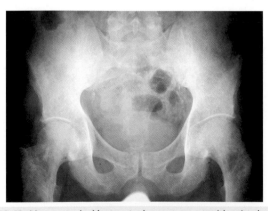

Fig. 13.63 Mastocytosis. Mastocytosis can present with mixed osteopenia and sclerosis, as in this 50-year-old man. The sclerosis can be either diffuse (as in this patient) or focal.

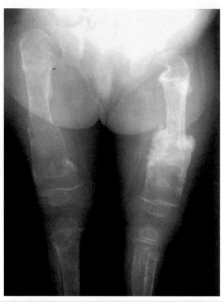

Fig. 13.64 Mastocytosis. Radiographic manifestations of mastocytosis include diffuse osteopenia, as seen in this 4-month-old child who has already sustained multiple fractures. (Image used with permission from BJ Manaster, MD, from the American College of Radiology Learning File.)

Paget's Disease of Bone

Paget's disease is not a metabolic disease per se, but it shares with many metabolic bone diseases a disturbance of osteoblast and osteoclast equilibrium.

First described as 'osteitis deformans' by Sir James Paget in 1877.

Paget's disease is a disease of osteoclasts. Normal osteoclasts are large and multinucleated. Osteoclasts in Paget's disease are larger and contain more nuclei than normal. These osteoclasts are activated, causing rapid osteolysis. The frantic osteoblastic response produces bone that is disordered and weak.

Key Concepts

Paget's Disease

Mechanism: Activated osteoclasts
Three sequential phases: Lytic, mixed lytic and sclerotic, and sclerotic

Imaging

Hallmarks: Bone expansion, cortical, and trabecular bone thickening
Leading edge of lytic phase: 'Blade-of-grass' = 'flame-shaped' margin; equivalent finding in skull: Osteoporosis circumscripta
Later phases: Spine: picture-frame vertebrae; skull: 'cotton wool' diploe

Complications

Osteoarthritis
Bone deformity ('bone softening'): Basilar skull invagination, insufficiency fractures, protrusio acetabuli, and proximal femoral varus
Cranial nerve palsies
Osteomyelitis
High-output cardiac failure possible in extensive disease
Malignant transformation (new-onset pain); look for new lytic lesion; poor prognosis
Giant cell tumors

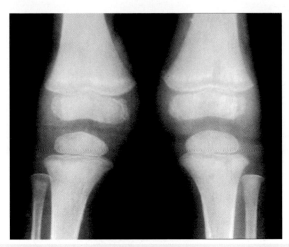

Fig. 13.65 Leukemic lines. AP radiograph of the knees in a child with acute myeloid leukemia shows lucent metaphyseal bands.

ASSOCIATIONS

- Genetic:
  - British ancestry.
  - Specific genetic mutations, some involved with osteoclast activity have been identified.
  - Slightly more common in men.
- Older age. Rare before 40.
- Environmental factors:
  - Slow virus infection has been hypothesized but not proven. Inclusion bodies resembling paramyxoviral inclusion bodies have been observed in pagetic osteoclasts. Canine distemper, respiratory syncytial, and measles virus have been proposed.
  - Disease prevalence and severity is decreasing and onset age is increasing. This might be related to improved sanitary conditions with decreased human exposure. However, this is speculation.
- Paget's disease manifests in three sequential, although often coexistent stages:
  - *Stage I: osteolytic phase*, also termed the *hot phase*. Rapid osteolysis.
  - *Stage II: mixed lytic and blastic phase*; corresponds to the onset of osteoblastic activation in response to osteoclastic bone resorption.
  - *Stage III: sclerotic phase*. Eventually a new equilibrium is established between bone production and bone lysis. The rapid, disordered bone resorption and production results in an abnormal, mosaic-like histologic appearance of osteoid and bone that is disordered and weak.
- *Labs*: Serum phosphorus and calcium levels usually are normal, but serum alkaline phosphatase and hydroxyproline are elevated, reflecting increased bone production and resorption, respectively.
- Most frequent sites of bone involvement: skull, spine, pelvis, femur, tibia, and humerus.

IMAGING OF PAGET'S DISEASE

Characteristic imaging findings of Paget's disease are demonstrated in Figures 13.66 through 13.72.

Stage 1:
- Long bones: usually begins at one end and extends roughly 1 cm per year, potentially eventually involving the entire bone. (Rarely, Paget's disease begins in the diaphysis; this occurs most frequently in the tibia.)
- The *leading edge* represents the osteolytic phase and usually has a sharply defined wedge-shaped margin between the normal and involved bone, a feature that is not characteristic of neoplasia (see Fig. 13.66). The long-bone leading-edge lysis is often described as having a '*flame-shaped*' or '*blade-of-grass*' appearance (see Fig. 13.67).
- Skull: The equivalent finding in the skull is termed *osteoporosis circumscripta*, which describes sharply marginated bone demineralization during the lytic phase of disease (see Fig. 13.68).

Stage 2:
- Following the lytic leading edge, mixed lytic, and sclerotic phase, disease develops in a frequently disorganized pattern.

Stage 3:
- Findings are often pathognomonic for Paget's disease: bone expansion, cortical thickening, and trabecular bone thickening or 'coarsening' (see Fig. 13.71).
- 'Picture-frame vertebra' in the spine (see Fig. 13.69A).

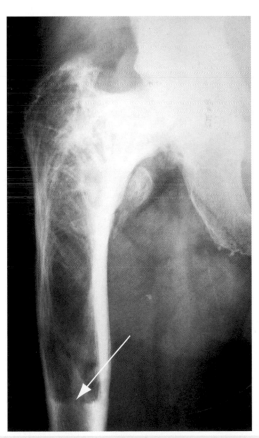

Fig. 13.66 Paget's disease. AP radiograph shows a sharp linear transition between pagetic and normal bone *(arrow)*. This finding is highly uncharacteristic of neoplasm. Moderate bone expansion, increased cortical thickness, and trabecular bone thickening assure the diagnosis of Paget's disease.

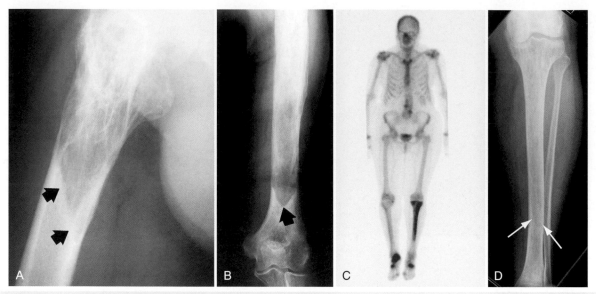

Fig. 13.67 Paget's disease, long bones: blade of grass. **(A)** Lateral radiograph of the right proximal femur shows the mixed lytic and sclerotic phase in the proximal aspect of pagetic bone and the lytic phase in the distal portion of pagetic bone. This indicates that the advancing front of Paget's disease is in the distal aspect of pagetic bone. The sharp, bladelike appearance of the margin between pagetic and normal bone *(arrows)* is shown, a feature that would be highly uncharacteristic for neoplasm. **(B)** AP view of the humerus in a different patient shows a flame-shaped distal margin of Paget's disease with an abrupt transition to normal bone *(arrow)*. Note the mixed phase of Paget's disease in the more proximal humerus, with bone expansion, cortical bone thickening, and trabecular bone thickening. At the flame-shaped margin, the appearance of Paget's disease is purely lytic. **(C)** Paget's disease discovered as an incidental finding on bone scan. Note the typical intense tracer uptake in the left tibia and right calcaneus related to hyperactive bone remodeling. Radiograph of this patient's tibia **(D)** shows findings similar to A and B, including flame-shaped leading edge *(arrows)*.

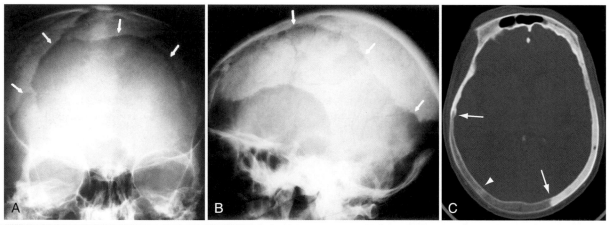

Fig. 13.68 Paget's disease, lytic phase, skull: osteoporosis circumscripta. AP **(A)** and lateral **(B)** skull films show a broad calvarial lytic region with sharp margins *(arrows)* between pagetic and normal bone in the acute, lytic phase of disease. **(C)** CT scan in a different patient shows a similar lucent region of Paget's disease *(arrowhead)* with characteristic sharp margins *(arrows)*.

- 'Cotton wool' in the skull (see Fig. 13.70).
- CT findings reflect those of radiographs, with trabecular thickening, mixed lysis, and sclerosis, depending on disease stage and bone expansion.
- Bone scanning: extremely hot in stages 1 and 2, hot in stage 3 (see Fig. 13.67C).
- MRI shows marrow signal that is highly heterogeneous and often bizarre and chaotic, with prominent areas of bright T2 signal being a common finding (see Fig. 13.68C and D). Fat signal is variably present but usually is prominent in chronic Paget's disease. Additional clues to the diagnosis are bone expansion, thickening of low-signal cortex and trabeculae, and bone deformity.
- Paget's disease may be asymptomatic.

Sample X-Ray Report

'Proximal half of the femur is expanded with cortical thickening and coarsened trabecula. Sharply marginated lucency is noted between the proximal femur and the normal-appearing distal femur. These findings are characteristic of Paget's disease. No fracture or concerning lytic lesion'.

PAGET'S DISEASE COMPLICATIONS

- Pagetic bone is 'soft' and prone to fracture and deformity (Fig. 13.73).
- Weight-bearing bones tend to deform in typical patterns.
  - Hip protrusio.

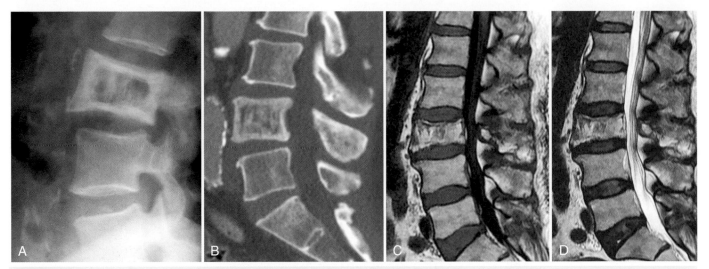

Fig. 13.69 Paget's disease, mixed and sclerotic phase, spine. **(A)** Lateral radiograph of the lumbar spine shows a picture-frame appearance of the L3 vertebral body. Note the increased density of the vertebral body, with greater density at the margins, trabecular bone thickening, and overall bone expansion. **(B)** CT sagittal reconstruction in a different patient shows similar findings. (C and D) Sagittal T1-weighted **(C)** and T2-weighted **(D)** MR images obtained in a different patient show typical highly heterogeneous marrow signal, with areas of increased T2 signal. Also note spinal stenosis caused by vertebral body and posterior element expansion and endplate deformity related to 'bone softening'. (A, Image used with permission from BJ Manaster, MD, from the American College of Radiology Learning File.)

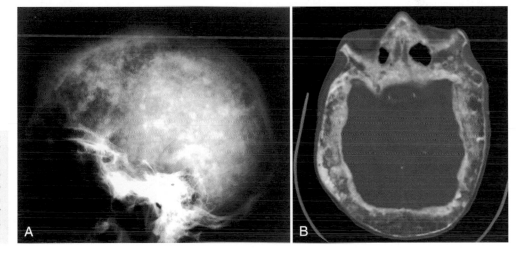

Fig. 13.70 Paget's disease, mixed lytic and sclerotic phase, "cotton wool" skull. **(A)** Lateral radiograph of the skull shows a cotton wool appearance due to the mixed lytic and sclerotic phase of Paget's disease. **(B)** Axial CT image in a different patient shows the patchy sclerosis, with thickening of the tables of the skull.

- ▪ Femur lateral bowing.
- ▪ Tibia anterior bowing.
- ■ Fractures of long bones generally begin as incomplete transverse fractures on the convex side of the bone, which often are multiple ('banana fracture', see Fig. 13.73A).
- ■ Within a joint, weakened subchondral bone leads to OA, which occurs in 50–96% of patients with Paget's disease (see Fig. 13.71A).
- ■ Basilar skull impression is common, occurring in one third of patients. Neurologic complications related to osseous expansion include sensorineural and conductive hearing loss and spinal stenosis.
- ■ Neoplastic transformation, most commonly osteosarcoma, occurs in less than 1% of patients with Paget's disease (Fig. 13.74). In the skull, however, giant cell tumor is the most common form of neoplastic transformation. *Paget's sarcoma* usually occurs in patients with widespread Paget's disease. New-onset pain in a

patient with Paget's disease should alert the clinician to the possibility of sarcomatous transformation. These are aggressive sarcomas and have a poor prognosis (11% 5-year survival).
- ■ Osteomyelitis is more common in patients with Paget's disease, related to the hypervascularity of affected bones and the subsequent increased risk of organisms such as *Staphylococcus aureus* seeding these areas.
- ■ Crystal deposition diseases such as gout and calcium pyrophosphate dihydrate deposition disease occur with greater frequency in patients with Paget's disease, possibly because of increased calcium mobilization in these patients.
- ■ Extramedullary hematopoiesis.
- ■ High-output cardiac failure is a rare complication, due to the high vascularity of pagetic bone. Occurs only with extensive disease, often with coexistent cardiac disease.
- ■ Osteoporosis is more commonly related to decreased weight-bearing and can occur rapidly due to the osteoclast activation.

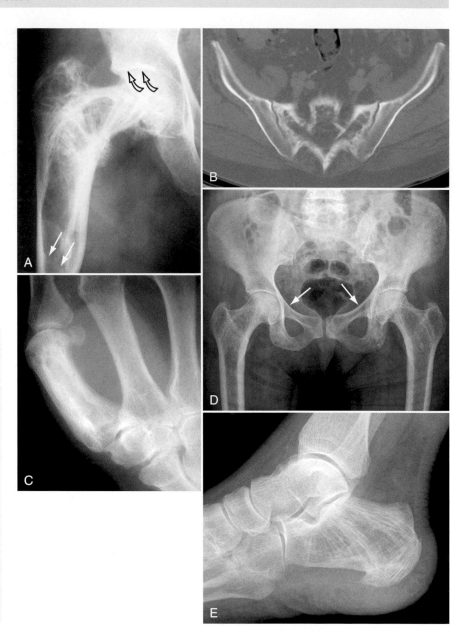

Fig. 13.71 The essential features of Paget's disease are bone expansion, cortical bone thickening, and trabecular bone thickening. **(A)** AP radiograph of the right hip shows bone expansion, cortical bone thickening, and trabecular bone thickening. Note also the abrupt transition to normal bone *(straight arrows)*. In addition, there is moderate osteoarthritis of the hip *(curved arrows)*, a common complication of Paget's disease adjacent to a joint. **(B)** Axial CT image of the pelvis shows sacral bone expansion, cortical bone thickening, and trabecular bone thickening. Symmetry may make the findings easy to overlook. **(C)** Paget's disease of thumb metacarpal; no matter what the bone, enlargement with trabecular thickening and mixed lysis and sclerosis should bring the diagnosis of Paget's disease to mind. **(D)** Subtle example of bilateral proximal femur and left hemipelvis Paget's disease. Note the thicker iliopubic cortex of the involved left pelvis compared with the normal right *(arrows)*. **(E)** Calcaneus. This is the same patient as in Fig. 13.67C. Any bone can be involved with Paget's disease, although fibular involvement for some reason is extremely rare.

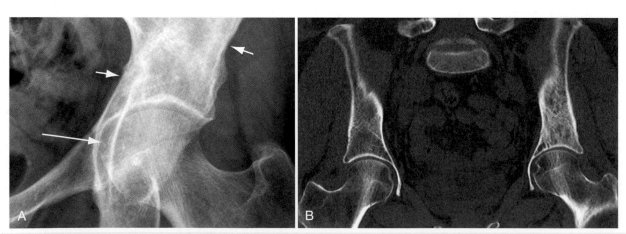

Fig. 13.72 Typical appearance of Paget's disease. **(A)** AP radiograph demonstrates mild expansion of the supraacetabular region of the pelvis *(short arrows)*. The normally lucent triangular region of the superior acetabulum is replaced by mixed lytic and sclerotic density. No distinct cortical thickening is seen, but there is protrusio of the acetabulum *(long arrow)*, typically seen in Paget's disease because the involved bone is softened and deforms with weight-bearing. **(B)** Coronal CT image of the same case shows the mild expansion of the left acetabulum relative to the normal right side, with the differences in bone density readily apparent.

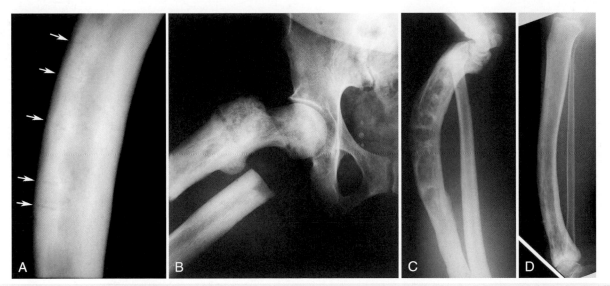

Fig. 13.73 Complications of Paget's disease. **(A)** Detail of a femur radiograph shows 'banana fractures' *(arrows)*, which are distraction insufficiency fractures on the convex side of a long bone curved by Paget's disease. **(B)** Frog-leg lateral radiograph of the right hip shows insufficiency fracture of the subtrochanteric femur and features of Paget's disease at and proximal to the fracture site. **(C)** Lateral radiograph of the left forearm shows substantial bone expansion in the radius associated with cortical and trabecular bone thickening, with angular deformity of the radius due to multiple healed insufficiency fractures. **(D)** Lateral radiograph of the leg shows Paget's disease of the distal tibia with anterior bowing. Note that the leading edge is well defined but subtler than the examples in Fig. 28.2. Also note the varus of the proximal femur in Fig. 13.71A, termed *shepherd's crook deformity*, which is a common deformity.

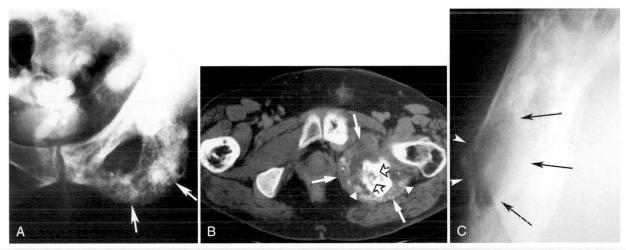

Fig. 13.74 Paget's sarcoma. **(A)** AP radiograph of left pelvis shows bone expansion, cortical bone thickening, and trabecular bone thickening in pubic bone, diagnostic for Paget's disease. In the ischium, however, there is an ill-defined mix of lysis and sclerosis *(arrows)* that is suspicious for sarcomatous transformation. **(B)** Axial CT image shows pagetic left ischium with cortical bone thickening and slight bone expansion. However, the ischium is surrounded by a large soft tissue mass *(closed arrows)* with associated fluffy matrix calcifications *(arrowheads)*. Similar calcifications are shown centrally in the ischium *(open arrows)*. The diagnosis at surgery was osteosarcoma with background of Paget's disease. **(C)** Sarcomatous transformation in a different patient. Proximal humerus radiograph shows Paget's disease and a lytic lesion *(arrows)* with lateral cortical destruction *(arrowheads)* that was a new finding. This was a high-grade osteosarcoma.

DIFFERENTIAL DIAGNOSIS

- Skull: hyperostosis frontalis interna, fibrous dysplasia.
- Long bones: findings are usually pathognomonic.

MANAGEMENT

- No cure.
- Bisphosphonates, which inhibit osteoclast-mediated bone resorption.
- Calcitonin is also used (second-line drug).

- Surgery for correction of complications. Bleeding during procedures such as hip arthroplasty is more common due to the high vascularity of pagetic bone.

Sources and Suggested Readings

Blomlie V, Rofstad E, Skjonsberg A, et al. Female pelvic bone marrow: serial MR imaging before, during, and after radiation therapy. *Radiology.* 1995;194:537–543.

Chan BY, Gill KG, Rebsamen SL, Nguyen JC. MR imaging of pediatric bone marrow. *Radiographics.* 2016;36:1911–1930.

Chan SS, Rosenberg ZS, Chan K, Capeci C. Subtrochanteric femoral fractures in patients receiving long-term alendronate therapy: imaging features. *AJR Am J Roentgenol*. 2010;194(6):1581–1586.

Chang CY, Rosenthal DI, Mitchell DM, et al. Imaging findings of metabolic bone disease. *Radiographics*. 2016;36:1871–1887.

Fidler JL, Murthy NS, Khosla S, et al. Comprehensive assessment of osteoporosis and bone fragility with CT colonography. *Radiology*. 2016;278: 172–180.

Guglielmi G, Muscarella S, Bazzocchi A. Integrated imaging approach to osteoporosis: state-of-the-art review and update. *Radiographics*. 2011;31:1343–1364.

Jang S, Graffy PM, Ziemlewicz TJ. Opportunistic osteoporosis screening at routine abdominal and thoracic CT: normative L1 trabecular attenuation values in more than 20000 adults. *Radiology*. 2019;291: 360–367.

Kopecky K, Braunstein E, Brandt K, et al. Apparent avascular necrosis of the hip: appearance and spontaneous resolution of MR findings of renal allograft recipients. *Radiology*. 1991;179:523–527.

Laor T, Jaramillo D. MR imaging insights into skeletal maturation: what is normal? *Radiology*. 2009;250:28–38.

Link TM. Osteoporosis imaging: state of the art and advanced imaging. *Radiology*.

Maclachlan J, Gough-Palmer A, Hargunani R, et al. Haemophilia imaging: a review. *Skeletal Radiol*. 2009;38(10):949–957.

Murphey MD, Foreman KL, Kalssen-Fischer MK. From the radiologic pathology archives imaging of osteonecrosis: radiologic-pathologic correlation. *Radiographics*. 2014;34:1003–1028.

Sidhu HS, Venkatanarasimha N, Bhatnagar G, et al. Imaging features of therapeutic drug-induced musculoskeletal abnormalities. *Radiographics*. 2012;32:105–127.

Stevens S, Moore S, Amylon M. Repopulation of marrow after transplantation: MR imaging with pathologic correlation. *Radiology*. 1990;175: 213–218.

Swischuck LE, Hayden CK. Rickets: a roentgenographic scheme for diagnosis. *Pediatr Radiol*. 1979;8:203–208.

14 *Musculoskeletal Infection*

Introduction

Infection can be one of the true musculoskeletal imaging emergencies. Infection is common, and radiologists should be familiar with its typical and atypical manifestations. Imaging appearance depends on the anatomic location, infecting organism, host response, and imaging modality used. Infection can mimic other conditions on imaging studies, so one should always consider the diagnosis as part of the differential for an unknown condition.

The musculoskeletal system can be contaminated by three principal routes:

- *Hematogenous.*
  - This is the most common mechanism of osteomyelitis in children and discitis-osteomyelitis in adults.
- *Contiguous spread.*
  - Example: Osteomyelitis and abscess near a decubitus ulcer in a bedridden patient.
- *Direct implantation.*
  - Example: Infection following penetrating injury such as a human bite.

Use of different imaging modalities in the setting of clinically suspected infection is somewhat flexible and varies with the specific situation as well as local expertise and scanner availability. Therefore, use of imaging modalities will be incorporated into each section of this chapter when relevant.

This chapter first reviews bacterial musculoskeletal infections, which are the most common in the developed world.

Musculoskeletal infection with non bacterial 'atypical' organisms is reviewed later in the chapter. Awareness of both types of infection is essential knowledge for practicing radiologists.

Types of Bacterial Infection and Imaging Findings

CELLULITIS

- *Cellulitis* is acute infection of the dermis and subcutaneous tissues.

Imaging Characteristics

- Radiographs, computed tomography (CT):
  - Skin thickening and subcutaneous fat edema.
  - Radiographs may show poor definition of the muscle–subcutaneous fat interface.
- Magnetic resonance imaging (MRI):
  - Classic findings: Edema and uniform mild enhancement in the infected subcutaneous fat, without abscess.
  - Edema is highly sensitive for cellulitis but not specific.
  - Uniform mild enhancement is more specific.
  - T1 signal loss within fat, while not always present, can be highly specific for infection:
    - Some infections, whether in soft tissue or bone, can result in metabolization of fat by certain organisms, with reduced T1 signal.

- A combination of low T1 signal, high T2 signal, and enhancement within fat (be it subcutaneous fat or marrow fat) in an appropriate clinical setting is specific for infection (Fig. 14.1).
  - Because it takes some time for this fat metabolism to occur, in the early stages of infection (in both cellulitis and osteomyelitis), T1 signal may be normal or only minimally decreased. Note that absence of loss of fat signal does not exclude infection as many infectious organisms do not metabolize or dissolve fat.
- Edema without enhancement:
  - Noninflammatory edema, for example dependent edema or bland edema without infection, demonstrates no more enhancement than the surrounding tissues, even when the edema is extensive.
  - Alternatively, soft tissue devitalization (early necrosis) shows no enhancement; this is important because these regions will not be effectively treated with antibiotic therapy (Fig. 14.2). These regions are often sharply demarcated, often (but not always) edematous, and surrounded by intense enhancement.
- Contrast enhancement is also useful on MRI to identify abscesses and sinus tracts that characteristically rim-enhance, and to assess for inflammation in muscle and fascia.

ABSCESS

- An *abscess* is a localized collection of necrotic tissue, inflammatory cells, and neutrophils, walled off by a highly vascular and typically irregular inflammatory pseudocapsule.
- Surrounding soft tissue edema and enhancement can vary widely from none or little to extensive. This variation reflects both infectious agent virulence and host response, which are usually but not always concordant.
- Solid or complex inflammatory tissue prior to liquefaction is referred to as a *phlegmon*, seen as a focal inflammatory region of the subcutaneous or deep soft tissues with mass effect but without a discrete, nonenhancing fluid collection.

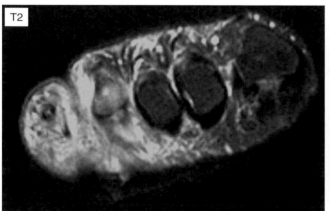

Diffuse edema on T2; inflammatory tissue is obscured

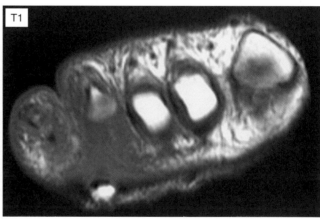

Replacement of subcutaneous fat signal on T1

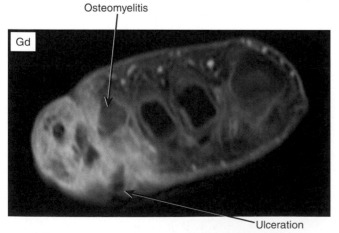

Contrast uptake delineates region of inflammation

Fig. 14.1 Cellulitis of the forefoot on MRI. Cellulitis replaces fat signal on T1-weighted images, with edema on fluid-sensitive sequences and enhancement of the inflamed region following gadolinium-based contrast administration. Postcontrast images better define the inflammatory tissue compared to the fluid sequences. (From Morrison W. *Problem Solving in Musculoskeletal Imaging.* Philadelphia: Elsevier; 2010.)

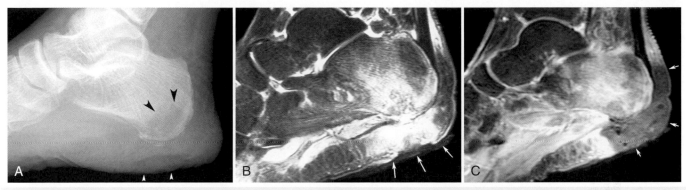

Fig. 14.2 Diabetic patient with plantar heel ulcer. **(A)** Lateral radiograph of the calcaneus shows plantar ulcer *(small white arrowheads)*, bone loss in the adjacent calcaneus *(black arrowheads)*, and destruction of the adjacent cortex. Sagittal fat-suppressed T2-weighted **(B)** and fat-suppressed contrast-enhanced T1-weighted **(C)** MR images show intense marrow edema and enhancement in the posterior calcaneus. T1-weighted images (not shown) showed low signal intensity, also consistent with osteomyelitis. Also note lack of soft tissue enhancement plantar and posterior to the calcaneus *(arrows in C)* that is more extensive than the pus and edema in and around the plantar ulcer *(arrows in B)*. This was devitalized tissue, not yet liquefied, that was debrided at surgery.

- With maturation, the infected tissue undergoes necrosis and liquefaction, thus becoming a mature abscess, with a peripheral hypercellular and hypervascular zone, particularly in the acute phase.

Imaging Characteristics

- On MRI, abscess collections typically show fluid signal on T2-weighted or short-tau inversion recovery (STIR) images with a variable surrounding degree of adjacent soft tissue edema. This edema may be quite intense, and the abscess may blend with surrounding tissue inflammation.
  - On MRI, abscesses may have variable signal related to hemorrhagic and proteinaceous contents.
  - The central cavity of an abscess is typically iso- or hypointense on T1-weighted images (to muscle) and may not be apparent since signal can be similar to that of adjacent cellulitis or muscle.
    - The abscess cavity has high signal on diffusion weighted imaging (DWI) MRI sequences due to the restricted diffusion in pus.
  - The abscess margin is composed of hypervascular inflammatory tissue that is seen on MRI as a thick rind of enhancement following intravenous contrast administration. Abscess wall margins may be smooth or irregular. The central portion does not enhance, making the abscess cavity conspicuous on fat-suppressed postcontrast images (Figs. 14.3 and 14.4).
  - The multiplanar capability of MRI and soft tissue contrast make it the ideal modality in planning prior to surgery or percutaneous drainage.
  - A potential mimic of phlegmon and abscess on MRI is the early phases of heterotopic ossification and myositis ossificans, as seen in spinal cord injury and following trauma or surgery.
    - These lesions are also often T2 hyperintense and rim-enhance after gadolinium-based administration.
    - CT is helpful for detecting subtle marginal calcifications seen in early heterotopic ossification (Fig 14.5).

- Contrast-enhanced CT is an alternative to MRI for abscess detection and evaluation.
  - CT with contrast can delineate rim-enhancement at the margins of the abscess; this appearance is similar to that on contrast-enhanced MR images, but often less conspicuous.
  - Without contrast, an abscess may be only faintly visible or isodense on CT with standard soft tissue windows. Adjusting window and level settings to increase contrast can improve detection.
- Ultrasound (US) is excellent for detection of more superficial fluid collections, and color and power Doppler can identify the hyperemia of the pseudocapsule and surrounding tissues that results in rim-enhancement on other modalities.
- As noted previously, US is the modality of choice for image-guided aspiration of superficial abscesses.
  - However, US is limited compared to contrast-enhanced MRI and CT in evaluating deep abscesses and in larger patients.
- A careful search for abscess is warranted in paralyzed patients who might be scanned for some unrelated reason, as these patients are at increased risk of decubitus ulcers and abscess formation.
- Sinus tracts and abscesses that communicate with the skin may also fill with air, and portions may be visible based on this finding.

PYOMYOSITIS

- Pyomyositis = bacterial muscle infection (Fig. 14.6).
- Occurs mainly in the lower extremities, particularly the thigh, and is often multifocal.
- Usually via contiguous spread: for example, adjacent cellulitis.
- Hematogenous muscle infection is uncommon, but contiguous spread as a cause is common. Example: psoas abscesses from discitis-osteomyelitis via small communicating veins.
- Pyomyositis also may be caused by penetrating injury.

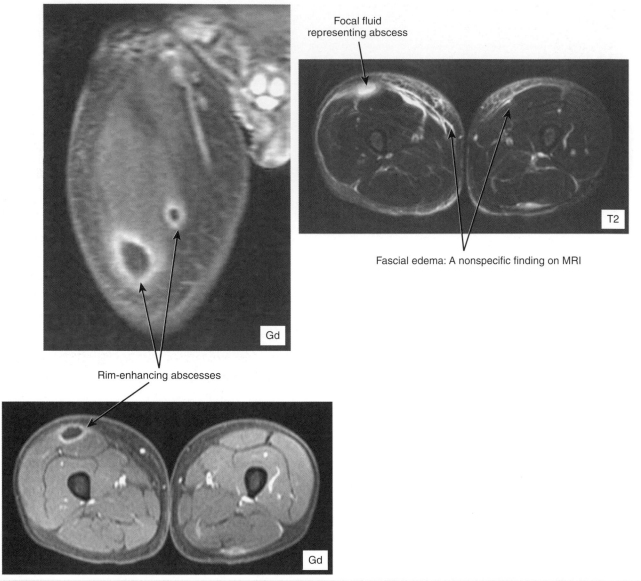

Focal fluid
representing abscess

T2

Fascial edema: A nonspecific finding on MRI

Gd

Rim-enhancing abscesses

Gd

Fig. 14.3 Soft tissue abscesses related to hematogenous spread in a patient with endocarditis. Postcontrast MR images (on left) show rim-enhancement of the collections. T2-weighted image (upper right) shows fluid collection and fascial edema (which can be reactive, not necessarily representing infectious fasciitis). (From Morrison W. *Problem Solving in Musculoskeletal Imaging.* Philadelphia: Elsevier; 2010.)

- In the past was unusual outside of the tropics (*tropical pyomyositis* or 'myositis tropicans').
- Pyomyositis incidence has increased in temperate climates due to immunosuppression (e.g., organ transplantation, bone marrow transplantation, chemotherapy), methicillin-resistant *Staphylococcus aureus* (MRSA), and intravenous drug abuse.
- Muscle injury (for example, due to trauma or rhabdomyolysis) is also a risk factor.

Imaging Characteristics

- Radiographs and noncontrast CT may show only nonspecific soft tissue swelling and obscured tissue planes due to edema.
- US can show hypoechogenicity within the affected muscle diffusely, with fluid collection(s) if abscess(es) is/are present (see Fig. 14.4). Doppler evaluation is useful to show hyperemia.

- MRI is highly sensitive, with hyperintensity on fluid-sensitive (fat-suppressed T2-weighted or STIR) images, initially diffuse.
  - On T1-weighted images the muscle may appear enlarged and intramuscular fat (when present) may become effaced, though signal may appear relatively normal.
  - Perifascial edema may be seen on T1- and T2-weighted sequences.
  - Postcontrast images show diffuse enhancement in the early stages and help separate this process from other entities such as diabetic myonecrosis (which resembles abscesses). However, in later stages superimposed necrosis may also occur, resulting in heterogeneous enhancement.
  - With disease progression, more focal fluid collections representing abscesses may become evident. Postcontrast images demonstrate rim-enhancement around abscesses.

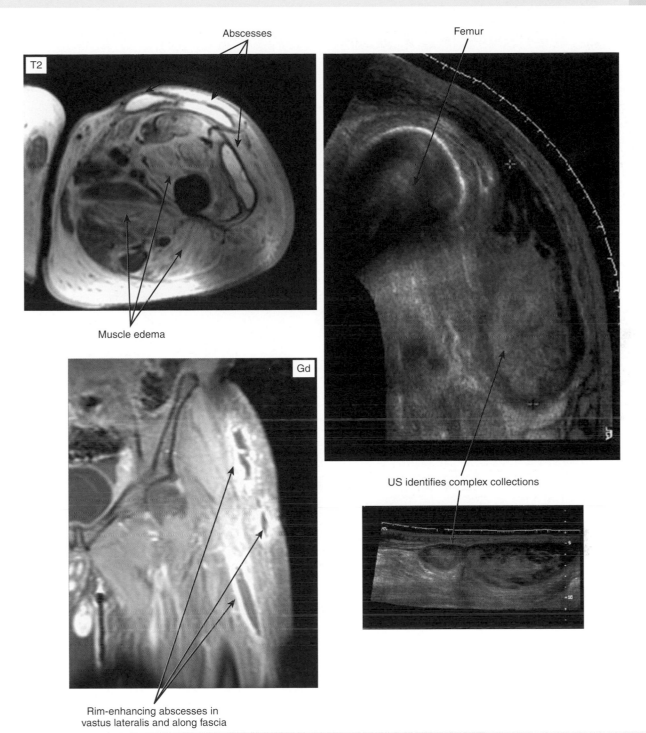

Fig. 14.4 Soft tissue abscess of the thigh on MRI and US. MRI shows complex fluid signal on T2-weighted images (upper left) with thick, irregular rim-enhancement on post-contrast images (lower left). US (on right) shows a localized collection with internal complexity. (From Morrison W. *Problem Solving in Musculoskeletal Imaging.* Philadelphia: Elsevier; 2010.)

- Areas of abscess and necrosis often require debridement. Contrast-enhanced sequences on MRI or contrast-enhanced CT can provide the surgeon with a road map for treatment.

Note: Muscle edema on MRI is nonspecific, with many differential diagnostic possibilities including overuse injury, contusion, denervation, rhabdomyolysis, infarction, diabetic myonecrosis, autoimmune myositis, and tumor. Therefore, clinical correlation is essential.

INFECTIOUS FASCIITIS

- *Infectious fasciitis* varies in severity depending on the organisms and immune response.
  - MRI:
    - Very sensitive for evaluation of fascial inflammation.
    - Also look for edema and fluid collections in adjacent tissues including subcutaneous fat and skin, which are evidence of a more severe infection.

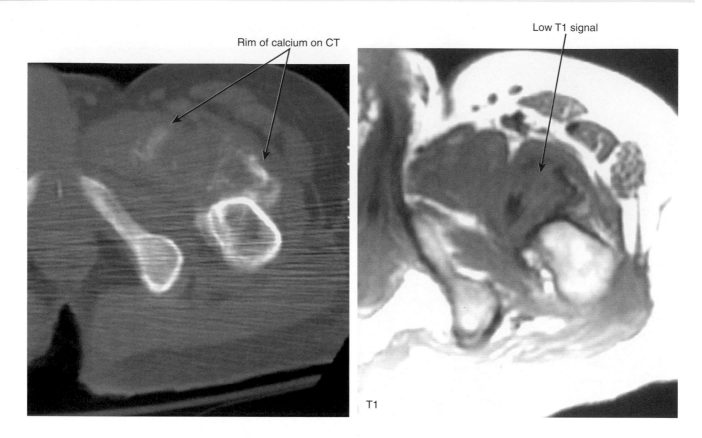

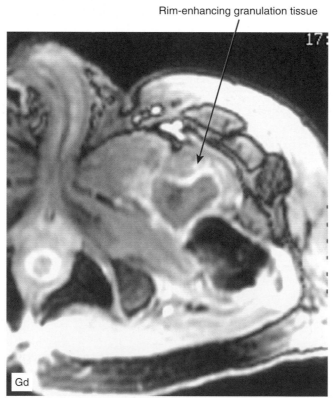

Fig. 14.5 Early heterotopic ossification simulating soft tissue abscess with rim-enhancement on post-contrast MRI (lower image). CT (upper left) shows marginal calcification corresponding to low T1 signal on MRI (upper right). (From Morrison W. *Problem Solving in Musculoskeletal Imaging*. Philadelphia: Elsevier; 2010.)

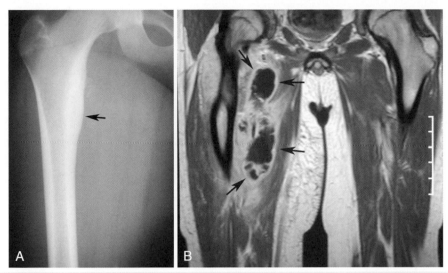

Fig. 14.6 Soft tissue infection. **(A)** AP radiograph of the thigh in a 16-year-old patient who had reported pain for 6 months. The radiograph demonstrates diffuse soft tissue swelling and thick, solid periosteal new bone formation in the medial subtrochanteric femur *(arrow)*. **(B)** Coronal T1-weighted MR image following intravenous administration of gadolinium-based contrast demonstrates a multiloculated intramuscular abscess with thick enhancing rim and adjacent edema *(arrows)*. The underlying bone was normal with the exception of thick cortical reaction as is seen on the radiograph. This is the usual appearance of a soft tissue abscess, but the bone reaction is more exaggerated than usually is seen because the condition had been present for so long.

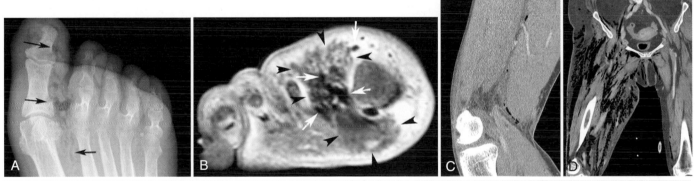

Fig. 14.7 Soft tissue gas/air associated with necrotizing infection. **(A)** Frontal radiograph of the foot of a diabetic patient shows mottled air density centered between the first and second metatarsal heads, extending into the lateral first toe *(arrows)*. **(B)** Short-axis fat-suppressed contrast-enhanced T1-weighted MR image through the metatarsal heads shows the air as signal voids *(white arrows)* within a nonenhancing area of necrosis *(black arrowheads)*. In a diabetic patient with ulceration, soft tissue air is common due to communication with necrotic areas. **(C)** Subtle gas along tissue planes in another patient with necrotizing infection. **(D)** Extensive soft tissue gas related to a gas-forming organism in a different patient with florid necrotizing fasciitis.

- Can demonstrate the extent of infection and presence of underlying abscess, septic arthritis, and osteomyelitis.
- *Necrotizing fasciitis* is the most severe form and caused by aggressive, toxin-producing bacteria.
  - Most cases are polymicrobial in patients with diabetes or other immune compromise.
  - This is a true surgical emergency, requiring immediate debridement, decompression, and aggressive antibiotic therapy.
  - The patient may go directly to surgery without delay for imaging.
  - Fascial gas is a specific finding, best detected with CT followed by radiographs (Figs. 14.7 through 14.9). Gas can be subtle on MRI.
    - *Gas may not be present and the absence of fascial gas does not exclude necrotizing fasciitis!.*

- CT or MRI with contrast can demonstrate enhancement and/or fluid along fascial planes, myonecrosis, and necrosis and liquefaction of adjacent fat.
  - IV contrast may be contraindicated if rhabdomyolysis is present.
- Note that fascial edema as an isolated finding is not specific for clinically aggressive fascial infection (Fig. 14.10).
- Also note that not all soft tissue gas is a sign of infection with a gas-forming organism or infectious fasciitis.
  - A skin ulcer can allow air to penetrate through sinus tracts into areas of necrosis.
  - Other potential causes of fascial gas include recent arthroplasty (especially hip), and air leak in intubated patients (especially neck, pectoralis muscles), and penetrating injury.

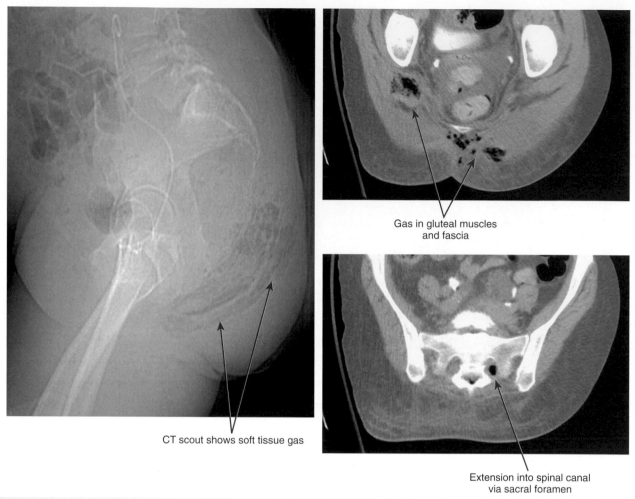

CT scout shows soft tissue gas

Gas in gluteal muscles
and fascia

Extension into spinal canal
via sacral foramen

Fig. 14.8 Necrotizing fasciitis of the buttocks on CT. Scout image (left) and axial images (right) nicely demonstrate gas in the soft tissues, in this case related to infection by a gas-forming organism. Under pressure, the infection can spread rapidly along fascial planes. (From Morrison W. *Problem Solving in Musculoskeletal Imaging.* Philadelphia: Elsevier; 2010.)

SEPTIC BURSITIS

- Bursitis due to infection.
  - As opposed to other causes such as trauma or crystal deposition disease.
- Imaging studies show synovial inflammation, usually with bursal effusion. Septic bursitis shares many features with septic arthritis, discussed in the following section.
- Radiographs: Focal soft tissue swelling in the region of an anatomic bursa or over a bony prominence may indicate septic bursitis.
- Ultrasonography (US) and MRI: Synovial thickening and hyperemia, often with effusion and adjacent soft tissue edema.

SEPTIC ARTHRITIS

- *Septic arthritis* is infection of a joint.
- Usually hematogenous spread.
- Pathogens:
  - *Staphylococcus aureus* is the most common pathogen overall.
  - Gonorrhea is the most common cause in younger, sexually active patients.

- Multiple other pathogens.
- Increasing incidence with greater use of immunosuppressive drugs, IV drug abuse, arthroplasties, and in elderly patients.
- Frequently coexists with adjacent osteomyelitis in children up to about 18 months.
- Joint effusion is a hallmark of septic arthritis, and usually the initial manifestation.
- Synovial inflammation causes hyperemia. In general, hyperemia causes 'rarefaction' of adjacent bone, that is, bone demineralization with decreased density on radiographs and CT. The corresponding finding on MRI is subchondral marrow edema (Figs. 14.11 through 14.13).
- Joint infection also causes pannus (inflamed, thickened synovium). Erosions begin at the margins of the joint, similar to rheumatoid arthritis, but as the infection progresses frank destruction of the articular surfaces may occur (Figs. 14.14 and 14.15).
- Chondrolytic enzymes are released by activated neutrophils and *S. aureus.* Associated articular cartilage destruction can be rapid and eventually results in joint space narrowing, radiographically visible in later stages.

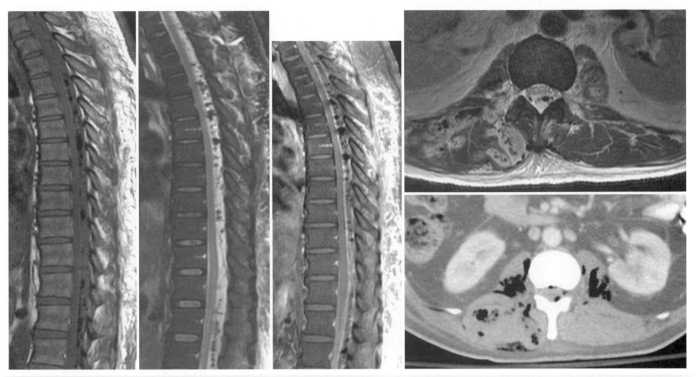

Fig. 14.9 Necrotizing infection involving the epidural space. MRI (upper row, left to right: T1, T2 and post-contrast) show foci of low signal in the epidural space representing gas, with diffuse edema and enhancement of the dura consistent with infection. Axial images (lower row: T2-weighted MRI on left, contrast-enhanced CT on right) show gas extending along the paraspinal musculature and within the epidural space. (From Morrison W. *Problem Solving in Musculoskeletal Imaging* Philadelphia: Elsevier; 2010.)

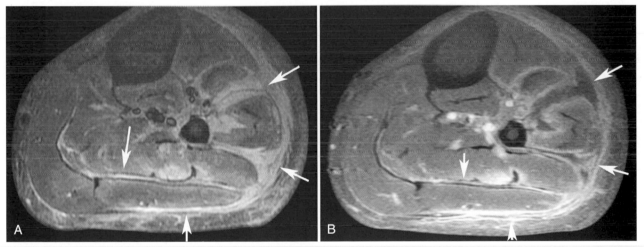

Fig. 14.10 Infectious fasciitis. Axial inversion recovery **(A)** and fat-suppressed contrast-enhanced T1-weighted **(B)** MR images show edema, fluid, and enhancement along fascial planes *(arrows)* of the lateral and posterior leg.

- Gonococcal arthritis is less pyogenic, so cartilage loss occurs much less quickly.
- Late changes include findings related to secondary osteomyelitis, including frank destruction of bone, and adjacent thick, smooth periosteal reaction.
- US is excellent for depiction of joint effusion with color or power Doppler showing synovial and adjacent soft tissue hyperemia.
- MRI typically shows a complex joint effusion.
  - Complex fluid is also a characteristic of other inflammatory but noninfectious arthropathies such as

rheumatoid arthritis, gout, psoriasis, and to a lesser degree even osteoarthritis, and unless clinical information is available, it may be impossible to determine the cause.
- Whenever a monoarticular arthropathy is encountered, infection should be excluded.
- The thickened synovium of an infected joint can have irregular contours and enhances, similar to the pseudocapsule of an abscess.
- A band of subchondral bone marrow edema is common on MRI in septic arthritis. This can be reactive,

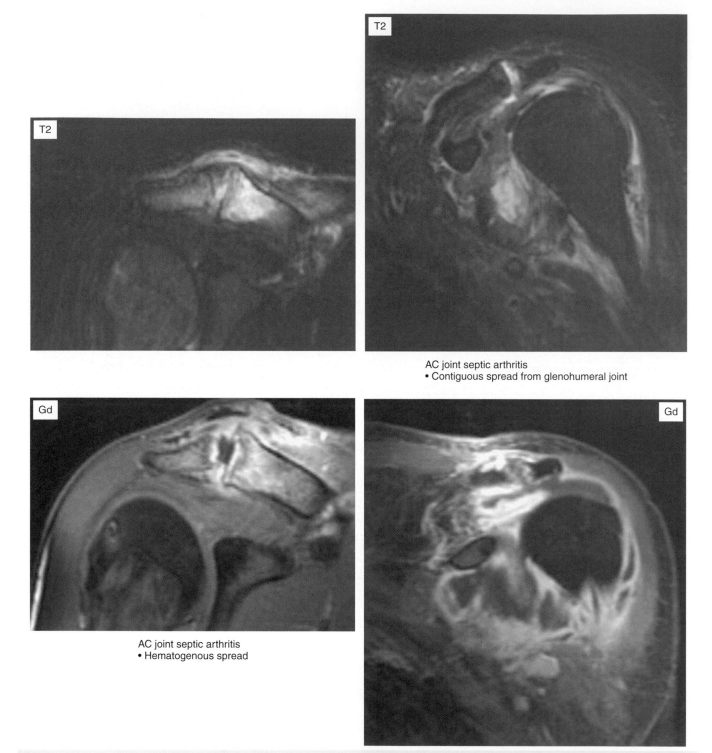

Fig. 14.11 Septic arthritis of the acromioclavicular (AC) joint on MRI. Left images show effusion, edema, and enhancement in a patient with hematogenous implantation of infection. Right images from a different patient show septic arthritis of the glenohumeral joint with spread to the AC joint through a full-thickness rotator cuff tear. Septic arthritis typically demonstrates significant periarticular edema and enhancement 'angry' effusion that helps separate this diagnosis from other arthropathies. *From Morrison W. Problem Solving in Musculoskeletal Imaging.* Philadelphia: Elsevier; 2010.)

without osteomyelitis. However, when the edema or enhancement extends beyond the subchondral bone deeper into the medullary cavity, osteomyelitis should be suspected.
- Septic arthritis in the sacroiliac (SI) joint has a different imaging appearance related to joint anatomy.

- Radiographs are insensitive. The erosions, cartilage loss, and (tiny) effusion are difficult to see on radiographs.
  - Tip: Carefully inspect the inferior aspect of the SI joint (the synovial portion) for loss of the thin white line of subchondral bone, reflecting hyperemia and erosion.

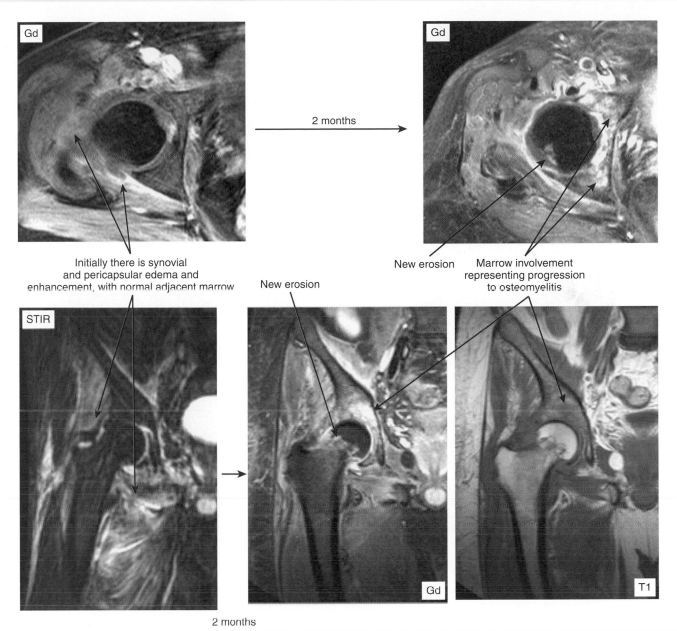

Fig. 14.12 Septic arthritis with progression to osteomyelitis on MRI. MRI of the hip initially shows a small joint effusion with periarticular edema and enhancement (left images). Follow-up MR images after 2 months (right images) show new marrow enhancement with replacement of normal fat signal representing osteomyelitis. (From Morrison W. *Problem Solving in Musculoskeletal Imaging.* Philadelphia: Elsevier; 2010.)

- MRI is much more sensitive.
  - Early findings can be subtle.
  - Look for bulging joint capsule with soft tissue edema and fluid adjacent to the joint. These findings are more often seen anterior reflecting the normal joint anatomy (thinner anterior capsule). In more advanced cases, adjacent abscess or abscesses are seen.
  - Marrow edema and erosions develop next and may simulate the inflammatory sacroiliitis of seronegative spondyloarthropathy.
  - However, seronegative spondyloarthropathies do not show the adjacent soft tissue changes, which are fairly specific for infection.

- Potential pitfall: After arthroscopic or other joint surgery, transient soft tissue and bone marrow alterations can simulate infection in imaging studies:
  - Hyperemic synovium.
  - Effusion and synovial proliferation.
  - Surrounding soft tissues are often very edematous, and periarticular fluid collections can also be seen depending on the surgical approach and extent.
  - Some implants, especially bioabsorbable components (screws, anchors, sutures, etc.) can incite an inflammatory response. MRI shows a very complex effusion and subchondral marrow edema. One clue that a bioabsorbable screw or anchor was used is that there is focal low signal in the marrow in an

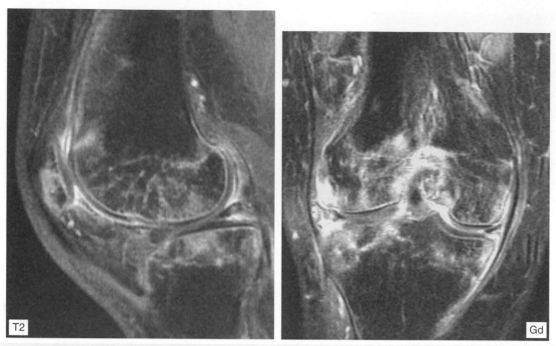

Fig. 14.13 Septic arthritis of the knee with hyperemia demonstrated on MRI. T2-weighted image (left) and post-contrast image (right) show edema and enhancement along the vascular supply of the distal femur and proximal tibia centered at the margins of the joint and the subchondral bone representing hyperemia. (From Morrison W. *Problem Solving in Musculoskeletal Imaging*. Philadelphia: Elsevier; 2010.)

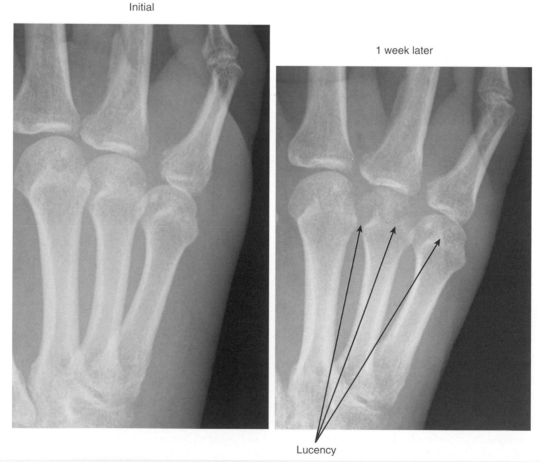

Fig. 14.14 Progression of septic arthritis on radiographs. Follow-up a week after onset of infection of 4th and 5th metacarpophalangeal joints shows rarefaction of bone at the joint margins reflecting hyperemia and early erosion. (From Morrison W. *Problem Solving in Musculoskeletal Imaging*. Philadelphia: Elsevier; 2010.)

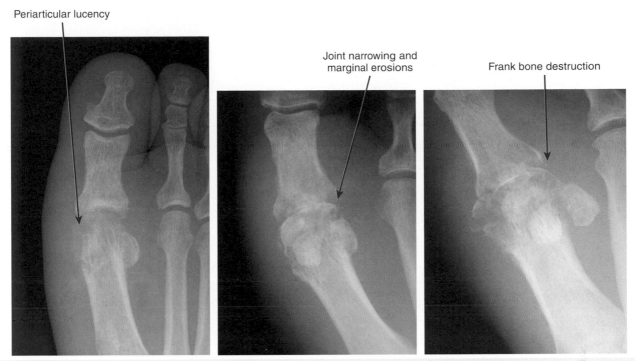

Periarticular lucency

Joint narrowing and
marginal erosions

Frank bone destruction

Fig. 14.15 Progression of septic arthritis to osteomyelitis. Radiographs over time show periarticular lucency (left image) progressing to joint space narrowing and marginal erosion (middle image) and eventually frank bone destruction (right image) as osteomyelitis ensues. (From Morrison W. *Problem Solving in Musculoskeletal Imaging.* Philadelphia: Elsevier; 2010.)

expected location without any metallic artifact. The bioabsorbable components are invisible on radiographs, and without provided history, surgical changes are subtle and may be overlooked.

- Labeled white blood cell (WBC) nuclear medicine scan can be used to help identify infection in the postoperative setting, but if there is clinical suspicion of infection, joint aspiration is the gold standard for diagnosis.
- MRI can be useful to exclude medullary marrow edema or enhancement associated with osteomyelitis (Fig. 14.16).

- After surgery, unless there has been extensive medullary drilling or exposure, typically the marrow signal abnormality is limited to the immediate surgical zone.
  - For example, shortly after anterior cruciate ligament (ACL) reconstruction there will be marrow edema limited to immediately around the tunnels and in the subchondral bone.
  - Signal abnormality involving bone marrow remote from the surgical sites should be considered suspicious (Fig. 14.17).

Pediatric Considerations in Septic Arthritis

- In neonates and infants, osteomyelitis frequently coexists with septic arthritis, in part because of the frequency of epiphyseal osteomyelitis in children under 2 years.
- Extension of osteomyelitis into an adjacent joint is especially common in the hip in children of all ages, as the metaphysis of the femur is within the hip joint capsule. (As discussed in the following text, the metaphysis is the most common site of osteomyelitis in the skeletally immature.)

- Two dilemmas are frequently encountered when a child presents with a clinically suspected septic hip.
  - The first issue is whether a joint effusion is present, because joint infection by pyogenic organisms is almost invariably associated with an effusion. Radiographs may show an increased distance between the teardrop and the femoral metaphysis or bulging fat planes in a perfectly aligned anteroposterior (AP) radiograph. These findings are suggestive of a joint effusion but not as reliable as US or MRI. Producing a vacuum phenomenon in the joint with traction on the hip rules out an effusion and septic hip. US is far more sensitive and specific in diagnosis of a hip joint effusion in a child (Fig. 14.18). It can be performed quickly and requires no sedation. MRI also is very accurate and allows detection of osteomyelitis (Fig. 14.19); however, it may require sedation.
  - The second dilemma arises if a hip effusion is present. Not all effusions indicate joint infection. *Transient synovitis (toxic synovitis)* is a noninfectious hip joint inflammation with clinical and imaging findings that may be indistinguishable from those of a septic hip. Transient synovitis is self-limited, likely post-viral or post-traumatic in etiology, and requires no therapy. If there is any real clinical suspicion of a septic hip, it should be regarded as an emergency and hip aspiration should be performed.

OSTEOMYELITIS

- *Osteomyelitis* is inflammation of the medullary space due to infection.

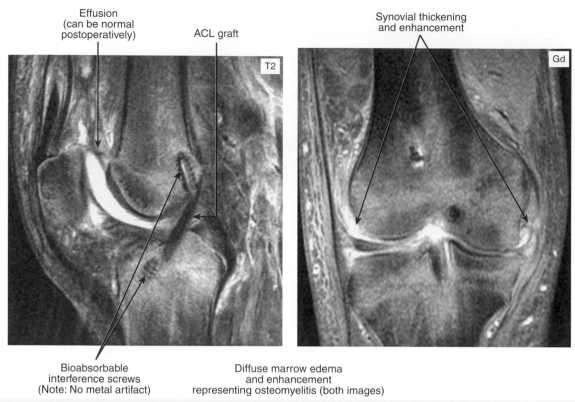

Effusion
(can be normal
postoperatively)

ACL graft

Synovial thickening
and enhancement

T2

Gd

Bioabsorbable
interference screws
(Note: No metal artifact)

Diffuse marrow edema
and enhancement
representing osteomyelitis (both images)

Fig. 14.16 Septic arthritis of the knee following ACL reconstruction. T2-weighted (left) and post-contrast (right) images show effusion with periarticular edema and enhancement, as well as marrow edema and enhancement concerning for progression to osteomyelitis. (From Morrison W. *Problem Solving in Musculoskeletal Imaging*. Philadelphia: Elsevier; 2010.)

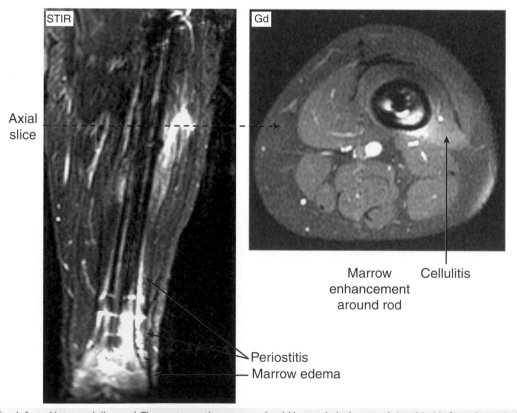

STIR

Gd

Axial
slice

Marrow
enhancement
around rod

Cellulitis

Periostitis
Marrow edema

Fig. 14.17 MRI of an infected intramedullary rod. The postoperative marrow should have relatively normal signal (aside from the underlying fracture); in these images of the femur there is bone marrow edema and enhancement with periosteal reaction, suspicious for infection. (From Morrison W. *Problem Solving in Musculoskeletal Imaging*. Philadelphia: Elsevier; 2010.)

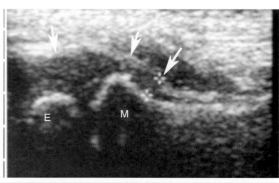

Fig. 14.18 Septic hip in a child. Sagittal US image of the hip in a 13-month-old with septic hip shows low-echogenicity joint effusion with elevation of the anterior joint capsule *(arrows)*. Note the capital femoral epiphysis (E) and the proximal femur metaphysis (M) separated by the hypoechoic physis.

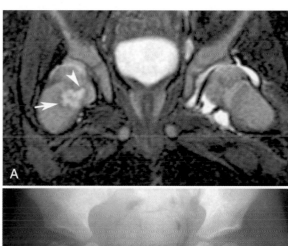

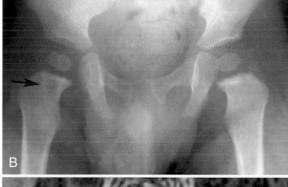

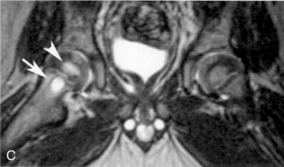

Fig. 14.19 Osteomyelitis in an infant. **(A)** Coronal inversion recovery MR image shows right proximal femur osteomyelitis. Note increased signal intensity in the epiphysis *(arrowhead)* and proximal metaphysis *(arrow)*. Also note the left hip joint effusion, which required diagnostic aspiration but did not show infection in this case. **(B)** AP radiograph of the hips in a different child, 13 months old, shows a well-circumscribed lytic lesion in the proximal metaphysis *(arrow)*. **(C)** Coronal T2-weighted MR image in the same child shows high signal in the metaphyseal abscess *(arrow)* and in the epiphysis *(arrowhead)* due to osteomyelitis.

- Most prevalent in children (peak 6 years, M>F) and older adults.
- Frequent sites include the feet of diabetic patients, the hips and bony pelvis in bedridden patients, the spine, and the long bones in children.
- Osteomyelitis is becoming more common and virulent due to MRSA, diabetes, and immune suppression.
- Important complications include bone destruction, osteonecrosis, growth disturbance in children, and infection of adjacent joints and soft tissues.
- The main imaging modalities are MRI and radiographs, but CT, US, and nuclear medicine also are useful.

Osteomyelitis can be classified by the mode of infection: *hematogenous, continuous spread,* or *direct inoculation.*

Osteomyelitis can also be classified as *acute, subacute,* or *chronic.* These terms can overlap, and some authors use only acute and chronic.

Modes of Infection

Hematogenous Spread
- The most common mode in children.
- Metaphyses have a rich vascular supply, especially during growth. The metaphyseal blood vessels in the growing skeleton adjacent to the physis (metaphyseal sinusoids) are prone to bacterial implantation due to their anatomy.
- Pattern of infection varies with age (Fig. 14.20).
  - Neonates and infants up to about 18 months: some vessels cross the physis. This anatomy allows osteomyelitis originating in the metaphysis easy access to the epiphysis, with subsequent potential decompression into the joint causing secondary septic arthritis, most commonly the hip. Less commonly, this may allow osteomyelitis to start in the epiphysis.
  - Children/adolescents: The vessels crossing the physis involute, theoretically protecting the epiphysis.
    - Septic joint accompanying osteomyelitis is much less common after age 2 years, but does still occur, especially in the hip where the metaphysis is

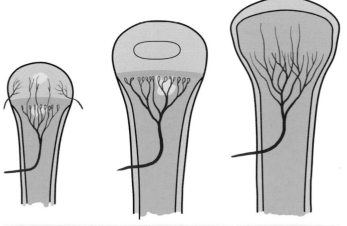

Fig. 14.20 Changes in epiphyseal blood flow during growth. (Left image) Neonates up to about 18 months. Osteomyelitis sites are the metaphysis and epiphysis. (Middle image) Older children. Osteomyelitis initiation site is the metaphysis (see text). (Right image) Adults. Hematogenous osteomyelitis can begin in the epiphysis.

intraarticular. The physis is a relative barrier to spread of infection, but in clinical practice it is common to see osteomyelitis on both sides of the physis in children of all ages.

- Adults: After the physis closes epiphyseal–metaphyseal vascular connections are reestablished, allowing for epiphyseal seeding with potential secondary septic joint. However, hematogenous osteomyelitis is less common than infection by continuous spread in adults.

Contiguous Spread

- Spread from an ulcer, adjacent soft tissue infection or septic joint.
- Examples include:
  - Paralyzed patients (especially pelvis—sacrum, ischium, greater trochanters).
  - Diabetic patients (feet/ankles—breakdown of callus).
  - Patients with peripheral vascular disease.

Direct Implantation

- Direct inoculation of tissues from an external source.
- Examples include:
  - Penetrating injury (i.e., knife injury, stepping on a nail, human bite).
  - Open fracture.
  - Surgery/intervention (notably spinal fusion or hip replacement, and needle-based procedures such as discography, epidural injection, or joint injection); uncommon with surgical/sterile technique, occasionally tracked to contaminated material from vendor. Root cause analysis is required to determine origin.

Acute Osteomyelitis

Entry of bacteria into bone by hematogenous spread or direct inoculation causes an immune response with influx of WBCs. Pus accumulates in the medullary cavity and cavity pressure increases.

- The elevated pressure can compromise blood supply, causing osteonecrosis.
- Pus can decompress through the cortex via the Haversian system. This can disrupt periosteal blood supply to the marrow, increasing the risk of osteonecrosis, as well as physeal injury and growth disturbance in children.
- If not successfully treated, additional complications include:
  - Bone destruction.
  - Adjacent soft tissue, tendon sheath, and joint infection.
  - Development of a sinus tract to the skin.
  - Chronic osteomyelitis.

Osteomyelitis caused by contiguous spread from infected adjacent soft tissues basically reverses the first steps described earlier.

Imaging Acute Osteomyelitis

- Radiography is often the first-line test for osteomyelitis, although it is not sensitive.
  - Acute osteomyelitis is first demonstrated radiographically by blurring or obliteration of soft tissue fat planes (Fig. 14.21); adjacent soft tissue swelling is nonspecific and may not be seen at all in deep tissues.

Late: Destruction

Early: Soft tissue swelling

Mid: Rarefaction

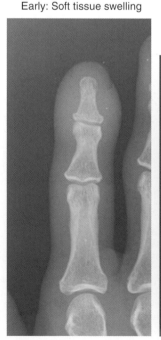
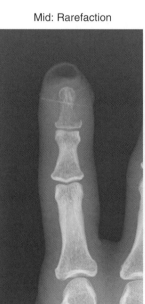
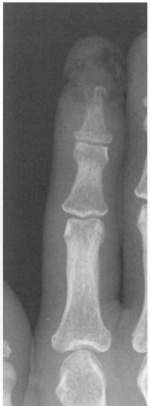

Fig. 14.21 Natural history of osteomyelitis, depicted in the terminal tuft of a digit. AP views of the finger over time initially show soft tissue swelling only (left image). This is followed by rarefaction (lucency) of bone (middle image); in later stages there is frank bone destruction (right image). (From Morrison W. *Problem Solving in Musculoskeletal Imaging.* Philadelphia: Elsevier; 2010.)

- Even this radiographic change lags behind the clinical onset of infection by 1–2 weeks.
- Cortical rarefaction or resorption is next seen as a region of decreased cortical density or a permeative pattern of bone loss in the cortex. By the time frank cortical destruction is seen, the infectious process is well established and generally quite extensive.
- The classic radiographic appearance is a lytic, permeative process, resembling 'small round cell' neoplasms. Radiographs are still useful as the first test to exclude other pathology, and to obtain a baseline exam.
- These osseous changes may appear highly aggressive in the acute phase of osteomyelitis and may be difficult to differentiate from an aggressive neoplasm (Fig. 14.22). Knowing the time course of the disease may be helpful, because an acute osteomyelitis causes osseous destruction much more rapidly than does a tumor.
- As infection becomes more established, periosteal reaction ensues. The periosteal new bone is typically thick, unbroken, and wavy, characteristic of a benign process. Less commonly, periosteal reaction can be intermediately aggressive (lamellated, or 'onion skin') or even aggressive (such as Codman triangle).
- MRI is the test of choice in most settings.
  - Initial finding is marrow edema, which can begin as early as the first 2 days of infection.
  - On MRI the classic sign of osteomyelitis is replacement of marrow fat on T1-weighted images, with marrow edema and enhancement on fluid-sensitive and postcontrast images (Fig. 14.23).
  - Normal marrow signal on T1- and STIR or fat-suppressed T2-weighted sequences makes osteomyelitis highly unlikely.

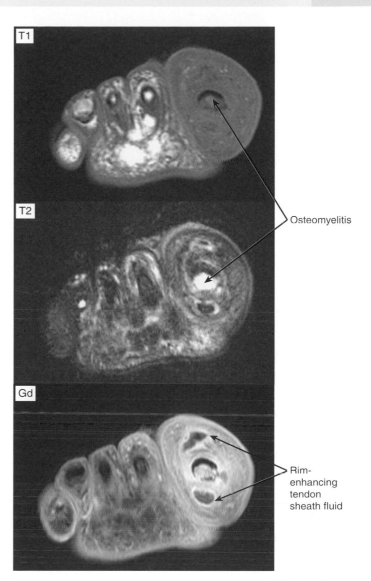

Fig. 14.23 Osteomyelitis of the great toe with septic tenosynovitis. Coronal (short-axis) MR images show rim-enhancement of the tendon sheaths of the great toe representing septic tenosynovitis. The underlying bone demonstrates marrow edema with low T1 signal and enhancement consistent with osteomyelitis. (From Morrison W. *Problem Solving in Musculoskeletal Imaging*. Philadelphia: Elsevier; 2010.)

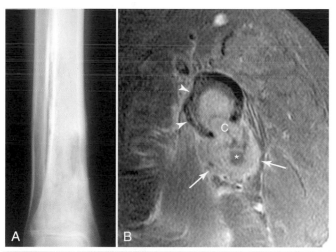

Fig. 14.22 Osteomyelitis with periosteal reaction. **(A)** The osseous destruction is highly aggressive in this case, with a moth-eaten pattern. Osteomyelitis can have a radiographic appearance that is highly aggressive, appearing similar to a malignant tumor. However, smooth periosteal reaction suggests infection rather than tumor. **(B)** Humeral shaft in a different patient, an adult intravenous drug user with *Staphylococcus aureus* infection by direct inoculation. Axial fat-suppressed contrast-enhanced T1-weighted MR image shows intense marrow and cortical enhancement *(arrowheads)*, a large cloaca ('C') with adjacent marrow enhancement, and soft tissue enhancement *(arrows)* surrounding a small abscess *(asterisk)*.

- However, remember that when present, these findings are not specific for infection and can be seen in a wide variety of disease and injury.
- Periosteal reaction can be seen as increased T2 signal at the cortical margin.
- In addition to its high sensitivity and specificity, MRI facilitates medical and surgical treatment planning by detecting abscesses, septic arthritis and tenosynovitis, sinus tracts, and can accurately define soft tissue and osseous extent of involvement.
- The MRI report should always describe presence of any nonenhancing tissue representing necrosis, which usually requires debridement.
- Additional considerations in generating a differential diagnosis include the following:
  - Review lab values related to infection (WBC count, erythrocyte sedimentation rate, C-reactive protein) as

well as those that may shed light on the underlying disease (glucose: diabetes; creatinine: renal failure).

- CT usually mirrors the appearance of the radiograph but with greater sensitivity for bone destruction. Contrast enhancement assists in identifying associated abscess.
- Tc-99m-methyl diphosphonate (MDP) three-phase bone scan has high sensitivity for detection of osteomyelitis, if there is adequate blood flow to distribute radiotracer.
  - Classically, osteomyelitis presents as rapid uptake on the early inflow phase due to hyperemia, with persistent activity on the second, blood pool phase, and concentration of activity within bone on the delayed phase acquired hours later, indicating increased bone turnover (Fig. 14.24).
  - Uptake on all phases suggests osteomyelitis in the appropriate clinical setting, but these findings can be seen in other inflammatory, traumatic, and neoplastic conditions, as well as neuropathic arthropathy. Increased specificity has been reported with acquisition of a 'fourth' phase, obtained after 24 hours.
  - Normal tracer uptake in pediatric physes complicates interpretation.
  - Note: In some pediatric osteomyelitis cases, no radiotracer uptake is observed due to increased marrow cavity pressure and associated ischemia. This may delay diagnosis and result in increased morbidity. MRI is more reliable.

Periostitis

- Periostitis (reactive periosteal new bone formation) is a well-known finding in osteomyelitis, especially of long bones. On radiographs the periostitis associated with infection is typically in a nonaggressive, continuous, thick, undulating pattern (see Fig. 14.22).
- On MRI periostitis appears as linear edema and enhancement along the outer cortex, wrapping around the bone. Radiographs and CT better demonstrate and characterize periosteal new bone.
- Periostitis is not specific for infection. Numerous other conditions such as stress fracture, tumor, and osteonecrosis can also show periosteal reaction.
- Periostitis is not seen in carpal and tarsal bones, and usually is subtle in the flat bones of the pelvis or scapula (Fig. 14.25).

Soft tissue Findings

- Evaluation of adjacent soft tissues is very important in evaluation of possible infection seen on MRI (Figs. 14.23, 14.26, and 14.27).
- Hematogenous infection to joints or bone typically creates an inflammatory reaction in the adjacent soft

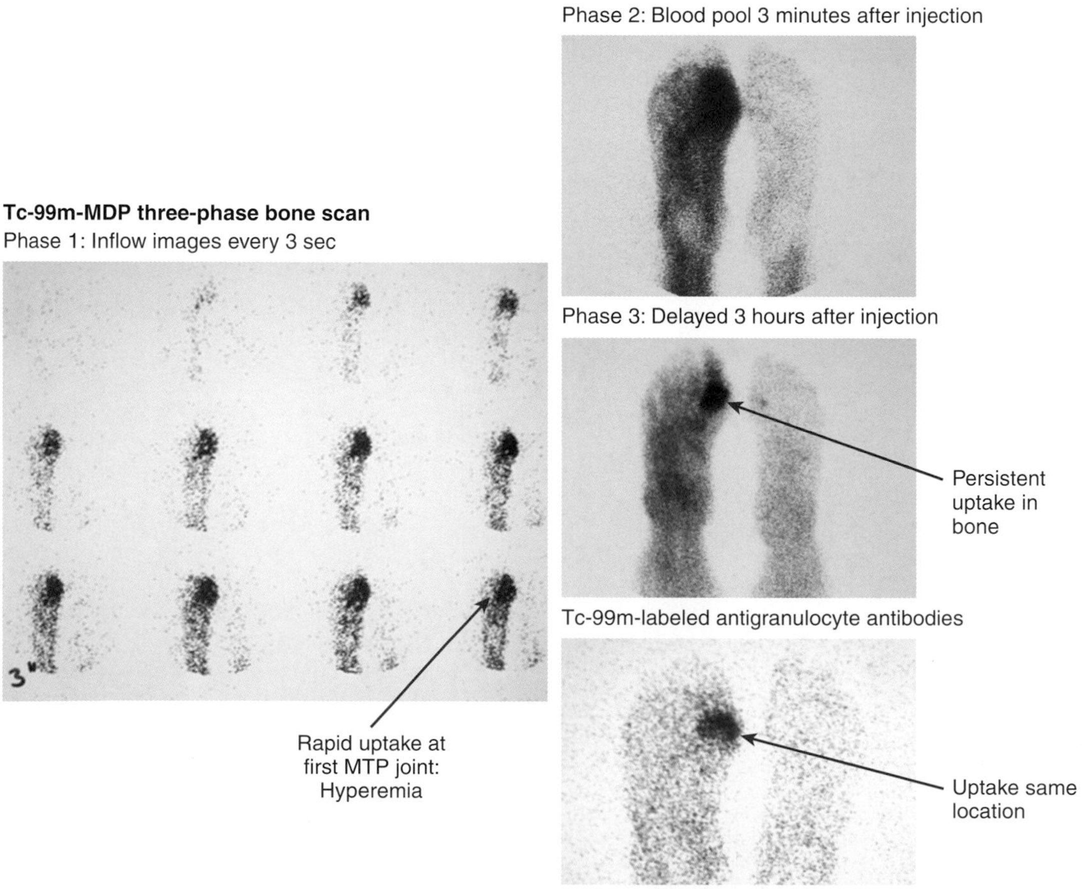

Tc-99m-MDP three-phase bone scan
Phase 1: Inflow images every 3 sec

Rapid uptake at first MTP joint: Hyperemia

Phase 2: Blood pool 3 minutes after injection

Phase 3: Delayed 3 hours after injection

Persistent uptake in bone

Tc-99m-labeled antigranulocyte antibodies

Uptake same location

Fig. 14.24 Diagnosis of osteomyelitis of the great toe using nuclear medicine. Vascular phase of Tc-99m-MDP three-phase bone scan (left image) shows increased uptake at the great toe. Blood pool and delayed images (right top and middle images) show concentration of radiotracer in the bone. A separate injection of Tc-99m labeled antigranulocyte antibodies demonstrates inflammatory activity in the great toe. (Courtesy of Hans Ledermann, MD, Basel, Switzerland.)

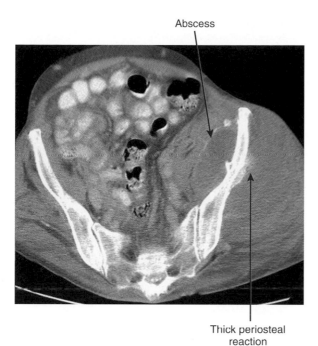

Abscess

Thick periosteal
reaction

Fig. 14.25 Osteomyelitis with adjacent abscess. Axial CT image through the pelvis shows thick periosteal reaction at the iliac bone reflecting underlying osteomyelitis. Fluid density under the iliacus muscle with mass effect represents abscess formation. (From Morrison W. *Problem Solving in Musculoskeletal Imaging.* Philadelphia: Elsevier; 2010.)

tissues. This appears as an 'angry' joint effusion, with associated synovial hypertrophy and edema and periarticular soft tissue edema. In the absence of trauma, such findings should be considered suspicious for septic arthritis (see Fig. 14.11).

- Sinus tracts and abscesses may arise from the infected bone/joint.
- In some situations, normal soft tissues adjacent to edematous bone marrow can steer the diagnosis away from osteomyelitis. For example, osteomyelitis in the feet of diabetics and the pelvis of paralyzed patients usually is by contiguous spread. In this setting, if there is a marrow abnormality and the adjacent subcutaneous fat is preserved, other etiologies such as neuropathic disease should be considered.

Additional Practical Tips

- Imaging findings are often ambiguous, neither normal nor pathognomonic for osteomyelitis, especially in complex cases such as the feet of diabetics. Our experience in such cases is that more intense marrow edema near a diabetic foot ulcer is more likely to be osteomyelitis than is mild edema, which is often seen as a reactive finding.
- A way to communicate the degree of suspicion in indeterminate cases is to apply the terms *high likelihood* or *low likelihood* of osteomyelitis based on severity of imaging findings.

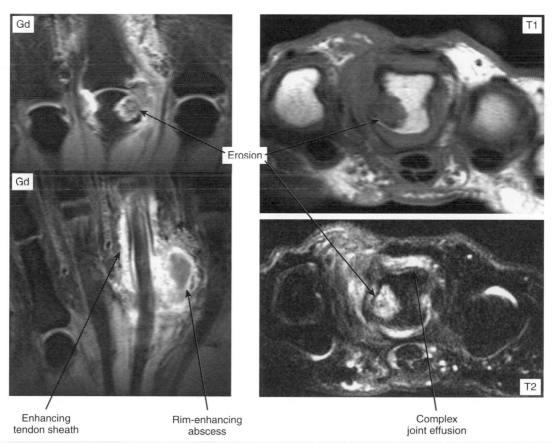

Enhancing
tendon sheath

Rim-enhancing
abscess

Erosion

Complex
joint effusion

Fig. 14.26 Septic arthritis and tenosynovitis of the hand. MRI shows metacarpophalangeal joint effusion with synovial enhancement on post-contrast images. Note erosion at the joint margin. Enhancement extends along the adjacent tendon sheath representing septic tenosynovitis. This pattern is especially common following a fight, with laceration over the knuckles sustained by punching someone in the teeth. (From Morrison W. *Problem Solving in Musculoskeletal Imaging.* Philadelphia: Elsevier; 2010.)

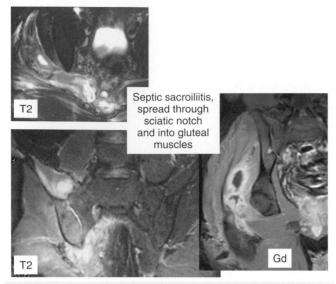

Septic sacroiliitis, spread through sciatic notch and into gluteal muscles

T2

T2

Gd

Fig. 14.27 Septic sacroiliitis on MRI. T2-weighted images (on left) show unilateral right sacroiliac (SI) joint effusion with edema and fluid in the periarticular soft tissues including the sciatic notch and gluteus muscles. Post-contrast image (right) demonstrates rim-enhancement of the intramuscular abscess. Patients with septic sacroiliitis often present with rapid onset of sciatica due to proximity of the SI joint with the sciatic notch. (From Morrison W. *Problem Solving in Musculoskeletal Imaging.* Philadelphia: Elsevier; 2010.)

- Clinical presentation and exam can be helpful and should be reviewed:
  - Are the symptoms minimal compared to the extent of imaging findings? If so, maybe neuropathic arthropathy, amyloidosis, or a chronic inflammatory arthropathy should be considered rather than infection.
  - Are symptoms greater than the imaging findings? If so, consider gout, which is extremely painful.
- Patterns of spread of infection: Normal or abnormal communications can hasten spread of infection. Some patterns of spread are predicable, based on location and orientation of fascial planes:
  - Lumbar spine infection spreads along the psoas muscle(s).
  - Sacroiliac infection spreads along the ipsilateral iliacus muscle and into the sciatic notch and gluteus muscles (Fig. 14.27).
  - Sternoclavicular (SC) infection spreads into the retrosternal space, the lower neck, and pectoralis major.
  - Infections of the hands and feet may spread along tendon sheaths.
  - Septic arthritis can spread along tendon sheaths, especially if the tendon communicates with the joint (long head of the biceps and the glenohumeral joint; flexor hallucis longus and ankle/subtalar joint; popliteus and knee joint).
  - Joints may communicate (tibiotalar and subtalar joints; wrist compartments through ligament tears).
  - Joints and bursae may communicate (the hip joint and the iliopsoas bursa; the glenohumeral joint and the subacromial-subdeltoid bursa and acromioclavicular (AC) joint through a rotator cuff tear).

- If there is disruption of the articular cartilage, for example due to rheumatoid arthritis, joint infection may spread more easily into the underlying bone.
- Infection readily crosses synovial joints and discs, but these represent a relative barrier to tumor. Thus a process that crosses a joint is unlikely to be tumor.
  - However, some aggressive tumors can cross joints, especially joints with extensive ligamentous connections such as the sacroiliac joint, which provides a route for migration of tumor cells.
- MRI should not be used to determine the aggressiveness of a lesion, and tumor should always be considered in the back of your mind if infection is the primary diagnosis, especially if the clinical scenario does not fit the imaging findings.

Key Concepts

Imaging of Acute Osteomyelitis

Radiography useful as screening but insensitive
Nuclear imaging: Tc-99m-MDP three-phase bone scanning, tagged leukocyte scanning, PET-CT, PET-MRI
Magnetic resonance imaging with contrast usually best test
Marrow edema and enhancement
Search for: Abscesses, sinus tract, skin ulcers

Some common variations of acute osteomyelitis are discussed in the following sections.

Hematogenous Osteomyelitis in a Child

- Most are *S. aureus*, often community-acquired MRSA.
- Periosteum is loosely attached in children and can be elevated by pus, except at the physis where it is tightly attached. Subperiosteal abscess is an excellent target for aspiration and should be noted in MRI or US reports (Figs. 14.28 and 14.29).
- Complications include bone destruction and physeal injury, with subsequent growth disturbance.
- Younger than 18 months:
  - As noted earlier, epiphyseal spread from the metaphysis and septic joint is a common association before age 18 months due to vessels crossing the physis.
  - Septic joint in a child 18 months or younger is often associated with unsuspected osteomyelitis.
- In older children, involvement of both sides of the growth plate is less frequent, but is still commonly seen (Fig. 14.30).
- In older children, associated septic joint occurs by far most frequently in the hip (metaphysis is intraarticular).
  - Key differential diagnosis is *transient (toxic) synovitis*; see previous discussion.
- In younger children, intravenous contrast is very helpful to detect or exclude infection of unossified cartilage.
- Osteomyelitis is included in the differential diagnosis of lytic epiphyseal lesions in children along with chondroblastoma and Langerhans cell histiocytosis (eosinophilic granuloma) (Fig. 14.31).
- Treatment is antibiotics, sometimes also surgical debridement.

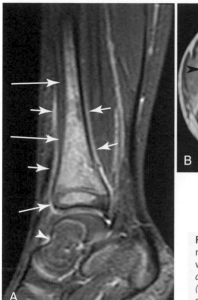

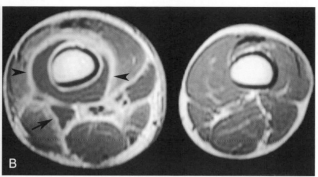

Fig. 14.28 Early acute osteomyelitis. **(A)** Sagittal short-tau inversion recovery (STIR) MR image shows intense marrow edema in the tibia diaphysis and metaphysis *(long arrows)* and epiphysis *(medium arrow)*; contrast with normal marrow signal in the talus *(arrowhead)*. Also note periosteal edema and mild elevation *(short arrows)*. **(B)** Postcontrast T1-weighted axial MR image in a different child shows periosteal abscess *(arrowheads)* and adjacent soft tissue abscess *(arrow)*, each with thick enhancing rim. Fluid-sensitive sequences (not shown) showed marrow edema. This was a staphylococcal osteomyelitis.

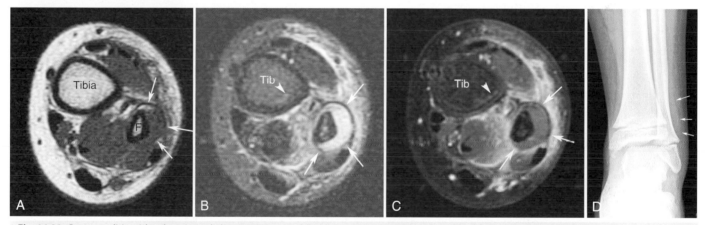

Fig. 14.29 Osteomyelitis with subperiosteal abscess. A 9-year-old with acute osteomyelitis of the distal fibula. **(A, B,** and **C)** Axial T1w **(A)**, STIR **(B)**, and postcontrast T1 **(C)** images. Note the low-signal periosteum *(arrows)* elevated by pus. The pus has high T2 signal and does not enhance. Also note the subtle marrow edema in the distal lateral tibia *(arrowhead* in B), which is reactive and does not indicate osteomyelitis. **(D)** The periosteal elevation is also faintly visible on the AP radiograph *(arrows) Tib,* tibia; *F,* fibula.

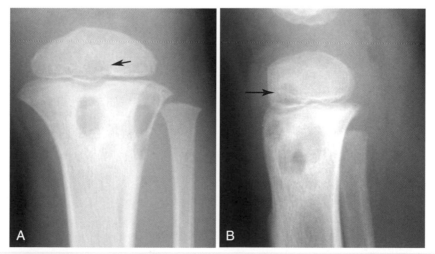

Fig. 14.30 Epiphyseal osteomyelitis in a toddler. AP **(A)** and lateral **(B)** radiographs demonstrate multiple well-defined lytic lesions, predominantly in the metaphysis but also involving the epiphysis *(arrow)*. Physeal injury with growth disturbance may result.

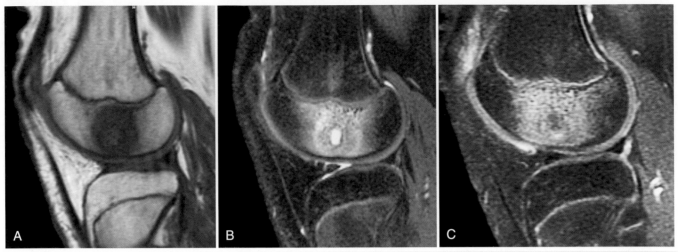

Fig. 14.31 Epiphyseal osteomyelitis in a child. Sagittal T1-weighted MR image **(A)**, fat-suppressed T2-weighted MR image **(B)**, and fat-suppressed contrast-enhanced T1-weighted MR image **(C)** in a child with an epiphyseal abscess in the distal femur show small fluid signal–intensity region surrounded by intense edema and enhancement.

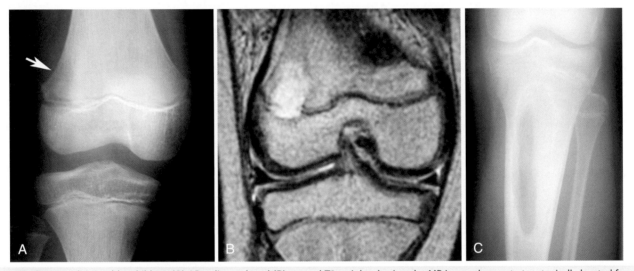

Fig. 14.32 Osteomyelitis in older children. **(A)** AP radiograph and **(B)** coronal T2-weighted spin-echo MR image demonstrate a typically located focus of osteomyelitis in the metaphysis of the lateral femoral condyle (*arrow* in A), not crossing into the epiphysis, in an 8-year-old child. **(C)** Brodie abscess. The well-defined oval metaphyseal lytic lesion with a sclerotic margin and thick periosteal reaction is a classic pattern in a child. This example is larger than usual.

Hematogenous Osteomyelitis in a Neonate

- Neonatal period is first 30 days.
- Most common agents are *S. aureus, Group B Streptococcus*, Gram negative bacteria.
- More common in neonatal intensive care unit (NICU) babies/premies.
- Osteomyelitis in neonates and very young infants is often multifocal and frequently accompanied by septic arthritis.
- Bone scan has limited sensitivity. Whole-body MRI can be helpful in identifying all sites.

Hematogenous Osteomyelitis in an IV Drug Abuser

- AC, SC, and SI joints (the 'letter joints') infected more frequently than in other patients (see Figs. 14.11 and 14.27).
- Infectious agent may be unusual, for example *Pseudomonas aeruginosa*.

BRODIE ABSCESS

A *Brodie abscess* is an intraosseous abscess in children usually caused by *S. aureus* and represents a subacute or chronic infection.

- Usually found in the metaphysis (Fig. 14.32A and B).
- Typical radiographic appearance is a geographic lytic lesion with a well-defined, often broad, sclerotic margin (Fig. 14.32C).
- It is usually oval, with the long axis parallel to the long axis of the bone, and typically borders the growth plate.
- Brodie abscess often appears radiographically nonaggressive, unlike acute osteomyelitis.
- On MRI the lesion appears as ovoid fluid signal in the metaphysis abutting the physis (Fig. 14.33). There is typically surrounding ill-defined bone marrow edema, and often periosteal reaction reflecting its inflammatory nature.

Brodie abscess

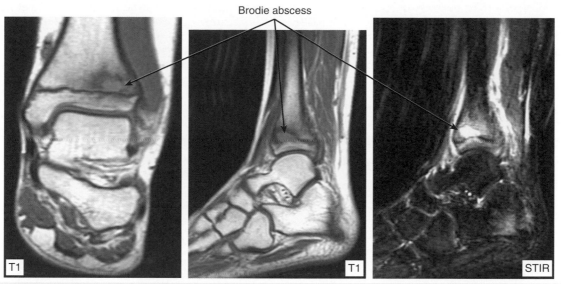

Fig. 14.33 MRI of an adolescent patient with a Brodie abscess. MRI of the ankle shows a fluid collection abutting the physeal plate representing an intraosseous (Brodie) abscess. There is surrounding bone marrow edema and periosteal reaction along the tibial shaft. (From Morrison W. *Problem Solving in Musculoskeletal Imaging.* Philadelphia: Elsevier; 2010.)

- Clinically, patients with Brodie abscess may not have associated fever or elevated erythrocyte sedimentation rate.
- Occasionally a Brodie abscess is cortically-based, where it may elicit significant sclerosis and periosteal reaction. These cortically-based infections with significant reactive bone formation can have an appearance similar to that of a cortically-based osteoid osteoma or reactive bone formation around a subacute stress fracture.

CHRONIC OSTEOMYELITIS

Chronic osteomyelitis is bone infection of at least 4–6 weeks duration. Chronic infection can have a varied appearance. A combination of sclerosis and bone destruction is common. If unsuccessfully treated, some distinctive features such as sequestrum and involucrum can develop, as described in the following text. The transition from acute to chronic osteomyelitis is indistinct. 'Subacute' can be used

for infection with features of both, for example a Brodie abscess, although some authors do not use this term.

- Chronic osteomyelitis is commonly seen in paralyzed patients, in feet of diabetics, and occasionally following an open fracture or orthopedic hardware implantation; it can also occur in immunocompromised patients, atypical organism infections, and chronically untreated/mistreated infections. The infection may smolder for many years, occasionally presenting with drainage through sinus tracts and acute-on-chronic osteomyelitis.
- Necrotic bone caused by the acute phase or prior fracture provides a haven for bacteria.
- A *sequestrum* represents a segment of necrotic bone that is separated from living bone by granulation tissue (Fig. 14.34).
  - The sequestrum acts as a persistent nidus of infection; due to its devitalization, antibiotics and WBCs cannot penetrate this tissue and bacteria can remain present for long periods of time in a dormant state, periodically reactivating infection.

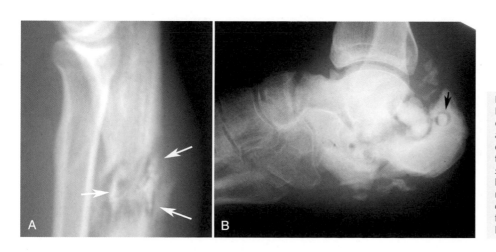

Fig. 14.34 Sequestrum in osteomyelitis. **(A)** Lateral radiograph of a proximal ulna shows osteomyelitis that has developed following an open fracture. There is permeative bone destruction, as well as an H-shaped dense fragment of necrotic bone *(arrows)*, termed a *sequestrum.* **(B)** Lateral radiograph in a diabetic patient with neuropathic foot shows a round sequestrum *(arrow)* in the posterior calcaneus. (A, Image used with permission from BJ Manaster, MD, from the American College of Radiology Learning File.)

- The sequestrum may be seen on CT as a focus of dense bone surrounded by lucent granulation tissue, and on MRI as a focus or region of hypointensity on all sequences, surrounded by edematous inflammatory tissue.
- Often colonized with organisms even after effective treatment.
- Must be debrided to avoid reemergence of active infection.

- Infected orthopedic hardware can act like a sequestrum.
- An *involucrum* denotes a layer of viable bone that has formed about the dead bone (Fig. 14.35).
- Infected tissue can decompress into adjacent soft tissues through a hole in the bone, termed a *cloaca* (Figs. 14.22, 14.36, and 14.37).
- A *sinus tract*, if present, extends to the skin, eventually draining pus and necrotic material.

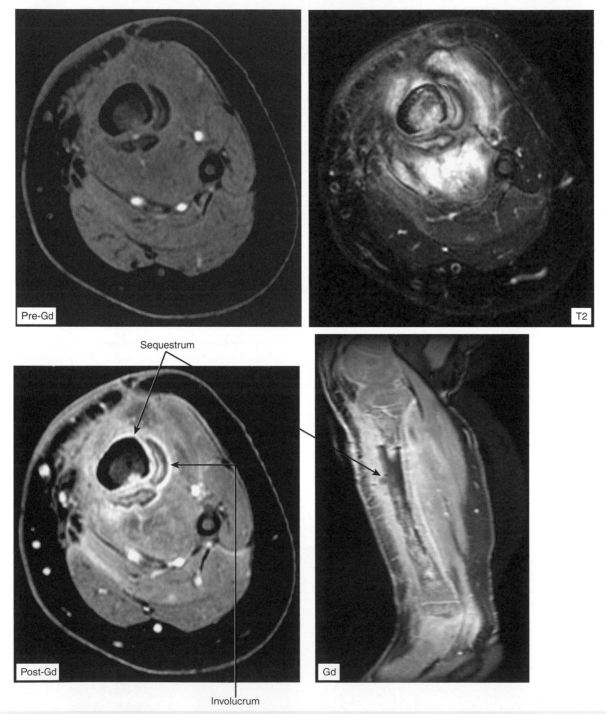

Fig. 14.35 MRI of chronic osteomyelitis of the tibia in a 6-year-old boy. T2-weighted image (upper right) shows bone marrow and soft tissue edema representing osteomyelitis and cellulitis; precontrast (upper left) and postcontrast (lower row) images show nonenhancement of the edematous tibia representing devitalized bone (sequestrum). The enhancing new bone formation surrounding the sequestrum is called the involucrum. (From Morrison W. *Problem Solving in Musculoskeletal Imaging.* Philadelphia: Elsevier; 2010.)

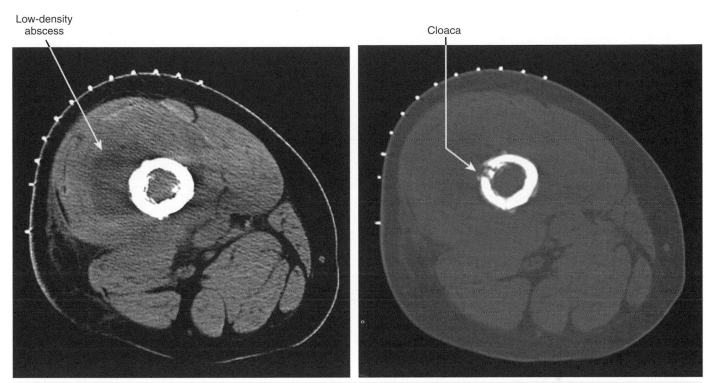

Fig. 14.36 Osteomyelitis with cloaca. Axial CT images of the femur using soft tissue (left) and bone (right) windowing show an abscess in the soft tissues next to the femoral shaft with an opening in the cortex of the infected bone, referred to as a cloaca, through which the marrow cavity infection decompresses into adjacent soft tissues. (From Morrison W. *Problem Solving in Musculoskeletal Imaging.* Philadelphia: Elsevier; 2010.)

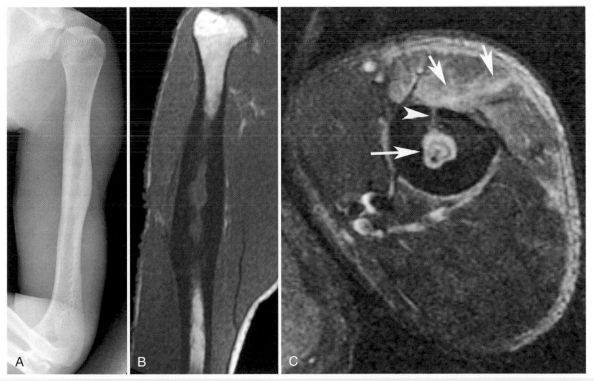

Fig. 14.37 Chronic osteomyelitis with draining sinus tract. (A–C) A 29-year-old man who had sustained an open humerus fracture several years previously, now with a draining sinus in the upper lateral arm. Radiograph **(A)** shows cortical thickening and mild expansion of the humeral midshaft. Sagittal T1-weighted MR image **(B)** shows similar findings, as well as abnormal, low marrow signal intensity in the humeral midshaft. Axial fat-suppressed contrast-enhanced T1-weighted MR image **(C)** shows intense enhancement in the marrow cavity *(long arrow)*, cloaca *(arrowhead)*, and sinus tract *(short arrows)* in the deltoid muscle.

- Usually T2-hyperintense. May have 'tram track'-like enhancement.
- Chronic osteomyelitis of the tibia or femur often is associated with a chronically draining sinus tract. If the drainage occurs over many years (usually decades), the tract may develop a squamous cell carcinoma. This tumor may be superficial and clinically apparent or may be located deeper along the sinus tract; it may be suspected because of new pain and detected by evidence of bone destruction on radiographs or visualization of the mass on MRI.
- In most developed regions musculoskeletal infection is diagnosed in the early stages, on clinical grounds and by imaging, before reaching these 'classic' advanced stages.
    - Therefore, these classically described findings in chronic osteomyelitis are unusual and can even be considered 'atypical'
- Nevertheless, classic findings exist in isolated cases as well as in rural and disadvantaged populations; associated imaging findings should be recognized by radiologists for their uncommon yet important presentation.

A different pattern of chronic osteomyelitis is a mixed pattern of lysis and sclerosis with cortical thickening or thick, wavy periosteal reaction.

- *Sclerosing osteomyelitis of Garre* is a manifestation of this process.
- The sclerosis is typically low signal on both T1- and T2-weighted images, with granulation tissue representing active infection demonstrating hyperintensity on T2-weighted images and enhancement on contrast-enhanced images (Figs 14.38 through 14.40).

Key Concepts

Hematogenous Osteomyelitis in Children

Vascular anatomy predisposes to seeding in the distal metaphysis
Neonates:
- Group B Streptococcus most common
- Multifocal

Less than 2 years:
- Epiphyseal involvement frequent due to patent vessels across the physis
- Most cases begin in the metaphysis
- Frequent association with septic joint

Older than 2 years:
- Usually *Staph A*, often MRSA
- Originates in the metaphysis (vessels connecting to the epiphysis closed), but epiphyseal involvement still occurs
- Septic joint association less frequent, but still frequent in the hip (metaphysis is intraarticular), less often shoulder, elbow, and ankle (but not the knee)
- Pus elevates periosteum (subperiosteal abscess—good site for aspiration)
    - Bone and joint destruction
    - High intraosseous pressure and periosteal elevation reduce marrow blood supply—osteonecrosis
    - Physis injury, growth deformity
    - Infection in adjacent tissues
- Can progress to Brodie abscess in older children (distal metaphyseal lucent lesion with dense surrounding bone), and chronic osteomyelitis with sequestrum, etc.

Key Concepts

Chronic Osteomyelitis

Infection longer than 4–6 weeks
Sclerosis, cloaca, sequestrum
Sinus tract (may develop squamous cell carcinoma if present for many years)
May be quiescent for years, then reactivate
MRI for abscess, sinus tract, cloaca, and marrow edema and enhancement
Tagged leukocyte scanning for detection, localization

Key Concepts

Musculoskeletal Infection Terminology

Cellulitis: Infected soft tissue with ill-defined margins
Phlegmon: Solid infected/inflamed tissue. Vascular supply intact. May progress to abscess
Abscess: Pus-filled cavity lined with granulation tissue
Sinus tract: Soft tissue channel between two compartments or to the skin. Pus drains through it
Cloaca: Cortical and periosteal opening, potentially communicating with the skin. Pus drains through it
Sequestrum: Fragment of infected necrotic bone. Potential source of chronic infection
Involucrum: New bone formed around sequestrum.

SOME COMMON VARIATIONS OF CHRONIC OSTEOMYELITIS

Infection in Paralyzed Patients

- Paralyzed and bedridden patients are prone to pressure ulceration and contiguous spread of infection (Figs. 14.41 through 14.43). This is most commonly seen at the pelvis (at the ischeal tuberosities, the greater trochanters, and sacrum/coccyx), the posterior calcanei, and the knees over the condylar prominences.
- Typically a deep ulcer is seen extending to the bone, with underlying acute or chronic osteomyelitis.
    - The ulcer and associated wide sinus tract is thick walled, with marked surrounding enhancement representing chronic granulation tissue and acute inflammation.
    - Chronic osteomyelitis and hyperemia often result in bone resorption, especially at the ischia which can be small or even absent. The ischia remaining bone is often sclerotic.
    - In acute infection septic arthritis of an adjacent joint is common, and the joint may contain air extending through the tract from the skin; abscess formation occurs in the adjacent soft tissues, and can extend far from the site of inoculation, spreading along fascial planes. For example, it is common in acute infections arising from ischeal decubitus ulcers to see inflammation and abscess extending into the obturator region and pubis anteriorly, through the sciatic notch to the gluteus region, and superiorly to the sacrum and lumbar spine.

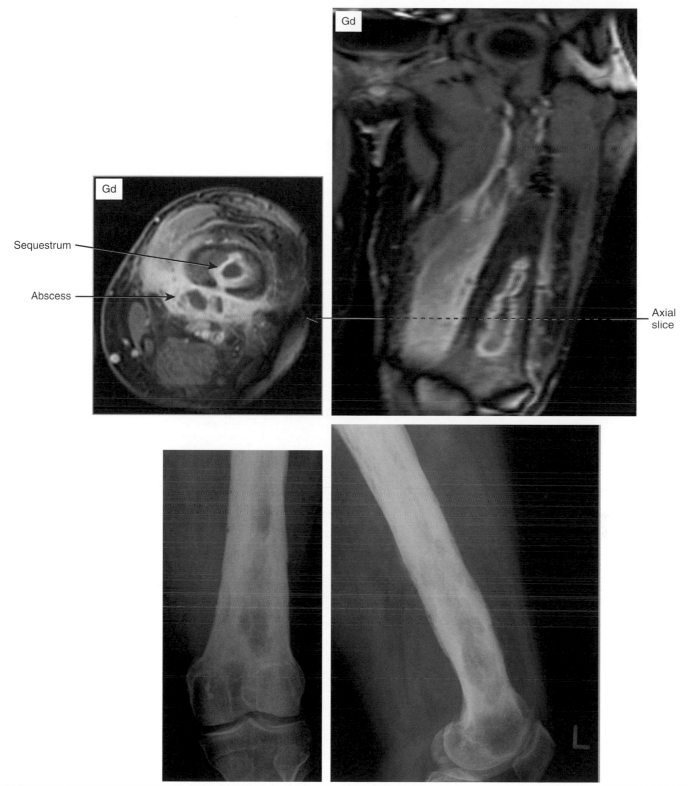

Fig. 14.38 Acute-on-chronic osteomyelitis. Sclerosis and periosteal thickening of the femoral shaft is consistent with a long-standing process. Active infection is suggested by areas of enhancement in the bone and adjacent soft tissue. Bone infarction within the distal femoral shaft acts as a sequestrum, serving as a nidus for persistent infection. (From Morrison W. *Problem Solving in Musculoskeletal Imaging.* Philadelphia: Elsevier; 2010.)

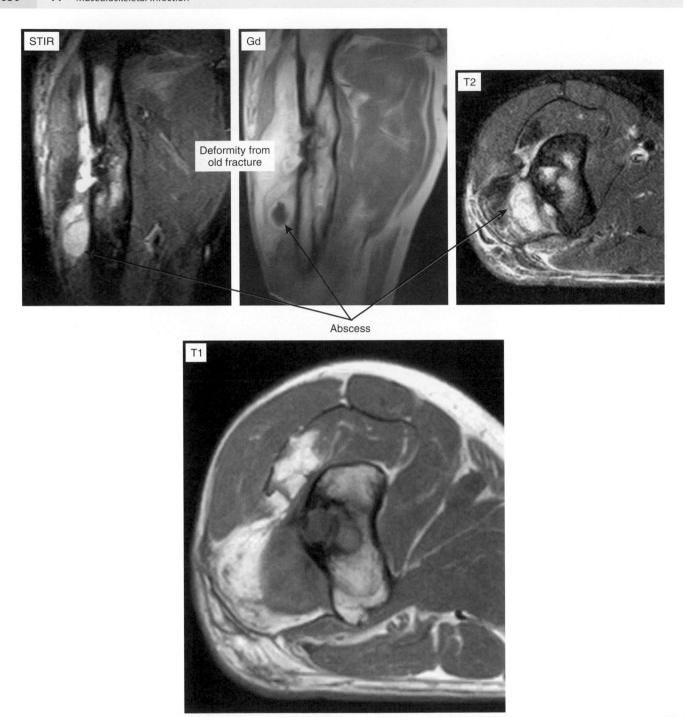

Fig. 14.39 Acute-on-chronic osteomyelitis following a fracture. MRI shows edema and enhancement of the marrow and adjacent soft tissue, with a focal abscess. (From Morrison W. *Problem Solving in Musculoskeletal Imaging*. Philadelphia: Elsevier; 2010.)

FEET OF DIABETICS

- Impaired WBC function, circulation, and pain sensation allow skin breakdown with soft tissue infection and osteomyelitis by contiguous spread.
  - Typically with multiple organisms.
- Neuropathic arthropathy (Charcot arthropathy) also afflicts the feet of diabetics.
- These conditions may have similar clinical and imaging features but are treated differently.

- If neuropathic change is present, the specificity of MRI for osteomyelitis is reduced.
- Nuances of imaging neuropathic joints without and with infection are discussed in greater detail in the following sections.
- A brief summary of findings favoring osteomyelitis:
  - Location—toes, distal metatarsals.
  - Asymmetry—one side of the foot.
  - Nearby skin ulcer.

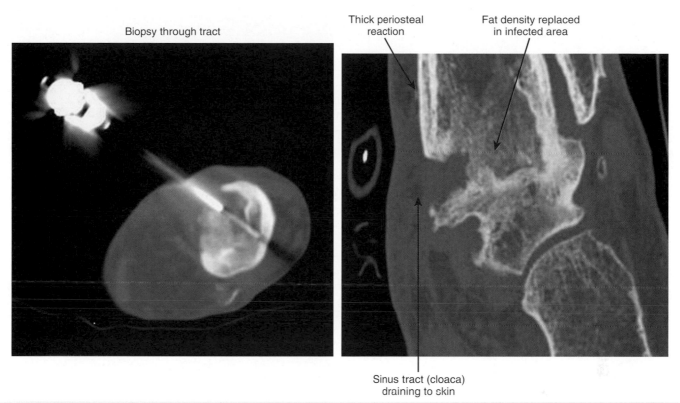

Biopsy through tract

Thick periosteal reaction

Fat density replaced in infected area

Sinus tract (cloaca) draining to skin

Fig. 14.40 Biopsy for chronic osteomyelitis. Lytic areas typically represent more active regions of inflammation and are targeted for sampling. (From Morrison W. *Problem Solving in Musculoskeletal Imaging*. Philadelphia: Elsevier; 2010.)

- Sinus tract.
- Abscess.

Neuropathic Arthropathy (Charcot Arthropathy) Versus Infection

- Evaluation of diabetic patients with clinically suspected pedal infection is a common indication for medical imaging.
- There are two basic clinical scenarios resulting in referral for imaging:
  - A patient with early neuropathic arthropathy (e.g., little to no deformity) who presents with a warm, swollen erythematous foot, the question being: *is the condition infection or a noninfectious manifestation of neuropathy?*
  - A patient with chronic neuropathic disease and deformity presenting with ulceration or swelling, the question being: *is superimposed infection present?*
- A common characteristic of diabetic feet on MRI is diffuse soft tissue edema and muscle atrophy, which is seen in early phases as T2 hyperintensity. This finding remains sensitive for infection but has poor specificity in diabetic feet, and may be misinterpreted as infection when none is present.

Early Neuropathic Arthropathy (Figs. 14.44 and 14.45)

- In the early phase of neuropathic disease, radiographs have low sensitivity.
  - On radiographs the soft tissues typically appear swollen, but the underlying bones show few findings.

There may be a subtle malalignment at an involved joint; at the tarsometatarsal (Lisfranc) joint, which is most commonly affected by neuropathic disease in diabetics, the second metatarsal base migrates dorsally and laterally.

- CT can better document subtle malalignment. However, although subluxation is a hallmark of early neuropathic disease, it is not specific.
- Tc-99m-MDP three-phase bone scan is typically hot on all phases due to the marked hyperemia and reactive bone formation resulting from the joint injury and instability.
- A labeled WBC scan can be useful; lack of uptake in an area hot on the delayed phase of a bone scan is strong evidence that no infection is present. However, the labeled WBC scan must be interpreted in conjunction with the bone scan, since lack of uptake could alternatively imply lack of blood flow; also, uptake can be seen with cellulitis or abscess, so the finding must correlate with focal bone uptake on the three-phase bone scan in order to support osseous involvement.
  - Presence of inflammatory cells in noninfected neuropathic joints can result in occasional false-positive exams in patients with early neuropathic disease. This is especially true with a Gallium-67 scan; a labeled WBC scan is more specific.
- MRI in noninfected early neuropathic arthropathy shows diffuse soft tissue edema that generally shows little enhancement, reflecting lack of inflammation.
  - Bone marrow edema/enhancement is pronounced and is often diffuse; effusions are common.

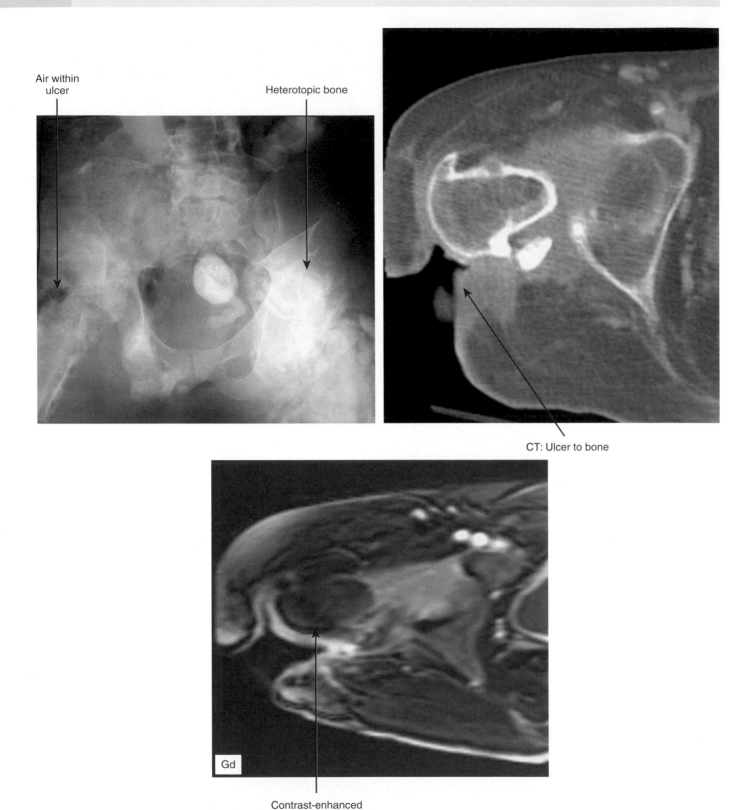

Fig. 14.41 Imaging of the pelvis in a paralyzed patient. AP radiograph (upper left) shows extensive heterotopic ossification at the left hip, with lucency adjacent to the right hip representing decubitus ulceration. CT (upper right) and post-contrast MRI (lower image) show the ulceration extending to the bone. Marrow signal is normal indicating lack of osteomyelitis. (From Morrison W. *Problem Solving in Musculoskeletal Imaging*. Philadelphia: Elsevier; 2010.)

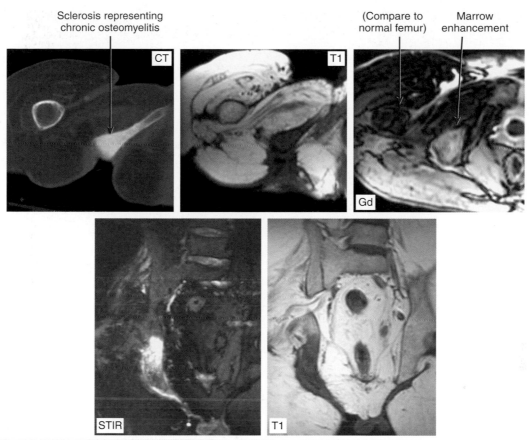

Fig. 14.42 Paralyzed patient with decubitus ulcer and chronic osteomyelitis. CT of the lower pelvis (upper left) shows ulceration extending to the ischium with sclerosis of the bone consistent with chronic osteomyelitis. Corresponding MRI shows edema and enhancement of the bone representing active infection. (From Morrison W. *Problem Solving in Musculoskeletal Imaging*. Philadelphia: Elsevier; 2010.)

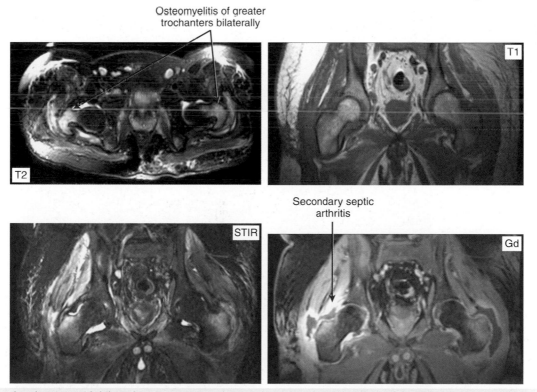

Fig. 14.43 Paralyzed patient with bilateral septic greater trochanteric bursitis and septic arthritis of the right hip joint. Bone marrow edema in the adjacent greater trochanters is consistent with osteomyelitis. (From Morrison W. *Problem Solving in Musculoskeletal Imaging*. Philadelphia: Elsevier; 2010.)

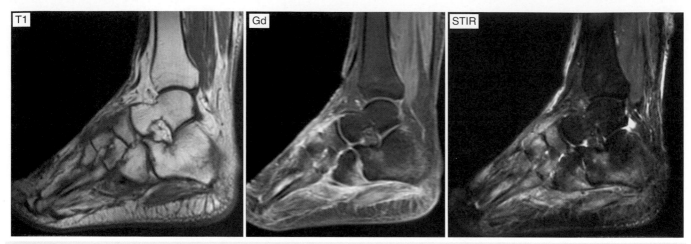

Fig. 14.44 Early neuropathic arthropathy of the foot on MRI. Note subchondral and periarticular edema and enhancement throughout the midfoot and hindfoot, without apparent deformity. There is no ulceration to suggest contiguous spread of infection. (From Morrison W. *Problem Solving in Musculoskeletal Imaging*. Philadelphia: Elsevier; 2010.)

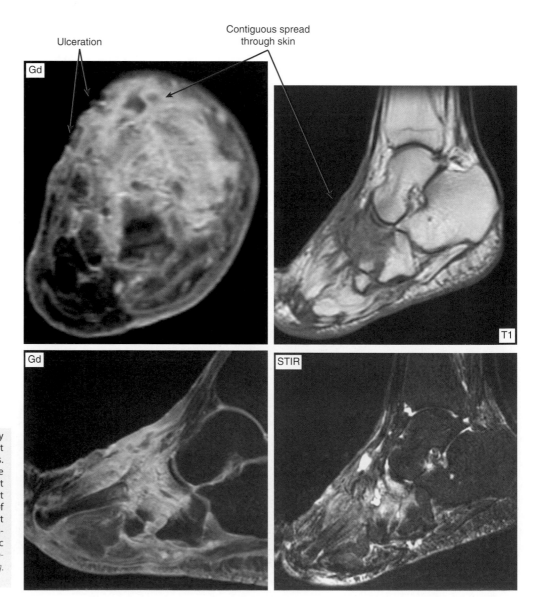

Fig. 14.45 Neuropathic arthropathy at the midfoot of a diabetic patient with superimposed osteomyelitis. MRI shows soft tissue and bone marrow edema and enhancement at the midfoot with ulceration at the dorsal aspect. Demonstration of contiguous spread helps document that marrow findings represent osteomyelitis rather than neuropathic disease only. (From Morrison W. *Problem Solving in Musculoskeletal Imaging*. Philadelphia: Elsevier; 2010.)

- Presence of a fracture in the setting of neuropathic disease causes intense, diffuse marrow edema and enhancement (Fig. 14.46).
- Marrow edema and enhancement at this stage is a pitfall that is easily misinterpreted as infection.

Neuropathic Arthropathy with Superimposed Infection

- Radiographic and CT signs of infection superimposed on neuropathic disease include bone lysis, periostitis, and joint erosions, although these findings can be seen with chronic neuropathic disease as well.
- Tc-99m-MDP three-phase bone scan can be misleading:
  - False-negative exams can be seen in the setting of ischemia, which is common in this population.
  - False-positive exams are seen since ulceration and cellulitis cause early-phase uptake while chronic joint disease leads to delayed uptake.
- Gallium-67 scan is nonspecific and can show uptake in infection and neuropathic disease.
- Labeled WBC scan is more specific and is useful in differentiating severe noninfected neuropathic disease from superimposed infection.
- On MRI there are some rules of thumb one may use to help determine if infection is present. These guidelines are based on the fact that osteomyelitis of the foot and ankle is by far most commonly related to contiguous spread from the skin.
  - A bone marrow abnormality without adjacent skin ulceration, sinus tract, or soft tissue inflammation is less likely to represent infection.
    - This concept is especially useful when there are extensive bone marrow signal abnormalities; in this setting infection is unlikely if the subcutaneous tissues are uninvolved.

- Conversely, if there is a marrow abnormality next to an ulcer or sinus tract, osteomyelitis is likely (Fig. 14.47).
- Diffuse soft tissue edema on T2-weighted or STIR images is nonspecific, seen in many patients related to vascular insufficiency, friction from shoes, trauma, and especially in diabetic patients.
  - However, if the edema is associated with replacement of fat signal and enhancement, it is more likely to represent cellulitis, which next to a marrow signal abnormality would suggest osteomyelitis.
- Another consideration is that neuropathic arthropathy is a predominantly articular process; because it is a manifestation of instability, often multiple joints in a region are similarly affected (e.g., the entire Lisfranc joint, Chopart joint, or multiple adjacent metatarsophalangeal joints).
  - This finding and other articular manifestations of neuropathic disease (subluxation, cysts, necrotic debris) are not as common in infection.
- Also, marrow changes associated with neuropathic arthropathy can be extensive (especially at the midfoot), but tend to be centered at a joint and subarticular bone, and are present on both sides of the joint fairly symmetrically.
- Osteomyelitis shows more diffuse marrow involvement, and unless there is primary septic arthritis, the marrow changes are generally greater on one side of the joint.
- Location of disease is also important.
  - Osteomyelitis occurs predominantly at the metatarsal heads, the toes, the calcaneus, and the malleoli, a distribution which mirrors that of friction, callus, and ulceration.
  - Neuropathic arthropathy by far is most common at the Lisfranc and Chopart joints. However, if

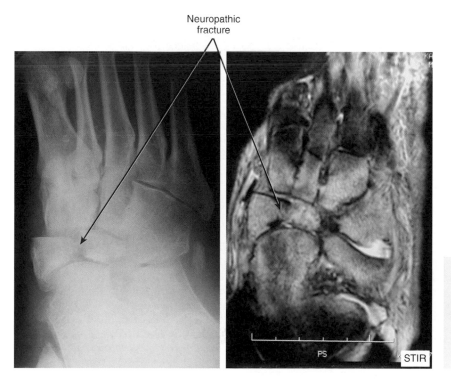

Neuropathic fracture

Fig. 14.46 Neuropathic fracture. Oblique radiograph of the foot and corresponding MRI show fracture of the navicular bone. There is marked soft tissue and bone marrow edema throughout the hindfoot. Fractures can occur in the setting of neuropathic disease, resulting in tremendous edema as the patient continues to walk on the insensate foot. (From Morrison W. *Problem Solving in Musculoskeletal Imaging.* Philadelphia: Elsevier; 2010.)

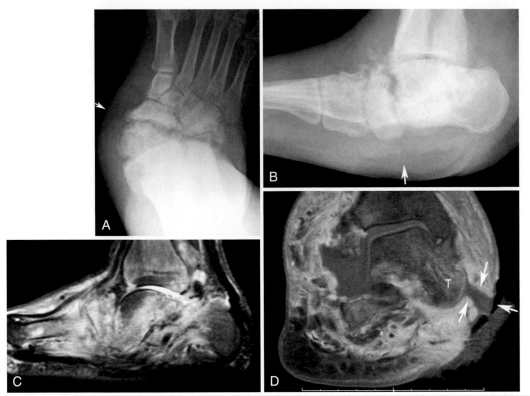

Fig. 14.47 Osteomyelitis in diabetic neuropathic foot. (A and B) AP **(A)** and lateral **(B)** radiographs show classic neuropathic changes in the midfoot and hindfoot with increased bone density, collapse of the arch, and severe degenerative changes. There is a medial plantar ulcer adjacent to the medially subluxed talar head *(arrow)*. **(C)** Sagittal inversion recovery MR image shows diffuse marrow edema and effusions, which are an expected finding given the severe neuropathic changes and are not specific for osteomyelitis. **(D)** Short-axis contrast-enhanced fat-suppressed T1-weighted MR image obtained through the distal hindfoot shows marrow enhancement, a large fluid collection, and a sinus tract extending from the talar head (T) to the lateral ulcer *(arrows)*. The sinus tract increases the MRI specificity for diagnosis of osteomyelitis.

there is foot deformity, contiguous spread of infection can occur at atypical sites (e.g., the cuboid in cases of 'rocker-bottom' deformity).

- Culture results of percutaneous bone biopsy specimens in pedal infection may be unreliable due to contamination from adjacent infected or colonized soft tissues.
  - If percutaneous biopsy of bone is performed, the needle route should be planned away from the area of soft tissue infection. This is done for two reasons: to avoid a false positive culture, and to avoid potentially inoculating noninfected bone.

Sample Report

Exam Type: MRI FOOT LEFT WO CONTRAST
Exam Date and Time: DATE/TIME
Indication: 65-year-old female diabetic with wound at great
   toe, rule out osteomyelitis
Comparison: Left foot radiographs from 1 day prior

IMPRESSION:
1. *Early osteomyelitis of the great toe involving the distal phalanx and proximal phalanx head, with associated first interphalangeal joint septic arthritis and overlying soft tissue ulcer.*
2. *Postoperative changes of the third digit amputation at the level of the distal interphalangeal joint, with normal appearance of the resection margin.*
3. *Denervation edema/atrophy throughout the intrinsic musculature of the forefoot.*

Sample Report—cont'd

TECHNIQUE:
MRI of the left foot was performed on a 1.5-Tesla system using a standard noncontrast protocol in three planes (axial, sagittal, and coronal).

FINDINGS:
There is a soft tissue ulcer at the plantar aspect of the great toe. There is intense marrow edema in the subjacent first distal phalanx and proximal phalanx head, with associated subtle replacement of normal T1 marrow signal, consistent with early osteomyelitis and first interphalangeal joint septic arthritis. No additional sites of osteomyelitis are identified. No organized fluid collection is identified to suggest abscess.

There are postoperative changes consistent with amputation of the third digit at the level of the distal interphalangeal joint. The resection margin appears normal. No fractures are identified. There is no significant midfoot neuropathic (Charcot) arthropathy.

There is diffuse nonspecific circumferential soft tissue swelling about the forefoot. There is severe denervation edema throughout the intrinsic musculature of the forefoot with moderate fatty infiltration. A small ganglion cyst is interposed between the proximal fourth and fifth metatarsals.

Visualized portions of the flexor, extensor, and peroneal tendons are intact. The Lisfranc ligament complex is intact.

Recurrent Infection After Amputation

- Decades ago the treatment for osteomyelitis of the foot in diabetic patients was amputation, leaving a functional stump (transmetatarsal, Lisfranc, Chopart, Symes [entire foot resected], or below-the-knee amputation [BKA]).
- Due to improvement in revascularization procedures and recognition that amputation results in acceleration of disease in the contralateral extremity due to shift of weight-bearing, the surgical goal over the past decade has been to preserve as much tissue (and function) as possible and only resect the infected bone.
- The new postoperative challenge has been to heal the surgical site in an ischemic foot, and to leave no infected bone that would result in recurrent disease.
- If there is concern for persistent/recurrent infection, MRI is the imaging modality of choice.
  - After amputation, regardless of time course, the marrow should have no edema or enhancement. There are exceptions, of course: for example, if the patient is stressing the stump with an ill-fitting prosthesis or due to lack of sensation, edema may be

seen. However, as a rule, any bone marrow edema at the amputation site should be considered suspicious for infection (Fig. 14.48).
  - It can also be helpful to review the preoperative MRI to see whether all infected bone was removed.
  - Rim-enhancing fluid collections and sinus tracts are useful secondary signs (Fig. 14.49).

Infection Around Metal Implants (Figs. 14.17, 14.50 through 14.52)

- Assessment of the postoperative patient, especially post joint replacement, can be difficult.
- Radiographs are the recommended screening exam; these may show signs of loosening such as lucency at the bone–cement or bone–implant interface, subsidence (component 'sinking into' the underlying bone), and/or periosteal reaction.
  - Radiographic findings appear late in the course of infection and are relatively insensitive.
- Metal artifact may limit evaluation with MR or CT. Increasing tube current (mAs) and kilovoltage peak (kVp)

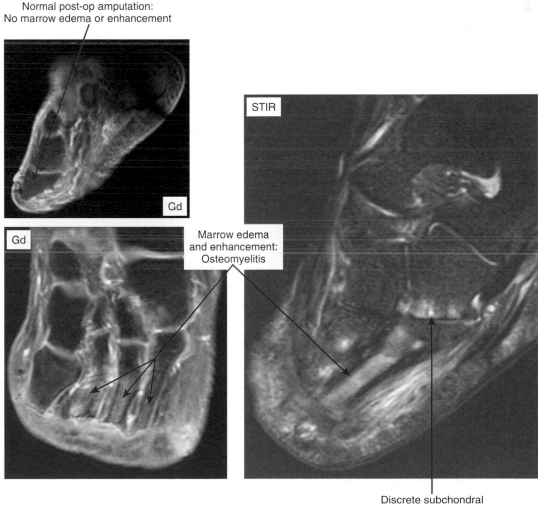

Fig. 14.48 Postoperative transmetatarsal amputation for diabetic pedal infection. Post-contrast MRI of a patient without recurrent infection (upper left) shows normal bone marrow signal without enhancement. MRI of a different patient (lower images) shows marrow edema and enhancement representing recurrent infection of the residual metatarsal bones. (From Morrison W. *Problem Solving in Musculoskeletal Imaging*. Philadelphia: Elsevier; 2010.)

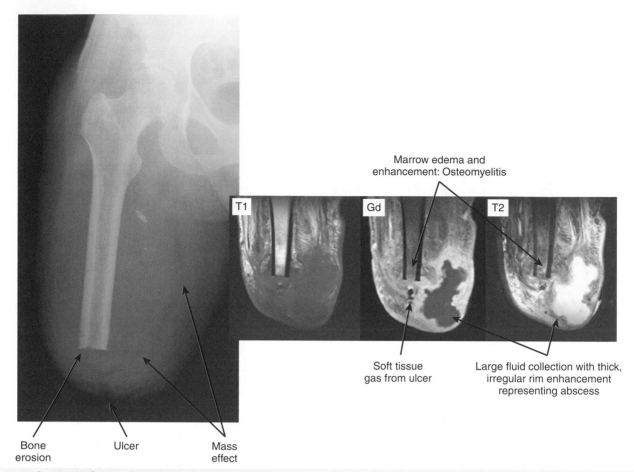

Marrow edema and
enhancement: Osteomyelitis

T1   Gd   T2

Soft tissue
gas from ulcer

Large fluid collection with thick,
irregular rim enhancement
representing abscess

Bone
erosion   Ulcer   Mass
effect

Fig. 14.49 Recurrent infection of a residual limb following above-the-knee amputation. Radiograph (left image) shows ulceration, soft tissue swelling, and erosion of the bone. MRI (right images) reveals a large abscess with adjacent bone marrow edema and enhancement representing osteomyelitis. (From Morrison W. *Problem Solving in Musculoskeletal Imaging*. Philadelphia: Elsevier; 2010.)

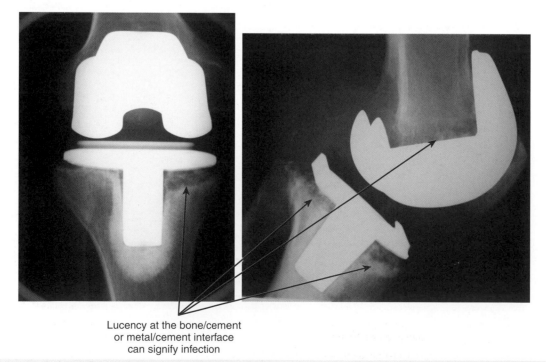

Lucency at the bone/cement
or metal/cement interface
can signify infection

Fig. 14.50 Total knee replacement with infection. Lucency at the interface with bone could indicate infection or loosening. Clinical correlation is needed and aspiration may be required. (From Morrison W. *Problem Solving in Musculoskeletal Imaging*. Philadelphia: Elsevier; 2010.)

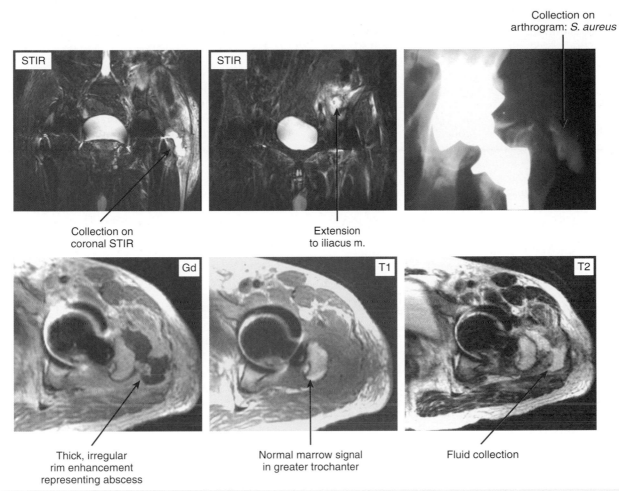

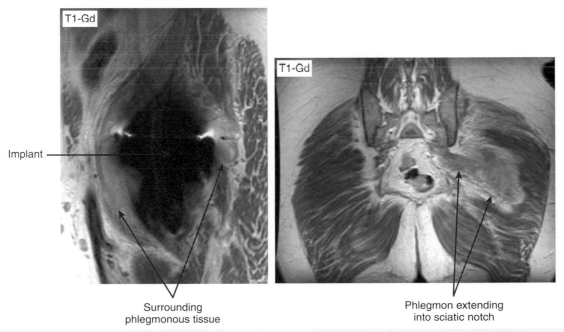

Fig. 14.51 Hip prosthesis infection on MRI. STIR sequences (upper left, center) show a fluid collection at the greater trochanteric bursa extending under the iliacus muscle; axial images (lower row) demonstrate communication with the prosthetic joint. This is confirmed on joint aspiration followed by injection of contrast, showing opacification of the bursa (top right image). (From Morrison W. *Problem Solving in Musculoskeletal Imaging.* Philadelphia: Elsevier; 2010.)

Fig. 14.52 Hip prosthesis infection. Following total hip replacement, this patient developed fever and symptoms of sciatic nerve irritation. Post-contrast MRI shows enhancing phlegmonous tissue extending from the hip into the sciatic notch. (From Morrison W. *Problem Solving in Musculoskeletal Imaging.* Philadelphia: Elsevier; 2010.)

and using specialized reconstruction algorithms on CT, and metal artifact reduction techniques on MRI can be helpful, as reviewed in Chapter 1 – Introduction to Musculoskeletal Imaging and Chapter 10 – Arthroplasty.

- On CT, focal lucency around the implants and adjacent fluid collections are associated with infection.
- On MRI adjacent marrow edema and enhancement can be detected occasionally.
  - Fluid collection or collections with thick, enhancing rims near the implant are present, which suggests infection.
  - Contrast arthrography can be used to detect the presence of communication with the joint.
  - MRI can also serve an adjunctive role, diagnosing fluid collections far from the implants that may need to be drained during surgery.
- Bone scan can show increased uptake in the areas of infection, and labeled WBC scanning is also useful.
- Ultimately, however, aspiration with culture and fluid analysis may be needed to document presence or absence of infection (see Chapter 16 – Musculoskeletal Procedure and Techniques).

Bacterial Infection of the Spine

Spine infection deserves special consideration; this is a relatively common clinical condition that can result in serious morbidity. This discussion is focused on disc and bone infection.

- *Discitis* represents infection of the intervertebral disc.
- If the infection extends beyond the endplate into the medullary space, it is referred to as *discitis-osteomyelitis*, or *infectious spondylitis*.
- Recognition of early radiographic and MRI manifestations are extremely important to avoid serious complications.

MODES OF SPINE INFECTION

The three modes of musculoskeletal infection previously described also apply to the spine: hematogenous, contiguous spread, and direct implantation.

Hematogenous

Most spine infection is hematogenous.

- Arterial: Spread occurs via paired arteries that course along the posterior margin of the vertebral bodies.
  - One branch enters the posterior vertebral body and supplies the posterior-central aspect.
  - Another branch passes through the neural foramen and forms an anastomotic network of vessels surrounding the metaphyseal aspect of the vertebral body margin (adjacent to the endplates), with end-arterioles in the periphery of the anterior-lateral vertebral body next to the endplates.
- Venous: Spread occurs via Batson's plexus.
  - *Batson's plexus*: a valveless venous complex responsible for draining blood from the pelvis, lumbar spine, and the lower thoracic spine.
  - Direction of flow is away from the vertebral column in most situations, but with increased intraabdominal

pressure the direction can reverse and blood from the pelvis can flow in retrograde fashion into the vertebral bodies.
- The plexus penetrates each vertebra at the central aspect of the posterior vertebral body margin, with a Y-shaped channel within the vertebra that branches out to anastomotic vessels at the periphery.
- Patients with pelvic infection can acquire secondary vertebral infection; most commonly seen with *Mycobacterium tuberculosis* (TB; where genitourinary involvement is common), with discitis-osteomyelitis occurring at the thoracolumbar junction.
- Both arterial and venous patterns of spread result in inoculation of the endplate first in adults.
  - Therefore, the most common source of disc infection is considered to be direct spread from the adjacent endplate.
  - The disc is composed of mucoproteinaceous material that offers a rich supply of nutrients for the infecting organism, and extension of infection through the disc and into the opposite endplate is rapid.
  - This causes the classic pattern of involvement of the disc and adjacent endplates commonly seen in discitis-osteomyelitis.
- Although the intervertebral disc is considered avascular, children and some young adults have vessels penetrating into the discs from the endplates, a distribution that has been theorized to explain the incidence of primary discitis in children.
- In older adults with degenerative disc disease, the discs may become revascularized, which can explain reports of increased incidence of infection in degenerated discs.

Contiguous Spread

From an extraspinal source to the vertebral column is relatively uncommon. Some of the more common sources include:

- Parapharyngeal infection extending to the cervical spine.
- Pulmonary infection extending to the thoracic spine.
- Extension of SI joint infection proximally to the lower lumbar spine.
- Extension of pelvic infection or sinus tracts from bowel to the adjacent sacrum or lumbar spine.
- Paralyzed patients with decubitus ulcers where infection spreads contiguously to the spine more cephalad.

Direct Implantation

- Spine surgery and percutaneous procedures such as discography, vertebral augmentation, and pain injections.

IMAGING OF BACTERIAL INFECTIOUS SPONDYLITIS

- Radiographs are typically the first study obtained as part of the radiologic workup of suspected infection.
- Early manifestations of pyogenic discitis-osteomyelitis on radiographs include disc space narrowing, vertebral endplate osteolysis or irregularity, and paraspinal soft tissue mass effect (Fig. 14.53).

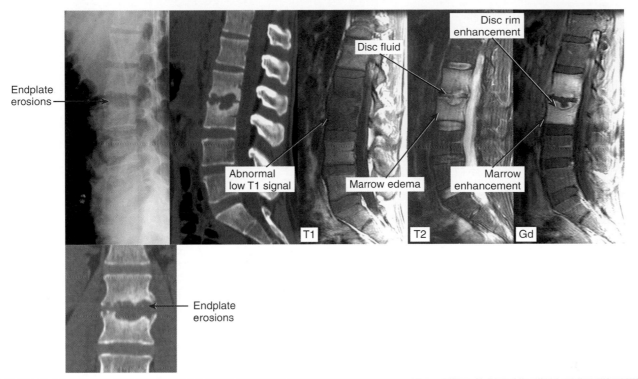

Fig. 14.53 Imaging characteristics of bacterial discitis-osteomyelitis. Radiographs and CT (left three images) show erosion of the disc endplates. MRI (right three images) reveals adjacent vertebral bone marrow edema and enhancement with fluid signal in the disc. (From Morrison W. *Problem Solving in Musculoskeletal Imaging.* Philadelphia: Elsevier; 2010.)

- Eventually, there may be gross destruction of the endplates, collapse of the vertebral body, deformity, and sclerosis.
- In most cases with bacterial infection, only one disc level is involved. In more severe or chronic cases, spread to adjacent vertebral levels can occur along paravertebral ligaments or fascial planes.
- Mycobacterial infection can have a different appearance than bacterial infection, noted for paravertebral spread with sparing of the disc, multilevel involvement, bone destruction, and deformity.

MR Imaging

- MRI is the primary modality for establishing the diagnosis of discitis-osteomyelitis. High sensitivity (ranging from 90 to 100%) and specificity (ranging from 80 to 95%), combined with anatomic detail, allows accurate diagnosis as well as delineation of extent of involvement and identification of paraspinal and epidural abscess (Fig. 14.54).
- The infected disc demonstrates low signal on T1-weighted images and high signal (approximating fluid) on T2-weighted images (Fig. 14.53).
- Fat-suppression technique is recommended on the T2-weighted images in order to best demonstrate associated endplate edema.
- On T1- and T2-weighted sagittal images, the endplates may be irregular, with loss of the normal low-signal cortical line.
- Administration of intravenous gadolinium-based contrast in conjunction with a fat-suppressed T1-weighted imaging sequence can aid diagnostic confidence; the

infected disc demonstrates rim-enhancement along the disc margins, with enhancement of the adjacent vertebral endplates.
- Initially, vertebral body enhancement is adjacent to the disc, but frequently the entire vertebral body above and below the affected disc level will enhance diffusely.
- T2-weighted images and fat-suppressed T1-weighted contrast-enhanced images are particularly useful for identification of paraspinal or epidural abscess.
  - Abscesses are typically longitudinally oriented, extending along paraspinal ligaments or fascial planes, often distant from the original site of infection.
  - MRI is ideal for identification of location and extent of involvement, as well as level and degree of compromise of the spinal canal for operative planning.

NONINFECTIOUS MIMICS OF INFECTIOUS SPONDYLITIS

Certain noninfectious conditions can result in radiologic findings which can mimic those of discitis-osteomyelitis.

Degenerative Disease

- Like infection, degenerative disc disease results in disc narrowing, with associated endplate irregularity and sclerosis.
- Although soft tissue mass effect is absent with degenerative disc disease (except for disc bulge/herniation), this is not a reliable discriminator on radiographs or CT.
- Disc degeneration is commonly associated with a vacuum phenomenon, which is nearly 100% specific for degenerative disc disease and virtually excludes infection.

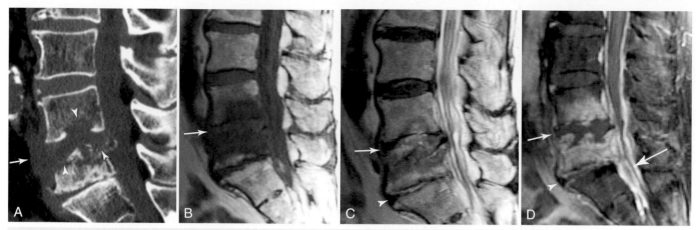

Fig. 14.54 Adult lumbar discitis-osteomyelitis with epidural abscess. **(A)** Sagittal CT reconstruction shows endplate destruction at L4-L5 *(arrowheads)* and anterior soft tissue attenuation *(arrow)*. (B–D) Sagittal T1-weighted **(B)**, T2-weighted **(C)**, and postcontrast fat-suppressed T1-weighted **(D)** MR images show edematous L4-L5 *(arrow)* and L5-S1 *(arrowhead)* discs, intense marrow edema and enhancement in L4 and L5 adjacent to the L4-L5 disc and loss of the normal low-signal cortical line of the vertebral endplates. Also note intense enhancement around an epidural abscess posterior to S1 in D *(long arrow)*.

Flexion   Extension

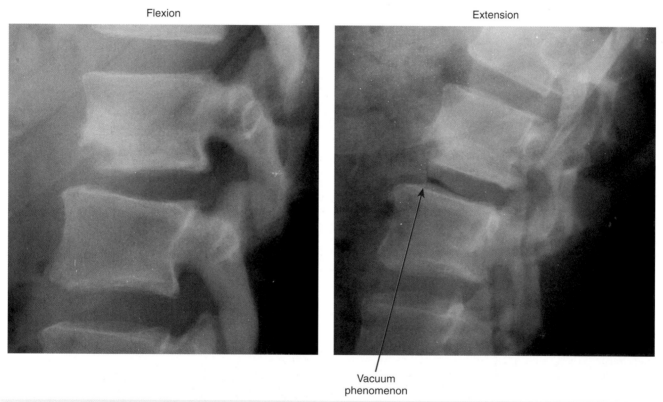

Vacuum
phenomenon

Fig. 14.55 Segmental instability simulating discitis-osteomyelitis. Lateral radiographs of the upper lumbar spine show disc narrowing and what appears to be erosion of an adjacent endplate. However, flexion and extension views show excess motion at the disc level, with appearance of a vacuum on extension. Presence of a vacuum disc is common in segmental instability but rare in the setting of infection. (From Morrison W. *Problem Solving in Musculoskeletal Imaging.* Philadelphia: Elsevier; 2010.)

As a result, this sign should be sought in cases of suspected infection; lateral radiographs in flexion and extension can aid in identification of vacuum phenomenon (Fig. 14.55). CT is highly sensitive for detection of subtle vacuum phenomenon.

- On MRI, Modic type 1 degenerative endplate changes can mimic infection, with decreased T1 signal and increased T2 signal. However, the associated disc itself will show low signal on T1- and T2-weighted images if degenerated, versus high T2 signal seen in infection.
  - There is some evidence that a subset of symptomatic discs with Modic 1 changes are infected with low-virulence organisms, although has not been confirmed.
- MRI can also detect paraspinal edema and mass effect which are absent in degenerative disc disease. Facet

osteoarthritis, like other arthritic joints, can exhibit adjacent bone marrow edema and should not be confused for infection.

- Schmorl nodes (intravertebral disc herniation) cause the appearance of endplate irregularity, and in early stages show marrow edema on MRI (Fig. 14.56), which can falsely suggest infection.

Segmental Instability/Neuropathic Disease
(Figs. 14.57 and 14.58)

- Instability and neuropathic disease of the spine radiographically appears as aggressive degenerative disc disease, often with subluxation (spondylolisthesis), debris and disorganization, and preservation of bone density characteristically seen in other joints with neuropathic arthropathy.
  - Endplate irregularity can be marked, associated with disc narrowing, resembling an infectious etiology. Again, identification of a vacuum phenomenon is the best discriminator; fortunately, vacuum phenomena are common in situations of instability and neuropathy.
  - Facet joint involvement is common in segmental instability; it is rare in discitis-osteomyelitis.
  - On MR images, segmental instability can appear similar to infection; the unstable level can demonstrate high T2 signal in the disc, as well as edema in the adjacent vertebral bodies, and paraspinal edema and mass effect.
- In some cases, it can be difficult to differentiate segmental instability from infection, and aspiration/biopsy may be necessary.

Dialysis-Associated Spondyloarthropathy

- Long-term hemodialysis results in retention and accumulation of beta-2 microglobulin, which forms a type of amyloid.

- The amyloid can accumulate in joints where it simulates inflammatory arthritis, and in the intervertebral discs where it is painful and resembles discitis-osteomyelitis on imaging (Fig. 14.59).
  - More than one disc level is commonly involved.
  - Look for evidence of renal failure and secondary hyperparathyroidism.
  - Amyloid deposition in the appendicular skeleton can present as paraarticular soft tissue masses or juxtaarticular lucent lesions.
  - A clue to the diagnosis is that on MRI amyloid usually appears as low-signal material on T1- and T2-weighted sequences. Although helpful, this is not a completely reliable sign.
  - In some situations, differentiation from infection can be difficult, prompting aspiration/biopsy.
    - If amyloid is suspected, the pathologist should be alerted; Congo red stain is utilized to detect amyloid.
- Amyloid is discussed further in Chapter 9 – Arthritis and Chapter 13 – Bone Marrow and Metabolic Bone Disease.

Postoperative Changes

- Unfortunately, it can be difficult to differentiate recent postoperative changes from such procedures as discectomy or fusion from those of superimposed infection.
  - High disc T2 signal, diffuse enhancement, and fluid collections can all be seen in the postoperative period.
  - Follow-up MRI examinations may provide useful information, as postoperative changes should gradually subside.
    - MRI can identify suspicious sites of enhancement or fluid collections to aspirate for culture. In this situation, a nuclear medicine scan utilizing labeled WBCs may also be useful.

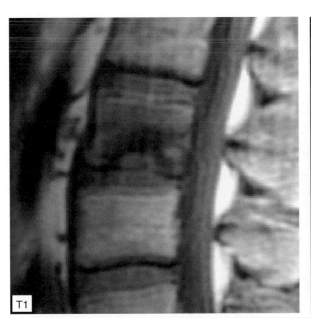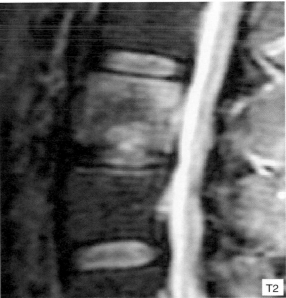

Fig. 14.56 Acute traumatic Schmorl node. Herniation of disc material through the vertebral endplate is often accompanied by bone marrow edema in the early stages, which can simulate infection. Caution should be exercised, however, because Schmorl nodes can form in bone weakened by tumor and other causes. (From Morrison W. *Problem Solving in Musculoskeletal Imaging.* Philadelphia: Elsevier; 2010.)

No surrounding
edge

Anterolisthesis

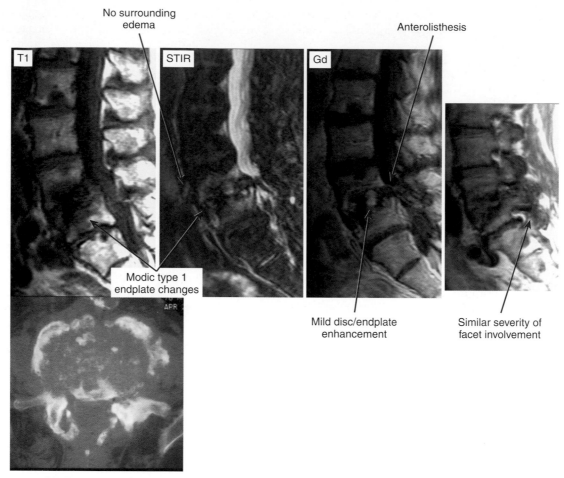

Modic type 1
endplate changes

Mild disc/endplate
enhancement

Similar severity of
facet involvement

CT: Bone proliferation

Fig. 14.57 Segmental instability of the spine on MRI and CT. MR images (upper row) show anterolisthesis, disc narrowing, and Modic type I degenerative endplate changes. Note similar severity of degenerative changes at the facet joints. CT (lower image) of a different patient with segmental instability related to laminectomy shows bony proliferation and fragmentation reminiscent of neuropathic arthropathy. (From Morrison W. *Problem Solving in Musculoskeletal Imaging*. Philadelphia: Elsevier; 2010.)

Screw in
disc

Low T1
signal

Endplate
erosions

Disc fluid

Marrow
enhancement

Disc rim
enhancement

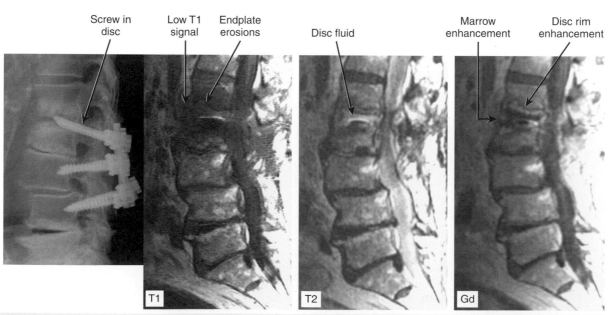

Fig. 14.58 Segmental instability related to failure of spinal fusion. Lateral radiograph (on left) shows posterior metallic fixation with migration of the upper pedicle screw into the adjacent disc. Resultant disc narrowing and erosion of the endplate can simulate infection, with edema and enhancement on MRI. (From Morrison W. *Problem Solving in Musculoskeletal Imaging*. Philadelphia: Elsevier; 2010.)

Rugger jersey spine

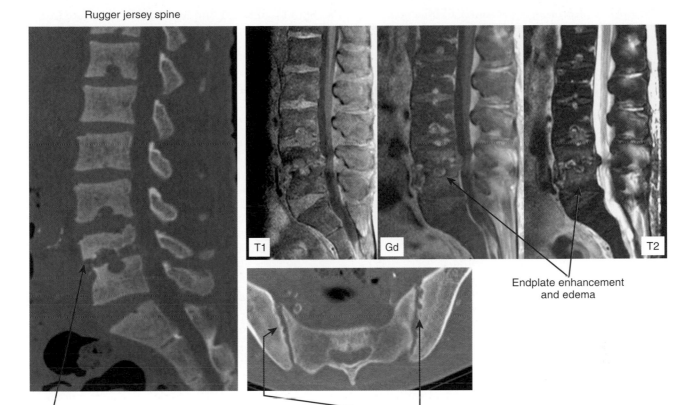

T1

Gd

T2

Endplate enhancement
and edema

Endplate
erosions

Resorption
at the sacroiliac joints

Fig. 14.59 Renal failure and secondary hyperparathyroidism simulating infection. CT (left and lower image) show bone resorption at the sacroiliac joints and erosion at the vertebral endplates. MRI (upper right) shows endplate erosions with edema and enhancement. (From Morrison W. *Problem Solving in Musculoskeletal Imaging*. Philadelphia: Elsevier; 2010.)

Histology/Culture

- Bone biopsy is performed if clinical and radiological evaluation is not conclusive or if microbial diagnosis is needed for selecting antibiotic coverage.
- Definitive diagnosis of osteomyelitis relies on positive culture results of causative organisms from a biopsy sample or characteristic histological findings, including aggregates of inflammatory cells (including neutrophils, lymphocytes, histiocytes, and plasma cells), erosions of trabecular bone, and marrow changes that range from loss of normal marrow fat in acute osteomyelitis to fibrosis and reactive bone formation in chronic osteomyelitis.
- Limitations of percutaneous and surgical bone biopsy include: sampling error, false-negative cultures (especially in patients receiving antibiotics), difficulties in distinguishing other osteopathy from osteomyelitis histologically, and the risk of introducing contaminating uninfected bone after passing the needle through a soft tissue infection.
- Culture results of percutaneous bone biopsy specimens in pedal infection may be unreliable due to contamination from adjacent infected soft tissue; also, in diabetic feet, multiorganism infections predominate.
- Bone biopsy cultures in osteomyelitis in general may be falsely negative in up to 50% of cases. If antibiotics have been used, the false negative result can be as high as 80%.

- Adding histopathologic diagnosis improves sensitivity for detection of osteomyelitis.
  - Therefore, bone biopsy should always include a histology evaluation as well as culture. Aspiration alone may not provide the diagnosis.

Common Organisms in Bacterial Osteomyelitis

- Acute osteomyelitis is usually caused by pyogenic bacteria.
- Common pathogens of acute osteomyelitis vary with the age of the patient.
  - In neonates *S. aureus*, group B *Streptococcus*, and *Escherichia coli* are most common.
  - In children *S. aureus*, often MRSA, is most common.
  - Children with sickle cell disease may also be infected with *Salmonella*.
  - In adults *Staphylococcus* and enteric pathogens predominate.
  - Intravenous drug users are often infected with Gram-negative species such as *Pseudomonas* and *Klebsiella*.
- *S. aureus* is the most common bacterium cultured in cases of septic arthritis and osteomyelitis. Less common are *Streptococcus*, *Klebsiella*, *Pseudomonas* species, and others.

- When chronic ulceration is the source of infection, multiple organisms are often cultured.
- Mycobacterial infections are becoming more common in the general population as resistant strains emerge.
  - Mycobacterial infection is discussed in greater detail later in this chapter.
- Parasitic and fungal infections are relatively rare, but prevalence depends on the region and travel history as well as clinical factors.
  - Residence in or travel to the southwest U.S. should raise suspicion for coccidioidomycosis. An immunocompromised state increases the incidence of opportunistic infections such as fungi.
- Seasonal variations can also occur; for instance, a child presenting with a monoarticular inflammatory arthritis during tick season in endemic regions should prompt consideration of Lyme disease.
- Some specific types of osteomyelitis deserve special mention.
  - *Congenital syphilis* osteomyelitis initially demonstrates metaphyseal irregularity and a widened zone of provisional calcification, occasionally resulting in slipped epiphyses. It may progress to invade the diaphysis and elicit periosteal reaction (Fig. 14.60).
  - Congenital syphilis is in the differential diagnosis for neonates and infants with generalized periosteal reaction. Other conditions to be considered include nonaccidental trauma, tumor, other infections, and metabolic diseases.
  - Acquired tertiary syphilis osteomyelitis presents as a chronic infection, with periostitis and endosteal reaction resulting in an enlarged bowed bone with mixed lytic and sclerotic areas. The flat bones and cranium may be involved with syphilis osteomyelitis. When the tibia is involved, it tends to develop an anterior bowing deformity that has been termed the *saber shin deformity*. Another manifestation of syphilis is neuropathic arthropathy, especially involving the knees.

- Skin breakdown and injuries are associated with soft tissue and bone infection, which are often multiorganism.
  - In the hand, metacarpals and phalanges are at risk for infection from a human bite, which is usually acquired by punching an adversary in the mouth.
  - A finger or toe may develop a *felon* or infection in the terminal pulp that may progress to osteomyelitis of the tuft.
  - A stubbed great toe with a nail bed injury may result in osteomyelitis of the distal phalanx because the periosteum is immediately adjacent to the nail bed (Fig. 14.61). Soft tissue infection of the hand or foot may spread along tendon sheaths and fascial planes, so that a site of osteomyelitis may be distant from the site of soft tissue injury.
  - Foreign bodies in the hand or foot may lead to infection (see Fig. 1.75).

Atypical Manifestations of Bacterial Infection

INFECTION SUPERIMPOSED ON UNDERLYING DISORDERS

- Underlying metabolic disorders can alter marrow signal on MRI and uptake on bone scan, leading to errors in interpretation.
  - Examples include marrow-packing disorders such as Gaucher's disease or marrow hyperplasia such as from severe anemia or colony-stimulating factor treatment (both of which can result in diffusely increased T2 signal), as well as hemosiderin deposition (e.g., numerous blood transfusions or hemochromatosis) and marrow fibrosis (resulting in diffusely low signal on MRI).
  - Osteonecrosis also causes a diagnostic dilemma (Fig. 14.62). Acute osteonecrosis in the metaphysis

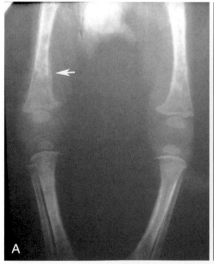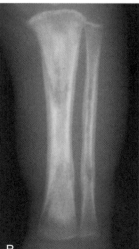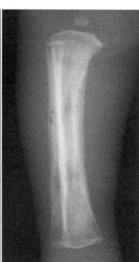

Fig. 14.60 Congenital syphilis osteomyelitis. **(A)** AP radiograph of the lower extremities shows periosteal reaction *(arrow)* and lucent metaphyses. **(B)** AP and lateral leg radiographs show similar findings. Also note the diaphyseal lucencies and anterior bowing of the tibia in B. (Part B Only From Morrison W. *Problem Solving in Musculoskeletal Imaging.* Philadelphia: Elsevier; 2010.)

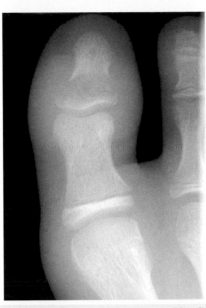

Fig. 14.61 Osteomyelitis in the stubbed great toe. AP radiograph demonstrates soft tissue swelling about the great toe and lysis of the distal phalanx. This 13-year-old had a history of stubbed toe and nail bed injury. The great toe nail bed is contiguous with the proximal dorsal periosteum of the distal phalanx, which provides a route of bacterial entry. (Image used with permission from BJ Manaster, MD, from the American College of Radiology Learning File.)

or diaphysis (often termed a *bone infarct*) can cause an appearance of periosteal reaction on radiographs, marrow edema on MRI, and reactive bone turnover as well as migration of inflammatory cells with abnormal uptake on nuclear medicine scans.

- Chronic bone infarcts usually have characteristic appearance on various modalities (discussed in Chapter 13 – Bone Marrow and Metabolic Bone Disease). However, imaging findings may overlap, and osteomyelitis and osteonecrosis can coexist.
- Secondary signs of infection on MRI such as fluid collections, sinus tracts, and overlying cellulitis can be helpful, as well as gadolinium-based contrast enhancement, which would not be expected in infarcted tissue.
- Occasionally imaging cannot distinguish infection from these underlying disorders, and biopsy is indicated.

NONINFECTIOUS BONE REACTION TO ADJACENT SOFT TISSUE INFLAMMATION

In response to chronic ulceration and/or cellulitis, the periosteum can focally lay down new bone, forming what has been termed an *ulcer osteoma*, or *inflammatory exostosis* (Figs. 14.6 and 14.63).

A corresponding MRI pattern: Adjacent to soft tissue inflammation, adjacent cortex may become hyperemic and demonstrate subcortical edema and enhancement on MR images (*reactive changes*).

- This has been previously termed *osteitis* implying inflammation of the cortex to distinguish it from inflammation of the marrow cavity (*osteomyelitis*) (Figs. 14.29 and 14.64).

- However, this finding may represent early osteomyelitis.
- The main clinical question is presence or absence of osteomyelitis.
- Thus it is now recommended that the report be phrased to incorporate level of concern for osteomyelitis (i.e., 'low likelihood' vs. 'high likelihood' of osteomyelitis) as well as recommendations for follow-up.
    - Also recommended is to avoid using the term *osteitis* altogether, given its variable application (osteitis pubis, osteitis condensans ilii, and others) and variable MRI features used to describe it.

Musculoskeletal Infection with 'Atypical' Organisms

- Imaging appearance of the so-called 'atypical infections', that is, with fungal, mycobacterial, or parasitic agents, can differ from those of routine bacterial infections described earlier.
- Additionally, unlike bacterial infections, clinical systemic manifestations and laboratory values may not immediately suggest infection.
- Radiological manifestations of bacterial infections stem from common characteristics such as rapid course, metabolization and destruction of cartilage and fat, immune response resulting in generation of debris and inflammatory infiltrate (pus), and reactive bone response. Atypical organisms often proceed slowly and survive on different materials, altering the imaging appearance and immune response.
    - For example, infective bacteria, (especially *S. aureus*), in synovial joints or intervertebral discs rapidly metabolize proteoglycan matrix that is composed of hyaline cartilage and disc material, resulting in rapid joint/disc narrowing and destruction. Mycobacteria have different nutritional preferences and therefore tend to spare articular cartilage and disc material early on, instead presenting as indolent infections and preferring to spread along paraspinal fascial planes along multiple levels rather than through the disc at one level.
    - However, many mycobacterial infections resemble typical bacterial infections.

MYCOBACTERIUM TUBERCULOSIS INFECTION

- Mycobacterial infections, especially *M. tuberculosis* (TB), can infect the spine (Figs. 14.65 through 14.67).
- Early descriptions were made by Pott in 1779. Evidence of tuberculous spondylitis has been observed in skeletons of prehistoric humans.
- Advent of modern antibiotic therapy initially made the disease relatively rare.
- In more recent years, there has been a resurgence of TB cases caused by drug-resistant strains and due to an increasing prevalence of immunocompromised individuals.
- TB is typically spread via a hematogenous route, although some cases in the thoracic spine have been

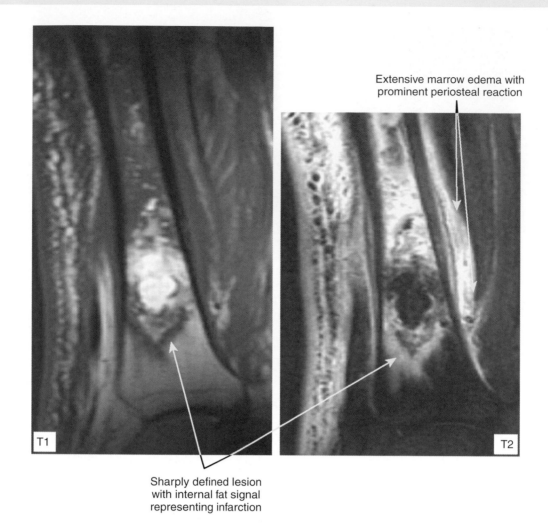

Extensive marrow edema with
prominent periosteal reaction

Sharply defined lesion
with internal fat signal
representing infarction

Cloaca in cortex

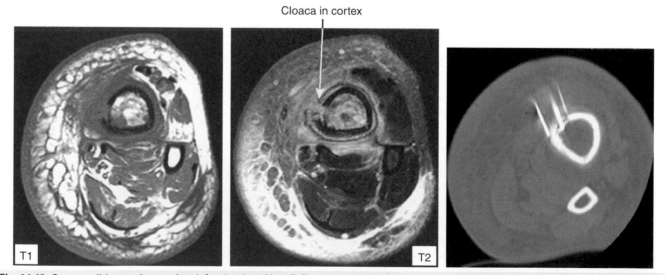

Fig. 14.62 Osteomyelitis superimposed on infarction in sickle cell disease. Acute infarction can resemble infection on radiographs and CT (with periosteal reaction), MRI (with diffuse edema), and bone scan (surrounding tracer uptake). Some differentiating features include sinus tract, rim-enhancing fluid collection, and diffuse marrow enhancement. However, contrast may be contraindicated in acute sickle crisis. Periosteal reaction, diffuse edema, and cloaca (opening in the cortex) suggested infection, confirmed at biopsy (lower right image). (From Morrison W. *Problem Solving in Musculoskeletal Imaging*. Philadelphia: Elsevier; 2010.)

Axial slices

Ulcer osteoma

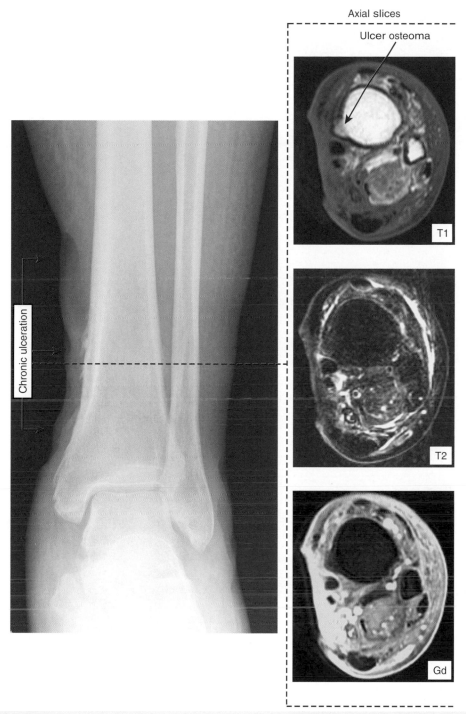

Fig. 14.63 Ulcer osteoma. Bone formation can occur adjacent to chronic ulceration, simulating periosteal reaction and bone infection. MRI is useful to confirm normal marrow signal. See also Fig. 14.6. (From Morrison W. *Problem Solving in Musculoskeletal Imaging*. Philadelphia: Elsevier; 2010.)

related to contiguous spread from pulmonary parenchymal and pleural disease.

- The majority of patients with skeletal involvement have primary involvement of other organ systems, especially pulmonary or genitourinary.
- Clinically, tuberculous spondylitis can present insidiously, with progressive back pain, occasionally with neurologic symptoms.
- Fever may be low grade or not present, and the WBC count may be mildly elevated or normal. Involvement

of other organ systems may not be readily apparent clinically.

- A purified protein derivative (PPD) skin test is generally positive, although it can be negative during overwhelming infection.
- The most common imaging presentation in the spine and appendicular skeleton is the same as routine bacterial infection.
- However, especially in untreated chronic cases, 'classic' features develop, including preservation of the disc or

Normal T1 signal

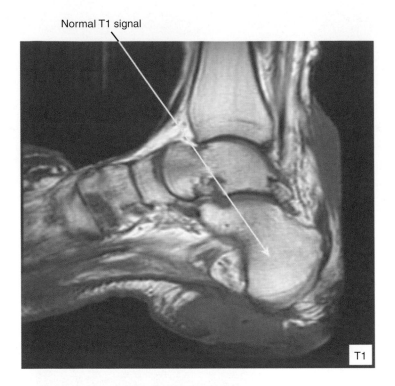

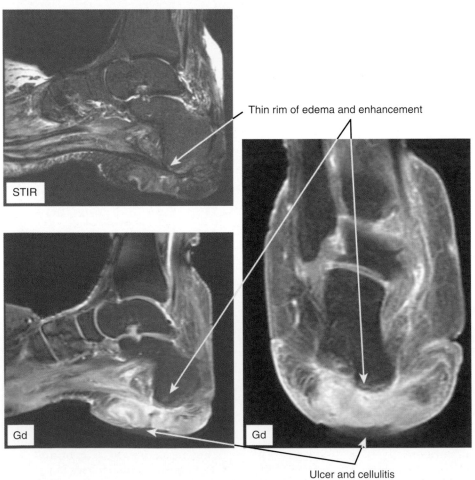

Thin rim of edema and enhancement

Ulcer and cellulitis

Fig. 14.64 Mild subcortical edema can be reactive to adjacent soft tissue infection without bone infection. In this example, early osteomyelitis is not excluded, but this is of low probability for osteomyelitis. Follow-up imaging can be helpful if there is ongoing clinical concern for osteomyelitis. (From Morrison W. *Problem Solving in Musculoskeletal Imaging*. Philadelphia: Elsevier; 2010.)

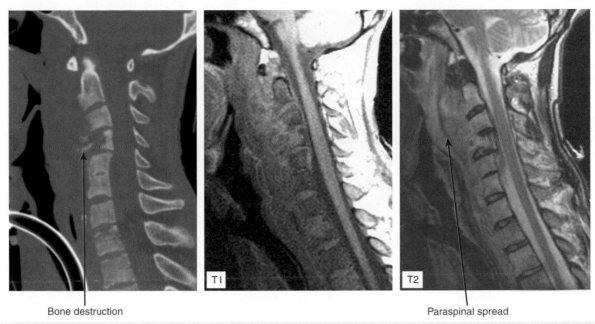

Bone destruction   Paraspinal spread

Fig. 14.65 Tuberculosis of the cervical spine. Spinal involvement in tuberculous infection can spare the disc initially, spreading along the paraspinal soft tissues to other vertebral levels. Bone destruction and deformity may ensue in later stages. (From Morrison W. *Problem Solving in Musculoskeletal Imaging*. Philadelphia: Elsevier; 2010.)

articular cartilage, paraspinal spread, extensive bone destruction, deformity, and adjacent soft tissue calcification (see Figs. 14.66 and 14.67).

Key Concepts

Tuberculous Versus Bacterial Spine Infection

BACTERIAL	TUBERCULOUS
Aggressive	Indolent
Rapid onset	Slow onset
Single spinal level	Multiple spinal levels
Spread through disc to endplates	Paraspinal spread around discs
Paraspinal, epidural abscesses	Paraspinal, epidural abscesses
No calcification	Paraspinal calcification
Endplate destruction, erosion	Masslike destruction of bone; collapse
Minimal/no deformity (rapid onset)	Kyphotic deformity ('Gibbus' deformity)

- *Phemister's triad* is the 'classic' appearance of tuberculous arthritis and consists of juxtaarticular osteopenia, preservation of the joint space, and erosions (Fig. 14.68).

OTHER MYCOBACTERIAL INFECTIONS

- Other atypical mycobacterial infections may also involve the musculoskeletal system, including *Mycobacterium kansasii*, *Mycobacterium scrofulaceum*, and *Mycobacterium avium-intracellulare* (MAI).
- There are no specific musculoskeletal imaging features, but the diagnosis can be suspected based on typical

involvement of other organs (e.g., lung with MAI, lymph nodes with scrofula).
- *Mycobacterium leprae* is the causative agent in leprosy; it is endemic in Africa, South America, and Asia.
  - The organism exhibits a long incubation period, which may be over many years.
  - Direct involvement of the musculoskeletal system can result in bone destruction. Peripheral nerve involvement (visible occasionally as nerve calcification) results in atrophic neuropathic disease.
  - Ultimately this may result in a mutilating condition of the distal extremities and face.

OTHER 'ATYPICAL' INFECTIONS

- These infections are uncommon in developed countries. However, if the patient population is prone to certain infections (e.g., immigrants from countries where these organisms are commonplace), it is important for the radiologist to be aware of the manifestations of atypical infections prevalent in their population (Figs. 14.69 through 14.71; see Fig 14.60).
- One characteristic appearance that suggests an atypical infection is presence of one or more destructive masses. This finding is seen in some mycobacterial, fungal, and parasitic infections and, although not specific, suggests something other than routine bacterial infection.
- More commonly unless there are systemic findings or history suggesting infection, these lesions masquerade as primary bone tumors or metastatic lesions.
- Whenever a bone biopsy is performed for a tumor, one must keep in mind the possibility of atypical infection.
- An immunocompromised state may also alter the imaging appearance of an infection or result in infection with atypical organisms.

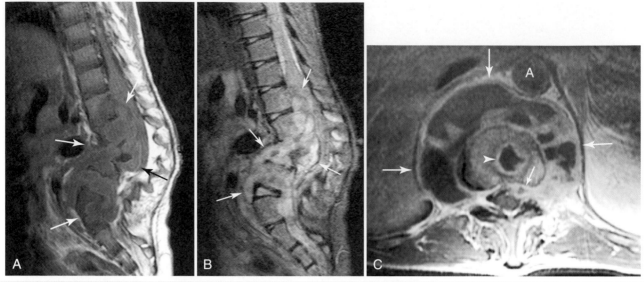

Fig. 14.66 Spine tuberculosis. MR image of active disease. (A and B) Sagittal T1-weighted **(A)** and inversion recovery **(B)** MR images show multilevel vertebral body and disc infiltration with a large surrounding mass *(arrows)*, representing discitis-osteomyelitis and large phlegmon. Note the lumbar kyphosis (gibbus deformity). **(C)** Pott disease in a different patient. Axial contrast-enhanced T1-weighted MR image at L1 shows a massive abscess *(large arrows)*, small vertebral abscess *(arrowhead)*, and epidural abscess *(small arrow)*. A, Aorta.

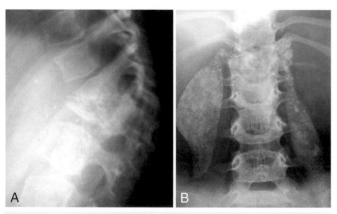

Fig. 14.67 Tuberculosis of the spine, late radiographic findings. **(A)** Lateral and **(B)** AP radiographs demonstrate destruction of much of the vertebral bodies and disc spaces of T11, T12, and L1. There is a gibbus deformity, as well as densely calcified abscesses in the psoas muscles bilaterally, as seen on the AP view. (Images used with permission from BJ Manaster, MD, from the American College of Radiology Learning File.)

Those that may be seen along with distinguishing imaging features, if any, are listed in Table 14.1.

Chronic Recurrent Multifocal Osteomyelitis

- Chronic recurrent multifocal osteomyelitis (CRMO) is also termed *chronic nonbacterial osteomyelitis* (CNO).
- Rare condition seen in adolescents and children characterized by a prolonged or fluctuating course of infectious-like processes involving various bones.
- Involved bones have radiological findings typical of osteomyelitis and/or Brodies abscess (Fig. 14.73).
- Typically multifocal, with spontaneous remission and recurrence or onset at new locations subsequently.

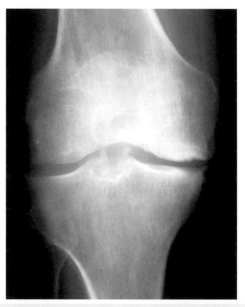

Fig. 14.68 Tuberculosis arthritis. AP radiograph demonstrates osteopenia and small cortical erosions but nearly normal cartilage thickness. This combination is typical of tuberculosis or fungal arthritis.

- Although the imaging and histologic appearance of bone and clinical features suggest infection, no causative organism has been identified. Cultures are negative, and there is no associated abscess or fistula.
- Rather, current understanding is that CRMO is autoinflammatory (direct immune attack on bone), analogous to inflammatory bowel disease (IBD).
- Can be associated with psoriasis and IBD.
- Diagnosis of exclusion.
- Can cause growth disturbances.
- Treatment is with antiinflammatory meds. More severe cases are treated with methotrexate or biologic agents.

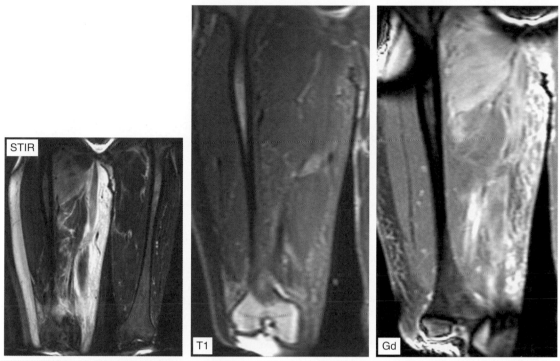

Fig. 14.69 Candida myositis of the thigh in a human immunodeficiency virus (HIV)-positive patient with acquired immunodeficiency syndrome (AIDS). Note diffuse edema and enhancement in the medial musculature. Fungal infections are more common in immunocompromised patients. (From Morrison W. *Problem Solving in Musculoskeletal Imaging*. Philadelphia: Elsevier; 2010.)

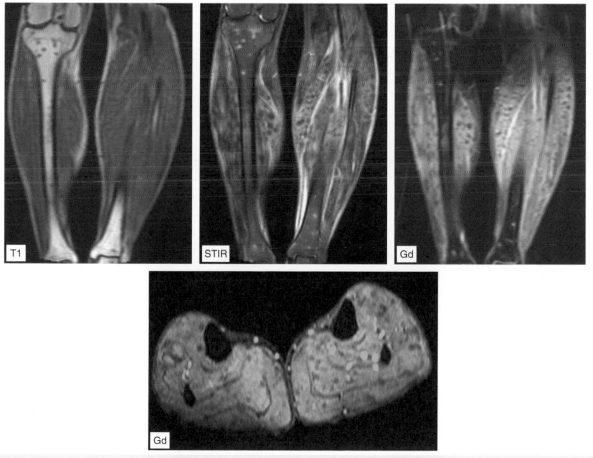

Fig. 14.70 Disseminated fungal infection on MRI of the lower legs. Note innumerable foci in bone and muscle. (From Morrison W. *Problem Solving in Musculoskeletal Imaging*. Philadelphia: Elsevier; 2010.)

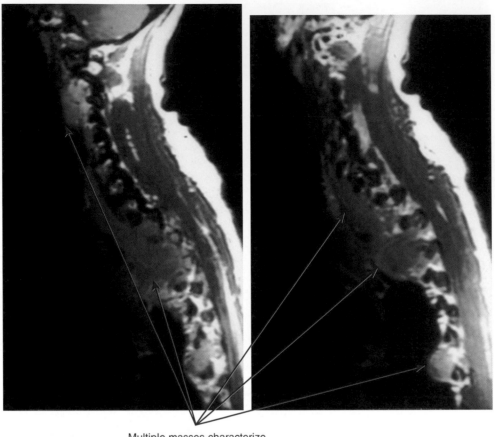

Multiple masses characterize
many disseminated atypical
infections and are easily confused
with metastatic disease

Fig. 14.71 Disseminated infection with coccidioidomycosis presenting on MRI as multiple masses. (From Morrison W. *Problem Solving in Musculoskeletal Imaging.* Philadelphia: Elsevier; 2010.)

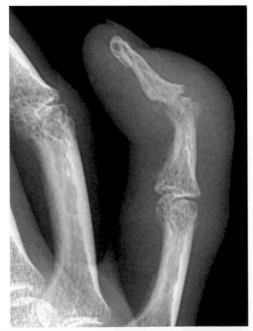

Fig. 14.72 Coccidioides septic arthritis in a 40-year-old man. The joint infection was by hematogenous spread from a primary pulmonary infection. Fungal infections also can occur from direct inoculation.

Sarcoidosis

- Sarcoidosis is a systemic granulomatous disorder. Sarcoidosis is not known to be an infectious process but is included in this chapter because it shares some imaging features with atypical infections.
- Patients with sarcoidosis frequently have muscle and joint pain.
- Lung abnormalities, including hilar adenopathy, pulmonary infiltrates and fibrosis, and apical bullous disease are present in most patients (80–90%).
- Nodular liver disease with hepatosplenomegaly may be present as well, as may ocular abnormalities such as uveitis and iritis.
- Sarcoidosis is seen in young adults without gender predominance. Black patients are affected more frequently than either white or Asian patients.
- Radiographic osseous abnormalities are seen in about 10% of patients with sarcoidosis because of granulomatous infiltration, most frequently lacy lytic lesions usually found in the middle or distal phalanges (Fig. 14.74).
  - Other, less frequent, radiographic osseous manifestations include generalized osteopenia, sclerosis of phalangeal tufts, and focal or generalized sclerosis.

Table 14.1 'Atypical' infection

LYME DISEASE (LYME BORRELIOSIS)

- Tick vector illness most common in the late spring and early summer in the northeastern U.S. and upper Midwest but present throughout much of the northern hemisphere throughout local tick season
- Caused by bacterium *Borrelia burgdorferi*, transmitted by the deer tick (*Ixodes scapularis*)
- Circular rash can simulate fungal infection
- Systemic symptoms (flu-like illness, fever, weight loss)
- Can result in arthralgias and 'unexplained' joint effusion, and can simulate oligoarticular juvenile idiopathic arthritis in children

BRUCELLOSIS

- Endemic in Midwestern U.S., Saudi Arabia, South America, southern Europe
- From infected milk/meat ingestion
- Causes septic arthritis, osteomyelitis, discitis-osteomyelitis; spine involvement relatively common
- May appear 'atypical' on imaging, like TB; however, no specific manifestations

ACTINOMYCOSIS

- Most common sites: mandible, spine, ribs, pelvis
- Often begins as lung infection that grows through the rib cage ('empyema necessitans')

CAT SCRATCH DISEASE

- Caused by *Bartonella henselae*, a fastidious Gram-negative bacterium
- Causes swelling, enlargement of lymph nodes near the area of skin inoculation
- A cause of swelling of the epitrochlear lymph node at the medial elbow; can simulate a soft tissue mass

BACILLARY ANGIOMATOSIS

- Infection with a *Bartonella* in an immunocompromised state can result in a skin lesion with prominent vascularity
- Seen in AIDS patients
- Lesions appear similar to Kaposi sarcoma
- Underlying bone can become involved with a permeative pattern

FUNGAL INFECTIONS (see Fig. 14.70)

Aspergillosis

- Various forms: localized destruction of bone, often with soft tissue mass; disseminated
- Lung involvement common
- Underlying immunosuppression common

Coccidioidomycosis (see Figs. 14.71 and 14.72)

- Endemic in southwest U.S. and parts of northern Mexico; travel history common in nonresidents
- Localized destructive lesion and/or soft tissue mass
- Disseminated form with multiple masses
- Can simulate metastasis or soft tissue sarcoma

Candidiasis (see Fig. 14.69)

- Typically associated with immunosuppression; may appear as disseminated abscesses

Sporotrichosis

- 'Rose thorn disease'
- Fungus called Sporothrix lives throughout the world in soil and on plant matter such as moss, rose bushes, and hay
- Saprophyte on vegetation
- Enters body through cut; enters lymphatic system
- Extremity infection with lymph node involvement
- Presents as nodal mass on imaging (especially epitrochlear node at the elbow from inoculation of the hand)

Mucormycosis

- Sinus involvement; bone destruction on imaging

Histoplasmosis

- *Histoplasma capsulatum* is endemic in the U.S.
- Lung/mediastinal involvement; bone involvement rare
- *Histoplasma dubosii* in Africa, bone involvement more common

Mycetoma
- Various organisms; tropical climates, India, Africa, South America
- Chronic granulomatous infection, invasive, foot most common (Madura foot)

PARASITIC INFECTION

Echinococcus

- *Echinococcus granulosus* versus *Echinococcus multilocularis*
- Parasitic cysts can look like abscesses on CT and MRI, with calcification
- Involvement of bone is rare but can result in lytic, 'blowout' lesions

Table 14.1 'Atypical' infection—cont'd

Cysticercosis

■ Involvement of muscles with small multifocal elongated T2-hyperintense cystic lesions oriented parallel with surrounding muscle fibers. Late stage: lesions calcify

Filariasis

■ Involvement of lymphatic channels, resulting in obstruction/valvular incompetence and extremity swelling (elephantiasis)

SYPHILIS

■ Spirochete infection
■ Adult infection with destructive lesions in tertiary form
■ Congenital form (see Fig. 14.60): maternal-fetal transmission
  ■ Diffuse sclerosis, bone destruction, and periosteal reaction
  ■ Metaphyseal irregularity
  ■ Widened physes

HIV

■ Musculoskeletal manifestations—mostly related to opportunistic infections, which often become disseminated due to immunocompromised state (see Fig. 14.69). Also susceptible to neoplasia including lymphoma and Kaposi sarcoma. Patients with acquired immunodeficiency syndrome (AIDS) and chronic wasting may also develop *serous atrophy* also termed *gelatinous transformation* of the bone marrow, discussed in Chapter 13 – Marrow and Metabolic Disease, with metabolism of marrow fat resulting in low T1 and intermediate-to-high T2 marrow signal. This is not seen in human immunodeficiency virus (HIV)-positive patients taking effective medication.

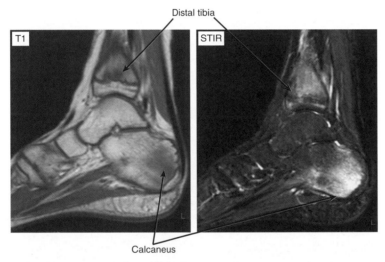

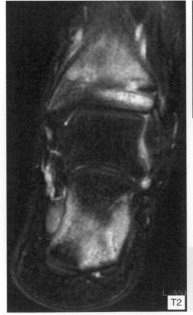

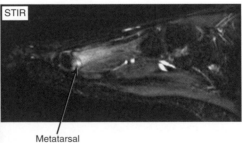

Distal tibia

Calcaneus

Brodies abscess–type pattern at multiple sites

Metatarsal

Fig. 14.73 Chronic recurrent multifocal osteomyelitis. Note multiple lesions in the foot and ankle resembling Brodie abscesses in this adolescent patient. (From Morrison W. *Problem Solving in Musculoskeletal Imaging.* Philadelphia: Elsevier; 2010.)

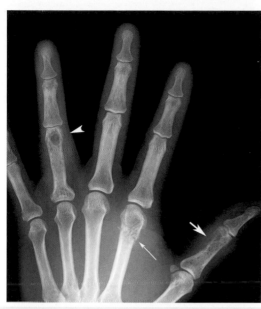

Fig. 14.74 Sarcoidosis. PA hand radiograph shows lytic lesions *(arrowhead)*, some so small that they produce a 'lacelike' appearance in the thumb proximal phalanx *(thick arrow)*. Note the pathologic fracture through a lesion in the distal second metacarpal *(thin arrow)*.

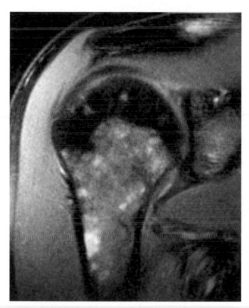

Fig. 14.75 Sarcoidosis, marrow disease. Coronal fat-suppressed T2-weighted MR image shows multiple small high-signal masses that are sarcoid granulomas. Marrow involvement with sarcoidosis is often extensive, but may be detected only with MRI or biopsy. (Courtesy of Sandra Moore, MD.)

- The granulomas are seen as nodules of various sizes or as infiltration, with high T2 signal, intermediate T1 signal, and enhancement with gadolinium-based contrast. This appearance can easily lead to a false diagnosis of metastatic disease.
- Chronic sarcoidosis causes granulomatous arthritis. MRI may show synovial thickening and enhancement in joints and tendon sheaths.

- Muscular sarcoidosis is uncommon. Discrete enhancing nodules are occasionally seen on MRI, classically with a low-signal-intensity spiculated central region. Generalized sarcoid myositis is more common. This resembles polymyositis clinically and on MRI and can lead to proximal muscle fatty atrophy if not controlled with steroids. Steroid therapy for sarcoidosis also can cause fatty muscle atrophy.

Sources and Suggested Readings

Browne LP, Guillerman RP, Orth RC, et al. Community-acquired staphylococcal musculoskeletal infection in infants and young children: necessity of contrast-enhanced MRI for the diagnosis of growth cartilage involvement. *AJR Am J Roentgenol.* 2012;198(1):194–199.

Chaudhry AA, Baker KS, Gould ES, Gupta R. Necrotizing fasciitis and its mimics: what radiologists need to know. *AJR Am J Roentgenol.* 2015;204: 128–139.

Crockett MT, Kelly BS, van Baarsel S, Kavanagh EC. Modic type 1 vertebral endplate changes: injury, inflammation, or infection? *AJR Am J Roentgenol.* 2017;209:167–170.

Collins M, Schaar M, Wenger D, Mandrekar J. T1-weighted MRI characteristics of pedal osteomyelitis. *AJR Am J Roentgenol.* 2005;185: 386–393.

Fayad LM, Carrino JA, Fishman EK. Musculoskeletal infection: role of CT in the emergency department. *Radiographics.* 2007;27(6): 1723–1736.

Gilbertson-Dahdal D, Wright JE, Krupinski E, et al. Transphyseal involvement of pyogenic osteomyelitis is considerably more common than classically taught. *AJR Am J Roentgenol.* 2014;203:190–195.

Harish S, Chiavaras MM, Kotnis N, Rebello R. MR imaging of skeletal soft tissue infection: utility of diffusion-weighted imaging in detecting abscess formation. *Skeletal Radiol.* 2011;40(3):285–294.

Jaramillo D. Infection: musculoskeletal. *Pediatr Radiol.* 2011;41(suppl 1): S127–S134.

Khanna G, Sato TS. Imaging of chronic recurrent multifocal osteomyelitis. *Radiographics.* 2009;29(4):1159–1177.

Kim KT, Kim YJ, Lee JW, et al. Can necrotizing infectious fasciitis be differentiated from nonnecrotizing infectious fasciitis with MR imaging? *Radiology.* 2011;259(3):816–824.

Morrison WB, Schwietzer ME, Batte WG, et al. Osteomyelitis of the foot: relative importance of primary and secondary MR imaging signs. *Radiology.* 1988;207:625–652.

Morrison WB, Schwietzer ME, Bock GE, et al. Diagnosis of osteomyelitis: utility of fat-suppressed contrast-enhanced MR imaging. *Radiology.* 1993;189:251–257.

Morrison WB, Schwietzer ME, Wapner KL, et al. Osteomyelitis in feet of diabetics: clinical accuracy, surgical utility and cost effectiveness of MR imaging. *Radiology.* 1995;196:557–564.

Santiago Restrepo C, Lemos D, Gordillo H, et al. Imaging findings in musculoskeletal complications of AIDS. *Radiographics.* 2004;24: 1029–1049.

Steinbach L, Tehrawzadeh J, Fleckenstein J, et al. Human immunodeficiency virus infection: musculoskeletal manifestations. *Radiology.* 1993; 186:833–838.

- Patients with sarcoidosis experience polyarticular arthralgias. Early in the disease this symptom is reactive and imaging studies are normal or may show only an effusion.
- MRI shows that widespread marrow involvement by granulomas is much more common than is suggested by radiographs or bone scan (Fig. 14.75).

15 Congenital and Developmental Conditions

This chapter reviews various maladies that affect the growing skeleton.

Scoliosis

- The normal infant spine is straight. The normal adult pattern of cervical lordosis, thoracic kyphosis, and lumbar lordosis develops after infancy.
- Normally, no curvature is present in the coronal plane.
- *Scoliosis* is spinal curvature in the coronal plane.
- Mild scoliosis is common. Nearly 4% of the population has a curve of 10 degrees or greater, but most are less than 20 degrees.
- Abnormal spinal alignment can cause cosmetic deformities, and severe scoliosis may decrease the size of the thorax with consequent restriction of pulmonary and cardiac function.
- Management decisions are complex but generally depend on:
  - The cause of the scoliosis, which is the single most important issue.
  - The degree of abnormal curvature.
  - The child's age and how much additional spinal growth may be expected.
  - Whether the curvature is increasing over time, and if increasing, how rapidly.

Causes of Scoliosis

- Idiopathic (up to 85%).
- Leg-length discrepancy.
- Congenital:
  - Spinal segmentation anomalies.
  - Unilateral tethering bar or bone.
- Neuromuscular:
  - Neural tube defects, cerebral palsy, Chiari malformation, tethered cord.
- Syndromes, dysostoses, and connective-tissue disorders:
  - Notably (but not exclusively) NF1, Marfan, achondroplasia, Ehlers–Danlos, osteogenesis imperfecta (OI).
- Trauma.
- Tumors:
  - Osteoid osteoma most common.
- Radiation therapy:
  - Uncommon today.

IDIOPATHIC SCOLIOSIS

- By far the most common form of scoliosis.
  - Diagnosis of exclusion (Box 15.1).
- Infantile, juvenile, and adolescent forms:
  - *Infantile*: early onset, familial, M>F, some have associated CNS abnormalities.
    - Mild cases may resolve spontaneously, but progressing or more severed curves may compromise ventilation and may be fatal if untreated.
    - Most are convex left.
  - *Juvenile*: onset between 4 and 10 years of age, some have associated CNS abnormalities (syrinx, Chiari, tether cord, spina bifida).
    - F>M.

Box 15.1   Clues That Scoliosis May Not Be Idiopathic

Present at birth
Deformities of vertebral bodies
Multiple limb deformities (arthrogryposis, chromosomal abnormalities)
Convex left thoracic curve (associated with syringomyelia and spinal cord tumors)
Long, C-shaped curve (neuromuscular conditions)
Focal, sharp curve (trauma; focal bony bar; neurofibromatosis, often with kyphosis and vertebral body dysplasia)
History of radiation therapy
Pelvic tilt (leg-length discrepancy)
Pain (osteoid osteoma or other tumor; fracture; infection)

- Often convex right.
- Usually requires treatment.
- *Adolescent*: onset age 10–18 years.
  - F> M 7:1. Also tends to be more severe in girls.
  - Positive family history is common (30%).
  - Most are convex right.

IMAGING OF SCOLIOSIS

The following discussion is focused on adolescent idiopathic scoliosis, but the imaging techniques and concepts apply in varying degrees to any type of scoliosis.

- Radiography is the main imaging modality in idiopathic scoliosis.
- Long-cassette radiographs, patient standing.
  - Smaller images can be stitched together to create a single image (Fig. 15.1).
- Correct patient positioning is essential for accurate measurements and comparing with prior studies.
- Posteroanterior (PA) rather than anteroposterior (AP) reduces breast and thyroid exposure.
- Gonadal shielding has fallen out of favor (well intentioned but ineffective). Local customs vary.
- An optimal image extends from the skull base to the proximal femurs, although a more focused exam from C7 to the upper sacrum is sometimes obtained on follow-up to reduce patient radiation exposure.

Spine Malalignment Terminology and Measurement

The following review uses terminology in the *Lenke system* for describing and classifying adolescent idiopathic scoliosis. This system has become popular with spine surgeons. There are other systems.

- *Scoliosis* is curvature of the spine in the coronal plane.
  - Convex toward the right: convex right scoliosis, *dextroscoliosis*, or right scoliosis.
  - Convex toward the left: convex left scoliosis, *levoscoliosis*, or left scoliosis.
  - Measured with *Cobb angle*: for each curve, measured from the upper endplate of the most cephalad vertebral body and the lower endplate of the most caudad body (the *end vertebrae*). If an endplate is not well seen, then use the pedicles.

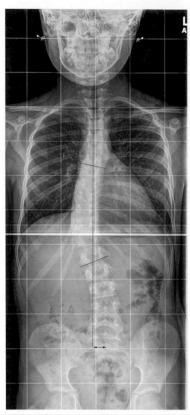

Fig. 15.1 Scoliosis. Composite image created by combining images of the upper and lower spine. Sample report describing this image:
History: 11-year 6-month-old female with scoliosis
Standing PA view of the entire spine.
Brace: none
Curves:
Major: T6-L1 29 degree convex right, apex T10. Minimal rotational component
Minor: C7-T6 7 degrees convex left
Minor: L1-L5 21 degrees convex left
Coronal balance: C7 is 21mm to the right of S1
Vertebral anomalies: None apparent
Leg-length discrepancy: none
Risser stage: 0
Change since prior exams: (*prior exams not shown*)
Additional Findings: none

- Cobb angle > 10 degrees = scoliosis.
- *Abnormal kyphosis* or *lordosis* is abnormal alignment in the sagittal plane. Measured in a manner similar to the Cobb angle, but on a lateral radiograph.
- *Rotatory deformity* is vertebral rotation along the long axis of the spine.
  - Seen as a shift of the pedicles on frontal view.
- These deformities may occur together, for example, *kyphoscoliosis, rotoscoliosis*.

Primary (Major) Curve
- Largest curve.
- Usually convex away from the descending aorta in adolescent idiopathic scoliosis (i.e., convex right in most patients).
  - If convex left, look for a right aortic arch. If the descending aorta is on the left, magnetic resonance imaging (MRI) may be obtained to search for potential neuraxis lesion such as a syrinx.

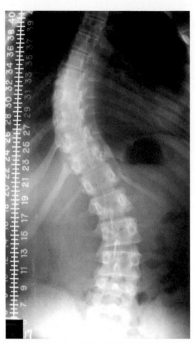

Fig. 15.2 Idiopathic scoliosis with a double major curve.

- In addition to reporting the end vertebrae and measuring the Cobb angle, report the *apex*, that is, the vertebra or disc deviated farthest right or left.
- More than one major curve may be present ('double major' scoliosis, Fig. 15.2).
- Usually contains a rotational component.

Minor Curve(s)
- Curves other than the major curve(s).
- *Compensatory curve* attempts to correct the malalignment caused by the major curve.

Balance is the relationship of C7 to the midline upper sacrum.

- Balance is increasingly recognized to be an important concept in scoliosis evaluation.
- Normally the neck base is centered over the pelvis. Displacement in scoliosis leads to greater patient discomfort and worsened cosmesis.
- *Sagittal balance* is the relationship of the head with the pelvis in the sagittal plane (anterior or posterior shift).
  - Measured by drawing a vertical line ('plumb line') from the center of the C7 vertebral body to the posterior superior margin of the S1 body on a standing lateral view.
  - *Positive sagittal balance* is present if C7 is >2 cm anterior to posterior superior S1.
  - *Negative sagittal balance* is present if C7 is >2 cm posterior to posterior superior S1.
  - Alternatively, simply report anterior or posterior position of C7 relative to S1.
- *Coronal balance* is relationship of C7 with the pelvis in the coronal plane (rightward or leftward shift).
  - Measured by drawing a vertical line from the center of the C7 vertebral body to the sacrum on a standing frontal view.

- *Positive coronal balance* is present if C7 is >2 cm right lateral to the midsacrum (Fig. 15.1).
- *Negative coronal balance* is present if C7 is >2 cm left lateral to the midsacrum.
- Alternatively, simply report rightward or leftward position of C7 relative to S1.

Fixed Versus Flexible Curves

- Assessed with frontal right and left-side bending views (Fig. 15.3).
- *Fixed curves* cannot be corrected with right- and left-side bending.
- *Flexible curves* can be corrected with bending.
- Many curves are a combination of fixed and flexible, i.e., can be partially but not fully corrected with bending.
- Curves that start as flexible may become completely or partially fixed over time.

Structural Versus Nonstructural Curves

- A modification of fixed versus flexible used in surgical planning in the Lenke system.
- Also measured on frontal right and left bending images.
- Structural:
  - Major curve with a 25-degree or greater fixed component.
  - Minor curve with a 10-degree or greater fixed component.
- Nonstructural: curves with milder fixed component.

Rotatory Deformity

- Vertebral rotation moves the pedicles toward the concave side of a curve.
- The degree of rotation can be described by the shift of the pedicles as seen on a frontal radiograph.
- A *neutral vertebra* is a vertebra with no rotational deformity. Often found between curves.

Additional Considerations

- Make sure to note if the patient was wearing a brace.
- Spine surgeons usually make their own measurements, and some might request that their radiology reports not include measurements, rather just descriptive terminology.

MANAGEMENT OF IDIOPATHIC SCOLIOSIS

- Idiopathic scoliosis frequently progresses over time. Curves may progress rapidly during the adolescent growth spurt.
- Mild curves usually stop progressing after skeletal maturity is reached.
- A brace is used for a scoliosis of about 25 degrees or greater, or in a younger child with less severe curvature that is rapidly progressing.
  - The goal of bracing is to halt progression of the scoliosis until spinal maturity is reached.
- Severe curves greater than 40 degrees generally require surgery to prevent respiratory and other complications.

Surgery is most successful if delayed until after skeletal maturity is reached. Therefore critical management decisions require knowledge of the skeletal maturity of the spine and specifically when completion of spinal growth may be expected.

- Fusion of the spinal ring apophyses (Fig. 15.4) is not a reliable indicator of completion of spinal growth.
- The Risser method described earlier in Chapter 1 – Introduction to Musculoskeletal Imaging is a preferred method for determining spinal maturity in adolescents (Fig. 15.5).
  - The adolescent growth spurt occurs during Risser stages 0–2, mostly during 0
  - Risser 4 or 5 can be used as a marker for spinal maturity.
- Surgeons sometimes use an additional bone age determination such as Greulich and Pyle or Tanner Whitehouse.

Surgical Options

- The goal is to improve alignment and prevent further progression.
- Most combine fixation hardware with fusion of either the posterior elements (posterior fusion) or across the disc spaces (anterior fusion).
- Successful bony fusion is essential because the hardware eventually may fail or loosen if spinal fusion is not achieved, potentially resulting in a pseudarthrosis.

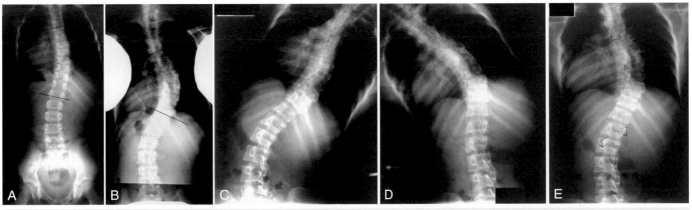

Fig. 15.3 Idiopathic scoliosis. Orthopedic surgeons prefer to view spine radiographs the same way they examine the spine—from the back. **(A)** Standing view in an adolescent girl shows a convex right curve from T5 to L1 that measures 25 degrees. The child was treated with a brace. **(B)** Standing PA view obtained 3 years later shows that the curve has progressed despite the bracing and now measures almost 50 degrees. Right **(C)** and left **(D)** bending views reveal that the primary curve is partially but not completely correctable. **(E)** Preoperative standing radiograph shows the surgeon's planned placement of laminar hooks (*arrows drawn on the radiograph*) as part of spinal fixation.

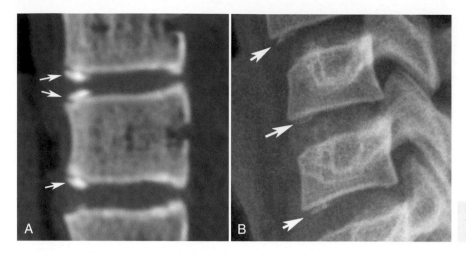

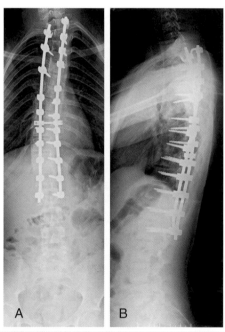

Fig. 15.4 Spinal ring apophyses (*arrows*) in the thoracic spine (**A,** sagittal CT reconstruction) and cervical spine (**B**).

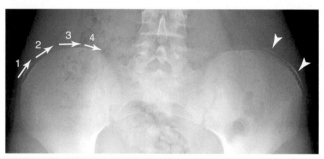

Fig. 15.5 Risser classification for estimation of spinal maturity. This system is based on the ossification of the iliac crest apophysis, which begins laterally and proceeds medially, followed by fusion of the apophysis to the iliac wing. Stage 0: no ossification of the iliac crest apophysis; stage 1: ossification of the lateral one-fourth of the iliac crest apophysis; stage 2: ossification of the lateral half of the iliac crest apophysis; stage 3: ossification of the lateral three-fourths of the iliac crest apophysis; stage 4: ossification of the entire iliac crest apophysis, without fusion to the iliac crest; stage 5: fusion of the iliac crest apophysis. Risser 4 and 5 coincide with completion of spinal growth. This child is Risser stage 2 (*arrowheads*).

Fig. 15.6 (A and **B)** Pedicle screw and spinal rod instrumentation. This is a common current surgical technique, with laminar hooks at the cranial terminus of the pedicle screw and spinal rod construct.

Posterior Spinal Fusion

Most posterior fusion today uses pedicle screws fixed to paired, custom-fitted spinal rods (Fig. 15.6), often in combination with laminar hooks at the superior end of the construct. This provides the best control of each vertebra to optimize curve correction. Preoperative computed tomography (CT) is sometimes obtained to evaluate pedicle size and suitability for pedicle screw placement.

Other fixation techniques include a single distracting spinal rod or custom-fitted spinal rod or rods, often in left and right side pairs, fixed with laminar wires or hooks (Fig. 15.7).

- Historical note: The famous early instrumentation for scoliosis was the *Harrington rod* (Fig. 15.7A). A single straight spinal rod is placed along the concave side of the curve. The rod is fixed to the spine by two hooks: one under the inferior margin of the vertebral lamina at the upper end of the curve, and one over the superior margin of the vertebral lamina at the lower end of the curve. The hooks are distracted (spread apart), resulting in straightening of the curve. Curve correction is limited by the amount of force that can be safely applied to just two

laminae. This approach also has the undesired side effect of straightening normal thoracic kyphosis and lumbar lordosis. Harrington rods were vulnerable to rod fracture owing to their distinctive shape. Newer applications of the distracting rod technique tend to use smooth or threaded distracting rods and/or modern alloys that are less vulnerable to rod failure.

Anterior Spinal Fusion

Uses vertebral body screws and a cable or rod linkage. The screws are placed transversely in the vertebral bodies, with portions projecting laterally along the convex side of the scoliotic curve. The screws are linked together by a rod, a plate, or a cable. These systems are used most often for treating neuromuscular or congenital scoliosis.

Each system has advantages and disadvantages, and the surgeon's preference often determines which system is used. Because surgical hardware and technique are constantly

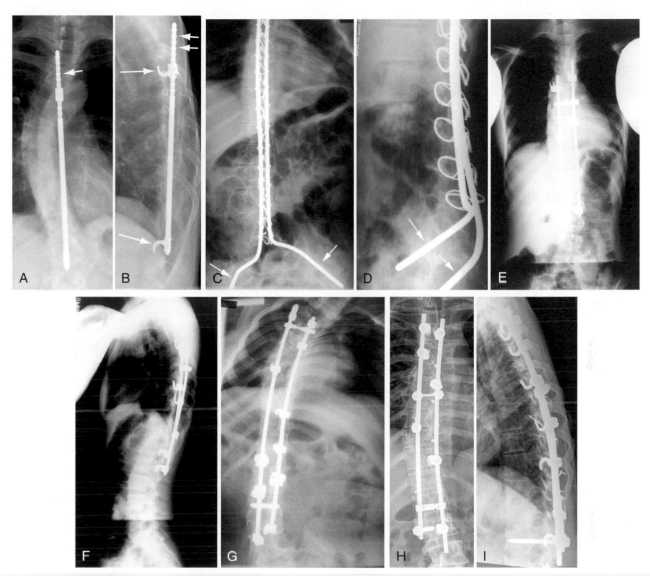

Fig. 15.7 Other instrumentation techniques. **(A** and **B)** Harrington spinal distracting rod. Note the laminar hooks (*long arrows* in B) and the distinctive serrated contour of the superior portion of the rod *(short arrows)*. **(C** and **D)** Laminar wires. The custom curved spinal rods are fixed to the laminae at multiple levels by wires. Note the extension of the spinal rods into the iliac bones *(arrows)*, which is no longer preferred. When needed, pelvic fixation currently is achieved with screws. **(E** and **F)** Laminar hook and spinal rod hardware. Same patient as in Fig. 15.3. Note the significant improvement in the scoliosis. Also note that the primary curve was not corrected beyond the fixed curve revealed in the preoperative bending views **(C)**. This is because further straightening of the spine would injure the paraspinal supporting soft tissues. **(G)** Similar instrumentation in a different patient better demonstrates the appearance of this hardware. **(H** and **I)** Hybrid instrumentation combining pedicle screws, laminar hooks, and laminar wires.

evolving, the reader is cautioned not to be dogmatic in naming the hardware system seen when interpreting radiographs. In particular, not all rods are Harrington rods! In fact, almost none are today. It is preferable to use generic terms such as *spinal rod* unless the radiologist is certain of the system that has been implanted.

Potential Complications

There are many potential complications of scoliosis surgery. These are some that are detected with radiography:
- Hardware fracture.
- Loss of hardware purchase on the spine:
  - Pedicle screw loosening—look for lucency around the screw.
  - Laminar hook no longer fixed to the spine.
- Fracture.

- Worsened deformity, which may occur with hardware failure, failed fusion, or if the surgery was performed before spinal maturity.

OTHER CAUSES OF SCOLIOSIS

Leg-length discrepancy

- Leg length inequality, i.e., unequal leg length; considered to be significant if greater than 1–2 cm. There are numerous causes:
- Unilateral leg shortening:
  - Physis injury (trauma, infection).
  - Proximal femur and hip disorders.
    - Developmental dysplasia of the hip (DDH).
    - Slipped capital femoral epiphysis (SCFE).

- Proximal focal femoral deficiency (PFFD).
- Neurologic conditions such as cerebral palsy.
- Unilateral leg lengthening:
  - Any condition that causes hyperemia near a physis has the potential to accelerate growth at that physis, for example, inflammatory arthritis, high-flow vascular malformation, and fracture.
  - Hemihypertrophy.

Imaging of leg-length discrepancy:

- Pelvic tilt on standing radiograph with unequal femoral head heights.
- Leg length measurement:
  - Long-cassette radiography.
  - 'Sliding table' technique (Fig. 15.8).
  - CT AP scanogram. Uses the least amount of ionizing radiation.
- Measurement landmarks: femurs: top of femoral head, distal medial femoral condyle; tibias: medial tibial plateau, tibial plafond (above talar dome).

Orthopedic intervention for leg-length discrepancy consists of unilateral lengthening of the short leg (Fig. 15.9), or shortening of the longer leg by *epiphysiodesis* (fusion of a physis to prevent further growth; Fig. 15.10).

Congenital Scoliosis

- Due to congenital vertebral body deformity, specifically abnormalities of formation or segmentation of the vertebra during the first trimester of gestation.
- Each vertebra (segment) normally forms from three main ossification centers: one for the vertebral body and

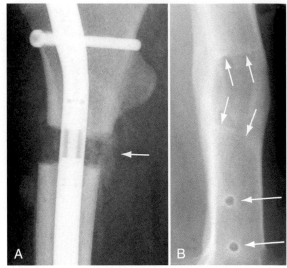

Fig. 15.9 Surgical leg lengthening. **(A)** Spot image less than 3 months after proximal femur osteotomy and fragment distraction *(arrow)*. The periosteum is left intact and is contributing to new bone formation. Note the internal fixation hardware (only partially shown) and early new bone formation in the gap *(arrow)*. The gap is widened slowly, about 1 mm/day, to allow for nerve growth. **(B)** Late findings at a different site. *Short arrows* mark the old distal femur osteotomy margins. Mature bone spans the old defect. Note the old external fixation pin tracts *(long arrows)*.

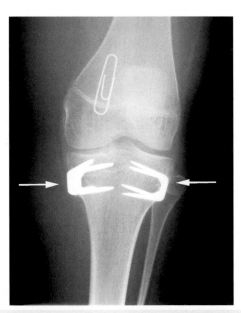

Fig. 15.10 Leg shortening by epiphysiodesis. The proximal tibial physis was fused (epiphysiodesis) by fixation with staples *(arrows)* over 1 year previously to allow the shorter contralateral leg (not shown) to catch up. (The paper clip is an artifact.) Note that the distal femoral physis is closing, indicating the completion of growth of both legs. Limbs can also be shortened by resection of a segment of a long bone with internal fixation.

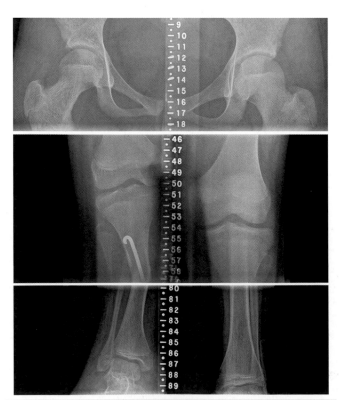

Fig. 15.8 Leg-length discrepancy. Scanogram in a child with right lower extremity hypoplasia.

disc, and one for each side of the posterior elements. One of these ossification centers may fail to form or may aberrantly fuse to a center from an adjacent segment. (Note: vertebra contain additional ossification centers, e.g., for the transverse processes, but these generally are not potential sources of significant spinal deformity.)

- Resulting deformities include misshapen vertebrae (for example, hemivertebrae), or a bone or fibrous bar that tethers part of one vertebral body to another (Fig. 15.11).

Congenital scoliosis associations:

- **VACTERL** (vertebral, anorectal, cardiac, tracheoesophageal fistula, renal, and limb anomalies; see Fig. 15.11D).
  - Renal ultrasound recommended.
- Spinal cord anomalies such as tethered cord or *diastematomyelia*.
  - Spine MRI should be considered.
    - Including a coronal inversion recovery or T2-weighted sequence helps to delineate the misshapen vertebrae from the discs because the discs in children have high T2 signal.

Treatment of congenital scoliosis is frequently surgical to provide stabilization and to prevent further deformity caused by asymmetric growth.

Neuromuscular Scoliosis

- Paraspinal muscle imbalance as a result of spasticity or flaccidity with resulting scoliosis.

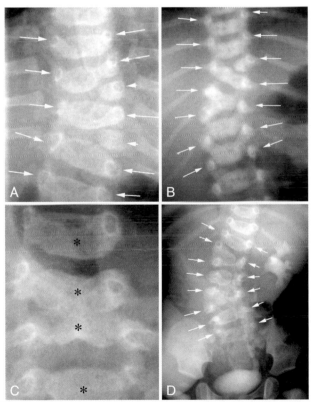

Fig. 15.11 Vertebral segmentation anomalies. **(A)** Hemivertebrae. The pedicles are marked with *arrows*. Note the hemivertebrae *(short arrows)* with associated scoliosis. **(B)** Segmentation anomalies with fusion abnormalities, hemivertebrae, and scoliosis. The pedicles are marked with *arrows*. **(C)** Failure of segmentation. The vertebral bodies are marked with *asterisks*. Note the fusion of the two bodies at the center of the image. **(D)** Failure of formation and the VACTERL association (vertebral, anorectal, cardiac, tracheoesophageal fistula, renal, and limb anomalies). The pedicles are marked with *arrows*. Note the greater number of pedicles on the right than the left, with associated scoliosis. The intravenous urogram shows unilateral right renal agenesis. (D courtesy of Stephanie Spottswood, MD.)

- Neuromuscular scoliosis tends to be long and C-shaped, without compensatory curves above or below (Fig. 15.12).
- Causes include cerebral palsy, muscular dystrophy, paralysis, and arthrogryposis.
- Frequent association: dysplasia or dislocation of one or both hips.

Neurofibromatosis 1 (NF1)

Mesodermal dysplasia results in weak bones, including vertebra, that are prone to deformity.

Scoliosis in NF1 has two forms:

- A sharply angled midthoracic kyphoscoliosis (*dystrophic form*, Fig. 15.13).
  - Has potential for rapid progression to severe angulation and subluxation that can lead to paralysis.
  - Difficult to manage, fusions often fail.

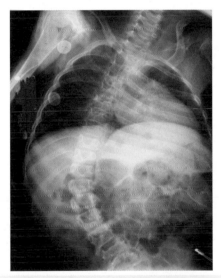

Fig. 15.12 Long C-shaped scoliosis caused by a neuromuscular condition. (Courtesy of L. Das Narla, MD.)

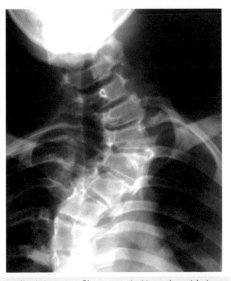

Fig. 15.13 Scoliosis in neurofibromatosis. Note the wide interpediculate distance (transverse distance between pedicles) caused by dural ectasia.

- A longer curve that is similar to idiopathic scoliosis, but tends to occur earlier and has greater risk of progression.

Look for other spine findings associated with NF1: *dural ectasia* (posterior vertebral body scalloping, enlarged neural foramina) and rib abnormalities (twisted, narrow 'ribbon ribs'). The musculoskeletal manifestations of neurofibromatosis are further discussed later in this chapter.

Connective-tissue disorders such as Marfan syndrome and Ehlers–Danlos syndrome frequently cause scoliosis. These conditions are reviewed in later in this chapter.

Spine trauma may result in scoliosis. Instrumentation may be required to maintain stability.

Painful scoliosis should prompt a search for an underlying tumor of the spine or spinal cord, stress fracture, or infection.

Vertebral Osteoid Osteoma

- Most common tumor to cause scoliosis.
- Usually occurs in the posterior elements.
- The scoliosis is concave toward the side of the nidus because of ipsilateral muscle spasm.
- Radionuclide bone scanning will reveal intense tracer uptake around the tumor.
- CT is the preferred technique for characterization and precise localization of the nidus before resection.

Radiation therapy for pediatric tumors near the spine such as Wilms tumor commonly resulted in scoliosis in the past, as the radiated side of the spine stopped growing, or muscle injury resulted in muscle imbalance. Modern therapies minimize this risk.

Miscellaneous Spine Disorders

JUVENILE KYPHOSIS AND SCHEUERMANN DISEASE

Juvenile kyphosis is greater than 40 degrees of kyphotic curvature from T3 to T12. Juvenile kyphosis may be caused by any of the many causes of scoliosis or may be idiopathic.

Idiopathic forms:

- Postural kyphosis (prolonged slouching), occurs without associated abnormalities.
- *Scheuermann disease* (Fig. 15.14):
    - Thoracic vertebral body wedging, disk space narrowing, endplate irregularity in adjacent vertebrae with exaggerated kyphosis.
    - Compensatory exaggerated lumbar lordosis.
    - Frequently painful.
    - The cause is unknown. There are several theories (partial vertebral growth disturbance due to congenital endplate weakness, focal osteonecrosis, trauma).
    - Autosomal dominant inheritance.
    - M=F, peak incidence at age 13–16 years, preferentially affects the lower thoracic spine.

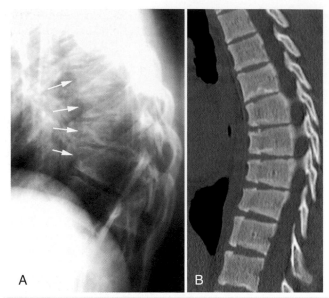

Fig. 15.14 Scheuermann disease. **(A)** This teenage boy had painful, clinically evident kyphosis. Note the wedging of several adjacent mid-thoracic vertebral bodies *(arrows)* with irregular vertebral body end plates. **(B)** Sagittal CT reconstruction in a different teenager shows similar findings.

LUMBAR SPONDYLOLYSIS

- Spectrum of stress reaction, fracture, and spondylolisthesis classically involving the pars interarticularis of the posterior elements (Figs. 15.15 through 15.18).
- Stress fractures of the posterior elements may occur at sites other than the pars interarticularis, notably the pedicles (Fig. 15.19).
- Occurs more frequently in adolescent athletes who participate in activities with repetitive lumbar flexion and extension, such as gymnastics, football, soccer, and numerous other sports.
- There also appears to be a genetic predisposition in some cases.
- Rare causes include tumor and congenital posterior element deformities (Fig. 15.20).
- L5 is the most commonly affected level.
- May be symptomatic.
- Conservative treatment usually allows the fractures to heal. Bracing is sometimes used.
- Bilateral spondylolysis may result in *spondylolisthesis* (anterior displacement of the affected vertebral body relative to the body below, also termed *anterolisthesis*).
    - Graded by the degree of displacement:
        - Grade 1 spondylolisthesis is anterior displacement of the superior vertebral body by up to 25% of the AP dimension of the endplate.
        - Grade 2: 25–50%.
        - Grade 3: 50–75%.
        - Grade 4: 75–100%.
        - Grade 5: > 100% (*spondyloptosis*, complete loss of contact between the vertebral bodies).
    - Also described by kyphosis between the bodies, when present (*slip angle*).
        - A larger slip angle is greater kyphosis = greater risk of spondylolithesis progression.

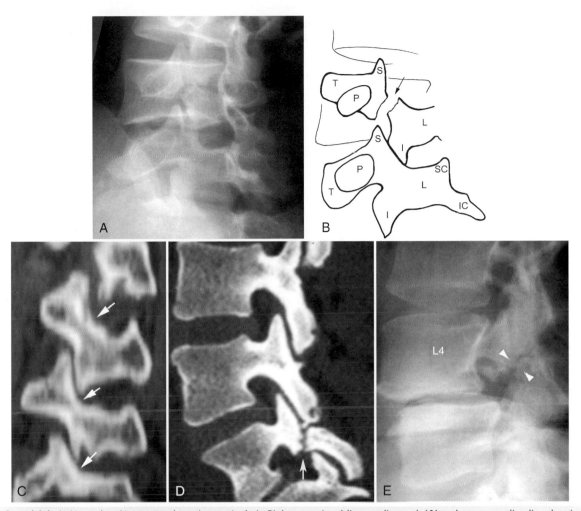

Fig. 15.15 Spondylolysis. Normal and interrupted pars interarticularis. Right posterior oblique radiograph **(A)** and corresponding line drawing **(B)** show an intact right pars interarticularis at L5 and a right pars defect with a collar around the 'Scottie dog's' neck at L4 (*arrow* in B). **(C)** Oblique sagittal CT reconstruction in a normal patient. Note the intact pars interarticularis *(arrows)*. **(D)** Sagittal CT reformat in a different patient shows a pars defect in L5 *(arrow)*. **(E)** Bilateral L4 pars defects *(arrowheads)* with grade 1 anterolisthesis at L4-L5. Bilateral pars defects are often easy to see on a lateral view. *I,* Inferior articulating facet (the Scottie dog's front leg); *IC,* contralateral inferior articulating facet (rear leg); *L,* lamina (body); *P,* pedicle (eye); *S,* superior articulating facet (ear); *SC,* contralateral superior articulating facet (tail); *I,* transverse process (nose).

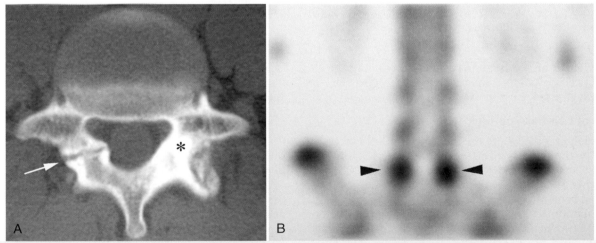

Fig. 15.16 (A) Axial CT image of unilateral spondylolysis. Note the spondylolysis on the right *(arrow)*. Also note the sclerosis of the contralateral pars interarticularis *(asterisk)*. This nonspecific finding may indicate that left-sided adaptive changes caused increased stress because of the right-sided pars defect, or an impending left pars stress fracture. **(B)** Tc99m MDP bone scan of bilateral L5 pars defects in a different patient. Coronal single-photon emission (SPECT) image obtained through the posterior elements shows increased tracer bilaterally at L5 *(arrowheads)*. CT scan (not shown) was needed to confirm bilateral defects, because a unilateral defect with adaptive hypertrophy on the contralateral side could have similar bone scan findings.

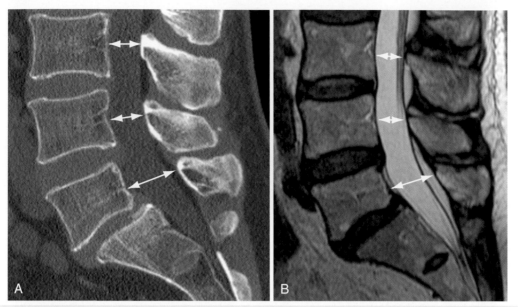

Fig. 15.17 Bilateral L5 spondylolysis with grade 1 spondylolisthesis at L5-S1. Sagittal CT scan **(A)** and T2-weighted MR image **(B)** show the characteristic AP dimension enlargement of the spinal canal above the slip *(double arrows)*. In contrast, the common finding on lumbar spine MRI of spondylolisthesis caused by facet degeneration without spondylolysis does not show this finding. Regardless of the cause of spondylolisthesis, foraminal stenosis is a frequent associated finding.

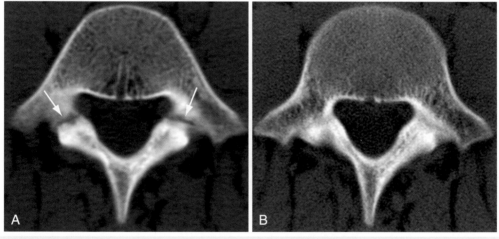

Fig. 15.18 Healing of pars defects. **(A)** CT shows bilateral L4 pars defects *(arrows)* in a 16-year-old girl. She was treated with a brace and cessation of athletic activity. **(B)** Repeat CT 6 months later shows the defects have healed.

Spondylolisthesis tends not to progress after about age 20 but may become painful after that age. Spinal fusion is sometimes required.

Imaging of Lumbar Spondylolysis

Oblique radiographs, where the defect is seen as a break in the neck of the famous 'Scottie dog' (see Fig. 15.15). The dog's nose points to the patient's affected side. *Bilateral spondylolysis* often may be appreciated on a coned lateral radiograph centered at the affected level.

CT is superior to radiographs for detection and characterization and can be accomplished with low-dose technique.

Radionuclide bone scanning may reveal increased tracer uptake at the affected side in a subacute or healing defect, at the contralateral side because of increased mechanical stress or an additional impending spondylolysis, or bilaterally. Single-photon emission CT imaging (SPECT)

helps to localize the tracer uptake to the posterior elements. Bone scan may be cold in a chronic complete pars defect.

Fluid-sensitive MR images often show marrow edema in the pars and, like bone scan, can show an impending fracture before it becomes apparent on CT or radiographs. This sensitivity, combined with absence of ionizing radiation and the ability of MRI to identify or exclude other causes of back pain such as disc disease, has increased the role of MRI in the initial evaluation of suspected pars defect.

TRANSITIONAL SEGMENTATION

A spectrum of spinal abnormalities may result from abnormal formation and segmentation of the vertebral bodies, as noted earlier in the discussion of congenital scoliosis.

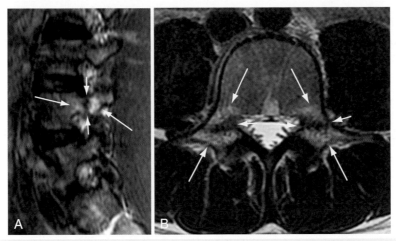

Fig. 15.19 Pedicle stress fractures, MR diagnosis. Sagittal STIR **(A)** and axial T2-weighted **(B)** MR images show low-signal stress fractures traversing the bilateral L4 pedicles *(short arrows)* with surrounding marrow edema *(long arrows)*.

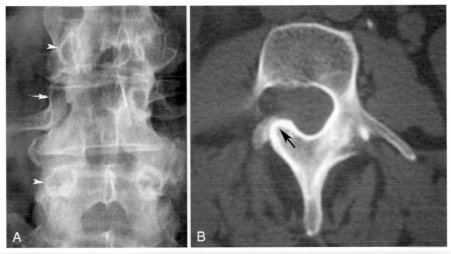

Fig. 15.20 Congenital absence of a pedicle. **(A)** AP radiograph shows absent right lumbar pedicle *(arrow)*. Contrast with normal ring shadow of normal pedicles *(arrowheads)*. **(B)** Axial CT shows intact cortex *(urrow)* adjacent to the defect.

Transitional segmentation refers to congenital variation from the standard arrangement of 7 cervical, 12 thoracic, and 5 lumbar vertebrae and 5 sacral segments.

- Occurs most frequently in the lumbosacral spine.
- Numerous variations may be seen.
- A common form of transitional segmentation is a transitional lumbosacral segment, with morphologic features intermediate between a lumbar vertebra and a sacral segment (Fig. 15.21).
- Assigning a numeric level to each vertebra (e.g., L1, L2) can be somewhat arbitrary. Consistency is essential when correlating different studies to direct spine surgery to the intended level.
- Guidelines to assist in assigning numbers to lumbar vertebrae are based on findings in 'normal' spines: a chest radiograph usually shows 12 rib pairs but may show 11 or 13 rib pairs; a line connecting the top of the iliac crests usually passes through L4-L5; the widest transverse processes usually occur at L3, and the left renal vein is usually located anterior to L1-L2.

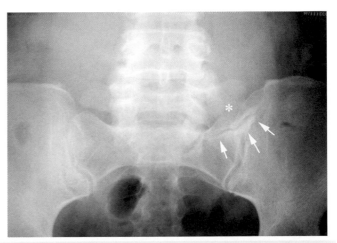

Fig. 15.21 Transitional lumbosacral segmentation. AP radiographic view of the lower lumbar spine shows wide transverse process of the lowest lumbar segment *(asterisk)*, with a false joint formation with the sacrum. Note the sclerosis along this joint *(arrows)*. This form of otherwise normal variant transitional segmentation may be painful.

KLIPPEL–FEIL SYNDROME

- Failure of cervical segmentation at multiple levels, with a short neck with low hairline (Fig. 15.22).
- Cervical motion is limited owing to the paucity of normally formed disks and facet joints. Associated findings may include renal, spinal cord, and inner, middle, and outer ear abnormalities.
- Approximately one-third of patients with Klippel–Feil syndrome have *Sprengel deformity* (Fig. 15.24).
  - *Sprengel deformity* is the tethering of the scapula to the cervical spine by a fibrous band or an anomalous bone *(omovertebral bone)* that results in a high position of the scapula and reduced shoulder mobility.
- The term *Klippel–Feil* is also often used less narrowly to describe any congenital fusion anomaly encountered in the cervical spine (Fig. 15.23).

- Such abnormalities most frequently are isolated to a single-disk level and are asymptomatic. The congenitally fused segments tend to be short in the AP dimension.

CAUDAL REGRESSION SYNDROME (CAUDAL DYSPLASIA SEQUENCE)

- A spectrum of caudal axial skeletal and associated neurologic and soft tissue defects caused by an insult to the caudal mesoderm and ectoderm early in the first trimester.
- Ranges from subtle partial sacral agenesis to complete absence of the sacrum, lumbar spine, and caudal thoracic spine (Fig. 15.25).
- Other axial skeletal findings may include spina bifida, spinal stenosis, an angular, wedge-shaped conus medullaris, and presacral (anterior) meningocele.

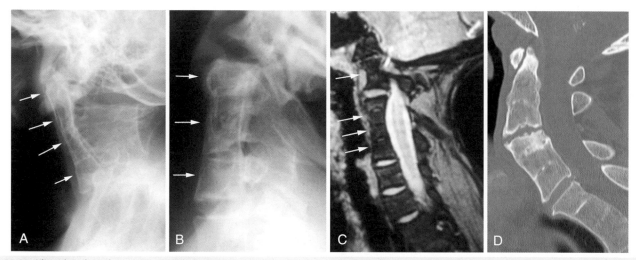

Fig. 15.22 Klippel–Feil syndrome. **(A)** Lateral cervical spine radiograph shows absent segmentation of several cervical segments *(arrows)*. **(B)** Different patient with similar findings *(arrows)* on a lateral radiograph. **(C)** Sagittal T2-weighted MR image in a different patient with similar findings *(arrows)*. **(D)** Sagittal CT reconstruction in a different patient. Note the degenerative changes at the C3-C4 disk, which must handle the motion and forces normally distributed across several disks.

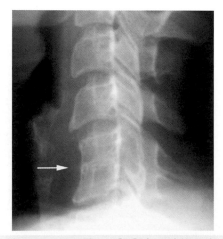

Fig. 15.23 Absent segmentation at C5-C6 *(arrow)*. Note the narrow AP dimension of the fused vertebral bodies, which distinguishes this finding from a mature surgical fusion. Juvenile rheumatoid arthritis could have a similar appearance but would involve more levels.

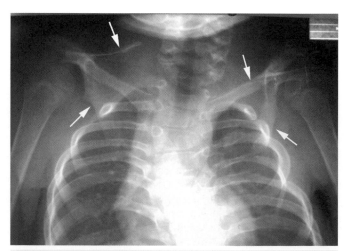

Fig. 15.24 Sprengel deformity. Compare the position of the scapulae *(arrows)*, with the right higher than the left. Also note the upper thoracic spinal segmentation anomalies with associated scoliosis.

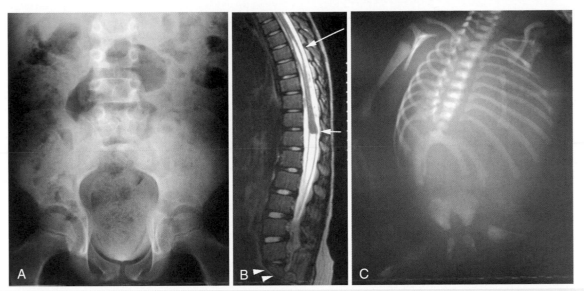

Fig. 15.25 Sacral agenesis (caudal regression syndrome). **(A)** This radiograph was obtained after intravenous urography (note the contrast medium in the bladder). Note the absence of the midsacrum and lower sacrum. Also note the large amount of stool in the colon because of related colon dysfunction. **(B)** Sagittal T2-weighted MR image shows the characteristic angular contour of the conus medullaris *(short arrow)*. This finding is not always present in sacral agenesis, however. Note the syrinx *(long arrow)*, a finding that can occur in association with caudal regression. Also note the small sacrum *(arrowheads)*. **(C)** Severe case. Note the complete absence of the lumbar spine and sacrum.

- Clinical findings also are highly varied, ranging from mild leg weakness to bowel and bladder control difficulties to anorectal atresia, renal aplasia, and pulmonary hypoplasia.
- The caudal regression syndrome is much more frequent in children of diabetic mothers, but most cases are sporadic.

Caudal regression syndrome has been associated with congenital fusion of the lower extremities (*sirenomelia*; Fig. 15.26), but these most likely are unrelated conditions. *Sirenomelia* is associated with severe oligohydramnios. This condition is named after the Greek mythical creatures called sirens, who lured sailors to their deaths on rocky reefs and coastlines with their sweet songs.

Torsion of The Femur and Tibia

- *Torsion* is rotation around the long axis of a bone. The term is most frequently applied to describe abnormal twisting along the long axis of the femur or tibia.
- Unlike other bone deformities, torsion is not as easily evaluated with radiographs, and the concept can be confusing at first. Imagine that you are looking down the long axis of the femur. Femoral torsion is determined by the angle formed by a line through the femoral neck and a line drawn across the posterior margins of the femoral condyles (Fig. 15.27). If the femoral head is anterior to the plane containing the femoral condyles, then *antetorsion* is present. The synonymous term *anteversion* is more frequently used for the femur. If the femoral head projects posterior to this plane, then *retrotorsion*, or *retroversion*, is present.
- The terminology used to characterize tibial torsion is slightly different. *Medial* or *internal tibial torsion* results

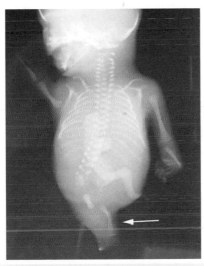

Fig. 15.26 Sirenomelia. Note the fused, dysplastic lower extremities *(arrow)*.

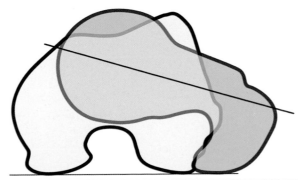

Fig. 15.27 Femoral anteversion. 'Bird's eye' view of the femur. Anteversion is the angle formed by the femoral neck *(blue shading)* and a line connecting the posterior margins of the femoral condyles *(yellow shading)*.

in internal rotation-like twisting of the distal tibia (pigeon-toed). *Lateral* or *external tibial torsion* is the opposite (penguin-footed).

- Femoral anteversion and tibial torsion can be assessed by limited low-dose CT or MRI. Axial images are limited to the femoral neck and condyles, and their relative angle is determined (Fig. 15.28).
  - Note that this measurement in the femur can be falsely reduced if the hip is flexed. Measuring off oblique axial images reformatted perpendicular to the femoral shaft on a lateral scout image can avoid this pitfall.
- Normal femoral torsion is 30+ degrees anteversion at birth, decreasing to about 16 degrees by age 16, and to 10 degrees by adulthood.
  - Excessive femoral anteversion causes gait and hindfoot abnormalities and contributes to hip dysplasia.
  - Excessive femoral anteversion occurs in DDH, Legg–Calvé–Perthes disease, and neurologic and neuromuscular conditions.
- Excessive anteversion frequently resolves spontaneously during growth, but surgery may be needed. Surgical treatment is *femoral derotation osteotomy*: The proximal femoral shaft femur is transversely divided, alignment is improved, and the fragments are fixed with orthopedic hardware and allowed to heal with casting (Fig. 15.28C).
  - A distal femoral osteotomy is preferred when genu valgum or varum is also present to simultaneously correct the abnormal knee alignment (Fig. 15.29).
- Radiographs can estimate torsion, but CT or MRI is used when a higher degree of precision is needed.
- Excessive internal tibial torsion frequently occurs in association with congenital foot deformities or genu varum. Toddlers with excessive internal tibial torsion will have bowlegs and a pigeon-toed gait. Excessive lateral torsion causes a penguin-footed gait.
  - Abnormal tibial torsion usually resolves during growth.

Congenital and Developmental Hip Disorders

Key Concepts

Developmental Dysplasia of the Hip

Deformity and subluxation of the hip, or more frequently *neonatal potential to develop dysplasia* and possibly dislocation later in infancy and childhood
True congenital dislocation is rare
Most cases are completely curable if diagnosed and treated early
Delayed diagnosis leads to decreased joint mobility, pain, and early osteoarthritis.
Radiographs are of limited utility in neonates
Ultrasound is highly sensitive but in most cases is best performed after about age 4 weeks because of potential for false-positive findings in neonates

DEVELOPMENTAL DYSPLASIA OF THE HIP

DDH is a spectrum of hip pathology that includes hip dysplasia or dislocation at birth, or more frequently *the potential to develop dysplasia* and possibly dislocation later in infancy and childhood.

The most frequent form of neonatal hip dysplasia is merely mild hip laxity and/or a shallow acetabulum at birth. This seemingly innocuous situation can be difficult or impossible to detect with physical exam, but has the potential to progress over a period of months and years to significant hip dysplasia, early osteoarthritis, and occasionally hip dislocation.

Congenital hip dislocation was formerly used for DDH. This term should be reserved for cases where the hip is dislocated or dislocatable at birth, which is uncommon.

- Some otherwise normal infants have severe neonatal hip laxity with a hip that is easily dislocated or relocated. This is in the DDH spectrum.

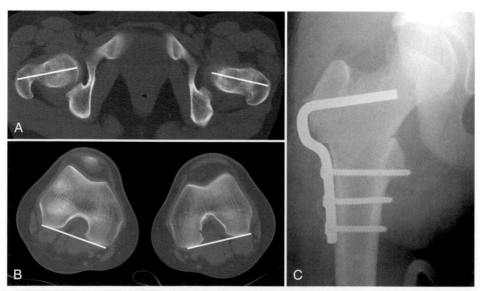

Fig. 15.28 **(A** and **B)** Axial CT images obtained through the femoral necks **(A)** and condyles **(B)** without change in position of the patient allow accurate measurement of femoral anteversion. In this 13-year-old girl femoral anteversion is 33 degrees on the right and 26 degrees on the left. Bilateral proximal femoral derotation osteotomies were performed. **(C)** Postoperative appearance of the right hip. Note the blade plate and the osteotomy.

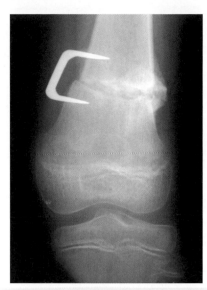

Fig. 15.29 Distal femoral osteotomy performed to correct excessive anteversion in a child.

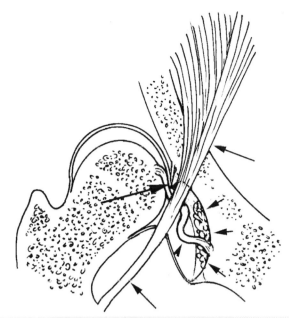

Fig. 15.30 Chronic hip subluxation or dislocation: associated soft tissue changes. Pulvinar *(short arrows)*. Elongated ligamentum teres *(arrowhead)*. Labrum flipped medially ('inverted limbus', *large long arrow)*. Tight psoas tendon stretched across the anterior joint capsule *(small long arrows)*.

■ *Teratogenic* (or *pathologic*) *dislocation* is congenital dislocation due to severe congenital deformity, such as *arthrogryposis* or *Chiari II malformation*. Pathologic dislocations are usually readily detected at birth by physical examination and confirmed with radiographs.

DDH Associations

■ DDH is relatively common (1 case per 1000 births). Roughly one-third are bilateral.
■ F > M 6:1, thought to be due to increased sensitivity by females to maternal hormones that relax ligaments.
■ Intrauterine positioning, notably breech presentation that tends to lever the femoral head out of the acetabulum. Routine screening of breech deliveries with ultrasonography (US) is now advocated.
■ Left hip is more frequently affected because the fetal spine is usually to the maternal left in a fetus in vertex presentation. This places the fetal left knee against the unyielding maternal spine, which tends to lever the left femoral head out of the acetabulum.
■ Genetic—family history.
■ Rare in children of African descent.
■ 'Tight' intrautine environment.
  ■ Olighydramnios.
  ■ Firstborn.
  ■ Congenital torticollis.
■ Contralateral hip dysplasia.
■ Scoliosis (pelvic tilt uncovers one femoral head).
■ Ehlers–Danlos syndrome (generalized joint laxity).
■ Neuromuscular imbalance (e.g., cerebral palsy).
■ The practice in some cultures of papoosing infants with the hips adducted and extended increases the risk for DDH.

How DDH Develops

In a normal hip, the femoral head and acetabulum grow together, in concert. The enlarging spherical femoral head serves as a mold for the growing acetabulum, and the acetabulum contains the femoral head.

The initiating factor in DDH is neonatal ligamentous laxity related to maternal hormone effects (which are greater in female infants), uterine 'packaging' risk factors (breech, firstborn, oligohydramnios), and genetics. The femoral head may become 'decentered' relative to the acetabulum, typically anterior and lateral at first. The acetabulum adapts to the abnormal femoral head mobility by becoming wider and shallower (*acetabular dysplasia*) as it attempts to accommodate the abnormal range of motion of the femoral head. A vicious cycle of increasing femoral head subluxation and increasing acetabular dysplasia may ensue, with progressive hip subluxation and potentially eventual dislocation. Soft tissues around the hip eventually tighten, limiting further femoral head displacement, but at the expense of mobility.

Femoral anteversion increases (the femoral neck angles anteriorly). The acetabulum becomes shallow with increased anteversion (increased anterior orientation). In advanced chronic cases the femoral head dislocates completely and flattens along its superomedial margin as it abuts the lateral aspect of the ilium. A shallow concavity may develop on the lateral ilium adjacent to a chronically dislocated femoral head, termed *pseudoacetabulum*.

Chronic subluxation or dislocation creates potential impediments to successful reduction (Fig. 15.30):

■ Fibrofatty tissue, termed *pulvinar* (pillow), can fill the acetabulum.
■ The acetabular labrum may flip inferiorly against the medial margin of the subluxed femoral head and overgrow, termed an *inverted limbus*, or *inverted labrum*.
■ A ridge of cartilage may grow medial to the labrum, termed *limbus* or *neolimbus* and sometimes *inverted limbus* in the orthopedic literature. (Note the potential confusion of terminology.)

- A tight psoas tendon may stretch across the hip joint medial to the laterally displaced femoral head, resulting in an hourglass configuration of the joint capsule.
- The adductor muscles are shortened by the superior migration of the proximal femur.
- The ligamentum teres, which extends from the femoral head to the center of the acetabulum, becomes elongated and redundant.

Pain and early osteoarthritis are late complications, even in comparatively mild cases. Hip replacement surgery may be required as early as the fourth decade of life.

DDH Imaging

Physical exam findings may be subtle or absent in early DDH. Imaging is indispensable.

Radiography and US are the cornerstones of imaging of DDH.

- US: First-line test in neonates up to 4 months, and can be used up to 6 months in many infants.
- Radiography after 4 months.
- CT, MRI, MR arthrography, and intraoperative arthrography are used in advanced DDH and are discussed in the following text.

Ultrasonography in DDH

- Provides excellent visualization of the cartilaginous femoral head and unossified acetabulum (Fig. 15.31).
- Allows for dynamic assessment of hip joint stability.
- Can sometimes be used after age 6 months, depending on the degree of femoral head ossification.
- Mild technical difficulty.
- No ionizing radiation.

Historical note: The initial application of US to infants with DDH emphasized static coronal imaging, simulating an AP radiograph. An elaborate system of measurements and categories was developed, termed the *Graf system* in honor of the Austrian orthopedic surgeon Reinhard Graf, MD, who developed this approach. The subsequent application of real-time US by the American pediatric radiologist H. Theodore Harcke, MD, and others pioneered the dynamic assessment of hip stability. Posteriorly oriented stress, similar to the Barlow maneuver used in screening newborns for hip dislocation, can detect hip laxity in infants with a subluxable or a dislocatable hip that might be normally located on static images.

Current practice of infant hip US usually incorporates features of both approaches (Figs. 15.32 and 15.33), although some institutions prefer to emphasize the detailed morphologic assessment of the Graf system, whereas others emphasize the dynamic assessment of hip stability. An overview of a popular hybrid approach is described in the appendix at the end of this chapter.

Regardless of the radiologist's preferred technique, complete US assessment of the infant hip always documents:

- Position of the femoral head relative to the acetabulum.
  - Cartilagenous femoral head coverage by the osseous portion of the acetabular roof (normal is at least 50%).
- Contour of the acetabular roof:
  - Should be straight or gently concave, matching the contour of the cartilaginous femoral head.

- Cortex of the roof of the acetabulum and the lateral ilium should meet at a sharp angle that is not rounded.
- If the hip is dislocated or subluxed, potential impediments to successful reduction (e.g., pulvinar or limbus as discussed earlier).
- The *alpha angle* is formed by the acetabular roof and the lateral ilium (see Fig. 15.31B).
  - Normal is 60 degrees or greater, although lower values (as low as 50–55 degrees) may be accepted in young infants up to 6 months of age if there are no other findings to suggest DDH.
- Presence or absence of abnormal hip laxity.
  - Stress maneuver: Gentle posterior force is applied with the hip flexed and adducted, similar to the Barlow maneuver.
- Trace laxity can be normal.
- The *beta angle* is part of the Graf system, not routinely measured or reported unless the complete Graf system is used.
  - Beta angle is the angle formed by inferior continuation of the lateral ilium line and the inferior surface of the echogenic labrum (see Fig. 15.31B). Normal is roughly 55 degrees or less. If the femoral head is subluxed laterally, the beta angle will be greater than 55 degrees.

Limitations of US in DDH

- Operator dependence.
- Limited visualization of the acetabulum in older infants caused by shadowing from the ossifying capital femoral epiphysis.
- Potential for false-positive findings in the immediate neonatal period.
  - Neonates' hips are frequently transiently lax. False-positive neonatal scans can result in unnecessary follow-up examinations, parental anxiety, and overtreatment. Therefore it is generally recommended that the first US examination be delayed until the child is at least 4–6 weeks old to avoid such false-positive results. Exception: when physical exam findings are more concerning, for example, for truly dislocated or dislocatable hip.

Radiographic Evaluation of DDH (see Fig. 15.33)

Radiography in neonates and young infants is reserved for pathologic dislocation. Otherwise, it is not used until age 4 months, after the capital femoral epiphysis has begun to ossify.

- Requires a well-positioned AP radiograph.
  - The symphysis pubis and coccyx should be superimposed or very nearly superimposed on a properly positioned AP radiograph (assuming that neither is deformed).

Radiographic Assessment of DDH

Note that many of these measurements are also used in evaluation of femoracetabular impingement. See also the appendix at the end of Chapter 5 – Pelvis and Hips

The *Hilgenreiner line* (think 'H for horizontal', also called the Y-Y line) is drawn horizontally through the center or top of the bilateral radiolucent triradiate cartilages. The

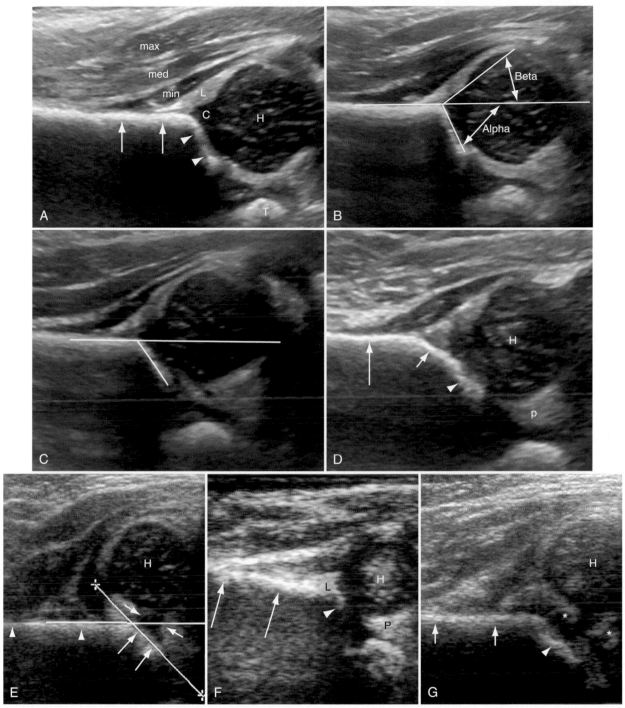

Fig. 15.31 US of developmental dysplasia of the hip (DDH): Coronal images. **(A)** Normal. The lateral margin of the ilium *(arrows)* is seen as an echogenic line with posterior acoustic shadowing. Note the osseous roof of the acetabulum *(arrowheads)*, the unossified (cartilaginous) portion of the acetabular roof *(C)*, and adjacent hyperechoic labrum and capsule *(L)*, the cartilaginous femoral head *(H)*, hypoechoic triradiate with deeper echoes from the pelvis *(T)*, and the overlying gluteus minimus *(min)*, medius *(med)*, and maximus *(max)*. **(B)** Alpha and beta angles. The alpha angle is formed by the osseous acetabular roof and the lateral ilium. The beta angle is formed by the extension of the lateral ilium line and the inferior surface of the labrum. The beta angle is highly variable and less widely used. **(C)** Mild DDH. The hip is normally located, but the alpha angle is less than 60 degrees and the acetabulum is shallow, seen as the acetabular roof covers less than 50% of the hypoechoic femoral head. This infant was treated conservatively, and the hip became normal by age 4 months. **(D)** More severe DDH with a long gentle curve *(short arrow)* between the acetabular roof *(arrowhead)* and the lateral ilium *(long arrow)*. Note echogenic pulvinar *(p)* deep to the femoral head *(H)*. **(E)** Severe DDH. The femoral head *(H)* is subluxed superiorly and laterally (i.e., toward the transducer). Note the very shallow angle formed by the ilium *(arrowheads)* and the steep osseous acetabular roof *(arrows)* and the hypoechoic inverted limbus (between *short arrows*): the echogenic capsule and labrum are interposed between the femoral head and the acetabulum *(long arrows* mark the acetabular roof, *arrowheads* mark the lateral ilium). **(F** and **G)** Severe DDH in different infants. *Arrows* mark the lateral ilium; *arrowheads* mark the acetabular roof; *H* is the femoral head. Pulvinar *(P)* as echogenic tissue filling the acetabulum medial to the femoral head in F. Note the extensive soft tissues interposed between the acetabulum and femoral head in G *(asterisks)*.

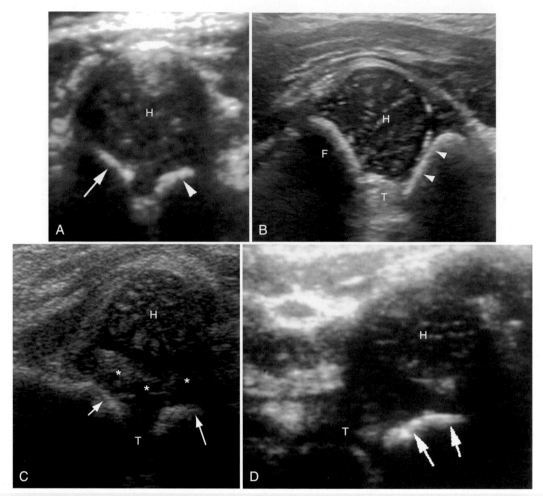

Fig. 15.32 US of developmental dysplasia of the hip (DDH): axial images. (A and **B)** Transverse US images, with anterior to the viewer's left, in two different 5-week-old girls. **(A)** Hip extended. **(B)** Hip flexed. Note the round femoral head *(H)*, echogenic ischium cortex at the posterior acetabulum *(arrowheads)*, pubis at the anterior acetabulum in A *(arrow)*, and bright echoes *(T)* medial to the triradiate cartilage. The anterior acetabulum is obscured by the ossified proximal femur *(F)* in B. **(C)** Severe DDH. Same infant as in Fig. 15.31G. Femoral head *(H)* is displaced laterally (toward the transducer), separated from the pubis and ischium *(arrows)* and triradiate cartilage *(T)* by interposed soft tissues *(asterisks)*. **(D)** Severe DDH, oblique axial image. The transducer was angled to include the triradiate cartilage at the center of the acetabulum, and the subluxed femoral head. The femoral head is subluxed superiorly, laterally, and posteriorly over the ilium *(arrows)*.

triradiate cartilage is the confluence of the ilium, ischium, and pubis slightly anterior to the center of the acetabulum. It is formed by cartilage of the three bones that make up the pelvis, hence its name.

The *Perkin line* is drawn perpendicular to the Hilgenreiner line (think 'P for perpendicular') through the superolateral corner of the acetabular roof. The ossified portion of the capital femoral epiphysis should be entirely or nearly entirely medial to this line. Compare each side. Deficient acetabular coverage of the ossified portion of the femoral heads by as little as 2–3 mm can be significant.

The *center-edge angle* is formed by the Perkin line and a line drawn through the anterior inferior iliac spine and the center of the capital femoral epiphysis. Like the Perkin line, it is a measure of lateral femoral head subluxation and is used in a variety of hip conditions. A normal center-edge angle is about 20 degrees in infancy and 26–30 degrees in adolescence.

Acetabular angle or acetabular index: A fourth line is drawn between the triradiate cartilage and the anterior inferior iliac spine of each hip. The angle formed by this line and the

Hilgenreiner line is the acetabular angle. A useful simplification is that the acetabular angle should be 30 degrees or less. The acetabular angle normally decreases as the child grows by on an average of about 2 degrees per year. Usually it is greater in girls than in boys.

Note that a truly horizontal or nearly horizontal acetabular roof is abnormal and is usually part of a syndrome or skeletal dysplasia.

The *Reimers migration index* is a common measurement of hip dysplasia in children with cerebral palsy, whose dysplasia is not DDH but rather caused by muscle imbalance. The migration index is the percentage of the transverse width of the ossified capital femoral epiphysis lateral to the Perkin line.

The *Shenton line* is an arc drawn along the medial and superior obturator foramen and medial proximal femur. This arc is interrupted or elongated if the femoral head is subluxed.

Some hips with DDH have a smaller ossified capital femoral epiphysis on the affected side. This is a nonspecific finding because some asymmetry may be normal.

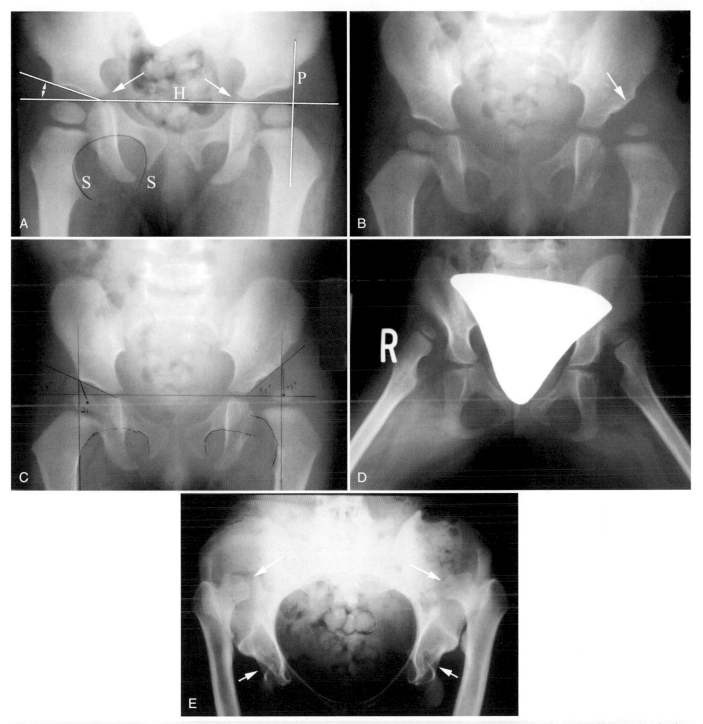

Fig. 15.33 Radiography of developmental dysplasia of the hip (DDH). **(A)** Normal hips. *Arrows* mark the triradiate cartilages. *Double arrow* marks the acetabular angle (acetabular index). Note that the femoral heads are symmetric in size and are nearly completely covered by the acetabular roofs. The acetabular angle is less than 30 degrees. *H,* Hilgenreiner line; *P,* Perkin line; *S,* Shenton line *(arc* drawn in black). **(B)** Left DDH. Note the shallow acetabular roof, early pseudoacetabulum *(arrow),* superolateral subluxation of the left femoral head, and small size of the left femoral epiphysis compared with the normal right side. **(C)** Same radiograph as in B, after review by an orthopedic surgeon. The lines shown on A have been marked on the film, as well as the center-edge angle. The normal right acetabular angle is 24 degrees. The dysplastic left hip acetabular angle is 42 degrees. The right center-edge angle is 21 degrees (normal), and the left is −3 degrees. Also note the discontinuity of the Shenton line on the left. **(D)** Bilateral hip dislocations in a child with cerebral palsy. **(E)** Untreated DDH: late sequelae in a 35-year-old woman with bilateral, severe, untreated DDH. Note the superior bilateral femoral head dislocations *(long arrows).* Also note the dysplastic acetabula *(short arrows).* This patient was able to ambulate but was developing progressive hip pain that required bilateral hip arthroplasties.

DDH may not be discovered until adolescence or adulthood. Early osteoarthritis is a classic late finding. Radiographic findings in mild cases can be subtle. Femoral head coverage by the acetabulum is less on the affected side. The fovea capitus often is higher than normal (*fovea alta*).

Limitations of Radiography in DDH

- Limited assessment of the hips of neonates because the capital femoral epiphyses are not ossified at birth.
- Potential for incorrect acetabular angle measurements if the radiograph is improperly positioned.
- Lack of dynamic imaging.
- Ionizing radiation.

Preoperative Planning

- CT with three-dimensional reconstruction is sometimes used in assessment of dysplastic acetabulum before surgical modification (*acetabuloplasty*; see discussion in the following text).
- Arthrography, MRI, and MR arthrography allow visualization of the femoral head, articular cartilage, labral tears, and potential soft tissue impediments to reduction such as pulvinar, inverted labrum and limbus tight psoas tendon, and redundant ligamentum teres.
- Intraoperative arthrography is usually performed by an orthopedic surgeon during closed or open reduction of a chronically subluxed or dislocated hip (Fig. 15.34).

DDH Management

The main goal of the orthopedic surgeon is to return the femoral head to the center of the acetabulum and keep it there with a brace, cast, or surgical modification of the proximal femur or acetabulum.

- Very mild dysplasia in a neonate may resolve spontaneously without treatment.
- Pavlik harness:
  - Used in neonates and young infants up to about 6 months.
  - Hip must be reducible.
  - Holds the hips in flexion, mild abduction, and mild external rotation (Fig. 15.35).
  - This position keeps the femoral head within the center of the acetabulum, which breaks the vicious cycle of increasing subluxation and dysplasia, allowing healthy acetabular growth.
  - Well tolerated by infants and parents.
  - US can be performed with the harness in place.
  - High success rate (Fig. 15.36).
  - If unsuccessful, a rigid brace may be applied.
- Closed or open reduction followed by hip spica casting:
  - For older children aged 6–18 months, or failed Pavlik harness.
  - Open is more aggressive and more likely to be used in older children or failed closed reduction and casting.
  - Done under general anesthesia.
  - Hip is reduced under fluoroscopy with intraoperative arthrography to evaluate potential impediments to reduction (e.g., pulvinar and inverted limbus, Figs. 15.30 and 15.34).
  - A cast is applied holding the hips in flexion and abduction.

Imaging is obtained immediately following open or closed reduction and casting for confirmation of satisfactory reduction:

- MRI or low-dose CT (Fig. 15.37).
  - CT: 30 mAs, coverage limited to the femoral heads.

The feared complication of reduction and casting is impaired femoral head blood supply with risk of subsequent osteonecrosis (avascular necrosis [AVN]).

- Early identification of femoral head ischemia can avert this complication.
- Subtraction precontrast and postcontrast MRI can demonstrate diminished femoral head perfusion.
- Maximum enhancement occurs 5–10 minutes after injection.

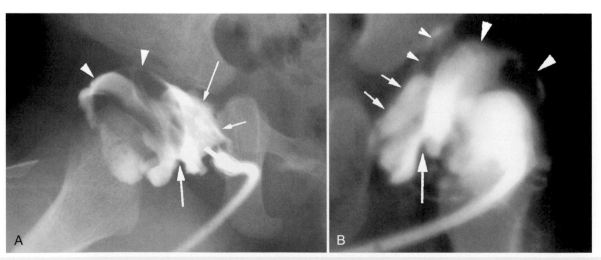

Fig. 15.34 Developmental dysplasia of the hip: arthrography. Compare to Fig. 15.30. **(A and B)** Both studies show the radiolucent cartilaginous femoral head *(arrowheads)*, filling defect from pulvinar *(small arrows)*, and hourglass shape of the capsule *(large arrow)*. **(B)** Arthrogram also shows an inverted limbus *(small arrowheads)*.

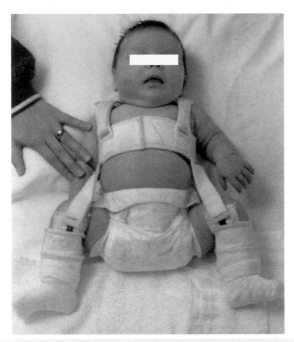

Fig. 15.35 Pavlik harness.

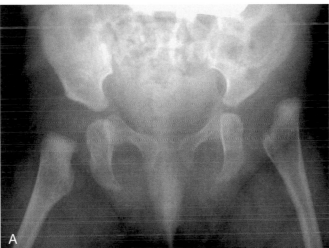

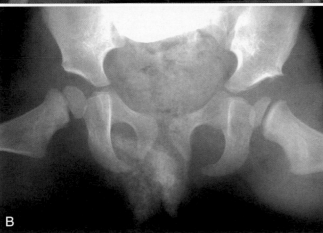

Fig. 15.36 Successful treatment with a Pavlik harness. **(A)** Radiograph during the first week of life shows a left hip dislocation and shallow left acetabulum. The right is normal. **(B)** Radiograph at approximately age 8 months shows near-normal left hip.

Later osteonecrosis radiographic findings:

- Delayed appearance of femoral head ossification.
- If the femoral head was already partially ossified, no further ossification.
- Later: broadening of the femoral neck (coxa magna), femoral head fragmentation.

Surgical Modification of the Proximal Femur and/or Acetabulum

- For more advanced dysplasia in children older than about 2 years.
- CT with three-dimensional reconstruction is sometimes used in preoperative assessment.

Proximal Femur Surgery

- *Varus derotation osteotomy* (VDRO, Fig. 15.38):
  - Proximal femoral shaft osteotomy that produces varus alignment of the femoral neck and corrects the excessive femoral anteversion that is a frequent complication of advanced DDH

Pelvic Surgeries

- Several options (Fig. 15.39), depending on the patient age, morphologic features of the acetabulum, and preference of the surgeon.
- All increase acetabular coverage of the femoral head.

Late-stage DDH in adults causes early osteoarthritis. Hip arthroplasty may be complicated by altered anatomy. CT, MRI, or MR arthrography are sometimes used for preoperative planning.

PROXIMAL FOCAL FEMORAL DEFICIENCY

- A spectrum of congenital deficiency (hypoplasia or aplasia) of the proximal femur (Fig. 15.40).
- Can be bilateral.
- The abnormalities in proximal focal femoral deficiency tend to be centered roughly at the intertrochanteric femur.
- Mild cases: hypoplasia of a short segment of intertrochanteric femur, with a normal femoral head and hip joint. The hypoplastic segment may be composed of unossified cartilage or bone.
- More severe cases: may have hypoplasia of the femoral head with resulting acetabular dysplasia, or absence of the proximal femoral shaft, resulting in a gap (deficiency) in the femur between the head and shaft with overall femoral shortening.
- The most severe cases: absence of nearly the entire femur (see Fig. 15.40C).
- Associated abnormalities: congenital absence of the ipsilateral fibula and foot deformities.
- Most cases are evident at birth because the affected leg is short.

Imaging

- Radiographs.
- US and MRI can assist in characterizing the femoral deficiency and the status of the hip joint.

The goal of treatment is to maximize function of the affected limb. Mild cases do not benefit from surgery.

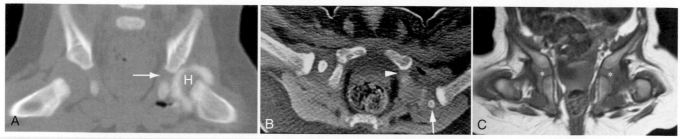

Fig. 15.37 Developmental dysplasia of the hip (DDH): imaging after closed reduction and casting. **(A)** Good reduction of left DDH. Coronal CT arthrogram through the hip joints shows the left femoral head *(H)* to be adjacent to the triradiate cartilage *(arrow)*. Note the shallow left acetabulum compared with the right. **(B)** Poor reduction of left DDH. Axial CT image shows the left femoral head *(arrow)* is subluxed posteriorly relative to the triradiate cartilage *(arrowhead)*. The right hip is normal. The left capital femoral epiphysis ossification center is smaller than the normal right side, a frequent finding in DDH. **(C)** Poor reduction of bilateral DDH. Coronal T1-weighted MR image obtained through the triradiate cartilages *(asterisks)* should also show both femoral heads, but neither is seen. Axial images (not shown) revealed both femoral heads to be posteriorly dislocated.

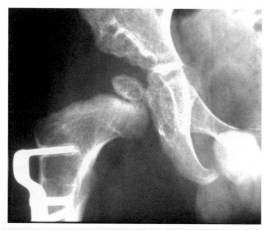

Fig. 15.38 Varus derotation osteotomy. A blade plate and screws (not completely shown) were used to fix the varus-producing osteotomy. This procedure directs the femoral head more directly into the acetabulum.

COXA VARA AND COXA VALGA

The angle formed by the femoral neck and shaft is normally 150 degrees at birth and decreases throughout development to reach an average angle of about 125 degrees in normal adults.

- Increase in this angle is *coxa valga*.
- A decrease is *coxa vara*.
  Coxa vara occurs in several forms:

Congenital Coxa Vara

- Probably results from a limb bud insult during the first trimester of gestation.
- Rare.
- Similar to proximal focal femoral deficiency, and both may occur in the same patient.
- A fixed defect that worsens little, if at all, after birth (Fig. 15.41).

Developmental (Infantile) Coxa Vara

- Abnormal ossification in the medial femoral neck.
- Painless limp in a preschooler.
- Can be bilateral.
- Progresses as the child grows, with potential resulting limb-length discrepancy.
- Often managed surgically.

Acquired Coxa Vara

- In children: Proximal femoral physis injury, slipped capital femoral epiphysis, infection, metabolic conditions that cause bone softening (notably rickets and osteomalacia), tumors, certain rare syndromes.
- Later onset: fibrous dysplasia, Paget's disease.

Coxa valga in children is most often due to decreased tone of the muscles that cross the hip and decreased ambulation. Occurs commonly in neuromuscular conditions such as cerebral palsy and spinal dysraphic defect (Fig. 15.42).

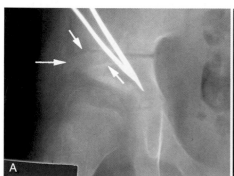
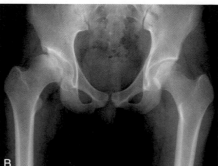
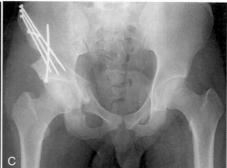

Fig. 15.39 Acetabular osteotomy for developmental dysplasia of the hip (DDH). **(A)** Salter osteotomy. The ilium has been divided transversely, a wedge opened and fixed with a bone plug *(arrows)*, resulting in a more horizontal alignment of the acetabular roof. **(B)** Woman with DDH and early secondary osteoarthritis. **(C)** Ganz osteotomy was performed. This procedure rotates the entire acetabulum to contain the femoral head.

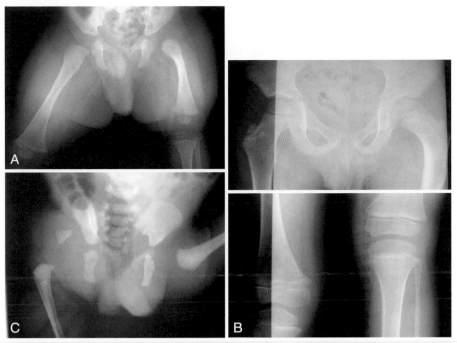

Fig. 15.40 Proximal focal femoral deficiency: spectrum of abnormalities. **(A)** Mild case in a 2-month-old. Note the normal left acetabulum, which indicates that the femoral head is present. **(B)** Same patient at age 4 years. The proximal femur has ossified but is short and dysplastic. **(C)** Severe case with presence only of the most distal right femur. Note the shallow acetabulum, which indicates that there is no right femoral head.

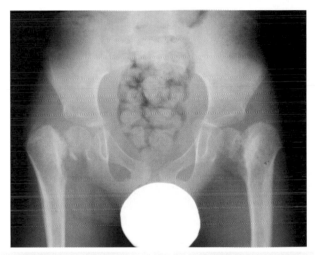

Fig. 15.41 Congenital coxa vara. The findings in this 4-year-old were unchanged from birth.

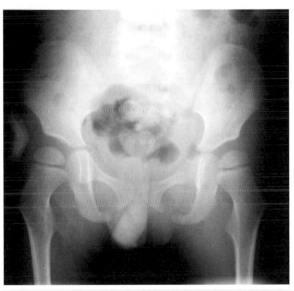

Fig. 15.42 Bilateral coxa valga in a child with cerebral palsy.

Blount's Disease (Tibia Vara)

- Growth disturbance of the medial and posteromedial proximal tibial metaphysis with pathologic genu varum (knee varus) centered at the medial proximal tibia.
- Two forms are recognized: infantile and adolescent.

INFANTILE BLOUNT'S DISEASE

- Onset age 2–5 years.
- Progressive tibia vara.
- More common in early walkers, overweight and large children, and children of African descent. A genetic component likely also is present.

- Some genu varum can be physiologic up to age 2 years. This places greater compressive force on the medial proximal tibial physis. This mechanical force in a genetically susceptible child can slow, alter, or completely stop new bone formation in the medial physis.
- May be unilateral but frequently is bilateral.
- Usually progressive, but milder cases may resolve spontaneously.
- Severe cases may progress to a physeal bar.
- Imaging (Fig. 15.43):
  - Medial and posteromedial proximal epiphysis downslope distally, often with obvious deformity including varus and apex anterior angulation.

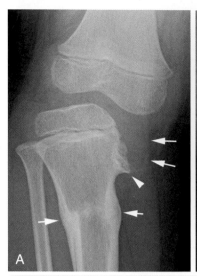
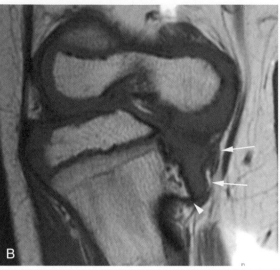
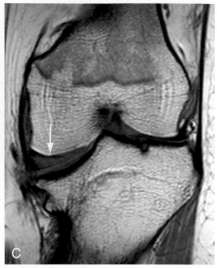

Fig. 15.43 Blount's disease. **(A and B)** Radiograph **(A)** and coronal T1-weighted MR image **(B)** in a 5-year-old with infantile Blount's disease. Note the inferior displacement of unossified cartilage *(arrows)*, varus alignment, and the beak-like contour of the ossified medial metaphysis *(arrowhead)*. The radiograph shows a healed proximal tibial valgus-producing osteotomy (between *short arrows*) that did not succeed in preventing further deformity. **(C)** In this milder case in an older child, medial growth and ossification was slowed, but not stopped *(arrow)*. Note that the 'beak' in this case is formed both by the epiphysis and metaphysis.

- *Beak sign*: deformed proximal medial tibial metaphysis resembles a beak.
- Delayed or absent medial cartilage ossification may be seen.
- Tibial internal torsion is increased. This can be measured with CT or MRI.
- Femur typically is normal.
- Treatment is with bracing and reduced weight-bearing to unload the medial tibia.
- Valgus-producing proximal tibial osteotomy is used in more severe cases.

ADOLESCENT BLOUNT'S DISEASE

- Onset at age 10 or later.
- Unilateral and painful.
- Tends to have milder tibial deformity than the infantile form.
- Caused by medial tibial growth plate injury from trauma or infection, often with bone bar across the physis.
- Femur often abnormal, in contrast with infantile Blount's disease.

Common Congenital Foot Deformities

The most common foot deformities can be described in a straightforward manner, using descriptors and occasional measurement of only three parameters (Box 15.2):

- Hindfoot equinus.
- Hindfoot varus or valgus.
- Forefoot varus or valgus.

Imaging: Foot deformities should be evaluated on AP and lateral weight-bearing radiographs, or with equivalent position in infants.

UNDERSTANDING HINDFOOT EQUINUS

- Evaluated on a lateral weight-bearing radiograph.
- Normally the calcaneus is dorsiflexed relative to the plantar surface of the foot. If measurement is desired, the angle between the longitudinal axis of the tibia and the calcaneus (measured along its base) ranges between 60 and 90 degrees (Fig. 15.44).
- Another way of measuring the alignment of the calcaneus is *calcaneal pitch*, where on a lateral view a line drawn along the base of the calcaneus should slant upward from the horizontal surface by 20–30 degrees.

Box 15.2   Congenital Foot Deformity

Weight-bearing radiographs
Hindfoot equinus: Calcaneus plantar flexed
Hindfoot calcaneus: Calcaneus is excessively dorsiflexed (calcaneal-tibial angle is less than 60 degrees)
Hindfoot varus: Talocalcaneal angle less than 15 degrees (AP radiograph)—talus and calcaneus look parallel
Hindfoot valgus: Talocalcaneal angle greater than 40 degrees (AP radiograph)
Forefoot varus: Forefoot is inverted and often slightly supinated. Metatarsals parallel in AP and lateral radiographs.
Forefoot valgus: Forefoot is everted and often pronated. First metatarsal most plantar on lateral radiograph.
Clubfoot: Hindfoot equinus, hindfoot varus, and forefoot varus
Congenital vertical talus (rocker-bottom foot): Talus in extreme plantar flexion with dorsal dislocation of the navicular, hindfoot equinus, valgus hindfoot, dorsiflexed, and valgus forefoot
Flexible flatfoot deformity (pes planovalgus): Hindfoot valgus, forefoot valgus, but no equinus. Weight-bearing radiographs definitely required!
Pes cavus: High-arched foot (hindfoot calcaneus) with compensatory plantar flexion of the forefoot
Metatarsus adductus: Forefoot adduction, normal hindfoot

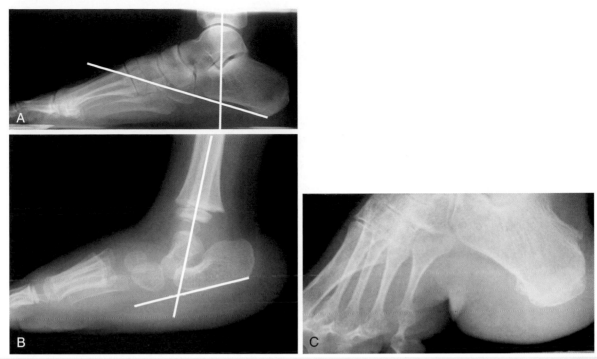

Fig. 15.44 Evaluation of equinus. **(A)** Normal tibiocalcaneal angle, with normal dorsiflexion of the calcaneus. **(B)** Equinus with calcaneotibial angle greater than 90 degrees and plantar flexion of the calcaneus. **(C)** Hindfoot calcaneus, with abnormal dorsiflexion of the calcaneus (in this case caused by a bound foot in a Chinese woman).

- Plantar flexion of the calcaneus such that the calcaneal-tibial angle is greater than 90 degrees represents *hindfoot equinus* (see Fig. 15.44B).
  - Hindfoot equinus is seen in clubfoot and congenital vertical talus.
  - The opposite occurs with *hindfoot calcaneus*, where the calcaneus is excessively dorsiflexed such that the calcaneal-tibial angle is less than 60 degrees (see Fig. 15.44C). Hindfoot calcaneus is seen in cavus and spastic deformities.

UNDERSTANDING HINDFOOT VARUS AND VALGUS

- Both AP and lateral weight-bearing radiographs are used for this evaluation.
- Conceptually, the talus may be considered the point of reference because it may be assumed to be fixed relative to the lower leg. Although this is not exactly correct, for the purpose of this discussion let us assume that the calcaneus rotates medially (internally) or laterally (externally) with respect to a fixed talus. On an AP view the talocalcaneal angle is described by lines drawn through the longitudinal axis of the talus and calcaneus. The AP talocalcaneal angle normally measures 15–40 degrees (30–50 degrees in newborns). Note also that in the normal foot the midtalar line passes through or slightly medial to the base of the first metatarsal. The midcalcaneal line passes through the base of the fourth metatarsal (Fig. 15.45).
  Hindfoot varus: If you presume then that the talus is fixed and the calcaneus internally rotates, the talocalcaneal angle decreases to less than 15 degrees, to the point that in some cases the talocalcaneal angle may

approach 0 degrees or parallelism of those bones. A talocalcaneal angle less than 15 degrees is hindfoot varus (see Fig. 15.45B). In classic cases the angle is 0 degrees. Note that in a hindfoot varus deformity the talus ends up pointing lateral to the first metatarsal because the entire foot is swung medially.
  Hindfoot valgus: The opposite occurs when the calcaneus externally rotates relative to the talus. A talocalcaneal angle greater than 40 degrees is hindfoot valgus. Note also that with this increased talocalcaneal angle, the talus points medial to the first metatarsal because the calcaneus and the entire foot swing laterally (Fig. 15.45C).

Hindfoot varus or valgus is also evaluated on the lateral view. Normally the lateral talocalcaneal angle (also termed 'the Kite angle') is measured by a line bisecting the talus and a line along the base of the calcaneus, measuring 25–45 degrees (50 degrees in newborns). The calcaneus is dorsiflexed, as already discussed, and the talus is mildly plantar flexed to produce this angle (Fig. 15.46).

In hindfoot varus, the calcaneus internally rotates. With the anterior portion of the calcaneus moving into a position beneath the head of the talus, the talus can no longer be as plantar flexed. This results in a decrease in the talocalcaneal angle on the lateral view, with the two bones approaching parallelism (see Fig. 15.46B). **Thus on both the AP and lateral views, with a hindfoot varus deformity, the talocalcaneal angles decrease and the bones approach parallel**.

In hindfoot valgus, the calcaneus externally rotates, as seen on the AP view in Fig. 15.45C. With external rotation of the calcaneus, the anterior calcaneus no longer supports

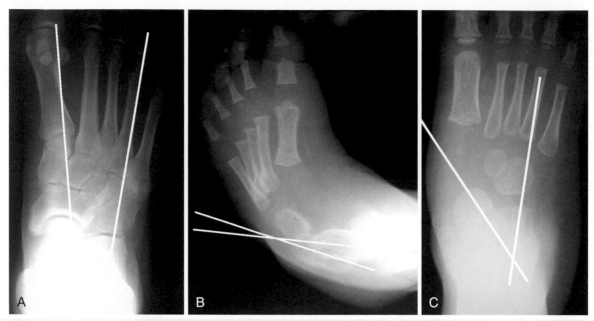

Fig. 15.45 AP radiographic evaluation of the hindfoot. **(A)** Normal AP talocalcaneal angle, with the midtalar line passing through the base of the first metatarsal and the midcalcaneal line passing through the base of the fourth metatarsal. **(B)** AP evaluation of hindfoot varus, with a decreased talocalcaneal angle and the talus pointing lateral to the first metatarsal base. **(C)** AP evaluation of hindfoot valgus, with an increased talocalcaneal angle and the talus pointing medially to the first metatarsal base.

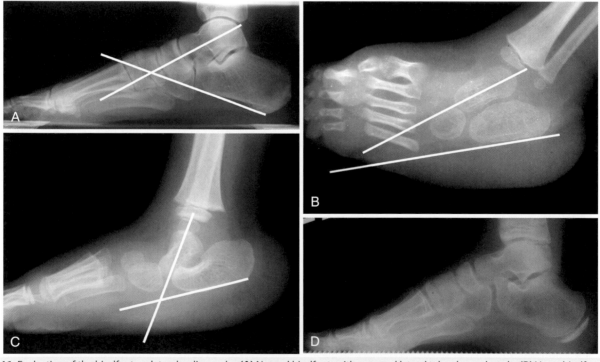

Fig. 15.46 Evaluation of the hindfoot on lateral radiography. **(A)** Normal hindfoot, with a normal lateral talocalcaneal angle. **(B)** Varus hindfoot, with a decreased talocalcaneal angle. **(C)** Valgus hindfoot, with an increased talocalcaneal angle. **(D)** Pes cavus (hindfoot valgus, high longitudinal arch).

the head of the talus and the talus is allowed to further plantar flex. On the lateral view, then, we see increased plantar flexion of the talus, which results in an increased talocalcaneal angle (see Fig. 15.46C). This is the appearance of hindfoot valgus on the lateral view. **Thus, with hindfoot valgus there is an increased talocalcaneal angle on both AP and lateral radiographs**.

UNDERSTANDING FOREFOOT VARUS AND VALGUS

- This is a much more qualitative and subjective evaluation. On the AP radiograph the metatarsals normally converge proximally with slight overlap at the bases (Fig. 15.47A).

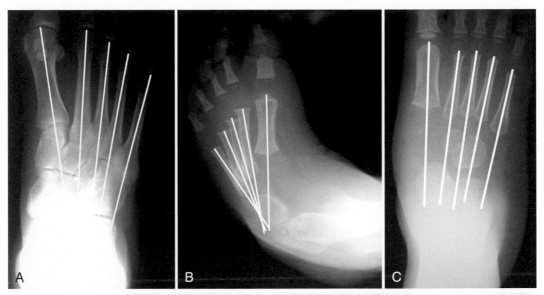

Fig. 15.47 AP evaluation of the forefoot. **(A)** The normal appearance of convergence with slight overlap at the bases of the metatarsals. **(B)** Forefoot varus, with abnormally increased convergence at the bases of the metatarsals. **(C)** Forefoot valgus, with divergence or at least a decrease in the overlap at the bases of the metatarsals.

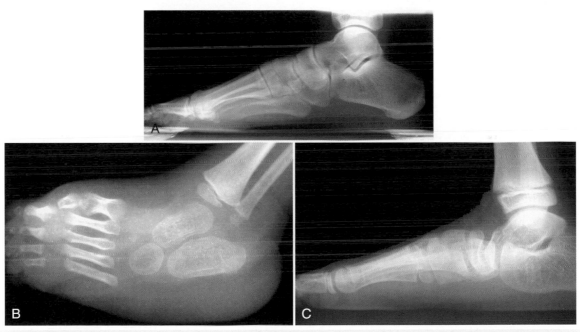

Fig. 15.48 Lateral radiographic evaluation of the forefoot. **(A)** Normal, with partial superimposition of the metatarsals and the fifth in the plantar position (same image as in Fig. 15.46A). **(B)** Varus forefoot, with a ladderlike configuration of the metatarsals, fifth in the plantar position (same image as in Fig. 15.46B). **(C)** Forefoot valgus, with superimposition of the metatarsals on the lateral view and the first in the most plantar position.

- With forefoot varus, the forefoot is inverted and often slightly supinated. On the AP radiograph, then, the forefoot would appear narrowed, with an increased convergence at the bases of the metatarsals (Fig. 15.47B).
- With forefoot valgus, the forefoot is everted and often pronated. With this change in position, on the AP radiograph the forefoot is seen to be broadened with a decrease in overlap at the metatarsal bases (Fig. 15.47C).
- Consider now the appearance of the forefoot on the lateral view. Normally the metatarsals are partially superimposed, with the fifth metatarsal in the most plantar position (Fig. 15.48A).
- With forefoot varus (inversion, often with supination), the metatarsals on the lateral view have a more ladderlike arrangement, with the first metatarsal in the most dorsal position and the fifth metatarsal in the most plantar position (Fig. 15.48B).
- On the other hand, with forefoot valgus (eversion and pronation), the metatarsals are usually more superimposed on one another on the lateral radiograph, and the first metatarsal is in the most plantar position (Fig. 15.48C).

CLUBFOOT (*TALIPES EQUINOVARUS*)

- *Talipes* is deformity of the foot involving the talus.
- Occurs in 1 in 1000 births, M>F 2:1 to 3:1.
- The cause of the clubfoot deformity is unclear, but possible contributing factors include ligamentous laxity, muscle imbalance, intrauterine position deformity, and persistence of an early normal fetal alignment.
- The radiographic findings of a clubfoot deformity are hindfoot equinus, hindfoot varus, and forefoot varus (Fig. 15.49).
- Most are sporadic. A positive family history is present in about 25%. Also associated with several rare syndromes.

CONGENITAL VERTICAL TALUS (ROCKER-BOTTOM FOOT)

- The talus is in extreme plantar flexion with dorsal dislocation of the navicular, locking the talus into plantar flexion.
- Radiographs: equinus deformity, valgus hindfoot, dorsiflexed and valgus forefoot, and abnormal talus with dislocated navicular (Fig. 15.50A and B).
- Congenital vertical talus clinically presents as a rigid flatfoot, may occur in isolation or as part of a variety of syndromes, and frequently is associated with myelomeningocele.

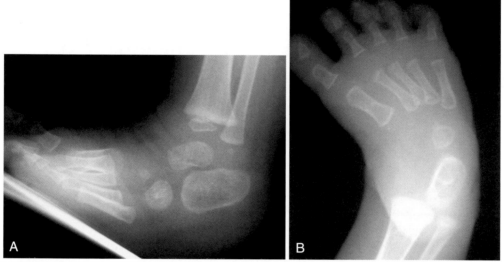

Fig. 15.49 Clubfoot. Lateral radiographic view **(A)** demonstrates equinus of the hindfoot. Both AP **(B)** and lateral views show a varus hindfoot (decreased talocalcaneal angle, with the bones nearly parallel). Both views show forefoot varus. Lateral view is obtained with dorsiflexion force (the equivalent of a weight-bearing view in an infant), which diminishes the apparent forefoot varus. See Fig. 15.48B for the appearance of the forefoot in clubfoot without application of dorsiflexion stress.

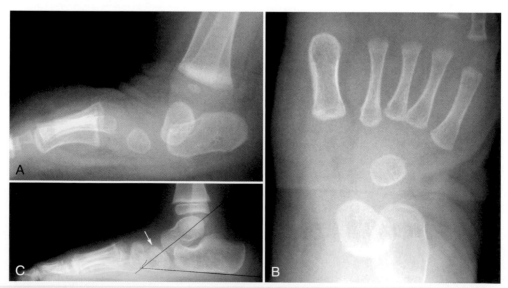

Fig. 15.50 Congenital vertical talus (rocker-bottom foot) and planovalgus. Both have hindfoot valgus. **(A and B)** Congenital vertical talus. Note the hindfoot equinus and hindfoot valgus (increased talocalcaneal angle), with the talus being nearly vertical on the lateral view. Both views show forefoot valgus. Note that the navicular is dorsal relative to the talar head. **(C)** Planovalgus. Hindfoot valgus is present with forefoot valgus, like congenital vertical talus, but the hindfoot is not in equinus and the navicular *(arrow)* is aligned with the talus.

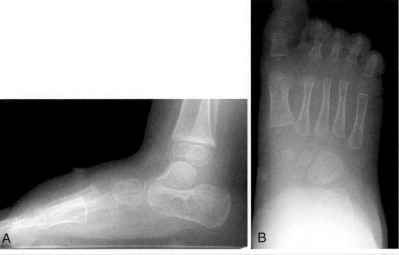

Fig. 15.51 Flexible flatfoot deformity. Lateral **(A)** and AP **(B)** weight-bearing radiographic views demonstrate no hindfoot equinus but do show hindfoot and forefoot valgus. Non–weight-bearing radiographs (not shown) would depict a normal alignment of both the hindfoot and forefoot. (Images used with permission from BJ Manaster, MD, from the American College of Radiology Learning File.)

FLEXIBLE FLATFOOT DEFORMITY (*PES PLANOVALGUS*)

- Relatively common, affecting 4% of the population.
- An important part of the diagnosis is that it is indeed flexible; the abnormality is seen only on weight-bearing radiographs, and the deformity is reduced with non–weight-bearing radiographs.
- Hindfoot valgus and forefoot valgus, but no equinus (Figs. 15.47C and 15.51). The valgus deformities are usually subtler than those of a congenital vertical talus.

PES CAVUS

High-arched foot (*hindfoot calcaneus*) with compensatory plantar flexion of the forefoot. Seen in patients with upper motor neuron lesions (*Friedreich ataxia*), lower motor neuron lesions (polio), vascular ischemia as in Volkmann contracture, and the neuropathy Charcot–Marie–Tooth disease.

METATARSUS ADDUCTUS

The most common structural abnormality of the foot, seen in infancy 10 times more frequently than clubfoot.

- Radiologists do not see it as frequently because it usually is not imaged.
- Usually bilateral and more common in females than in males.
- Forefoot adduction, with a normal hindfoot (Fig. 15.52).

BUNION DEFORMITY

- Common, acquired.
- First metatarsal varus and hallux (great toe) valgus, often with bony overgrowth of the medial first metatarsal head.
- Although this is an adult condition, it probably begins in many cases during the teenage years. Ill-fitting shoes are a main cause, and women outnumber men.

Other foot deformities that combine varus and valgus hindfoot and forefoot deformities are usually caused by spastic neuromuscular conditions such as cerebral palsy.

Coalitions

- Failure of prenatal segmentation into the normal osseous anatomy occurs most commonly in the wrist, foot, and spine.
- Spectrum from complete osseous fusion, partial osseous fusion, fibrous or cartilaginous coalition, or an incompletely formed joint that is prone to degeneration.
- The most common clinically important coalitions occur in the foot and spine. Spine coalitions (Klippel–Feil and segmentation anomalies) were discussed earlier this chapter.

UPPER EXTREMITY COALITIONS

Congenital Carpal Coalitions

- The most common carpal bone coalition is lunate-triquetrum (alternative term is *lunotriquetral*, Fig. 15.53A), followed by capitate-hamate (capitohamate, Fig. 15.53B).
- F>M 2:1.
- In the US, much more common in African Americans.
- Almost never clinically significant.
- Multiple coalitions occur in some rare syndromes.

Symphalangism

- Congenital coalition of phalanges (Fig. 15.54). Metacarpals may also be involved. May also occur in the toes.
- The condition is variable and frequently is familial.

Congenital Radioulnar Synostosis

- Congenital fusion of the ulna and radius (Fig 15.55).
- Caused by failure of segmentation of the proximal radius and ulna in early intrauterine limb development.

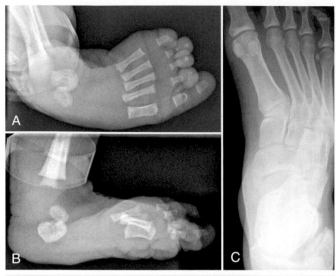

Fig. 15.52 Metatarsus adductus. AP **(A)** and lateral **(B)** radiographs in a newborn with normal hindfoot alignment and forefoot adduction. **(C)** Mild case in an adult shows adduction of the forefoot.

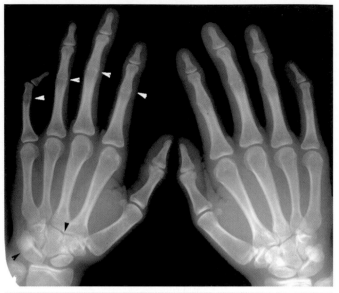

Fig. 15.54 Symphalangism. This mild case involves only the PIP joints *(white arrowheads)*. Also note the lunotriquetral and trapezoid-capitate carpal coalitions *(black arrowheads)*.

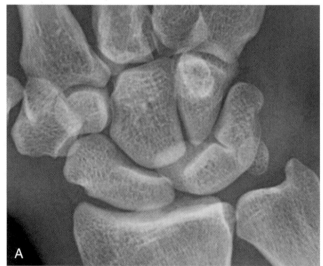

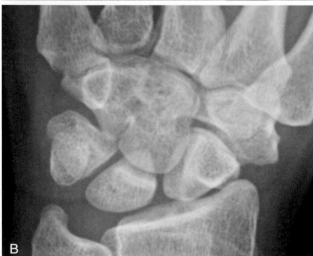

Fig. 15.53 Carpal coalition. **(A)** Lunate-triquetrum. **(B)** Capitate-hamate. Both are partial osseous coalitions.

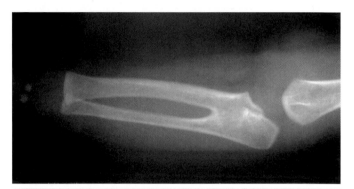

Fig. 15.55 Congenital radioulnar synostosis. The proximal fusion is typical.

- The proximal radius is often posteriorly displaced, and the radius is often bowed laterally.
- Can occur as an isolated abnormality, as a familial condition, or in association with a variety of rare syndromes, such as abnormal karyotypes (XXXY, XXYY).
- Acquired radioulnar synostosis can occur after trauma, surgery, infection, or Caffey disease (infantile cortical hyperostosis).

Key Concepts

Tarsal Coalition

Fibrous, cartilaginous, or osseous
May be bilateral
CT or MRI for diagnosis if radiographs negative or indeterminate, and for therapy planning
Subtalar: Medial facet; talar beak
Calcaneonavicular coalition: 'Anteater sign' on oblique or lateral radiograph
Other patterns: Talonavicular, calcaneocuboid, cubonavicular

CONGENITAL TARSAL COALITIONS

- Involve bones of the hindfoot and/or midfoot.
- Occur in 1% of the population and is bilateral in about one-fourth of these patients.
- Fibrous and cartilaginous coalitions show close approximation of the bones with irregular cortical margins, bone deformity, sclerosis, and, on fluid-sensitive MRI sequences, adjacent marrow edema.
- Rarely, tarsal coalitions may be seen as a part of various rare syndromes.
- Clinical: Although the condition is congenital, symptoms usually do not develop until the second decade of life, when a combination of greater activity and more advanced replacement of flexible cartilage with rigid bone makes a previously asymptomatic coalition painful.
- A teenager or young adult who presents with limited subtalar motion, pes planus, and shortening or persistent or intermittent spasm of the peroneal muscles is a classic presentation.

Imaging

- Plain films show many coalitions, or at least secondary signs.
- CT and MRI are highly accurate.
  - Both feet may be imaged because tarsal coalitions of any type can be bilateral.

Calcaneonavicular Coalition

- Most common tarsal coalition.
- Best seen on an oblique radiograph where either the solid osseous coalition or the abnormal joint is visible.
- The elongated anterior process of the calcaneus resembles the long snout of an anteater on a lateral radiograph 'anteater sign', (Fig. 15.56).
- CT or MRI are generally not needed for diagnosis but can better assess the anatomic features before surgery.

Talocalcaneal (Subtalar) Coalition

- Second most common tarsal coalition.
- Often more complex than calcaneonavicular coalition (Figs. 15.57 and 15.58).
- Usually occurs at the middle facet between the talus and the sustentaculum tali of the calcaneus.
- More extensive cases also involve the posterior facet, but anterior facet involvent is uncommon.
- CT and MRI are definitive.
- Radiographic findings can be subtle. The normal middle facet usually is seen on a weight-bearing lateral

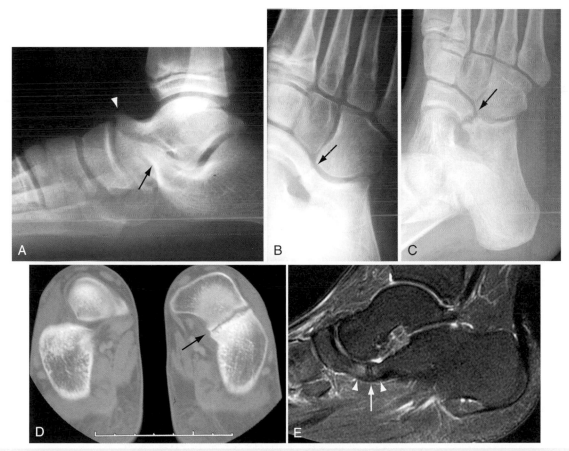

Fig. 15.56 Calcaneonavicular tarsal coalition, spectrum of disease. **(A)** Lateral radiograph in a 14-year-old boy demonstrates a small talar beak *(arrowhead)* and an elongated anterior extension of the calcaneus *(arrow; 'anteater' sign)*. **(B)** Oblique view shows the calcaneonavicular coalition to be osseous except for a subtle radiolucent cleft *(arrow)*. **(C–E)** Fibrous coalitions. Oblique radiograph **(C)** shows broad calcaneonavicular articulation with irregular adjacent cortex *(arrow)*. CT image **(D)** in a different patient shows broad and irregular left calcaneonavicular joint *(arrow)*. **(E)** Sagittal fat-suppressed T2-weighted MR image in another patient shows findings similar to those seen in D. The coalition *(arrow)* is almost continuous bone. Note the adjacent bone marrow edema *(arrowheads)*.

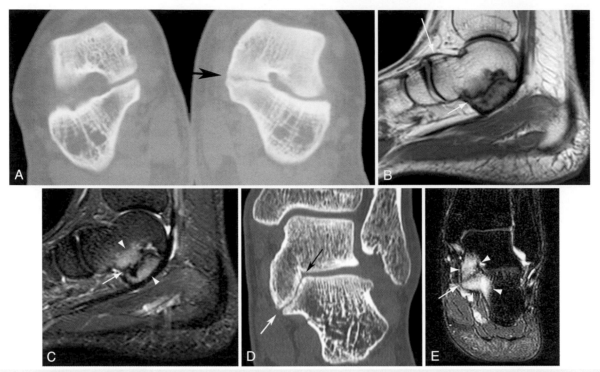

Fig. 15.57 Fibrous talocalcaneal (subtalar) coalition. **(A)** Direct coronal CT image shows typical appearance of a fibrous coalition of the left medial facet joint *(arrow)*, in contrast to normal medial facet joint on the right. **(B** and **C)** Sagittal T1-weighted **(B)** and fat-suppressed T2-weighted **(C)** MR images in a different patient show talar beak *(long arrow* in B) and irregular middle facet joint *(short arrow* in B and C). Note adjacent bone marrow edema *(arrowheads)* in C. **(D)** Coronal CT reconstruction in a different patient. Note the oblique orientation of the dysplastic middle facet *(arrows)*, which is a frequent finding in fibrous subtalar coalition. **(E)** Coronal fat-suppressed T2-weighted MR image in a different patient also shows irregular, oblique middle facet *(arrow)* with extensive adjacent bone marrow edema *(arrowheads)*.

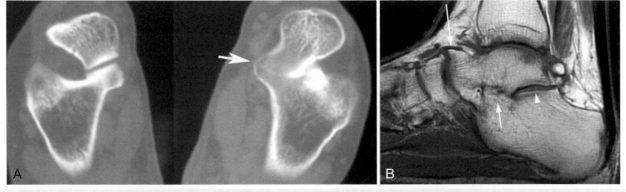

Fig. 15.58 Osseous subtalar coalition. **(A)** Direct coronal CT image shows continuous bone across the left middle facet joint *(arrow)*, in contrast with the normal right middle facet. The posterior facets (not shown) were normal bilaterally. **(B)** Sagittal T1-weighted MR image in a different patient shows continuous bone marrow fat signal between the calcaneus and talus *(short arrow)*. Also note intact posterior facet joint *(arrowhead)* and talar beak *(long arrow)*.

radiograph, but failure to visualize this joint may be a result of x-ray obliquity to the joint rather than a coalition.

- A Harris (skier's) view can detect a talocalcaneal coalition because it profiles the sustentaculum and middle facet joint.
- Indirect radiographic signs:
  - *Talar beak* is a large, broad spur extending dorsally from the talar head (Fig. 15.59).
    - Caused by excessive motion at the talonavicular joint resulting from restriction in the other hindfoot/midfoot joints.

- Talar beak may also be seen with other coalitions, including *calcaneonavicular coalition*.
- *C sign*.
  - Caused by continuous bone across the middle facet on the lateral view, resembling the letter 'C', open anteriorly (Fig. 15.59).

Other Tarsal Coalitions

- Coalitions also occur in other patterns: talonavicular, calcaneocuboid, and cubonavicular. Any or all of the hindfoot and hindfoot/midfoot joints may be fused.

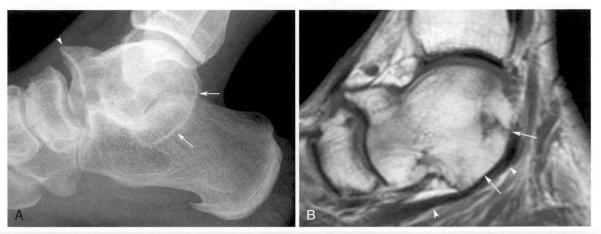

Fig. 15.59 Talar beak and C signs in subtalar coalition. Both the middle and posterior facets are extensively fused in this young adult. **(A)** Lateral radiograph shows a dorsal spur at the distal talus, known as a talar beak *(arrowhead)*. This radiograph also shows the less common and less reliable C sign, formed by continuous bone across the posterior margin of the middle facet *(arrows)*. **(B)** Sagittal T1-weighted MR image shows continuous marrow between the talus and calcaneus. *Arrows* mark the posterior cortex of the fused middle and posterior facets. Note the flexor hallucis longus tendon coursing below the sustentaculum tali *(arrowheads)*. The talar beak finding is more commonly seen with subtalar coalition, but sometimes neither is present.

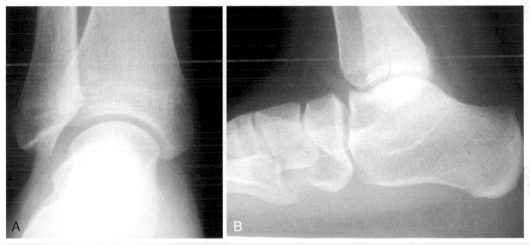

Fig. 15.60 Tarsal coalition: ball-and-socket joint. AP **(A)** and lateral **(B)** radiographs show a spherical contour of the tibiotalar joint, allowing a ball-and-socket type of motion. The talus and calcaneus are completely fused, with no definition of the normal subtalar joints.

- When there is a substantial coalition with multiple fusions, the patient may develop a *ball-and-socket ankle*, as seen on an AP radiograph (Fig. 15.60).
  - Converting the tibiotalar joint from a hinge joint to a ball-and-socket joint provides the inversion-eversion motion that is restricted at the coalesced hindfoot.

Tarsal coalition can be acquired following trauma or infection.

Treatment of tarsal coalitions is tailored to each case. Treatment options include casting, surgical resection of the coalition, or arthrodesis.

Skeletal Dysplasias

Over 400 distinct skeletal dysplasias (or more precisely *osteochondrodysplasias*) and syndromes that cause skeletal deformity and/or impair normal skeletal function have been identified. Many are constitutional diseases of bones, caused by errors in bone formation or remodeling.

Understanding of skeletal dysplasias has been revolutionized in recent decades by advances in genetics and molecular biology and continues to evolve. Classification formerly was based on clinical and radiographic features, but is now based on the affected gene, receptor, or protein in most cases. From the radiologist's perspective, this new knowledge has had two major effects: the first is easing the formerly heavy emphasis on radiologic diagnosis (though radiologists are still involved with diagnosis and assessment of disease penetrance and complications); second, the taxonomy of dysplasias has been revised, with the revised taxonomy groups joining together conditions that have in common a defective receptor or protein.

Most dysplasias present at or even before birth, although some dysplasias can be mild and clinically silent at birth and beyond. The genetics and inheritance patterns (autosomal dominant or recessive, X-linked dominant or recessive, etc.) are now known for most dysplasias. Precise diagnosis allows for genetic counseling of the parents and siblings.

Dysplasia diagnosis begins with physical exam and genetic testing of umbilical cord blood.

When radiographs are requested, this is a sample screening protocol:

- Lateral skull.
- AP and lateral thoracolumbar spine.
- Frontal chest (including the shoulders).
- AP pelvis and hips.
- AP view of a single upper extremity.
- AP view of a single lower extremity.
- PA hand detail view.

Interpreting radiographs in skeletal dysplasias can be very challenging. Here is a suggested approach:

- Break down the findings by location and other features *before* turning to one of the dysplasia radiology references.
- A dysplasia may affect all or only parts of the skeleton. Try to identify which of the following categories of bones are abnormal: skull, spine, thorax, pelvis, and/or limbs.
- If the limbs are abnormal, try to localize the findings to the epiphyses, metaphyses, or diaphyses.

USEFUL TERMINOLOGY

- If the vertebrae are abnormal, the syndrome's name may contain the prefix 'spondylo'.
- If the limbs are short, is it proportionate or disproportionate? If disproportionate, try to identify if the shortening is most severe in the humeri and femurs (*rhizomelic* shortening; *rhizo*, root), forearms and legs (*mesomelic* shortening), or hands and feet (*acromelic* shortening).
- If the epiphyses are abnormal, for example, with delayed ossification or fragmented into small 'punctate' or irregular ossicles, the syndrome may be an epiphyseal dysplasia.

- If the metaphyses are abnormal, especially adjacent to the physis, for example, wide or deformed, the syndrome may be a metaphyseal dysplasia.
- If the diaphyses are abnormally narrow or wide, or with cortical thickening, the syndrome may be a diaphyseal dysplasia.
- More than one area may be abnormal, for example, a *spondyloepiphyseal* dysplasia.
- Finger abnormalities:
    - Brachydactyly = short fingers.
    - Arachnodactyly = long, slender fingers.
    - Polydactyly = more than five fingers.
    - Syndactyly = two or more fingers fused together.
    - Clinodactyly = deformity in the coronal plane, usually the fifth finger with valgus.
    - Camptodactyly = flexion deformity, usually at the fifth proximal interphalangeal (PIP) joint.
- Gamuts can be useful, such as for short ribs or horizontal acetabular roofs.

The following text includes some of the more common or distinctive skeletal dysplasias. Some are very rare but are included because the ABR has listed them as potential core exam content.

ACHONDROPLASIA

- Rhizomelic short-limbed dwarfism.
- By far the most common skeletal dysplasia (1 in 26,000 live births).
- Autosomal dominant. Most cases are spontaneous mutations.
- Caused by a mutation of fibroblast growth factor receptor 3 (FGFR3).
- Causes defective enchondral bone formation.
- Normal intelligence and near-normal life span.

Radiologic Features of Achondroplasia (Fig. 15.61)

- Large cranium.
- Long bones are short and wide, with flared metaphyses.

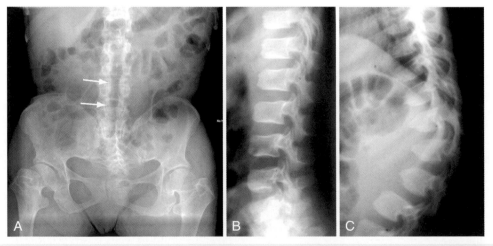

Fig. 15.61 Achondroplasia and hypochondroplasia. **(A)** AP spine shows narrow interpediculate distance in the lower lumbar spine *(arrows)*. The lower lumbar spinal processes are absent because a decompressive laminectomy was performed to relieve spinal stenosis. **(B)** Lateral lumbar spine. Note the posterior vertebral body scalloping, mild anterior beaking, and short pedicles. **(C)** Lateral spine, more severe dysplasia. Note the thoracolumbar kyphosis with prominent anterior beaking.

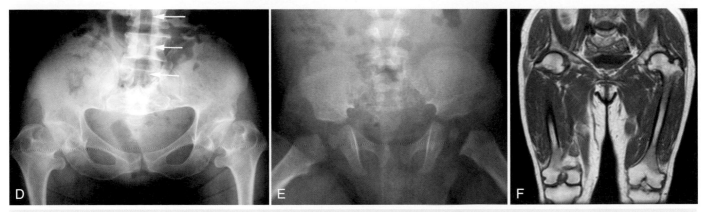

Fig. 15.61, cont'd **(D)** Pelvis in an adult. Note the prior lumbar laminectomy *(arrows).* **(E)** Pelvis in an infant with hypochondroplasia also shows narrow interpediculate distance, but the pelvis is relatively spared, because the iliac wings are less 'squared' and the champagne glass configuration is less apparent. **(F)** Coronal T1-weighted MR image of the thighs in an adult shows the 'short, squat' overtubulated appearance of long bones. (B courtesy of Stephanie Spottswood, MD.)

- Spine:
  - The vertebral bodies are bullet shaped in infancy and become mildly flattened in adulthood.
  - Thoracolumbar kyphosis.
  - Exaggerated lumbar lordosis.
  - Lumbar stenosis develops, with narrow interpediculate distance and short pedicles.
- Pelvis: squared iliac wings, horizontal acetabular roofs, and a narrow pelvic inlet that has been likened to a champagne glass.
- Short ribs.
- Hands: 'trident' configuration because of equal length of the second, third, and fourth digits.
- The major cause of morbidity is neurologic impingement caused by the spinal and foramen magnum stenosis.

Achondroplasia is the most common member of a group of dysplasias that result from fibroblast growth factor receptor 3 (FGFR 3) mutations. The others vary widely in severity, but not surprisingly share some imaging features. Here are two examples from this group:

- **Hypochondroplasia** has clinical and radiographic features that are similar to but much milder than achondroplasia. Notably the skull and pelvis are relatively spared in hypochondroplasia (see Fig. 15.61E).
- **Thanatophoric dysplasia** (or dwarfism) is the most severe form (Fig. 15.62).
  - Lethal short-limbed dwarfism.
  - May be diagnosed by prenatal US.
  - The skull has a cloverleaf deformity caused by global synostosis.
  - The ribs are severely shortened, and the chest is small.
  - The spine has *platyspondyly* (flat vertebral bodies) with U-shaped vertebral bodies and narrow interpediculate distance. Overall spine length is normal because the disc spaces are wide.
  - The iliac wings are squared, and the acetabular roofs are horizontal. The limbs are severely shortened, and the femurs are characteristically curved (*telephone-receiver femurs*).

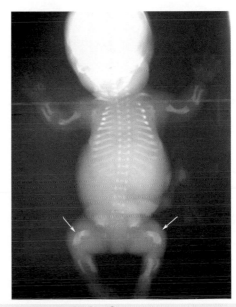

Fig. 15.62 Thanatophoric dwarfism. Note the short, bowed femurs *(arrows)* and the flat, U-shaped vertebral bodies with wide disc spaces. The rhizomelic dwarfisms achondroplasia, achondrogenesis, and thanatophoric dwarfism share many morphologic and radiologic features and can be considered as a spectrum, with achondroplasia on the mild end and thanatophoric dysplasia on the severe end.

CLEIDOCRANIAL DYSPLASIA (CLEIDOCRANIAL DYSOSTOSIS, PELVICOCLEIDOCRANIAL DYSPLASIA)

- Results from abnormal development of membranous bones.
- Autosomal dominant, with about one-third of cases caused by spontaneous mutations. Variable expression.
- Clinical and radiographic manifestations are usually evident at birth and may be detected prenatally.
- Clinical manifestations: small face, wide head with hypertelorism, and generalized joint laxity. After the newborn period, dental dysplasia (too many or too few teeth, abnormal teeth), drooping shoulders, and an abnormal gait may become evident.

■ Radiographic findings reflect the abnormal development of membranous bone (Fig. 15.63):

■ Skull: delayed closure of the cranial sutures and fontanelles, including a persistent metopic suture, *wormian bones* (*intrasutural ossicles*, Box 15.3).

■ Partial or complete absence of the clavicle, and occasional apparent pseudarthroses caused by discontinuous ossification. The middle or lateral third of the

clavicle is most likely to be absent, probably because these portions are formed by intramembranous ossification. When the lateral third of the clavicle is absent, this finding may simulate other causes of an absent distal clavicle (Box 15.4).

■ Scoliosis.

■ Coxa vara or valga, genu varum.

■ Wide symphysis pubis (Box 15.5).

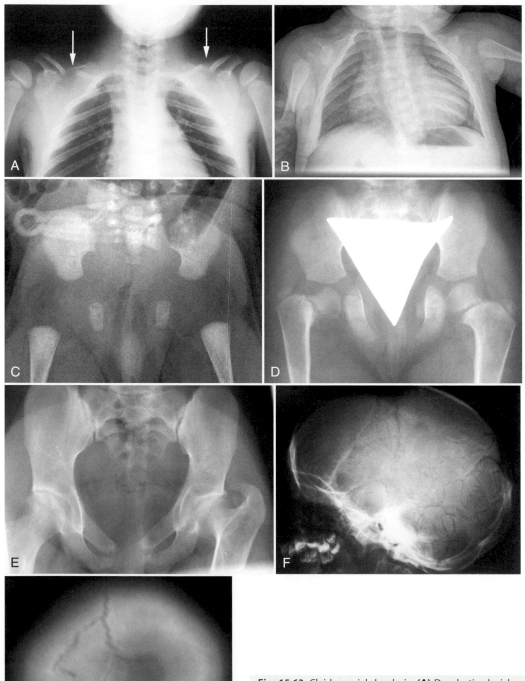

Fig. 15.63 Cleidocranial dysplasia. **(A)** Dysplastic clavicles with absent middle segments *(arrows)*. **(B)** Newborn with absent clavicles. **(C)** Newborn pelvis, with absent ossification of most of the pubic bones. **(D)** Pelvis in a child shows no pubis ossification and unusually shaped capital femoral epiphyses. **(E)** Pelvis in an adult shows absence of ossification around the symphysis pubis and bilateral hip dysplasia with early secondary osteoarthritis. **(F)** Wormian bones (sutural ossicles). **(G)** Head CT in a different child also shows sutural ossicles.

Box 15.3   Wormian Bones (Sutural Bones)

Hypothyroidism
Hypophosphatasia
Cleidocranial dysplasia
Pyknodysostosis
Osteogenesis imperfecta
Zellweger syndrome (autosomal recessive, seizures, mental retardation, microcystic renal disease, death in infancy)
Menkes syndrome (males, fragile bones, abnormal copper metabolism)

Box 15.4   Absent Distal Clavicle

Trauma: Posttraumatic osteolysis (weightlifters)
Metastases/myeloma
Infection
Surgery
Rheumatoid arthritis
Hyperparathyroidism
Cleidocranial dysplasia

Box 15.5   Wide Symphysis Pubis

Trauma
Metastases/myeloma
Infection
Surgery
Hyperparathyroidism
Cleidocranial dysplasia
Epispadius/bladder exstrophy/prune-belly syndrome spectrum

OSTEOGENESIS IMPERFECTA

Key Concepts

Osteogenesis Imperfecta

A group of heritable, debilitating conditions characterized by weak bones with frequent fractures that often result in severe deformity
Blue sclerae, osteoporosis, and wormian bones (intrasuteral ossicles) are frequently present

Osteogenesis imperfecta is a group of disorders of collagen synthesis that result in abnormal bone formation with radiolucent bones that are easily fractured (Fig. 15.64; see Fig. 1.80).

Current understanding is that there are at least eight or more subtypes depending on specific classifications. All result in deficient quantity and/or quality of type 1 collagen. Most forms are autosomal dominant spontaneous mutations. Autosomal recessive forms also occur.

The severity of skeletal manifestations varies (Fig. 15.64).

- Mild forms have only relatively mild bone fragility that may not be diagnosed until late childhood or adulthood.
- Intermediate forms result in multiple fractures that can cause deformity manifesting as short-limbed dwarfism. Healing fractures often exhibit exuberant callus formation (Box 15.6). Hearing loss caused by

otic bone fractures, gray teeth (*dentinogenesis imperfecta*), and blue sclerae are seen in 90% of cases. Basilar invagination with brainstem compression and arterial dissections may occur.

- The most severe forms result in multiple fractures in utero and are incompatible with life.

Distinguishing Osteogenesis Imperfecta From Child Abuse

The main differential diagnosis in an infant or child with multiple fractures of different ages is child abuse and OI. (Several extremely rare conditions, such as *Caffey disease* and *Menkes syndrome*, also may resemble child abuse.) Child abuse is much more frequent than all forms of OI combined. OI can usually be diagnosed or excluded by a combination of clinical and radiographic findings prior to completion of genetic testing. Note that a small subset of children with OI do not have blue sclerae, abnormal dentition, or juvenile hearing loss.

- The pattern and extensiveness of fractures in OI tend to differ from child abuse.
- Fractures in OI more typically involve the shafts of long bones and result in deformity.
- Certain fracture patterns are highly specific for child abuse, including posterior rib fractures and the classic metaphyseal lesion. These were reviewed in Chapter 1 – Introduction to Musculoskeletal Imaging.

Treatment of OI is supportive and includes fracture casting and internal fixation. Bisphosphonate therapy can improve bone density and strength, reducing the frequency of fractures.

SCLEROSING BONE DYSPLASIAS

A large and heterogeneous group of conditions that have radiographically dense bones as a cardinal feature. Several dozen are listed in the dysplasia and syndrome textbooks. Many of these conditions result from a failure of osteoclasts to resorb bone during remodeling. Some are incidental and asymptomatic, whereas others have fragile bones that are easily fractured. Some of the most common or distinctive sclerosing bone dysplasias are discussed in this section.

Other potential causes of diffusely increased bone density include renal osteodystrophy, and, less commonly, myelofibrosis, hypothyroidism, chronic infections (including intrauterine infections, notably rubella and less typically syphilis), and heavy metal poisoning.

Osteopetrosis

A group of conditions characterized by diffusely very dense but brittle bones, caused by diminished osteoclast function. Genetic defects limit osteoclast ability to generate acid, which is essential to normal osteoclast function. Four clinically and radiographically distinct subtypes of osteopetrosis are recognized. Radiographic and clinical features reflect the variable impaired osteoclast dysfunction (Fig. 15.65).

Malignant Infantile Osteopetrosis

- Presents in neonates.
- Autosomal recessive.

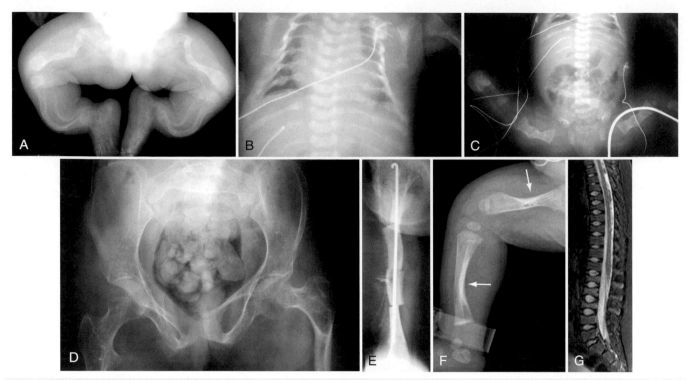

Fig. 15.64 Osteogenesis imperfecta. **(A)** Osteogenesis imperfecta type 3, with severe bowing. **(B)** In a newborn, with multiple rib fractures. **(C)** Lower body in the same patient as in B. There are numerous fractures, but the bones are not bowed. **(D)** Pelvis in an older child shows osteopenia, deformity caused by prior fractures, and gracile and deformed proximal femurs. **(E)** Surgical intervention for a bowed femur. Multiple osteotomies were performed with intramedullary pin fixation. **(F)** Osteogenesis imperfecta type 1. Neonate with deformity of the femur and tibia *(arrows)*. **(G)** Sagittal inversion recovery MR image shows multiple spinal compression fractures in a young child with osteogenesis imperfecta. (E courtesy of Stephanie Spottswood, MD.)

Box 15.6   Excessive Callus Formation

Corticosteroids (exogenous, Cushing)
Neuropathic joint
Congenital insensitivity to pain
Paralysis
Osteogenesis imperfecta
Renal osteodystrophy
Burn patients
Subperiosteal bleed in scurvy

- Absent corticomedullary differentiation (i.e., the cortical thickening is so severe that there is almost no medullary space).
- Bone-within-a-bone appearance of vertebra, pelvis, skull, and long bones.
- Normal marrow components are displaced and diminished.
- *Pancytopenia.*
- *Hepatosplenomegaly* is usually present.
- Treatment is stem cell transplantation; otherwise, it is fatal.

Autosomal Dominant Osteopetrosis (Albers-Schönberg disease)

- Variable severity.
- Mild forms may not be discovered until later in life owing to a fracture or mild anemia, or as an incidental finding on a chest radiograph.

- Radiographs of long bones:
  - Dense bones with markedly thickened cortices. Corticomedullary differentiation is preserved, in contrast with the infantile form.
  - Broad, dense metaphyseal bands or a bone-within-a-bone appearance on radiographs. Note: The radiographic finding of 'bone within a bone' is not specific to osteopetrosis and may be seen as a transient normal finding during periods of rapid growth, especially in very young children (Fig. 15.66).
  - Wide metaphyses/undertubulation.
  - Long bone fractures tend to be transverse, as with many pathologic fractures.
- Radiographs of the spine:
  - Scoliosis.
  - 'Sandwich' appearance of vertebral bodies on radiographs with dense endplates with prominent posterior vascular notches.
- Additional features:
  - Failure to remodel around cranial foramina during growth causes stenosis with blindness and hearing loss in the more severe forms.
  - Dental dysplasia and infections are frequent.

Intermediate Recessive Osteopetrosis

- Presents in childhood.
- Autosomal recessive.
- Pancytopenia.

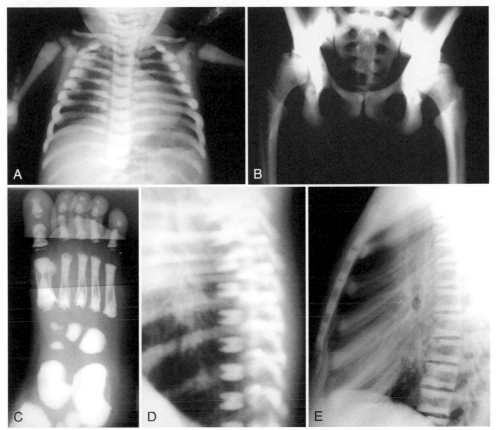

Fig. 15.65 Osteopetrosis. **(A)** Infantile-type osteopetrosis. The bones are diffusely dense, and the medullary space is obliterated. **(B)** Adult-type osteopetrosis. The bones are dense with thick cortices, but the medullary space is not obliterated. **(C)** 'Bone within a bone' within the metatarsals, with diffusely dense bones. **(D)** 'Sandwich vertebrae' in a young child. The vertebral body end plates are very dense. **(E)** Sandwich vertebrae in an adult.

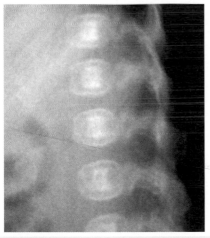

Fig. 15.66 'Bone within a bone' of thoracic and lumbar vertebral bodies as a normal finding in a former premature infant. Nutritional and metabolic factors associated with prematurity often lead to this appearance, which will eventually remodel to a normal appearance.

- Clinical and radiographic features intermediate between the infantile and adult types.
- Rare.

Osteopetrosis Associated With Renal Tubular Acidosis

- Cerebral calcifications, frequent intellectual disability.
- Lymphedema.
- Immune deficiency.

Pyknodysostosis (Pycnodysostosis)

- Rare short-limbed dwarfism (Fig. 15.67).
- Diffuse osteosclerosis.
- Long bones resemble osteopetrosis. Frequent transverse fractures.
- Skull: Wormian bones (intrasutural ossicles; see Box 15.3), preservation of the anterior fontanelle into adulthood.
- Acroosteolysis and sclerosis of distal phalanges and occasionally fragmentation of the distal phalanges.
- Mandible angle is increased, almost straight.
- Scoliosis.
- The distal clavicles may be resorbed (see Box 15.4).
- Rare. Autosomal recessive.
- The French painter Toulouse-Lautrec is believed to have had pyknodysostosis. The condition is sometimes named after him.

Melorheostosis

- Rare condition with distinctive radiographic findings.
- Classic appearance: dense bone deposited along the cortex of otherwise normal bones, usually along one side of a single extremity, in an irregular, elongated, wavy pattern that is likened to dripping candle wax (Fig. 15.68). However, many cases have a different appearance, notably more localized ossification or streaky increased bone density resembling osteopathia striata.

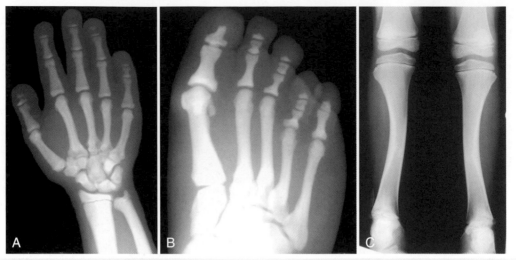

Fig. 15.67 Pyknodysostosis. **(A)** Hand. **(B)** Foot. **(C)** Legs. Note the diffuse osteosclerosis; short, tapered distal phalanges with acro-osteolysis; and mild bowing deformity of the tibias caused by prior insufficiency fractures.

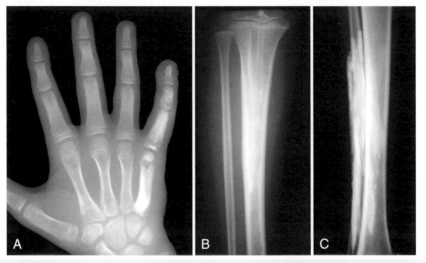

Fig. 15.68 Melorheostosis. **(A)** Hand. **(B** and **C)** Tibias (all different patients). Note the dense new bone formation in a pattern similar to 'candle wax dripping' of the fifth ray of the hand in A and the tibias in B and C.

- The distribution tends to follow a *sclerotome* (i.e., a portion of the skeleton innervated by a single spinal nerve).
- The added bone is usually periosteal but may be endosteal. It is histologically similar to cortical (compact) bone.
- Caused by a somatic mutation, not heritable.
- Although life expectancy is not shortened in patients with melorheostosis, significant morbidity can occur, especially when the condition presents in childhood.
- Clinical features include pain, progressive contractures with reduced joint mobility, and overlying skin changes (erythema, tense, shiny).
- Severe cases may simulate arthrogryposis multiplex. Premature physeal closure can occur in an affected limb, resulting in growth disturbance and limb-length discrepancy. Orthopedic intervention may be required to manage these complications.

Osteopoikilosis

- Multiple bone islands clustered around joints (Fig. 15.69).

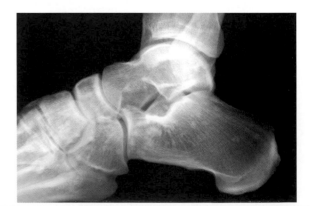

Fig. 15.69 Osteopoikilosis. Multiple bone islands are centered on the joints.

- The number of bone islands may increase during childhood but tends to stabilize after skeletal maturity is reached.

- Autosomal dominant.
- One in four patients also have Buschke–Ollendorff syndrome.
    - Autosomal dominant syndrome with numerous small subcutaneous connective-tissue nevi.
    - Melorrheostosis may also occur in this syndrome.
- How to distinguish osteopoikilosis from multiple blastic metastases:
    - The individual 'lesions' of osteopoikilosis are bone islands, which have characteristic findings of uniform density, continuity with the surrounding bony trabeculae, and orientation parallel to the alignment of the surrounding bony trabeculae. Osteopoikilosis bone islands all look alike.
    - Osteopoikilosis bone islands are most numerous in the epiphyses, whereas metastases are uncommon in epiphyses, as they more often occur in red marrow.
    - Bone islands tend to have higher CT attenuation than blastic metastases.

Osteopathia Striata (*Voorhoeve Disease*)

- Uniform, dense, linear striations in the metaphyses of the long bones, 2–3mm wide.
    - The striations are oriented parallel to the long axis of the long bones (Fig. 15.70).
- If the striations occur in the ilium, they radiate from the acetabulum in a 'sunburst' pattern.
- Clinically benign.

Mixed Sclerosing Bone dysplasia

Osteopathia striata, melorheostosis, and/or osteopoikilosis rarely occur simultaneously in some patients, for example in Buschke–Ollendorff syndrome as noted earlier.

OSTEO-ONYCHODYSPLASIA (*NAIL-PATELLA SYNDROME, FONG SYNDROME*)

- Rare autosomal dominant condition with multiple skeletal abnormalities (Fig. 15.71).

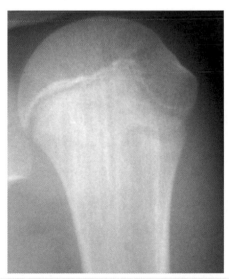

Fig. 15.70 Osteopathia striata. Note the longitudinally oriented dense striations in the metaphysis of the proximal humerus.

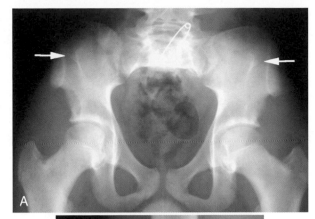

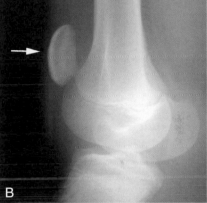

Fig. 15.71 Osteo-onychodysplasia (Fong syndrome). **(A)** Pelvis shows characteristic laterally oriented posterior iliac horns *(arrows)*. **(B)** Lateral knee radiograph shows hypoplastic patella *(arrow)*.

- The most distinctive feature is posterior iliac horns, a pathognomonic finding that is present in most cases.
- The knees are dysplastic with absent or hypoplastic patellae, hypoplastic lateral femoral condyles, and associated valgus alignment (genu valgum).
- The elbows also are dysplastic, with a hypoplastic capitellum and associated radial head dislocation.
- The fifth metacarpals may be short.
- Clinical features include dysplastic fingernails, especially of the thumb and index fingers, clinodactyly (curvature of a finger in the coronal plane, typically the fifth finger with valgus), and renal disease.

Radial Dysplasias

Congenital absence, partial aplasia, or hypoplasia of the radius occurs in association with numerous syndromes and as part of the VACTERL association (**v**ertebral, **a**norectal, **c**ardiac, **t**rache**o**esophageal **f**istula, **r**enal, and **l**imb anomalies).

MADELUNG DEFORMITY (FIG. 15.72)

- Abnormal growth of the distal radius results in bowing that orients the distal radius in a volar and ulnar direction.
- Radius is shortened, resulting in ulnar positive variance.
- The distal ulna may be dorsally dislocated.
- Associations:
    - Trauma (female gymnasts) most common.

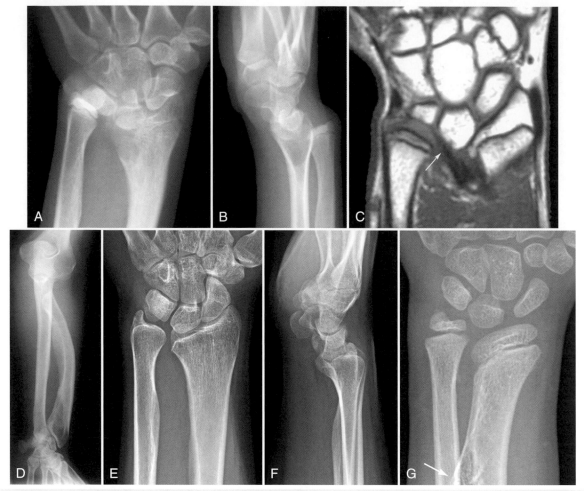

Fig. 15.72 Madelung deformity. AP **(A)** and lateral **(B)** radiographs in a child with Madelung deformity show short radius, with more severe shortening medially, wide distal radioulnar joint, and dorsal subluxation of the distal ulna. **(C)** Coronal T1-weighted MR image. Note the elongated low-signal triangular fibrocartilage *(arrow)*, a common finding. **(D)** Radiograph of the forearm in a young adult with dyschondrosteosis demonstrates the basic deformity in Madelung deformity: dorsolateral bowing of the radius caused by deficient growth at the distal volar medial radius. **(E–G)** Mimics. **(E** and **F)** Distal radius deformity resembling Madelung deformity caused by a childhood growth plate injury. PA view **(E)** resembles a true Madelung deformity, but lateral view **(F)** does not show the classic volar orientation of the distal radius or distal radioulnar joint dislocation. **(G)** Distal radius deformity in a child with multiple hereditary osteochondromas. Note the partially seen sessile osteochondroma in the medial radial shaft *(arrow)*.

- Multiple osteochondromas or enchondromas.
- Turner syndrome.
- Can be familial (autosomal dominant).
- As part of the rare skeletal dysplasia *dyschondrosteosis* (Léri–Weill disease).

HOLT–ORAM SYNDROME

- Association of congenital heart disease (classically atrial septal defect) and thumb or radius abnormalities.
- The classic osseous finding is triphalangeal thumbs (Fig. 15.72A), but a spectrum of thumb abnormalities can occur, ranging from absence to hypoplasia to bifid.
- The radius may be absent, hypoplastic, or normal.
- Inheritance is autosomal dominant.

TAR SYNDROME (THROMBOCYTOPENIA–ABSENT RADIUS)

- Association of congenital radial anomalies and severe thrombocytopenia.

- The classic skeletal findings are absence of the radius and shortening of the ulna with the hand oriented at a 90-degree angle to the forearm (Fig. 15.73B).
- The radii are often absent bilaterally, but the thumbs are typically present.
- Rare.

RADIAL CLUBHAND

- Radiologically similar to the deformity in the TAR syndrome, but the term usually also implies that the thumb and scaphoid are also absent (Fig. 15.73C).

FANCONI ANEMIA

- Association of brown pigmentation of the skin and late childhood pancytopenia. Congenital radial ray and thumb anomalies are present in about half of the cases, classically a hypoplastic thumb.
- A variety of congenital renal anomalies may occur as well.

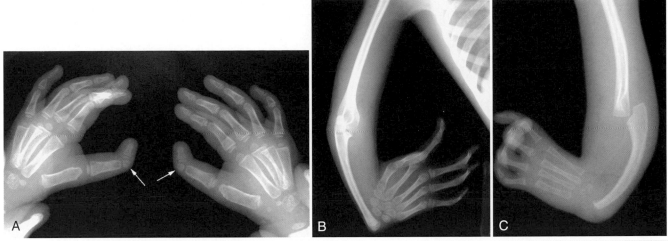

Fig. 15.73 Radial ray dysplasias. **(A)** Holt–Oram syndrome. Note the triphalangeal thumbs *(arrows).* **(B)** TAR syndrome (thrombocytopenia–absent radius). The radius is absent, but the thumb and scaphoid are present. **(C)** Radial clubhand. In contrast with B, the thumb is absent.

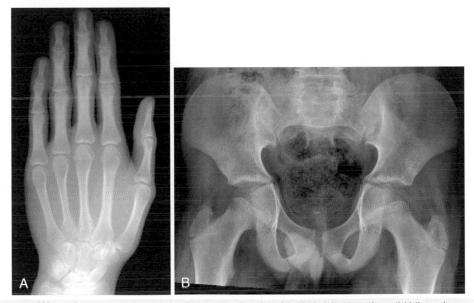

Fig. 15.74 Marfan syndrome. **(A)** Hand. Note the long, slender fingers (arachnodactyly). **(B)** Pelvis. Note the mild bilateral protrusio acetabuli.

Connective-Tissue Disorders

MARFAN SYNDROME

- Autosomal dominant connective-tissue disorder with high penetrance but variable expression.
- A genetic defect results in a collagen abnormality. Most cases are inherited; some occur as spontaneous mutations.
- Patients with Marfan syndrome are tall and have disproportionate lengthening of the distal aspects of the extremities (*arachnodactyly,* Fig. 15.74A).
- Skeletal findings include kyphoscoliosis, joint hypermobility, early osteoarthritis, protrusio acetabuli (Fig. 15.74B), spondylolysis of L5, posterior scalloping of the vertebral bodies caused by dural ectasia (especially prominent at L5 and S1 compared with normal), and pectus excavatum. Bone mineral density is normal.

- Important extraosseous complications include ocular lens dislocation, retinal detachment, and cystic medial degeneration of the proximal ascending aorta and pulmonary artery. The cardiovascular lesions may lead to aortic dissection or rupture, or to aortic or pulmonic valve insufficiency.

HOMOCYSTINURIA

- Autosomal recessive inborn error of metabolism—cystathionine synthetase deficiency.
- Accumulation of homocysteine in the serum and urine.
- Causes defective collagen synthesis by an unknown mechanism.
- Morphologically and radiographically similar to Marfan syndrome.
  - Both conditions are associated with scoliosis, posterior vertebral body scalloping, pectus excavatum, and

arachnodactyly (uniformly present in Marfan syndrome, variably present in homocystinuria).

- Differences between homocystinuria and Marfan:
  - Homocystinuria causes osteopenia, with resultant vertebral compression fractures.
  - The lens dislocations of Marfan syndrome and homocystinuria tend to occur in different directions.
  - Patients with homocystinuria also have intellectual disability, seizures and joint contractures, which are not usual features of Marfan syndrome.

EHLERS–DANLOS SYNDROME

A spectrum of mostly autosomal dominant conditions, each caused by a defect in collagen synthesis that have the following in common:

- Exceptionally lax skin that is easily injured and heals poorly.
- Musculoskeletal features overlap with those seen in Marfan syndrome and homocystinuria.
- Hypermobile joints that are prone to contractures in old age.
- Kyphoscoliosis, posterior vertebral scalloping, arachnodactyly, and spondylolysis are seen, as well as marked joint hypermobility leading to dislocations, flat feet, and early osteoarthritis.
- In some forms, the great vessels are prone to aneurysm, dissection, and tortuosity. Angiography is dangerous owing to the fragility of the vessels.
- Easy bleeding because of fragile blood vessels.
  - Hemarthroses may occur after minimal trauma.
  - Subcutaneous bleeding and fat necrosis from minimal trauma, resulting in phlebolith-like subcutaneous calcifications, especially in the forearms and shins.
  - The presence of such calcifications combined with a history of skin hyperelasticity helps to make the diagnosis of Ehlers–Danlos syndrome.

Gigantism and Hypoplasia

- Abnormalities of size and shape may affect only a small portion of the body (*focal gigantism*), an entire extremity (*macromelia*), or half of the body (*hemihypertrophy*).
- Only one or two organ systems may be affected (e.g., the lymphatics or the blood vessels), or every tissue may be involved.
- Chronically increased blood flow, regardless of the cause, can cause accelerated growth at adjacent physes. Potential causes include vascular malformation, chronic synovial inflammation (as in juvenile idiopathic arthritis), or hemophilia.
- *Hemihypertrophy* is overgrowth of half (or nearly half) of the body. A variety of syndromes and malignancies are associated with hemihypertrophy, most notably Beckwith–Wiedemann syndrome and Wilms tumor.
- *Hemiatrophy* is usually an acquired condition caused by asymmetric neurologic and neuromuscular conditions that cause severe unilateral muscle atrophy.
- *Hemihypotrophy* may be considered congenital hemiatrophy. This rare condition is associated with intrauterine growth retardation and chromosomal abnormalities.

- A leg-length discrepancy resulting from any of these conditions may require orthopedic intervention.

MACRODYSTROPHIA LIPOMATOSA

- Rare and distinctive form of localized gigantism of unknown cause.
- Overgrowth of adipose and periosteal osteoblasts.
- Fingers and toes are most frequently involved with this condition.
- Discussed further in Chapter 12 (Fig. 12.17).

KLIPPEL–TRÉNAUNAY SYNDROME (KLIPPEL–TRÉNAUNAY–WEBER SYNDROME)

- Macromelia associated with a cutaneous capillary hemangioma (port-wine stain, nevus flameous) and dilated and tortuous superficial veins.
- A lower extremity is the usual site of involvement (Fig. 12.12 and Fig. 15.75).
- The limb overgrowth becomes most apparent during the growth spurt at puberty.
- It is speculated that the abnormalities are caused by increased flow through a persistent fetal superficial vascular system that failed to regress during gestation.
- The normal deep venous system of the affected extremity is not present.
- The resulting vascular abnormalities cause chronically increased blood flow that may contribute to the limb overgrowth.

Chromosomal Abnormalities

TRISOMY 21 (*DOWN SYNDROME*)

- Cervical spine anomalies (Fig. 15.76).
  - Atlantoaxial subluxation in 10–20% of cases.
  - The posterior arch of C1 is often hypoplastic.
- 11 rib pairs.
- Two manubrial ossification centers rather than the usual single ossification center.

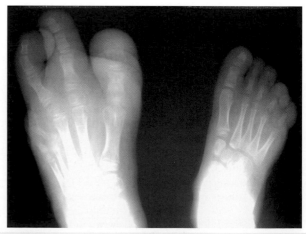

Fig. 15.75 Klippel–Trénaunay–Weber syndrome. In addition to the foot overgrowth evident on this image, most of the right lower extremity was overgrown (not shown).

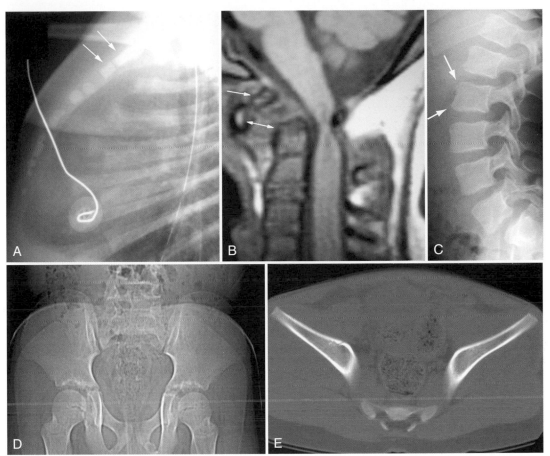

Fig. 15.76 Trisomy 21. **(A)** Lateral sternum shows multiple ossification centers, including two manubrial ossification centers *(arrows)*. **(B)** Atlantoaxial subluxation. Sagittal T1-weighted MR image obtained with voluntary neck flexion shows severe cord compression. Note the ununited ossiculum terminale *(arrow)* and the wide interval between the anterior arch of C1 and C2 *(double arrow)*. Atlantoaxial instability is present in 10–20% of children with trisomy 21. **(C)** Lateral lumbar spine shows rounded anterior vertebral bodies *(arrows)*. **(D and E)** Pelvis. CT scout **(D)** and axial image **(E)** show low acetabular angles, coronal plane orientation of the iliac wings with rounded appearance on the frontal view, and inferior tapering of the ischia.

- Short tubular bones of the hands and fingers with fifth-finger clinodactyly (abnormal angulation of a finger in the coronal plane) because of a short and broad fifth-finger middle phalanx.
- Flared iliac wings with nearly horizontal acetabular roofs.
- Hip dysplasia.
- Patellar dislocations.
- Variety of foot anomalies.

TRISOMY 18

- Abnormalities of multiple organ systems, notably severe congenital heart disease.
- Characteristic skeletal manifestations that may be detected on prenatal US:
  - 'Rocker-bottom feet'.
  - Clenched hand with an adducted thumb and a short first metacarpal.

TURNER SYNDROME

- 45X0, deletion of one X chromosome.
- Short stature, webbed neck, and abnormalities of many organ systems, including congenital heart disease, horseshoe kidney, and streak ovaries.

- Aortic root dilation and dissection is an uncommon but potentially catastrophic association.
- Skeletal findings.
  - Short fourth metacarpals (a finding that is also seen in pseudohypoparathyroidism and pseudopseudo-hypoparathyroidism).
  - Depression of the medial tibial plateau.
  - Tarsal coalitions.
  - Diffuse osteopenia.
  - Madelung deformity (discussed earlier).

Mucopolysaccharidoses

Mucopolysaccharidoses (MPSs) are a group of conditions caused by inborn errors of mucopolysaccharide metabolism that result in accumulation of mucopolysaccharides (glycosaminoglycans) in the bone marrow, brain, liver, lens, and other sites. The MPSs are distinguished by differences in clinical manifestations, biochemistry, and inheritance.

Short stature is invariably present in all forms.

They share a set of radiographic features termed *dysostosis multiplex* (Fig. 15.77). Not all features of dysostosis

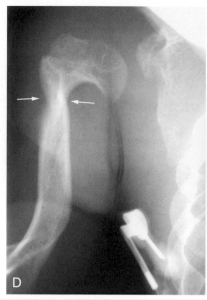
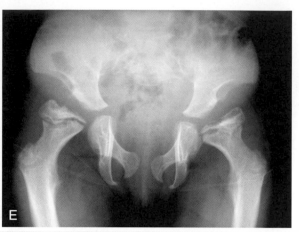

Fig. 15.77 Dysostosis multiplex. **(A)** Lateral thoracic and lumbar spine and ribs (mucopolysaccharidosis [MPS] IV). Note the broad 'oarlike' ribs *(short arrows)* and the thoracolumbar kyphosis with small inferior beaks *(long arrows)*. **(B)** Lateral thoracolumbar spine (MPS IH). The vertebral bodies are shaped differently than in MPS IV **(A)** but also have a short AP size and an inferior beak in a thoracolumbar junction vertebral body *(arrow)*. **(C)** Chest (MPS IV). Note the wide ribs, with focal constrictions at the costovertebral junctions *(arrowheads)*. **(D)** Humerus (MPS IV). The long bones are generally expanded and may be bowed. Note the characteristic focal constriction in the proximal diaphysis *(arrows)*. **(E)** Pelvis (MPS IH). The iliac wings are narrowed inferiorly. The femoral heads are flat, and the hips are dysplastic.

multiplex are found in each type of MPS, but each type of MPS exhibits several of these features:

- Expanded bones (packed with accumulated mucopolysaccharides).
  - Long bones are short with wide metaphyses and diaphyses.
  - Wide, oar-shaped ribs with focal narrowing at the costovertebral junction.
- Spine: platyspondyly (flat vertebral bodies) with an anterior beak or spur.
- Thoracolumbar focal kyphosis (gibbous deformity).
- Epiphyseal dysplasia and delayed ossification (especially in Morquio).
- Focal narrowing of the proximal humeral diaphysis.
- Fanlike or 'bullet-shaped' metacarpals.
- Wide iliac wings, narrow inferior iliac bones.

The following is a brief overview of four of the most common MPSs. Several additional forms are recognized.

MORQUIO SYNDROME (MPS IV)

- Only MPS with normal intelligence.
- Accumulates keratan sulfate, which interferes with enchondral ossification and bone formation.
- Epiphyseal dysplasia is a dominant finding, with delayed ossification of the epiphyses and fragmented epiphyses.
- Dens hypoplasia with atlantoaxial instability, expansion of C2, and displacement of the posterior arch of C1 into the foramen magnum that can cause spinal cord compression. Surgical stabilization may be required.
- The vertebral bodies have midanterior beaking. Platyspondyly (flat vertebral bodies) can be prominent.

HURLER SYNDROME (MPS 1H)

- Most severe MPS.
- Accumulates dermatan sulfate and heparan sulfate. These are not as toxic to enchondral ossification, so epiphyseal findings are mild, in contrast with Morquio.
- Early and severe appearance of other findings of dysostosis multiplex beginning by about 1 year of age.
- Anterior vertebral body beaks at the *inferior* endplates around the focal thoracolumbar gibbous deformity.
- J-shaped sella turcica.
- C1-C2 instability in some patients.

HUNTER SYNDROME (MPS II)

- X-linked recessive enzyme defect (males only).
- As with Hurler accumulates of dermatan sulfate and heparan sulfate, but clinically less severe.
- Radiography:
  - Dysostosis multiplex (see previous text), with relative sparing of epiphyses.
  - Macrocranium with a J-shaped sella turcica.
  - Upper cervical instability in a minority.

SANFILLIPO SYNDROME (MPS III)

Autosomal recessive enzyme defect leads to accumulation of heparan sulfate.

Additional forms of MPS are recognized.

Other storage diseases, such as the *mucolipidoses* and *Gaucher disease*, also can have some features of dysostosis multiplex. As with the MPSs, the clinical and radiographic changes caused by these conditions are not present at birth but rather take years to develop as the abnormal metabolites accumulate. As with the MPSs, diagnosis of these conditions is based primarily on clinical and laboratory findings.

Gaucher Disease

- The most common lysosomal storage disease.
- Three types, all autosomal recessive inborn errors of metabolism that result in accumulation of lipid-laden macrophages called Gaucher cells in the reticuloendothelial system, including the marrow.
- The Gaucher cells enlarge over time and fill the marrow space, replacing normal marrow elements and increasing intramedullary pressure, resulting in intramedullary venous occlusion and osteonecrosis.
- The most common form develops in later childhood or young adulthood and is associated with a normal life span. This form of Gaucher disease most often occurs in Ashkenazi Jews and can usually be managed successfully with enzyme replacement therapy.
- Radiographic findings:
  - Hepatosplenomegaly.
  - Expansion of the distal femur with Erlenmeyer flask deformity (Fig. 15.78, Box 13.4). This expansion is caused by marrow infiltration and is present in 40–50% of patients.
  - The marrow replacement causes generalized osteoporosis with increased risk of fracture and osteomyelitis.
  - Bone infarction with focal sclerosis and occasional bone-within-bone appearance or focal cyst-like lucent lesions.

- The vertebral endplates may fracture in an H-shaped pattern, as is seen in sickle cell disease, related to osteonecrosis.
- Femoral head osteonecrosis is common.
- Any of these abnormalities, seen in conjunction with hepatosplenomegaly, should suggest the diagnosis of Gaucher disease.
- MRI findings:
  - Low T1 and T2 signal in the infiltrated marrow. The infiltration may be patchy or diffuse.
  - Severe cases may show transcortical extension of the Gaucher cell infiltration.
  - Osteonecrosis is frequent, especially in the femoral head.
  - MRI can be used to monitor response to enzyme replacement therapy. The marrow, liver, and spleen of successfully treated patients show a dramatic response, attaining a near-normal appearance.

Additional Conditions

NEUROFIBROMATOSIS (NF1, VON RECKLINGHAUSEN DISEASE)

- Skeletal involvement is frequent (Fig. 15.79).
- Mesodermal dysplasia results in weak bones that are prone to remodeling into abnormal shapes.
- Extrinsic compression by a neurofibroma may also cause bone deformity.
- Scoliosis (see Fig. 15.13):
  - May resemble routine idiopathic scoliosis.
  - Dystrophic form: short segment (4–6 vertebrae), abrupt thoracic kyphoscoliosis. May become unstable

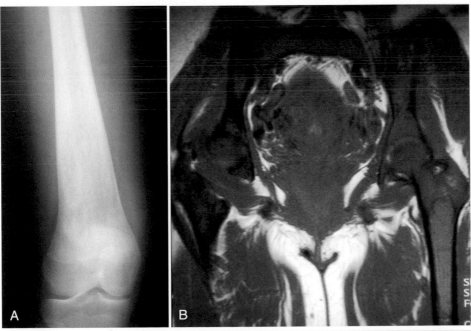

Fig. 15.78 Gaucher disease. **(A)** AP radiograph of the femur in an 18-year-old woman with Gaucher disease shows widening of the distal femur metadiaphysis (Erlenmeyer flask deformity) because of marrow packing with Gaucher cells, which are reticuloendothelial cells filled with the abnormal metabolites of Gaucher disease (glucocerebrosides). Note the cortical thinning, also a typical finding. **(B)** Coronal T1-weighted MR image in a different patient shows diffuse marrow low signal, also because of marrow packing. MRI is so sensitive to the marrow disease burden that it can be used to guide enzyme replacement therapy. Successful therapy with enzyme replacement will return the marrow signal to normal or near-normal.

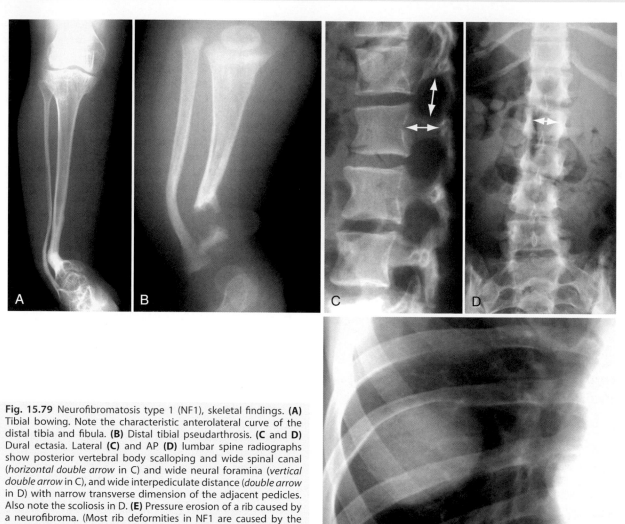

Fig. 15.79 Neurofibromatosis type 1 (NF1), skeletal findings. **(A)** Tibial bowing. Note the characteristic anterolateral curve of the distal tibia and fibula. **(B)** Distal tibial pseudarthrosis. **(C** and **D)** Dural ectasia. Lateral **(C)** and AP **(D)** lumbar spine radiographs show posterior vertebral body scalloping and wide spinal canal (*horizontal double arrow* in C) and wide neural foramina (*vertical double arrow* in C), and wide interpediculate distance (*double arrow* in D) with narrow transverse dimension of the adjacent pedicles. Also note the scoliosis in D. **(E)** Pressure erosion of a rib caused by a neurofibroma. (Most rib deformities in NF1 are caused by the skeletal dysplasia, not pressure erosion.) See also Fig. 15.13.

with pseudoarthrosis. Surgical stabilization can be difficult, requiring reoperation.

- Dural ectasia: enlarged neural foramina and posterior vertebral body scalloping.
- Cranial osseous abnormalities include hypoplastic or absent cranial bones (sphenoid wing, posterosuperior orbital wall, mastoid), macrocranium, and enlarged cranial neural foramina caused by neurofibromas.
- Anterior distal tibial bowing, often with pseudarthrosis that may develop characteristic tapered margins, may be seen at birth or develop during childhood. These pseudarthroses are frequently resistant to healing despite orthopedic fixation, and a short leg can result.
- Multiple nonossifying fibromas also may be seen.
  - A finding of multiple nonossifying fibromas in any patient should suggest the diagnosis of neurofibromatosis.
- Twisted, narrow, irregular 'ribbon ribs' reflects the mesodermal dysplasia more frequently than extrinsic compression from adjacent neurofibromas.
- The plexiform neurofibromas found in NF1 often reveal a 'target sign' appearance on T2-weighted MRI, with low signal intensity centrally and high signal intensity peripherally.

Skeletal manifestations are prominent in phakomatoses other than NF1.

- The findings of Klippel–Trénaunay–Weber syndrome are discussed in this chapter in the review of focal gigantism (Fig. 15.75) and in Chapter 12 – Soft Tissue Tumors.
- *Tuberous sclerosis* causes patchy bone sclerosis and cystlike changes in the bones of the hands and feet (Fig. 15.80). These bone findings are not clinically significant.
- *Gorlin syndrome* (basal cell nevus syndrome) of basal cell carcinomas and palmar skin pits also causes mandible cysts, patchy and bone-island–like bone sclerosis, and scoliosis.

ARTHROGRYPOSIS (ARTHROGRYPOSIS MULTIPLEX CONGENITA)

- Rare, sporadic condition characterized by severe joint abnormalities that include fixed flexion deformities, dislocations, radiographically dense joint capsules, long scoliosis (neuromuscular pattern), muscle and soft tissue atrophy, and osteoporotic bones (from disuse) that are prone to insufficiency fracture (Fig. 15.81).
- Clubfeet and clubhands may be present.

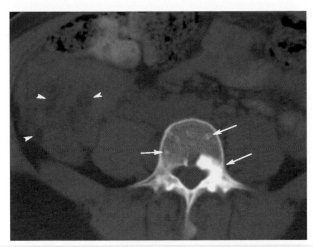

Fig. 15.80 Tuberous sclerosis. Unenhanced axial CT image shows sclerotic regions in the lumbar spine *(arrows)*. Numerous fat attenuation angiomyolipomas can be seen in the lower pole of the enlarged right kidney *(arrowheads)*.

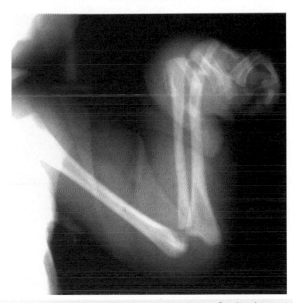

Fig. 15.81 Arthrogryposis. The upper extremity was fixed in this position.

- Soft tissue webs may fix joints in flexion.
- The lower extremities are almost always involved, particularly the distal limbs; the upper extremities may be involved.
- Intelligence is normal.
- The cause is unknown. There may be many different causes. Lack of fetal motion in utero is a likely cause. Some cases are associated with oligohydramnios and associated restricted fetal movement.

AMNIOTIC BAND SYNDROME

- Congenital amputations and soft tissue defects caused by entanglement of the fetus by aberrant bands of amniotic membrane that traverse the gestational sac.
- Abnormalities range from minimal amputations or focal syndactyly to major cranial or body wall defects (Fig. 15.82).

- Focal soft tissue constrictions may occur that may result in chronic lymphedema. Surgery is often required to minimize loss of function and to improve appearance.

FIBROMATOSIS COLLI

- Nonneoplastic, masslike, focal or diffuse enlargement of a sternocleidomastoid muscle in an infant (Fig. 15.83).
- Probably results from birth injury to the sternocleidomastoid muscle.
- Associated with forceps delivery.
- The affected sternocleidomastoid muscle often shortens, which may result in torticollis.
- Imaging studies reveal focal, often fusiform enlargement of the affected muscle but are especially useful in excluding another cause of a neck mass, such as adenopathy, neoplasm, branchial cleft cyst, or cystic hygroma.
- Typically presents at about 2 weeks of age and may enlarge before spontaneously resolving over a period of months.
- Most cases respond to physical therapy with passive stretching of the shortened sternocleidomastoid muscle. Surgery is rarely required for refractory torticollis.

CEREBRAL PALSY

- Brain injury due to prematurity, anoxia, trauma, or prenatal insult such as infection.
- 1 5:1000.
- Wide spectrum of clinical features.
- Contractures.
- Scoliosis: long 'C'-shaped curve.
  - May be convex left and M>F, in contrast with idiopathic scoliosis.
  - Harder to manage than routine idiopathic scoliosis due to earlier onset, faster progression, curve rigidity, delayed skeletal maturation in CP, pelvic tilt due to muscle imbalance, and patient fragility.
  - Larger curves and curves in less mobile children are most likely to progress.
- Hips: coxa valga, hip dysplasia, dislocation (Fig. 15.42).
- Various foot abnormalities: hindfoot equinus most common, also vertical talus, others.

CAFFEY DISEASE (*INFANTILE CORTICAL HYPEROSTOSIS*)

- Exuberant periosteal new bone in infants, especially around the mandible (Fig. 15.84).
- Elevated inflammatory markers (ESR, CRP) and alkaline phosphatase (high bone turnover).
- Soft tissue swelling, irritability.
- Rare.
- Autosomal dominant, variable penetrance.
- Self-limited.
- May cause deformities, including synostosis of adjacent affected ribs or long bones.
- Rare prenatal form is lethal.

CONGENITAL SYPHILIS

- Maternal–fetal transmission.
- Targets include the CNS, liver, and bones.

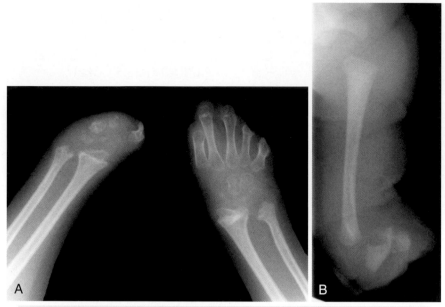

Fig. 15.82 (A and B) Amniotic band syndrome. Note the amputations of the extremities.

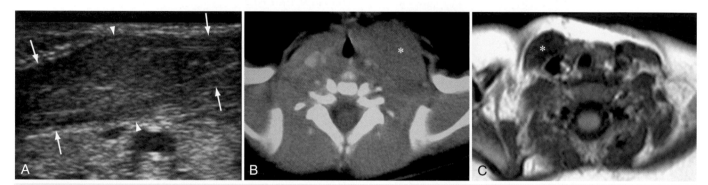

Fig. 15.83 Fibromatosis colli in three different infants. **(A)** Longitudinal ultrasound image shows typical focal fusiform enlargement of the sternocleido-mastoid muscle belly (between *arrowheads*), compared with the normal muscle above and below (between *arrows*). Axial CT **(B)** and axial T1-weighted MR **(C)** images in different infants show unilateral enlargement of a sternocleidomastoid muscle (*asterisk*). Except for the enlargement, the affected muscle resembles normal muscle on all three modalities. (B and C courtesy of Fred Laine, MD.)

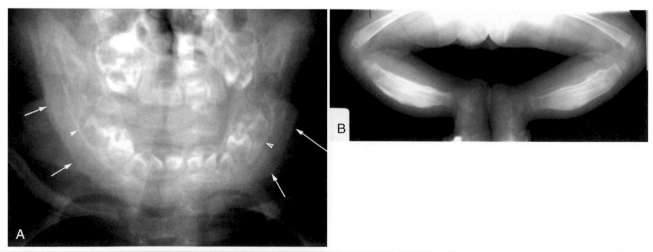

Fig. 15.84 Caffey disease (infantile cortical hyperostosis). **(A)** Prominent expansion of the mandible because of periosteal new bone formation *(arrows)*. Note the underlying mandible cortex *(arrowheads)*. **(B)** Legs show bilateral prominent periosteal new bone formation in the tibias. (B courtesy of L. Das Narla, MD.)

- Early versus late presentation.
- Early: present within the first 2 years of life.
  - Periosteal new bone formation (*periostitis*) on diaphyses, often also metaphyses (see list of causes of periosteal new bone formation in children in the Gamuts section of Chapter 11 – Bone Tumors and Fig. 14.60A).
  - Heterogeneous bone density related to osteomyelitis and healing.
  - Physis widened and irregular.
  - *Wimberger sign*: multifocal, bilateral metaphyseal lysis. Highly specific for congenital syphilis. (Not to be confused with *Wimberger ring*, which is a sharply defined sclerotic ring around an osteopenic epiphysis seen in scurvy.)
- Late: children and adolescents.
  - As with early presentation, periosteal new bone formation and mixed bone density.
  - Focal lytic lesions due to osteomyelitis.
- Bone softening can lead to bone deformity in weight-bearing bones. In very severe cases, bone deformity is detected on prenatal US.
  - Anterior tibial bowing: '*saber shins*'.
  - Pathologic fractures.

Appendix: Infant Hip Ultrasonography for DDH: Technique

GENERALIZATIONS

This section briefly reviews how to obtain ultrasonography (US) images of the infant hip. The pathophysiology and interpretation of US findings of development dysplasia of the hip were reviewed earlier in this chapter.

The US technique emphasized here is based on a popular and widely accepted approach to infant hip US. It must be emphasized that this is not the only way to reliably detect and follow developmental dysplasia of the hip. Many experienced ultrasonographers have developed slightly or even widely different approaches that have stood the test of time. For example, the Graf system (Table Appendix 15.1) of careful measurements of static coronal images is popular in many centers, at least as part of a hybrid approach. If your institution does it differently, this description is not intended as a criticism of your technique.

Scans are easiest to obtain when the child is relaxed and quiet. The temperature and lighting should be comfortable for an infant, and the gel should be warmed. Feeding the child before or during the examination helps the child to relax. Glucose water will suffice if no milk or formula is available. Enlist the parent's help in feeding, calming, and positioning the baby. Beware of male infants, because they will urinate on your shoes. An appropriately placed towel or washcloth can avoid this problem. Stress maneuvers are best left until the end of the examination, because this forceful handling may irritate the infant.

A high-frequency linear array transducer, at least 5 MHz, is used. Occasionally a wide array transducer is used to obtain the 'big picture' of a dislocated hip and can better show the relationship of the dislocated femoral head and acetabulum. If the child is in a cast placed to maintain reduction of a previously dislocated hip, the available window may be too small for anything other than a small footprint sector array transducer. Be creative.

If the child is in a Pavlik harness, do not remove it or perform stress maneuvers unless so instructed by the ordering orthopedic surgeon. The harness will not impede the examination.

A routine examination includes both hips. The examination is often easiest to perform from a lateral approach with the child in a decubitus or oblique decubitus position, scanning the upside hip. If using the Graf system, images are obtained with the hips extended. Otherwise, the hips may be flexed or extended.

Table Appendix 15.1   The Graf Classification of Infant Hip Dysplasia

Hip Type	Bony Roof*	Angle†	Alpha Angle (Degrees)	Beta Angle (Degrees)
Ia: Mature hip	Good	Sharp	≥60	<55
Ib: Transitional form	Good	Blunt	≤60	>55
IIa: Physiologically immature (<3 months of age)	Sufficient	Round	50–59	>55
IIb: Delayed ossification (>3 months of age)	Deficient	Round	50–59	>55
IIc: Critical range (any age, normal labrum)	Deficient	Round or flat	43–49	<77
IId: Subluxed hip	Severely def.	Round or flat	43–49	>77
IIIa: Dislocated hip (any age, no structural alteration of the acetabular roof)	Poor	Flat	<43	>77
IIIb: Dislocated hip (any age, with structural alteration of the acetabular roof)	Poor	Flat	<43	>77
IV: Severely dislocated hip (any age, with inverted labrum between femoral head and acetabulum)	Poor	Flat	<43	>77

* Bony roof, coverage of femoral head. Good is ≥50%.
† Junction of osseous ilium and osseous acetabular roof.
Modified from Graf R, Wilson B. *Sonography of the Infant Hip and Its Therapeutic Implications*. London: Chapman and Hall; 1995; and Laor T, Jarmillo D, Oestereich AE. Musculoskeletal system. In: Kirks DR, Griscom NT, eds. *Practical Pediatric Imaging*. 3rd ed. Philadelphia: Lippincott-Raven; 1998.

Landmarks

Major landmarks of hip US include the femoral head, triradiate cartilage, lateral ilium, and acetabular roof (Figs. 15.32 and 15.33).

The *cartilaginous femoral head* is round and hypoechoic and contains speckled internal echoes. Ossification of the femoral head begins as early as the third month as a central small, round hyperechoic focus with posterior acoustic shadowing (Figs. Appendix 15.1 and 15.2). Such ossification provides a convenient landmark for localizing the center of the femoral head. In younger infants, adjust the transducer position to maximize the diameter of the femoral head on each image. This technique guarantees that the center of the femoral head is in the image.

The hypoechoic *triradiate cartilage* is located anterior and superior to the center of the acetabulum. The goal is to have this landmark in the images. Placing the triradiate cartilage at the center of the images requires angling the transducer slightly forward from a slightly posterior approach. A few echoes medial to the triradiate cartilage assist in locating this landmark (see Fig. Appendix 15.1). On axial images the triradiate cartilage is located between the pubic bone anteriorly and the slightly longer ischium posteriorly.

The *lateral cortex of the ilium*, like the other ossified bones, is seen as a well-defined hyperechoic line with dense posterior acoustic shadowing. The lateral ilium is continuous with the osseous acetabular roof. The angle formed by the lateral ilium and the acetabular roof is the *alpha angle*, not to be confused with the alpha angle used in femoroacetabular impingement (Fig. 15.32).

The *acetabular labrum* and adjacent capsule form an echogenic triangle lateral to the acetabular roof (Fig. 15.32A).

Images

Scans are obtained in the coronal and transverse planes. The hips may be flexed or extended.

Optimal coronal images have the following features (see Fig. 15.32 and Fig. Appendix 15.1):

1. The lateral cortex of the ilium is displayed as a straight line parallel to the transducer.
2. The acetabular roof is clearly displayed. The alpha angle is formed by the lateral ilium and the acetabular roof (see Fig. 15.32).
3. The center of the femoral head is in the image.
4. The triradiate cartilage is in the image. The triradiate cartilage is so named because it includes portions of all three pelvic bones: the ilium, the ischium, and the pubis. It provides a landmark to enhance image reproducibility. The triradiate cartilage is located just anterior to the center of the acetabulum. Thus, in a normally aligned hip the femoral head is centered slightly posterior to the triradiate cartilage. Obtaining images with the femoral head centered over the triradiate cartilage requires moving the transducer slightly posteriorly and angling anteriorly.
5. The labrum is seen as an echogenic triangle lateral to the acetabular roof.

An image with these qualities is termed *the standard plane* in the Graf system and is the only image that this system requires.

Displaying the lateral ilium as a straight line parallel to the transducer is usually straightforward. If the lateral ilium has a concave contour, then the transducer is too far posterior (see Fig. Appendix 15.1). If the lateral ilium flares laterally toward the transducer, then the transducer is too far anterior (see Fig. Appendix 15.2). Angling the transducer slightly is often needed to fine-tune the image.

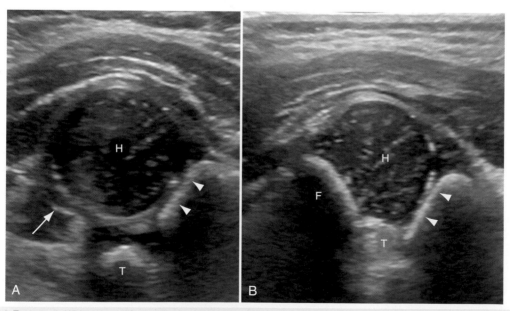

Fig. Appendix 15.1 Transverse US images, with anterior to the viewer's left, in two different 5-week-old girls. **(A)** Hip extended. **(B)** Hip flexed. Note the round femoral head (*H*), echogenic ischium cortex at the posterior acetabulum (*arrowheads*), pubis at the anterior acetabulum in A (*arrow*), and bright echoes (*T*) medial to the triradiate cartilage. The anterior acetabulum is obscured by the ossified proximal femur (*F*) in B. Maximize the size of the femoral head to make sure the scan is through the center of the head.

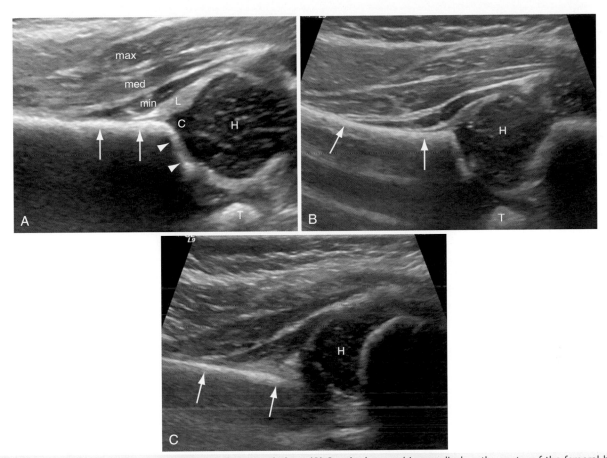

Fig. Appendix 15.2 Optimizing transducer position in the coronal plane. **(A)** Standard coronal image displays the center of the femoral head (*H*) achieved by maximizing the size of the head, triradiate cartilage (*T*), and lateral ilium (*long arrows*) displayed as a straight line. Note the normal straight or slightly concave contour of the osseous acetabular roof (*arrowheads*). Also note the hypoechoic cartilaginous acetabulum (*C*) and hyperechoic labrum (*L*) *max*, Gluteus maximus; *med*, gluteus medius; *min*, gluteus minimus. **(B)** Transducer anterior. This image is adequate but not optimal. The scan is aligned with the triradiate cartilage (*T*), but the femoral head (*H*) is not maximized in size and is not round in cross section, and the lateral ilium curves toward the transducer (*arrows*). **(C)** Transducer too far posterior. The lateral ilium has a straight contour (*arrows*), but the triradiate cartilage is not seen and the head is small. This image incorrectly simulates DDH.

Including both the center of the femoral head and the center of the triradiate cartilage in the image requires some dexterity. One approach is to first find the lateral ilium, then, while keeping the ilium in proper alignment, find the center of the femoral head. Next is the hard part: while keeping the ilium and femoral head in proper alignment, find the hypoechoic triradiate cartilage to complete the image. These maneuvers require sliding the transducer over the hip while constantly adjusting the angle. Slight rotation off of true coronal is often helpful.

Obtain the coronal image at least twice to document that the alpha angle is reproducible.

Transverse scans are obtained with and without posterior subluxing stress. The acetabulum is demarcated by the echogenic pubic bone anteriorly, the slightly longer, echogenic ischium posteriorly, and the hypoechoic triradiate cartilage between them. An optimal axial image in a normal hip will extend through both the center of the femoral head and the center of the triradiate cartilage. If the hip is flexed and the scan is obtained parallel to the femur, the ossified femoral shaft will obscure some of the pubis (see Fig. Appendix 15.1). The greater trochanter and sometimes the femoral shaft will be included on routine transverse views with the hip in flexion. Obtaining

axial scans with the hip flexed and extended also can be performed. A modified Barlow maneuver is performed with the hip flexed and adducted. Posterior force is applied to the femur, and the relationship of the femoral head and acetabulum is observed. A subluxable hip is displaced posteriorly and laterally by this maneuver. When performing this stress maneuver, you may find it helpful to hold the transducer between your thumb and index and middle fingers while placing your remaining fingers against the infant's sacrum. This allows force to be directed to the hip joint, rather than simply displacing the entire infant posteriorly. Start gently and observe closely. If no subluxation is evident during application of light force, push a little more firmly. A millimeter or two of subluxation with firm pressure is normal in neonates. (How much force is enough? The amount of force to apply is somewhat subjective, and experience is helpful. Several experienced ultrasonographers have demonstrated to one of the authors the amount of pressure they apply. Most apply a force in the range of 2–5 kg, but sometimes more. Practice on your bathroom scale.)

A minimum set of images obtained in a routine screening examination will include at least two coronal images that document reproducible measurement of the alpha angle (and the beta angle if you use the Graf system), and axial images with and without stress. Remember to scan both hips. Compare the hips to each other and to any prior studies. A complete examination will document the size and symmetry of the cartilaginous femoral heads and the ossific femoral nuclei (if present), the shape of the acetabular roof (concave is normal, straight is a gray zone between normal and abnormal, wavy is abnormal), the femoral head coverage by the osseous acetabular roof (should be at least 50% covered), the position of the labrum (should not be flipped medially), and hip stability if stress views were obtained.

Scans of a dislocated hip are different. If the femoral head is subluxed or frankly dislocated, it is important to document whether alignment is improved by altering the position of the femur. This can be assessed by moving the femur through a range of motion under direct US observation. Note what you see because this information will assist the orthopedic surgeon. Chronically subluxed or dislocated hips may demonstrate potential impediments to reduction such as a displaced labrum, cartilage overgrowth of the acetabular roof, or overgrowth of fat in the deep acetabulum.

Interpretation of properly obtained images is relatively straightforward, except in the most dysplastic hips. In contrast, performing the study has a learning curve. There is no substitute for experience. Advice to residents: Take advantage of any opportunity offered to obtain the scan yourself, particularly under the direction of an experienced ultrasonographer who can assist and guide you toward obtaining reproducible and accurate images.

Sources and Suggested Readings

Beltran L, Rosenberg ZS, Mayo JD, et al. Imaging evaluation of developmental hip dysplasia in the young adult. *AJR Am J Roentgenol.* 2013;200(5):1077–1088.

Dwek JR. A framework for the radiologic diagnosis of skeletal dysplasias and syndromes as revealed by molecular genetics. *Pediatric Radiology.* 2019;49:1576–1586.

Elgenmark O. Normal development of the ossific centers during infancy and childhood: clinical, roentgenologic and statistical study. *Acta Pediatr.* 1946;33(suppl):1–79.

Gerscovich EO. Practical approach to ultrasound of the hip in developmental dysplasia. *Radiologist.* 1998;5:23–33.

Graf R. *Guide to Sonography of the Infant Hip.* New York: Thieme; 1987.

Greenspan A. Sclerosing bone dysplasias: a target sign approach. *Skeletal Radiol.* 1991;20:561–583.

Greulich WW, Pyle SI. *Radiographic Atlas of Skeletal Development of the Hand and Wrist.* 2nd ed. Stanford: Stanford University Press; 1959.

Habermann CR, Weiss F, Shoder V, et al. MR evaluation of dural ectasia in Marfan syndrome: reassessment of the established criteria in children, adolescents and young adults. *Radiology.* 2005;234:535–541.

Harcke HT, Grisson LE. Performing dynamic sonography of the infant hip. *AJR Am J Roentgenol.* 1990;155:834–844.

Harcke HT. Screening newborns for developmental dysplasia of the hip: the role of sonography. *AJR Am J Roentgenol.* 1994;162:395–397.

Keats TE. *Atlas of Roentgenographic Measurement.* 6th ed. St. Louis: Mosby-Yearbook; 1990.

Keats TE, Anderson MW. *An Atlas of Normal Roentgen Variants That May Simulate Disease.* 5th ed. St. Louis: Mosby; 1992.

Keats TE, Smith TH. *An Atlas of Normal Developmental Roentgen Anatomy.* 2nd ed. Chicago: Year Book Medical Publishers; 1988.

Kilcoyne R, Rych S, Gloch H. Radiological measurement of congenital and acquired foot deformities. *Appl Radiol.* 1993:35–41:December.

Kim H, Kim SH, Kim S, et al. Scoliosis imaging: what radiologists should know. *Radiographics.* 2010;30(7):1823–1842.

Lachman RS. *Taybi and Lachman's Radiology of Syndromes, Metabolic Disorders, and Skeletal Dysplasias.* 5th ed. St. Louis: Mosby; 2006.

Laor T, Jaramillo D. MR imaging insights into skeletal maturation: what is normal? *Radiology.* 2009;250:28–38.

Laor T, Jaramillo D, Oesterreich AE. Musculoskeletal system. In: Kirks DR, Griscom NT, eds. *Practical Pediatric Imaging.* Philadelphia: Lippincott-Raven; 1998.

Laor T, Zbojniewicz AM, Eismann EA, Wll EJ. Juvenile osteochondritis dissecans: is it a growth disturbance of the secondary physis of the epiphysis? *AJR Am J Roentgenol.* 2012;199(5):1121–1128.

Lenke LG, Betz RR, Harms J, et al. Adolescent idiopathic scoliosis: a new classification to determine extent of spinal arthrodesis. *J Bone Joint Surg Am.* 2001;83-A(8):1169–1181.

Leone A, Cianfoni A, Cerase A, et al. Lumbar spondylolysis: a review. *Skeletal Radiol.* 2010;40:683–700.

Malfair, Flemming AK, Dvorak MF, et al. Radiographic evaluation of scoliosis: review. *AJR Am J Roentgenol.* 2010;194:S8-S22.

McAlister WH, Heman TE. Osteochondrodysplasias, dysostoses, chromosomal aberrations, mucopolysaccharidoses, and mucolipidoses. In: Resnick D, ed. *Diagnosis of Bone and Joint Disorders.* Philadelphia: Saunders; 1995:4163–4244.

Meyers AB. Physeal bridges: causes, diagnosis, characterization and post-treatment imaging. *Pediatric Radiology.* 2019;49:1595–1609.

Morvan G, Guerini H, Vuillemin V. Femoral torsion: impact of femur position on CT and stereoradiography measurements. *AJR Am J Roentgenol.* 2017;209(2):W93–W99.

Oesterreich AE. Systematic evaluation of bone dysplasias by the paediatric radiologist. *Pediatr Radiol.* 2010;40(6):975–977.

Ozonoff MB. *Pediatric Orthopaedic Radiology.* 2nd ed. Philadelphia: Saunders; 1992.

Patel NB, Stacy GS. Musculoskeletal manifestations of neurofibromatosis Type 1. *AJR Am J Roentgenol.* 2012;199(1):W99–W106.

Reimers J. The stability of the hip in children: a radiological study of the results of muscle surgery in cerebral palsy. *Acta Orthop Scand Suppl.* 1980;184:1–100.

Resnick D, ed. *Diagnosis of Bone and Joint Disorders.* Philadelphia: Saunders; 2002.

Sontag LW, Snell D, Anderson M. Rate of appearance of ossification centers from birth to the age of five years. *Am J Dis Child.* 1939;58:949–956.

Spranger JW, Brill PW, Poznanski A. *Bone Dysplasias.* 2nd ed. Philadelphia: Saunders; 2002.

Starr V, Ha BY. Imaging update on developmental dysplasia of the hip with the role of MRI. *AJR Am J Roentgenol.* 2014;203(6):1324–1335.

West EY, Jaramillo D. Imaging of osteochondrosis. *Pediatric Radiology.* 2019;49:1610–1611.

Zonoobi D, Hareendranathan A, Mostofi E, et al. Developmental hip dysplasia diagnosis at three-dimensional US: a multicenter study. *Radiology.* 2018; 287(3):1003–1015.

Zucker EJ, Lee EY, Restrepo R, Eisenberg RL. Hip disorders in children. *AJR Am J Roentgenol.* 2013;201(6):W776–W796.

16 *Musculoskeletal Procedures and Techniques*

Biopsy

INTRODUCTION

- Percutaneous image-guided biopsy for soft tissue and bone tumors is a safe and effective method for determination of histopathologic diagnosis prior to treatment.
  - Image-guided biopsy is often performed at the request of and in consultation with the orthopedic oncologist.
  - It is important to first assess whether a biopsy is indicated, which is usually determined when a lesion is not definitively (or highly likely to be) benign by imaging.
- Primary musculoskeletal tumors often require more tissue than is provided by *fine-needle aspiration* (FNA) for evaluating both diagnosis and grade of the lesion.
  - *Core needle biopsy* (CNB) samples are usually obtained for both bone and soft tissue tumors.
  - Unlike FNA, CNB generally does not require the presence of a pathologist in the biopsy suite to evaluate sample adequacy.
- Biopsy samples must be adequate and representative of the lesion; it is crucial to biopsy an active, viable portion of the tumor.
  - Imaging features such as enhancement pattern on magnetic resonance imaging (MRI) and activity on 18F-fluorodeoxyglucose (18F-FDG) positron emission tomography/computed tomography (PET-CT) can identify active portions of the tumor, which are neither hemorrhagic nor necrotic.
  - Targeting such areas on image-guided biopsy will maximize diagnostic yield.
  - For soft tissue masses, color Doppler flow on ultrasound (US) can be helpful for targeting viable tumor.

- Osseous lesions may occasionally be apparent on MRI or PET-CT, but not well seen on CT.
  - In such cases, the expected region of the lesion can be targeted under CT guidance by using anatomic landmarks (Fig. 16.1).
  - MRI guidance can also be used if available.
- Rare malignant transformation of a benign bone lesion into a sarcoma is usually seen as an area of bone destruction and/or some other change in appearance of the underlying original lesion.
  - In such cases, biopsy should be targeted to the aggressive or worrisome region.
- A major factor in the planning algorithm for biopsy of a potentially malignant musculoskeletal neoplasm is whether the lesion could represent a primary sarcoma.
  - Biopsy of primary bone and soft tissue sarcomas requires special consideration for potential seeding of the biopsy track, which affects definitive surgical management.

BIOPSY OF KNOWN OR SUSPECTED PRIMARY SARCOMA

- If the lesion is known to be or might be a primary sarcoma rather than metastasis or myeloma, the approach must avoid potential contamination of tissue compartments that may be needed if limb-salvage surgery is considered.
  - Because the entire needle track must be resected as part of sarcoma curative surgery, the biopsy plan must include consideration of which tissue will be needed for reconstruction.
  - Thus, it is crucial that the case be reviewed and discussed in detail with the surgeon providing definitive treatment to determine an acceptable biopsy approach.

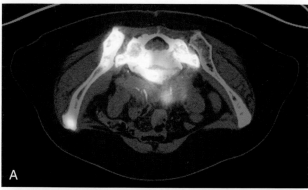

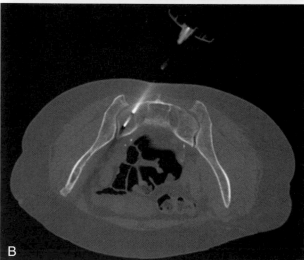

Fig. 16.1 Bone biopsy of osseous metastatic disease in a patient with primary breast carcinoma. **(A)** Axial 18F-FDG PET/CT image through the pelvis demonstrates FDG-avid osseous metastases in the sacrum and iliac bone. **(B)** Intraprocedure image obtained during CT-guided biopsy of the sacrum. The osseous lesions are much more subtle on CT but can be targeted based on anatomic landmarks.

■ The article by Liu et al. listed under Sources and Suggested Readings provides excellent guidance in optimal approaches to various biopsy sites.
■ CNB is strongly preferred to FNA when primary sarcoma is suspected.
   ■ Coaxial technique, in which the outer cannula remains outside of the tumor, reduces but does not eliminate the possibility of needle track seeding with tumor.
■ If possible (it usually is), the needle approach should enter only one anatomic compartment, neurovascular bundles must be avoided, and joints must be avoided.
■ Contamination of the physis should be avoided in skeletally immature patients.
■ Baseline MRI of the lesion should be performed *prior to* biopsy.
   ■ Biopsy may result in hemorrhage, which can obscure the true extent of tumor.

BIOPSY OF METASTASES OR MULTIPLE MYELOMA

■ If a bone lesion is suspected to be a metastasis or multiple myeloma (i.e., suspected primary tumor identified

or multiple lesions detected), then the principles of protecting tissues that may be used for limb-salvage surgery are no longer applicable.
■ For technically challenging biopsies, a screening procedure such as bone scan, radiographs of symptomatic long bones, and/or CT of chest, abdomen, and pelvis should be obtained before biopsy, as there may be other sites that are easier and safer to biopsy.
■ Metastatic renal cell and thyroid carcinomas have a greater propensity for bleeding after biopsy.
   ■ One may choose a smaller biopsy needle, less aggressive biopsy technique, or prebiopsy embolization when such primary lesions are suspected.
   ■ Gelatin sponge material can be injected along the biopsy track to help reduce post-biopsy bleeding.
■ FNA may be adequate for diagnosis of metastases or multiple myeloma, but core biopsy is usually preferred for a more accurate histopathologic analysis.

SITE-SPECIFIC CONSIDERATIONS

Listed in the following are some site-specific tips to consider when planning biopsy of a suspected primary sarcoma.

■ *Shoulder.*
   ■ If at all possible, the biopsy approach should be through the anterior third of the deltoid.
   ■ The deltopectoral groove should be avoided so as to not compromise the use of the pectoralis muscle for reconstruction.
   ■ The posterior deltoid should be avoided because deltoid innervation is from posterior to anterior, so posterior deltoid resection leaves the anterior deltoid denervated and therefore functionless.
■ *Humeral shaft.*
   ■ The ulnar, median, musculocutaneous, and radial nerves course through the arm.
   ■ When a percutaneous biopsy of the humerus is performed, these nerves may be avoided by choosing an anterolateral approach.
■ *Pelvis.*
   ■ Avoid the gluteal muscles, as these are most often used for reconstruction.
■ *Thigh.*
   ■ Avoid the rectus femoris and other quadriceps muscles and tendons, as they are required for functional limb-sparing surgery. Note that the rectus femoris is in a separate compartment from the other quadriceps muscles. If the quadriceps compartment is contaminated, preserving the rectus femoris is essential.
■ *Knee.*
   ■ Avoid contaminating the joint; remember that the suprapatellar recess is large and extends far proximally and medial-to-lateral from the patella.
   ■ If the patient has a complex posterior mass, consider US to make certain that it is not highly vascular and to avoid the popliteal vessels.
■ *Tibia.*
   ■ The best approach is through the anteromedial cortex as there is no significant soft tissue to contaminate through this approach.

NEEDLES

- Needle choice is to some degree a matter of personal preference.
  - Larger-gauge core biopsy needles (>18-gauge) generally provide better-quality biopsy samples with greater tissue volume.
  - Bone biopsy systems have various stylets to penetrate through cortical or sclerotic bone, including trocar- and diamond-tipped.
  - Biopsy needles typically have a bone-cutting or trephined needle, which has a crown-shaped cylindrical tip that cuts a cylindrical defect around a core specimen.
  - Battery-powered drill systems may be used for both bone marrow aspirations and bone biopsies, providing easier access and decreased procedure time, although may degrade sample quality compared to manual techniques.
- In our practices, typically at least three core biopsy samples are obtained for bone lesions and four core biopsy samples are obtained for soft tissue lesions, though this may be limited by lesion size and accessibility.
  - For bone biopsies, we typically use an 11-gauge or 13-gauge coaxial biopsy system, which consists of a trocar-tip stylet, outer cannula, and trephine-tip biopsy needle.
  - For soft tissue biopsies, we typically use a 14-gauge spring-loaded biopsy system, with a coaxial introducer for deeper lesions.
  - Different gauge biopsy devices may be dictated by biopsy needle length and lesion depth.

IMAGING GUIDANCE

- Modalities utilized for image-guided biopsy include CT, US, and even MRI in some centers.

- Image guidance is used to localize the tumor, avoid vital structures, and maintain needle visualization throughout the entire procedure.
- User preference and 'whatever works best' usually make this determination.
- US allows for real-time imaging of the advancing needle and is often used for biopsy of soft tissue masses.
  - Deeper soft tissue lesions that are poorly visualized by US may require CT guidance.
- CT is usually used for bone biopsies; in some cases, combining US with CT can assist in avoiding vascular structures.

BONE BIOPSY

- Observe the general principles described previously when choosing the biopsy approach.
- If there is an accompanying soft tissue mass, it may be easier to obtain tissue from that site rather than the osseous site.
- Bone biopsies are typically performed under conscious sedation; infiltrating the densely innervated periosteum liberally with a local anesthetic will also substantially reduce patient discomfort.
- If the osseous lesion is entirely lytic, a spring-loaded device may be required to obtain adequate core samples; in such cases, the coaxial introducer can be placed through an area of cortical destruction or through a small corticotomy made with a traditional bone biopsy device (Fig. 16.2).
- If a lesion is sclerotic or you must drill through dense cortex to get to a lesion, it may take a great deal of strength; it can help to stand on a stool for leverage or use a powered drill system.
- Once the biopsy system is positioned near the lesion, the stylet is removed from the outer cannula and the bone-cutting biopsy needle is used to obtain core samples.

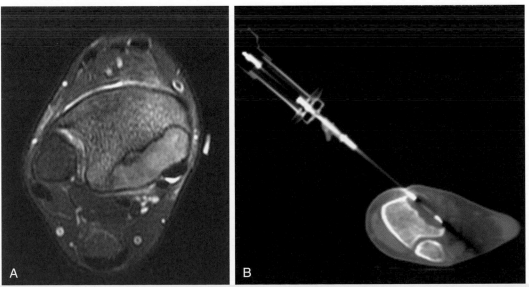

Fig. 16.2 Bone biopsy of a lytic bone tumor in the ankle. **(A)** Axial T2-weighted fat-suppressed MR image of the ankle demonstrates a large lesion at the posteromedial aspect of the distal tibia with extensive surrounding bone marrow edema. **(B)** Intraprocedure image obtained during CT-guided biopsy with the ankle in the lateral position. A 14-gauge spring-loaded biopsy system was used due to the purely lytic nature of the lesion, easily placed through the markedly thinned tibial cortex. Histopathology was consistent with giant cell tumor of bone.

- Bone biopsy needles are designed to retain the core sample within the needle tip, though sometimes it may be difficult to retain the sample for softer lesions; in such cases, it can be helpful to connect a syringe to the biopsy needle hub to generate negative pressure while withdrawing the needle.
- Treat each core carefully; use the obturator to carefully back it out of the coring needle in order to reduce crush artifact.
- Obtaining three or more samples of a bone lesion maximizes diagnostic yield.
- Consider whether percutaneous biopsy of a cartilage lesion is indicated, as there are special considerations for such lesions.
  - Chondrosarcoma is the most likely of all osseous tumors to recur in a biopsy track because cartilage does not need to establish a blood supply to grow.
  - It is extremely difficult to distinguish an enchondroma from an atypical enchondroma or low-grade chondrosarcoma both on imaging and histopathologically based solely on core biopsy samples.
  - Interval follow-up MRIs may be recommended for suspected low-grade chondroid lesions to document lesion stability.

SOFT TISSUE BIOPSY

- Observe the general principles described previously when choosing the biopsy approach.
- Infiltrate the skin and subcutaneous tissues with a local anesthetic, up to the margin of the lesion.
- Using a spring-loaded biopsy system can help penetrate through a firm or mobile soft tissue mass by firing the biopsy tray at a high velocity through the lesion (Fig. 16.3).
- A coaxial introducer may be used for deeper lesions to decrease trauma to surrounding tissues (Fig. 16.4).
- Obtaining four or more samples of a soft tissue lesion maximizes diagnostic yield.
- For heterogeneous lesions, cores should be obtained from several different sites within the tumor, for the best chance of obtaining representative tissue.

- Peripheral nerve sheath tumors can be exquisitely painful when biopsied; consider a regional anesthetic block or conscious sedation when prebiopsy imaging suggests this diagnosis.

SAMPLE PREPARATION

- Samples are usually placed either in formalin fixative or in a sterile container on a saline-moistened gauze pad.
- Formalin fixation prevents ancillary testing, such as flow cytometry or cytogenetics, and should be avoided when there is clinical concern for possible lymphoma.
- Bone samples are decalcified prior to processing by the pathology laboratory to allow sectioning.
- If in doubt, consult with your pathologist prior to performing biopsy.

Arthrography and Aspiration

Intraarticular needle placement is one of the basic skills of musculoskeletal and general radiologists. Similar needle placement techniques are used for both joint injection and aspiration. This section first reviews general principles, followed by specific techniques for commonly injected joints.

GENERAL PRINCIPLES

Direct arthrography is the technique of injecting contrast solution into a joint, which was historically performed in combination with conventional radiographs, termed *conventional arthrography*. Though conventional arthrography is rarely used anymore, *direct arthrography* is now combined with advanced imaging modalities, namely MRI and CT. Direct MR arthrography is performed with far greater frequency than direct CT arthrography. MR arthrography requires imaging on a high field strength scanners (1.5 or 3 Tesla). Intraarticular instillation of contrast solution distends the joint capsule and provides better visualization of the intraarticular structures on imaging immediately following injection. *Indirect MR arthrography* using intravenous contrast can also be performed when a radiologist is

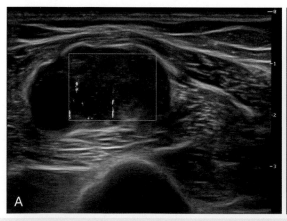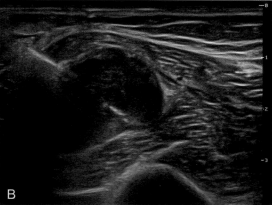

Fig. 16.3 Soft tissue biopsy of an intramuscular thigh mass. **(A)** Transverse US image with color Doppler flow overlay demonstrates a hypoechoic mass with internal vascularity in the vastus medialis muscle. **(B)** Intraprocedural image obtained during US-guided biopsy shows the biopsy needle positioned within the mass. Several core needle biopsy samples were obtained by placing the biopsy needle through an outer cannula, which is positioned just outside of the tumor. Histopathology was consistent with intramuscular myxoma; prebiopsy MRI for this patient is presented in Fig. 12.35.

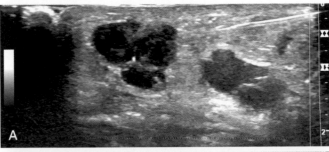
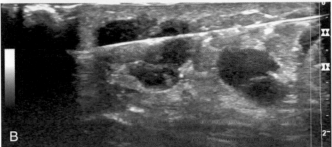

Fig. 16.4 Soft tissue biopsy of subcutaneous melanoma metastases. Pre- **(A)** and postfire **(B)** images of a spring-loaded biopsy device obtained during US-guided biopsy of small hypoechoic subcutaneous masses. Using a spring-loaded biopsy needle can help penetrate small or mobile soft tissue masses by firing the biopsy tray through the lesion at a high velocity.

not available to perform an injection, but is generally regarded as inferior due to lack of joint distention. Arthrograms are most commonly performed under fluoroscopic or US guidance to confirm intraarticular positioning of the needle, though x-ray, CT, and even MRI guidance can be used. Identical techniques can be used for image-guided joint injections of corticosteroid performed for pain.

Joint aspirations are performed by a radiologist most commonly when there is concern for septic arthritis in a joint that needs imaging to enter reliably. Septic arthritis in a native joint is an orthopedic emergency treated with urgent surgical intervention, and aspiration is thus requested and performed expeditiously. Aspiration may also be requested on an outpatient basis to evaluate for an inflammatory or crystalline arthropathy, or to assess for indolent infection of an implanted prosthesis. The technique for joint aspiration is generally similar to arthrography, though a larger-gauge needle is used due to increased viscosity of infected synovial fluid. Specifically, an 18-gauge needle is recommended for joint aspiration when infection is suspected. This larger needle requires greater local anesthesia than smaller gauge needles used for joint injection. Using US guidance may be helpful to reliably identify and successfully aspirate joint fluid, particularly if loculated or pooled dependently.

Informed Consent

- Be certain that the patient understands the reason his or her clinician has requested the examination, and describe the procedure step by step.
- For MR arthrography, verify the patient has no contraindication to MRI.
- Verify the patient has no known allergy to the contrast material(s) being administered.

- Confirm the patient's identity, target joint, and laterality.
- Inform the patient of the minimal risks associated with the procedure, including bleeding or bruising around the injection site, damage to adjacent structures, introducing infection (risk is less than 1 in 10,000 to 20,000), and extremely small risk of anaphylactic contrast reaction (1 in 100,000).
  - Contrast reactions during MR arthrography are extremely rare due to the small amount of contrast utilized and low systemic concentrations achieved following injection.
- Inform the patient that the most painful portion of the examination is usually the initial introduction of local anesthesia.
  - For injection of large joints, distention of the joint itself is usually not painful.
    - The major exception to this generalization is injection of the wrist, where distention to full capacity can be painful.
    - Mixing anesthetic into the contrast solution reduces discomfort associated with the injection.
  - Joint aspiration for septic arthritis is typically more painful than arthrogram injection due to larger needle gauge and inflammation around the joint.
- Unless the patient has unusual anatomy (e.g., significant hip protrusio), none of the standard approaches for joint access places the needle close to a neurovascular bundle, so these structures are not at risk.

Patient Preparation

- Position the patient in a comfortable position that also provides access to the joint via the planned approach.
- Mark the ideal needle placement on the skin; this is determined for x-ray or fluoroscopic-guided procedures by taking an image with a radiopaque marker on the skin surface.
- Clean the skin using a sterile antiseptic solution (e.g., a chlorhexidine gluconate and isopropyl alcohol skin prep solution) and place a sterile drape over the injection site.
- At the planned needle entry site, infiltrate the skin and subcutaneous tissues with a local anesthetic: 1–2% lidocaine, ideally buffered with sodium bicarbonate.

Needle Selection

- Joint injection (arthrogram contrast or medication for pain injection):
  - The smaller the needle gauge, the less painful for the patient.
  - A 25-gauge needle causes less tissue injury than a 22-gauge needle and is less painful; however, a 22- or 20-gauge needle is more rigid and thus easier to direct.
  - A 20- or 22-gauge needle also allows better tactile distinction of low-resistance intraarticular flow versus high-resistance extraarticular needle tip positioning.
  - A 25-gauge needle is typically used for small joints (wrist, hand, foot).
  - A 22- to 25-gauge needle may be used for intermediate joints (elbow, ankle).
  - A 20- or 22-gauge needle is usually used for large joints (shoulder, hip, knee).

- Joint aspiration:
  - Inflammatory exudates increase the viscosity of joint fluid, which may not flow through a small-gauge needle.
  - We routinely use an 18-gauge needle when joint infection is suspected.
  - Using a 22- or even 20-gauge needle may result in a false-negative "dry tap".
- Needle length is chosen based on the target joint but may be modified according to patient size.

Contrast Volume

- Contrast solution volume depends on the joint injected (see specific joints included later in this chapter).
- Achieving adequate joint distention is especially important in MR and CT arthrography, but paradoxically, injecting more contrast may defeat this goal by causing contrast leakage into adjacent tissues and decompression of the joint, analogous to over-inflating a balloon.
- Consistently excellent MR and CT arthrography images are obtained with adequate (not maximal) joint distention; sometimes, less is more.

Contrast Solution for MR Arthrography

- Gadolinium contrast agents differ in relaxivity and T1 shortening effects.
- For most contrast agents, a 1:200 to 1:400 dilution factor provides optimal imaging.
- If a joint effusion is suspected (for example, following a shoulder dislocation) or observed (i.e., spontaneous return of joint fluid into the needle hub upon entering the joint), joint aspiration may be performed before injection of contrast to avoid overdistention of the joint and underconcentration of the gadolinium-based contrast agent. Alternatively, a higher concentration of gadolinium-based contrast agent can be used in this situation.
- Standard injection ingredients include normal saline, gadolinium contrast agent, and anesthetic.
  - For x-ray or fluoroscopic-guided injections, iodinated contrast is used to confirm intraarticular needle placement.
    - We prefer to separate iodinated contrast from the gadolinium contrast, as a combined mixture may degrade the imaging study if initial needle placement was outside or only partially within the joint.
    - Some radiologists prefer to mix the iodinated contrast with the gadolinium contrast into a single solution to simplify the procedure and decrease the potential for introducing air into the joint.
    - Iodinated contrast detracts from MR image quality, as it reduces the T1 shortening effects of gadolinium and also results in T2 shortening causing lower signal intensity on all sequences, especially with 3 Tesla scanners; the gadolinium agent should therefore be diluted primarily with normal saline.
  - For US-guided injections, intraarticular needle tip is confirmed visually and does not require use of iodinated contrast.
  - Anesthetic is often added to the contrast solution mixture to reduce patient discomfort and thereby reduce motion artifact on subsequently obtained MR images.
    - Anesthetic can also be used as an adjunct to help differentiate between intraarticular and extraarticular sources of pain by performing an examination of the affected joint before and following injection.
    - Lidocaine or ropivacaine is typically used rather than bupivacaine, which has been shown to have chondrotoxic effects in vitro.
- MR arthrography can also be performed after saline injection, using T2-weighted sequences rather than T1-weighted sequences to highlight the intraarticular structures.
  - We prefer gadolinium MR arthrography because of the potential for superior spatial and contrast resolution with T1-weighted sequences.
  - If the patient is allergic to gadolinium, saline MR arthrography is an acceptable alternative.
  - If the patient has a known allergy to iodinated contrast, the patient can be premedicated, or the injection can be performed under x-ray or fluoroscopy by an experienced radiologist by injecting only dilute gadolinium based on tactile sensation.
  - US guidance is also a useful alternative to avoid the use of iodinated contrast.
  - If the patient has a known allergy to gadolinium contrast, normal saline can be injected and the joint imaged via saline MR arthrography using T2-weighted sequences.

Contrast Solution for CT Arthrography

- Although MR arthrography is generally preferred to CT arthrography, there are circumstances that dictate the need for CT arthrography, such as contraindication to MRI, patient size, and presence of metallic orthopedic hardware near the target joint.
- CT arthrography can provide excellent spatial resolution, superior to MR arthrography in certain cases.
- On modern scanners, full-strength high-density non-ionic contrast (300 mg/mL) provides excellent-quality images.
- Iodinated contrast may be diluted with of anesthetic to reduce discomfort associated with the procedure, similar to MR arthrography.

Injection

- Needle placement is specific to each joint (see specific joints included later in this chapter).
- In most joints a 'straight-down' approach is used with x-ray and fluoroscopic guidance; needle approach under US guidance is more flexible and open to radiologist preference.
- One should avoid injection of air bubbles because they may simulate or obscure small intraarticular bodies on MR arthrography. This is less of a concern on CT arthrography, but many musculoskeletal radiologists prefer that introduction of intra-articular gas still should be avoided.
- For x-ray and fluoroscopic-guided injection, confirm intraarticular needle tip position by injecting a small amount of iodinated contrast solution.

- If the placement is intraarticular, contrast will flow away from the needle, often in a particular pattern that is unique to the joint.
  - If needle placement is extraarticular, injected contrast will pool around the needle tip or dissect along tissue planes.
  - Resistance to injection is higher with extraarticular positioning, with a notable exception being the knee joint.
- If resistance is met and contrast does not flow freely, try simply rotating the needle 90 or 180 degrees and repeating the injection attempt.
- If initial needle positioning is unsuccessful and intraarticular flow of contrast is not confirmed, the needle should be repositioned.
- Once the needle is in proper position, inject the recommended volume, which varies by joint.
- Do not over-distend the joint (e.g., if you feel resistance) because doing so may result in contrast extravasation into adjacent soft tissues, decompressing the joint and possibly confusing interpretation.

Postprocedure Assessment

- Before the patient sits up, take the time to assess the patient.
- Vasovagal symptoms are occasionally seen with arthrography; it is easier to recover patients on the table than after standing up.

SHOULDER

- *Primary indication*: glenoid labrum tears.
- *Secondary indications*: undersurface and full-thickness rotator cuff tears, rotator cuff re-tears following repair, articular cartilage lesions.
- *Technique*:
  1. **Patient position**: patient supine with arm positioned at the side, palm up (external rotation of the

humerus); a sandbag may be used to hold the hand in external rotation. External rotation of the humerus is key to a successful injection. If the humeral head does not resemble a club, work with the patient to achieve better positioning.
  2. **Approach**: place the needle through the rotator interval over the superomedial humeral head (lateral to the base of the coracoid process) and advance straight-down onto bone (Figs. 16.5 and 16.6).
     - This approach is easy, fast, and virtually painless, in contrast with the previously popular more inferior approach that punctures the subscapularis tendon.
     - For US-guided injection, a posterior approach is often preferred.
  3. **Needle**: 20- or 22-gauge, 1.5–3.5″ in length.
  4. **Intraarticular flow**: away from the needle, often immediately outlining the humeral head or first appearing in the superior subscapularis recess.
     - If contrast does not flow, try spinning the needle or gently internally rotate the humeral head until the needle advances.
  5. **Volume**: 10–15 mL.
     - Overdistention may result in contrast leakage into the soft tissues, usually decompressing along the subscapularis muscle.

ELBOW

- *Primary indication*: ulnar collateral ligament (UCL) tears.
- *Secondary indications*: radial collateral ligament (RCL) complex tears, articular cartilage and osteochondral lesions, intraarticular bodies.
- *Technique*:
  1. **Patient position**:
     - *Option 1*: patient prone with arm over the head, elbow flexed 90 degrees with the thumb up; elevate the elbow with a rolled towel or pad to provide a true lateral view and easier access.

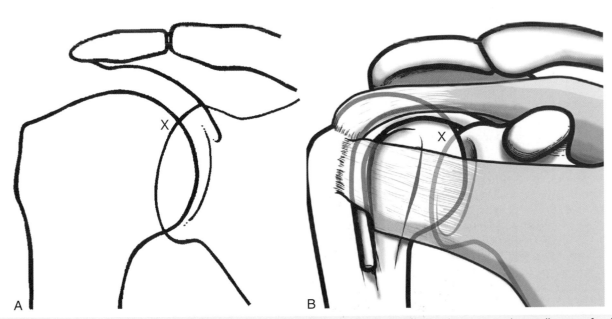

Fig. 16.5 Rotator interval approach for shoulder injection. Line drawing **(A)** and anatomic diagram **(B)** demonstrate the needle target for shoulder injection (*X* in both) using a rotator interval approach. The needle is advanced straight-down onto bone, avoiding the subscapularis tendon.

- *Option 2*: patient sitting in a chair with arm placed on a table, elbow flexed 90 degrees with the thumb up; this approach may be useful if the patient has difficulty abducting the shoulder.

2. **Approach:**

Posterior transtriceps approach (preferred):

- Palpate the distal triceps tendon just proximal to the olecranon process, between the medial and lateral epicondyles, and advance the needle horizontal to the table through the triceps tendon, into the olecranon fossa and onto bone (Figs. 16.7 and 16.8A).

- This is the easiest approach, is virtually painless for the patient, and does not disturb the structures of interest.

Lateral radiocapitellar approach:

- Advance the needle perpendicular to the table, straight down into the radiocapitellar articulation (see Figs. 16.7 and 16.8B).

- It is sometimes difficult to appreciate when the needle has entered the joint, which may result in iatrogenic infiltration of the RCL complex and common extensor muscle/tendon group when contrast is injected; this approach should

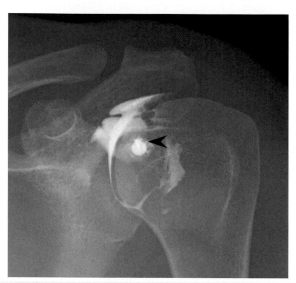

Fig. 16.6 Shoulder arthrogram injection. Intraprocedure AP radiograph of the shoulder immediately following injection of iodinated contrast to confirm intraarticular needle placement demonstrates contrast outlining the humeral head and extending into the joint recesses. The needle is advanced straight-down onto the humeral head via a rotator interval approach *(arrowhead)*.

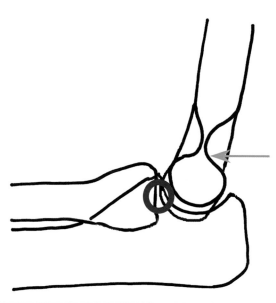

Fig. 16.7 Lateral radiocapitellar and posterior transtriceps approaches for elbow injection. For the lateral radiocapitellar approach, the needle is advanced straight down into the radiocapitellar joint *(red circle)*. For the posterior transtriceps approach, the needle is advanced from the posterior elbow into the olecranon fossa *(blue arrow)*.

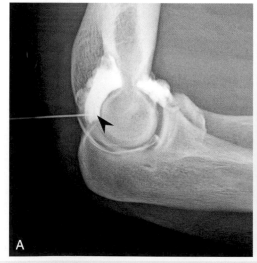
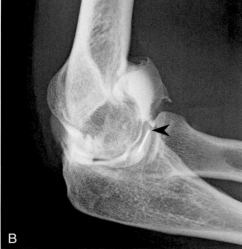

Fig. 16.8 Elbow arthrogram injection. **(A)** Intraprocedural lateral radiograph of the elbow immediately following injection of iodinated contrast to confirm intraarticular needle placement demonstrates contrast outlining the ulnotrochlear articulation, extending into the anterior and posterior joint recesses, and outlining the radial head. The needle is advanced via a posterior transtriceps approach with needle tip positioned in the olecranon fossa *(arrowhead)*. **(B)** Intraprocedural lateral radiograph of the elbow immediately following injection of iodinated contrast in a different patient demonstrates contrast outlining the ulnotrochlear articulation and extending into the anterior joint recess. The needle is advanced straight-down via a lateral approach with needle tip positioned in the radiocapitellar articulation *(arrowhead)*.

be avoided if there is clinical concern for injury of the lateral elbow structures.

- *Oblique posterolateral* (not shown on the diagram).
    - Palpate these landmarks: olecranon process and lateral epicondyle.
- Just anterior to a line between these landmarks is a palpable fat pad that provides easy and near painless access to the joint. Even in obese patients, this site rarely is far from the joint.
    - With the elbow flexed 90 degrees and in lateral projection (patient supine, ipsilateral hand on belly, elbow elevated by towels or similar to achieve true lateral projection).
    - 25g 1.5" needle. After injecting the skin with analgesic, advance the needle towards the radial head - capitellum articulation. Injected contrast will outline the elbow joint, confirming successful needle placement.

3. **Needle**: 22- to 25-gauge, 1.5" in length.
4. **Intraarticular flow**: away from needle, usually flows into the anterior and posterior joint recesses or around the radial neck.
5. **Volume**: 6–8 mL.
    - Overdistention may result in contrast leakage into the soft tissues, usually decompressing along the distal triceps muscle.

WRIST (RADIOCARPAL)

- *Primary indications*: triangular fibrocartilage complex (TFCC), scapholunate ligament (SLL), and lunotriquetral ligament (LTL) tears.
- *Technique*:
    1. **Patient position**:
        - *Option 1*: patient prone with arm over the head, palm down with wrist mildly flexed and ulnar deviated; this can be facilitated with a rolled towel placed under the wrist.
        - *Option 2*: patient supine with arm positioned at the side, palm down with wrist mildly flexed and ulnar deviated (again, using a rolled towel); this approach may be useful if the patient has difficulty abducting the shoulder.
    2. **Approach**: place the needle over the proximal scaphoid, just distal to the radiocarpal joint space, and advance at a slightly distal-to-proximal angle down into the radioscaphoid articulation (Figs. 16.9 and 16.10).
        - Angling the needle from distal to proximal allows one to avoid the dorsal lip of the distal radius.
        - Alternatively, the radial aspect of the radioscaphoid articulation can be targeted in a straight-down approach (see Fig. 16.9).
        - For US-guided injection, the dorsal recess of the radiocarpal joint is targeted.
    3. **Needle**: 25-gauge, 1.5" in length.
    4. **Intraarticular flow**: contrast may initially fill dorsal or volar recesses or flow into the radial or ulnar recesses.
        - Watch for flow from the radiocarpal joint into the distal radioulnar joint (DRUJ), indicating a TFCC, or flow into the midcarpal joint, indicating an SLL or LTL tear.

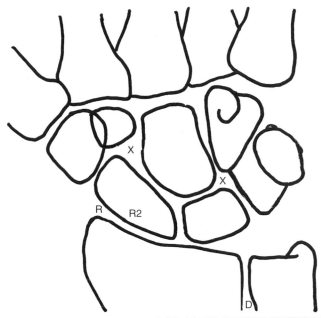

Fig. 16.9 Dorsal approach for wrist injection. There are three synovial compartments of the wrist. All are injected using a dorsal approach. *R* and *R2* mark injection site options for the radiocarpal joint; the wrist is positioned palm down with wrist mildly flexed and ulnar deviated, which can be accomplished by placing a rolled towel or small pad under the wrist. Each *X* marks an acceptable injection site for the midcarpal compartment. *D* marks an injection site for the distal radioulnar joint.

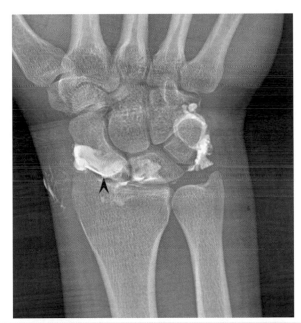

Fig. 16.10 Wrist (radiocarpal) arthrogram injection. Intraprocedural PA radiograph of the wrist immediately following injection of iodinated contrast to confirm intraarticular needle placement demonstrates contrast outlining the recesses of the radiocarpal joint. The needle is advanced at a slight distal-to-proximal angle with needle tip positioned in the radioscaphoid articulation *(arrowhead)*.

- Serial fluoroscopic image captures may document the site of abnormal contrast flow between compartments that is not evident on static fluoroscopic or CT or MR images obtained later.

5. **Volume**: 3–5 mL.
   - Overdistention may be painful and result in contrast leakage into the soft tissues, which may decompress dorsally along the needle track or into the extensor tendon sheaths, limiting evaluation of these structures.
6. **Special considerations:**
   - Although the single radiocarpal injection is usually sufficient for diagnosis of intrinsic ligament tears, particularly when MR arthrography is being performed, arthrogram injection into the midcarpal joint or DRUJ may occasionally be requested (see Fig. 16.9 for injection sites).
   - These injections may be performed if a tiny one-way 'ball-valve' perforation is suspected or if intraarticular details of those joints are desired (such as evaluation of the undersurface of the central TFCC articular disc).
   - Since the advent of MRI, midcarpal and DRUJ arthrogram injections are rarely performed.

HIP

- *Primary indication*: acetabular labrum tears, therapeutic injection, joint aspiration.
- *Secondary indications*: diagnostic evaluation with an anesthetic to determine intra- versus extraarticular source of hip pain, articular cartilage lesions, and intraarticular bodies.
- *Technique*:
   1. **Patient position**: supine, hip straight, leg internally rotated; a sandbag may be used to hold the foot in internal rotation.
   2. **Approach**: place the needle straight down onto the superolateral femoral head–neck junction (Figs. 16.11 and 16.12).
      - The hip capsule extends distally, nearly to the intertrochanteric line; thus the target for successful injection is large.

- Targeting the center of the femoral neck is also a commonly used technique (see Fig. 16.11), though this may 'pinch' the capsule onto bone, resulting in higher rates of extraarticular or capsular infiltration. Before injecting contrast, wait a moment to observe if joint fluid flows from the needle hub. If so, removing some joint fluid can make the subsequent injection less painful.
3. **Needle**: 20- or 22-gauge, 3.5″ in length (may need longer needle for particularly large patients).
4. **Intraarticular flow**: into the redundant portion of the joint, usually 'ringing' the femoral neck.
   - Specifically, it should not pool around the needle tip or flow in a linear pattern along the superoinferior path of the iliopsoas bursa.
5. **Volume**: 10–15 mL.
6. **Special considerations:**
   - If placing a needle for aspiration of a suspected infected hip arthroplasty, a direct anterior approach onto the prothsetic femoral head or neck portion of the prosthesis may be used. Alternatively, an anterolateral approach (advancing lateral-to-medial from above the greater trochanter) onto the femoral head/neck may be used (Fig. 16.13); there will be a distinct 'metal-on-metal' feel when the needle contacts the prosthesis.
   - Because fluid in the hip may be in a dependent position (behind the prosthesis), moving the hip into internal rotation and flexing the hip and knee while aspirating may allow return of fluid in a difficult case; alternatively, US guidance may be used to detect and aspirate fluid.
   - If aspiration attempts are initially unsuccessful, proof of intraarticular placement is made by injection of a small amount of iodinated contrast (this is only weakly bacteriostatic), followed by lavage of the joint with 10 mL of nonbacteriostatic saline

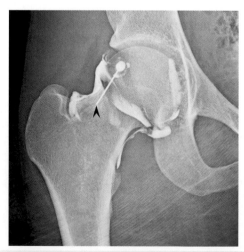

Fig. 16.12 Hip arthrogram injection. Intraprocedural AP radiograph of the hip immediately following injection of iodinated contrast to confirm intraarticular needle placement demonstrates contrast outlining the femoral head and neck in a ringlike fashion. The needle is advanced via an anterior approach onto bone, with the tip positioned at the superolateral femoral head–neck junction *(arrowhead)*. Note that the hip joint capsule (outlined by contrast) extends distally, nearly to the intertrochanteric line.

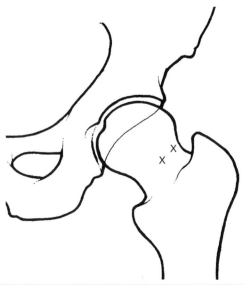

Fig. 16.11 Anterior approach for hip injection. The *X*s mark two injection sites preferred by the authors.

and attempted reaspiration; this process may be repeated until fluid is aspirated.

- Iodinated contrast may also be injected (usually 10-15 mL is sufficient) following successful hip aspiration to evaluate for abnormal communication or fistulization to the surrounding soft tissues (Fig. 16.14).

KNEE

- *Primary indication*: evaluate for meniscal re-tear in the postoperative setting.
- *Technique*:
  1. **Patient position:**
     - *Option 1*: patient supine, with the knee slightly flexed over a pillow, quadriceps relaxed.
     - *Option 2*: patient in the lateral decubitus 'running man' position, knee slightly flexed.
  2. **Approach:**
     Lateral patellofemoral approach
     - Palpate the patella and advance the needle between the patella and lateral femoral condyle (Fig. 16.15A).
     Medial patellofemoral approach
     - Similar technique to the lateral approach; requires traversing the vastus medialis obliquus and can be more painful.
     Anterior 'arthroscopic' approach
     - Mimics approach of placing an arthroscopic portal; needle placed medial or lateral to the

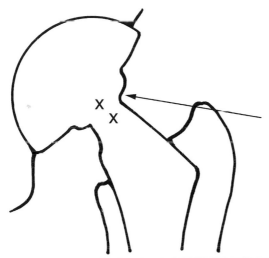

Fig. 16.13 Hip arthroplasty aspiration. The *X*s mark acceptable needle placement sites if an anterior approach is used. *Arrow* marks the needle track using an anterolateral approach, advancing lateral-to-medial from above the greater trochanter and aiming for the prosthetic femoral head. There will be a distinct 'metal-on-metal' feel when the needle contacts the prosthesis.

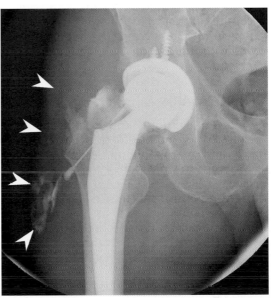

Fig. 16.14 Hip arthroplasty infection. AP radiographic exposure obtained following fluoroscopic-guided aspiration of pus from an infected hip prosthesis. Injection of iodinated contrast into the joint demonstrates abnormal communication with a large fluid and gas containing collection in the lateral thigh *(arrowheads)*.

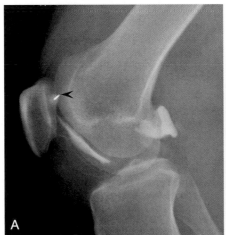 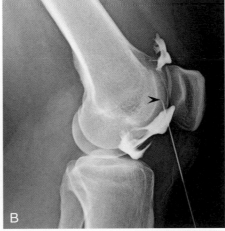

Fig. 16.15 Knee arthrogram injection. **(A)** Intraprocedural lateral fluoroscopic image of the knee immediately following injection of iodinated contrast to confirm intraarticular needle placement demonstrates contrast extending into the anterior and posterior joint recesses. The needle is advanced via a lateral patellofemoral approach between the patella and femoral condyle *(arrowhead)*. **(B)** Intraprocedural lateral radiograph of the knee immediately following injection of iodinated contrast in a different patient demonstrates contrast extending into the anterior and suprapatellar joint recesses. The needle is advanced via an anterior arthroscopic approach with needle angled cephalad and tip directed toward the central trochlea *(arrowhead)*.

patellar tendon and angled cephalad and toward the central aspect of the femoral trochlea (Fig. 16.15B).

3. **Needle**: 20- or 22-gauge, 1.5–3.5″ in length (depending on the approach).
4. **Intraarticular flow**: away from the needle, into the anterior, posterior, or suprapatellar joint recesses.
   ▪ Pooling of contrast around the needle tip may indicate positioning within one of the anterior knee fat pads.
5. **Volume**: 20–30 mL.
6. **Special considerations:**
   ▪ The suprapatellar recess is potentially very large (easily holding 40–60 mL); therefore, in the presence of a joint effusion, it is important to aspirate as much joint fluid as possible before injection of contrast to avoid dilution.
   ▪ Squeezing or 'milking' the suprapatellar recess while aspirating a knee joint effusion can be helpful.

ANKLE (TIBIOTALAR)

▪ *Primary indication*: not routinely indicated; occasionally requested for impingement syndromes, articular cartilage and osteochondral lesions, intraarticular bodies, therapeutic injection.
▪ *Technique*:
  1. **Patient position**: patient lying on side, ankle in the lateral position.
  2. **Approach**: palpate dorsalis pedis artery and anterior tendons (to avoid them), advance needle from an anterior approach into the tibiotalar joint (Figs. 16.16 and 16.17).
  3. **Needle**: 22- to 25-gauge, 1.5″ in length.
  4. **Intraarticular flow**: directly into the tibiotalar joint.
  5. **Volume**: 4–8 mL.

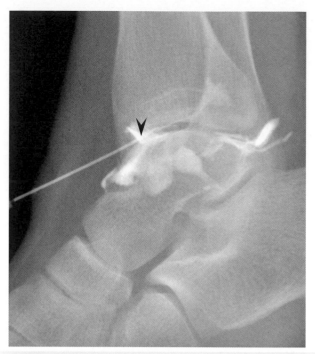

Fig. 16.17 Ankle arthrogram injection. Intraprocedural lateral fluoroscopic image of the ankle immediately following injection of iodinated contrast to confirm intraarticular needle placement demonstrates contrast extending into the recesses of the tibiotalar joint. The needle is advanced via an anterior approach with the tip positioned in the tibiotalar joint *(arrowhead)*.

Sources and Suggested Readings

Cerezal L, Llopis E, Canga A, et al. MR arthrography of the ankle: indications and technique. *Radiol Clin North Am*. 2008;46(6):973–994, v.

Dépelteau H, Bureau NJ, Cardinal E, et al. Arthrography of the shoulder: a simple fluoroscopically guided approach for targeting the rotator cuff interval. *AJR Am J Roentgenol*. 2004;182(2):329–332.

Espinosa LA, Jamadar DA, Jacobson JA, et al. CT-guided biopsy of bone: a radiologist's perspective. *AJR Am J Roentgenol*. 2008;190(5):W283–W289.

Kheterpal AB, Bunnell KM, Husseini JS, et al. Value of response to anesthetic injection during hip MR arthrography to differentiate between intra- and extra-articular pathology. *Skeletal Radiol*. 2020;49(4):555–561.

Lee RK, Ng AW, Griffith JF. CT-guided bone biopsy with a battery-powered drill system: preliminary results. *AJR Am J Roentgenol*. 2013;201(5):1093–1095.

Liu PT, Valadez SD, Chivers FS, et al. Anatomically based guidelines for core needle biopsy of bone tumors: implications for limb-sparing surgery. *Radiographics*. 2007;27(1):189–205; discussion 206.

Lohman M, Borrero C, Casagranda B, et al. The posterior transtriceps approach for elbow arthrography: a forgotten technique? *Skeletal Radiol*. 2009;38(5):513–516.

Meek RD, Mills MK, Hanrahan CJ, et al. Pearls and pitfalls for soft tissue and bone biopsies: a cross-institutional review. *Radiographics*. 2020;40(1):266–290.

Oliveira MP, Lima PM, da Silva HJ, et al. Neoplasm seeding in biopsy tract of the musculoskeletal system. A systematic review. *Acta Ortop Bras*. 2014;22(2):106–110.

Rastogi AK, Davis KW, Ross A, et al. Fundamentals of joint injection. *AJR Am J Roentgenol*. 2016;207(3):484-494. doi: 10.2214/AJR.16.16243. Epub 2016 Jun 8.

Shortt CP, Morrison WB, Roberts CC, et al. Shoulder, hip, and knee arthrography needle placement using fluoroscopic guidance: practice patterns of musculoskeletal radiologists in North America. *Skeletal Radiol*. 2009;38(4):377–385.

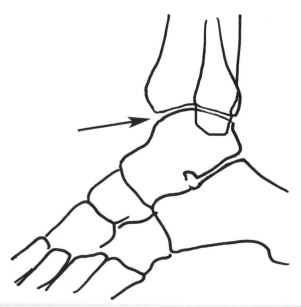

Fig. 16.16 Anterior approach for ankle (tibiotalar) injection. *Arrow* marks the needle track using an anterior approach with lateral x-ray or fluoroscopy.

Note: Page numbers followed by *f* refer to figures, by *t* to tables, and by *b* to boxes.